D1162038

SEVENTH EDITION

Clinical Chemistry

Principles, Techniques, and Correlations

Michael L. Bishop, MS, MLS(ASCP)^{CM}
Senior Learning Consultant
Organization Learning
Duke Clinical Research Institute
Duke University Medical Center
Durham, North Carolina

Edward P. Fody, MD
Clinical Professor
Department of Pathology, Microbiology
  and Immunology
Vanderbilt University School of Medicine
Nashville, Tennessee
and
Medical Director
Department of Pathology
Holland Hospital
Holland, Michigan

Larry E. Schoeff, MS, MT(ASCP)
Professor, Medical Laboratory Science Program
Department of Pathology
University of Utah School of Medicine
Salt Lake City, Utah

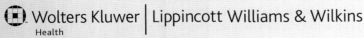
Wolters Kluwer | Lippincott Williams & Wilkins
Health
Philadelphia · Baltimore · New York · London
Buenos Aires · Hong Kong · Sydney · Tokyo

Acquisitions Editor: David Troy
Product Manager: Michael Egolf
Marketing Manager: Shauna Kelley
Designer: Stephen Druding
Compositor: Integra Software Services

Copyright © 2013, 2010, 2005, 2000, 1996, 1992, 1985, by LIPPINCOTT WILLIAMS & WILKINS, a WOLTERS KLUWER business.

Two Commerce Square
2001 Market Street
Philadelphia, PA 19103 USA
LWW.com

All rights reserved. This book is protected by copyright. No part of this book may be reproduced or transmitted in any form or by any means, including as photocopies or scanned-in or other electronic copies, or utilized by any information storage and retrieval system without written permission from the copyright owner, except for brief quotations embodied in critical articles and reviews. Materials appearing in this book prepared by individuals as part of their official duties as U.S. government employees are not covered by the above-mentioned copyright. To request permission, please contact Lippincott Williams & Wilkins at Two Commerce Square, 2001 Market Street, Philadelphia, PA 19103, via email at permissions@lww.com, or via website at lww.com (products and services).

9 8 7 6 5 4 3 2 1

Printed in China

Library of Congress Cataloging-in-Publication Data

Clinical chemistry : principles, techniques, and correlations/[edited by] Michael L. Bishop, Edward P. Fody, Larry E. Schoeff.—7th ed.
   p. cm.
 ISBN 978-1-4511-1869-8
 1. Clinical chemistry. I. Bishop, Michael L. II. Fody, Edward P. III. Schoeff, Larry E.
  RB40.C576 2013
  616.07'56—dc23

                  2012036179

Care has been taken to confirm the accuracy of the information presented and to describe generally accepted practices. However, the authors, editors, and publisher are not responsible for errors or omissions or for any consequences from application of the information in this book and make no warranty, expressed or implied, with respect to the currency, completeness, or accuracy of the contents of the publication. Application of this information in a particular situation remains the professional responsibility of the practitioner; the clinical treatments described and recommended may not be considered absolute and universal recommendations.

The authors, editors, and publisher have exerted every effort to ensure that drug selection and dosage set forth in this text are in accordance with the current recommendations and practice at the time of publication. However, in view of ongoing research, changes in government regulations, and the constant flow of information relating to drug therapy and drug reactions, the reader is urged to check the package insert for each drug for any change in indications and dosage and for added warnings and precautions. This is particularly important when the recommended agent is a new or infrequently employed drug.

Some drugs and medical devices presented in this publication have Health Canada clearance for limited use in restricted research settings. It is the responsibility of the health care provider to ascertain the Health Canada status of each drug or device planned for use in his or her clinical practice.

Visit Lippincott Williams & Wilkins on the Internet: http://www.lww.com. Lippincott Williams & Wilkins customer service representatives are available from 8:30 am to 6:00 pm, EST.

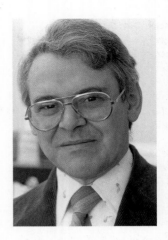

In memory of the University of Vermont Emeritus Professor René C. Lachapelle for going the extra mile to ensure his students and colleagues succeeded.

and

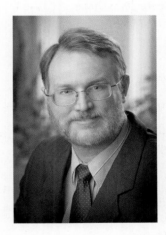

In memory of the University of Utah Professor Dr. William Roberts, internationally recognized clinical pathologist and clinical chemist.

and

To my parents, Stewart and Betty Bishop, for their guidance and encouragement.

and

To Sheila, Chris, and Carson for their support and patience.

MLB

Foreword

You should not be surprised to learn that the delivery of health care has been undergoing major transformation for several decades. The clinical laboratory has been transformed in innumerable ways as well. At one time the laboratory students' greatest asset was motor ability. That is not the case any longer. Now the need is for a laboratory professional who is well educated, an analytical thinker and problem solver, and one who can add value to the information generated in the laboratory regarding a specific patient.

This change impacts the laboratory professional in a very positive manner. Today the students' greatest asset is their mental skill; their ability to acquire and apply knowledge. The laboratory professional is now considered a knowledge worker, and a student's ability to successfully become this knowledge worker depends on their instruction and exposure to quality education. Herein lies the need for the seventh edition of *Clinical Chemistry: Principles, Techniques, and Correlations*. It contributes to the indispensable solid science foundation in medical laboratory sciences and the application of its principles in improving patient outcomes needed by the laboratory professional of today. This edition provides not only a comprehensive understanding of clinical chemistry but also the foundation upon which all the other major laboratory science disciplines can be further understood and integrated. It does so by providing a strong discussion of organ function and a solid emphasis on pathophysiology, clinical correlations, and differential diagnosis. This information offers a springboard to better understand the many concepts related to the effectiveness of a particular test for a particular patient.

Reduction of health care costs, while ensuring quality patient care, remains the goal of health care reform efforts. Laboratory information is a critical element of such care. It is estimated that $65 billion is spent each year to perform more than 4.3 billion laboratory tests. This impressive figure has also focused a bright light on laboratory medicine, and appropriate laboratory test utilization is now under major scrutiny. The main emphasis is on reducing costly overutilization and unnecessary diagnostic testing; however, the issue of under- and misutilization of laboratory tests must be a cause for concern as well. The role of laboratorians in providing guidance to clinicians regarding appropriate test utilization is becoming not only accepted but also welcomed as clinicians try to maneuver their way through an increasingly complex and expensive test menu. These new roles lie in the pre- and post-analytic functions of laboratorians. The authors of this text have successfully described the importance of these phases as well as the more traditional analytic phase. It does not matter how precise or accurate a test is during the analytic phase if the sample has been compromised, or if an inappropriate test has been ordered on the patient. In addition, the validation of results with respect to a patient's condition is an important step in the post-analytic phase. Participation with other health care providers in the proper interpretation of test results and appropriate follow-up will be important abilities of future graduates as the profession moves into providing greater consultative services for a patient-centered medical delivery system. Understanding these principles is a necessary requirement of the knowledge worker in the clinical laboratory. This significant professional role provides effective laboratory services that will improve medical decision making and thus patient safety while reducing medical errors. This edition of *Clinical Chemistry: Principles, Techniques, and Correlations* is a crucial element in graduating such professionals.

Diana Mass, MA, MT(ASCP)
Clinical Professor and Director (Retired)
Clinical Laboratory Sciences Program
Arizona State University
Tempe, Arizona
President
Associated Laboratory Consultants
Valley Center, California

Make no mistake: There are few specialties in medicine that have a wider impact on today's health care than laboratory medicine. For example, in the emergency room, a troponin result can not only tell an ER physician if a patient with chest pain has had a heart attack but also assess the likelihood of that patient suffering an acute myocardial infarction in 30 days. In the operating room during a parathyroidectomy, a parathyroid hormone assay can tell a surgeon that it is appropriate to close the procedure because he has successfully removed all of the affected glands, or go back and look for more glands to excise. In labor and delivery, testing for pulmonary surfactants from amniotic fluid can tell an obstetrician if a child can be safely delivered or if the infant is likely to develop life-threatening respiratory distress syndrome. In the neonatal intensive care unit, measurement of bilirubin in a premature infant is used to determine when the ultraviolet lights can be turned off. These are just a handful of the thousands of medical decisions that are made each day based on results from clinical laboratory testing.

Despite our current success, there is still much more to learn and do. For example, there are no good laboratory tests for the diagnosis of stroke or traumatic brain injury. The work on Alzheimer's and Parkinson's disease prediction and treatment is in the early stages. And when it comes to cancer, while our laboratory tests are good for monitoring therapy, they fail in the detection of early cancer, essential for improving treatment and prolonging survival. Finally, personalized medicine including pharmacogenomics will play an increasingly important role in the future. Pharmacogenomic testing will be used to select the right drug at the best dose for a particular patient in order to maximize efficacy and minimize side effects.

If you are reading this book, you are probably studying to be a part of the field. As a clinical chemist for over 30 years, I welcome you to our profession.

Alan H. B. Wu, PhD, DABCC
Director, Clinical Chemistry Laboratory, San Francisco
General Hospital
Professor, Laboratory Medicine, University of
California, San Francisco
San Francisco, California

Preface

Clinical chemistry continues to be one of the most rapidly advancing areas of laboratory medicine. Since the publication of the first edition of this textbook in 1985, many changes have taken place. New technologies and analytical techniques have been introduced, with a dramatic impact on the practice of clinical chemistry and laboratory medicine. In addition, the healthcare system is constantly changing. There is increased emphasis on improving the quality of patient care, individual patient outcomes, financial responsibility, and total quality management. Now, more than ever, clinical laboratorians need to be concerned with disease correlations, interpretations, problem solving, quality assurance, and cost-effectiveness; they need to know not only the *how* of tests but more importantly the *what, why, and when*. The editors of *Clinical Chemistry: Principles, Techniques, and Correlations* have designed the seventh edition to be an even more valuable resource to both students and practitioners.

Now 35 plus years since the initiation of this effort, the editors have had the privilege of completing the seventh edition with another diverse team of dedicated clinical laboratory professionals. In this era of focusing on metrics, the editors would like to share the following information. The 295 contributors in the 7 editions represent 65 clinical laboratory science programs, 77 clinical laboratories, 13 medical device companies, 4 government agencies, and 1 professional society. One hundred and twenty contributors were clinical laboratory scientists with advanced degrees. With today's global focus, the text has been translated into six languages. By definition, a profession is a calling requiring specialized knowledge and intensive academic preparation to define its scope of work and produce its own literature. The profession of Clinical Laboratory Science has evolved significantly over the past four decades.

Like the previous six editions, the seventh edition of *Clinical Chemistry: Principles, Techniques, and Correlations* is comprehensive, up-to-date, and easy to understand for students at all levels. It is also intended to be a practically organized resource for both instructors and practitioners. The editors have tried to maintain the book's readability and further improve its content. Because clinical laboratorians use their interpretative and analytic skills in the daily practice of clinical chemistry, an effort has been made to maintain an appropriate balance between analytic principles, techniques, and the correlation of results with disease states.

In this seventh edition, the editors have made several significant changes in response to requests from our readers, students, instructors, and practitioners. Key Terms and Chapter Objectives have been introduced at the beginning of each chapter. Ancillary materials have been updated and expanded. Chapters now include current, more frequently encountered case studies and practice questions or exercises. To provide a thorough, up-to-date study of clinical chemistry, all chapters have been updated and reviewed by professionals who practice clinical chemistry and laboratory medicine on a daily basis. The basic principles of the analytic procedures discussed in the chapters reflect the most recent or commonly performed techniques in the clinical chemistry laboratory. Detailed procedures have been omitted because of the variety of equipment and commercial kits used in today's clinical laboratories. Instrument manuals and kit package inserts are the most reliable reference for detailed instructions on current analytic procedures. All chapter material has been updated, improved, and rearranged for better continuity and readability. **thePoint**✳, a web site with additional case studies, review questions, teaching resources, teaching tips, additional references, and teaching aids for instructors and students is available from the publisher to assist in the use of this textbook.

Michael L. Bishop

Edward P. Fody

Larry E. Schoeff

Acknowledgments

A project as large as this requires the assistance and support of many individuals. The editors wish to express their appreciation to the contributors of this seventh edition of *Clinical Chemistry: Principles, Techniques, and Correlations*—the dedicated laboratory professionals and educators whom the editors have had the privilege of knowing and exchanging ideas with over the years. These individuals were selected because of their expertise in particular areas and their commitment to the education of clinical laboratorians. Many have spent their professional careers in the clinical laboratory, at the bench, teaching students, or consulting with clinicians. In these frontline positions, they have developed a perspective of what is important for the next generation of clinical laboratorians.

We extend appreciation to our students, colleagues, teachers, and mentors in the profession who have helped shape our ideas about clinical chemistry practice and education. Also, we want to thank the many companies and professional organizations that provided product information and photographs or granted permission to reproduce diagrams and tables from their publications. Many Clinical and Laboratory Standards Institute (CLSI) documents have also been important sources of information. These documents are directly referenced in the appropriate chapters.

The editors would like to acknowledge the contribution and effort of all individuals to previous editions. Their efforts provided the framework for many of the current chapters. We also want to thank Dr. Özgür Aydin for reviewing the manuscript of this edition for accuracy. Finally, we gratefully acknowledge the cooperation and assistance of the staff at Lippincott Williams & Wilkins for their advice and support.

The editors are continually striving to improve future editions of this book. We again request and welcome our readers' comments, criticisms, and ideas for improvement.

Contributors

Dev Abraham, MD
Professor of Medicine
Division of Endocrinology
University of Utah
Salt Lake City, UT

Josephine Abraham, MD
Professor of Medicine
Division of Nephrology
University of Utah
Salt Lake City, UT

John J. Ancy, MA, RRT
Senior Clinical Consultant
Instrumentation Laboratory
Bedford, MA

Nadia Ayala, MLS(ASCP)
Department of Pharmacology and Toxicology
Michigan State University
East Lansing, MI

Elzbieta (Ela) Bakowska, PhD
Technical Director
Elba Elemental Consulting
Corning, NY

Laura M. Bender, PhD
Clinical Chemistry Fellow, Pathology and Laboratory
Medicine
University of North Carolina Hospital
Chapel Hill, NC

Michael J. Bennett, PhD
Director of Metabolic Disease
Children's Hospital of Philadelphia
Philadelphia, PA

Maria G. Boosalis, PhD, MPH, RD, LD
Director, Division of Clinical Nutrition
College of Health Sciences
University of Kentucky
Lexington, KY

Raffick A. R. Bowen, PhD
Associate Director, Clinical Chemistry and Immunology
Laboratory
Stanford University Medical Center
Stanford, CA

Larry A. Broussard, PhD
Department Head, Clinical Laboratory Sciences
Louisiana State University Health Sciences Center
New Orleans, LA

Janetta Bryksin, PhD
Clinical Chemistry Fellow, Pathology
Emory University School of Medicine
Atlanta, GA

Dean C. Carlow, MD, PhD
Director of Clinical Chemistry
Children's Hospital of Philadelphia
Philadelphia, PA

Eileen Carreiro-Lewandowski, MS, CLS
Professor, Medical Laboratory Science
University of Massachusetts – Dartmouth
Dartmouth, MA

Janelle M. Chiasera, PhD
Department Chair, Clinical and Diagnostic Sciences
University of Alabama – Birmingham
Birmingham, AL

Steven W. Cotten, PhD, DABCC, NRCC
Associate Director of Toxicology and Special Functions
Wexner Medical Center
Assistant Professor
The Ohio State University
Columbus, OH

Julia C. Drees, PhD, DABCC
Clinical Research and Development Scientist
Kaiser Permanente Regional Laboratory
Berkeley, CA

Michael Durando, MD/PhD Candidate
School of Medicine
Boston University
Boston, MA
and
Graduate College
University of North Carolina
Chapel Hill, NC

Sharon S. Ehrmeyer, PhD
Professor, Pathology and Laboratory Medicine
University of Wisconsin – Madison
Madison, WI

Corinne R. Fantz, PhD
Director, Point-of-Care Testing, Pathology &
Laboratory Medicine
Emory University Hospital Midtown
Atlanta, GA

Edward P. Fody, MD
Clinical Professor
Department of Pathology, Microbiology and Immunology
Vanderbilt University School of Medicine
Nashville, TN
and
Medical Director
Department of Pathology
Holland Hospital
Holland, MI

Elizabeth L. Frank, PhD
Associate Professor, Department of Pathology
University of Utah School of Medicine
Salt Lake City, UT
and
Medical Director, Analytic Biochemistry and Calculi
ARUP Laboratories, Inc.
Salt Lake City, UT

Vicki S. Freeman, PhD, MLS(ASCP)^CM SC, FACB
Department Chair, Clinical Laboratory Sciences
University of Texas Medical Branch
Galveston, TX

Linda S. Gorman, PhD
Medical Laboratory Science
Education Coordinator
Associate Professor
University of Kentucky
Lexington, KY

Ryan W. Greer, MS, I&C(ASCP)
Assistant Vice President, Group Manager Chemistry
Group III, Technical Operations
ARUP Laboratories, Inc.
Salt Lake City, UT

Marissa Grotzke, MD
Assistant Professor
Internal Medicine
University of Utah
Salt Lake City, UT

Mahima Gulati, MD
Fellow
Division of Endocrinology, Diabetes, and Metabolism
University of Utah Hospital
Salt Lake City, UT

George A. Harwell, EdD
Chairman, Clinical Laboratory Science
Winston-Salem State University
Winston-Salem, NC

Matthew P. A. Henderson, PhD
Clinical Biochemist, Division of Biochemistry
The Ottawa Hospital
Ottawa, ON

Brian C. Jensen, MD
Assistant Professor
Department of Medicine
Division of Cardiology
University of North Carolina Hospitals
Chapel Hill, NC

Kamisha L. Johnson-Davis, PhD, DABCC, FACB
Assistant Professor, Pathology
University of Utah
Salt Lake City, UT

Robert E. Jones, MD
Professor of Medicine
Division of Endocrinology
University of Utah
Salt Lake City, UT

Deborah E. Keil, PhD, MLS(ASCP), DABT
Associate Professor
Program of Medical Laboratory Science
Department of Microbiology
Montana State University
Bozeman, MT

Louann W. Lawrence, DrPH
Professor Emeritus, Clinical Laboratory Sciences
Louisiana State University Health Sciences Center
New Orleans, LA

Kara L. Lynch, PhD
Associate Division Chief, Chemistry and Toxicology
Laboratory
San Francisco General Hospital
San Francisco, CA

Jack M. McBride, Jr, MD
Fellow, Geriatric Medicine
University of North Carolina Health Care
Chapel Hill, NC

Christopher R. McCudden, PhD
Clinical Biochemist, Pathology and Laboratory Medicine
The Ottawa Hospital
Ottawa, ON

Shashi Mehta, PhD
Department of Clinical Laboratory Sciences
School of Health Related Professions
University of Medicine and Dentistry
of New Jersey
Newark, NJ

A. Wayne Meikle, MD
Professor, Medicine and Pathology
University of Utah School of Medicine
Salt Lake City, UT

T. Creighton Mitchell, MD
Fellow
Division of Endocrinology, Metabolism,
and Diabetes
University of Utah
Salt Lake City, UT

Lillian A. Mundt, EdD
Medical Laboratory Scientist
Adventist Hinsdale Hospital
Hinsdale, IL

Matthew S. Petrie, PhD
Clinical Chemistry Fellow, Department of
Laboratory Medicine
University of California San Francisco
San Francisco, CA

Alan T. Remaley, MD, PhD
Senior Staff, Department of Laboratory
Medicine
National Institutes of Health
Bethesda, MD

William L. Roberts, MD, PhD
Professor, Pathology
University of Utah
Salt Lake City, UT

Alan L. Rockwood, PhD
Associate Professor, Clinical Chemistry
University of Utah School of Medicine
Salt Lake City, UT

Michael W. Rogers, MT(ASCP), MBA
Quality Management Specialist
McLendon Clinical (Core) Laboratories
University of North Carolina Hospitals
Chapel Hill, NC

Amar A. Sethi, PhD
Chief Scientific Officer, Research and Development
Pacific Biomarkers
Seattle, WA

Kristy Shanahan, MS, MLS(ASCP)
Assistant Professor, College of Pharmacy
Rosalind Franklin University
North Chicago, IL

Joely A. Straseski, PhD
Assistant Professor, Pathology
University of Utah
Salt Lake City, UT

Frederick G. Strathmann, PhD
Assistant Medical Director, Toxicology
ARUP Laboratories
Salt Lake City, UT

Tolmie E. Wachter, MBA/HCM, SLS(ASCP)
Director of Corporate Safety
ARUP Laboratories
Salt Lake City, UT

G. Russell Warnick, MS, MBA
Chief Scientific Officer
Health Diagnostic Laboratory
Richmond, VA

Monte S. Willis, MD, PhD, FAHA, FCAP, FASCP
Director, Campus Health Sciences Laboratory
Associate Director, McLendon Clinical (Core)
Laboratories
Associate Professor
University of North Carolina
Chapel Hill, NC

Alan H. B. Wu, PhD, DABCC
Director, Clinical Chemistry Laboratory, San Francisco
General Hospital
Professor, Laboratory Medicine, University of
California, San Francisco
San Francisco, CA

Xin Xu, MD, PhD, MLS(ASCP)
Division of Pulmonary, Allergy, and Critical Care
Medicine
Department of Medicine
University of Alabama at Birmingham
Birmingham, AL

Contents

Basic Principles and Practice of Clinical Chemistry

Basic Principles and Practices

EILEEN CARREIRO-LEWANDOWSKI

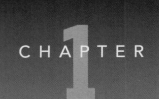

CHAPTER OUTLINE

Chapter Objectives

Upon completion of this chapter, the clinical laboratorian should be able to do the following:

- Convert results from one unit format to another using the SI and traditional systems.
- Describe the classifications used for reagent grade water.
- Identify the varying chemical grades used in reagent preparation and indicate their correct use.
- Define primary standard, standard reference materials, and secondary standard.
- Describe the following terms that are associated with solutions and, when appropriate, provide the respective units: percent, molarity, normality, molality, saturation, colligative properties, redox potential, conductivity, and specific gravity.
- Define a buffer and give the formula for pH and pK calculations.
- Use the Henderson-Hasselbalch equation to determine the missing variable when given either the pK and pH or the pK and concentration of the weak acid and its conjugate base.

- List and describe the types of thermometers used in the clinical laboratory.
- Classify the type of pipet when given an actual pipet or its description.
- Demonstrate the proper use of a measuring and volumetric pipet.
- Describe two ways to calibrate a pipetting device.
- Define a desiccant and discuss how it is used in the clinical laboratory.
- Describe how to properly care for and balance a centrifuge.
- Correctly perform the laboratory mathematical calculations provided in this chapter.
- Identify and describe the types of samples used in clinical chemistry.
- Outline the general steps for processing blood samples.
- Apply Beer's law to determine the concentration of a sample when the absorbance or change in absorbance is provided.
- Identify the preanalytic variables that can adversely affect laboratory results as presented in this chapter.

KEY TERMS

Analyte
Anhydrous
Arterial blood
Beer's law

Buffer
Buret
Centrifugation
Cerebrospinal fluid (CSF)
CLSI

Colligative property
Conductivity
Deionized water
Deliquescent substances
Delta absorbance
Density
Desiccant
Desiccator
Dialysis
Dilution
Dilution factor
Distilled water
Equivalent weight
Erlenmeyer flasks
Filtrate
Filtration
Graduated cylinder
Griffin beaker
Hemolysis
Henderson-Hasselbalch equation
Hydrate
Hygroscopic
Icterus
International unit
Ionic strength
Lipemic
Mantissa
Molality
Molarity

Normality
One-point calibration
Osmotic pressure
Oxidized
Oxidizing agent
Percent solution
pH
Pipet
Primary standard
Ratio
Reagent grade water
Redox potential
Reduced
RO water
Secondary standard
Serial dilution
Serum
Significant figures
Solute
Solution
Solvent
Specific gravity
Standard
Standard reference materials (SRMs)
Système International d'Unités (SI)
Thermistor
Ultrafiltration
Valence
Whole blood

The primary purpose of a clinical chemistry laboratory is to facilitate the correct performance of analytic procedures that yield accurate and precise information, aiding patient diagnosis and treatment. The achievement of reliable results requires that the clinical laboratory scientist be able to correctly use basic supplies and equipment and possess an understanding of fundamental concepts critical to any analytic procedure. The topics in this chapter include units of measure, basic laboratory supplies, and introductory laboratory mathematics, plus a brief discussion of specimen collection, processing, and reporting.

UNITS OF MEASURE

Any meaningful *quantitative* laboratory result consists of two components: the first component represents the number related to the actual test value, and the second is a label identifying the units. The unit defines the physical quantity or dimension, such as mass, length, time, or volume.[1] Not all laboratory tests have well-defined units, but whenever possible, the units used should be reported.

Although several systems of units have traditionally been utilized by various scientific divisions, the Système International d'Unités (SI), adopted internationally in 1960, is preferred in scientific literature and clinical laboratories and is the only system employed in many countries. This system was devised to provide the global scientific community with a uniform method of describing physical quantities. The SI system units (referred to as *SI units*) are based on the metric system. Several subclassifications exist within the SI system, one of which is the *basic unit*. There are seven basic units (Table 1-1), with length (meter), mass (kilogram), and quantity of a substance (mole) being the units most frequently encountered. Another set of SI-recognized units is termed *derived units*. A derived unit, as the name implies, is a derivative or a mathematical function describing one of the basic units. An example of a SI-derived unit is meters per second (m/s), used to express velocity. However, some non-SI units are so widely used that they have become acceptable for use with SI basic or SI-derived units (Table 1-1). These include certain longstanding units such as hour, minute, day, gram, liter, and plane angles expressed as degrees. These units, although widely used, cannot technically be categorized as either basic or derived SI units.

The SI uses standard *prefixes* that, when added to a given basic unit, can indicate decimal fractions or multiples of that unit (Table 1-2). For example, 0.001 liter can be expressed using the prefix *milli*, or 10^{-3}, and since

TABLE 1-1	SI UNITS	
BASE QUANTITY	**NAME**	**SYMBOL**
Length	Meter	m
Mass	Kilogram	kg
Time	Second	s
Electric current	Ampere	A
Thermodynamic temperature	Kelvin	K
Amount of substance	Mole	mol
Luminous intensity	Candela	cd
SELECTED DERIVED		
Frequency	Hertz	Hz
Force	Newton	N
Celsius temperature	Degree Celsius	°C
Catalytic activity	Katal	kat
SELECTED ACCEPTED NON-SI		
Minute (time)	(60 s)	min
Hour	(3,600 s)	h
Day	(86,400 s)	d
Liter (volume)	($1\ dm^3 = 10^{-3}\ m^3$)	L
Angstrom	($0.1\ nm = 10^{-10}\ m$)	Å

TABLE 1-2	PREFIXES USED WITH SI UNITS		
FACTOR	**PREFIX**	**SYMBOL**	**SELECT DECIMALS**
10^{-18}	atto	a	—
10^{-15}	femto	f	—
10^{-12}	pico	p	—
10^{-9}	nano	n	—
10^{-6}	micro	μ	0.000001
10^{-3}	milli	m	0.001
10^{-2}	centi	c	0.01
10^{-1}	deci	d	0.1
10^{0}	Liter, meter, gram	Basic unit	1.0
10^{1}	deka	da	10.0
10^{2}	hecto	h	100.0
10^{3}	kilo	k	1,000.0
10^{4}	mega	M	—
10^{9}	giga	G	—
10^{12}	tera	T	—
10^{15}	peta	P	—
10^{18}	exa	E	—

Prefixes are used to indicate a subunit or multiple of a basic SI unit.

it requires moving the decimal point three places to the right, it can then be written as 1 milliliter, or abbreviated as 1 mL. It may also be written in scientific notation as 1×10^{-3} L. Likewise, 1,000 liters would use the prefix of kilo (10^3) and could be written as 1 kiloliter or expressed in scientific notation as 1×10^3 L.

It is important to understand the relationship these prefixes have to the basic unit. The highlighted upper portion of Table 1-2 indicates that these prefixes are all smaller than the basic unit and frequently used expressions in clinical laboratories. When converting between prefixes, simply note the relationship between them based on whether you are changing to a smaller or larger prefix and the incremental factor between them. For example, if converting from one liter (1.0×10^0 or 1) to milliliters (1.0×10^{-3} or 0.001), the starting unit is larger than the desired unit by a factor of 1,000 or 10^3. This means that the decimal place would be moved to the *right* of one (1) three places, so 1.0 liter (L) equals 1,000 milliliters (mL). When changing 1,000 milliliter (ml) to 1 liter (L), the process is reversed and decimal point would be moved three places to the left to become 1 L. Note that the SI term for mass is *kilogram*; it is the only basic unit that contains a prefix as part of its naming convention. Generally, the standard prefixes for mass use the term *gram* rather than *kilogram*.

Example 1: Convert 1 L to mL
1 L (1×10^0) = ? mL (milli = 10^{-3}); move the decimal place three places to the right and it becomes 1,000 mL; reverse the process to determine the expression in L (move the decimal three places to the left of 1,000 mL to get 1 L). However, 1 mL (smaller) = ? L (larger by 10^3); move the decimal to the left by three places and it becomes 0.001 L.

Example 2: Convert 50 mL to L
50 mL (milli = 10^{-3} and is smaller) = ? L (larger by 10^3); move the decimal by three places to the left and it becomes 0.050 L. Using the illustration, the # substituted would be "50" in this example.

Example 3: Convert 5 dL to mL
5 dL (deci = 10^{-1} and is larger) = ? mL (milli = 10^{-3} and is smaller by 10^{-2}); move the decimal place two places to the right and it becomes 500 mL. Note that in this case the # substituted would be "5."

Reporting of laboratory results is often expressed in terms of substance concentration (e.g., moles) or the mass of a substance (e.g., mg/dL, g/dL, g/L, mmol/L, and IU) rather than in SI units. These familiar and traditional units can cause confusion during interpretation. It has been recommended that analytes be reported using moles of solute per volume of solution (substance concentration) and that the liter be used as the reference volume.[2] Appendix D (on the companion web site), *Conversion of Traditional Units to SI Units for Common Clinical Chemistry Analytes*, lists both reference and SI units together with the conversion factor from traditional to SI units for common analytes. As with other areas of industry, the laboratory and the rest of medicine is moving toward adopting universal standards promoted by the International Organization for Standardization, often referred to as ISO. This group develops standards of practice, definitions, and guidelines that can be adopted by everyone in a given field, providing for more uniform terminology and less confusion. As with any transition, clinical laboratory scientists should be familiar with all the terms currently used in their field.

REAGENTS

In today's highly automated laboratory, there seems to be little need for reagent preparation by the clinical laboratory scientist. Most instrument manufacturers make the reagents in ready-to-use form or in a "kit" form (i.e., all necessary reagents and respective storage containers are prepackaged as a unit) requiring only the addition of water or buffer to the prepackaged reagent components for reconstitution. A heightened awareness of the hazards of certain chemicals and the numerous regulatory agency requirements has caused clinical chemistry laboratories to readily eliminate massive stocks of chemicals and opt instead for the ease of using prepared reagents. Periodically, especially in hospital laboratories involved in research and development, biotechnology applications, specialized analyses, or method validation, the laboratorian may still face preparing various reagents or solutions. As a result of reagent deterioration, supply and demand, or the institution of cost-containment programs,

---

SI CONVERSIONS

To convert between SI units, move the decimal by the difference between the exponents represented by the prefix either to the right (from a larger to a smaller unit) or to the left (from a smaller to a larger one) of the number given:

decimal point

◄── 000 #.000 ──►

smaller to larger unit   larger to smaller unit

Convert to larger unit: smaller to larger unit—move to the left

Convert to a smaller unit: larger to smaller—move to the right

= the numeric value given

the decision may be made to prepare reagents in-house. Therefore, a thorough knowledge of chemicals, standards, solutions, buffers, and water requirements is necessary.

Chemicals

Analytic chemicals exist in varying grades of purity: analytic reagent (AR); ultrapure, chemically pure (CP); United States Pharmacopeia (USP); National Formulary (NF); and technical or commercial grade.[3] A committee of the American Chemical Society (ACS; www.acs.org) established specifications for AR grade chemicals, and chemical manufacturers will either meet or exceed these requirements. Labels on reagents state the actual impurities for each chemical lot or list the maximum allowable impurities. The labels should be clearly printed with the percentage of impurities present and either the initials *AR* or *ACS* or the term *For laboratory use* or *ACS Standard-Grade Reference Materials*. Chemicals of this category are suitable for use in most analytic laboratory procedures. Ultrapure chemicals have been put through additional purification steps for use in specific procedures such as chromatography, atomic absorption, immunoassays, molecular diagnostics, standardization, or other techniques that require extremely pure chemicals. These reagents may carry designations of HPLC (high-performance liquid chromatography) or chromatographic (see later) on their labels.

Because USP and NF grade chemicals are used to manufacture drugs, the limitations established for this group of chemicals are based only on the criterion of not being injurious to individuals. Chemicals in this group may be pure enough for use in most chemical procedures; however, it should be recognized that the purity standards are not based on the needs of the laboratory and, therefore, may or may not meet all assay requirements.

Reagent designations of CP or pure grade indicate that the impurity limitations are not stated and that preparation of these chemicals is not uniform. Melting point analysis is often used to ascertain the acceptable purity range. It is not recommended that clinical laboratories use these chemicals for reagent preparation unless further purification or a reagent blank is included. Technical or commercial grade reagents are used primarily in manufacturing and should never be used in the clinical laboratory.

Organic reagents also have varying grades of purity that differ from those used to classify inorganic reagents. These grades include a practical grade with some impurities; CP, which approaches the purity level of reagent grade chemicals; spectroscopic (spectrally pure) and chromatographic (minimum purity of 99% determined by gas chromatography) grade organic reagents, with purity levels attained by their respective procedures; and reagent grade (ACS), which is certified to contain impurities below certain levels established by the ACS. As in

any analytic method, the desired organic reagent purity is dictated by the particular application.

Other than the purity aspects of the chemicals, laws related to the Occupational Safety and Health Administration (OSHA)[4] require manufacturers to clearly indicate the lot number, plus any physical or biologic health hazard and precautions needed for the safe use and storage of any chemical. A manufacturer is required to provide technical data sheets for each chemical manufactured on a document called a Material Safety Data Sheet (MSDS). A more detailed discussion of this topic may be found in Chapter 2.

Reference Materials

Unlike other areas of chemistry, clinical chemistry is involved in the analysis of biochemical by-products found in *biological* fluids, such as serum, plasma, or urine, making purification and a known *exact* composition of the material almost impossible. For this reason, traditionally defined standards used in analytical chemistry do not readily apply in clinical chemistry.

Recall that a **primary standard** is a highly purified chemical that can be measured directly to produce a substance of *exact* known concentration and purity. The ACS purity tolerances for primary standards are 100 ± 0.02%. Because most biologic constituents are unavailable within these limitations, the National Institute of Standards and Technology (NIST; http://ts.nist.gov)–certified **standard reference materials** (SRMs) are used instead of ACS primary standard materials.[5-9]

The NIST developed certified reference materials/SRMs for use in clinical chemistry laboratories. They are assigned a value after careful analysis, using state-of-the-art methods and equipment. The chemical composition of these substances is then certified; however, they may not possess the purity equivalent of a primary standard. Because each substance has been characterized for certain chemical or physical properties, it can be used in place of an ACS primary standard in clinical work and is often used to verify calibration or accuracy/bias assessments. Many manufacturers use a NIST SRM when producing calibrator and standard materials, and in this way, these materials are considered "traceable to NIST" and may meet certain accreditation requirements. There are SRMs for a number of routine analytes, hormones, drugs, and blood gases, with others being added.[10]

A **secondary standard** is a substance of lower purity, with its concentration determined by comparison with a primary standard. The secondary standard depends not only on its composition, which cannot be directly determined, but also on the analytic reference method. Once again, because physiologic primary standards are generally unavailable, clinical chemists do not by definition have "true" secondary standards. Manufacturers of secondary standards will list the SRM or primary standard used for comparison. This information may be needed during laboratory accreditation processes.

Water Specifications[11]

Water is the most frequently used reagent in the laboratory. Because tap water is unsuitable for laboratory applications, most procedures, including reagent and standard preparation, use water that has been substantially purified. Water solely purified by distillation results in distilled water; water purified by ion exchange produces deionized water. Reverse osmosis, which pumps water across a semipermeable membrane, produces RO water. Water can also be purified by ultrafiltration, ultraviolet light, sterilization, or ozone treatment. Laboratory requirements generally call for reagent grade water that, according to the Clinical and Laboratory Standards Institute (CLSI), is classified into one of six categories based on the specifications needed for its use rather than the method of purification or preparation.[12] These categories include clinical laboratory reagent water (CLRW), special reagent water (SRW), instrument feed water, water supplied by method manufacturer, autoclave and wash water, and commercially bottled purified water. Laboratories need to assess whether the water meets the specifications needed for its application. Most water monitoring parameters include at least microbiological count, pH (related to the hydrogen ion concentration), resistivity (measure of resistance in ohms and influenced by the number of ions present), silicate, particulate matter, and organics. Each category has a specific acceptable limit. A long-held convention for categorizing water purity was based on three types, I through III, with type I water having the most stringent requirements and generally suitable for routine laboratory use.

Prefiltration can remove particulate matter from municipal water supplies before any additional treatments. Filtration cartridges are composed of glass; cotton; activated charcoal, which removes organic materials and chlorine; and submicron filters (≤0.2 mm), which remove any substances larger than the filter's pores, including bacteria. The use of these filters depends on the quality of the municipal water and the other purification methods used. For example, hard water (containing calcium, iron, and other dissolved elements) may require prefiltration with a glass or cotton filter rather than activated charcoal or submicron filters, which quickly become clogged and are expensive to use. The submicron filter may be better suited after distillation, deionization, or reverse osmosis treatment.

Distilled water has been purified to remove almost all organic materials, using a technique of distillation much like that found in organic chemistry laboratory distillation experiments in which water is boiled and vaporized. The vapor rises and enters into the coil of a condenser, a glass tube that contains a glass coil. Cool water surrounds this condensing coil, lowering the temperature of the water vapor. The water vapor returns to a liquid state, which is then collected. Many impurities do not rise in the water vapor, remaining in the boiling apparatus. The water collected after condensation has less contamination. Because laboratories use thousands of liters of water each day, stills are used instead of small condensing apparatuses; however, the principles are basically the same. Water may be distilled more than once, with each distillation cycle removing additional impurities.

Deionized water has some or all ions removed, although organic material may still be present, so it is neither pure nor sterile. Generally, deionized water is purified from previously treated water, such as prefiltered or distilled water. Deionized water is produced using either an anion or a cation exchange resin, followed by replacement of the removed ions with hydroxyl or hydrogen ions. The ions that are anticipated to be removed from the water will dictate the type of ion exchange resin to be used. One column cannot service all ions present in water. A combination of several resins will produce different grades of deionized water. A two-bed system uses an anion resin followed by a cation resin. The different resins may be in separate columns or in the same column. This process is excellent in removing dissolved ionized solids and dissolved gases.

Reverse osmosis is a process that uses pressure to force water through a semipermeable membrane, producing water that reflects a filtered product of the original water. It does not remove dissolved gases. Reverse osmosis may be used for the pretreatment of water.

Ultrafiltration and nanofiltration, like distillation, are excellent in removing particulate matter, microorganisms, and any pyrogens or endotoxins. Ultraviolet oxidation (removes some trace organic material) or sterilization processes (uses specific wavelengths), together with ozone treatment, can destroy bacteria but may leave behind residual products. These techniques are often used after other purification processes have been used.

Production of reagent grade water largely depends on the condition of the feed water. Generally, reagent grade water can be obtained by initially filtering it to remove particulate matter, followed by reverse osmosis, deionization, and a 0.2 mm filter or more restrictive filtration process. Type III/autoclave wash water is acceptable for glassware washing but not for analysis or reagent preparation. Traditionally, type II water was acceptable for most analytic requirements, including reagent, quality control, and standard preparation, while type I water was used for test methods requiring minimum interference, such as trace metal, iron, and enzyme analyses. Use with HPLC may require less than a 0.2 mm final filtration step and falls into the SRW category. Some molecular diagnostic or mass spectrophotometric techniques may require special reagent grade water; some reagent grade water should be used immediately, so storage is discouraged because the resistivity changes. Depending on the application, CLRW should be stored in a manner that reduces any chemical or bacterial contamination and for short periods.

Testing procedures to determine the quality of reagent grade water include measurements of resistance, pH, colony counts (for assessing bacterial contamination) on selective and nonselective media for the detection of coliforms, chlorine, ammonia, nitrate or nitrite, iron, hardness, phosphate, sodium, silica, carbon dioxide, chemical oxygen demand, and metal detection. Some accreditation agencies[13] recommend that laboratories document culture growth, pH, and specific resistance on water used in reagent preparation. Resistance is measured because pure water, devoid of ions, is a poor conductor of electricity and has increased resistance. The relationship of water purity to resistance is linear. Generally, as purity increases, so does resistance. This one measurement does not suffice for determination of true water purity because a nonionic contaminant may be present that has little effect on resistance. Note that reagent water meeting specifications from other organizations, such as the ASTM, may not be equivalent to those established for each type by the CLSI, and care should be taken to meet the assay procedural requirements for water type requirements.

Solution Properties

In clinical chemistry, substances found in biologic fluids are measured (e.g., serum, plasma, urine, and spinal fluid). A substance that is dissolved in a liquid is called a **solute**; in laboratory science, these biologic solutes are also known as *analytes*. The liquid in which the solute is dissolved—in this instance, a biologic fluid—is the **solvent**. Together they represent a **solution**. Any chemical or biologic solution is described by its basic properties, including concentration, saturation, colligative properties, redox potential, conductivity, density, pH, and ionic strength.

Concentration

Analyte concentration in solution can be expressed in many ways. Routinely, concentration is expressed as percent solution, molarity, molality, or normality, and because these non-SI expressions are so widely used, they will be discussed here. Note that the SI expression for the amount of a substance is the mole.

Percent solution is expressed as equal parts per hundred or the amount of solute per 100 total units of solution. Three expressions of percent solutions are weight per weight (w/w), volume per volume (v/v), and, most commonly, weight per volume (w/v). For v/v solutions, it is recommended that grams per deciliter (g/dL) be used instead of percent or % (v/v).

Molarity (M) is expressed as the number of moles per 1 L of solution. One mole of a substance equals its gram molecular weight (gmw), so the customary units of molarity (M) are moles/liter. The SI representation for the traditional molar concentration is moles of solute per volume of solution, with the volume of the solution given in liters. The SI expression for concentration should be represented as moles per liter (mol/L), millimoles per liter (mmol/L), micromoles per liter (μmol/L), and nanomoles per liter (nmol/L). The familiar concentration term *molarity* has not been adopted by the SI as an expression of concentration. It should also be noted that molarity depends on volume, and any significant physical changes that influence volume, such as changes in temperature and pressure, will also influence molarity.

Molality (m) represents the amount of solute per 1 kg of solvent. Molality is sometimes confused with molarity; however, it can be easily distinguished from molarity because molality is always expressed in terms of weight per weight or moles per kilogram and describes moles per 1,000 g (1 kg) of solvent. Note that the common abbreviation (m) for molality is a lower case "m," while the upper case (M) refers to molarity. However, the preferred expression for molality is moles per kilogram (mol/kg) to avoid any confusion. Unlike molarity, molality is not influenced by temperature or pressure because it is based on mass rather than volume.

Normality is the least likely of the four concentration expressions to be encountered in clinical laboratories, but it is often used in chemical titrations and chemical reagent classification. It is defined as the number of gram equivalent weights per 1 L of solution. An **equivalent weight** is equal to the gmw of a substance divided by its valence. The **valence** is the number of units that can combine with or replace 1 mole of hydrogen ions for acids and hydroxyl ions for bases and the number of electrons exchanged in oxidation–reduction reactions. It is the number of atoms/elements that can combine for a particular compound; therefore, the equivalent weight is the gram combining weight of a material. Normality is always equal to or greater than the molarity of that compound. Normality was previously used for reporting electrolyte values, such as sodium [Na^+], potassium [K^+], and chloride [Cl^-], expressed as milliequivalents per liter (mEq/L); however, this convention has been replaced with the more familiar units of millimoles per liter (mmol/L).

Solution saturation gives little specific information about the concentration of solutes in a solution.

Temperature, as well as the presence of other ions, can influence the solubility constant for a solute in a given solution and thus affect the saturation. Routine terms in the clinical laboratory that describe the extent of saturation are *dilute*, *concentrated*, *saturated*, and *supersaturated*. A *dilute solution* is one in which there is relatively little solute or one which has been made to a lower solute concentration per volume of solvent as when making a dilution. In contrast, a *concentrated solution* has a large quantity of solute in solution. A solution in which there is an excess of undissolved solute particles can be referred to as a *saturated solution*. As the name implies, a *supersaturated solution* has an even greater concentration of undissolved solute particles than a saturated solution of the same substance. Because of the greater concentration of solute particles, a supersaturated solution is thermodynamically unstable. The addition of a crystal of solute or mechanical agitation disturbs the supersaturated solution, resulting in crystallization of any excess material out of solution. An example is seen when measuring serum osmolality by freezing point depression.

Colligative Properties

The behavior of particles or solutes in solution demonstrates four repeatable properties based only on the relative number of each kind of molecule present. The properties of osmotic pressure, vapor pressure, freezing point, and boiling point are called **colligative properties**. *Vapor pressure* is the pressure at which the liquid solvent is in equilibrium with the water vapor. *Freezing point* is the temperature at which the vapor pressures of the solid and liquid phases are the same. *Boiling point* is the temperature at which the vapor pressure of the solvent reaches one atmosphere.

Osmotic pressure is the pressure that opposes osmosis when a solvent flows through a semipermeable membrane to establish equilibrium between compartments of differing concentration. The osmotic pressure of a dilute solution is proportional to the concentration of the molecules in solution. The expression for concentration is the osmole. One osmole of a substance equals the molarity or molality multiplied by the number of particles, not the kind, at dissociation. If molarity is used, the resulting expression would be termed osmolarity; if molality is used, the expression changes to osmolality. Osmolality is preferred since it depends on the weight rather than volume and is not readily influenced by temperature and pressure changes. When a solute is dissolved in a solvent, these colligative properties change in a predictable manner for each osmole of substance present; the freezing point is lowered by −1.86°C, the boiling point is raised by 0.52°C, the vapor pressure is lowered by 0.3 mm Hg or torr, and the osmotic pressure is increased by a factor of 1.7×10^4 mm Hg or torr. In the clinical setting, freezing point and vapor pressure depression can be measured as a function of osmolality. Freezing point is preferred since vapor pressure measurements can give inaccurate readings when some substances, such as alcohols, are present in the samples.

Redox Potential

Redox potential, or *oxidation–reduction potential*, is a measure of the ability of a solution to accept or donate electrons. Substances that donate electrons are called *reducing agents*; those that accept electrons are considered **oxidizing agents**. The pneumonic—LEO (lose electrons **oxidized**) the lion says GER (gain electrons **reduced**)—may prove useful when trying to recall the relationship between reducing/oxidizing agents and redox potential.

Conductivity

Conductivity is a measure of how well electricity passes through a solution. A solution's conductivity quality depends principally on the number of respective charges of the ions present. *Resistivity*, the reciprocal of conductivity, is a measure of a substance's resistance to the passage of electrical current. The primary application of resistivity in the clinical laboratory is for assessing the purity of water. Resistivity or resistance is expressed as ohms and conductivity is expressed as $ohms^{-1}$ or mho.

pH and Buffers

Buffers are weak acids or bases and their related salts that, as a result of their dissociation characteristics, minimize changes in the hydrogen ion concentration. Hydrogen ion concentration is often expressed as pH. A lowercase *p* in front of certain letters or abbreviations operationally means the "negative logarithm of" or "inverse log of" that substance. In keeping with this convention, the term **pH** represents the negative or inverse log of the hydrogen ion concentration. Mathematically, pH is expressed as

$$pH = \log\left(\frac{1}{[H^+]}\right)$$
$$pH = -\log[H^+] \qquad \textbf{(Eq. 1-1)}$$

where $[H^+]$ equals the concentration of hydrogen ions in moles per liter.

The pH scale ranges from 0 to 14 and is a convenient way to express hydrogen ion concentration.

A buffer's capacity to minimize changes in pH is related to the dissociation characteristics of the weak acid or base in the presence of its respective salt. Unlike a strong acid or base, which dissociates almost completely, the dissociation constant for a weak acid or base solution tends to be very small, meaning little dissociation occurs.

The ionization of acetic acid (CH_3COOH), a weak acid, can be illustrated as follows:

$$[HA] \leftrightarrow [A^-] + [H^+]$$
$$[CH_3COOH] \leftrightarrow [CH_3COO^-] + [H^+] \quad \text{(Eq. 1-2)}$$

where HA is a weak acid, A^- is a conjugate base, H^+ represents hydrogen ions, and [ ] signifies concentration of anything in the bracket. Sometimes the conjugate base, A^-, will be referred to as a "salt" since, physiologically, it will be associated with some type of cation such as sodium (Na^+).

Note that the dissociation constant, K_a, for a weak acid may be calculated using the following equation:

$$K_a = \frac{[A^-][H^+]}{[HA]} \quad \text{(Eq. 1-3)}$$

Rearrangement of this equation reveals

$$[H^+] = K_a \times \frac{[HA]}{[A^+]} \quad \text{(Eq. 1-4)}$$

Taking the log of each quantity and then multiplying by minus 1 (−1), the equation can be rewritten as

$$-\log[H^+] = -\log K_a \times -\log \frac{[HA]}{[A^-]} \quad \text{(Eq. 1-5)}$$

By convention, lower case p means "negative log of"; therefore, $-\log[H^+]$ may be written as pH, and $-K_a$ may be written as pK_a. The equation now becomes

$$pH = pK_a - \log \frac{[HA]}{[A^-]} \quad \text{(Eq. 1-6)}$$

Eliminating the minus sign in front of the log of the quantity $\frac{[HA]}{[A^-]}$ results in an equation known as the Henderson-Hasselbalch equation, which mathematically describes the dissociation characteristics of weak acids (pK_a) and bases (pK_b) and the effect on pH:

$$pH = pK_a + \log \frac{[A^-]}{[HA]} \quad \text{(Eq. 1-7)}$$

When the ratio of $[A^-]$ to $[HA]$ is 1, the pH equals the pK and the buffer has its greatest buffering capacity. The dissociation constant K_a, and therefore the pK_a, remains the same for a given substance. Any changes in pH are solely due to the ratio of base/salt $[A^-]$ concentration to weak acid $[HA]$ concentration.

Ionic strength is another important aspect of buffers, particularly in separation techniques. Ionic strength is the concentration or activity of ions in a solution or buffer. It is defined[14] as follows:

$$\mu = I = \frac{1}{2}\Sigma C_i Z_i^2 \text{ or}$$
$$\frac{\Sigma\{(C_i) \times (Z_i)^2\}}{2} \quad \text{(Eq. 1-8)}$$

where C_i is the concentration of the ion, Z_i is the charge of the ion, and Σ is the sum of the quantity $(C_i)(Z_i)^2$ for each ion present. In mixtures of substances, the degree of dissociation must be considered. Increasing ionic strength

increases the ionic cloud surrounding a compound and decreases the rate of particle migration. It can also promote compound dissociation into ions effectively increasing the solubility of some salts, along with changes in current, which can also affect electrophoretic separation.

CLINICAL LABORATORY SUPPLIES

Many different supplies are required in today's medical laboratory; however, several items are common to most facilities, including thermometers, pipets, flasks, beakers, burets, desiccators, and filtering material. The following is a brief discussion of the composition and general use of these supplies.

Thermometers/Temperature

The predominant practice for temperature measurement uses the Celsius (°C) or centigrade scale; however, Fahrenheit (°F) and Kelvin (°K) scales are also used.[15,16] The SI designation for temperature is the Kelvin scale. Table 1-3 gives the conversion formulas between Fahrenheit and Celsius scales and Appendix C (on the companion web site) lists the various conversion formulas between them all.

All analytic reactions occur at an optimal temperature. Some laboratory procedures, such as enzyme determinations, require precise temperature control, whereas others work well over a wide range of temperatures. Reactions that are temperature dependent use some type of heating/cooling cell, heating/cooling block, or water/ice bath to provide the correct temperature environment. Laboratory refrigerator temperatures are often critical and need periodic verification. Thermometers are either an integral part of an instrument or need to be placed in the device for temperature maintenance. The three major types of thermometers discussed include liquid-in-glass, electronic thermometer or thermistor probe, and digital thermometer; however, several other types of temperature-indicating devices are in use. Regardless of which is being used, all temperature reading devices must be calibrated to ascertain accuracy. Liquid-in-glass thermometers use a colored liquid (red or other colored material), or at one time mercury, encased in plastic or glass material with a bulb at one end and a graduated

TABLE 1-3	COMMON TEMPERATURE CONVERSIONS
Celsius (Centigrade) to Fahrenheit	°C (9/5) + 32 (Multiply Celsius temperature by 9; divide the answer by 5, then add 32)
Fahrenheit to Celsius (Centigrade)	(°F − 32)5/9 (Subtract 32 and divide the answer by 9; then multiply that answer by 5)

stem. They usually measure temperatures between 20°C and 400°C. Partial immersion thermometers are used for measuring temperatures in units such as heating blocks and water baths and should be immersed to the proper height as indicated by the continuous line etched on the thermometer stem. Total immersion thermometers are used for refrigeration applications, and surface thermometers may be needed to check temperatures on flat surfaces, such as in an incubator or heating oven. Visual inspection of the liquid-in-glass thermometer should reveal a continuous line of liquid, free from separation or gas bubbles. The accuracy range for a thermometer used in clinical laboratories is determined by the specific application, but generally, the accuracy range should equal 50% of the desired temperature range required by the procedure.

Liquid-in-glass thermometers should be calibrated against an NIST-certified or NIST-traceable thermometer for critical laboratory applications.[17] NIST has an SRM thermometer with various calibration points (0°C, 25°C, 30°C, and 37°C) for use with liquid-in-glass thermometers. Gallium, another SRM, has a known melting point and can also be used for thermometer verification.

As automation advances and miniaturizes, the need for an accurate, fast-reading electronic thermometer (thermistor) has increased and is now routinely incorporated in many devices. The advantages of a thermistor over the more traditional liquid-in-glass thermometers are size and millisecond response time. Similar to the liquid-in-glass thermometers, the thermistor can be calibrated against an SRM thermometer or the gallium melting point cell.[18,19] When the thermistor is calibrated against the gallium cell, it can be used as a reference for any type of thermometer.

Glassware and Plasticware

Until recently, laboratory supplies (e.g., pipets, flasks, beakers, and burets) consisted of some type of glass and could be correctly termed *glassware*. As plastic material was refined and made available to manufacturers, plastic has been increasingly used to make laboratory utensils. Before discussing general laboratory supplies, a brief summary of the types and uses of glass and plastic commonly seen today in laboratories is given. (See Appendices G, H, and I on the book's companion web site.) Regardless of design, most laboratory supplies must satisfy certain tolerances of accuracy and fall into two classes of precision tolerance, either Class A or Class B as given by the American Society for Testing and Materials (ASTM; www.astm.org).[20,21] Those that satisfy Class A ASTM precision criteria are stamped with the letter "A" on the glassware and are preferred for laboratory applications. Class B glassware generally have twice the tolerance limits of Class A, even if they appear identical,

and are often found in student laboratories where durability is needed. Vessels holding or transferring liquid are designed either to contain (TC) or to deliver (TD) a specified volume. As the names imply, the major difference is that TC devices do not deliver that same volume when the liquid is transferred into a container, whereas the TD designation means that the labware will deliver that amount.

Glassware used in the clinical laboratory usually fall into one of the following categories: Kimax/Pyrex (borosilicate), Corex (aluminosilicate), high silica, Vycor (acid and alkali resistant), low actinic (amber colored), or flint (soda lime) glass used for disposable material.[22] Whenever possible, routinely used clinical chemistry glassware should consist of high thermal borosilicate or aluminosilicate glass and meet the Class A tolerances recommended by the NIST/ASTM/ISO 9000. The manufacturer is the best source of information about specific uses, limitations, and accuracy specifications for glassware.

Plasticware is beginning to replace glassware in the laboratory setting. The unique high resistance to corrosion and breakage, as well as varying flexibility, has made plasticware most appealing. Relatively inexpensive, it allows most items to be completely disposable after each use. The major types of resins frequently used in the clinical chemistry laboratory are polystyrene, polyethylene, polypropylene, Tygon, Teflon, polycarbonate, and polyvinyl chloride. Again, the individual manufacturer is the best source of information concerning the proper use and limitations of any plastic material.

In most laboratories, glass or plastic that is in direct contact with biohazardous material is usually disposable. If not, it must be decontaminated according to appropriate protocols. Should the need arise, however, cleaning of glass or plastic may require special techniques. Immediately rinsing glass or plastic supplies after use, followed by washing with a powder or liquid detergent designed for cleaning laboratory supplies and several distilled water rinses, may be sufficient. Presoaking glassware in soapy water is highly recommended whenever immediate cleaning is impractical. Many laboratories use automatic dishwashers and dryers for cleaning. Detergents and temperature levels should be compatible with the material and the manufacturer's recommendations. To ensure that all detergent has been removed from the labware, multiple rinses with appropriate grade water is recommended. Check the pH of the final rinse water and compare it with the initial pH of the prerinse water. Detergent-contaminated water will have a more alkaline pH as compared with the pH of the appropriate grade water. Visual inspection should reveal spotless vessel walls. Any biologically contaminated labware should be disposed of according to the precautions followed by that laboratory.

Some determinations, such as those used in assessing heavy metals or assays associated with molecular testing, require scrupulously clean or disposable glassware. Some applications may require plastic rather than glass because glass can absorb metal ions. Successful cleaning solutions are acid dichromate and nitric acid. It is suggested that disposable glass and plastic be used whenever possible.

Dirty reusable pipets should be placed immediately in a container of soapy water with the pipet tips up. The container should be long enough to allow the pipet tips to be covered with solution. A specially designed pipet soaking jar and washing/drying apparatus are recommended. For each final water rinse, fresh reagent grade water should be provided. If possible, designate a pipet container for final rinses only. Cleaning brushes are available to fit almost any size glassware and are recommended for any articles that are washed routinely.

Although plastic material is often easier to clean because of its nonwettable surface, it may not be appropriate for some applications involving organic solvents or autoclaving. Brushes or harsh abrasive cleaners should not be used on plasticware. Acid rinses or washes are not required. The initial cleaning procedure described in Appendix J (on the book's companion web site) can be adapted for plasticware as well. Ultrasonic cleaners can help remove debris coating the surfaces of glass or plasticware. Properly cleaned laboratory ware should be completely dried before using.

Laboratory Vessels

Flasks, beakers, and graduated cylinders are used to hold solutions. Volumetric and Erlenmeyer flasks are two types of containers in general use in the clinical laboratory.

A Class A *volumetric flask* is calibrated to hold one exact volume of liquid (TC). The flask has a round, lower portion with a flat bottom and a long, thin neck with an etched calibration line. Volumetric flasks are used to bring a given reagent to its final volume with the prescribed diluent and should be Class A quality. When bringing the bottom of the meniscus to the calibration mark, a pipet should be used when adding the final drops of diluent to ensure maximum control is maintained and the calibration line is not missed.

Erlenmeyer flasks and **Griffin beakers** are designed to hold different volumes rather than one exact amount. Because Erlenmeyer flasks and Griffin beakers are often used in reagent preparation, flask size, chemical inertness, and thermal stability should be considered. The Erlenmeyer flask has a wide bottom that gradually evolves into a smaller, short neck. The Griffin beaker has a flat bottom, straight sides, and an opening as wide as the flat base, with a small spout in the lip.

Graduated cylinders are long, cylindrical tubes usually held upright by an octagonal or circular base. The cylinder has calibration marks along its length and is used to measure volumes of liquids. Graduated cylinders do not have the accuracy of volumetric labware. The sizes routinely used are 10, 25, 50, 100, 500, 1,000, and 2,000 mL.

All laboratory utensils used in critical measurement should be Class A whenever possible to maximize accuracy and precision and thus decrease calibration time. (Fig. 1-1 illustrates representative laboratory glassware.)

Pipets

Pipets are glass or plastic utensils used to transfer liquids; they may be reusable or disposable. Although pipets may transfer any volume, they are usually used for volumes of 20 mL or less; larger volumes are usually transferred or dispensed using automated pipetting devices or jar-style pipetting apparatus. Table 1-4 outlines the classification applied here.

Similar to many laboratory utensils, pipets are designed to contain (TC) or to deliver (TD) a particular volume of liquid. The major difference is the amount of liquid needed to wet the interior surface of the ware and the amount of any residual liquid left in the pipet tip.

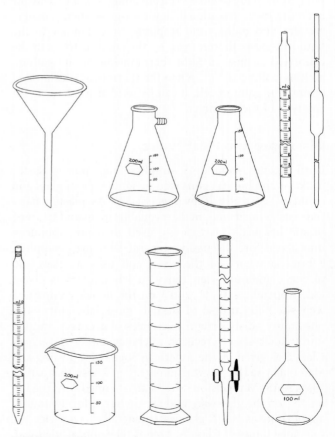

FIGURE 1-1 Laboratory glassware.

TABLE 1-4	PIPET CLASSIFICATION

I. Design
   A. To contain (TC)
   B. To deliver (TD)

II. Drainage characteristics
   A. Blowout
   B. Self-draining

III. Type
   A. Measuring or graduated
      1. Serologic
      2. Mohr
      3. Bacteriologic
      4. Ball, Kolmer, or Kahn
      5. Micropipet
   B. Transfer
      1. Volumetric
      2. Ostwald-Folin
      3. Pasteur pipets
      4. Automatic macropipets or micropipets

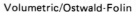

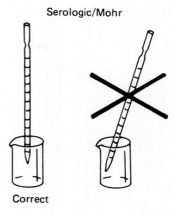

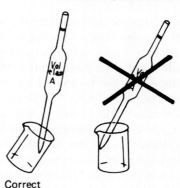

FIGURE 1-2 Correct and incorrect pipet positions.

Most manufacturers stamp *TC* or *TD* near the top of the pipet to alert the user as to the type of pipet. Like other TC-designated labware, a TC pipet holds or contains a particular volume but does not dispense that exact volume, whereas a TD pipet will dispense the volume indicated. When using either pipet, the tip must be immersed in the intended transfer liquid to a level that will allow the tip to remain in solution after the volume of liquid has entered the pipet—without touching the vessel walls. The pipet is held upright, not at an angle (Fig. 1-2). Using a pipet bulb or similar device, a slight suction is applied to the opposite end until the liquid enters the pipet and the meniscus is brought above the desired graduation line (Fig. 1-3A), suction is then stopped. While the meniscus level is held in place, the pipet tip is raised slightly out of the solution and wiped with a laboratory tissue of any adhering liquid. The liquid is allowed to drain until the bottom of the meniscus touches the desired calibration mark (Figs. 1-2B and 1-3). With the pipet held in a vertical position and the tip against the side of the receiving vessel, the pipet contents are allowed to drain into the vessel (e.g., test tube, cuvet, and flask). A *blowout pipet* has a continuous etched ring or two small, close, continuous rings located near the top of the pipet. This means that the last drop of liquid should be expelled into the receiving vessel. Without these markings, a pipet is *self-draining*, and the user allows the contents of the pipet to drain by gravity. The tip of the pipet should not be in contact with the accumulating fluid in the receiving vessel during drainage. With the exception of the Mohr pipet, the tip should remain in contact with the side of the vessel for

several seconds after the liquid has drained. The pipet is then removed. Various pipet bulbs are illustrated in Figure 1-4.

Measuring or graduated pipets are capable of dispensing several different volumes. Because the graduation lines located on the pipet may vary, they should be indicated on the top of each pipet. For example, a 5 mL pipet can be used to measure 5, 4, 3, 2, or 1 mL of liquid, with further graduations between each milliliter. The pipet is designated as 5 in 1/10 increments (Fig. 1-5) and could deliver any volume in tenths of a milliliter, up to 5 mL. Another pipet, such as a 1 mL pipet, may be designed to dispense 1 mL and have subdivisions of hundredths of a milliliter. The markings at the top of a

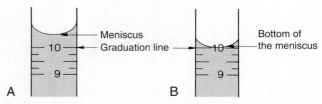

FIGURE 1-3 Pipetting technique. **(A)** Meniscus is brought above the desired graduation line. **(B)** Liquid is allowed to drain until the bottom of the meniscus touches the desired calibration mark.

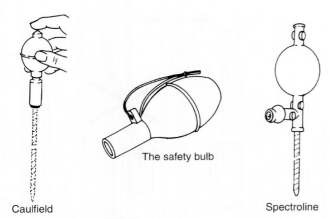

Caulfield   Spectroline

The safety bulb

FIGURE 1-4 Type of pipet bulbs.

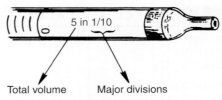

5 in 1/10

Total volume   Major divisions

FIGURE 1-5 Volume indication of a pipet.

measuring or graduated pipet indicate the volume(s) it is designed to dispense. The subgroups of measuring or graduated pipets are Mohr, serologic, and micropipets. A *Mohr pipet* does not have graduations to the tip. It is a self-draining pipet, but the tip should not be allowed to touch the vessel while the pipet is draining. A *serologic pipet* has graduation marks to the tip and is generally a blowout pipet. A *micropipet* is a pipet with a total holding volume of less than 1 mL; it may be designed as either a Mohr or a serologic pipet. Measuring pipets are used to transfer reagents and to make dilutions and can be used to repeatedly transfer a particular solution.

The next major category is the *transfer pipets*. These pipets are designed to dispense one volume without further subdivisions. *The bulblike enlargement in the pipet stem easily distinguishes the Ostwald-Folin and volumetric subgroups.* Ostwald-Folin pipets are used with biologic fluids having a viscosity greater than that of water. They are blowout pipets, indicated by two etched continuous rings at the top. The volumetric pipet is designed to dispense or transfer aqueous solutions and is always self-draining. This type of pipet usually has the greatest degree of accuracy and precision and should be used when diluting standards, calibrators, or quality-control material. They should only be used once. *Pasteur pipets* do not have calibration marks and are used to transfer solutions or biologic fluids without consideration of a specific volume. These pipets should not be used in any quantitative analytic techniques.

The *automatic pipet* is the most routinely used pipet in today's clinical chemistry laboratory. The term *automatic*, as used here, implies that the mechanism that draws up and dispenses the liquid is an integral part of the pipet. It may be a fully automated/self-operating, semiautomatic, or completely manually operated device. Automatic and semiautomatic pipets have many advantages, including safety, stability, ease of use, increased precision, the ability to save time, and less cleaning required as a result of the contaminated portions of the pipet (e.g., the tips) often being disposable. Figure 1-6 illustrates many

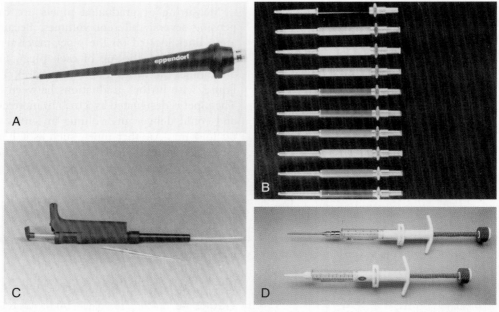

FIGURE 1-6 (A) Fixed volume, ultramicrodigital, air-displacement pipettes with tip ejector. **(B)** Fixed-volume air-displacement pipet. **(C)** Digital electronic positive-displacement pipets. **(D)** Syringe pipets.

common automatic pipets. A pipet associated with only one volume is termed a *fixed* volume, and models able to select different volumes are termed *variable*; however, only one volume may be used at a time. The available range of volumes is 1 μL to 5,000 mL. The widest volume range usually seen in a single pipet is 0 to 1 mL. A pipet with a pipetting capability of less than 1 mL is considered a *micropipet*, and a pipet that dispenses greater than 1 mL is called an *automatic macropipet*.

In addition to classification by volume delivery amounts, automatic pipets can also be categorized according to their mechanism: air-displacement, positive-displacement, and dispenser pipets. An *air-displacement pipet* relies on a piston for creating suction to draw the sample into a disposable tip that must be changed after each use. The piston does not come in contact with the liquid. A *positive-displacement pipet* operates by moving the piston in the pipet tip or barrel, much like a hypodermic syringe. It does not require a different tip for each use. Because of carryover concerns, rinsing and blotting between samples may be required. *Dispensers* and *dilutor/dispensers* are automatic pipets that obtain the liquid from a common reservoir and dispense it repeatedly. The dispensing pipets may be bottle-top, motorized, handheld, or attached to a dilutor. The dilutor often combines sampling and dispensing functions. Figure 1-7 provides examples of different types of automatic pipetting devices. These pipets should be used according to the individual manufacturer's directions. Many automated pipets use a wash between samples to eliminate carryover problems. However, to minimize carryover contamination with manual or semiautomatic pipets, careful wiping of the tip may remove any liquid that adhered to the outside of the tip before dispensing

any liquid. Care should be taken to ensure that the orifice of the pipet tip is not blotted, drawing sample from the tip. Another precaution in using manually operated semiautomatic pipets is to move the plunger in a continuous and steady manner.

Disposable one-use pipet tips are designed for use with air-displacement pipets. The laboratory scientist should ensure that the pipet tip is seated snugly onto the end of the pipet and free from any deformity. Plastic tips used on air-displacement pipets can vary. Different brands can be used for one particular pipet but they do not necessarily perform in an identical manner. Plastic burrs may be present on the interior of the tip that cannot always be detected by the naked eye. A method using a 0.1% solution of phenol red in distilled water has been used to compare the reproducibility of different brands of pipet tips.[23] When using this method, the pipet and the operator should remain the same so that variation is only a result of changes in the pipet tips.

Tips for positive-displacement pipets are made of straight columns of glass or plastic. These tips must fit snugly to avoid carryover and can be used repeatedly without being changed after each use. As previously mentioned, these devices may need to be rinsed and dried between samples to minimize carryover.

Class A pipets, like all other Class A labware, do not need to be recalibrated by the laboratory. Automatic pipetting devices, as well as non–Class A materials, do need recalibration. A gravimetric method (see Box 1-1) can accomplish this task by delivering and weighing a solution of known specific gravity, such as water. A currently calibrated analytic balance and at least Class 2 weights should be used. A pipet should be used only if it is within ±1.0% of the expected value.

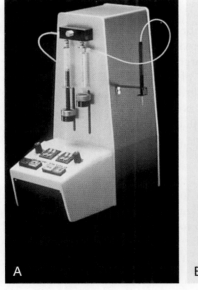 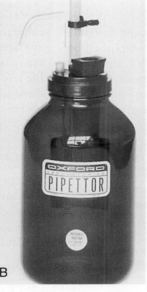 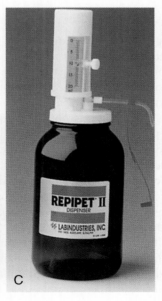

FIGURE 1-7 (A) Digital dilutor/dispenser. **(B, C)** Dispenser.

BOX 1-1 GRAVIMETRIC PIPET CALIBRATION

Materials

Pipet
10 to 20 pipet tips, if needed
Balance capable of accuracy and resolution to ±0.1% of dispensed volumetric weight
Weighing vessel large enough to hold volume of liquid
Type I/CLRW
Thermometer and barometer

Procedure

1. Record the weight of the vessel. Record the temperature of the water. It is recommended that all materials be at room temperature. Obtain the barometric pressure.
2. Place a small volume (0.5 mL) of the water into the container. To prevent effects from evaporation, it is desirable to loosely cover each container with a substance such as Parafilm. Avoid handling of the containers.
3. Weigh each container plus water to the nearest 0.1 mg *or* set the balance to zero.
4. Using the pipet to be tested, draw up the specified amount. Carefully wipe the outside of the tip. Care should be taken not to touch the end of the tip; this will cause liquid to be wicked out of the tip, introducing an inaccuracy as a result of technique.
5. Dispense the water into the weighed vessel. Touch the tip to the side.
6. Record the weight of the vessel.
7. Subtract the weight obtained in step 3 from that obtained in step 6. Record the result.
8. If plastic tips are used, change the tip between each dispensing. Repeat steps 1 to 6 for a minimum of nine additional times.
9. Obtain the average or mean of the weight of the water. Multiply the mean weight by the corresponding density of water at the given temperature and pressure. This may be obtained from the *Handbook of Chemistry and Physics*.[6] At 20°C, the density of water is 0.9982.
10. Determine the accuracy or the ability of the pipet to dispense the expected (selected or stated) volume according to the following formula:

$$\frac{\text{Mean volume}}{\text{Expected volume}} \times 100\% \qquad \text{(Eq. 1-9)}$$

The manufacturer usually gives acceptable limitations for a particular pipet, but they should not be used if the value differs by more than 1.0% from the expected value.

Precision can be indicated as the percent coefficient of variation (%CV) or standard deviation (SD) for a series of repetitive pipetting steps. A discussion of %CV and SD can be found in Chapter 3. The equations to calculate the SD and %CV are as follows:

$$SD = \sqrt{\frac{\Sigma(x - \bar{x})^2}{n - 1}}$$
$$\%CV = \frac{SD}{\bar{x}} \times 100 \qquad \text{(Eq. 1-10)}$$

Required imprecision is usually ±1 SD. The %CV will vary with the expected volume of the pipet, but the smaller the %CV value, the greater the precision. When *n* is large, the data are more statistically valid.[21,24]

Although gravimetric validation is the most desirable method, pipet calibration may also be accomplished by using photometric methods, particularly for automatic pipetting devices. When a spectrophotometer is used, the molar extinction coefficient of a compound, such as potassium dichromate, is obtained. After an aliquot of diluent is pipetted, the change in concentration will reflect the volume of the pipet. Another photometric technique used to assess pipet accuracy compares the absorbances of dilutions of potassium dichromate, or another colored liquid with appropriate absorbance spectra, using Class A volumetric labware versus equivalent dilutions made with the pipetting device.

These calibration techniques are time consuming and, therefore, impractical for use in daily checks. It is recommended that pipets be checked initially and subsequently three or four times per year, or as dictated by the laboratory's accrediting agency. Many companies offer calibration services; the one chosen should also satisfy any accreditation requirements. A quick, daily check for many larger volume automatic pipetting devices involves the use of volumetric flasks. For example, a bottle-top dispenser that routinely delivers 2.5 mL of reagent may be checked by dispensing four aliquots of the reagent into a 10 mL Class A volumetric flask. The bottom of the meniscus should meet with the calibration line on the volumetric flask.

Burets
A buret looks like a wide, long, graduated pipet with a stopcock at one end. A buret's usual total volume ranges from 25 to 100 mL of solution and is used to dispense a particular volume of liquid during a titration (Fig. 1-8).

Syringes
Syringes are sometimes used for transfer of small volumes (less than 500 μL) in blood gas analysis or in separation

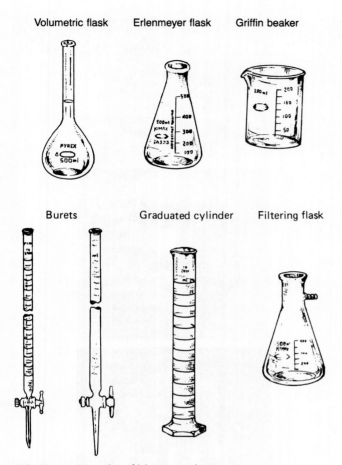

Volumetric flask   Erlenmeyer flask   Griffin beaker

Burets   Graduated cylinder   Filtering flask

FIGURE 1-8 Examples of laboratory glassware.

are called **deliquescent substances**. Closed and sealed containers, referred to as **desiccators**, that contain desiccant material may be used to store more hygroscopic substances. Many sealed packets or shipping containers, often those that require refrigeration, include some type of small packet of desiccant material to prolong storage.

Balances

A properly operating balance is essential in producing high-quality reagents and standards. However, because many laboratories discontinued in-house reagent preparation, balances may no longer be as widely used. Balances are classified according to their design, number of pans (single or double), and whether they are mechanical or electronic or classified by operating ranges, as determined by precision balances (readability ≈2 μg), analytic balances (readability ≈0.001 g), or microbalances (readability ≈0.1 μg; Fig. 1-9).

Analytic and electronic balances are currently the most popular in the clinical laboratory. Analytic balances are required for the preparation of any primary standard. The mechanical analytic balance is also known as a *substitution balance*. It has a single pan enclosed by sliding transparent doors, which minimize environmental influences on pan movement. The pan is attached to a series of calibrated weights that are counterbalanced by a single weight at the opposite end of a knife-edge fulcrum. The operator adjusts the balance to the desired mass and

techniques such as chromatography or electrophoresis. The syringes are glass and have fine barrels. The plunger is often made of a fine piece of wire. Tips are not used when syringes are used for injection of sample into a gas chromatographic system. In electrophoresis work, however, disposable Teflon tips may be used. Expected inaccuracies for volumes less than 5 μL are 2%, whereas for greater volumes, the inaccuracy is approximately 1%.

Desiccators and Desiccants

Many compounds combine with water molecules to form loose chemical crystals. The compound and the associated water are called a hydrate. When the water of crystallization is removed from the compound, it is said to be anhydrous. Substances that take up water on exposure to atmospheric conditions are called hygroscopic. Materials that are very hygroscopic can remove moisture from the air as well as from other materials. These materials make excellent drying substances and are sometimes used as desiccants (drying agents) to keep other chemicals from becoming hydrated. If these compounds absorb enough water from the atmosphere to cause dissolution, they

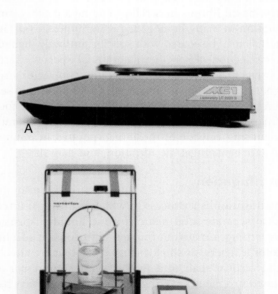

FIGURE 1-9 (A) Electronic top-loading balance. **(B)** Electronic analytic balance with printer.

places the material, contained within a tared weighing vessel, on the sample pan. An optical scale allows the operator to visualize the mass of the substance. The weight range for certain analytic balances is from 0.01 mg to 160 g.

Electronic balances are single-pan balances that use an electromagnetic force to counterbalance the weighed sample's mass. Their measurements equal the accuracy and precision of any available mechanical balance, with the advantage of a fast response time (less than 10 seconds).

Test weights used for calibrating balances should be selected from the appropriate ANSI/ASTM Classes 1 through 4.[25] This system has replaced the former NIST Class S standards used prior to 1993. Class 1 weights provide the greatest precision and should be used for calibrating high-precision analytic balances in the weight range of 0.01 to 0.1 mg. Former NBS S standard weights are equivalent to ASTM Class 2 (0.001 to 0.01 g), and S-1 is equivalent to ASTM Class 3 (0.01 to 0.1 g). The frequency of calibration is dictated by the accreditation/licensing guidelines for a specific laboratory. Balances should be kept scrupulously clean and be located in an area away from heavy traffic, large pieces of electrical equipment, and open windows. The level checkpoint should always be corrected before weighing occurs.

BASIC SEPARATION TECHNIQUES

Contemporary modifications of filtration and dialysis use matrix-based fibrous material providing a mechanism of separation in many homogeneous immunoassays. These materials may be coated with specific antibody–ligand to foster selection of specific materials or species. Certain labels use magnetic particles in conjunction with strong magnets to effect separation. Further discussion of separation mechanisms used in immunoassays may be found in Chapters 8 and 9. Basic universally used separation mechanisms, outside of those incorporated in immunoassay, are centrifugation, filtration, and dialysis.

Centrifugation

Centrifugation is a process in which centrifugal force is used to separate solid matter from a liquid suspension. The *centrifuge* carries out this action. It consists of a head or rotor, carriers, or shields (Fig. 1-10) that are attached to the vertical shaft of a motor or air compressor and enclosed in a metal covering. The centrifuge always has a lid and an on/off switch; however, many models include a brake or a built-in tachometer, which indicates speed, and some centrifuges are refrigerated. Centrifugal force depends on three variables: mass, speed, and radius. The speed is expressed in revolutions per minute (rpm), and the centrifugal force generated is expressed in terms of relative centrifugal force (RCF) or gravities (g). The

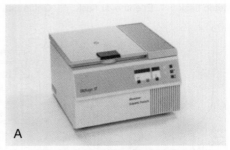

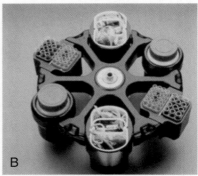

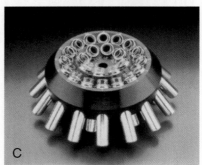

FIGURE 1-10 (A) Benchtop centrifuge. (B) Swinging-bucket rotor. (C) Fixed-head rotor.

speed of the centrifuge is related to the RCF by the following equation:

$$RCF = 1.118 \times 10^{-5} \times r \times (rpm)^2 \quad \text{(Eq. 1-11)}$$

where 1.118×10^{-5} is a constant, determined from the angular velocity, and r is the radius in centimeters, measured from the center of the centrifuge axis to the bottom of the test tube shield or bucket. The RCF value may also be obtained from a nomogram similar to that found in Appendix F on the book's companion web site. Centrifuge classification is based on several criteria, including benchtop or floor model, refrigeration, rotor head (e.g., fixed, hematocrit, swinging-bucket, or angled; Fig. 1-10), or maximum speed attainable (i.e., ultracentrifuge). Centrifuges are generally used to separate serum or plasma from the blood cells as the blood samples are being processed; to separate a supernatant from a precipitate during an analytic reaction; to separate two immiscible liquids, such as a lipid-laden sample; or to expel air.

Centrifuge care includes daily cleaning of any spills or debris, such as blood or glass, and ensuring that the centrifuge is properly balanced and free from any excessive vibrations. Balancing the centrifuge load is critical (Fig. 1-11). Many newer centrifuges will automatically decrease their speed if the load is not evenly distributed, but more often, the centrifuge will shake and vibrate or make more noise than expected. A centrifuge needs to be balanced based on equalizing both the volume and weight distribution across the centrifuge head. Many laboratories will make up "balance" tubes that approximate routinely used volumes and tube sizes, including the stopper on phlebotomy tubes, which can be used to match those needed from patient samples. A good rule of thumb is one of even placement and one of "opposition." Exact positioning of tubes depends on the design of the centrifuge holders.

The centrifuge cover should remain closed until the centrifuge has come to a complete stop to avoid any aerosol contamination. It is recommended that the timer, brushes (if present), and speed be periodically checked. The brushes, which are graphite bars attached to a retainer spring, create an electrical contact in the motor. The specific manufacturer's service manual should be consulted for details on how to change brushes and on lubrication requirements. The speed of a centrifuge is easily checked using a tachometer or strobe light. The hole located in the lid of many centrifuges is designed for speed verification using these devices but may also represent an aerosol biohazard. Accreditation agencies require periodic verification of centrifuge speeds.

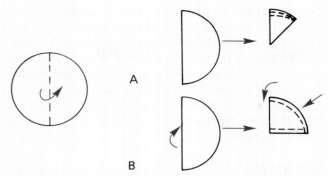

FIGURE 1-12 Methods of folding a filter paper. **(A)** In a fan. **(B)** In fourths.

Filtration

Filtration can be used instead of centrifugation for the separation of solids from liquids. However, paper filtration is only occasionally used in today's laboratory and, therefore, only the basics are discussed here. Filter material is made of paper, cellulose and its derivatives, polyester fibers, glass, and a variety of resin column materials. Traditionally, filter paper was folded in a manner that allowed it to fit into a funnel. In method A, round filter paper is folded like a fan (Fig. 1-12A); in method B, the paper is folded into fourths (Fig. 1-12B).

Filter papers differ in pore size and should be selected according to separation needs and associated flow rate for given liquids. Filter paper should not be used when using strong acids or bases. When the filter paper is placed inside the funnel, the solution slowly drains through the filter paper within the funnel and into a receiving vessel. The liquid that passes through the filter paper is called the filtrate.

Dialysis

Dialysis is another method for separating macromolecules from a solvent or smaller substances. It became popular when used in conjunction with the Technicon AutoAnalyzer system in the 1970s. Basically, a solution is put into a bag or is contained on one side of a semipermeable membrane. Larger molecules are retained within the sack or on one side of the membrane, while smaller molecules and solvents diffuse out. This process is very slow. The use of columns that contain a gel material has replaced manual dialysis separation in most analytic procedures.

LABORATORY MATHEMATICS AND CALCULATIONS

Significant Figures

Significant figures are the minimum number of digits needed to express a particular value in scientific notation without loss of accuracy. The number 814.2 has

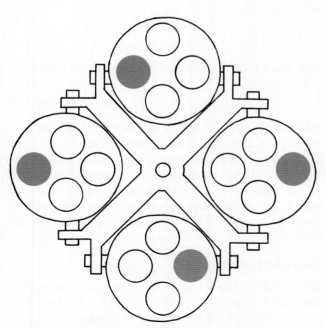

FIGURE 1-11 Properly balanced centrifuge. *Colored circles* represent counterbalanced positions for sample tubes.

four significant figures, because in scientific notation it is written as 8.142×10^2. The number 0.000641 has three significant figures, because the scientific notation expression for this value is 6.41×10^{-4}. The zeros are merely holding decimal places and are not needed to properly express the number in scientific notation. However, by convention, zeros following a decimal point are considered significant. For example, 10.00 has four significant figures.

Logarithms

The base 10 *logarithm* (log) of a positive number N greater than zero is equal to the exponent to which 10 must be raised to produce N. Therefore, it can be stated that N equals 10^x, and the log of N is equal to x. The number N is the antilogarithm (antilog) of x.

The logarithm of a number, which is written in *decimal* format, consists of two parts: the character, or characteristic, and the mantissa. The characteristic is the number to the left of the decimal point in the log and is derived from the exponent, and the mantissa is that portion of the logarithm to the right of the decimal point and is derived from the number itself. Although several approaches can be taken to determine the log, one approach is to write the number in scientific notation. The number 1,424 expressed in scientific notation is 1.424×10^3, making the characteristic value a 3. The characteristic can also be determined by adding the number of significant figures and then subtracting 1 from the sum. The mantissa is derived from a log table or calculator having a log function for the remainder of the number. For 1.424, a calculator would give a mantissa of 0.1535. Certain calculators with a log function do not require conversion to scientific notation. This would give a log value of 3.1535 (3 + 0.1535).

To determine the original number from a log value, the process is done in reverse. This process is termed the *antilogarithm*. If given a log of 3.1535, most calculators require that you enter this value, use an inverse or secondary/shift function, and enter log, and the resulting value should be 1.424×10^3. Consult the specific manufacturer's directions to become acquainted with the proper use of these functions.

pH (Negative Logarithms)

The characteristic of a log may be positive or negative, but the mantissa is always positive. In certain circumstances, the laboratory scientist must deal with negative logs. Such is the case with pH or pK_a. As previously stated, the pH of a solution is defined as minus the log of the hydrogen ion concentration. The following is a convenient formula to determine the negative logarithm when working with pH or pK_a:

$$\frac{pH}{pK_a} = x - \log N \qquad \text{(Eq. 1-12)}$$

where x is negative exponent base 10 expressed without the minus sign and N is the decimal portion of the scientific notation expression.

For example, if the hydrogen ion concentration of a solution is 5.4×10^{-6}, then $x = 6$ and $N = 5.4$. Substitute this information into Equation 1-12, and it becomes

$$pH = 6 - \log 5.4 \qquad \text{(Eq. 1-13)}$$

The logarithm of N (5.4) is equal to 0.7324, or 0.73. The pH becomes

$$pH = 6 - 0.73 = 5.27 \qquad \text{(Eq. 1-14)}$$

The same formula can be applied to obtain the hydrogen ion concentration of a solution when only the pH is given. Using a pH of 5.27, the equation becomes

$$5.27 = x - \log N \qquad \text{(Eq. 1-15)}$$

In this instance, the x term is always the next largest whole number. For this example, the next largest whole number is 6. Substituting for x, the equation becomes

$$5.27 = 6 - \log N \qquad \text{(Eq. 1-16)}$$

A shortcut is to simply subtract the pH from x (6 − 5.27 = 0.73) and take the antilog of that answer 5.73. The final answer is 5.73×10^{-6}. Note that rounding, while allowed, can alter the answer. A more algebraically correct approach follows in Eqs. 1-17 through 1-19. Multiply all the variables by −1:

$$(-1)(5.27) = (-1)(6) - (-1)(\log N)$$
$$-5.27 = -6 + \log N \qquad \text{(Eq. 1-17)}$$

Solve the equation for the unknown quantity by adding a positive 6 to both sides of the equal sign and the equation becomes

$$6 - 5.27 = \log N$$
$$0.73 = \log N \qquad \text{(Eq. 1-18)}$$

The result is 0.73, which is the antilogarithm value of N, which is 5.37, or 5.4:

$$\text{Antilog } 0.73 = N; N = 5.37 = 5.4 \qquad \text{(Eq. 1-19)}$$

The hydrogen ion concentration for a solution with a pH of 5.27 is 5.4×10^{-6}. Many scientific calculators have an inverse function or syntax that allows for more direct calculation of negative logarithms. It is important, however, to fully understand the proper use of the many calculator functions available, keeping in mind that the specific steps vary between manufacturers.

Concentration

A detailed description of each concentration term (e.g., molarity and normality) may be found at the beginning of this chapter. The following discussion focuses on the basic mathematical expressions needed to prepare reagents of a stated concentration.

Percent Solution

A percent solution is determined in the same manner regardless of whether weight/weight, volume/volume, or weight/volume units are used. *Percent* implies "parts per 100," which is represented as percent (%) and is independent of the molecular weight of a substance.

Example 1-1 Weight/Weight (w/w)

To make up 100 g of a 5% aqueous solution of hydrochloric acid (using 12 M HCl), multiply the total amount by the percent expressed as a decimal. The calculation becomes

$$5\% = \frac{5}{100} = 0.050 \qquad \textbf{(Eq. 1-20)}$$

Therefore,

$$0.50 \times 100 \text{ g} = 5 \text{ g of 12 M HCl} \qquad \textbf{(Eq. 1-21)}$$

Another way of arriving at the answer is to set up a ratio so that

$$\frac{5}{100} = \frac{x}{100}$$
$$x = 5 \qquad \textbf{(Eq. 1-22)}$$

Example 1-2 Weight/Volume (w/v)

The most frequently used term for a percent solution is weight per volume, which is often expressed as grams per 100 mL of the diluent. To make up 1,000 mL of a 10% (w/v) solution of NaOH, use the preceding approach. The calculations become

$$10/100 = 0.10 \quad \times \quad 1{,}000 = 100 \text{ g}$$
$$\text{(\% expressed as a decimal)} \qquad \text{(total amount)}$$

or

$$\frac{10}{100} = \frac{x}{1{,}000}$$
$$x = 100 \qquad \textbf{(Eq. 1-23)}$$

Therefore, add 100 g of 10% NaOH to a 1,000 mL volumetric Class A flask and dilute to the calibration mark with reagent grade water.

Example 1-3 Volume/Volume (v/v)

Make up 50 mL of a 2% (v/v) concentrated hydrochloric acid solution.

$$2/100 = 0.02 \times 50 = 1 \text{ mL}$$

or

$$\frac{2}{100} = \frac{x}{50}$$
$$x = 1 \qquad \textbf{(Eq. 1-24)}$$

Therefore, add 40 mL of water to a 50 mL Class A volumetric flask, add 1 mL of concentrated HCl, mix, and dilute up to the calibration mark with reagent grade water. Remember, always add acid to water!

Molarity

Molarity (M) is routinely expressed in units of moles per liter (mol/L) or sometimes millimoles per milliliter (mmol/mL). Remember that 1 mol of a substance is equal to the gmw of that substance. When trying to determine the amount of substance needed to yield a particular concentration, initially decide what final concentration *units* are needed. For molarity, the final units will be moles per liter (mol/L) or millimoles per milliliter (mmol/mL). The second step is to consider the existing units and the relationship they have to the final desired units. Essentially, try to put as many units as possible into "like" terms and arrange so that the same units cancel each other out, leaving only those wanted in the final answer. To accomplish this, it is important to remember what units are used to define each concentration term. It is key to understand the relationship between molarity (moles/liter), moles, and gmw. While molarity is given in these examples, the approach for molality is the same except that one molal is expressed as one mole of solute per kilogram of solvent. For water, one kilogram is proportional to one liter, so molarity and molality are equivalent.

Example 1-4

How many *grams* are needed to make 1 L of a 2 M solution of HCl?

Step 1: Which *units* are needed in the final answer? *Answer:* Grams per liter (g/L).

Step 2: Assess other mass/volume terms used in the problem. In this case, moles are also needed for the calculation: How many grams are equal to 1 mole? The gmw of HCl, which can be determined from the periodic table, will be equal to 1 mole. For HCl, the gmw is 36.5, so the equation may be written as

$$\frac{36.5 \text{ g HCl}}{\text{mol}} \times \frac{2 \text{ mol}}{1} = \frac{73 \text{ g HCl}}{1} \qquad \textbf{(Eq. 1-25)}$$

Cancel out like units, and the final units should be grams per liter. In this example, 73 grams HCl per liter is needed to make up a 2 M solution of HCl.

Example 1-5

A solution of NaOH is contained within a Class A 1 L volumetric flask filled to the calibration mark. The content label reads 24 g of NaOH. Determine the molarity.

Step 1: What *units* are ultimately needed? *Answer:* Moles per liter (mol/L).

Step 2: The units that exist are grams and 1 L. NaOH may be expressed as moles and grams. The gmw of NaOH is calculated to equal 40 g/mol. Rearrange the equation so that grams can be canceled and the remaining units reflect those needed in the answer, which are mole/L.

Step 3: The equation becomes

$$\frac{24 \text{ g NaOH}}{1} \times \frac{1 \text{ mol}}{40 \text{ g NaOH}} = 0.6 \frac{\text{mol}}{\text{L}} \qquad \textbf{(Eq. 1-26)}$$

By canceling out like units and performing the appropriate calculations, the final answer of 0.6 M or 0.6 mol/L is derived.

Example 1-6

Make up 250 mL of a 4.8 M solution of HCl.

Step 1: *Units* needed? *Answer*: Grams (g).

Step 2: Determine the gmw of HCl (36.5 g), which is needed to calculate the molarity.

Step 3: Set up the equation, cancel out like units, and perform the appropriate calculations:

$$\frac{36.5 \text{ g HCl}}{\text{mol}} \times \frac{4.8 \text{ mol HCl}}{L} \times \frac{250 \text{ mL} \times 1 L}{1,000 \text{ mL}}$$

$$= 43.8 \text{ g HCl} \qquad \text{(Eq. 1-27)}$$

In a 250 mL volumetric flask, add 200 mL of reagent grade water. Add 43.8 g of HCl and mix. Dilute up to the calibration mark with reagent grade water.

Although there are various methods to calculate laboratory mathematical problems, this technique of canceling like units can be used in most clinical chemistry situations, regardless of whether the problem requests molarity, normality, or exchanging one concentration term for another. However, it is necessary to recall the interrelationship between all the units in the expression.

Normality

Normality (N) is expressed as the number of equivalent weights per liter (Eq/L) or milliequivalents per milliliter (mmol/mL). Equivalent weight is equal to gmw divided by the valence (V). Normality has often been used in acid–base calculations because an equivalent weight of a substance is also equal to its combining weight. Another advantage in using equivalent weight is that an equivalent weight of one substance is equal to the equivalent weight of any other chemical.

Example 1-7

Give the equivalent weight, in grams, for each substance listed below.

1. NaCl (gmw = 58 g, valence = 1)

$$58/1 = 58 \text{ g per equivalent weight} \qquad \text{(Eq. 1-28)}$$

2. HCl (gmw = 36, valence = 1)

$$36/1 = 36 \text{ g per equivalent weight} \qquad \text{(Eq. 1-29)}$$

3. H_2SO_4 (gmw = 98, valence = 2)

$$98/2 = 49 \text{ g per equivalent weight} \qquad \text{(Eq. 1-30)}$$

A. What is the normality of a 500 mL solution that contains 7 g of H_2SO_4? The approach used to calculate molarity could be used to solve this problem as well.

Step 1: Units needed? *Answer*: Normality expressed as equivalents per liter (Eq/L).

Step 2: Units you have? *Answer*: Milliliters and grams. Now determine how they are related to equivalents per liter. (Hint: There are 49 g per equivalent—see Equation 1-30 above.)

Step 3: Rearrange the equation so that like terms cancel out, leaving Eq/L. This equation is

$$\frac{7 \text{ g } H_2SO_4}{500 \text{ mL}} \times \frac{1 \text{ Eq}}{49 \text{ g } H_2SO_4} \times \frac{1,000 \text{ mL}}{1 L}$$

$$= 0.285 \text{ Eq/L} = 0.285 \text{ N} \qquad \text{(Eq. 1-31)}$$

Because 500 mL is equal to 0.5 L, the final equation could be written by substituting 0.5 L for 500 mL, eliminating the need to include the 1,000 mL/L conversion factor in the equation.

B. What is the normality of a 0.5 M solution of H_2SO_4? Continuing with the previous approach, the final equation is

$$\frac{0.5 \text{ mol } H_2SO_4}{L} \times \frac{98 \text{ g } H_2SO_4}{\text{mol } H_2SO_4} \times \frac{1 \text{ Eq } H_2SO_4}{49 \text{ g } H_2SO_4}$$

$$= 1 \text{ Eq/L} = 1 \text{ N} \qquad \text{(Eq. 1-32)}$$

When changing molarity into normality or vice versa, the following conversion formula may be applied:

$$M \times V = N \qquad \text{(Eq. 1-33)}$$

where V is the valence of the compound. Using this formula, Example 1-7.3 becomes

$$0.5 \text{ M} \times 2 = 1 \text{ N} \qquad \text{(Eq. 1-34)}$$

Example 1-8

What is the molarity of a 2.5 N solution of HCl? This problem may be solved in several ways. One way is to use the stepwise approach in which existing units are exchanged for units needed. The equation is

$$\frac{2.5 \text{ Eq HCl}}{L} \times \frac{36 \text{ g HCl}}{1 \text{ Eq}} \times \frac{1 \text{ mol HCl}}{36 \text{ g HCl}}$$

$$= 2.5 \text{ mol/L HCl} \qquad \text{(Eq. 1-35)}$$

The second approach is to use the normality-to-molarity conversion formula. The equation now becomes

$$M \times V = 2.5 \text{ N}$$

$$V = 1$$

$$M = \frac{2.5 \text{ N}}{1} = 2.5 \text{ N} \qquad \text{(Eq. 1-36)}$$

When the valence of a substance is 1, the molarity will equal the normality. As previously mentioned, normality either equals or is greater than the molarity.

Specific Gravity

Density is expressed as mass per unit volume of a substance. The specific gravity is the ratio of the density of a material when compared with the density of pure water at a given temperature and allows the laboratory scientist a means of expressing density in terms of volume.

The units for density are grams per milliliter. Specific gravity is often used with very concentrated materials, such as commercial acids (e.g., sulfuric and hydrochloric acids).

The density of a concentrated acid can also be expressed in terms of an assay or percent purity. The actual concentration is equal to the specific gravity multiplied by the *assay* or *percent purity value* (expressed as a decimal) stated on the label of the container.

Example 1-9

A. What is the actual weight of a supply of concentrated HCl whose label reads specific gravity 1.19 with an assay value of 37%?

$$1.19 \text{ g/mL} \times 0.37 = 0.44 \text{ g/mL of HCl} \qquad \text{(Eq. 1-37)}$$

B. What is the molarity of this stock solution? The final units desired are moles per liter (mol/L). The molarity of the solution is

$$\frac{0.44 \text{ g HCl}}{\text{mL}} \times \frac{1 \text{ mol HCl}}{36.5 \text{ g HCl}} \times \frac{1,000 \text{ mL}}{\text{L}}$$

$$= 12.05 \text{ mol/L or 12 M} \qquad \text{(Eq. 1-38)}$$

Conversions

To convert one unit into another, the same approach of crossing out like units can be applied. In some instances, a chemistry laboratory may report a given analyte using two different concentration units—for example, calcium. The recommended SI unit for calcium is millimoles per liter. The better known and more traditional units are milligrams per deciliter (mg/dL). Again, it is important to understand the relationship between the units given and those needed in the final answer.

Example 1-10

Convert 8.2 mg/dL calcium to millimoles per · liter (mmol/L). The gmw of calcium is 40 g. So, if there are 40 g per mol, then it follows that there are 40 mg per mmol. The units wanted are mmol/L. The equation becomes

$$\frac{8.2 \text{ mg}}{\text{dL}} \times \frac{1 \text{ dL}}{100 \text{ mL}} \times \frac{1,000 \text{ mL}}{\text{L}} \times \frac{1 \text{ mmol}}{40 \text{ mg}}$$

$$= \frac{2.05 \text{ mmol}}{\text{L}} \qquad \text{(Eq. 1-39)}$$

Once again, the systematic stepwise approach of deleting similar units can be used for this conversion problem.

A frequently encountered conversion problem or, more precisely, a dilution problem occurs when a weaker concentration or different volume is needed than the stock substance available, but the concentration *terms* are the same. The following formula is used:

$$V_1 \times C_1 = V_2 \times C_2 \qquad \text{(Eq. 1-40)}$$

This formula is useful only if the concentration and volume units between the substances are the *same* and if three of four variables are known.

Example 1-11

What volume is needed to make 500 mL of a 0.1 M solution of Tris buffer from a solution of 2 M Tris buffer?

$$V_1 \times 2 \text{ M} = 0.1 \text{ M} \times 500 \text{ mL}$$

$$(V_1)(2 \text{ M}) = (0.1 \text{ M})(500 \text{ mL}); (V_1)(2 \text{ M}) = 50$$

$$\text{therefore } V_1 = 50/2 = 25 \text{ mL} \qquad \text{(Eq. 1-41)}$$

It requires 25 mL of the 2 M solution to make up 500 mL of a 0.1 M solution. This problem differs from the other conversions in that it is actually a dilution of a stock solution. While this approach will provide how much stock is needed when making the solution, the laboratory scientist must subtract that volume from the final volume to determine the amount of diluent needed, in this case 475 mL. A more involved discussion of dilution problems follows.

Dilutions

A dilution represents the ratio of concentrated or stock material to the total final volume of a solution and consists of the volume or weight of the concentrate plus the volume of the diluent, with the concentration units remaining the same. This ratio of concentrated or stock solution to the total solution volume equals the dilution factor. Because a dilution is made by adding a more concentrated substance to a diluent, the dilution is always less concentrated than the original substance. The relationship of the dilution factor to concentration is an inverse one; thus, the *dilution factor* increases as the *concentration decreases*. To determine the dilution factor, simply take the concentration needed and divide by the stock concentration, leaving it in a reduced-fraction form.

Example 1-12

What is the dilution factor needed to make a 100 mmol/L sodium solution from a 3,000 mmol/L stock solution? The dilution factor becomes

$$\frac{100}{3,000} = \frac{1}{30} \qquad \text{(Eq. 1-42)}$$

The dilution factor indicates that the ratio of stock material is 1 part stock made to a *total volume* of 30. To actually make this dilution, 1 mL of stock is added to 29 mL of diluent. Note that the dilution factor indicates the parts per total amount; however, in *making* the dilution, the sum of the amount of the stock material plus the amount of the diluent must equal the total volume or dilution fraction denominator. The dilution factor may be correctly written as either a fraction or a ratio.

Confusion arises when distinction is not made between a ratio and a dilution, which by its very nature is a ratio of stock to diluent. A ratio is always expressed using a colon; a dilution can be expressed as either a fraction or a ratio.[26] Many directions in the laboratory are given orally. For example, making a "1-in-4" dilution means adding one part stock to a total of four parts. That is, one part of stock would be added "to" three parts of diluent. The dilution factor would be 1/4. Analyses performed on the diluted material would need to be multiplied by 4 to get the final concentration. That is very different from saying make a "1-to-4" dilution! In this instance, the dilution factor would be 1/5! It is important during procedures that you fully understand the meaning of these expressions. Patient sample or stock dilutions should be made using reagent grade water, saline, or method-specific diluent using Class A glassware. The sample and diluent should be thoroughly mixed before use. It is not recommended that sample dilutions be made in smaller volume sample cups or holders. Any total volume can be used as long as the fraction reduces to give the dilution factor.

Example 1-13

If in the preceding example 150 mL of the 100 mmol/L sodium solution was required, the dilution ratio of stock to total volume must be maintained. Set up a ratio between the desired total volume and the dilution factor to determine the amount of stock needed. The equation becomes

$$\frac{1}{30} = \frac{x}{150}$$
$$x = 5 \qquad \text{(Eq. 1-43)}$$

Note that 5/150 reduces to the dilution factor of 1/30. To make up this solution, 5 mL of stock is added to 145 mL of the appropriate diluent, making the ratio of *stock volume* to *diluent volume* equal to 5/145. Recall that the dilution factor includes the total volume of *both* stock plus diluent in the denominator and differs from the amount of diluent to stock that is needed.

Example 1-14

Many laboratory scientists like using $(V_1)(C_1) = (V_2)(C_2)$ for simple dilution calculations. This is fine, as long as you recall that you will need to subtract the stock volume from the total final volume for the correct *diluent* volume.

$$(V_1)(C_1) = (V_2)(C_2)$$
$$(x)(3{,}000) = (150)(100)$$
$$x = 5; \ 150 - 5 = 145 \text{ mL of diluent}$$
should be added to 5 mL of stock   **(Eq. 1-44)**

Simple Dilutions

When making a *simple dilution*, the laboratory scientist must decide on the total volume desired and the amount of stock to be used.

Example 1-15

A 1:10 (1/10) dilution of serum can be achieved by using any of the following approaches. A ratio of 1:9—one part serum and nine parts diluent (saline):

A. 100 μL of serum added to 900 μL of saline.
B. 20 μL of serum added to 180 μL of saline.
C. 1 mL of serum added to 9 mL of saline.
D. 2 mL of serum added to 18 mL of saline.

Note that the sum of the ratio of serum to diluent (1:9) needed to make up each dilution satisfies the dilution factor (1:10 or 1/10) of stock material to total volume. When thinking about the stock to diluent volume, subtract the parts of stock needed from the total volume or parts to get the number of diluent "parts" needed. Once the volume of each part, usually stock, is available, multiply the diluent parts needed to obtain the correct volume.

Example 1-16

You have a 10 g/dL stock of protein standard. You need a 2 g/dL standard. You only have 0.200 mL of 10 g/dL stock to use. The procedure requires 0.100 mL.
   Solution:

$$\frac{2 \text{ g/dL}}{10 \text{ g/dL}} = \frac{1}{5} = \text{Dilution factor} \qquad \text{(Eq. 1-45)}$$

You will need 1 part or volume of stock of a total of 5 parts or volumes. Subtracting 1 from 5 yields that 4 parts or volumes of diluent is needed (Fig. 1-13). In this instance, you need at least 0.100 mL for the procedure. You have 0.200 mL of stock. You can make the dilution in various ways, as seen in Example 1-17. This is a personal decision and often reflects the volumes of available pipets, etc.

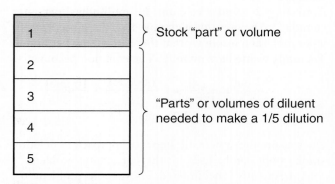

FIGURE 1-13 Simple dilution. Consider this diagram depicting a substance having a 1/5 dilution factor. The dilution factor represents that 1 part of stock is needed from a total of 5 parts. To *make* this dilution, you would determine the volume of 1 "part," usually the stock or patient sample. The remainder of the "parts" or total would constitute the amount of diluent needed, or four times the volume used for the stock.

Example 1-17

There are several ways to make a 1/5 dilution having only 0.200 mL of stock and needing a total minimum volume of 0.100 mL.

(a) Add 0.050 mL stock (1 part) to 0.200 mL of diluent (4 parts × 0.050 mL).
(b) Add 0.100 mL of stock (1 part) to 0.400 mL of diluent (4 parts × 0.100 mL).
(c) Add 0.200 mL of stock (1 part) to 0.800 mL of diluent (4 parts × 0.200 mL).

The dilution factor is also used to determine the final concentration of a dilution by multiplying the original concentration by the inverse of the dilution factor or the dilution factor denominator when it is expressed as a fraction.

Example 1-18

Determine the concentration of a 200 μmol/mL human chorionic gonadotropin (hCG) standard that was diluted 1/50. This value is obtained by multiplying the original concentration, 200 μmol/mL hCG, by the dilution factor, 1/50. The result is 4 μmol/mL hCG. Quite often, the concentration of the original material is needed.

Example 1-19

A 1:2 dilution of serum with saline had a creatinine result of 8.6 mg/dL. Calculate the actual serum creatinine concentration.
Dilution factor: 1/2
Dilution result = 8.6 mg/dL

Because this result represents 1/2 of the concentration, the actual serum creatinine value is

$$2 \times 8.6 = 17.2 = 17.2 \text{ mg/dL} \qquad \textbf{(Eq. 1-46)}$$

Serial Dilutions

A serial dilution may be defined as multiple progressive dilutions ranging from more concentrated solutions to less concentrated solutions. Serial dilutions are extremely useful when the volume of concentrate or diluent is in short supply and needs to be minimized or a number of dilutions are required, such as in determining a titer. The volume of patient sample available to the laboratory may be small (e.g., pediatric samples), and a serial dilution may be needed to ensure that sufficient sample is available. The serial dilution is initially made in the same manner as a simple dilution. Subsequent dilutions will then be made from each preceding dilution. When a serial dilution is made, certain criteria may need to be satisfied. The criteria vary with each situation but usually include such considerations as the total volume desired, the amount of diluent or concentrate available, the dilution factor, the final concentration needed, and the support materials required.

Example 1-20

A sample is to be diluted 1:2, 1:4, and, finally, 1:8. It is arbitrarily decided that the total volume for each dilution is to be 1 mL. Note that the least common denominator for these dilution factors is 2. Once the first dilution is made (1/2), a 1:2 (least common denominator between 2 and 4) dilution of it will yield

$$1/2 \times 1/2 = 1/4$$

(initial dilution factor)(next dilution factor)

$$= \text{(final dilution factor)} \qquad \textbf{(Eq. 1-47)}$$

By making a 1:2 dilution of the first dilution, the second dilution factor of 1:4 is satisfied. Making a 1:2 dilution of the 1:4 dilution will result in the next dilution (1:8). To establish the dilution factor needed for subsequent dilutions, it is helpful to solve the following equation for (x):

$$\text{Stock/preceding concentration} \times (x)$$

$$= \text{(final dilution factor)} \qquad \textbf{(Eq. 1-48)}$$

To make up these dilutions, three test tubes are labeled 1:2, 1:4, and 1:8, respectively. One milliliter of diluent is added to each test tube. To make the primary dilution of 1:2, 1 mL of serum is added to test tube no. 1. The solution is mixed, and 1 mL of the primary dilution is removed and added to test tube no. 2. After mixing, this solution contains a 1:4 dilution. Then 1 mL of the 1:4 dilution from test tube no. 2 is added to test tube no. 3. Mix, and the resultant dilution in this test tube is 1:8, satisfying all of the previously established criteria. Refer to Figure 1-14 for an illustration of this serial dilution.

Example 1-21

Another type of serial dilution combines several dilution factors that are not multiples of one another. In our previous example, 1:2, 1:4, and 1:8 dilutions are all related to one another by a factor of 2. Consider the situation when 1:10, 1:20, 1:100, and 1:200 dilution factors are required. There are several approaches to solving this type of dilution problem. One method is to treat the 1:10 and 1:20 dilutions as one serial dilution problem, the 1:20 and 1:100 dilutions as a second serial dilution, and the 1:100 and 1:200 dilutions as the last serial dilution.

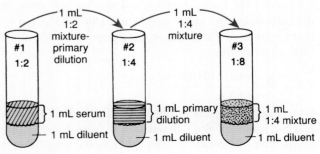

FIGURE 1-14 Serial dilution.

Another approach is to consider what dilution factor of the concentrate is needed to yield the final dilution. In this example, the initial dilution is 1:10, with subsequent dilutions of 1:20, 1:100, and 1:200. The first dilution may be accomplished by adding 1 mL of stock to 9 mL of diluent. The total volume of solution is 10 mL. Our initial dilution factor has been satisfied. In making the remaining dilutions, 2 mL of diluent is added to each test tube.

$$\text{Initial/preceding dilution} \times (x) = \text{dilution needed}$$

Solve for (x).

Using the dilution factors listed above and solving for (x), the equations become

$$1:10 \times (x) = 1:20$$
$$\text{where } (x) = 2 (\text{or 1 part stock to 1 part diluent})$$
$$1:20 \times (x) = 1:100$$
$$\text{where } (x) = 5 (\text{or 1 part stock to 4 parts diluent})$$
$$1:100(x) = 1:200$$
$$\text{where } (x) = 2 (\text{or 1 part stock to 1 part diluent})$$

(Eq. 1-49)

In practice, the 1:10 dilution must be diluted by a factor of 2 to obtain a subsequent 1:20 dilution. Because the second tube already contains 2 mL of diluent, 2 mL of the 1:10 dilution should be added (1 part stock to 1 part diluent). In preparing the 1:100 dilution from this, a 1:5 dilution factor of the 1:20 mixture is required (1 part stock to 4 parts diluent). Because this tube already contains 2 mL, the volume of diluent in the tube is divided by its parts, which is 4; thus, 500 μL, or 0.500 mL, of stock should be added. The 1:200 dilution is prepared in the same manner using a 1:2 dilution factor (1 part stock to 1 part diluent) and adding 2 mL of the 1:100 to the 2 mL of diluent already in the tube.

Water of Hydration

Some compounds are available in a hydrated form. To obtain a correct weight for these chemicals, the attached water molecule(s) must be included.

Example 1-22

How much $CuSO_4 \cdot 5H_2O$ must be weighed to prepare 1 L of 0.5 M $CuSO_4$? When calculating the gmw of this substance, the water weight must be considered so that the gmw is 250 g rather than gmw of $CuSO_4$ alone (160 g). Therefore,

$$\frac{250 \, \cancel{g} \, CuSO_4 \cdot 5H_2O}{\cancel{mol}} \times \frac{0.5 \, \cancel{mol}}{1 \, \cancel{L}} = 125 \text{ g/L} \quad \text{(Eq. 1-50)}$$

Cancel out like terms to obtain the result of 125 g/L. A reagent protocol often designates the use of an anhydrous form of a chemical; frequently, however, all that is available is a hydrated form.

Example 1-23

A procedure requires 0.9 g of $CuSO_4$. All that is available is $CuSO_4 \cdot 5H_2O$. What weight of $CuSO_4 \cdot 5H_2O$ is needed? Calculate the percentage of $CuSO_4$ present in $CuSO_4 \cdot 5H_2O$. The percentage is

$$\frac{160}{250} = 0.64, \text{ or } 64\% \quad \text{(Eq. 1-51)}$$

Therefore, 1 g of $CuSO_4 \cdot 5H_2O$ contains 0.64 g of $CuSO_4$, so the equation becomes

$$\frac{0.9 \text{ g } CuSO_4 \text{ needed}}{0.64 \, CuSO_4 \text{ in } CuSO_4 \cdot 5H_2O}$$
$$= 1.41 \text{ g } CuSO_4 \cdot 5H_2O \text{ required} \quad \text{(Eq. 1-52)}$$

Graphing and Beer's Law

The Beer-Lambert law (Beer's law) mathematically establishes the relationship between concentration and absorbance in many photometric determinations. Beer's law is expressed as

$$A = abc \quad \text{(Eq. 1-53)}$$

where A is absorbance; a is the absorptivity constant for a particular compound at a given wavelength under specified conditions of temperature, pH, and so on; b is the length of the light path; and c is the concentration.

If a method follows Beer's law, then absorbance is proportional to concentration as long as the length of the light path and the absorptivity of the absorbing species remain unaltered during the analysis. In practice, however, there are limits to the predictability of a linear response. Even in automated systems, adherence to Beer's law is often determined by checking the linearity of the test method over a wide concentration range. The limits of linearity often represent the reportable range of an assay. This term should not be confused with the reference ranges associated with clinical significance of a test. Assays measuring absorbance generally obtain the concentration results by using a Beer's law graph, known as a standard graph or curve. This graph is made by plotting absorbance versus the concentration of known standards (Fig. 1-15). Because most photometric assays set the initial absorbance to zero (0) using a reagent blank, the initial data points are 0,0. Graphs should be labeled properly and the concentration units must be given. The horizontal axis is referred to as the x-axis, whereas the vertical line is the y-axis. It is not important which variable (absorbance or concentration) is assigned to an individual axis, but it is important that the values assigned to them are uniformly distributed along the axis. By convention, in the clinical laboratory, concentration is usually plotted on the x-axis. On a standard graph, only the standard and their associated absorbances are plotted.

Once a standard graph has been established, it is permissible to run just one standard, or calibrator, as long as the system remains the same. One-point calculation

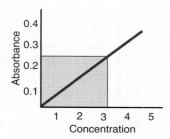

Unknown absorbance = 0.250
Concentration from graph = 3.2

FIGURE 1-15 Standard curve.

or calibration refers to the calculation of the comparison of the known standard/calibrator concentration and its corresponding absorbance to the absorbance of the unknown value according to the following ratio:

$$\frac{\text{Concentration of standard } (C_s)}{\text{Absorbance of standard } (A_s)}$$
$$= \frac{\text{Concentration of unknown } (C_u)}{\text{Absorbance of unknown } (A_u)} \quad \textbf{(Eq. 1-54)}$$

Solving for the concentration of the unknown, the equation becomes

$$C_u = \frac{(A_u)(C_s)}{A_s} \qquad \textbf{(Eq. 1-55)}$$

Example 1-24
The biuret protein assay is very stable and follows Beer's law. Rather than make up a completely new standard graph, one standard (6 g/dL) was assayed. The absorbance of the standard was 0.400, and the absorbance of the unknown was 0.350. Determine the value of the unknown in g/dL.

$$C_u = \frac{(0.350)(6 \text{ g/dL})}{(0.400)} = 5.25 \text{ g/dL} \quad \textbf{(Eq. 1-56)}$$

This method of calculation is acceptable as long as everything in the system, including the instrument and lot of reagents, remains the same. If anything in the system changes, a new standard graph should be done. Verification of linearity and/or calibration is required whenever a system changes or becomes unstable. Regulatory agencies often prescribe the condition of verification as well as how often the linearity needs to be checked.

Enzyme Calculations
Another application of Beer's law is the calculation of enzyme assay results. When calculating enzyme results, the *rate of absorbance change* is often monitored continuously during the reaction to give the difference in absorbance, known as the delta absorbance, or ΔA. Instead of using a standard graph or a one-point calculation, the molar absorptivity of the product is used. If the absorptivity constant and absorbance, in this case ΔA, is given,

Beer's law can be used to calculate the enzyme concentration directly without initially needing a standard graph, as follows:

$$A = abC$$
$$C = \frac{A}{ab} \qquad \textbf{(Eq. 1-57)}$$

When the absorptivity constant (a) is given in units of grams per liter (moles) through a 1 centimeter (cm) light path, the term *molar absorptivity* (ε) is used. Substitution of ε for a and ΔA for A produces the following Beer's law formula:

$$C = \frac{\Delta A}{\varepsilon} \qquad \textbf{(Eq. 1-58)}$$

Units used to report enzyme activity have traditionally included weight, time, and volume. In the early days of enzymology, method-specific units (e.g., King Armstrong, Caraway) were all different and confusing. In 1961, the Enzyme Commission of the International Union of Biochemistry recommended using one unit, the international unit (IU), for reporting enzyme activity. The IU is defined as the amount of enzyme that will catalyze 1 µmol of substrate per minute per liter. These units were often expressed as units per liter (U/L). The designations IU, U, or IU/L were adopted by many clinical laboratories to represent the IU. Although the reporting unit is the same, unless the analysis conditions are identical, use of the IU does not standardize the actual enzyme activity, and therefore, results between different methods of the same enzyme do not result in equivalent activity of the enzyme. For example, an alkaline phosphatase performed at 37°C will catalyze more substrate than if it is run at lower temperature, such as 25°C, even though the unit of expression, U/L, will be the same. The SI recommended unit is the *katal*, which is expressed as moles per liter per second. Whichever unit is used, calculation of the activity using Beer's law requires inclusion of the dilution and, depending on the reporting unit, possible conversion to the appropriate term (e.g., µmol to mol, mL to L, minute to second, and temperature factors). Beer's law for the IU now becomes

$$C = \frac{(\Delta A)10^{-6} (\text{TV})}{(\varepsilon)(b)(\text{SV})} \qquad \textbf{(Eq. 1-59)}$$

where TV is the total volume of sample plus reagents in mL and SV is the sample volume used in mL. The 10^{-6} converts moles to µmol for the IU. If another unit of activity is used, such as the katal, conversion into liters and seconds would be needed, but the conversions to and from micromoles are excluded.

Example 1-25
The ΔA per minute for an enzyme reaction is 0.250. The product measured has a molar absorptivity of 12.2×10^3 at 425 nm at 30°C. The incubation and reaction temperature are also kept at 30°C. The assay calls for 1 mL of

reagent and 0.050 mL of sample. Give the enzyme activity results in international units.

Applying Beer's law and the necessary conversion information, the equation becomes

$$C = \frac{(0.250)(10^{-6})(1.050\,\text{mL})}{(12.2 \times 10^3)(1)(0.050\,\text{mL})} = 430\,\text{U} \quad \textbf{(Eq. 1-60)}$$

Note: b is usually given as 1 cm; because it is a constant, it may not be considered in the calculation.

SPECIMEN CONSIDERATIONS

The process of specimen collection, handling, and processing remains one of the primary areas of *preanalytic* error. Careful attention to each phase is necessary to ensure proper subsequent testing and reporting of meaningful results. All accreditation agencies require laboratories to clearly define and delineate the procedures used for proper collection, transport, and processing of patient samples and the steps used to minimize and detect any errors, along with the documentation of the resolution of any errors. The Clinical Laboratory Improvement Amendments Act of 1988 (CLIA 88)[27] specifies that procedures for specimen submission and proper handling, including the disposition of any specimen that does not meet the laboratories' criteria of acceptability, be documented.

Types of Samples

Phlebotomy, or *venipuncture*, is the act of obtaining a blood sample from a vein using a needle attached to a syringe or a stoppered *evacuated tube*. These tubes come in different volume sizes: from pediatric sizes (≈150 µL) to larger 7 mL tubes. The most frequent site for venipuncture is the antecubital vein of the arm. A tourniquet made of pliable rubber tubing or a strip with hook and loop tape (Velcro) at the end is wrapped around the arm, causing cessation of blood flow and dilation of the veins, making them easier to detect. The gauge of the needle is inversely related to the size of the needle; the larger the number, the smaller the needle bore and length. An intravenous (IV) infusion set, sometimes referred to as a butterfly because of the appearance of the setup, may be used whenever the veins are fragile, small, or hard to reach or find. The butterfly is attached to a piece of tubing, which is then attached to either a hub or a tube. Because of potential needle sticks, this practice may be discouraged. Sites adjacent to IV therapy should be avoided; however, if both arms are involved in IV therapy and the IV cannot be discontinued for a short time, a site *below* the IV site should be sought. The initial sample drawn (5 mL) should be discarded because it is most likely contaminated with IV fluid and only subsequent sample tubes should be used for analytic purposes.

In addition to venipuncture, blood samples can be collected using a skin puncture technique that customarily involves the outer area of the bottom of the foot (a heel stick), the fleshy part of the middle of the last phalanx of the third or fourth (ring) finger (finger stick), or possibly the fleshy portion of the earlobe. A sharp lancet is used to pierce the skin and a capillary tube (i.e., short, narrow glass tube) is used for sample collection.[28]

Analytic testing of blood involves the use of whole blood, serum, or plasma. Whole blood, as the name implies, uses both the liquid portion of the blood called *plasma* and the cellular components (red blood cells, white blood cells, and platelets). This requires blood collection into a vessel containing an anticoagulant. Complete mixing of the blood immediately following venipuncture is necessary to ensure the anticoagulant can adequately inhibit the blood's clotting factors. As whole blood sits, the cells fall toward the bottom, leaving a clear yellow supernate on top called *plasma*. If a tube does *not* contain an anticoagulant, the blood's clotting factors are active to form a clot incorporating the cells. The clot is encapsulated by the large protein fibrinogen. The remaining liquid is called serum rather than plasma (Fig. 1-16). Most testing in the clinical chemistry laboratory is performed on either plasma or serum. The major difference between plasma and serum is that serum does not contain fibrinogen (i.e., there is less protein in serum than plasma) and some potassium is released from platelets (serum potassium is slightly higher in serum than in plasma). It is important that serum samples be allowed to completely clot (≈20 minutes) before being centrifuged. Plasma samples also require centrifugation but do not need to allow for clotting time and their use can decrease turnaround time for reporting results.

Centrifugation of the sample accelerates the process of separating the plasma and cells. Specimens should be centrifuged for approximately 10 minutes at an RCF of 1,000g to 2,000g but should avoid mechanical destruction of red cells that can result in hemoglobin release, called hemolysis.

Arterial blood samples measure blood gases (partial pressures of oxygen and carbon dioxide) and pH. Syringes are used instead of evacuated tubes because of the pressure in an arterial blood vessel. The radial, brachial, and femoral arteries are the primary arterial sites. Arterial punctures are more difficult to perform because of inherent arterial pressure, difficulty in stopping bleeding afterward, and the undesirable development of a hematoma, which cuts off the blood supply to the surrounding tissue.[29]

Continued metabolism may occur if the serum or plasma remains in contact with the cells for any period. Evacuated tubes may incorporate plastic, gel-like material that serves as a barrier between the cells and the plasma or serum and seals these compartments from one another during centrifugation. Some gels can interfere with certain analytes, notably trace metals, and drugs such as the tricyclic antidepressants.

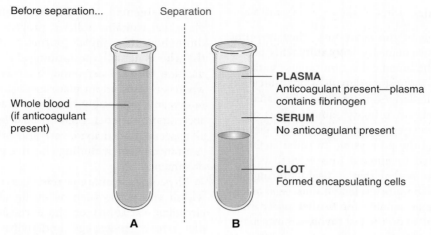

Before separation...   Separation

Whole blood
(if anticoagulant
present)

PLASMA
Anticoagulant present—plasma
contains fibrinogen

SERUM
No anticoagulant present

CLOT
Formed encapsulating cells

A   B

FIGURE 1-16 Blood sample.

Proper patient identification is the first step in sample collection. The importance of using the proper collection tube, avoiding prolonged tourniquet application, drawing tubes in the proper order, and proper labeling of tubes cannot be stressed strongly enough. Prolonged tourniquet application causes a stasis of blood flow and an increase in hemoconcentration and anything bound to proteins or the cells. Having patients open and close their fist during phlebotomy is of no value and may cause an increase in potassium and, therefore, should be avoided. IV contamination should be considered if a large increase occurs in the substances being infused, such as glucose, potassium, sodium, and chloride, with a decrease of other analytes such as urea and creatinine. In addition, the proper antiseptic must be used. Isopropyl alcohol wipes, for example, are used for cleaning and disinfecting the collection site; however, this is not the proper antiseptic for disinfecting the site when drawing blood alcohol levels.

Blood is not the only sample analyzed in the clinical chemistry laboratory. Urine is the next most common fluid for determination. Most quantitative analyses of urine require a timed sample (usually 24 hours); a complete sample (all urine must be collected in the specified time) can be difficult because many timed samples are collected by the patient in an outpatient situation. Creatinine analysis is often used to assess the completeness of a 24-hour urine sample because creatinine output is relatively free from interference and is stable, with little change in output within individuals. The average adult excretes 1 to 2 g of creatinine per 24 hours. Urine volume differs widely among individuals; however, a 4 L container is adequate (average output is ≈2 L). It should be noted that this analysis differs from the creatinine clearance test used to assess glomerular filtration rate, which compares urine creatinine output with that in the serum or plasma in a specified time interval and urine volume (often correcting for the surface area). The generic formula is

$$UV/P \qquad \text{(Eq. 1-61)}$$

where U represents the urine creatinine value in mg/dL, V is urine volume per unit of time expressed in mL/min, and P is the plasma or serum creatinine value in mg/dL. This formula expresses the creatinine clearance value in mL/min (see Chapter 27).

Other body fluids analyzed by the clinical chemistry laboratory include **cerebrospinal fluid (CSF)**, *paracentesis* fluids (pleural, pericardial, and peritoneal), and amniotic fluids. The color and characteristics of the fluid *before* centrifugation should be noted for these samples. *Before* centrifugation, a laboratorian should also verify that the sample is designated for clinical chemistry analysis *only* because a single fluid sample may be shared among several departments (i.e., hematology or microbiology) and centrifugation could invalidate certain tests in those areas.

CSF is an ultrafiltrate of the plasma and will, ordinarily, reflect the values seen in the plasma. For glucose and protein analysis (total and specific proteins), it is recommended that a blood sample be analyzed concurrently with the analysis of those analytes in the CSF. This will assist in determining the clinical utility of the values obtained on the CSF sample. This is also true for lactate dehydrogenase and protein assays requested on paracentesis fluids. All fluid samples should be handled immediately without delay between sample procurement, transport, and analysis.

Amniotic fluid is used to assess fetal lung maturity (L/S ratio), congenital diseases, hemolytic diseases, genetic defects, and gestational age. The laboratory scientist should verify the specific handling of this fluid with the manufacturer of the testing procedure(s).

Sample Processing

When samples arrive in the laboratory, they are processed. In the clinical chemistry laboratory, this means correctly matching the blood collection tube(s) with the appropriate analyte request and patient identification labels. This is a particularly sensitive area of preanalytic error. Bar code labels on primary sample tubes are a popular means to detect errors and to minimize clerical errors at this point of the processing. In some facilities, samples are numbered or entered into work lists or a second identification system that is useful during the analytic phase. The laboratory scientist must also ascertain if the sample is acceptable for further processing. The criteria used depend on the test involved but usually include volume considerations (i.e., is there sufficient volume for testing needs?), use of proper anticoagulants or preservatives, whether timing is clearly indicated and appropriate for timed testing, and whether the specimen is intact and has been properly transported (e.g., cooled or on ice, within a reasonable period, protected from light, and in a tube that is properly capped). Unless a whole blood analysis is being performed, the sample is then centrifuged as previously described and the serum or plasma should be separated from the cells if not analyzed immediately.

Once processed, the laboratory scientist should note the presence of any serum or plasma characteristics such as *hemolysis* and icterus (increased bilirubin pigment) or the presence of turbidity often associated with lipemia (increased lipids). Samples should be analyzed within 4 hours; to minimize the effects of evaporation, samples should be properly capped and kept away from areas of rapid airflow, light, and heat. If testing is to occur after that time, samples should be appropriately stored. For most, this means refrigeration at 4°C for 8 hours. Many analytes are stable at this temperature, with the exception of alkaline phosphatase (increases) and lactate dehydrogenase (decreases as a result of temperature labile fractions four and five). Samples may be frozen at −20°C and stored for longer periods without deleterious effects on the results. Repeated cycles of freezing and thawing, like those that occur in so-called frost-free freezers, should be avoided.

Sample Variables

Sample variables include physiologic considerations, proper patient preparation, and problems in collection, transportation, processing, and storage. Although laboratorians must include mechanisms to minimize the effect of these variables on testing and must document each preanalytic incident, it is often frustrating to try to control the variables that largely depend on individuals outside of the laboratory. The best course of action is to critically assess or predict the weak areas or links,

identify potential problems, and put an action plan in place that contains policies, procedures, or checkpoints throughout the sample's journey to the laboratory scientist who is actually performing the test. Good communication with all personnel involved helps ensure that whatever plans are in place meet the needs of the laboratory and, ultimately, the patient and physician. Most accreditation agencies require that laboratories consider all aspects of preanalytic variation as part of their quality assurance plans, including effective problem solving and documentation.

Physiologic variation refers to changes that occur within the body, such as cyclic changes (diurnal or circadian variation) or those resulting from exercise, diet, stress, gender, age, underlying medical conditions (e.g., fever, asthma, and obesity), drugs, or posture (Table 1-5). Most samples are drawn on patients who are fasting (usually overnight for at least 8 hours). Because overnight and fasting are relative terms, however, the length of time and what was consumed during that time should be determined before sample procurement for those tests most affected by diet or fasting. When fasting, many patients may avoid drinking water and they may become dehydrated, which can be reflected in higher than expected results. Patient preparation for timed samples or those requiring specific diets or other instructions must be well written and verbally explained to patients. Elderly patients often misunderstand or are overwhelmed by the directions given to them by physician office personnel. A laboratory information telephone number listed on these printed directions can often serve as an excellent reference for proper patient preparation.

Drugs can affect various analytes.[30] It is important to ascertain what, if any, medications the patient is taking that may interfere with the test. Unfortunately, many laboratorians do not have either the time for or access to this information and the interest in this type of interference only arises when the physician questions a result. Some frequently encountered influences are smoking, which causes an increase in glucose as a result of the action of nicotine; growth hormone; cortisol; cholesterol; triglycerides; and urea. High amounts or chronic consumption of alcohol causes hypoglycemia, increased triglycerides, and an increase in the enzyme gamma-glutamyltransferase and other liver function tests. Intramuscular injections increase the enzyme creatine kinase and the skeletal muscle fraction of lactate dehydrogenase. Opiates, such as morphine or meperidine, cause increases in liver and pancreatic enzymes, and oral contraceptives may affect many analytic results. Many drugs affect liver function tests. Diuretics can cause decreased potassium and hyponatremia. Thiazide-type medications can cause hyperglycemia and prerenal azotemia secondary to the decrease in blood volume. Postcollection variations are related to those factors

TABLE 1-5	VARIABLES AFFECTING SELECT CHEMISTRY ANALYTES
FACTOR	**EXAMPLES OF ANALYTES AFFECTED**
Age	Albumin, ALP ($\uparrow$ older), phosphorus (P), cholesterol
Gender	($\uparrow$ Males): Albumin, ALP, creatine, Ca^{2+}, uric acid, CK, AST, phosphate (PO_4), blood urea nitrogen, Mg^{2+}, bilirubin, cholesterol
	($\uparrow$ Females): Fe, cholesterol, γ-globulins, α-lipoproteins
Diurnal variation	$\uparrow$ in AM: ACTH, cortisol, Fe, aldosterone
	$\uparrow$ in PM: ACP, growth hormone, PTH, TSH
Day-to-day variation	$\geq$20% for ALT, bilirubin, Fe, TSH, triglycerides
Recent food ingestion	$\uparrow$ Glucose, insulin, triglycerides, gastrin, ionized Ca^{2+}
	$\downarrow$ chloride, phosphorus, potassium, amylase, ALP
Posture	$\uparrow$ When standing: albumin, cholesterol, aldosterone, Ca^{2+}
Activity	$\uparrow$ In ambulatory patients: CK
	$\uparrow$ With exercise: lactic acid, creatine, protein, CK, AST, LD
	$\downarrow$ With exercise: cholesterol, triglycerides
Stress	$\uparrow$ ACTH, cortisol, catecholamines
Race	TP $\uparrow$ (black), albumin $\downarrow$ (black); IgG 40% $\uparrow$, and IgA 20%$\uparrow$ (black male vs. white male); $\rightarrow$ CK/ LD $\uparrow$ black males; $\uparrow$ cholesterol and triglycerides > white >40 years old (glucose incidence diabetes in Asian, black, Native American, Hispanic)
Require fasting	Fasting blood sugar, glucose tolerance test, triglycerides, lipid panel, gastrin, insulin, aldosterone/renin
Anaerobic and require ICE slurry (immediate cooling)	Lactic acid, ammonia, blood gas (if not analyzed within 30 min = $\downarrow$ pH, and po_2), iCa^{+2} (heparinized whole blood if not analyzed within 30 min)
Hemolysis	$\uparrow$ K^+, ammonia, PO_4, Fe, Mg^{2+}, ALT, AST, LD, ALP, ACP, catecholamines, CK (marked hemolysis)

ALP, alkaline phosphatase; CK, creatine kinase; AST, aspartate aminotransferase; ACTH, adrenocorticotropic hormone; ACP, acid phosphatase; PTH, parathyroid hormone; TSH, thyroid-stimulating hormone; ALT, alanine aminotransferase; LD, lactate dehydrogenase; TP, total protein.

discussed under specimen processing. Clerical errors are the most frequently encountered, followed by inadequate separation of cells from serum, improper storage, and collection.

Chain of Custody

When laboratory tests are likely linked to a crime or accident, they become forensic in nature. In these cases, documented specimen identification is required at each phase of the process. Each facility has its own forms and protocols; however, the patient, and usually a witness, must identify the sample. It should have a tamper-proof seal. Any individual in contact with the sample must document receipt of the sample, the condition of the sample at the time of receipt, and the date and time it was received. In some instances, one witness verifies the entire process and cosigns as the sample moves along. Any analytic test could be used as part of legal testimony; therefore, the laboratory scientist should give each

sample—even without the documentation—the same attention given to a forensic sample.

Electronic and Paper Reporting of Results

Electronic transmission of laboratory data and the more routine use of an electronic medical record, coding, billing, and other data management systems have caused much debate regarding appropriate standards needed in terms of both reporting guidelines and safeguards to ensure privacy of the data and records. Complicating matters is that there are many different data management systems in use by health-care agencies that all use laboratory information. For example, the Logical Observation Identifiers Names and Codes (LOINC) system, International Federation of Clinical Chemistry/International Union of Pure and Applied Chemistry (IFCC/IUPAC), ASTM, Health Level 7 (HL7), and Systematized Nomenclature of Medicine, Reference Technology (SNOMED RT) are databases that use their own coding systems for laboratory observations. There are also additional proprietary systems in use, adding to the confusion. In an attempt to standardize these processes and to protect the confidentiality of patient information as required by the Health Insurance Portability and Accountability Act (HIPAA), the Healthcare Common Procedure Coding System (HCPCS) test and services coding system was developed to be recognized by all insurers for reimbursement purposes. The International Classification of Diseases (ICD) developed by the World Health Organization (WHO) uses codes identifying patient diseases and conditions. In the United States, ICD version 9 with clinical modifications (CM) will soon be replaced by ICD-10. The clinical modifications are maintained by the National Center for Health Statistics. Incorporated into the HCPCS system is the Current Procedural Terminology (CPT) codes, developed by the American Medical Association, that identify almost all laboratory tests and procedures. The CPT codes are divided into different subcategories, with tests or services assigned five-digit numbers followed by the name of the test or service. Together, these standard coding systems help patient data and tracking of disease transmission between all stakeholders such as physicians, patients, epidemiologists, and insurers.

Clinical laboratory procedures are found in CPT Category I with coding numbers falling between 80000 and 89000. There can be several codes for a given test based on the reason and type of testing and there are codes given for common profiles or array of tests that represent each test's separate codes. For example, blood glucose testing includes the codes 82947 (quantitative except for strip reading), 82948 (strip reading), and 82962 (self-monitoring by FDA cleared device) and the comprehensive metabolic panel (80053) includes albumin, alkaline phosphatase, total bilirubin, blood urea nitrogen, total calcium, carbon dioxide, chloride, creatinine, glucose, potassium, total protein, sodium, and alanine and aspartate transaminases and their associated codes. At a minimum, any system must include a unique patient identifier, test name, and code that relates back to the HCPCS and ICD databases. For reporting purposes, whether paper or electronic, the report should include the unique patient identifier and test name including any appropriate abbreviations, the test value with the unit of measure, date and time of collection, sample information, reference ranges, plus any other pertinent information for proper test interpretation. Results that are subject to autoverification should be indicated in the report. Table 1-6 lists the information that is often required by accreditation agencies.[31]

TABLE 1-6	MINIMUM ELEMENTS OF PAPER OR ELECTRONIC PATIENT REPORTS
Name and address of laboratory performing the analysis including any reference laboratories used	
Patient name and identification number or unique identifier	
Name of physician or person ordering the test	
Date and time of specimen collection	
Date and time of release of results (or available if needed)	
Specimen source or type	
Test results and units of measure if applicable	
Reference ranges, when available	
Comments relating to any sample or testing interferences that may alter interpretation	

For additional student resources please visit thePoint at **http://thepoint.lww.com**. **thePoint**

QUESTIONS

1. What is the *molarity* for a solution containing 100 g of NaCl made up to 500 mL with distilled water? Assume a gram molecular weight (from periodic table) of approximately 58 grams.
   - a. 3.45 M
   - b. 1.72 M
   - c. 290 M
   - d. 5.27 M

2. What is the *normality* for a solution containing 100 g of NaCl made up to 500 mL with distilled water? Assume a gram molecular weight (from periodic table) of approximately 58 grams.
   - a. 3.45
   - b. 0.86
   - c. 1.72
   - d. 6.9

3. What is the *percent (w/v)* for a solution containing 100 g of NaCl made up to 500 mL with distilled water?
   a. 20%
   b. 5%
   c. 29%
   d. 58%

4. What is the *dilution factor* for a solution containing 100 g of NaCl made up to 500 mL with distilled water?
   a. 1:5 or 1/5
   b. 5
   c. 50 or 1/50
   d. 10

5. What is the value in mg/dL for a solution containing 10 mg of $CaCl_2$ made with 100 mL of distilled water?
   a. 10
   b. 100
   c. 50
   d. Cannot determine without additional information

6. What is the molarity of a solution containing 10 mg of $CaCl_2$ made with 100 mL of distilled water? Assume a gram molecular weight from the periodic table of approximately 111 grams.
   a. 9×10^{-4}
   b. 1.1×10^{-3}
   c. 11.1
   d. 90

7. You must make 1 L of 0.2 M acetic acid (CH_3COOH). All you have available is concentrated glacial acetic acid (assay value, 98%; specific gravity, 1.05 g/mL). It will take _____ milliliters of acetic acid to make this solution. Assume a gram molecular weight of 60.05 grams.
   a. 11.7
   b. 1.029
   c. 3.42
   d. 12.01

8. What is the hydrogen ion concentration of an acetate buffer having a pH of 4.24?
   a. 5.75×10^{-5}
   b. 1.19×10^{-1}
   c. 0.62
   d. 0.76×10^{-4}

9. Using the Henderson-Hasselbalch equation, give the ratio of salt to weak acid for a Veronal buffer with a pH of 8.6 and a pK_a of 7.43.
   a. 14.7/1
   b. 1/8.6
   c. 1.17/1
   d. 1/4.3

10. The pK_a for acetic acid is 4.76. If the concentration of salt is 5 mmol/L and that of acetic acid is 10 mmol/L, what is the expected pH?
    a. 4.46
    b. 5.06
    c. 104
    d. 56

11. The hydrogen ion concentration of a solution is 0.0000937. What is the pH?
    a. 4.03
    b. 9.37×10^{-5}
    c. 9.07
    d. 8.03

12. Perform the following conversions:

    4×10^4 mg = ____ g

    1.3×10^2 mL = _____ dL

    0.02 mL = _____ μL

    5×10^{-3} mL = ___ μL

    5×10^{-2} L = ___ mL

    4 cm = _____ mm

13. What volume of 14 N H_2SO_4 is needed to make 250 mL of 3.2 M H_2SO_4 solution? Assume a gram molecular weight of 98.08 grams.
    a. 114 mL
    b. 1.82 mL
    c. 1.75 mL
    d. 7 mL

14. A 24-hour urine has a total volume of 1,200 mL. A 1:200 dilution of the urine specimen gives a creatinine result of 0.8 mg/dL. The serum value is 1.2 mg/dL. What is the final value of creatinine in mg/dL in the undiluted urine sample?
    a. 160
    b. 0.8
    c. 960
    d. 860

15. A 24-hour urine has a total volume of 1,200 mL. A 1:200 dilution of the urine specimen gives a creatinine result of 0.8 mg/dL. The serum value is 1.2 mg/dL. What is the result in terms of grams per 24 hours?
    a. 1.92
    b. 0.08
    c. 80
    d. 19

16. A new medical technologist was selecting analyte standards to develop a standard curve for a high-performance liquid chromatography (HPLC) procedure. This analyte must have a 100% purity level and must be suitable for HPLC. Which of the

following labels would be most appropriate for this procedure?
   a. ACS with no impurities listed
   b. USP
   c. NF
   d. CP
   e. ACS with impurities listed

17. When selecting quality control reagents for measuring an analyte in urine, the medical technologist should select:
   a. A quality control reagent prepared in a urine matrix.
   b. A quality control reagent prepared in a serum matrix.
   c. A quality control reagent prepared in deionized water.
   d. The matrix does not matter; any quality control reagent as long as the analyte of measure is chemically pure.

18. A patient's serum sample was placed on the chemistry analyzer and the output indicated "out of range" for the measurement of creatine kinase (CK) enzyme. A dilution of the patient serum was required. Which of the following should be used to prepare a dilution of patient serum?
   a. Deionized water
   b. Tap water
   c. Another patient's serum with confirmed, low levels of CK
   d. Type III water
   e. Type I water

19. True or False? Laboratory liquid in glass thermometers should be calibrated against an NIST-certified thermometer.

20. Which of the following containers is calibrated to hold only one exact volume of liquid?
   a. Volumetric flask
   b. Erlenmeyer flask
   c. Griffin beaker
   d. Graduated cylinder

21. Which of the following does NOT require calibration in the clinical laboratory?
   a. Electronic balance
   b. Liquid in glass thermometer
   c. Centrifuge
   d. Volumetric flask
   e. Air displacement pipet

22. Which of the following errors is NOT considered a preanalytical error?
   a. During a phlebotomy procedure, the patient is opening and clenching his fist multiple times.
   b. The blood was not permitted to clot and spun in a centrifuge after 6 minutes of collection.
   c. The patient was improperly identified leading to a mislabeled blood sample.
   d. The serum sample was diluted with tap water.
   e. During phlebotomy, the EDTA tube was collected prior to the red clot tube.

REFERENCES

1. National Institute of Standards and Technology (NIST). *Reference on Constants, Units, and Uncertainty*. Washington, DC: U.S. Department of Commerce; 1991/1993. http://physics.nist.gov/cuu/Units/introduction.html Accessed September 5, 2012. [Adapted from Special Publications (SP) Nos. 811 and 330.]
2. National Committee for Clinical Laboratory Standards (NCCLS)/CLSI. *The Reference System for the Clinical Laboratory: Criteria for Development and Credentialing of Methods and Materials for Harmonization and Results; Approved Guideline*. Wayne, PA: NCCLS; 2000. (NCCLS Document No. NRSCL 13-P.)
3. American Chemical Society (ACS). *Reagent Chemicals*. 9th ed. Washington, DC: ACS Press; 2000.
4. Department of Labor and Occupational Safety and Health Administration (OSHA). Occupational Exposure to Hazardous Chemicals in Laboratories. Washington, DC: OSHA; 1990. (Federal Register, 29 CFR, Part 1910.1450.)
5. National Institute of Standards and Technology (NIST). *Standard Reference Materials*. Washington, DC: U.S. Department of Commerce; 1991. (Publication No. 260.)
6. McNaught A, Wilkinson A, eds. International Union of Pure and Allied Chemistry (IUPAC). *Royal Society of Chemistry. Compendium of Chemical Terminology*. 2nd ed. Cambridge, UK: Blackwell Scientific; 1997.
7. Clinical and Laboratory Standards Institute (CLSI)/National Committee for Clinical Laboratory Standards (NCCLS). *How to Define and Determine Reference Intervals in the Clinical Laboratory; Approved Guideline*. 4th ed. Wayne, PA: CLSI; 2010. (Publication No. C28-A3c.)
8. International Organization for Standardization, European Committee for Standardization (ISO). *In Vitro Diagnostic Medical Devices—Measurement of Quantities in Samples of Biological Origin—Metrological Traceability of Values Assigned to Calibrators and Control Material*. Geneva, Switzerland: ISO; 2000. (Publication No. ISO/TC 212/WG2 N65/EN 17511.)
9. Lide DH, ed. *Handbook of Chemistry and Physics*. 88th ed. Boca Raton, FL: CRC Press; 2008.
10. National Institute of Standards and Technology (NIST). *Standard Reference Materials Program*. Washington, DC: U.S. Department of Commerce; 2008. http://www.nist.gov/srm/definitions.cfm. Accessed September 5, 2012.
11. Carreiro-Lewandowski E. Basic principles and practice of clinical chemistry. In: Bishop M, Schoeff L, Fody P, eds. *Clinical Chemistry, Principles, Procedures, and Correlations*. 6th ed. Baltimore, MD: Lippincott Williams & Wilkins; 2010:3-32.
12. Clinical Laboratory Standards Institute/National Committee for Clinical Laboratory Standards. *Preparation and Testing of Reagent Water in the Clinical Laboratory; Approved Guideline*. 4th ed. Wayne, PA: CLSI; 2006. (Publication No. C3-A4.)

13. College of American Pathologists (CAP). *General Laboratory Guidelines; Water Quality.* Northfield, IL: CAP; July 1999.
14. Skoog D, West D, Holler J, Crouch S, eds. *Analytical Chemistry: An Introduction.* 7th ed. Stamford, CT: Thompson/Brooks-Cole; 2000.
15. National Committee for Clinical Laboratory Standards (NCCLS)/ Clinical Laboratory Standards Institute. *Temperature Calibration of Water Baths, Instruments, and Temperature Sensors.* Villanova, PA: NCCLS; 1990. (Publication No. I2-A2.)
16. National Institute of Standards and Technology (NIST). *Calibration Uncertainties of Liquid-in-Glass Thermometers Over the Range from -20°C to 400°C.* Gaithersburg, MD: U.S. Department of Commerce; 2000.
17. Wise J. National Institute of Standards and Technology (NIST). *A Procedure for the Effective Recalibration of Liquid-in-Glass Thermometers.* Gaithersburg, MD: NIST; August 1991. (Publication No. SP 819.)
18. Bowers GN, Inman SR. The gallium melting-point standard. *Clin Chem.* 1977;23:733.
19. Bowie L, Esters F, Bolin J, et al. Development of an aqueous temperature-indicated technique and its application to clinical laboratory instruments. *Clin Chem.* 1976;22:449.
20. American Society for Testing and Materials (ASTM). *Standards Specification for Volumetric (Transfer) Pipets.* West Conshohocken, PA: ASTM; 1993:14.02:500-501. (Publication No. E969–83.)
21. American Society for Testing and Materials (ASTM). *Calibration of Volumetric Flasks.* West Conshohocken, PA: ASTM; 2003:14.04. (Publication No. E288–94.)
22. Seamonds B. Basic laboratory principles and techniques. In: Kaplan L, Pesce A, Kazmierczak S, eds. *Clinical Chemistry. Theory, Analysis, and Correlation.* 4th ed. St. Louis, MO: CV Mosby; 2003.
23. Bio-Rad Laboratories. *Procedure for Comparing Precision of Pipet Tips.* Hercules, CO: Bio-Rad Laboratories; 1993. (Product Information No. 81-0208.)
24. National Committee for Clinical Laboratory Standards (NCCLS). *Determining Performance of Volumetric Equipment.* Villanova, PA: NCCLS; 1984. (NCCLS Document No. 18-P.)
25. American Society for Testing and Materials (ASTM). *Standard Specification for Laboratory Weights and Precision Mass Standards.* West Conshohocken, PA: ASTM; 2003:14.04. (Publication No. E617–97.)
26. Campbell JB, Campbell JM. *Laboratory Mathematics: Medical and Biological Applications.* 5th ed. St. Louis, MO: CV Mosby; 1997.
27. Centers for Disease Control and Prevention, Division of Laboratory Systems. *Clinical Laboratory Improvement Amendments.* CFR Part 493, Laboratory requirements. http://wwwn.cdc.gov/clia/default.aspx. Accessed September 5, 2012.
28. Clinical Laboratory Standards Institute (CLSI)/National Committee for Clinical Laboratory Standards. *Procedures and Devices for the Collection of Diagnostic Blood Specimens by Skin Puncture.* Wayne, PA: CLSI; 2010.
29. Clinical Laboratory Standards Institute (CLSI)/National Committee for Clinical Laboratory Standards. *Procedures for the Handling and Processing of Blood Specimens.* 4th ed. Wayne, PA: CLSI; 2010. (Publication No. H18-A4 Vol. 30.)
30. Young DS. *Effects of Drugs on Clinical Laboratory Tests.* 5th ed. Washington, DC: AACC Press; 2000.
31. College of American Pathology; Commission On Laboratory Accreditation; Laboratory Accreditation Program Laboratory General Checklist Website. http://www.cap.org/apps/docs/laboratory_accreditation/checklists/laboratory. Accessed February 21, 2012.

Laboratory Safety and Regulations

TOLMIE E. WACHTER

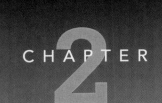

CHAPTER OUTLINE

Chapter Objectives

Upon completion of this chapter, the clinical laboratorian should be able to do the following:

- Discuss safety awareness for clinical laboratory personnel.
- List the responsibilities of employer and employee in providing a safe workplace.
- Identify hazards related to handling chemicals, biologic specimens, and radiologic materials.
- Choose appropriate personal protective equipment when working in the clinical laboratory.

- Identify the classes of fires and the types of fire extinguishers to use for each.
- Describe steps used as precautionary measures when working with electrical equipment, cryogenic materials, and compressed gases and avoiding mechanical hazards associated with laboratory equipment.
- Select the correct means for disposal of waste generated in the clinical laboratory.
- Outline the steps required in documentation of an accident in the workplace.

KEY TERMS

Airborne pathogens
Biohazard
Bloodborne pathogens
Carcinogen
Chemical hygiene plan

Corrosive chemical
Cryogenic material
Fire tetrahedron
Hazard communication standard
Hazardous material
High-efficiency particulate air (HEPA) filter
Laboratory standard

Safety Data Sheet (SDS)
Mechanical hazard
Medical waste
National Fire Protection Association (NFPA)
Occupational Safety and Health Act (OSHA)

Radioactive material
Reactive chemical
Teratogen
Universal precaution

LABORATORY SAFETY AND REGULATIONS

Clinical laboratory personnel, by the nature of the work they perform, are exposed daily to a variety of real or potential hazards: electric shock, toxic vapors, compressed gases, flammable liquids, radioactive material, corrosive substances, mechanical trauma, poisons, and the inherent risks of handling biologic materials, to name a few. Each clinician should develop an understanding of the risks associated with these hazards and must be "safety conscious" at all times.

Laboratory safety necessitates the effective control of all hazards that exist in the clinical laboratory at any given time. Safety begins with the recognition of hazards and is achieved through the application of common sense, a safety-focused attitude, good personal behavior, good housekeeping in all laboratory work and storage areas, and, above all, the continual practice of good laboratory technique. In most cases, accidents can be traced directly to two primary causes: unsafe acts (not always recognized by personnel) and unsafe environmental conditions. This chapter discusses laboratory safety as it applies to the clinical laboratory.

Occupational Safety and Health Act

Public Law 91-596, better known as the Occupational Safety and Health Act (OSHA), was enacted by the U.S. Congress in 1970. The goal of this federal regulation was to provide all employees (clinical laboratory personnel included) with a safe work environment. Under this legislation, the Occupational Safety and Health Administration (also known as OSHA) is authorized to conduct on-site inspections to determine whether an employer is complying with the mandatory standards. Safety is no longer only a moral obligation but also a federal law. In about half of the states, this law is administered by individual state agencies rather than by the federal OSHA. These states still fall within delineated OSHA regions, but otherwise they bear all administrative, consultation, and enforcement responsibilities. The state regulations must be at least as stringent as the federal ones, and many states incorporate large sections of the federal regulations verbatim.

OSHA standards that regulate safety in the laboratory include the Bloodborne Pathogen Standard, Formaldehyde Standard, Laboratory Standard, Hazard Communication Standard, Respiratory Protection Standard, Air Contaminants Standard, and Personal Protective Equipment Standard. Because laws, codes, and ordinances are updated frequently, current reference

materials should be reviewed. Assistance can be obtained from local libraries, the Internet, and federal, state, and local regulatory agencies. The primary standards applicable to clinical laboratory safety are summarized next.

Bloodborne Pathogens [29 CFR 1910.1030]

This standard applies to all exposure to blood or other potentially infectious materials in any occupational setting. It defines terminology relevant to such exposures and mandates the development of an *exposure control plan*. This plan must cover specific preventative measures including exposure evaluation, engineering controls, work practice controls, and administrative oversight of the program. Universal precautions and personal protective equipment (PPE) are foremost among these infection control measures. The *universal precautions* concept is basically an approach to infection control in which all human blood, tissue, and most fluids are handled as if known to be infectious for the human immunodeficiency virus (HIV), hepatitis B virus (HBV), and other bloodborne pathogens. The standard also provides fairly detailed directions for decontamination and the safe handling of potentially infectious laboratory supplies and equipment, including practices for managing laundry and infectious wastes. Employee information and training are covered regarding recognition of hazards and risk of infection. There is also a requirement for HBV vaccination or formal declination within 10 days of assuming duties that present exposure. In the event of an actual exposure, the standard outlines the procedure for postexposure medical evaluation, counseling, and recommended testing or postexposure prophylaxis.

Hazard Communication [29 CFR 1910.1200]

This subpart to OSHA's Toxic and Hazardous Substances regulations is intended to ensure that the hazards of all chemicals used in the workplace have been evaluated and that this hazard information is successfully transmitted to employers and their employees who use the substances. Informally referred to as the OSHA "HazCom Standard," it defines *hazardous substances* and provides guidance for evaluating and communicating identified hazards. The primary means of communication are through proper labeling, the development and use of safety data sheets (SDSs), and employee education.

Occupational Exposure to Hazardous Chemicals in Laboratories [29 CFR 1910.1450]

This second subpart to OSHA's Toxic and Hazardous Substances regulations is also known as the "OSHA Lab Standard." It was intended to address the shortcomings of the Hazard Communication Standard regarding its application peculiar to the handling of hazardous chemicals in laboratories, whose multiple small-scale manipulations differ from the industrial volumes and processes targeted by the original HazCom Standard. The Lab Standard requires the appointment of a *chemical hygiene officer* and the development of a *chemical hygiene plan* to reduce or eliminate occupational exposure to hazardous chemicals. This plan is required to describe the laboratory's methods of identifying and controlling physical and health hazards presented by chemical manipulations, containment, and storage. The chemical hygiene plan must detail engineering controls, PPE, safe work practices, and administrative controls, including provisions for medical surveillance and consultation, when necessary.

Other Regulations and Guidelines

There are other federal regulations relating to laboratory safety, such as the Clean Water Act, the Resource Conservation and Recovery Act (RCRA), and the Toxic Substances Control Act. In addition, clinical laboratories are required to comply with applicable local and state laws, such as fire and building codes. The Clinical and Laboratory Standards Institute (CLSI, formerly National Committee for Clinical Laboratory Standards [NCCLS]) provides excellent general laboratory safety and infection control guidelines in their documents GP17-A2 (*Clinical Laboratory Safety; Approved Guideline*, Second Edition) and M29-A3 (*Protection of Laboratory Workers from Occupationally Acquired Infections; Approved Guideline*, Third Edition).

Safety is also an important part of the requirements for initial and continued accreditation of health-care institutions and laboratories by voluntary accrediting bodies such as The Joint Commission (TJC; formerly the Joint Commission on Accreditation of Health Care Organizations [JCAHO]) and the Commission on Laboratory Accreditation of the College of American Pathologists (CAP). TJC publishes a yearly accreditation manual for hospitals and the *Accreditation Manual for Pathology and Clinical Laboratory Services*, which includes a detailed section on safety requirements. CAP publishes an extensive inspection checklist (*Laboratory General Checklist*) as part of their *Laboratory Accreditation Program*, which includes a section dedicated to laboratory safety.

Over the past decade, several new laws and directives have been emplaced regarding enhanced security measures for particular hazardous substances with potential for nefarious use in terrorist activities. These initiatives are typically promulgated by the Department of Homeland Security in cooperation with the respective agency regulating chemical, nuclear, or biological agents of concern. Although most laboratories do not store or use the large volumes of chemicals required to trigger chemical security requirements, many laboratories do surpass the thresholds for radiological and biological agents. Management and employees must be cognizant of security requirements for substances in quantities qualifying them for regulation under enhanced security measures for chemical (Chemical Facilities Anti-Terrorism Standards, 6 CFR 27), radiological (NRC *Security Orders* and *Increased Controls* for licensees holding sources above *Quantities of Concern*), and biological (Select Agents and Toxins, 42 CFR 73) agents. Most security measures involve restriction of access to only approved or authorized individuals, assessment of security vulnerabilities, secure physical containment of the agents, and inventory monitoring and tracking.

SAFETY AWARENESS FOR CLINICAL LABORATORY PERSONNEL

Safety Responsibility

The employer and the employee share safety responsibility. While the individual employee has an obligation to follow safe work practices and be attentive to potential hazards, the employer has the ultimate responsibility for safety and delegates authority for safe operations to laboratory managers and supervisors. In order to ensure clarity and consistency, safety management in the laboratory should start with a written safety policy. Laboratory supervisors, who reflect the attitudes of management toward safety, are essential members of the safety program.

Employer's Responsibilities

- Establish laboratory work methods and safety policies.
- Provide supervision and guidance to employees.
- Provide safety information, training, PPE, and medical surveillance to employees.
- Provide and maintain equipment and laboratory facilities that are free of recognized hazards and adequate for the tasks required.

The employee also has a responsibility for his or her own safety and the safety of coworkers. Employee conduct in the laboratory is a vital factor in the achievement of a workplace without accidents or injuries.

Employee's Responsibilities

- Know and comply with the established laboratory safe work practices.
- Have a positive attitude toward supervisors, coworkers, facilities, and safety training.
- Be alert and give prompt notification of unsafe conditions or practices to the immediate supervisor and ensure that unsafe conditions and practices are corrected.
- Engage in the conduct of safe work practices and use of PPE.

Signage and Labeling

Appropriate signs to identify hazards are critical, not only to alert laboratory personnel to potential hazards but

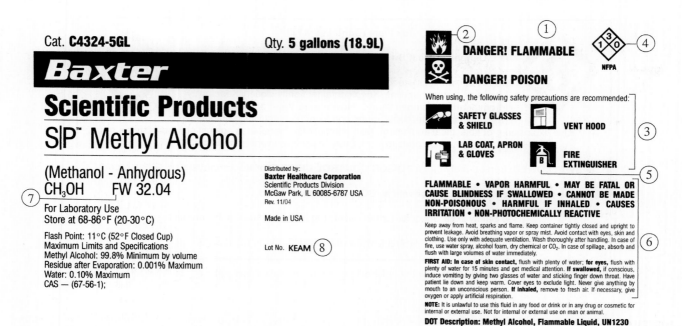

FIGURE 2-1 Sample chemical label: (**1**) statement of hazard; (**2**) hazard class; (**3**) safety precautions; (**4**) National Fire Protection Agency (NFPA) hazard code; (**5**) fire extinguisher type; (**6**) safety instructions; (**7**) formula weight; and (**8**) lot number. Color of the diamond in the NFPA label indicates hazard: Red = flammable. Store in an area segregated for flammable reagents. Blue = health hazard. Toxic if inhaled, ingested, or absorbed through the skin. Store in a secure area. Yellow = reactive and oxidizing reagents. May react violently with air, water, or other substances. Store away from flammable and combustible materials. White = corrosive. May harm skin, eyes, or mucous membranes. Store away from red-, blue-, and yellow-coded reagents. Gray = presents no more than moderate hazard in any of the categories. For general chemical storage. Exception = reagent incompatible with other reagents of same color bar. Store separately. Hazard code (**4**)—Following the NFPA use, each diamond shows a red segment (flammability), a blue segment (health; i.e., toxicity), and a yellow segment (reactivity). Printed over each color-coded segment is a black number showing the degree of hazard involved. The fourth segment, as stipulated by the NFPA, is left blank. It is reserved for special warnings, such as radioactivity. The numeric ratings indicate degree of hazard: 4 = extreme; 3 = severe; 2 = moderate; 1 = slight; and 0 = none according to present data. (Courtesy of Baxter International Inc.)

also to identify specific hazards that may arise because of emergencies such as fire or explosion. The National Fire Protection Association (NFPA) developed a standard hazard identification system (diamond-shaped, color-coded symbol), which has been adopted by many clinical laboratories. At a glance, emergency personnel can assess health hazards (blue quadrant), flammable hazards (red quadrant), reactivity/stability hazards (yellow quadrant), and other special information (white quadrant). In addition, each quadrant shows the magnitude of severity, graded from a low of 0 to a high of 4, of the hazards within the posted area. (Note the NFPA hazard code symbol in Fig. 2-1.)

Manufacturers of laboratory chemicals also provide precautionary labeling information for users. Information indicated on the product label includes statement of the hazard, precautionary measures, specific hazard class, first aid instructions for internal/external contact, the storage code, the safety code, and personal protective gear and equipment needed. This information is in addition to specifications on the actual lot analysis of the chemical constituents and other product notes (Fig. 2-1). Over the last two decades, there has been an effort to standardize hazard terminology and classification under an internationally recognized guideline,

titled the *Globally Harmonized System of Classification and Labeling of Hazardous Chemicals* (GHS). This system incorporates universal definitions and symbols to clearly communicate specific hazards in a single concise label format (Fig. 2-2). Although not yet law, or codified as a regulatory standard, OSHA is presently working to align the existing Hazard Communication Standard with provisions of the GHS and encourages employers to begin adopting the program.

All in-house prepared reagents and solutions should be labeled in a standard manner and include the chemical identity, concentration, hazard warning, special handling, storage conditions, date prepared, expiration date (if applicable), and preparer's initials.

SAFETY EQUIPMENT

Safety equipment has been developed specifically for use in the clinical laboratory. The employer is required by law to have designated safety equipment available, but it is also the responsibility of the employee to comply with all safety rules and to use safety equipment.

All laboratories are required to have safety showers, eyewash stations, and fire extinguishers and to periodically test and inspect the equipment for proper

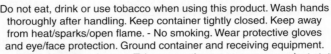

ToxiFlam (Contains: XYZ)

Danger! Toxic If Swallowed, Flammable Liquid and Vapor

Do not eat, drink or use tobacco when using this product. Wash hands
thoroughly after handling. Keep container tightly closed. Keep away
from heat/sparks/open flame. - No smoking. Wear protective gloves
and eye/face protection. Ground container and receiving equipment.
Use explosion-proof electrical equipment. Take precautionary measures against static discharge.
Use only non-sparking tools. Store in cool/well-ventilated place.

IF SWALLOWED: Immediately call a POISON CONTROL CENTER or doctor/physician. Rinse mouth.

In case of fire, use water fog, dry chemical, CO2, or "alcohol" foam.

See Safety Data Sheet for further details regarding safe use of this product.

MyCompany, MyStreet, MyTown NJ 00000, Tel: 111 222 3333

FIGURE 2-2 Example of a GHS inner container label (e.g., bottle inside a shipping box).

operation. It is recommended that safety showers deliver 30 to 50 gallons of water per minute at 20 to 50 pounds per square inch (psi) and be located in areas where corrosive liquids are stored or used. Eyewash stations must be accessible (i.e., within 100 feet or 10 s travel) in laboratory areas presenting chemical or biological exposure hazards. Other items that must be available for personnel include fire blankets, spill kits, and first aid supplies.

Mechanical pipeting devices must be used for manipulating all types of liquids in the laboratory, including water. Mouth pipeting is strictly prohibited.

Chemical Fume Hoods and Biosafety Cabinets

Fume Hoods

Fume hoods are required to contain and expel noxious and hazardous fumes from chemical reagents. Fume hoods should be visually inspected for blockages. A piece of tissue paper placed at the hood opening will indicate airflow direction. The hood should never be operated with the sash fully opened, and a maximum operating sash height should be established and conspicuously marked. Containers and equipment positioned within hoods should not block airflow. Periodically, ventilation should be evaluated by measuring the face velocity with a calibrated velocity meter. The velocity at the face of the hood (with the sash in normal operating position) should be 100 to 120 feet per minute and fairly uniform across the entire opening. Smoke testing is also recommended to locate no flow or turbulent areas in the working space. As an added precaution, personal air monitoring should be conducted in accordance with the chemical hygiene plan of the facility.

Biosafety Cabinets

Biological safety cabinets (BSCs) remove particles that may be harmful to the employee who is working with potentially infectious biologic specimens. The Centers for Disease Control and Prevention (CDC) and the National Institutes of Health have described four levels of biosafety, which consist of combinations of laboratory practices and techniques, safety equipment, and laboratory facilities. The biosafety level of a laboratory is based on the operations performed, the routes of transmission of the infectious agents, and the laboratory function or activity. Accordingly, biosafety cabinets are designed to offer various levels of protection, depending on the biosafety level of the specific laboratory (Table 2-1). BSCs should be periodically recertified to ensure continued optimal performance as filter occlusion or rupture can compromise their effectiveness.

Chemical Storage Equipment

Safety equipment is available for the storage and handling of hazardous chemicals and compressed gases. Safety carriers should always be used to transport glass bottles of acids, alkalis, or organic solvents in volumes larger than 500 mL, and approved safety cans should be used for storing, dispensing, or disposing of flammables in volumes greater than 1 quart. Steel safety cabinets with self-closing doors are required for the storage of flammable liquids, and only specially designed, explosion-proof refrigerators may be used to store flammable materials. Only the amount of chemical needed for that day should be available at the bench. Gas cylinder supports or clamps must be used at all times, and larger cylinders should be transported with valve caps on, using handcarts.

PPE and Hygiene

The parts of the body most frequently subject to injury in the clinical laboratory are the eyes, skin, and

TABLE 2-1	COMPARISON OF BIOSAFETY CABINET CHARACTERISTICS			
			APPLICATIONS	
BSC CLASS	FACE VELOCITY	AIRFLOW PATTERN	NONVOLATILE TOXIC CHEMICALS AND RADIONUCLIDES	VOLATILE TOXIC CHEMICALS AND RADIONUCLIDES
I	75	In at front through HEPA to the outside or into the room through HEPA	Yes	When exhausted outdoors
II, A1	75	70% recirculated to the cabinet work area through HEPA; 30% balance can be exhausted through HEPA back into the room or to outside through a canopy unit	Yes (minute amounts)	No
II, B1	100	30% recirculated, 70% exhausted. Exhaust cabinet air must pass through a dedicated duct to the outside through a HEPA filter	Yes	Yes (minute amounts)
I, B2	100	No recirculation; total exhaust to the outside through a HEPA filter	Yes	Yes (small amounts)
II, A2	100	Similar to II, A1, but has 100 lfm intake air velocity and plenums are under negative pressure to room; exhaust air can be ducted to the outside through a canopy unit	Yes	When exhausted outdoors (*formally* "B3") (minute amounts)

BSC, biological safety cabinet; HEPA, high-efficiency particulate air; lfm, linear feet per minute.
Adapted from *Biosafety in Microbiological and Biomedical Laboratories*. 5th ed. Revised December 2009.

respiratory and digestive tracts. Hence, the use of PPE and proper hygiene is very important. Safety glasses, goggles, visors, or work shields protect the eyes and face from splashes and impact. Contact lenses do not offer eye protection; it is strongly recommended that they not be worn in the clinical chemistry laboratory, unless additional protective eyewear is also utilized. If any solution is accidentally splashed into the eye(s), thorough irrigation is required.

Gloves and rubberized sleeves protect the hands and arms when using caustic chemicals. Gloves are required for routine laboratory use; however, polyvinyl or other nonlatex gloves are an acceptable alternative for people with latex allergies. Certain glove materials offer better protection against particular reagent formulations. Nitrile gloves, for example, offer a wider range of compatibility with organic solvents than do latex gloves. Laboratory coats, preferably with knit-cuffed sleeves, should be full length and buttoned and made of liquid-resistant material. When performing manipulations prone to splash hazards, the laboratory coat should be supplemented with an impermeable apron and/or sleeve

garters, constructed of suitable material to guard against the substances. Proper footwear is required; shoes constructed of porous materials, open-toed shoes, and sandals are considered ineffective against spilled hazardous liquids.

Respirators may be required for various procedures in the clinical laboratory. Whether used for biologic or chemical hazards, the correct type of respirator must be used for the specific hazard. Respirators with high-efficiency particulate air (HEPA) filters must be worn when engineering controls are not feasible, such as when working directly with patients with tuberculosis (TB) or when performing procedures that may aerosolize specimens of patients with a suspected or confirmed case of TB. Training, maintenance, and written protocol for use of respirators are required according to the respiratory protection standard.

Each employer must provide (at no charge) laboratory coats, gloves, or other protective equipment to all employees who may be exposed to biologic or chemical hazards. It is the employer's responsibility to clean and maintain any PPE used by more than one person.

All contaminated PPE must be removed and properly cleaned or disposed of before leaving the laboratory.

Hand washing is a crucial component of both infection control and chemical hygiene. After removing gloves, hands should be washed thoroughly with soap and warm water, even if glove breakthrough or contamination is not suspected. The use of antimicrobial soap is not as important as the physical action of washing the hands with water and any mild soap. After any work with highly toxic or carcinogenic chemicals, the face should also be washed.

BIOLOGIC SAFETY

General Considerations

All blood samples and other body fluids should be collected, transported, handled, and processed using universal precautions (i.e., presumed to be infectious). Gloves, gowns, and face protection must be used during manipulations or transfers when splashing or splattering is most likely to occur. Consistent and thorough hand washing is an essential component of infection control. Antiseptic gels and foams may be used at waterless stations between washes, but they should not take the place of an actual hand wash.

Centrifugation of biologic specimens produces finely dispersed aerosols that are a high-risk source of infection. Ideally, specimens should remain capped during centrifugation, or several minutes should be allowed to elapse after centrifugation is complete before opening the lid. As a preferred option, the use of a sealed-cup centrifuge is recommended.

Spills

Any blood, body fluid, or other potentially infectious material spill must be cleaned up, and the area or equipment must be disinfected immediately. Safe cleanup includes the following recommendations:

- Alert others in area of the spill.
- Wear appropriate protective equipment.
- Use mechanical devices to pick up broken glass or other sharp objects.
- Absorb the spill with paper towels, gauze pads, or tissue.
- Clean the spill site using a common aqueous detergent.
- Disinfect the spill site using approved disinfectant or 10% bleach, using appropriate contact time.
- Rinse the spill site with water.
- Dispose of all materials in appropriate biohazard containers.

Bloodborne Pathogens

In December 1991, OSHA issued the final rule for occupational exposure to **bloodborne pathogens**. To minimize employee exposure, each employer must have a written *exposure control plan*. The plan must be available to all employees whose duties may result in reasonably anticipated occupational exposure to blood or other potentially infectious materials. The exposure control plan must be discussed with all employees and be available to them while they are working. The employee must be provided with adequate training in all techniques described in the exposure control plan at initial work assignment and annually thereafter. All necessary safety equipment and supplies must be readily available and inspected on a regular basis.

Clinical laboratory personnel are knowingly or unknowingly in frequent contact with potentially biohazardous materials. In recent years, new and serious occupational hazards to personnel have arisen, and this problem has been complicated because of the general lack of understanding of the epidemiology, mechanisms of transmission of the disease, or inactivation of the causative agent. Special precautions must be taken when handling all specimens because of the continual increase in the proportion of infectious samples received in the laboratory. Therefore, in practice, specimens from patients with confirmed or suspected hepatitis, acquired immunodeficiency syndrome (AIDS), or other potentially infectious diseases should be handled no differently than other routine specimens. Adopting a universal precautions policy, which considers blood and other body fluids from all patients as potentially infective, is required.

Airborne Pathogens

Because of a global resurgence of TB, OSHA issued a statement in 1993 that the agency would enforce CDC Guidelines for Preventing the Transmission of Tuberculosis in Health Care Facilities. The purpose of the guidelines is to encourage early detection, isolation, and treatment of active cases. A TB exposure control program must be established, and risks to laboratory workers must be assessed. In 1997, a proposed standard (29 CFR 1910.1035, Tuberculosis) was issued by OSHA only to be withdrawn again when it was determined that existing CDC guidelines could be enforced by OSHA through its "general duty" clause and Respiratory Protection Standard. The CDC guidelines require the development of a *tuberculosis infection control program* by any facility involved in the diagnosis or treatment of cases of confirmed infectious TB. TB isolation areas with specific ventilation controls must be established in health-care facilities. Those workers in high-risk areas may be required to wear a respirator for protection. All health-care workers considered to be at risk must be screened for TB infection.

Other specific pathogens, including viruses, bacteria, and fungi, may be considered airborne transmission risks. Protective measures in the clinical laboratory generally involve work practice and engineering controls focused on prevention of aerosolization, containment/ isolation, and respiratory protection of N-95 (filtration of 95% of particles >0.3 μm) or better.

Shipping

Clinical laboratories routinely ship regulated material. The U.S. Department of Transportation (DOT) and the International Air Transport Association (IATA) have specific requirements for carrying regulated materials. There are two types of specimen classifications. Known or suspect infectious specimens are labeled *infectious substances* if the pathogen can be readily transmitted to humans or animals. *Diagnostic specimens* are those tested as routine screening or for initial diagnosis. Each type of specimen has rules and packaging requirements. The DOT guidelines are found in the *Code of Federal Regulations, Title 49, Subchapter C*; IATA publishes its own manual, *Dangerous Goods Regulations*.

CHEMICAL SAFETY

Hazard Communication

In the August 1987 issue of the *Federal Register*, OSHA published the new **Hazard Communication Standard** (Right to Know Law, 29 CFR 1910.1200). The Right to Know Law was developed for employees who may be exposed to hazardous chemicals in the workplace. Employees must be informed of the health risks associated with those chemicals. The intent of the law is to ensure that health hazards are evaluated for all chemicals that are produced and that this information is relayed to employees.

To comply with the regulation, clinical laboratories must

- Plan and implement a written hazard communication program.
- Obtain SDSs for each hazardous compound present in the workplace and have the SDSs readily accessible to employees.
- Educate all employees annually on how to interpret chemical labels, SDSs, and health hazards of the chemicals and how to work safely with the chemicals.
- Maintain hazard warning labels on containers received or filled on-site.

Safety Data Sheet

The SDS is a major source of safety information for employees who may use **hazardous materials** in their occupations. Employers are responsible for obtaining the SDS from the chemical manufacturer or developing an SDS for each hazardous agent used in the workplace. A standardized format is not mandatory, but all requirements listed in the law must be addressed. A summary of the SDS information requirements includes the following:

- Product name and identification
- Hazardous ingredients
- Permissible exposure limit
- Physical and chemical data
- Health hazard data and carcinogenic potential
- Primary routes of entry
- Fire and explosion hazards
- Reactivity data
- Spill and disposal procedures
- PPE recommendations
- Handling
- Emergency and first aid procedures
- Storage and transportation precautions
- Chemical manufacturer's name, address, and telephone number
- Special information section

The SDS must provide the specific compound identity, together with all common names. All information sections must be completed, and the date that the SDS was printed must be indicated. Copies of the SDS must be readily accessible to employees during all shifts.

The new GHS also addresses Safety Data Sheets and provides a more rigid format of 16 sections similar to those listed above.

OSHA Laboratory Standard

Occupational Exposure to Hazardous Chemicals in Laboratories (29 CFR 1910.1450), also known as the **laboratory standard**, was enacted in May 1990 to provide laboratories with specific guidelines for handling hazardous chemicals. This OSHA standard requires each laboratory that uses hazardous chemicals to have a written **chemical hygiene plan**. This plan provides procedures and work practices for regulating and reducing exposure of laboratory personnel to hazardous chemicals. *Hazardous chemicals* are those that pose a physical or health hazard from acute or chronic exposure. Procedures describing how to protect employees against **teratogens** (substances that affect cellular development in a fetus or embryo), carcinogens, and other toxic chemicals must be described in the plan. Training in the use of hazardous chemicals must be provided to all employees and must include recognition of signs and symptoms of exposure, location of SDS, the chemical hygiene plan, and how to protect themselves against hazardous chemicals. A chemical hygiene officer must be designated for any laboratory using hazardous chemicals. The protocol must be reviewed annually and updated when regulations are modified or chemical inventory changes. Remember that practicing consistent and thorough hand washing is an essential component of preventative chemical hygiene.

Toxic Effects from Hazardous Substances

Toxic substances have the potential of producing deleterious effects (local or systemic) by direct chemical action or interference with the function of body systems. They can cause acute or chronic effects related to the duration of exposure (i.e., short-term, or single contact, versus long-term, or prolonged, repeated contact). Almost any substance, even the most benign seeming, can pose risk of damage to a worker's lungs, skin, eyes, or mucous membranes following long- or short-term exposure and can be toxic in excess. Moreover, some chemicals are toxic at very low concentrations. Exposure to toxic agents can be through direct contact (absorption), inhalation, ingestion, or inoculation/injection.

In the clinical chemistry laboratory, personnel should be particularly aware of toxic vapors from chemical solvents, such as acetone, chloroform, methanol, or carbon tetrachloride, that do not give explicit sensory irritation warnings, as do bromide, ammonia, and formaldehyde. Air sampling or routine monitoring may be necessary to quantify dangerous levels. Mercury is another frequently disregarded source of poisonous vapors. It is highly volatile and toxic and is rapidly absorbed through the skin and respiratory tract. Mercury spill kits should be available in areas where mercury thermometers are used. Most laboratories are phasing out the use of mercury and mercury-containing compounds. Laboratories should have a policy on mercury reduction or elimination and a method for legally disposing of mercury. Several compounds, including formaldehyde and methylene chloride, have substance-specific OSHA standards, which require periodic monitoring of air concentrations. Laboratory engineering controls, PPE, and procedural controls must be adequate to protect employees from these substances.

Storage and Handling of Chemicals

To avoid accidents when handling chemicals, it is important to develop respect for all chemicals and to have a complete knowledge of their properties. This is particularly important when transporting, dispensing, or using chemicals that, when in contact with certain other chemicals, could result in the formation of substances that are toxic, flammable, or explosive. For example, acetic acid is incompatible with other acids such as chromic and nitric acid, carbon tetrachloride is incompatible with sodium, and flammable liquids are incompatible with hydrogen peroxide and nitric acid.

Arrangements for the storage of chemicals will depend on the quantities of chemicals needed and the nature or type of chemicals. Proper storage is essential to prevent and control laboratory fires and accidents. Ideally, the storeroom should be organized so that each class of chemicals is isolated in an area that is not used for routine work. An up-to-date inventory should be kept that indicates location of chemicals, minimum/maximum quantities required, and shelf life. Some chemicals deteriorate over time and become hazardous (e.g., many ethers and tetrahydrofuran form explosive peroxides). Storage should not be based solely on alphabetical order because incompatible chemicals may be stored next to each other and react chemically. They must be separated for storage, as shown in Table 2-2.

Flammable/Combustible Chemicals

Flammable and combustible liquids, which are used in numerous routine procedures, are among the most hazardous materials in the clinical chemistry laboratory because of possible fire or explosion. They are classified according to flash point, which is the temperature at which sufficient vapor is given off to form an ignitable mixture with air. A flammable liquid has a flash point below 37.8°C (100°F) and combustible liquids, by definition, have a flash point at or above 37.8°C (100°F). Some commonly used flammable and combustible solvents are acetone, benzene, ethanol, heptane, isopropanol, methanol, toluene, and xylene. It is important to remember that flammable or combustible chemicals also include certain gases, such as hydrogen, and solids, such as paraffin.

TABLE 2-2	STORAGE REQUIREMENTS
SUBSTANCE	**STORED SEPARATELY**
Flammable liquids	Flammable solids
Mineral acids	Organic acids
Caustics	Oxidizers
Perchloric acid	Water-reactive substances
Air-reactive substances	Others
Heat-reactive substances requiring refrigeration	
Unstable substances (shock-sensitive explosives)	

Corrosive Chemicals

Corrosive chemicals are injurious to the skin or eyes by direct contact or to the tissue of the respiratory and gastrointestinal tracts if inhaled or ingested. Typical examples include acids (acetic, sulfuric, nitric, and hydrochloric) and bases (ammonium hydroxide, potassium hydroxide, and sodium hydroxide). External exposures to concentrated corrosives can cause severe burns and require immediate flushing with copious amounts of clean water.

Reactive Chemicals

Reactive chemicals are substances that, under certain conditions, can spontaneously explode or ignite or that evolve heat or flammable or explosive gases. Some strong acids or bases react with water to generate heat (exothermic reactions). Hydrogen is liberated if alkali metals (sodium or potassium) are mixed with water or acids, and spontaneous combustion also may occur. The mixture of oxidizing agents, such as peroxides, and reducing agents, such as hydrogen, generates heat and may be explosive.

Carcinogenic Chemicals

Carcinogens are substances that have been determined to be cancer-causing agents. OSHA has issued lists of confirmed and suspected carcinogens and detailed standards for the handling of these substances. Benzidine is a common example of a known carcinogen. If possible, a substitute chemical or different procedure should be used to avoid exposure to carcinogenic agents. For regulatory (OSHA) and institutional safety requirements, the laboratory must maintain an accurate inventory of carcinogens.

Chemical Spills

Strict attention to good laboratory technique can help prevent chemical spills. However, emergency procedures should be established to handle any accidents. If a spill occurs, the first step should be to assist/evacuate personnel, and then confinement and cleanup of the spill can begin. There are several commercial spill kits available for neutralizing and absorbing spilled chemical solutions (Fig. 2-3). However, no single kit is suitable for all types of spills. Emergency procedures for spills should also include a reporting system.

RADIATION SAFETY

Environmental Protection

A radiation safety policy should include environmental and personnel protection. All areas where radioactive materials are used or stored must be posted with caution signs, and traffic in these areas should be restricted to essential personnel only. Regular and systematic monitoring must be emphasized, and decontamination of

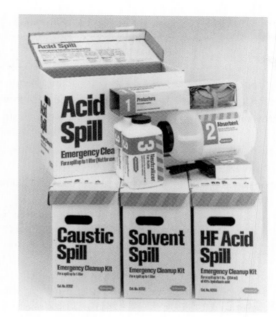

FIGURE 2-3 Spill cleanup kit.

laboratory equipment, glassware, and work areas should be scheduled as part of routine procedures. Records must be maintained as to the quantity of radioactive material on hand as well as the quantity that is disposed. A Nuclear Regulatory Commission (NRC) or agreement state license is required if the amount of radioactive material exceeds a certain level. The laboratory safety officer must consult with the institutional safety officer about these requirements.

Personal Protection

It is essential that only properly trained personnel work with radioisotopes. Good work practices must consistently be employed to ensure that contamination and inadvertent internalization are avoided. Users should be monitored to ensure that the maximal permissible dose of radiation is not exceeded. Radiation monitors must be evaluated regularly to detect degree of exposure for the laboratory employee. Records must be maintained for the length of employment plus 30 years.

Nonionizing Radiation

Nonionizing forms of radiation are also a concern in the clinical laboratory. Equipment often emits a variety of wavelengths of electromagnetic radiation that must be protected against through engineered shielding or use of PPE (Table 2-3). These energies have varying biologic effects, depending on wavelength, power intensity, and duration of exposure. Laboratorians must be knowledgeable regarding the hazards presented by their equipment to protect themselves and ancillary personnel.

TABLE 2-3	EXAMPLES OF NONIONIZING RADIATION IN CLINICAL LABORATORIES		
TYPE	**APPROXIMATE WAVELENGTH**	**SOURCE EQUIPMENT EXAMPLE**	**PROTECTIVE MEASURES**
Low frequency	>1 cm	Radiofrequency coil in inductively coupled plasma–mass spectrometer	Engineered shielding and posted pacemaker warning
Microwaves	3 m–3 mm	Energy beam microwave used to accelerate tissue staining in histology prep processes	Engineered shielding
Infrared	750 nm–0.3 cm	Heat lamps, lasers	Containment and appropriate warning labels
Visible spectrum	400–750 nm	General illumination and glare	Filters, diffusers, and nonreflective surfaces
Ultraviolet	4–400 nm	Germicidal lamps used in biologic safety cabinets	Eye and skin protection; UV warning labels

FIRE SAFETY

The Chemistry of Fire

Fire is basically a chemical reaction that involves the rapid oxidation of a combustible material or fuel, with the subsequent liberation of heat and light. In the clinical chemistry laboratory, all the elements essential for fire to begin are present—fuel, heat or ignition source, and oxygen (air). However, recent research suggests that a fourth factor is present. This factor has been classified as a reaction chain in which burning continues and even accelerates. It is caused by the breakdown and recombination of the molecules from the material burning with the oxygen in the atmosphere.

The fire triangle has been modified into a three-dimensional pyramid known as the fire tetrahedron (Fig. 2-4). This modification does not contradict established procedures in dealing with a fire but does provide additional means by which fires may be prevented or extinguished. A fire will extinguish if any of the three basic elements (heat, air, or fuel) are removed.

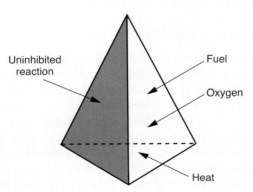

FIGURE 2-4 Fire tetrahedron.

Classification of Fires

Fires have been divided into four classes based on the nature of the combustible material and requirements for extinguishment:

Class A: ordinary combustible solid materials, such as paper, wood, plastic, and fabric
Class B: flammable liquids/gases and combustible petroleum products
Class C: energized electrical equipment
Class D: combustible/reactive metals, such as magnesium, sodium, and potassium

Types and Applications of Fire Extinguishers

Just as fires have been divided into classes, fire extinguishers are divided into classes that correspond to the type of fire to be extinguished. Be certain to choose the right type—using the wrong type of extinguisher may be dangerous. For example, do not use water on burning liquids or electrical equipment.

Pressurized water extinguishers, as well as foam and multipurpose dry-chemical types, are used for Class A fires. Multipurpose dry-chemical and carbon dioxide extinguishers are used for Class B and C fires. Halogenated hydrocarbon extinguishers are particularly recommended for use with computer equipment. Class D fires present special problems, and extinguishment is left to trained firefighters using special dry-chemical extinguishers (Fig. 2-5). Generally, all that can be done for a Class D fire in the laboratory is to try and isolate the burning metal from combustible surfaces with sand or ceramic barrier material. Personnel should know the location and type of portable fire extinguisher near their work area and know how to use an extinguisher before a fire occurs. In the event of a fire, first evacuate all personnel, patients, and visitors who are in immediate danger and then activate

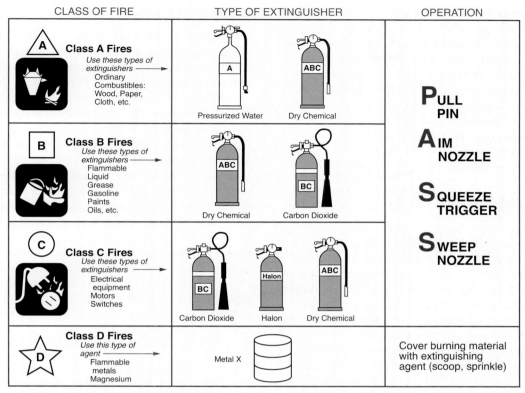

CLASS OF FIRE	TYPE OF EXTINGUISHER	OPERATION
Class A Fires *Use these types of extinguishers* → Ordinary Combustibles: Wood, Paper, Cloth, etc.	Pressurized Water Dry Chemical	**P**ULL PIN **A**IM NOZZLE **S**QUEEZE TRIGGER **S**WEEP NOZZLE
Class B Fires *Use these types of extinguishers* → Flammable Liquid Grease Gasoline Paints Oils, etc.	Dry Chemical Carbon Dioxide	
Class C Fires *Use these types of extinguishers* → Electrical equipment Motors Switches	Carbon Dioxide Halon Dry Chemical	
Class D Fires *Use this type of agent* → Flammable metals Magnesium	Metal X	Cover burning material with extinguishing agent (scoop, sprinkle)

FIGURE 2-5 Proper use of fire extinguishers. (Adapted from the Clinical and Laboratory Safety Department, The University of Texas Health Science Center at Houston.)

the fire alarm, report the fire, and, if possible, attempt to extinguish the fire. Personnel should work as a team to carry out emergency procedures. Fire drills must be conducted regularly and with appropriate documentation. Fire extinguishers must be inspected monthly to ensure that they are mounted, visible, accessible, and charged.

CONTROL OF OTHER HAZARDS

Electrical Hazards

Most individuals are aware of the potential hazards associated with the use of electrical appliances and equipment. Direct hazards of electrical energy can result in death, shock, or burns. Indirect hazards can result in fire or explosion. Therefore, there are many precautionary procedures to follow when operating or working around electrical equipment:

- Use only explosion-rated (intrinsically wired) equipment in hazardous atmospheres.
- Be particularly careful when operating high-voltage equipment, such as electrophoresis apparatus.
- Use only properly grounded equipment (three-prong plug).
- Check for frayed electrical cords.
- Promptly report any malfunctions or equipment producing a "tingle" for repair.
- Do not work on "live" electrical equipment.

- Never operate electrical equipment with wet hands.
- Know the exact location of the electrical control panel for the electricity to your work area.
- Use only approved extension cords in temporary applications and do not overload circuits. (Some local regulations prohibit the use of any extension cord.)
- Have ground, polarity, and leakage checks and other periodic preventive maintenance performed on outlets and equipment.

Compressed Gases Hazards

Compressed gases, which serve a number of functions in the laboratory, present a unique combination of hazards in the clinical laboratory: danger of fire, explosion, asphyxiation, or mechanical injuries. There are several general requirements for safely handling compressed gases:

- Know the gas that you will use.
- Store tanks in a vertical position.
- Keep cylinders secured at all times.
- Never store flammable liquids and compressed gases in the same area.
- Use the proper regulator, tubing, and fittings for the type of gas in use.
- Do not attempt to control or shut off gas flow with the pressure relief regulator.

- Keep removable protection caps in place until the cylinder is in use.
- Make certain that acetylene tanks are properly piped (the gas is incompatible with copper tubing).
- Do not force a "frozen" or stuck cylinder valve.
- Use a hand truck to transport large cylinders.
- Always check cylinders on receipt and then periodically for any problems such as leaks.
- Make certain that the cylinder is properly labeled to identify the contents.
- Empty tanks should be marked "empty."

Cryogenic Materials Hazards

Liquid nitrogen is probably one of the most widely used cryogenic fluids (liquefied gases) in the laboratory. There are, however, several hazards associated with the use of any cryogenic material: fire or explosion, asphyxiation, pressure buildup, embrittlement of materials, and tissue damage similar to that of thermal burns.

Only containers constructed of materials designed to withstand ultralow temperatures should be used for cryogenic work. In addition to the use of eye/face protection, hand protection to guard against the hazards of touching supercooled surfaces is recommended. The gloves, of impermeable material, should fit loosely so that they can be taken off quickly if liquid spills on or into them. Also, to minimize violent boiling/frothing and splashing, specimens to be frozen should always be inserted into the coolant very slowly. Cryogenic fluids should be stored in well-insulated but loosely stoppered containers that minimize loss of fluid resulting from evaporation by boil-off and that prevent plugging and pressure buildup.

Mechanical Hazards

In addition to physical hazards such as fire and electric shock, laboratory personnel should be aware of the mechanical hazards of equipment such as centrifuges, autoclaves, and homogenizers.

Centrifuges, for example, must be balanced to distribute the load equally. The operator should never open the lid until the rotor has come to a complete stop. Safety interlocks on equipment should never be rendered inoperable.

Laboratory glassware itself is another potential hazard. Agents, such as glass beads or boiling chips, should be added to help eliminate bumping/boilover when liquids are heated. Tongs or insulated gloves should be used to remove hot glassware from ovens, hot plates, or water baths. Glass pipets should be handled with extra care, as should sharp instruments such as cork borers, needles, scalpel blades, and other tools. A glassware inspection program should be in place to detect signs of wear or fatigue that could contribute to breakage or injury. All infectious *sharps* must be disposed in OSHA-approved containers to reduce the risk of injury and infection.

Ergonomic Hazards

Although increased mechanization and automation have made many tedious and repetitive manual tasks obsolete, laboratory processes often require repeated manipulation of instruments, containers, and equipment. These physical actions can, over time, contribute to repetitive strain disorders such as tenosynovitis, bursitis, and ganglion cysts. The primary contributing factors associated with repetitive strain disorders are position/posture, applied force, and frequency of repetition. Remember to consider the design of hand tools (e.g., ergonomic pipets), adherence to ergonomically correct technique, and equipment positioning when engaging in any repetitive task. Chronic symptoms of pain, numbness, or tingling in extremities may indicate the onset of repetitive strain disorders. Other hazards include acute musculoskeletal injury. Remember to lift heavy objects properly, keeping the load close to the body and using the muscles of the legs rather than the back. Gradually increase force when pushing or pulling, and avoid pounding actions with the extremities.

DISPOSAL OF HAZARDOUS MATERIALS

The safe handling and disposal of chemicals and other materials require a thorough knowledge of their properties and hazards. Generators of hazardous wastes have a moral and legal responsibility, as defined in applicable local, state, and federal regulations, to protect both the individual and the environment when disposing of waste. There are four basic waste disposal techniques: flushing down the drain to the sewer system, incineration, landfill burial, and recycling.

Chemical Waste

In some cases, it is permissible to flush water-soluble substances down the drain with copious quantities of water. However, strong acids or bases should be neutralized before disposal. The laboratory must adhere to institutional, local, and state regulations regarding the disposal of strong acids and bases. Foul-smelling chemicals should never be disposed of down the drain. Possible reaction of chemicals in the drain and potential toxicity must be considered when deciding if a particular chemical can be dissolved or diluted and then flushed down the drain. For example, sodium azide, which is used as a preservative, forms explosive salts with metals, such as the copper, in pipes. Many institutions ban the use of sodium azide due to this hazard. In all cases, check with the local water reclamation district or publicly owned treatment works for specific limitations before utilizing sewer disposal.

Other liquid wastes, including flammable solvents, must be collected in approved containers and segregated into compatible classes. If practical, solvents such as xylene and acetone may be filtered or redistilled for reuse. If recycling is not feasible, disposal arrangements should be made by specifically trained personnel. Flammable material can also be burned in specially designed incinerators with afterburners and scrubbers to remove toxic products of combustion.

Also, before disposal, hazardous substances that are explosive (e.g., peroxides) and carcinogens should be transformed to less hazardous forms whenever feasible. Solid chemical wastes that are unsuitable for incineration may be amenable to other treatments or buried in an approved, permitted landfill. Note that certain chemical wastes are subject to strict "cradle to grave" tracking under the RCRA, and severe penalties are associated with improper storage, transportation, and disposal.

Radioactive Waste

The manner of use and disposal of isotopes is strictly regulated by the NRC or NRC agreement states and depends on the type of waste (soluble or nonsoluble), its level of radioactivity, and the radiotoxicity and half-life of the isotopes involved. The radiation safety officer should always be consulted about policies dealing with radioactive waste disposal. Many clinical laboratories transfer radioactive materials to a licensed receiver for disposal.

Biohazardous Waste

On November 2, 1988, President Reagan signed into law The Medical Waste Tracking Act of 1988. Its purpose was to (1) charge the Environmental Protection Agency with the responsibility to establish a program to track medical waste from generation to disposal, (2) define medical waste, (3) establish acceptable techniques for treatment and disposal, and (4) establish a department with jurisdiction to enforce the new laws. Several states have implemented the federal guidelines and incorporated additional requirements. Some entities covered by the rules are any health-care–related facility including, but not limited to, ambulatory surgical centers; blood banks and blood drawing centers; clinics, including medical, dental, and veterinary; clinical, diagnostic, pathologic, or biomedical research laboratories; emergency medical services; hospitals; long-term care facilities; minor emergency centers; occupational health clinics and clinical laboratories; and professional offices of physicians and dentists.

Medical waste is defined as *special waste from healthcare facilities* and is further defined as solid waste that, if improperly treated or handled, "may transmit infectious diseases." (For additional information, see the TJC web site: http://www.jointcommission.org/). It comprises animal waste, bulk blood and blood products, microbiologic waste, pathologic waste, and sharps. The approved methods for treatment and disposition of medical waste are incineration, steam sterilization, burial, thermal inactivation, chemical disinfection, or encapsulation in a solid matrix.

Generators of medical waste must implement the following procedures:

- Employers of health-care workers must establish and implement an infectious waste program.
- All biomedical waste should be placed in a bag marked with the biohazard symbol and then placed into a leakproof container that is puncture resistant and equipped with a solid, tight-fitting lid. All containers must be clearly marked with the word biohazard or its symbol.
- All sharp instruments, such as needles, blades, and glass objects, should be placed into special puncture-resistant containers before placing them inside the bag and container.
- Needles should not be transported, recapped, bent, or broken by hand.
- All biomedical waste must then be disposed of according to one of the recommended procedures.
- Highly pathogenic waste should undergo preliminary treatment on-site.
- Potentially biohazardous material, such as blood or blood products and contaminated laboratory waste, cannot be directly discarded. Contaminated combustible waste can be incinerated. Contaminated noncombustible waste, such as glassware, should be autoclaved before being discarded. Special attention should be given to the discarding of syringes, needles, and broken glass that could also inflict accidental cuts or punctures. Appropriate containers should be used for discarding these sharp objects.

ACCIDENT DOCUMENTATION AND INVESTIGATION

Any accidents involving personal injuries, even minor ones, should be reported immediately to a supervisor. Manifestation of occupational illnesses and exposures to hazardous substances should also be reported. Under OSHA regulations, employers are required to maintain records of occupational injuries and illnesses for the length of employment plus 30 years. The record-keeping requirements include a first report of injury, an accident investigation report, and an annual summary that is recorded on an OSHA injury and illness log (Form 300).

The first report of injury is used to notify the insurance company and the human resources or safety department that a workplace injury has occurred. The employee and the supervisor usually complete the report, which contains information on the employer and injured person, as well as the time and place, cause, and nature of the injury. The report is signed and dated; then, it is forwarded to the institution's risk manager or insurance representative.

The investigation report should include information on the injured person, a description of what happened, the cause of the accident (environmental or personal), other contributing factors, witnesses, the nature of the injury, and actions to be taken to prevent a recurrence. This report should be signed and dated by the person who conducted the investigation.

Annually, a log and summary of occupational injuries and illnesses should be completed and forwarded to the U.S. Department of Labor, Bureau of Labor Statistics' OSHA injury and illness log (Form 300). The standardized form requests de-personalized information similar to the first report of injury and the accident investigation report. Information about every occupational death, nonfatal occupational illness, biologic or chemical exposure, and nonfatal occupational injury that involved loss of consciousness, restriction of work or motion, transfer to another job, or medical treatment (other than first aid) must be reported.

Because it is important to determine why and how an accident occurred, an accident investigation should be conducted. Most accidents can be traced to one of two underlying causes: environmental (unsafe conditions) or personal (unsafe acts). Environmental factors include inadequate safeguards, use of improper or defective equipment, hazards associated with the location, or poor housekeeping. Personal factors include improper laboratory attire, lack of skills or knowledge, specific physical or mental conditions, and attitude. The employee's positive motivation is important in all aspects of safety promotion and accident prevention.

It is particularly important that the appropriate authority be notified immediately if any individual sustains a contaminated needle puncture during blood collection or a cut during subsequent specimen processing or handling. For a summary of recommendations for the protection of laboratory workers, refer to *Protection of Laboratory Workers from Occupationally Acquired Infections; Approved Guideline, Third Edition*, M29-A3 (CLSI).

For additional student resources please visit thePoint at http://thepoint.lww.com. **thePoint**

QUESTIONS

1. Which of the following standards requires that SDSs are accessible to all employees who come in contact with a hazardous compound?
   a. Hazard Communication Standard
   b. Bloodborne Pathogen Standard
   c. CDC Regulations
   d. Personal Protection Equipment Standard

2. Chemicals should be stored
   a. According to their chemical properties and classification
   b. Alphabetically, for easy accessibility
   c. Inside a safety cabinet with proper ventilation
   d. Inside a fume hood, if toxic vapors can be released when opened

3. Proper PPE in the chemistry laboratory for routine testing includes
   a. Impermeable lab coat with eye/face protection and appropriate disposable gloves
   b. Respirators with HEPA filter
   c. Gloves with rubberized sleeves
   d. Safety glasses for individuals not wearing contact lenses

4. A fire caused by a flammable liquid should be extinguished using which type of extinguisher?
   a. Class B
   b. Halogen
   c. Pressurized water
   d. Class C

5. Which of the following is the proper means of disposal for the type of waste?
   a. Microbiologic waste by steam sterilization
   b. Xylene into the sewer system
   c. Mercury by burial
   d. Radioactive waste by incineration

6. What are the major contributing factors to repetitive strain injuries?
   a. Position/posture, applied force, and frequency of repetition
   b. Inattention on the part of the laboratorian
   c. Temperature and vibration
   d. Fatigue, clumsiness, and lack of coordination

7. Which of the following are examples of nonionizing radiation?
   a. Ultraviolet light and microwaves
   b. Gamma rays and x-rays
   c. Alpha and beta radiation
   d. Neutron radiation

8. One liter of 4 N sodium hydroxide (strong base) in a glass 1 L beaker accidentally fell and spilled on the laboratory floor. The first step is to:
   a. Call 911.
   b. Alert and evacuate those in the immediate area out of harms way.
   c. Throw some kitty litter on the spill.
   d. Squirt water on the spill to dilute the chemical.
   e. Neutralize with absorbing materials in a nearby spill kit.

9. Of the following, which is NOT reportable to the Department of Labor?
    a. A laboratorian with a persistent cough that is only triggered at work
    b. A laboratorian that experienced a chemical burn
    c. A laboratorian that tripped in the lab and hit her head on the lab bench rendering her unconscious
    d. A laboratorian that was stuck by a contaminated needle after performing phlebotomy on a patient
    e. A laboratorian that forgot to wear his lab coat and gloves while diluting patient serum

BIBLIOGRAPHY AND SUGGESTED READING

Allocca JA, Levenson HE. *Electrical and Electronic Safety*. Reston, VA: Reston Publishing Company; 1985.

American Chemical Society, Committee on Chemical Safety. Smith GW, ed. *Safety in Academic Chemistry Laboratories*. Washington, DC: American Chemical Society; 1985.

Boyle MP. Hazardous chemical waste disposal management. *Clin Lab Sci*. 1992;5:6.

Brown JW. Tuberculosis alert: an old killer returns. *MLO Med Lab Obs*. 1993;25:5.

Bryan RA. Recommendations for handling specimens from patients with confirmed or suspected Creutzfeldt-Jakob disease. *Lab Med*. 1984;15:50.

Centers for Disease Control and Prevention, National Institutes of Health. *Biosafety in Microbiological and Biomedical Laboratories*. 5th ed. Washington, DC: U.S. Government Printing Office; 2009.

Chervinski D. Environmental awareness: it's time to close the loop on waste reduction in the health care industry. *Adv Admin Lab*. 1994;3:4.

Clinical Laboratory Standards Institute (CLSI). *Clinical Laboratory Safety (Approved Guideline, GP17-A2)*. Wayne, PA: CLSI; 2004.

Clinical Laboratory Standards Institute (CLSI). *Protection of Laboratory Workers from Occupationally Acquired Infection (Approved Guideline, M29-A3)*. Wayne, PA: CLSI; 2005.

Clinical Laboratory Standards Institute (CLSI). *Clinical Laboratory Waste Management (Approved Guideline, GP05-A3)*. Wayne, PA: CLSI; 2011.

Committee on Hazardous Substances in the Laboratory, Assembly of Mathematical and Physical Sciences, National Research Council. *Prudent Practices for Handling Hazardous Chemicals in Laboratories*. Washington, DC: National Academies Press; 1981.

Furr AK. *Handbook of Laboratory Safety*. 5th ed. Boca Raton, FL: CRC Press; 2000.

Gile TJ. Hazard-communication program for clinical laboratories. *Clin Lab*. 1988;1:2.

Gile TJ. An update on lab safety regulations. *MLO Med Lab Obs*. 1995;27:3.

Gile TJ. *Complete Guide to Laboratory Safety*. Marblehead, MA: HCPro, Inc.; 2004.

Hayes DD. Safety considerations in the physician office laboratory. *Lab Med*. 1994;25:3.

Hazard communication. *Fed Regist*. February 1994;59:27.

Karcher RE. Is your chemical hygiene plan OSHA proof? *MLO Med Lab Obs*. 1993;25:7.

Le Sueur CL. A three-pronged attack against AIDS infection in the lab. *MLO Med Lab Obs*. 1989;21:37.

Miller SM. Clinical safety: dangers and risk control. *Clin Lab Sci*. 1992;5:6.

National Institute for Occupational Safety and Health (NIOSH). *NIOSH Pocket Guide to Chemical Hazards*. Atlanta, GA: Center for Disease Control; 2007.

National Institutes of Health, Radiation Safety Branch. *Radiation: The National Institutes of Health Safety Guide*. Washington, DC: U.S. Government Printing Office; 1979.

National Regulatory Committee, Committee on Hazardous Substances in the Laboratory. *Prudent Practices for the Handling of Hazardous Chemicals in Laboratories*. Washington, DC: National Academies Press; 1981.

National Regulatory Committee, Committee on Hazardous Substances in the Laboratory. *Prudent Practices for Disposal of Chemicals from Laboratories*. Washington, DC: National Academies Press; 1983.

National Regulatory Committee, Committee on the Hazardous Biological Substances in the Laboratory. *Biosafety in the Laboratory: Prudent Practices for the Handling and Disposal of Infectious Materials*. Washington, DC: National Academies Press; 1989.

National Safety Council (NSC). *Fundamentals of Industrial Hygiene*. 5th ed. Chicago, IL: NSC; 2002.

Occupational exposure to bloodborne pathogens; final rule. *Fed Regist*. December 1991;56:235.

Occupational Safety and Health Administration. Subpart Z 29CFR 1910.1000-1450.

Otto CH. Safety in health care: prevention of bloodborne diseases. *Clin Lab Sci*. 1992;5:6.

Pipitone DA. *Safe Storage of Laboratory Chemicals*. New York, NY: Wiley; 1984.

Rose SL. *Clinical Laboratory Safety*. Philadelphia, PA: JB Lippincott; 1984.

Rudmann SV, Jarus C, Ward KM, Arnold DM. Safety in the student laboratory: a national survey of university-based programs. *Lab Med*. 1993;24:5.

Stern A, Ries H, Flynn D, et al. Fire safety in the laboratory: part I. *Lab Med*. 1993;24:5.

Stern A, Ries H, Flynn D, et al. Fire safety in the laboratory: part II. *Lab Med*. 1993;24:6.

United Nations. *Globally Harmonized System of Classification and Labelling of Chemicals*. New York, NY; Geneva: United Nations; 2003.

Wald PH, Stave GM. *Physical and Biological Hazards of the Workplace*. New York, NY: Van Nostrand Reinhold; 1994.

Method Evaluation

MATTHEW P.A. HENDERSON, STEVEN W. COTTEN,
MIKE W. ROGERS, MONTE S. WILLIS,
CHRISTOPHER R. McCUDDEN

CHAPTER
3

CHAPTER OUTLINE

Chapter Objectives

Upon completion of this chapter, the clinical laboratorian should be able to do the following:

• Define the following terms: quality control, accuracy, precision, descriptive statistics, reference interval, random error, sensitivity, specificity, systematic error, and confidence intervals.
• Calculate the following: sensitivity, specificity, efficiency, predictive value, mean, median, range, variance, and standard deviation.
• Understand why statistics are needed for effective quality management.
• Read a descriptive statistics equation without fear.

• Understand the types, uses, and requirements for reference intervals.
• Understand the basic protocols used to verify or establish a reference interval.
• Appreciate how the test cutoff affects diagnostic performance.
• Evaluate laboratory data using multirules for quality control.
• Graph laboratory data and determine significant constant or proportional errors.
• Determine if there is a trend or a shift, given laboratory data.
• Discuss the processes involved in method selection and evaluation.
• Discuss proficiency testing programs in the clinical laboratory.
• Describe how a process can be systematically improved.

It is widely accepted that the majority of medical decisions are made using laboratory data. It is therefore critical that results generated by the laboratory be accurate. Determining and maintaining accuracy requires considerable effort and cost, entailing the use of a series of approaches depending on the complexity of the test. To begin, one must appreciate what *quality* is and how quality is measured. To this end, it is vital to understand basic statistical concepts that enable the laboratorian to measure quality. Before implementing a new test, it is important to determine if the test is capable of performing acceptably; *method evaluation* is used to verify the acceptability of new methods prior to reporting patient results. Once a method has been implemented, it is essential that the laboratory ensures it remains valid over time; this is achieved by a process known as quality control (QC). This chapter describes basic statistical concepts and provides an overview of the procedures necessary to implement a new method and ensure its continuing accuracy.

BASIC CONCEPTS

Each day, high–volume clinical laboratories generate thousands of results. This wealth of clinical laboratory data must be summarized to monitor test performance. The foundation for monitoring performance (known as QC) is descriptive statistics.

Descriptive Statistics: Measures of Center, Spread, and Shape

When examined closely, a collection of seemingly similar things always has at least slight differences for any given characteristic (e.g., smoothness, size, color, weight, volume, and potency). Similarly, laboratory data will have at least slight measurement differences. For example, if glucose on a given specimen is measured 100 times in a row, there would be a range of values obtained. Such differences in laboratory values can be a result of a variety of sources. Although measurements will differ, their values form patterns that can be visualized and analyzed collectively. Laboratorians view and describe these patterns using graphical representations and descriptive statistics (Fig. 3-1).

When comparing and analyzing collections or sets of laboratory data, patterns can be described by their center, spread, and shape. Although comparing the center of data is most common, comparing the spread can be even more powerful. Assessment of data dispersion, or spread, allows laboratorians to assess the predictability (and the lack of) in a laboratory test or measurement.

Measures of Center

The three most commonly used descriptions of the center of a dataset (Fig. 3-2) are the mean, the median, and the mode. The *mean* is most commonly used and often called

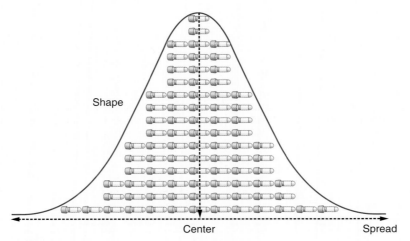

FIGURE 3-1 Basic measures of data include the center, spread, and shape.

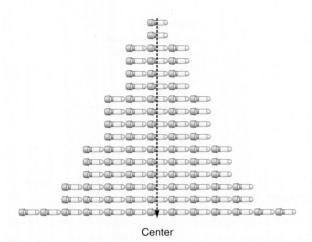

FIGURE 3-2 The center can be defined by the mean (x-bar character), median, or mode.

the *average*. The *median* is the "middle" point of the data and is often used with skewed data. The *mode* is rarely used as a measure of the data's center but is more often used to describe data that seem to have two centers (i.e., bimodal). The mean is calculated by summing the observations and dividing by the number of the observations.

$\sum$	Add up . . .
$\displaystyle\sum_{i=1}^{n} x_i$	the data points (the x's) and . . .
$\displaystyle\sum_{i=1}^{n} x_i/n$	divide by the total number of data points (n)

$$\bar{x} = \sum_{i=1}^{n} x_i/n \quad \text{to find the mean ("x bar")} \qquad \text{(Eq. 3-1)}$$

The summation sign, Σ, is an abbreviation for $(x_1 + x_2 + x_3 + \cdots + x_n)$ and is used in many statistical formulas. Often, the mean of a specific dataset is called $\bar{x}$, or "x bar."

The median is the middle of the data after the data have been rank ordered. It is the value that divides the data in half. To determine the median, values are rank ordered from least to greatest and the middle value is selected. For example, given a sample of 5, 4, 6, 5, 3, 7, 5, the rank order of the points is 3, 4, 5, 5, 5, 6, 7. Because there are an odd number of values in the sample, the middle value (median) is 5; the value 5 divides the data in half. Given another sample with an even number of values 5, 4, 6, 8, 9, 7, the rank order of the points is 4, 5, 6, 7, 8, 9. The two "middle" values are 6 and 7. Adding them yields 13 (6 + 7 = 13); division by 2 provides the median (13/2 = 6.5). The median value of 6.5 divides the data in half.

The mode is the most frequently occurring value in a dataset. Although it is seldom used to describe data, it is referred to when in reference to the shape of data, a bimodal distribution, for example. In the sample 3, 4, 5, 5, 5, 6, 7, the value that occurs most often is 5. The mode of this set is then 5. The dataset 3, 4, 5, 5, 5, 6, 7, 8, 9, 9, 9 has two modes, 5 and 9.

After describing the center of the dataset, it is very useful to indicate how the data are distributed (spread). The spread represents the relationship of all the data points to the mean (Fig. 3-3). There are three commonly used descriptions

---

BOX 3-1 SOURCES OF ANALYTIC VARIABILITY

Operator technique	Environmental conditions (e.g., temperature, humidity)
Instrument differences	Reagents
Test accessories	Power surges
Contamination	Matrix effects (hemolysis, lipemia, serum proteins)

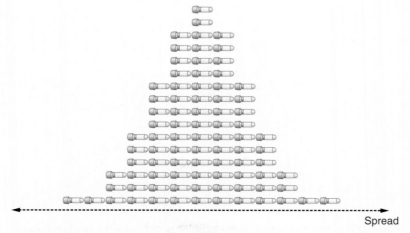

Spread

FIGURE 3-3 Spread is defined by the standard deviation and coefficient of variation.

of spread: (1) range, (2) standard deviation (SD), and (3) coefficient of variation (CV). The easiest measure of spread to understand is the range. The range is simply the largest value in the data minus the smallest value, which represents the extremes of data one might encounter. Standard deviation (also called "s," SD, or σ) is the most frequently used measure of variation. Although calculating SD can seem somewhat intimidating, the concept is straightforward; in fact, all of the descriptive statistics and even the inferential statistics have a combination of mathematical operations that are by themselves no more complex than a square root. The SD and, more specifically, the variance represent the "average" distance from the center of the data (the mean) and every value in the dataset. The CV allows a laboratorian to compare SDs with different units.

Range is one description of the spread of data. It is simply the difference between the highest and lowest data points: range = high − low. For the sample 5, 4, 6, 5, 3, 7, 5, the range is 7 − 3 = 4. The range is often a good measure of dispersion for small samples of data. It does have a serious drawback; the range is susceptible to extreme values or outliers.

To calculate the SD of a dataset, it is easiest to first determine the variance (s^2). Variance is similar to the mean in that it is an average. Variance is the average of the squared distances of all values from the mean:

$$s^2 = \sum_{i=1}^{n} (x_i - \bar{x})^2 / n - 1 \qquad \text{(Eq. 3-2)}$$

As a measure of dispersion, variance represents the difference between each value and the average of the data. Given the values 5, 4, 6, 5, 3, 7, 5, variance can be calculated as shown below:

$\bar{x}$	$(5 + 4 + 6 + 5 + 3 + 7 + 5)/7 = 5$
$(x_i - \bar{x})$	$(5 - 5) + (4 - 5) + (6 - 5)$ $+ (5 - 5) + (3 - 5)$ $+ (7 - 5) + (5 - 5)$
$(x_i - \bar{x})^2$	$(0)^2 + (-1)^2 + (1)^2 + (0)^2$ $+ (-2)^2 + (2)^2 + (0)^2$
$\sum_{i=1}^{n} (x_i - \bar{x})^2$	$0 + 1 + 1 + 0 + 4 + 4$ $+ 0 = 10$

$$\sum_{i=1}^{n} (x_i - \bar{x})^2 / n - 1 \qquad 10/(7-1) = 10/6$$

$$s^2 = \sum_{i=1}^{n} (x_i - \bar{x})^2 / n - 1 \qquad 1.67 \qquad \text{(Eq. 3-3)}$$

To calculate the SD (or "s"), simply take the square root of the variance:

$$s(\sigma) = \sqrt{s^2} = \sqrt{\sum_{i=1}^{n} (x_i - \bar{x})^2 / n - 1} \qquad \text{(Eq. 3-4)}$$

Although it is important to understand how these measures are calculated, many instruments, laboratory information systems, and software packages determine these automatically. SD describes the distribution of all data points around the mean.

Another way of expressing SD is in terms of the CV. The CV is calculated by dividing the SD by the mean and multiplying by 100 to express it as a percentage:

$$\text{CV (\%)} = \frac{100s}{x} \qquad \text{(Eq. 3-5)}$$

The CV simplifies comparison of SDs of test results expressed in different units and concentrations. As shown in Table 3-1, analytes measured at different concentrations can have a drastically different SD but a comparable CV. The CV is used extensively to summarize QC data. The CV of highly precise analyzers can be lower than 1%.

Measures of Shape

Although there are hundreds of different "shapes"—distributions—that datasets can exhibit, the most commonly discussed is the Gaussian distribution (also called normal distribution; Fig. 3-4). The Gaussian distribution describes many continuous laboratory variables and shares several unique characteristics: the mean, median, and mode are identical; the distribution is symmetric—meaning half the values fall to the left of the mean and the other half fall to the right—and the symmetrical shape is often called a "bell curve."

The total area under the Gaussian curve is 1.0, or 100%. Much of the area—68.3%—under the "normal" curve is between ±1 SD (μ ± 1σ) (Fig. 3-5A). Most of

TABLE 3-1	COMPARISON OF SD AND CV FOR TWO DIFFERENT ANALYTES					
FSH CONCENTRATION	**SD**	**CV**	**βHCG CONCENTRATION**	**SD**	**CV**
1	0.09	9.0	10	0.8	8.0
5	0.25	5.0	100	5.5	5.5
10	0.40	4.0	1,000	52.0	5.2
25	1.20	4.8	10,000	500.00	5.0
100	3.80	3.8	100,000	4,897.0	4.9

SD, standard deviation; CV, coefficient of variation; FSH, follicle-stimulating hormone; βhCG, β-human chorionic gonadotropin.

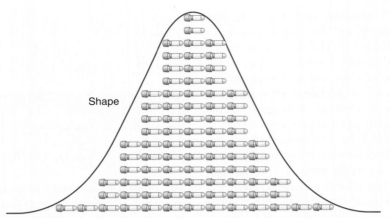

FIGURE 3-4 Shape is defined by how the distribution of data relates the center. This is an example of data that have "normal" or Gaussian distribution.

the area—95.4%—under the "normal" curve is between ±2 SDs (μ ± 2σ; Fig. 3-5B). And almost all of the area—99.7%—under the "normal" curve is between ±3 SDs (μ ± 3σ) (Fig. 3-5C).

The "68–95–99 Rule" summarizes the above relationships between the area under a Gaussian distribution and the SD. In other words, given any Gaussian distributed data, ≈68% of the data fall between ±1 SD from the mean; ≈95% of the data fall between ±2 SDs from the mean; and ≈99% fall between ±3 SDs from the mean. Likewise, if you selected a value in a dataset that is Gaussian distributed, there is a 0.68 chance of it lying between ±1 SD from the mean; there is a 0.95 likelihood of it lying between ±2 SDs; and a 0.99 probability of it lying between ±3 SDs. (Note: the terms "chance," "likelihood," and "probability" are synonymous in this example.)

As will be discussed in the reference interval section, most patient data are not normally distributed. These data may be skewed or exhibit multiple centers (bimodal, trimodal, etc.) as shown in Figure 3–6. Plotting data in

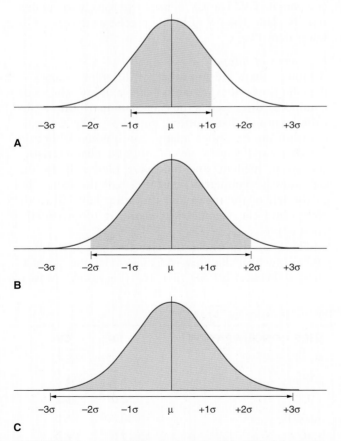

FIGURE 3-5 A normal distribution contains **(A)** ≈68% of the results within ±1 SD (1s or 1σ), **(B)** 95% of the results within ±2s (2σ), and **(C)** ≈99% of the results within ±3σ.

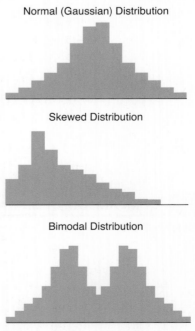

FIGURE 3-6 Examples of normal (Gaussian), skewed, and bimodal distributions. The type of statistical analysis that is performed to analyze the data depends on the distribution (shape).

histograms as shown in the figure is an useful and easy way to visualize distribution. However, there are also mathematical analyses (e.g., normality tests) that can confirm if data fit a given distribution. The importance of recognizing whether data are or are not normally distributed is related to the way it can be statistically analyzed.

Descriptive Statistics of Groups of Paired Observations

While the use of basic descriptive statistics is satisfactory for examining a single method, laboratorians frequently need to compare two different methods. This is most commonly encountered in comparison-of-methods (COM) experiments. A COM experiment involves measuring patient specimens by both an existing (reference) method and a new (test) method (described in the Reference Interval and Method Evaluation sections later). The data obtained from these comparisons consist of two measurements for each patient specimen. It is easiest to visualize and summarize the paired-method comparison data graphically (Fig. 3-7). By convention, the values obtained by the reference method are plotted on the x-axis and the values obtained by the test method are plotted on the y-axis.

In Figure 3-7, the agreement between the two methods is estimated from the straight line that best fits the points. Whereas visual estimation may be used to draw the line, a statistical technique known as **linear regression** analysis provides objective measures of the location and dispersion for the line. Three factors are generated in a linear regression—the slope, the y-intercept, and the correlation coefficient (r). In Figure 3-7, there is a linear relationship between the two methods over the entire range of values. The linear regression is defined by the equation $y = mx + b$. The slope of the line is described by m, and the value of the y-intercept (b) is determined by plugging $x = 0$ into the equation and solving for y. The correlation coefficient is a measure of the strength of the relationship between the two methods. The correlation coefficient can have values from -1 to 1, with the sign indicating the direction of relationship between the two variables. A positive r indicates that both variables increase and decrease together, whereas a negative r indicates that as one variable increases, the other decreases. An r value of 0 indicates no relationship, whereas $r = 1.0$ indicates a perfect relationship. Although many equate high positive values of r (0.95 or higher) with excellent agreement between the test and comparative methods, most

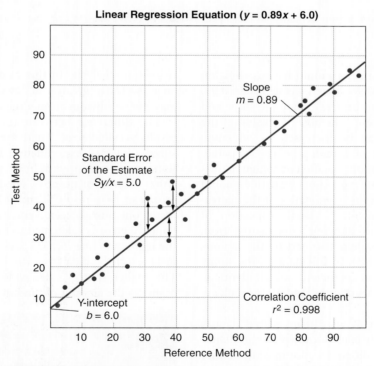

FIGURE 3-7 A generic example of a linear regression. A linear regression compares two tests and yields important information about systematic and random error. Systematic error is indicated by changes in the y-intercept (constant error) and the slope (proportional error). Random error is indicated by the standard error of the estimate ($S_{y/x}$); $S_{y/x}$ basically represents the distance of each point from the regression line. The correlation coefficient indicates the strength of the relationship between the tests.

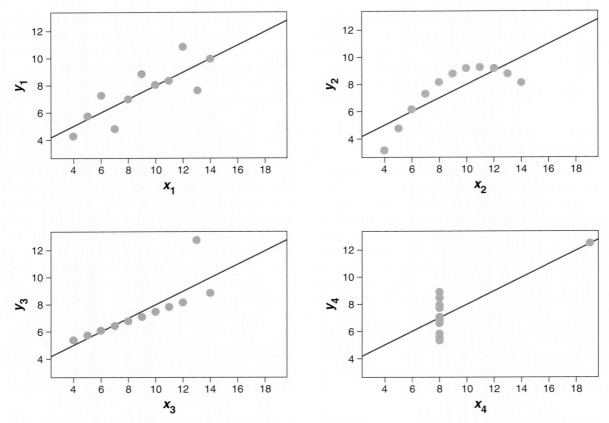

FIGURE 3-8 Anscombe's quartet demonstrates the need to visually inspect data. In each panel, $y = 0.5x + 3$, $r^2 = 0.816$, $S_{y/x} = 4.1$.

clinical chemistry comparisons should have correlation coefficients greater than 0.98. When r is less than 0.99, the regression formula can underestimate the slope and overestimate the y-intercept. The absolute value of the correlation coefficient can be increased by widening the concentration range of samples being compared. However, if the correlation coefficient remains less than 0.99, then alternate regression statistics should be used to derive more realistic estimates of the regression, slope, and y-intercept.[1,2] Visual inspection of data is essential prior to drawing conclusions from the summary statistics as demonstrated by the famous Anscombe quartet (Fig. 3-8). In this dataset, the slope, y-intercept, and correlation coefficients are all identical, yet visual inspection reveals that the underlying data are completely different.

An alternate approach to visualizing paired data is the difference plot, which is also known as the Bland-Altman plot (Fig. 3-9). A difference plot indicates either the percent or absolute bias (difference) between the reference and test method values over the average range of values. This approach permits simple comparison of the differences to previously established maximum limits. As is evident in Figure 3-9, it is easier to visualize any concentration-dependent differences than by linear

regression analysis. In this example, the percent difference is clearly greatest at lower concentrations, which may not be obvious from a regression plot.

The difference between test and reference method results is called *error*. There are two kinds of error measured in COM experiments: random and systematic. Random error is present in all measurements and can be either positive or negative. As described earlier, random error can be a result of many factors including instrument, operator, reagent, and environmental variations. Random error is calculated as the SD of the points about the regression line ($S_{y/x}$). $S_{y/x}$ essentially refers to average distance of the data from the regression line (Fig. 3-7). The higher the $S_{y/x}$, the wider is the scatter and the higher is the amount of random error.

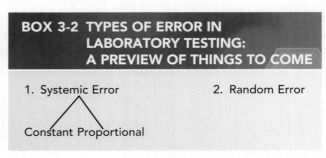

BOX 3-2 TYPES OF ERROR IN LABORATORY TESTING: A PREVIEW OF THINGS TO COME

1. Systemic Error   2. Random Error

Constant Proportional

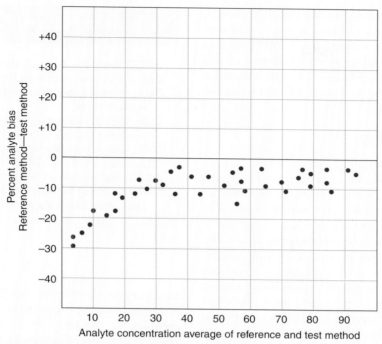

FIGURE 3-9 An example of a difference (Bland-Altman) plot. Difference plots are a useful tool to visualize concentration-dependent error.

$S_{y/x}$	Standard deviation of the regression line
$S_{y/x} = \Sigma$	Add up
$S_{y/x} = \Sigma(y_i - Y_i)$	The distance of each y-value from the regression line
$S_{y/x} = \Sigma(y_i - Y_i)^2$	Square each difference to make the sum a positive number
$S_{y/x} = [\Sigma(y_i - Y_i)^2/n - 2]$	Divide the sum of the squares by the number of points and subtract 2
$S_{y/x} = \text{sqrt } [\Sigma(y_i - Y_i)^2/n - 2]$	Take the square root

$$(Eq. 3-6)$$

In Figure 3-7, the $S_{y/x}$ is 5.0. If the points were perfectly in line with the linear regression, the $S_{y/x}$ would equal 0.0, indicating there would not be any random error. $S_{y/x}$ is also known as the standard error of the estimate S_E and is calculated according to Equation (3-6).

Systematic error influences observations consistently in one direction (higher or lower). The measures of slope and y-intercept provide estimates of the systematic error. Systematic error can be further broken down into constant error and proportional error. Constant systematic error exists when there is a continual difference between the test method and the comparative method values, regardless of the concentration. In Figure 3-7, there is a constant difference of 6.0 between the test

method values and the comparative method values. This constant difference, reflected in the y-intercept, is called *constant systematic error*. Proportional error exists when the differences between the test method and the comparative method values are proportional to the analyte concentration. Proportional error is present when the slope is 1. In the example, the slope of 0.89 represents the proportional error, where samples will be underestimated in a concentration-dependent fashion by the test method compared with the reference method; the error is proportional, because it will increase with the analyte concentration.

Inferential Statistics

The next level of complexity beyond paired descriptive statistics is inferential statistics. Inferential statistics are used to draw conclusions (inferences) regarding the means or SDs of two sets of data. Inferential statistical analyses are most commonly encountered in research studies, but can also be used in COM studies.

An important consideration for inferential statistics is the distribution of the data (shape). The distribution of the data determines what kind of inferential statistics can be used to analyze the data. Normally distributed (Gaussian) data are typically analyzed using what are known as "parametric" tests, which include a Student's t-test or analysis of variance (ANOVA). Data that are not normally distributed require a "nonparametric" analysis. Nonparametric tests are encountered in reference interval studies, where population data are often skewed. While many software packages are capable of performing either parametric or nonparametric analyses, it is important for the user to understand that the type of data (shape) dictates which statistical test is appropriate for the analysis. An inappropriate analysis of sound data can yield the wrong conclusion.

METHOD EVALUATION

The value of clinical laboratory service is based on its ability to provide reliable, accurate test results. At the heart of providing these services is the performance of a testing method. To maximize the usefulness of a test, laboratorians undergo a process in which a method is selected and evaluated for its usefulness to those who will be using the test. This process is carefully undertaken to produce results within medically acceptable error to help physicians maximally benefit their patients.

Currently, clinical laboratories more often select and evaluate methods that were commercially developed instead of developing their own. Most commercially developed tests have U.S. Food and Drug Administration (FDA) approval, only requiring a laboratory to provide a limited evaluation of a method to verify the manufacturer's performance claims and to see how well the method works specifically in your laboratory.

Regulatory Aspects of Method Evaluation (Alphabet Soup)

The Centers for Medicare and Medicaid Services (CMS) and the FDA are the primary government agencies that influence laboratory testing methods in the United States. The FDA regulates laboratory instruments and reagents, and the CMS regulates the Clinical Laboratory Improvement Amendments (CLIA).[3] Most large laboratories in the United States are accredited by the College of American Pathologists (CAP) and The Joint Commission (TJC; formerly the Joint Commission on Accreditation of Healthcare Organizations [JCAHO]), which impacts how method evaluations need to be performed. Professional organizations such as the National Academy of Clinical Biochemistry (NACB) and the American Association for Clinical Chemistry (AACC) also contribute important guidelines and method evaluations that influence how method evaluations are performed.

The FDA "Office of In Vitro Diagnostic Device Evaluation and Safety" (OIVD) regulates diagnostic tests. Tests are categorized into one of three groups: (1) waived, (2) moderate complexity, and (3) high complexity. Waived tests are cleared by the FDA to be so simple that they are most likely accurate and would pose negligible risk of harm to the patient if not performed correctly; these methods include dipstick tests and glucose monitors. Most automated methods are rated

<table>
<tr><td colspan="2">**DEFINITIONS BOX**</td></tr>
<tr><td colspan="2">**AACC:** American Association for Clinical Chemistry
CAP: College of American Pathologists
CLIA: Clinical Laboratory Improvement Amendments
CLSI: Clinical Laboratory and Standards Institute (formerly NCCLS)
CMS: Centers for Medicare and Medicaid Services
FDA: Food and Drug Administration
NACB: National Academy of Clinical Biochemistry
OIVD: Office of In Vitro Diagnostic Device Evaluation and Safety
TJC: The Joint Commission</td></tr>
</table>

as moderate complexity, while manual methods and methods requiring more interpretation are rated as high complexity. The CLIA final rule requires that waived tests simply follow the manufacturer's instructions. Both moderate- and high-complexity tests are validated on whether they are FDA approved or not. FDA-approved nonwaived tests must undergo a shorter validation process (Table 3-2), whereas a more extensive process is required for tests developed by laboratories (Table 3-2). While the major requirements for testing validation are driven by the CLIA, TJC and CAP essentially require the same types of experiments to be performed, with a few additions. It is these rules that guide the way tests in the clinical chemistry laboratory are selected and validated.

Method Selection

Evaluating a method is a labor-intensive costly process—so why select a new method? There are many reasons, including reducing costs, improving the quality of results, increasing client satisfaction, and improving efficiency. Selecting a test method starts with the collection of technical information about a particular test from colleagues, scientific presentations, and the scientific literature. Practical considerations should also be addressed at this point, such as the type and volume of specimen to be tested, the required throughput and turnaround time, your testing needs, cost, calibration, QC approach, space needs, disposal needs, personnel requirements, and safety considerations. Most importantly, the test should be able to meet the clinical task by having specific analytic performance standards that will accurately assist in the diagnosis of patients. Specific information that should be discovered about a test you might bring into the laboratory includes analytic sensitivity, analytic specificity, linear range, interfering substances, and estimates of imprecision and inaccuracy. The process of method

TABLE 3-2	GENERAL CLIA REGULATIONS OF METHOD VALIDATION
NONWAIVED FDA-APPROVED TESTS	1. Demonstrate test performance comparable to that established by the manufacturer. a. Accuracy b. Precision c. Reportable range
	2. Verify reference (normal) values appropriate for patient population
NONWAIVED FDA-APPROVED TESTS MODIFIED OR DEVELOPED BY LABORATORY	1. Determine a. Accuracy b. Precision c. Analytic sensitivity d. Analytic specificity (including interfering substances) e. Reportable range of test results f. Reference/normal ranges g. Other performance characteristics h. Calibration and control procedures

From Clinical Laboratory Improvement Amendments of 1988; final rule. *Fed Regist.* 7164 [42 CFR 493 1253]: Department of Health and Human Services, Centers for Medicare and Medicaid Services; 1992.

selection is the beginning of a process to bring in a new test for routine use (Fig. 3-10).

Method Evaluation

A short, initial evaluation should be carried out before the complete method evaluation. This preliminary evaluation should include the analysis of a series of *standards* to verify the linear range and the replicate analysis (at least eight measurements) of two controls to obtain estimates of short-term imprecision. If any results fall short of the specifications published in the method's product

information sheet (package insert), the method's manufacturer should be consulted. Without improvement in the method, more extensive evaluations are pointless.[4]

First Things First: Determine Imprecision and Inaccuracy

The first determinations (estimates) to be made in a method evaluation are the *imprecision* and *inaccuracy*, which should be compared with the maximum allowable error based on medical criteria. If the imprecision or inaccuracy exceeds the maximum allowable error, it

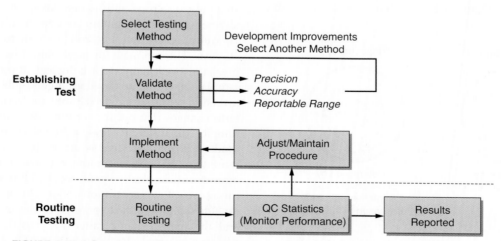

FIGURE 3-10 A flowchart on the process of method selection, evaluation, and monitoring. (Adapted from Westgard JO, Quam E, Barry T. *Basic QC Practices: Training in Statistical Quality Control for Healthcare Laboratories.* Madison, WI: Westgard Quality Corp.; 1998.)

DEFINITIONS BOX

Analytic sensitivity: Ability of a method to detect small quantities of an analyte.

Analytic specificity: Ability of a method to detect only the analyte it is designed to determine.

Specificity: Ability of a method to measure only the analyte of interest.

AMR (analytic measurement range): Also known as linear or dynamic range. Range of analyte concentrations that can be directly measured without dilution, concentration, or other pretreatment.

CRR (clinically reportable range): Range of analyte that a method can quantitatively report, allowing for dilution, concentration, or other pretreatment used to extend AMR.

LoD (limit of detection): Lowest amount of analyte accurately detected by a method.

SDI (standard deviation index): Refers to the difference between the measured value and the mean expressed as a number of SDs. An SDI = 0 indicates the value is accurate or in 100% agreement; an SDI = 3 is 3 SDs away from the target (mean) and indicates inaccuracy. SDI may be positive or negative.

DEFINITIONS BOX

Imprecision: Dispersion of repeated measurements about the mean due to analytic error.

Inaccuracy: Difference between a measured value and its true value due to systematic error, which can be either constant or proportional.

Systemic error: Error always in one direction.

Constant error: Type of systemic error in the sample direction and magnitude; the magnitude of change is constant and not dependent on the amount of analyte.

Proportional error: Type of systemic error where the magnitude changes as a percent of the analyte present; error dependent on analyte concentration.

Random error: Error varies from sample to sample. Causes include instrument instability, temperature variations, reagent variation, handling techniques, and operator variables.

Total error: Random error plus systemic error.

SDI: Standard deviation index. (Test method SD) − (Reference method SD)/(Reference method SD); analogous to Z-score.

---

is unacceptable and must be modified and reevaluated or rejected. Imprecision is the dispersion of repeated measurements around a mean (true level), as shown in Figure 3-11A with the mean represented as the bull's eye. Random analytic error is the cause of imprecision in a test. Imprecision is estimated from studies in which multiple aliquots of the same specimen (with a constant concentration) are analyzed repetitively. Inaccuracy, or the difference between a measured value and its actual value, is due to the presence of a systemic error, as represented in Figure 3-11B. Systemic error can be due

to constant or proportional error and is estimated from three types of study: (1) recovery, (2) interference, and (3) a COM study.

Measurement of Imprecision

Method evaluation begins with a precision study. This estimates the random error associated with the test method and detects any problems affecting its reproducibility. It is recommended that this study be performed over a 10- to 20-day period, incorporating one or two analytic runs (runs with patient samples or QC materials) per day.[5,6] A common precision study is a 2 × 2 × 10 study, where two controls are run twice a day for 10 days. The rationale for performing the evaluation of precision over many days is logical. Running multiple samples on the same day does a good job of estimating precision within a single day but underestimates long-term changes that occur over time. By running multiple samples on different days, a better estimation of the random error over time is given. It is important that more than one concentration be tested in these studies, with materials ideally spanning the clinically meaningful range of concentrations. For glucose, this might include samples in the hyperglycemic range (150 mg/dL) and the hypoglycemic range (50 mg/dL). After these data are collected, the mean, SD, and CV are calculated. An example of a precision study from our laboratory is shown in Figure 3-12.

Imprecision

Determined by:
Repeated analysis study

A

Inaccuracy

Determined by:
1) Recovery study
2) Interference study
3) Comparison of methods study

B

FIGURE 3-11 Graphic representation of **(A)** imprecision and **(B)** inaccuracy on a dartboard configuration with bull's eye in the center.

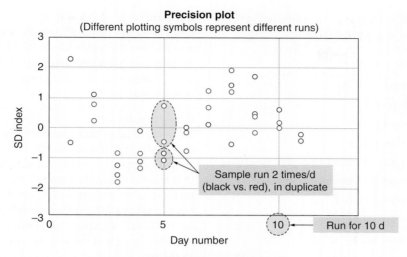

Precision plot
(Different plotting symbols represent different runs)

Sample run 2 times/d
(black vs. red), in duplicate

Run for 10 d

Precision estimate
User's Concentration: 76.78

	Within Run	Between Run	Between Day	Total	Medically Required	Verification Value (95%)	Pass/Fail
Std. Dev	1.06	0.45	1.37	**1.79**	**4.80**	6.2	Pass
% CV	1.4	0.6	1.8	**2.3**	6.3		
df	18	–	–	15			

FIGURE 3-12 An example of a precision study for vitamin B_{12}. The data represent analysis of a control sample run in duplicate twice a day (*red* and *black circles*) for 10 d (*x*-axis). Data are presented as standard deviation index (SDI). SDI refers to the difference between the measured value and the mean expressed as a number of SDs. An imprecision study is designed to detect random error.

The random error or imprecision associated with the test procedure is indicated by the SD and the CV. The within-run imprecision is indicated by the SD of the controls analyzed within one run. The total imprecision may be obtained from the SD of control data with one or two data points accumulated per day. The total imprecision is the most accurate assessment of performance that would affect the values a clinician might see and reflects differences in operators and pipettes and variations in environmental changes such as temperature. In practice, however, run imprecision is used more commonly than total imprecision. An inferential statistical technique, ANOVA, is then used to analyze the available precision data to provide estimates of the within-run, between-run, and total imprecision.[7]

Acceptable Performance Criteria: Imprecision Studies

During an evaluation of vitamin B_{12} in the laboratory, an imprecision study was performed for a new test method (Fig. 3-12). Several concentrations of vitamin B_{12} were run twice daily (in duplicate) for 10 days, as shown in Figure 3-12 (for simplicity, only one concentration is shown). The data are represented in the precision plot in Figure 3-12 (≈76 pg/mL). The amount of variability

between runs is represented by different colors, over 10 days (*x*-axis). The CV was then calculated for within-run, between-run, and between-days. The total SD, estimated at 2.3, is then compared with medical decision levels or medically required standards based on the analyte (Table 3-3). The acceptability of analytic error is based on how the test is to be used to make clinical interpretations.[8,9] In this case, the medically required SD limit is 4.8. The determination of whether long-term precision is adequate is based on the total imprecision being less than one-third of the total allowable error (total imprecision, in this case, 1.6; selection of one-third total allowable error for imprecision is based on Westgard[10]). In the case that the value is greater than the total allowable error (1.79 in our example), the test can pass as long as the difference between one-third total allowable error and the determined allowable error is not statistically significant. In our case, the 1.79 was not statistically different from 1.6 (1/3 × 4.8), and the test passed our imprecision studies (Fig. 3-12). The one-third of total error is a run of thumb; some laboratories may choose one-fourth of the total error. It is a bad idea to use all of the allowable error for imprecision (random error) as it leaves no room for systematic error (bias or inaccuracy).

TABLE 3-3	PERFORMANCE STANDARDS FOR COMMON CLINICAL CHEMISTRY ANALYTES AS DEFINED BY THE CLIA
Calcium, total	Target ±1.0 mg/dL
Chloride	Target ±5%
Cholesterol, total	Target ±10%
Cholesterol, HDL	Target ±30%
Glucose	Greater of target ±6 mg/dL or ±10%
Potassium	Target ±0.5 mmol/L
Sodium	Target ±4 mmol/L
Total protein	Target ±10%
Triglycerides	Target ±25%
Urea nitrogen	Greater of target ±2 mg/dL or ±9%
Uric acid	Target ±17%

Reprinted with permission from Centers for Disease Control and Prevention (CDC), Centers for Medicare and Medicaid Services (CMS), Health and Human Services. Medicare, Medicaid, and CLIA programs; laboratory requirements relating to quality systems and certain personnel qualifications. Final rule. *Fed Regist.* 2003;68:3639-3714.

DEFINITIONS BOX

Recovery: Ability of an analytic test to measure a known amount of analyte; a known amount of analyte is added to real sample matrices.
Interference: Effect of (a) compound(s) on the accuracy of detection of a particular analyte.
Interferents: Substances that cause interference.
Matrix: Body component (e.g., fluid and urine) in which the analyte is to be measured.

Estimation of Inaccuracy

Once method imprecision is estimated and deemed acceptable, the determination of accuracy can begin.[6] Accuracy is estimated using three different types of studies: (1) recovery, (2) interference, and (3) patient sample comparison.

Recovery Studies

Recovery studies will show whether a method is able to accurately measure an analyte. In a recovery experiment, a small aliquot of concentrated analyte is added (spiked) into a patient sample (matrix) and then measured by the method being evaluated. The amount recovered is the difference between the spiked sample and the patient sample (unmodified). The purpose of this type of study is to determine how much of the analyte can be detected (recovered) in the presence of all the other compounds in the matrix. The original patient samples (matrix) should not be diluted more than 10% so that the matrix solution is minimally affected. An actual example of a recovery study for total calcium is illustrated in Figure 3-13; the results are expressed as percentage recovered. The performance standard for calcium, defined by CLIA, is the target value ±1.0 mg/dL (see Table 3-3). Recovery of calcium in this example exceeds this standard at the two calcium levels tested (Fig. 3-13).

Interference Studies

Interference studies are designed to determine if specific compounds affect the accuracy of laboratory tests. Common interferences encountered in the laboratory include hemolysis (broken red blood cells and their contents), icterus (high bilirubin), and turbidity (particulate matter or lipids), which can affect the measurement of many analytes. Interferents often affect tests by absorbing or scattering light, but they can also react with the reagents or affect reaction rates used to measure a given analyte.

	Ca^{2+} Measured in Matrix	Ca^{2+} Added	Ca^{2+} Recovered	% Recovery
Baseline	7.5 mg/dL	NA	NA	NA
Sample 1	8.35 mg/dL	0.95 mg/dL	0.85 mg/dL	89%
Sample 2	9.79 mg/dL	2.38 mg/dL	2.29 mg/dL	96%

Calculation of % recovery

$$\% \text{ Recovered} = \frac{(\text{Measured in spike sample}) - (\text{Measured in baseline})}{\text{Concentration added}} \times 100$$

e.g., Calculation for Sample 1

$$\% \text{ Recovered} = \frac{(8.35 \text{ mg/dL}) - (7.5 \text{ mg/dL})}{0.95 \text{ mg/dL}} \times 100$$

% Recovered = 89%

FIGURE 3-13 An example of a sample recovery study for total calcium. A sample is spiked with known amounts of calcium in a standard matrix, and recovery is determined as shown. Recovery studies are designed to detect proportional error in an assay.

Interference experiments are typically performed by adding the potential interferent to patient samples.[11] If an effect is observed, the concentration of the interferent is lowered sequentially to determine the concentration at which test results are not affected (or minimally affected). It is common practice to flag results with unacceptably high levels of an interferent. Results may be reported with cautionary comments or not reported at all. An example of an interference study performed in one laboratory is shown in Figure 3-14. When designing a method validation study, potential interferents should be selected from literature reviews and specific references. Other excellent resources include Young[12] and Siest and Galteau.[13] Common interferences, such as hemolysis, lipemia, bilirubin, anticoagulant, and preservatives, are tested by the manufacturer. Glick and Ryder[14,15] published "interferographs" for clinical chemistry instruments, which relate analyte concentration measure to interferent concentration. They have also demonstrated that considerable expense can be saved by the acquisition of instruments that minimize hemoglobin, triglyceride, and bilirubin interference.[16] It is good laboratory practice and a regulatory requirement to consider interferences as part of any method validation.

COM Studies

A method comparison experiment examines patient samples by the method being evaluated (test method) with a reference method. It is used primarily to estimate systemic error in actual patient samples, and it may offer

the type of systematic error (proportional vs. constant). Ideally, the test method is compared with a standardized reference method (gold standard), a method with acceptable accuracy in comparison with its imprecision. Many times reference methods are laborious and time consuming, as is the case with the ultracentrifugation methods of determining cholesterol. Because most laboratories are not staffed to perform reference methods, most test methods are compared with those routinely used. These routine tests have their own particular inaccuracies, so it is important to determine what inaccuracies they might have that are documented in the literature. If the new test method is to replace the routine method, differences between the two should be well characterized.

To compare a test method with a comparative method, it is recommended by Westgard et al.[6] and CLIA[17] that 40 to 100 specimens be run by each method on the same day over 8 to 20 days (preferably within 4 hours), with specimens spanning the clinical range and representing a diversity of pathologic conditions. As an extra measure of QC, specimens should be analyzed in duplicate. Otherwise, experimental results must be checked by comparing test and comparative method results immediately after analysis. Samples with large differences should be repeated to rule out technical errors as the source of variation. Daily analysis of two to five patient specimens should be followed for at least 8 days if 40 specimens are compared and for 20 days if 100 specimens are compared in replication studies.[17]

A plot of the test method data (y-axis) versus the comparative method (x-axis) helps to visualize the data generated in a COM test (Fig. 3-15A).[18] As described earlier, if the two methods correlate perfectly, the data pairs plotted as concentration values from the reference method (x) versus the evaluation method (y) will produce a straight line ($y = mx + b$), with a slope of 1.0, a y-intercept of 0, and a correlation coefficient (r) of 1. Data should be plotted daily and inspected for outliers so that original samples can be reanalyzed as needed. While linearity can be confirmed visually in most cases, it may be necessary to evaluate linearity more quantitatively.[19]

Pooled TnI Concentration = 0.0295 ng/mL			
Sample #	Hemolysate (Hg) g/dL	TnI (ng/mL)	% Bias
1	<0.15	0.0295	
2	0.14	0.0255	−13.6
3	0.25	0.0220	−25.4
4	0.36	0.0205	−30.5
5	0.48	0.0200	−32.0
6	0.60	0.0180	−39.0

Calculation of Interference

$$\text{Interference} = \frac{\text{Concentration with interference added}}{\text{Concentration without interference}}$$

Bias =   Interference − concentration without interference
Bias % =   Bias x 100

FIGURE 3-14 An example of an interference study for troponin-I (TnI). Increasing amounts of hemolysate (lysed red blood cells, a common interference) were added to a sample with elevated TnI of 0.295 ng/mL. Bias is calculated based on the difference between the baseline and hemolyzed samples. The data are corrected for the dilution with hemolysate.

DEFINITIONS BOX

Deming regression analysis: Linear regression analysis (least squares analysis) used to compare two methodologies using the best fit line through the data points.

Deming plot: Graphical representation of the Deming regression analysis (see Figs. 3-24 and 3-25).

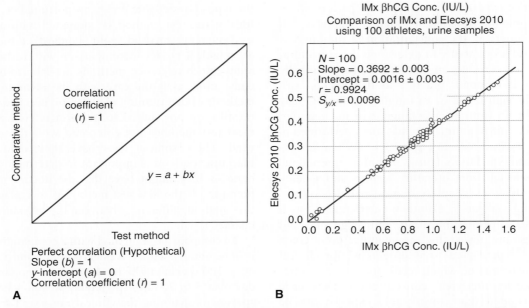

FIGURE 3-15 A comparison-of-methods experiment. **(A)** A model of a perfect method comparison. **(B)** An actual method comparison of beta-human chorionic gonadotropin (βhCG) between the Elecsys 2010 (Roche, Nutley, NJ) and the IMx (Abbott Laboratories, Abbott Park, IL). (Adapted from Shahzad K, Kim DH, Kang MJ. Analytic evaluation of the beta-human chorionic gonadotropin assay on the Abbott IMx and Elecsys2010 for its use in doping control. *Clin Biochem.* 2007;40:1259-1265.)

Statistical Analysis of COM Studies

The data used to plot the test method versus the comparative method can be further statistically analyzed using a linear regression. Linear regression generates statistical calculations of the slope (b), the y-intercept (a), the SD of the points about the regression line ($S_{y/x}$), and the correlation coefficient (r). An example of these calculations can be found in Figure 3-15, where a comparison of β-human chorionic gonadotropin (βhCG) concentrations on the IMx system and the Elecsys2010 is given. The reason for calculating statistics is to determine the types and amounts of error that a method has, to decide if the test is still valid to make clinical decisions. Several types of errors can be seen looking at a plot of test method versus comparative method (Fig. 3-16). When random errors occur (Fig. 3-16A), points randomly move about the mean. Increases in the $S_{y/x}$ statistic reflect random error. Constant error (Fig. 3-16B) is seen visually as a shift in the y-intercept; a t-test analysis can be used to determine if these differences are significant. Proportional error (Fig. 3-16C) is reflected in alterations in line slope and can also be analyzed with a t-test (see Fig. 3-1).

Interpretation of experimental data is performed by using the results of the paired t-test and the correlation coefficient. The paired t-test is used to compare the magnitude of the bias (the difference between the mean of the test and that of the comparative method) with that of the random error. The t-test indicates only whether a statistically significant difference exists between the two SDs or means, respectively. It does not provide information on the magnitude of the error compared in the context of clinically allowable limits of error.[20]

A linear regression is performed to analyze COM studies (see Fig. 3-15). Hypothetically, when two tests perfectly give the same results (as in the linear relationship in Fig. 3-15A), the correlation coefficient (r^2) = 1. The correlation coefficient used in COM studies should be 0.99 (or greater), indicating that the range of patient samples is adequate for the standard linear regression analysis (described in the section on Descriptive Statistics of Groups of Paired Observations). If r^2 is less than 0.99, then alternative analyses should be used.[21-23] Linear regression analysis is more useful than the t-test for evaluating COM studies,[20] as the constant systemic error can be determined by the y-intercept and the proportional systemic error can be determined by the slope. Random error can also be determined by the standard error of the estimate ($S_{y/x}$). Importantly, if a nonlinear relationship occurs between the test and comparative methods, linear regression analysis can be used only over the values in the linear range. To make accurate conclusions about the relationship between two tests, it is important to confirm that outliers are true outliers and not the result of technical errors.

To this point, we have described how we estimate error test methods in terms of imprecision and inaccuracy.

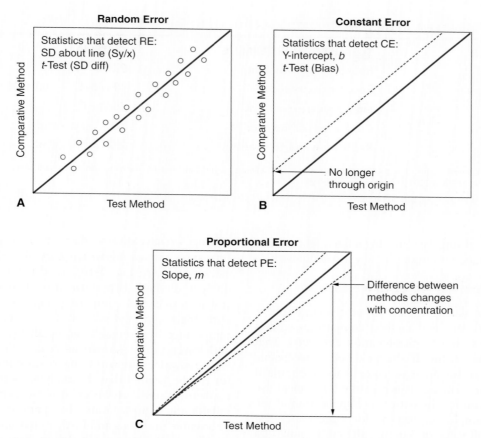

FIGURE 3-16 Examples of **(A)** random, **(B)** constant, and **(C)** proportional error using linear regression analysis. (Adapted from Westgard JO. *Basic Method Evaluation.* 2nd ed. Madison, WI: Westgard Quality Corp.; 2003.)

However, tests are performed to answer clinical questions, so to assess how this error might affect clinical judgments, it is assessed in terms of *allowable (analytic) error* (E_a).[24] This allowable error is determined for each test and is based on the amount of error that will not negatively affect clinical judgments. If both random and systemic error (total error) is less than E_a, then the performance of the test is considered acceptable. However, if the error is larger than E_a, corrections must be made to reduce the error or the method rejected. This process ensures that laboratory tests give accurate, clinically relevant information to physicians to manage their patients effectively.

Allowable Analytic Error

Probably the most important aspect of method evaluation is to determine if the random and systematic error (total error) is less than E_a. In the past, there have been several methodologies that have medically estimated E_a, including physiologic variation, multiples of the reference interval, and pathologist judgment.[25-28] The Clinical Laboratory Improvement Amendments of 1988 (CLIA 88) has published E_as for an array of clinical tests.[29] The E_a limits published by the CLIA specify the maximum

error allowable by federally mandated **proficiency testing** (see examples in Table 3-3). These performance standards are now being used to determine the acceptability of clinical chemistry analyzer performance.[30,31] The E_a is specifically calculated based on the types of studies described in the previous section (Table 3-4). While the specific mathematics are beyond the scope of this chapter, it is important to know that two sets of criteria are used in the evaluation of error: confidence interval criteria and single-value criteria.[9,24] An example of calculations made for the single-value criteria is shown in Table 3-4. Here, estimates of random and systematic error are calculated and then compared with the published allowable error at critical concentrations of the analyte. If the test does not meet the allowable error criteria, it must be modified to reduce error or rejected.

Comprehensive COM studies are demanding on personnel, time, and budgets. This has led to the description of abbreviated experiments that could be undertaken to estimate imprecision and inaccuracy.[32] CLIA has published guidelines for such an abbreviated application, which can be used by a laboratory to confirm that the precision and accuracy performance is consistent with the manufacturer's reported claims. These studies can be

TABLE 3-4	SINGLE-VALUE CRITERIA OF WESTGARD ET AL.	
TYPE OF ERROR	**TEST USED TO DETERMINE**	**CRITERIA**
Random error	Replication experiment	$2.58\ s < E_a$
Proportional error	Recovery experiment	$\mid (\text{Recovery} - 100) \times X_C/100 \mid < E_a$
Constant error	Interference experiment	$\mid \text{Bias} \mid < E_a$
Systemic error	Comparison of methods	$X0 \mid < E_a \mid (y_0 + mX_C)$
Total error	Replication and comparison	$2.58\ s + \mid y_0 + mX_C) - X_C \mid < E_a$

Based on National Committee for Clinical Laboratory Standards (NCCLS). *Approved Guideline for Handling and Processing of Blood Specimens.* 3rd ed. Villanova, PA: NCCLS; 2004 (Document no. H18-A3).

Medically acceptable error (E_a) based on performance standards set by CLIA, as shown in Table 3-12.

completed in 5 working days, making it likely laboratories will use these guidelines to set up new methodologies.

Method Evaluation Acceptance Criteria

Collectively, the data gathered in precision, linearity, interference, recovery, and method comparison studies are used to guide test implementation decisions. That is, the data do not define if a test method is acceptable by itself. Clinical judgment is required to determine if the analytical performance is acceptable for clinical use with consideration for the nature and application of the analyte. For example, imprecision for a pregnancy test around the cutoff value of 5 or 10 mIU/mL is more of a concern than it would be at 15,000 mIU/mL. Likewise, proportional bias for serum folate at a high concentration is of less concern than it is for a therapeutic drug near the clinical decision point. Thus, method evaluation studies and statistical analysis are necessary, but not sufficient to determine if a test is valid.

QUALITY CONTROL

QC in the laboratory involves the systematic monitoring of analytic processes to detect analytic errors that occur during analysis and to ultimately prevent the reporting of incorrect patient test results. In the context

DEFINITIONS BOX

Control limits: Threshold at which the value is statistically unlikely.

Control material: Material analyzed only for QC purposes.

Levey-Jennings control chart: Graphical representation of observed values of a control material over time in the context of the upper and lower control limits.

Multirule procedure: Decision criteria to determine if an analytic run is in control; used to detect random and systemic error over time.

of what we have discussed so far, QC is part of the performance monitoring that occurs after a test has been established (see Fig. 3-10). In general, monitoring of analytic methods is performed by assaying stable control materials and comparing their determined values with their expected values. The expected values are represented by intervals of acceptable values with upper and lower limits, known as *control limits*. When the expected values are within the control limits, the operator can be assured that the analytic method is properly reporting values. However, when observed values fall outside the control limits, the operator can be notified of possible problems and further analysis of the method can be made before potentially erroneously reporting patient results. The principles of statistically analyzing QC were initially applied to the clinical laboratory in the 1950s by Levey and Jennings.[33] Many important modifications have been made to these systems since that time, and they are discussed in general in this section.

Specimens analyzed for QC purposes are known as *QC materials*. These materials must be available in sufficient quantity to last at least a year and aliquoted in stable form. QC materials should be the same matrix as the specimens actually to be tested. For example, a glucose assay performed on serum should have QC materials that are prepared in serum. Variation between vials should be minimal so that differences seen over time can be attributed to the analytic method itself and not variation in the QC material. Control material concentrations should span the clinically important range of the analyte at appropriate decision levels. For example, sodium QC materials might be tested at 130 and 150 mmol/L, representing cutoff values for hyponatremia and hypernatremia, respectively. QC for general chemistry assays generally uses two levels of control, while immunoassays commonly use three. Today, laboratories more often purchase control materials from companies that manufacture products for QC, instead of preparing the materials themselves. These materials are often lyophilized (dehydrated to powder) for stability and can be reconstituted in specific diluents or matrices representing urine, blood, or cerebrospinal fluid (CSF). Control materials can be purchased with or without previously assayed ranges. Assayed materials give expected target ranges, often including the mean and SD using common analytic methods. While these products are more expensive because of the additional characterization, they allow another external check of method accuracy.

Because most commercially prepared control materials are lyophilized and require reconstitution before use, the diluent should be carefully added and mixed. Incomplete mixing yields a partition of supernatant liquid and underlying sediment and will result in incorrect control values. Frequently, the reconstituted material will be more turbid (cloudy) than the actual patient specimen. Stabilized frozen controls do not require reconstitution but may behave differently from patient specimens in some analytic systems. It is important to carefully evaluate these stabilized controls with any new instrument system.

QC Charts

A common method to assess the determination of control materials over time is by the use of a Levey-Jennings control chart (Fig. 3-17). Control charts graphically represent the observed values of a control material over time in the context of the upper and lower control limits. When the observed value falls with the control limits, it can be interpreted that the method is performed adequately. Points falling outside the control limits may suggest that problems may be developing. Control limits are expressed as the mean ± SD using formulas previously described in this chapter. Control charts can detect errors in accuracy and imprecision over time (Fig. 3-17A). Analytic errors that can occur can be separated into random and systematic errors as discussed in a previous chapter. The underlying rationale for running repeated assays is to detect random errors that affect precision (Fig. 3-17B, *middle*). Random errors may be caused by variations in technique. Systemic errors arise from factors that contribute to constant differences between measurements; these errors may be either positive or negative (Fig. 3-17B, *right*). Systemic errors may be due to several factors, including poorly made standards, reagents, and instrumentation problems or poorly written procedures.

Operation of a QC System

The QC system in the clinical laboratory is used to monitor the analytic variations that can occur. The QC program can be thought of as a three-stage process:

1. Establishing allowable statistical limits of variation for each analytic method
2. Using these limits as criteria for evaluating the QC data generated for each test

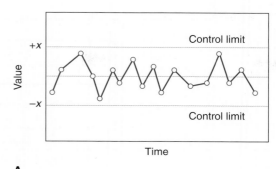

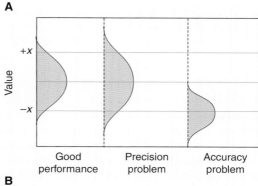

FIGURE 3-17 Levey-Jennings control chart. Data are plotted over time to identify quality control failures. (Adapted from Westgard JO, Klee GG. Quality management. In: Tietz NW, Burtis CA, Ashwood ER, Bruns DE, eds. *Tietz Textbook of Clinical Chemistry and Molecular Diagnostics.* 4th ed. St. Louis, MO: Elsevier Saunders; 2006: 485-529.)

3. Taking action to remedy errors when indicated

   a. Finding the cause(s) of error
   b. Taking corrective action
   c. Reanalyzing control and patient data

Establishment of a Statistical Quality Control

With a new instrument or with new lots of control material, the different levels of control material must be analyzed for 20 days. Exceptions include assays that are highly precise (CV < 1%), such as blood gases, where 5 days is adequate. Analysis of the control materials allows the determination of the mean and SD of control materials. Initial estimates of the mean and control limits may be somewhat inaccurate because of the low number of data points. Therefore, estimates of the mean and SDs should be frequently updated to include accumulated data to produce more reliable data. When changing to a new lot of similar material, laboratorians use the newly obtained mean as the target mean but retain the previous SD. As more data are obtained, all data should be averaged to derive the best estimates of the mean and SD.[34]

The distribution of error is assumed to be symmetrical and bell shaped (Gaussian) as shown in Figure 3-18. Control limits are set to include most observed values

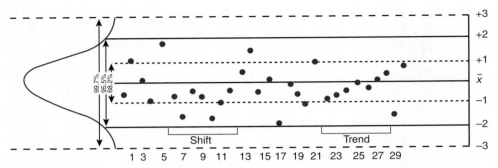

FIGURE 3-18 Control chart showing the relationship of control limits to the Gaussian distribution. Daily control values are graphed, and they show examples of a shift, an abrupt change in the analytic process, and a trend, a gradual change in the analytic process.

(95% to 99.7%), corresponding to the mean ±2 or 3 SDs. Observation of values in the distribution tails should therefore be rare (1/20 for 2 SDs; 3/1,000 for 3 SDs). Observations outside the control limits suggest changes in the analytic methods. If the process is in control, no more than 0.3% of the points will be outside the 3 SDs (3s) limits. Analytic methods are considered in control if a symmetrical distribution of control values about the mean is seen, and few values outside the 2 SDs (2s) control limits are observed. Some laboratories define a method out of control if a control value exceeds the 2s limits. Other laboratories use the 2s limit as a warning limit and the 3s limit as an error limit. In this particular case, a control point between 2s and 3s would alert the technologist to a potential problem, while a point greater than 3s would require a corrective action. The selection of control rules and numbers should be related to the goals set by the laboratory.[35] Understanding the problem of false rejections and its relationship to the control limits chosen for the Levey-Jennings plot is vital. False rejections can occur because of the control limits set and not actually identify a problem with the assay. The use of a 3s control limit reduces the false rejection problem, with a corresponding loss of error detection.

Multirules RULE!

The use of the statistical process control chart (Levey-Jennings) was pioneered by Shewhart in the 1920s. Multirules were formalized by the Western Electric Company and later applied to the clinical laboratory by Westgard and Groth.[36] Multirules establish a criterion for judging whether an analytic process is out of control. To simplify the various control rules, abbreviations are used to refer to the various control rules (Table 3-14). Control rules indicate the number of control observations per analytic run, followed by the control amount in subscript.[37] For example, the 1_{3s} rule indicates that a data point cannot exceed 3 SDs (3s). If the 1_{3s} rule is not triggered, the analytic run will be accepted (i.e., results will be reported). If the QC results are more than of 3 SDs (the 1_{3s} rule is violated), the run may be rejected and there will be additional investigation. The type of rule violated indicates what type of error exists. For example, a 1_{3s} rule violation may indicate a loss of precision or "random error" (Table 3-5).

Analogous to overlapping diseased and healthy patient results, it is important to consider that not every rule violation indicates that a process is out of control. The 1_{2s} rule, for example, will be outside the 2s limit in 5% of the runs with normal analytic variation (Fig. 3-19A). The 10_X rule is

TABLE 3-5	MULTIRULE PROCEDURES
• 1_{2s} One control observation exceeding the mean ±2s. A warning rule that initiates testing of control data by other rules.	
• 1_{3s} One control observation exceeding the mean ±3s. Allows high sensitivity to random error.	
• 2_{2s} Two control observations consecutively exceeding the same +2s or −2s. Allows high sensitivity to systemic error.	
• R_{4s} One control exceeding the +2s and another exceeding the −2s. Allows detection of random error.	
• 4_{1s} Four consecutive control observations exceeding +1s or −1s. This allows the detection of systemic error.	
• 10_X Ten consecutive control observations falling on one side or the other of the mean (no requirement for SD size). This allows the detection of systemic error.	

SD, standard deviation.

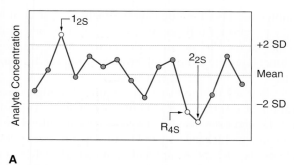

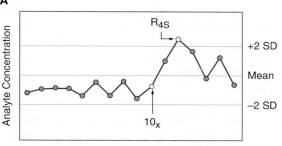

A

B

FIGURE 3-19 Application of multirule procedures. Multirules are used to identify errors while minimizing false-error detection. Multirules can help identify different types of errors that might occur (identified in *red*).

DEFINITIONS BOX

Proficiency test: Method used to validate a particular measurement process. The results are compared with other external laboratories to give an objective indication of test accuracy.
Proficiency samples: Specimens that have known concentrations of an analyte for the test of interest. The testing laboratory does not know the targeted concentration when tested.

violated if 10 consecutive control observations fall on one side or the other of the mean (Fig. 3-19B). The more levels of QC material analyzed, the higher the probability of a rule violation even in the absence of true error. When two controls are used, there is an approximately 10% chance that at least one control will be outside the 2s limits; when four controls are used, there is a 17% chance. For this reason, many laboratories use 2s limits as a warning rather than criteria for run rejection; laboratories may merely re-assay the controls rather than reject the entire run.

Proficiency Testing

In addition to daily QC practices, laboratories are required to participate in external proficiency testing programs. Acceptable performance in proficiency testing programs is required by the CAP, the CLIA, and TJC to maintain laboratory accreditation. Even more important, proficiency testing is another tool in the ongoing process of monitoring test performance.

The majority of clinical laboratories subscribe to the proficiency program provided by the CAP. The CAP program has been in existence for 50 years and it is the gold standard for clinical laboratory proficiency testing. In our laboratory, the majority of analytes are monitored with the CAP proficiency surveys. Other proficiency testing programs are often used when analytes of interest are not tested through CAP (e.g., esoteric tests) or as a means to supplement CAP proficiency testing programs. Additional proficiency programs used in our laboratory include the International Sirolimus Proficiency Testing Scheme (IST), the Binding Site, the American Proficiency Institute (API), and the Centers for Disease Control and Prevention (CDC). If there is no commercial proficiency testing program available for an analyte, the laboratory is required to implement a non–proficiency test scheme; this is reviewed at the end of this section.

For a proficiency test, a series of unknown samples are sent to the laboratory from the program offering this analysis, such as CAP. The samples are analyzed in the same manner as patient specimens, and the results are reported to the proficiency program. The program then compiles the results from all of the laboratories participating in the survey and sends a performance report back to each participating laboratory. Each analyte has a defined performance criteria (e.g., ±3 SDs to peer mean), where laboratories using the same method are graded by comparing them with the group. Some proficiency tests are not quantitative and are qualitatively compared with other laboratories. Areas of pathology other than clinical chemistry are also subjected to mandatory proficiency qualitative/

INDICATORS OF ANALYTIC PERFORMANCE

Proficiency testing
Internal quality control
Laboratory inspections (accreditation)
Quality assurance monitoring
Clinical utilization

EXAMPLE OF PROFICIENCY TEST RESULTS FOR βHCG

βhCG-08: CAP value = 75.58; SD = 4.80;
    CV = 6.4%; n = 47 peer laboratories
Evaluation criteria: Peer group ±3 SDs;
    acceptable range 65.7–85.2 mIU/mL
Testing laboratory value = 71.54; SDI = –0.84
    acceptable

interpretive testing, including anatomic pathology, clinical microbiology, and clinical microscopy.

An example of a hypothetical survey is shown in the text box above. The βhCG survey was the eighth sample sent in that year (βhCG-08). The mean of all the laboratories using the same method was 75.58 mIU/mL. The SD and CV are indicated, as is the number of laboratories that participate in that survey ($n = 47$). The acceptance criteria were that the test result was within ±3 SDs (i.e., between 65.7 and 85.2 mIU/mL). The laboratory's result was 71.54 mIU/mL, which is −0.84 SD from the mean and is within the acceptable limits.

When a laboratory performs proficiency testing, there are strict requirements as follows:

1. The laboratory must incorporate proficiency testing into its routine workflow as much as possible.
2. The test values/samples must not be shared with other laboratories at any time during the testing cycle.
3. Proficiency samples are tested by bench technical staff who normally conduct patient testing; there can be no unnecessary repeats or actions outside of how a patient sample would be tested and reported.
4. Testing should be completed within the usual time it would take for routine patient testing.

The bottom line is that the sample should be treated like a patient sample to yield a true indication of test accuracy. Unless a laboratory is in the practice of running every sample twice, they cannot do this for the proficiency sample.

The acceptability criteria for proficiency testing are provided by the proficiency program. For regulated analytes, these criteria are often the CLIA limits (see Table 3-3). For nonregulated analytes, acceptable criteria are often determined by the scientific community at large. For example, the acceptability criterion for lactate dehydrogenase is ±20% or 3 SDs (whichever is greater) based on peer group data.

Proficiency testing allows each laboratory to compare its test results with those of other laboratories that use the same or similar instruments and methods. Proficiency testing provides performance data for a given analyte at a specific point in time. Comparison of performance to a robust, statistically valid peer group is essential to identify areas for improvement. Areas of improvement that may be identified in a single proficiency testing event or over multiple events include variation from peer group results, imprecision, and/or results that trend above or below the mean consistently or at specific analyte concentrations. Use of these data allows laboratories to continuously improve their test performance. The proficiency testing samples also can serve as valuable troubleshooting aids when investigating problem analytes. In our hospital, proficiency

samples are also included in the technologist competency program. Proficiency tests can also be beneficial in validating the laboratory's measurement method, technical training, and uncertainty budgets for new tests.

Proficiency testing programs require thorough investigation of discrepant results for any analyte (i.e., failure). Laboratories may be asked to submit information that could include current and historical proficiency testing reports, QC and equipment monitoring, analysis and corrective action of the problem that caused the failure, and the steps taken to ensure the reliability of patient test results. If the laboratory cannot resolve analyte testing discrepancies, the testing facility may be at risk of losing the authority to perform patient testing for the analyte(s) in question.

To develop and manage a successful proficiency testing program for the clinical laboratory, it is important to understand the documented requirements from the two main accreditation bodies. A large proficiency testing program often requires considerable personnel resources and costs for the laboratory and is an essential factor in providing a quality management system. As an example of the scale and volume of proficiency tests, our laboratory (for a 700-bed hospital with outreach clinics) performed ≈9,000 proficiency tests in a year for ≈500 individual analytes. Besides meeting required accreditation standards, proficiency testing allows the laboratory to objectively ensure they report patient results accurately.

REFERENCE INTERVAL STUDIES

Laboratory test data are used to make medical diagnoses, assess physiologic function, and manage therapy. When interpreting laboratory data, clinicians compare the measured test result from a patient with a reference interval.

Reference intervals include all the data points that define the range of observations (e.g., if the interval is 5 to 10, a patient result of 5 would be considered within the interval). The upper and lower reference limits are set to define a specified percentage (usually 95%) of the values for a population; this means that a percentage (usually 5%) of patients will fall outside the reference interval in the absence of any condition or disease. Reference intervals are sometimes erroneously

DEFINITIONS BOX

Reference interval: A pair of medical decision points that span the limits of results expected for a defined healthy population.

called "normal ranges." While all normal ranges are in fact reference intervals, not all reference intervals are normal ranges. This is exemplified by the reference interval for therapeutic drug levels. In this case, a "normal" individual would not have any drug in their system, whereas a patient on therapy has a defined target range. Reference intervals are sometimes called reference ranges; the preferred term is reference interval because range implies the absolute maximum and minimum values.

The theory for the development of reference intervals was the work of two main expert committees.[38-41] These committees established the importance of standardizing collection procedures, the use of statistical methods for analysis of reference values and estimation of reference intervals, and the selection of reference populations. Reference intervals are usually established by the scientific community or the manufacturers of reagents and new methodologies. Developing reference intervals often has a financial impact on vendors and marketing of the laboratory products. Laboratorians must be aware of these scientific and economic forces when reviewing vendor data and determining the need for reference interval studies. The two main types of reference interval studies that are reviewed in this section are (1) establishing a reference interval and (2) verifying a reference interval.

The clinical laboratory is required by good laboratory practice and accreditation agencies (i.e., the CAP checklist) to either verify or establish reference intervals for any new tests or significant changes in methodology.

DEFINITIONS BOX

Establishing a reference interval: A new reference interval is established when there is no existing analyte or methodology in the clinical or reference laboratory with which to conduct comparative studies. It is a costly and labor-intensive study that will involve laboratory resources at all levels and may require from 120 to as many as ≈700 study individuals.

Verifying a reference interval (transference): This is done to confirm the validity of an existing reference interval for an analyte using the same (identical) type of analytic system (method and/or instrument). These are the most common reference interval studies performed in the clinical laboratory and can require as few as 20 study individuals.

The core protocols for both establishing and verifying reference ranges are reviewed in this section. Other terms are used for values or ranges that help the clinician determine the relationship of patients' test results to statistically determined values or ranges for the clinical condition under treatment.

BOX 3-3 EXAMPLES OF CAP CHECKLIST QUESTIONS REGARDING REFERENCE INTERVALS FOR LABORATORY INSPECTION

The laboratory establishes or verifies its reference intervals (normal values)

NOTE: Reference intervals are important to allow a clinician to assess patient results against an appropriate population. The reference range must be established or verified for each analyte and specimen source (e.g., blood, urine, and CSF), when appropriate. For many analytes (e.g., therapeutic drugs and CSF total protein), literature references or a manufacturer's package insert information may be appropriate.

Evidence of Compliance

Record of reference range study or records of verification of manufacturer's stated range when reference range study is not practical (e.g., unavailable normal population) or other methods approved by the laboratory director.[47-49]

The laboratory evaluates the appropriateness of its reference intervals and takes corrective action if necessary

Criteria for evaluation of reference intervals include the following:

1. Introduction of a new analyte to the test repertoire
2. Change of analytic methodology
3. Change in patient population

If it is determined that the range is no longer appropriate for the patient population, corrective action must be taken.[42-44]

Evidence of Compliance

Records of evaluation and corrective action, if indicated

Adapted with permission from Sarewitz SJ, ed. *Laboratory Accreditation Program Inspection Checklists.* Northfield, IL: College of American Pathologists; 2009.

DEFINITIONS BOX

Medical decision level: Value for an analyte that represents the boundary between different therapeutic approaches.

Normal range: Range of results between two medical decision points that correspond to the central 95% of results from a healthy patient population. Note: Of the results, 2.5% will be above the upper limit and 2.5% will be below the lower limit of the normal range.

Therapeutic range: Reference interval applied to a therapeutic drug. Reference intervals are needed for all tests in the clinical laboratory, and the provision of reliable reference intervals is an important task for clinical laboratories and test manufacturers. The dynamic review of existing reference intervals by the health care team (scientific community, manufacturers, and clinical laboratory) is crucial to meeting the challenges of providing optimal laboratory data for patient care.

TABLE 3-7 — βHCG AT DEFINED GESTATIONAL AGE

APPROXIMATE βHCG LEVELS AT DEFINED GESTATIONAL AGE UNITS MIU/ML (U/L)

WEEKS OF PREGNANCY	MEAN	RANGE	N
4	1,110	40–4,480	42
5	8,050	270–28,700	52
6	29,700	3,700–84,900	67
7	58,800	9,700–120,000	62
8	79,500	31,000–184,000	37
9	91,500	61,200–152,000	25
10	71,000	22,000–143,000	12
14	33,100	14,300–75,800	219
15	27,500	12,300–60,300	355
16	21,900	8,800–54,500	163
17	18,000	8,100–51,300	68
18	18,400	3,900–49,400	30
19	20,900	3,600–56,600	14

The application of reference intervals can be grouped into three main categories: diagnosis of a disease or condition (Table 3-6), monitoring of a physiologic condition (Table 3-7), or monitoring therapeutic drugs (Table 3-8). These different applications require different approaches for determination of a reference interval. Specifically, therapeutic drug targets are not derived from a healthy population and unique physiologically conditions require the appropriate reference population.

Tables 3-6, 3-7, and 3-8 also demonstrate the complexity of reference intervals when multiple levels (partitions) of reference intervals are required by the clinician. The framework for verifying or establishing reference intervals is one that can be overwhelming for the clinical laboratory. The costs, personnel, and resource requirements mandate that the reference interval experiment be well defined and structured in such a manner to provide accurate and timely reference intervals for optimal clinical use. Where possible, the clinical laboratory director may determine that a review of literature references or manufacturer's package inserts are appropriate in assigning reference intervals for an analyte or this additional information may allow for the shorter reference interval verification study (i.e., 20 study individuals).

Establishing Reference Intervals

The Clinical and Laboratory Standards Institute (CLSI, formerly National Committee for Clinical Laboratory Standards [NCCLS]) has published a preferred guideline/resource for establishing or verification of reference intervals.[45] A summary of the CLSI recommendations is given next.

TABLE 3-6 — THYROID-STIMULATING HORMONE (TSH) THYROID DISEASE

PATIENTS	AGE	TSH REFERENCE RANGES (µIU/ML)
Pediatric	0–3 d	1.00–20.00
	3–30 d	0.50–6.50
	31 d to 5 m	0.50–6.00
	6 m to 18 y	0.50–4.50
Adults, ambulatory, healthy	>18 y	0.60–3.30

Based on Dugaw KA, Jack RM, Rutledge J. Pediatric reference ranges for TSH, free T4, total T4 total T3 and T3 uptake on the vitros ECi analyzer. *Clin Chem.* 2001;47:A108.

TABLE 3-8 — THERAPEUTIC MANAGEMENT TARGETS FOR DIGOXIN

Normal	0.8–1.8 ng/mL (collected 6 h after dose)
Critical	>2.0 ng/mL

BOX 3-4 TO ESTABLISH A REFERENCE RANGE STUDY

1. Define an appropriate list of biological variations and analytic interferences from medical literature.
2. Choose selection and partition (e.g., age or gender) criteria.
3. Complete a written consent form and questionnaire to capture selection criteria.
4. Categorize the potential reference individuals based on the questionnaire findings.
5. Exclude individuals from the reference sample group based on exclusion criteria.
6. Define the number of reference individuals in consideration of desired confidence limits and statistical accuracy.
7. Standardize collection and analysis of reference specimens for the measurement of a given analyte consistent with the routine practice of patients.
8. Inspect the reference value data and prepare a histogram to evaluate the distribution of data.
9. Identify possible data errors and/or outliers and then analyze the reference values.
10. Document all of the previously mentioned steps and procedures.

BOX 3-5 EXAMPLE QUESTIONNAIRE

Creatinine Clearance Example
Time Urine Instructions Creatinine
Donor Number: _____
Sex: _____
Height: _____ Weight: _____
Exercise routine: _____
Pregnancy: Yes/No
Medications: _____

Selection of Reference Interval Study Individuals

The selection of individuals who can be included in a reference interval study requires defining detailed inclusion/exclusion criteria. Inclusion criteria define what factors (e.g., age and gender) are required to be used for the study, while exclusion criteria list factors that render individuals inappropriate for the study (Table 3-9). It is essential to select the appropriate individuals to obtain the optimal set of specimens with an acceptable level of confidence. Determination of the necessary inclusion and exclusion criteria for donor selection may require extensive literature searches and review with laboratory directors and clinicians. Initially, it must be exactly defined what is a "healthy"/"normal" donor for associated reference values. For example, for

a βhCG reference interval study, one would exclude pregnant women or those who may be pregnant, as well as individuals with βhCG-producing tumors. An important note to make is that laboratories are often challenged to locate donors outside the laboratory working environment, who may be largely females under 40 years of age. The use of donors who may not represent the population of interest has the potential to skew the evaluation data used to establish the reference interval. Inpatient samples should not be used for reference interval studies that are designed to reflect a population.

Capturing the appropriate information for the inclusion and exclusion criteria, such as donor health status, often requires a well-written confidential questionnaire and consent form. The following is an example of a questionnaire from a creatinine clearance reference interval study:

Another consideration when selecting individuals for a reference interval study is additional factors that may require partitioning individuals into subgroups (Table 3-10). These subgroups may require separate reference interval studies. Fortunately, a large number of laboratory tests do not require partitioning and can be used with only one reference interval that is not dependent on a variety of factors (Table 3-11). These real

TABLE 3-9	EXAMPLES OF POSSIBLE EXCLUSION FACTORS FOR A REFERENCE INTERVAL STUDY
Fasting or nonfasting	Pregnancy
Genetic factors	Illness, recent
Drugs: prescription or over the counter	Exercise pattern

TABLE 3-10	EXAMPLES OF POSSIBLE SUBGROUPS REQUIRING PARTITIONS FOR A REFERENCE INTERVAL STUDY
Age (adult and childhood)	Stage of pregnancy
Fasting or nonfasting	Sex
Diet	Tobacco use

TABLE 3-11	EXAMPLE OF A SIMPLE REFERENCE INTERVAL
Plasma potassium	3.5–5.0 mmol/L

examples are testimony to the complexity of conducting reference interval studies. The initial selection of individual donors is crucial to the successful evaluation of reference intervals.

Preanalytic and Analytic Considerations

Once individuals are selected for a reference interval study, it is important to consider both preanalytic and analytic variables that can affect specific laboratory tests (Table 3-12). Preanalytic and analytic variables must be controlled and standardized to generate a valid reference interval. To illustrate these points, we discuss establishing a reference interval for fasting glucose. An obvious preanalytic variable that should be addressed for this test is that individuals should not eat for at least 8 hours prior to sample collection. In terms of analytic factors, it is important to define acceptable levels of common interferences, such as hemolysis or lipemia. For fasting glucose, the laboratorian must define whether samples with excess hemolysis or lipemia will be included in the study; this depends, in part, on whether the interferences affect the methods (in this case, glucose). If specific interferences do affect the accuracy of the test, it is essential that interferences can be flagged, to appropriately deal with the results and interpretation. Hemolysis and lipemia can be detected automatically by large chemistry analyzers, but not small point-of-care tests; this could lead to errors when using point-of-care tests. It is also worth considering that some methods are more sensitive to interferences. Mass spectrometry, for example, can be relatively resistant to interferences, whereas chemical methods are at times highly sensitive to this problem. It is also necessary to consider what specific reagents are used in an assay. Changing to a new reagent lot in the middle of a reference study could widen the reference interval or change the data distribution (e.g., change from normal to bimodal). Thus, an effective reference interval study requires extensive knowledge of the analyte, analytic parameters, methodology, and instrumentation.

Determining Whether to Establish or Verify Reference Intervals

Whether to verify a reference interval or establish an entirely new reference interval for a new method/analyte depends on several factors, such as the presence of an existing reference interval for assay and on the results of a statistical analysis comparing the test method with the reference method. The most basic method comparison involves plotting a reference method against a test method and fitting a linear regression (described in Fig. 3-7). If the correlation coefficient is 1.0, slope is 1.000, and intercept is 0.000, the two methods agree and may not require new reference ranges. In this case, a simple reference interval verification study is all that may be required. Conversely, if the two methods differ considerably, then a new reference interval needs to be established.

Analysis of Reference Values

DEFINITIONS BOX

Nonparametric method: Statistical test that makes no specific assumption about the distribution of data. Nonparametric methods rank the reference data in order of increasing size. Because the majority of analytes are not normally (Gaussian) distributed (see Fig. 3-6), nonparametric tests are the recommended analysis for most reference range intervals.

Parametric method: Statistical test that assumes the observed values, or some mathematical transformation of those values, follow a (normal) Gaussian distribution (see Fig. 3-6).

Confidence interval: Range of values that include a specified probability, usually 90% or 95%. For example, consider a 95% confidence interval for slope = 0.972–0.988 from a method comparison experiment. If this same experiment were conducted 100 times, then the slope would fall between 0.972 and 0.988 in 95 of the 100 times. Confidence intervals serve to convey the variability of estimates and quantify the variability.

Bias: Difference between the observed mean and the reference mean. Negative bias indicates that the test values tend to be lower than the reference value, whereas positive bias indicates test values are generally higher. Bias is a type of constant systematic error.

TABLE 3-12	PREANALYTIC AND ANALYTIC CONSIDERATIONS FOR REFERENCE INTERVAL STUDIES
PREANALYTIC FACTORS	
Subject preparation	Sample storage
Prescription medications	Stress
Collection time	Food/beverage ingestion
ANALYTIC FACTORS	
Precision	Linearity
Accuracy	Interference
Lot-to-lot reagents	Recovery

Data Analysis to Establish a Reference Interval

To establish a reference interval, it is recommended that the study includes at least 120 individuals. This can be challenging and costly, but it may be necessary for esoteric and laboratory-developed tests. Once the raw data have been generated, the next step is to actually define the reference interval. The reference interval is calculated statistically using methods that depend on the distribution of the data. In the most basic sense, data may be either normally distributed (Gaussian) or skewed (non-Gaussian) (see Fig. 3-6). If reference data are normally distributed, the reference interval can be determined using a parametric method. A parametric method defines the interval by the mean ± 1.96 SDs; by centering on the mean, this formula will include the central 95% of values as given in the example in Figure 3-20A.

In reality, most analytes do not display a normal (Gaussian) distribution. For example, the distribution of

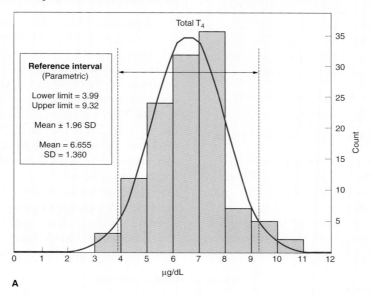

A

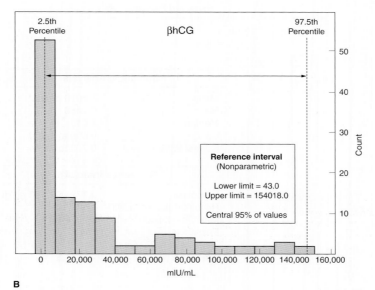

B

FIGURE 3-20 (A) Histogram of total thyroxine (TT_4) levels in a real population illustrating a shape indicative of a Gaussian distribution, which is analyzed by parametric statistics. The reference interval is determined from the mean ± 1.96 SDs. **(B)** Histogram of beta-human chorionic gonadotropin (βhCG) levels in a population of pregnant women demonstrating non-Gaussian data and nonparametric determination of the reference interval. The reference interval is determined from percentiles to include the central 95% of values. Although the selection of a wide range of gestational ages makes this a poor population for a reference interval study, it does demonstrate the application of nonparametric intervals.

βhCG in pregnant individuals over a range of gestational ages is skewed (Fig. 3-20B); although the selection of a wide range of gestational ages makes this a poor population for a reference interval study, it was selected as an example to emphasize the need for nonparametric intervals. Data that are not normally distributed (i.e., non-Gaussian) must be analyzed using nonparametric analyses. Nonparametric determination of the reference interval is analyzed using percentiles, which do not depend on the distribution. The reference interval is determined by using the central 95% of values; the reference range is therefore defined by the 2.5th to the 97.5th percentiles, as demonstrated in Figure 3-20B. To calculate the interval, values are ranked from lowest to highest and the 2.5th and 97.5th percentiles are then calculated as follows:

$$n = \text{number of reference specimens}$$
$$2.5\text{th percentile} = 0.025(n + 1)$$
$$97.5\text{th percentile} = 0.975(n + 1) \quad \textbf{(Eq. 3-7)}$$

Most reference interval analyses are determined using nonparametric analysis. This is because nonparametric analysis can be used on Gaussian distributed data and it is the CLSI-recommended method (Fig. 3-20B).[45]

With the development of statistical software packages such as EP Evaluator, Analyse-it, StatisPro, MedCalc, GraphPad Prism, Minitab, R, JMP, and SAS/STAT, reference intervals are rarely determined manually (hyperlinks to the software providers are supplied at the end of the chapter). However, it is important to understand how basic statistical concepts are used by the software to generate their analyses. For more information on these software programs, the interested reader can access the references and online resources listed at the end of the chapter.

Data Analysis to Verify a Reference Interval (Transference)

When possible, clinical laboratories rely on assay manufacturers or on published primary literature to determine reference intervals. This avoids the expensive and lengthy process of establishing a reference range interval on a minimum of 120 healthy people. The CLSI allows less vigorous studies to verify a reference interval with as few as 20 subject specimens.[45] Method verification studies can be used if the test method and study subjects are similar to the vendor's reference data and package insert information. The main assumption in using transference studies is that the reference method is of high quality and the subject populations are similar. The manufacturer's reported 95% reference limits may be considered valid if no more than 10% of the tested subjects fall outside the original reported limits. Figure 3-21 shows an example from our laboratory where we verify the manufacturer's

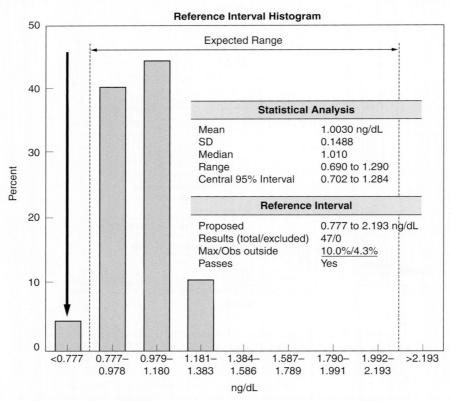

FIGURE 3-21 Reference verification test for free thyroxine (fT₄). Only 4.3% of the values are outside the expected range (*arrow*). The test passes because this is less than the allowable number of outlying samples (10%) (underlined in *red*).

reference range for free thyroxine (fT_4). In this example, fewer than 10% are outside the manufacturer's limits, enabling the reference interval to be adopted by the laboratory. If more than 10% of the values fall outside the proposed interval, an additional 20 or more specimens should be analyzed. If the second attempt at verification fails, the laboratorian should reexamine the analytic procedure and identify any differences between the laboratory's population and the population used by the manufacturer for their analysis. If no differences are identified, the laboratory may need to establish the reference interval using at least 120 individuals. Figure 3-22 demonstrates a simple algorithm to verify reference intervals.

Once a reference interval is determined, it needs to be communicated to the physicians interpreting test results at the time the test results are reported. This is important given the slight variations in reference intervals seen even among testing facilities using similar methodologies. It is considered good laboratory practice to monitor reference intervals regularly. Some common problems that occur when determining reference intervals are given in Table 3-13. To help identify reference interval problems, the clinical laboratorian should be aware of common flags. These flags often come in the form of an event or communication that alerts the laboratory that there is a potential problem with a test. Based on our observations, flags for reference intervals can include vendor notifications, clinician queries of a particular test, and **shifts/trends** in large average numbers of patients

TABLE 3-13	COMMON PROBLEMS ENCOUNTERED WHEN MONITORING REFERENCE INTERVALS
Changes in reagent formulations by the vendor (e.g., new antibody)	
Minor changes in reagents due to lot-to-lot variations	
Differences between reference interval and test populations—selection bias	

over time. Any of these or other related factors may warrant a review of existing reference intervals.

Not all analytes use population-based reference intervals. For example, therapeutic drugs are not found in healthy individuals, such that the target values are based either on toxicity limits or on minimum effective concentrations. The target limits are derived from clinical or pharmacological studies rather than the healthy population studies described above. In these situations, the need for analytical accuracy is essential. One cannot apply a clinical cutpoint for a test if the results do not agree with the method used to determine the cutpoint. Cholesterol and HbA1c are also used in the context of clinical outcomes rather than reflecting values in a healthy population. The quintessential example of this is vitamin D testing in extreme latitudes, where a healthy population will be deficient.

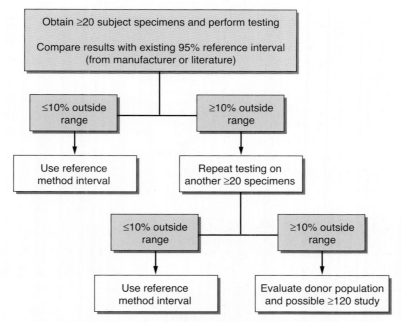

FIGURE 3-22 Algorithm to test whether a reference interval can be verified. A published reference interval (from a manufacturer or scientific literature) can be adopted if only a few samples fall outside the range. When possible, laboratory reference intervals are verified because of the time and expense of establishing a new interval.

DIAGNOSTIC EFFICIENCY

Ideally, healthy patients would have completely distinct laboratory values from patients with disease (Fig. 3-23A). However, the reality is that laboratory values usually overlap significantly between these populations (Fig. 3-23B). To determine how good a given test is at detecting and predicting the presence of disease (or a physiologic condition), there are a number of different parameters that are used. These parameters are broadly defined as *diagnostic efficiency*, which can be broken down into sensitivity, specificity, and predictive values.

DEFINITIONS BOX

Diagnostic sensitivity: Ability of a test to detect a given disease or condition.
Diagnostic specificity: Ability of a test to correctly identify the absence of a given disease or condition.
Positive predictive value: Chance of an individual having a given disease or condition if the test is abnormal.
Negative predictive value: Chance an individual does not have a given disease or condition if the test is within the reference interval.

Measures of Diagnostic Efficiency

Parameters of diagnostic efficiency are intended to quantify how useful a test is for a given disease or condition.[46] For example, βhCG is used as a test to diagnose pregnancy. While βhCG is excellent for this purpose, there are instances where βhCG may be increased because of other causes, such as cancer (trophoblastic tumors), or below the cutoff, as is the case very early in pregnancy.

It is important to recognize that there is both diagnostic and clinical sensitivity. Analytic sensitivity refers to the lower limit of detection for a given analyte (described in the Method Evaluation section), whereas clinical sensitivity refers to the proportion of individuals with that disease who test positively with the test. *Sensitivity* can be calculated from simple ratios (Fig. 3-24A). Patients with a condition who are correctly classified by a test to have the condition are called true positives (TPs). Patients with the condition who are classified by the test as not having the condition are called false negatives (FNs). Using the βhCG test as an example, sensitivity can be calculated as follows:

$$\text{Diagnostic sensitivity (\%)} = \frac{\text{(No. of pregnant with positive test)}}{\text{(No. of pregnant individuals tested)}}$$

$$(TP)/(TP + FN) \qquad \text{(Eq. 3-8)}$$

Another measure of clinical performance is diagnostic specificity. *Diagnostic specificity* is defined as the

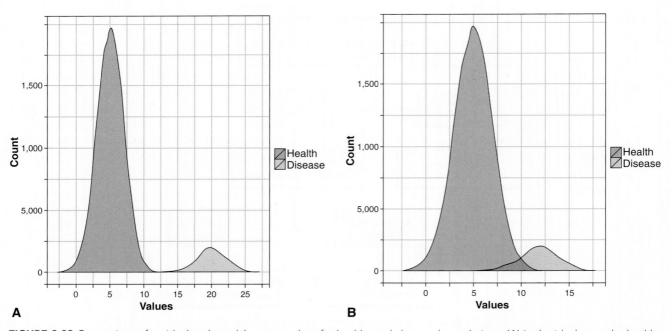

FIGURE 3-23 Comparison of an ideal and true laboratory values for healthy and abnormal populations. **(A)** In the ideal case, the healthy population is completely distinct from those with the condition. **(B)** In reality, values show significant overlap that affects the diagnostic efficiency of the test.

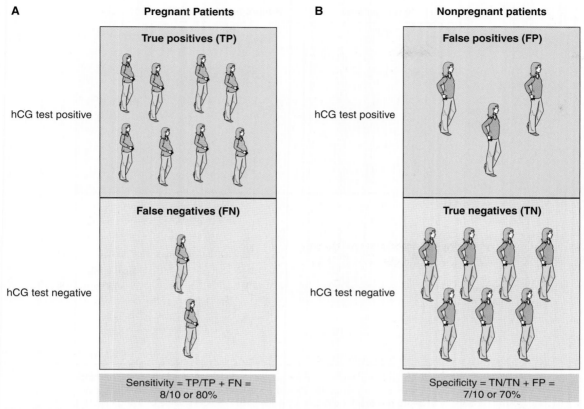

A   **Pregnant Patients**

True positives (TP)

hCG test positive

False negatives (FN)

hCG test negative

Sensitivity = TP/TP + FN =
8/10 or 80%

B   **Nonpregnant patients**

False positives (FP)

hCG test positive

True negatives (TN)

hCG test negative

Specificity = TN/TN + FP =
7/10 or 70%

FIGURE 3-24 The sensitivity and specificity of beta-human chorionic gonadotropin (βhCG) for pregnancy. **(A)** Sensitivity refers to the ability to detect pregnancy. **(B)** Specificity refers to the ability of the test to correctly classify nonpregnant women. FN, false negative; FP, false positive; TN, true negative; TP, true positive.

proportion of individuals without a condition who have a negative test for that condition (Fig. 3-24B). Note that there is also an analytic specificity (described in the Method Evaluation section), which refers to cross-reactivity with other substances. Continuing with βhCG as an example, diagnostic specificity refers to the percentage of nonpregnant individuals that have a negative test compared with the number of nonpregnant individuals tested. Patients who are not pregnant and have a negative βhCG test are called true negatives (TNs), whereas those who are incorrectly classified as pregnant by the test are called false positives (FPs). Clinical specificity can be calculated as follows:

$$\text{Specificity (\%)} = \frac{(\text{No. of nonpregnant with negative test})}{(\text{No. of nonpregnant individuals tested})}$$

$$(TN)/(TN + FP) \qquad \text{(Eq. 3-9)}$$

For example, a sensitivity of 100% plus a specificity of 100% means that the test detects every patient with disease and that the test is negative for every patient without the disease. Because of the overlap in laboratory values between people with and without disease, this is, of course, almost never the case (see Fig. 3-23B).

There are other measures of diagnostic efficiency such as predictive values. There are predictive values for both positive and negative test results. The predictive value of a positive (PPV) test refers to the probability of an individual having the disease if the result is abnormal ("positive" for the condition). Conversely, the predictive value of a negative (NPV) test refers to the probability that a patient does not have a disease if a result is within the reference range (test is negative for the disease) (Fig. 3-25). Predictive values are also calculated using ratios of TPs, TNs, FPs, and FNs as follows:

$$PPV = \frac{(\text{No. of pregnant with positive test})}{(\text{No. with positive test})}$$

$$(TP)/(TP + FP) \qquad \text{(Eq. 3-10)}$$

$$NPV = \frac{(\text{No. of nonpregnant with negative test})}{(\text{No. with negative test})}$$

$$(TN)/(TN + FN) \qquad \text{(Eq. 3-11)}$$

Using the data from Figure 3-25, if the βhCG test is "positive," there is a 72% chance the patient is pregnant; if the test is negative, then there is a 78% chance the

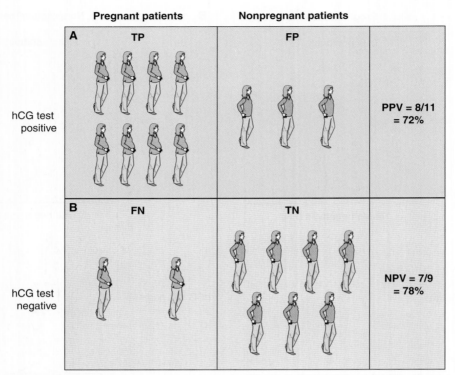

FIGURE 3-25 Positive and negative predictive values using beta-human chorionic gonado-tropin (βhCG) as a test for pregnancy. **(A)** Predictive value of a positive test (PPV) indicates the probability of being pregnant if the test is positive. **(B)** Predictive value of a negative test (NPV) refers to the probability of being nonpregnant if the test is negative. FN, false nega-tive; FP, false positive; TN, true negative; TP, true positive.

patient is not pregnant. It is important to understand that unlike sensitivity and specificity, predictive values depend on the prevalence of the condition in the popula-tion studied. Prevalence refers to the proportion of indi-viduals within a given population who have a particular condition. If one were testing for βhCG, the prevalence of pregnancy would be quite different between female Olympic athletes and young women shopping for baby clothes (Table 3-14). Accordingly, the predictive values would change drastically, while the sensitivity and speci-ficity of the test would remain unchanged.

Measures of diagnostic efficiency depend entirely on the distribution of test results for a population with and without the condition and the cutoff used to define abnormal levels. The laboratory does not have control of the overlap between populations but does have control of the test cutoff. Thus, we will consider what happens when the cutoff is adjusted. The test cutoff (also known as a "medical decision limit") is the analyte concentra-tion that separates a "positive" test from a "negative" one. For qualitative tests, such as a urine βhCG, the cutoff is defined by the manufacturer and can be visualized

TABLE 3-14	DEPENDENCE OF PREDICTIVE VALUE ON CONDITION PREVALENCE[a]		
POPULATION[b]	**PREVALENCE OF PREGNANCY**	**+PPV (%)**	**NPV (%)**
Olympic athletes	1/10,000	0.03	99.99
Ob/gyn clinic patients aged 18–35 y	1/50	5.16	99.42
Babies "R" Us shoppers	3/10	53.33	89.09

PPV, positive predictive value; NPV, negative predictive value.
[a]Based on a constant sensitivity of 80% and specificity of 70%.
[b]Hypothetical.

directly (Fig. 3-26). For quantitative tests, the cutoff is a concentration; in the case of pregnancy, a serum βhCG concentration greater than 5 mIU/mL could be considered "positive." By changing the cutoff, from 8 mIU/mL (Fig. 3-27A), to 5 mIU/mL (Fig. 3-27B), or 2 mIU/mL (Fig. 3-27C), it becomes apparent that the diagnostic efficiency changes. As the cutoff is lowered, the sensitivity of the test for pregnancy improves from 40% (Fig. 3-27A) to 90% (Fig. 3-27C). However, this occurs at the expense of specificity, which decreases from 80% (Fig. 3-27A) to 40% (Fig. 3-27C) at the same cutoff. The best test with the wrong cutoff would be clinically useless. Accordingly, it is imperative to use an appropriate cutoff for the testing purpose. In the most rudimentary sense, a high sensitivity is desirable for a screening test, whereas a high specificity is appropriate for confirmation testing.

To define an appropriate cutoff, laboratorians often use a graphical tool called the receiver operator characteristic (ROC).[47] ROC curves are generated by plotting the true-positive rate against the false-positive rate (sensitivity vs. 1 − specificity; Fig. 3-28). Each point on the curve represents an actual cutoff concentration. ROC curves can be used to determine the most efficient cutoff for a test and are an excellent tool for comparing two

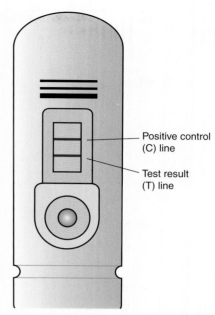

FIGURE 3-26 An example of a point-of-care device for beta-human chorionic gonadotropin. This is an example of a qualitative test, where the test line (T) represents whether the patient has a positive test, and the control (C) line is used to indicate that the test was successful.

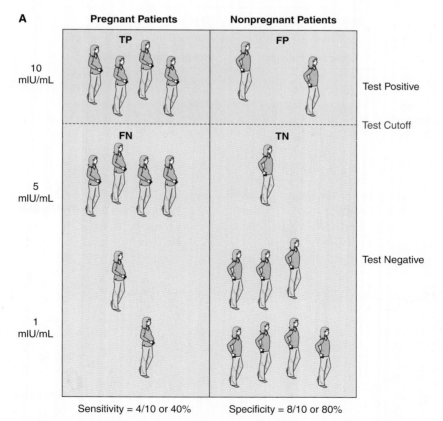

FIGURE 3-27 The effect of adjusting the beta-human chorionic gonadotropin test cutoff on sensitivity and specificity for pregnancy. **(A)** Using a high cutoff, sensitivity is low and specificity is high. **(B, C)** As the cutoff is lowered, the sensitivity improves at the expense of specificity. The predictive values also change as the cutoff is adjusted. TP, true positive; FP, false positive; FN, false negative; TN, true negative.

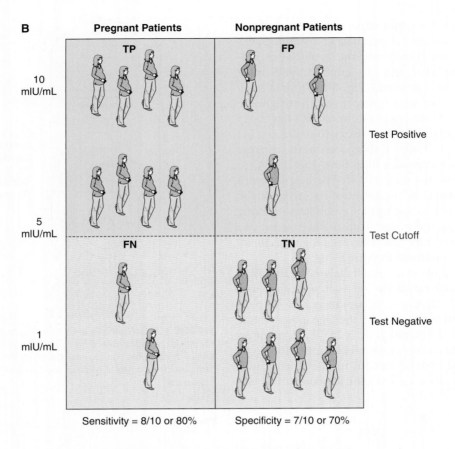

Sensitivity = 8/10 or 80%   Specificity = 7/10 or 70%

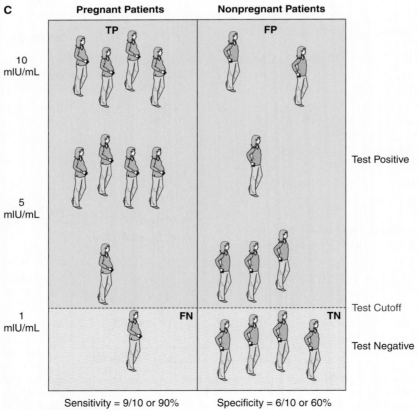

Sensitivity = 9/10 or 90%   Specificity = 6/10 or 60%

FIGURE 3-27 *(Continued)*

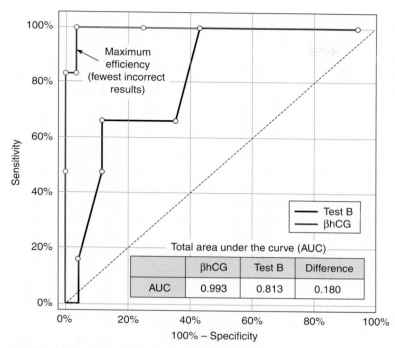

FIGURE 3-28 A receiver operator characteristic curve for beta-human chorionic gonadotropin (βhCG) and a hypothetical "test B." The area under the βhCG curve is greater than "test B" at all points, indicating that it is a superior test for pregnancy. The *thin dotted line* represents a test of no value (equal to diagnosis by a coin toss). The maximum (optimal) efficiency is indicated by the *arrow* and corresponds to the βhCG cutoff concentration with the fewest incorrect patient classifications.

different tests. The area under the curve represents the efficiency of the test, that is, how often the test correctly classifies individuals as having a condition or not. The higher the area under the ROC curve, the greater the efficiency. Figure 3-28 shows a hypothetical comparison of two tests used to diagnose pregnancy. The βhCG test has a larger area under the curve and has an overall higher performance than test B. Based on these ROC curves, βhCG represents a superior test compared with hypothetical test B, for diagnosing pregnancy.

ROC curves can also be used to determine the optimal cutoff point for a test. The optimal cutoff maximizes the number of correct tests (i.e., fewest FPs and FNs). A perfect test would have an area under the curve of 1.0 and reach the top-left corner of the graph (where sensitivity and specificity equal 100%). Clinical evaluations of diagnostic tests frequently use ROC curves to establish optimal cutoffs and compare different tests.[47] As with the other statistical measures described, there are many software applications that can be used to generate ROC curves.

In addition to sensitivity, specificity, and predictive values, there are a number of other measures of diagnostic efficiency. These include odds ratios, likelihood ratios, and multivariate analysis.[48,49] While these

have increasingly higher degrees of complexity, they all represent efforts to make clinical sense of data post-analytically. It is worth remembering the bigger picture, which is that laboratory values are not used in isolation. Laboratory tests are interpreted in the context of a patient's physical exam, symptoms, and clinical history to achieve a diagnosis.

PRACTICE PROBLEMS

Problem 3-1. Calculation of Sensitivity and Specificity

Urine hCG tests are commonly used to determine if someone is pregnant. Urine pregnancy tests qualitatively detect the presence of hCG in the urine. While manufacturers often state 99.99% accuracy, they are referring to the accuracy of a test in a patient who has a highly elevated urine hCG, effectively testing a positive control. The following data are based on population of women only a few weeks into pregnancy. Calculate the sensitivity, specificity, and efficiency of urine hCG for detecting pregnancy. Determine the predictive value of a positive urine hCG test.

NUMBER OF PREGNANCIES/INTERPRETATION OF hCG FINDINGS

PREGNANT?	POSITIVE URINE hCG	NEGATIVE URINE hCG	TOTAL
Yes	32	8	40
No	5	143	148
Total	37	151	188

Problem 3-2. A Quality Control Decision

GLUCOSE CONTROL VALUES

DAY	LOW	HIGH
1	86	215
2	82	212
3	83	218
4	87	214
5	85	220
6	81	217
7	88	223
8	83	224
9	82	217
10	85	222

1. Calculate the mean and standard deviation for the above dataset.
2. Plot these control data by day (one graph for each level, x-axis = day, y-axis = concentration). Indicate the mean and the upper and lower control limits (mean ±2 standard deviations) with horizontal lines (see Fig. 3-28).
3. You are working in the night shift at a community hospital and are the only person in the laboratory. You are running glucose quality control and obtain the following:

   Low control value = 90; High control value = 230
   Plot these controls on the process control chart (Levey-Jennings) you created above.

4. Are these values within the control limits? What do you observe about these control data?
5. What might be a potential problem?
6. What is an appropriate next step?

Problem 3-3. Precision (Replication)

For the following precision data, calculate the mean, SD, and CV for each of the two control solutions A and B. These control solutions were chosen because their concentrations were close to medical decision levels (X_C) for

glucose: 120 mg/dL for control solution A and 300 mg/dL for control solution B.

Control solution A was analyzed daily, and the following values were obtained:

118, 120, 121, 119, 125, 118, 122, 116, 124, 123, 117, 117, 121, 120, 120, 119, 121, 123, 120, and 122 mg/dL.

Control solution B was analyzed daily and gave the following results:

295, 308, 296, 298, 304, 294, 308, 310, 296, 300, 295, 303, 305, 300, 308, 297, 297, 305, 292, and 300 mg/dL.

Does the precision exceed the total allowable error defined by the CLIA?

Problem 3-4. Recovery

For the following tacrolimus immunosuppressant data, calculate the percent recovery for each of the individual experiments and the average of all the recovery experiments. The experiments were performed by adding two levels of standard to each of five patient samples (A through E) with the following results:

SAMPLE	0.9 mL BLOOD + 0.1 mL WATER	0.9 mL BLOOD + 0.1 mL 50 µg/L STD	0.9 mL BLOOD + 0.1 mL 100 µg/L STD
A	6.0	11.0	15.6
B	6.3	11.2	16.0
C	8.6	13.6	18.5
D	13.0	17.8	23.1
E	22.5	27.0	32.0

What do the results of this study indicate?

Problem 3-5. Interference

For the interference data that follow for glucose, calculate the concentration of bilirubin added, the interference for each individual sample, and the average interference for the group of patient samples. The experiments were performed by adding 0.1 mL of a 150 mg/dL ascorbic acid standard to 0.9 mL of five different patient samples (A through E). A similar dilution was prepared for each patient sample using water as the diluent. The results follow:

SAMPLE	GLUCOSE (mg/dL) 0.9 mL SERUM + 0.1 mL WATER	GLUCOSE (mg/dL) 0.9 mL SERUM + 0.1 mL 150 mg/dL BILIRUBIN STD
A	54	40
B	99	80
C	122	101
D	162	133
E	297	256

What do the results of this study indicate?

Problem 3-6. Sample Labeling

You receive an urine specimen in the laboratory with a request for a complete urinalysis. The cup is labeled and you begin your testing. You finish the testing and report the results to the ward. Several minutes later, you receive a telephone call from the ward informing you that the urine was reported on the wrong patient. You are told that the cup was labeled incorrectly before it was brought to the laboratory.

1. What is the problem in this case, and where did it occur?
2. Would your laboratory's QC system be able to detect or prevent this type of problem?

Problem 3-7. QC Program for POCT Testing

Your laboratory is in charge of overseeing the QC program for the glucometers (POCT) in use at your hospital. You notice that the ward staff is not following proper procedure for running QC. For example, in this case, the glucometer QC was rerun three times in a row in an effort to have the results in control. The first two runs were both 3 SD high. The last run did return to less than 2 SDs. Explain the correct follow-up procedure for dealing with the out-of-control results.

Problem 3-8. QC Rule Interpretation

Explain the R_{4s} rule, including what type of error it detects.

Problem 3-9. Reference Interval Study Design

You are asked to design a reference interval study for a new test. The results are known to be different in men and women and is affected by the consumption of aspirin, age, and time of day. Create a questionnaire to collect the appropriate information needed to perform a reference interval study. How would you account for these variables in the data collection?

For additional student resources please visit thePoint at http://thepoint.lww.com. **thePoint**

QUESTIONS

1. A Gaussian distribution is usually
   a. Bell-shaped
   b. Rectangular
   c. Uniform
   d. Skewed

2. The following chloride (mmol/L) results were obtained using a new analyzer:

106	111	104	106	112	110
115	127	83	110	108	109
83	119	105	106	108	114
120	100	107	110	109	102

What is the mean?
   a. 108
   b. 105
   c. 109
   d. 107

3. The following chloride (mmol/L) results were obtained using a new analyzer:

106	111	104	106	112	110
115	127	83	110	108	109
83	119	105	106	108	114
120	100	107	110	109	102

What is the median?
   a. 108.5
   b. 105
   c. 112
   d. 107

4. For a data value set that is Gaussian distributed, what is the likelihood (%) that a data point will be within ±1 SD from the mean?
   a. 68%
   b. 99%
   c. 95%
   d. 100%

5. The correlation coefficient
   a. Indicates the strength of relationship in a linear regression.
   b. Determines the regression type used to derive the slope and y-intercept.
   c. Is always expressed as "b."
   d. Expresses method imprecision.

6. If two methods agree perfectly in a method comparison study, the slope equals _____ and the y-intercept equals _____.
   a. 1.0, 0.0
   b. 0.0, 1.0

   c. 1.0, 1.0
   d. 0.0, 0.0
   e. 0.5, 0.5

7. Systematic error can best be described as consisting of
   a. Constant and proportional error.
   b. Constant error.
   c. Proportional error.
   d. Random error.
   e. Syntax error.

8. Examples of typical reference interval data distribution plots include all of the following except
   a. ROC
   b. Nonparametric
   c. Parametric
   d. Bimodal

9. A reference range can be verified by
   a. Testing as few as 20 normal donor specimens.
   b. Literature and vendor material review.
   c. Using samples from previously tested hospital patients.
   d. Using pharmacy-provided plasmanate spiked with target analyte concentrations.

10. Reference interval transference studies
   a. Are used to verify a reference interval.
   b. Are used to establish a reference interval.
   c. Require as many as 120 normal donors.
   d. Use a 68% reference limit for acceptability.

11. Diagnostic specificity is the
   a. Ability of a test to correctly identify the absence of a given disease or condition.
   b. Chance an individual does not have a given disease or condition if the test is within the reference interval.
   c. Chance of an individual having a given disease or condition if the test is abnormal.
   d. Ability of a test to detect a given disease or condition.

ONLINE RESOURCES

AACC	http://aacc.org
Centers for Disease Control and Prevention	http://www.cdc.gov
CLIA	http://www.cms.hhs.gov/clia
CLSI	http://www.clsi.org
College of American Pathologists	http://CAP.org
EP Evaluator	http://www.dgrhoads.com
FDA	http://www.FDA.gov
GraphPAD	http://www.graphpad.com
JMP	http://www.jmp.com
Labs Online	http://www.labtestsonline.org
McLendon Clinical Laboratories	http://labs.unchealthcare.org
OIVD	http://www.fda.gov/CDRH/oivd
R	http://www.r-project.org/
SAS	http://www.sas.com
Westgard Laboratory pages	http://www.westgard.com
	http://www.fda.gov/MedicalDevices

REFERENCES

1. Westgard JO, de Vos DJ, Hunt MR, et al. Concepts and practices in the evaluation of clinical chemistry methods. V. Applications. *Am J Med Technol.* 1978;44:803-813.
2. Wakkers PJ, Hellendoorn HB, Op de Weegh GJ, et al. Applications of statistics in clinical chemistry. A critical evaluation of regression lines. *Clin Chim Acta.* 1975;64:173-184.
3. Centers for Disease Control and Prevention (CDC), Centers for Medicare and Medicaid Services (CMS), Health and Human Services. Medicare, Medicaid, and CLIA programs; laboratory requirements relating to quality systems and certain personnel qualifications. Final rule. *Fed Regist.* 2003;68:3639-3714.
4. Westgard JO, de Vos DJ, Hunt MR, et al. Concepts and practices in the evaluation of clinical chemistry methods. I. Background and approach. *Am J Med Technol.* 1978;44:290-300.
5. National Committee for Clinical Laboratory Standards (NCCLS). *Approved Guideline for Precision Performance of Clinical Chemistry Devices.* Villanova, PA: NCCLS; 1999 (Document no. EP05-A).
6. Westgard JO, de Vos DJ, Hunt MR, et al. Concepts and practices in the evaluation of clinical chemistry methods. II. Experimental procedures. *Am J Med Technol.* 1978;44:420-430.
7. Krouwer JS, Rabinowitz R. How to improve estimates of imprecision. *Clin Chem.* 1984;30:290-292.
8. Westgard JO, Burnett RW. Precision requirements for cost-effective operation of analytic processes. *Clin Chem.* 1990;36:1629-1632.
9. Westgard JO, Carey RN, Wold S. Criteria for judging precision and accuracy in method development and evaluation. *Clin Chem.* 1974;20:825-833.
10. Westgard JO. *Basic Method Evaluation.* 2nd ed. Madison, WI: Westgard Quality Corp; 2003.
11. National Committee for Clinical Laboratory Standards (NCCLS). *Proposed Guideline for Interference Testing in Clinical Chemistry.* Villanova, PA: NCCLS; 1986 (Document no. EP07-A).
12. Young DS. *Effects of Drugs on Clinical Laboratory Tests.* 4th ed. Washington, DC: American Association of Clinical Chemistry; 2000.
13. Siest G, Galteau MM. *Drug Effects on Laboratory Tests.* Littleton, MA: PSG Publishing; 1988.
14. Glick MR, Ryder KW. Analytical systems ranked by freedom from interferences. *Clin Chem.* 1987;33:1453-1458.
15. Glick MR, Ryder KW, Jackson SA. Graphical comparisons of interferences in clinical chemistry instrumentation. *Clin Chem.* 1986;32:470-475.
16. Ryder KW, Glick MR. Erroneous laboratory results from hemolyzed, icteric, and lipemic specimens. *Clin Chem.* 1993;39:175-176.

17. National Committee for Clinical Laboratory Standards (NCCLS). *Approved Guideline for Method Comparison and Bias Estimation Using Patient Samples.* Villanova, PA: NCCLS; 2002 (Document no. EP09-A2).

18. Shahzad K, Kim DH, Kang MJ. Analytic evaluation of the beta-human chorionic gonadotropin assay on the Abbott IMx and Elecsys2010 for its use in doping control. *Clin Biochem.* 2007;40:1259-1265.

19. National Committee for Clinical Laboratory Standards (NCCLS). *Proposed Guideline for Evaluation of Linearity of Quantitative Analytical Methods.* Villanova, PA: NCCLS; 2001 (Document no. EP6-P2).

20. Westgard JO, Hunt MR. Use and interpretation of common statistical tests in method-comparison studies. *Clin Chem.* 1973;19:49-57.

21. Westgard JO. Precision and accuracy: concepts and assessment by method evaluation testing. *Crit Rev Clin Lab Sci.* 1981;13:283-330.

22. Cornbleet PJ, Gochman N. Incorrect least-squares regression coefficients in method-comparison analysis. *Clin Chem.* 1979;25:432-438.

23. Feldmann U, Schneider B, Klinkers H, et al. A multivariate approach for the biometric comparison of analytical methods in clinical chemistry. *J Clin Chem Clin Biochem.* 1981;19:121-137.

24. Westgard JO, de Vos DJ, Hunt MR, et al. Concepts and practices in the evaluation of clinical chemistry methods: IV. Decisions of acceptability. *Am J Med Technol.* 1978;44:727-742.

25. Barnett RN. Medical significance of laboratory results. *Am J Clin Pathol.* 1968;50:671-676.

26. Fraser CG. Data on biological variation: essential prerequisites for introducing new procedures? *Clin Chem.* 1994;40:1671-1673.

27. Fraser CG. *Biological Variation: From Principles to Practice.* Washington, DC: AACC Press; 2001.

28. Tonks DB. A study of the accuracy and precision of clinical chemistry determinations in 170 Canadian laboratories. *Clin Chem.* 1963;9:217-233.

29. Medicare, Medicaid and CLIA programs; regulations implementing the Clinical Laboratory Improvement Amendments of 1988 (CLIA)—HCFA. Final rule with comment period. *Fed Regist.* 1992;57:7002-7186.

30. Ehrmeyer SS, Laessig RH, Leinweber JE, et al. 1990 Medicare/CLIA final rules for proficiency testing: minimum intralaboratory performance characteristics (CV and bias) needed to pass. *Clin Chem.* 1990;36:1736-1740.

31. Westgard JO, Seehafer JJ, Barry PL. European specifications for imprecision and inaccuracy compared with operating specifications that assure the quality required by US CLIA proficiency-testing criteria. *Clin Chem.* 1994;40(7 pt 1):1228-1232.

32. Bland JM, Altman DG. Statistical methods for assessing agreement between two methods of clinical measurement. *Lancet.* 1986;1:307-310.

33. Levey S, Jennings ER. The use of control charts in the clinical laboratory. *Am J Clin Pathol.* 1950;20:1059-1066.

34. Westgard JO, Barry PL, Hunt MR, et al. A multi-rule Shewhart chart for quality control in clinical chemistry. *Clin Chem.* 1981;27:493-501.

35. Clinical and Laboratory Standards Institute (CLSI). *Statistical Quality Control for Quantitative Measurements: Principles and Definitions.* Wayne, PA: CLSI; 2006.

36. Westgard JO, Groth T. Power functions for statistical control rules. *Clin Chem.* 1979;25:863-869.

37. Westgard JO, Groth T, Aronsson T, et al. Performance characteristics of rules for internal quality control: probabilities for false rejection and error detection. *Clin Chem.* 1977;23:1857-1867.

38. Solberg HE. The IFCC recommendation on estimation of reference intervals. The RefVal program. *Clin Chem Lab Med.* 2004;42:710-714.

39. Solberg HE. International Federation of Clinical Chemistry. Scientific Committee, Clinical Section. Expert Panel on Theory of Reference Values and International Committee for Standardization in Haematology Standing Committee on Reference Values. Approved recommendation (1986) on the theory of reference values. Part 1. The concept of reference values. *Clin Chim Acta.* 1987;165:111-118.

40. Solberg HE. International Federation of Clinical Chemistry (IFCC), Scientific Committee, Clinical Section, Expert Panel on Theory of Reference Values, and International Committee for Standardization in Haematology (ICSH), Standing Committee on Reference Values. Approved Recommendation (1986) on the theory of reference values. Part 1. The concept of reference values. *J Clin Chem Clin Biochem.* 1987;25:337-342.

41. Standardization of blood specimen collection procedure for reference values. International Committee for Standardization in Haematology (ICSH). *Clin Lab Haematol.* 1982;4:83-86.

42. Clinical Laboratory Improvement Amendments of 1988; final rule. *Fed Regist.* 7164 [42 CFR 493.1213]: Department of Health and Human Services, Centers for Medicare and Medicaid Services; 1992.

43. van der Meulen EA, Boogaard PJ, van Sittert NJ. Use of small-sample-based reference limits on a group basis. *Clin Chem.* 1994;40:1698-1702.

44. National Committee for Clinical Laboratory Standards (NCCLS). *How to Define and Determine Reference Intervals in the Clinical Laboratory; Approved Guideline C28-A2.* Wayne, PA: NCCLS; 2000.

45. Clinical and Laboratory Standards Institute (CLSI). C28-A2: *How to Define and Determine Reference Intervals in the Clinical Laboratory; Approved Guideline.* 2nd ed. Villanova, PA: CLSI; 2008.

46. Galen RS, Gambino SR. *Beyond Normality: The Predictive Value and Efficiency of Medical Diagnoses.* New York, NY: Wiley; 1975.

47. Zweig MH, Campbell G. Receiver-operating characteristic (ROC) plots: a fundamental evaluation tool in clinical medicine [published erratum appears in *Clin Chem.* 1993;39:1589]. *Clin Chem.* 1993;39:561-577.

48. van der Helm HJ, Hische EA, Bolhuis PA. Bayes' theorem and the estimation of the likelihood ratio. *Clin Chem.* 1982;28:1250-1251.

49. Reibnegger G, Fuchs D, Hausen A, et al. Generalized likelihood ratio concept and logistic regression analysis for multiple diagnostic categories. *Clin Chem.* 1989;35:990-994.

Lean Six Sigma Methodology for Quality Improvement in the Clinical Chemistry Laboratory

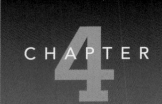

STEVEN W. COTTEN, CHRISTOPHER R. McCUDDEN,
MICHAEL W. ROGERS, MONTE S. WILLIS

CHAPTER OUTLINE

- ◆ LEAN SIX SIGMA METHODOLOGY
- ◆ ADOPTION AND IMPLEMENTATION OF LEAN SIX SIGMA
- ◆ PROCESS IMPROVEMENT
- ◆ MEASUREMENTS OF SUCCESS USING LEAN AND SIX SIGMA
- ◆ LEAN SIX SIGMA APPLICATIONS IN IHE LABORATORY AND THE GREATER HEALTH-CARE SYSTEM

- ◆ PRACTICAL APPLICATION OF SIX SIGMA METRICS
  Detecting Laboratory Errors
  Defining the Sigma Performance of an Assay
  Choosing the Appropriate Westgard Rules
- ◆ CONCLUSIONS
- ◆ ACKNOWLEDGMENTS
- ◆ QUESTIONS
- ◆ REFERENCES

Chapter Objectives

Upon completion of this chapter, the clinical laboratorian should be able to do the following:

- Discuss the basic concepts of Lean Six Sigma process improvement

- Apply the DMAIC methodology in laboratory process improvement projects
- Explain the role of Six Sigma Metrics in laboratory quality control

KEY TERMS

DMAIC
Lean Six Sigma

QC
Process Sigma
Quality control

LEAN SIX SIGMA METHODOLOGY

In the previous chapter, we discussed how laboratory tests are established by method evaluation and how quality control (QC) continuously monitors their processes. In this chapter, we expand on these ideas to discuss the concept of quality improvement (Fig. 4-1). Quality improvement goes beyond monitoring, detecting, and preventing errors. Quality improvement achieves new levels of performance, not otherwise realized through QC, and addresses chronic problems. Lean Six Sigma Methodology is the combination of Six Sigma quality management, developed by Motorola, with Lean manufacturing strategy, pioneered by Toyota, to provide tangible metrics for quality improvement. In its simplest form, Six Sigma asks the question, how can this process be improved? while Lean manufacturing asks the question, does this process (or step) need to exist?

Together as Lean Six Sigma, they are being increasingly used to reduce error (Six Sigma) and waste (Lean) within the health-care system.

ADOPTION AND IMPLEMENTATION OF LEAN SIX SIGMA

Effective adoption of Lean Six Sigma for process improvement requires an organization-wide dedication and support for a continuous process improvement culture. A pioneer in this field, Dr. J. M. Juran taught that continuous improvement does not make an organization distinctive or "excellent." Instead, it is the rate of improvement that distinguishes an organization.[1] Effecting change will not occur without support from senior members within the organization. These leaders select and assign quality improvement projects to teams within the organization.

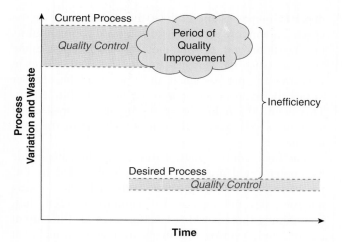

FIGURE 4-1 Quality improvement for a given process. Quality improvement seeks to eliminate inefficiencies in a process through reduction of variation and waste. The current process exhibits high variation and waste and quality control (QC) measures do not adequately manage the process. After a period of quality improvement, the desired process shows much smaller variation and waste and tighter control of the process using the new QC measures. Lean Six Sigma methodology seeks to identify, measure, and eliminate the large gaps of inefficiency in a process. Examples from the laboratory include data accuracy, turnaround times, and reagent inventory.

The three most common team roles are the project coaches/leaders (black belts), project team members (green belts), and project sponsors (blue belts). Black belts dedicate 100% of their time to quality improvement projects, proactively addressing process and quality problems. Green belts contribute 20% of their time to improvement projects while delivering their normal job functions. Blue belts are mid- to senior-level sponsors who review the project, remove organizational barriers, and encourage the team members. In the laboratory, a team may consist of expert or specialist technologists, supervisors, directors, and an expert consultant who will lead the process. Typically, a full Six Sigma improvement project takes 6 to 8 months to complete. Smaller scale improvement projects typically headed by purple belts use the same Lean Six Sigma principles condensed over 1 week to improve more focused and limited processes.

PROCESS IMPROVEMENT

All work is a dynamic process, and every process has variation, overlap, and waste. Variation results in unpredictable and undesirable outcomes. Waste results in increased cost and delays and thereby limiting efficiency. Lean Six Sigma uses a problem–cause–solution methodology to improve any process through waste elimination and variation reduction. The **DMAIC** (Define, Measure,

Analyze, Improve, and Control) methodology is the quality improvement team's project management road map (Fig. 4-2). The five phases allow for the identification of the root cause for error and waste through establishment of the following:

1. A universally accepted framework for quality improvement
2. Common language throughout the organization
3. A checklist to guide the process
4. Control measures for long-term monitoring

The Define phase explicitly describes the quality improvement issues. In the Measure phase, the team collects data to measure the process. That is, they determine the difference between the current process and the desired one. The Analyze phase searches for the root causes of inefficiencies in the process. In the Improve phase, the team pilots process changes that seek to remove the identified root problems. The Control phase continues to measure the process and ensures changes are maintained.

Let's apply the DMAIC methodology to a real life example in the laboratory. Assume that a high rate of mislabeled aliquot tubes continues to be a chronic problem in the hospital laboratory. Aliquots are currently poured off manually when each specimen arrives in the laboratory either through the tube system or specimen

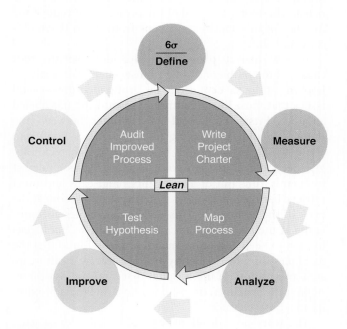

FIGURE 4-2 Integration of Six Sigma and Lean principles. The methodologies of Six Sigma manufacturing and Lean process optimization are combined to an iterative cycle of quality improvement. Applications of Lean Six Sigma are now being applied to all aspects of the laboratory and the health-care system as a whole.

drop-off window. The project would begin in the Define phase by setting a goal to reduce by 60%, for example, the number of mislabeled aliquot tubes when the specimens arrive within 2 months. By the end of the Define phase, both the project team and the management team have validated the "project charter." The project charter states the overall purpose and potential impact, the scope of the project (what is included and what is not), its resources (e.g., who is on the team and what resources are available to implement changes), and expectations—what will be delivered and when. This is a modifiable document intended to keep everyone involved focused on the problem and improving the outcomes.

The Measure phase maps, measures, and assesses the current process. For this example, the number of aliquot tubes made on each shift and the number of mislabeled aliquot tubes would be monitored. The data collected would allow the team to calculate the current percentage of mislabeled aliquot tubes that occurs on each shift. In doing so, the team will also map how the aliquots are made, including the number of specimens received, where labels are printed, where the aliquot tubes are stored, and how many technologists are involved in the process. In this laboratory, it is found that three technologists are responsible for making aliquots and they all share one common label printer. Bags of empty aliquot tubes and caps are stored in the laboratory's surplus room at the back of the laboratory. It is also found that 20 out of every 100 aliquot tubes are mislabeled. Therefore, the goal of the project is to reduce the number of mislabeled specimens from 20 to 8 samples for every shift.

In the Analyze phase, the team identifies the root causes of the problem through cause–effect data analysis. Looking at the data collected, the group identifies several issues that most likely contribute toward the mislabeled aliquots. First, the shared label printer between the three technologists making aliquots creates confusion about which printed label belongs to which technologist. Second, during high-volume times, the technologist frequently runs out of aliquot tubes and caps and must retrieve bags of empty tubes from the surplus room at the back of the laboratory. This results in samples accumulating at the aliquot station and causes the technologists to rush to keep up with demand. It is also found that the technologists are frequently interrupted by health-care staff and visitors in the hospital that stop and ask directions at the specimen drop-off window due to its proximity to a busy elevator.

The team next develops strategies that address each of these specific problems and pilots the changes in the Improve phase. Each technologist is given an aliquot label printer and storage is built around the bench that holds enough aliquot tubes and caps for an entire shift. The laboratory also requested that the hospital facilities

department post signs both at the elevator and at the specimen window with directions toward common units on the floor and provide hospital maps outside the elevator. Once the changes are implemented, the team measures the process again and finds that the number of mislabeled specimens that occur on each shift is four. This is an 80% reduction in the number of mislabeled aliquots, which exceeds the goals of 60% set by the project charter.

The final Control phase ensures that the gains made by implemented improvements are maintained by QC mechanisms. For this example, this includes stocking aliquot tubes and caps at the beginning of each shift, maintaining three working label printers for the aliquot station, and ensuring that maps are readily available at the elevator. The way the aliquots are made (poured off and labeled by hand) did not change. Instead, modifying the steps around the process was enough to improve the outcome to the level set by the project charter. Furthermore, these modifications included factors both inside and outside the laboratory. The DMAIC method (Fig. 4-2) was applied to a problem in the laboratory and allowed the team to quantitatively measure the error of the process, identify the root cause(s) of the problem, develop improvement strategies, and monitor the changes in a defined manner.

MEASUREMENTS OF SUCCESS USING LEAN AND SIX SIGMA

Originally, Lean and Six Sigma were separate ideas designed to improve two related metrics: time and error. Lean was designed to eliminate non–value-adding steps and Six Sigma aimed to reduce variation. The metrics for measuring quality improvement with Lean Six Sigma still reflect those original principles. Combination of these two ideas provides a positive synergistic impact on process and quality improvement.

The Lean approach seeks to streamline the process by eliminating duplication, excess, and barriers for a more optimized flow. The major measurement for Lean is generally time, but it can also include things such as cost, inventory, and distribution. A common method of Lean improvement is the concept of a Kaizen event. This is analogous to the DMAIC method used in Six Sigma but can be implemented on a smaller scale. The Kaizen event is 3 to 5 days of quality improvement by a cross-functional team that analyzes the current steps associated with a particular process and makes changes to improve its efficiency. With detailed study, most teams find unnecessary complexity in their process. This complexity often contributes to errors as well as delays. Teams typically find that only 5% of the activities in any process add value; this means that a vast majority of activities do not contribute to the process. Graphically,

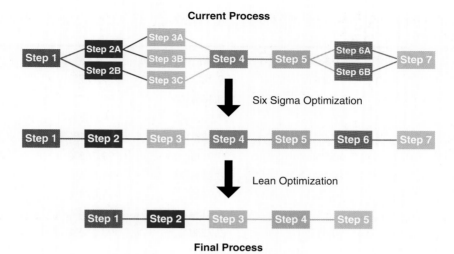

FIGURE 4-3 Application of Six Sigma and Lean methodologies toward process improvement. Steps in a process can have duplication, failure, and waste, all of which contribute to delay, increased cost, inefficiency, and longer turnaround times.

this might look like the redundant and nonlinear process shown in Figure 4-3. Lean Six Sigma measures the amount of non–value-adding steps in a process as part of its core metrics. The implemented solutions (based on charter goals) represented by the final process in Figure 4-3 where inefficiency has been removed illustrate a more streamlined, efficient process.

Six Sigma metrics seek to quantitatively measure the amount of error or variation that occurs within a system. A process sigma represents the capability of a process to meet (or exceed) its defined criteria for acceptability. In the laboratory, this could refer to assay performance, turnaround times, number of rejected samples, specimen transport, or relay of critical values. The process sigma is usually represented as the number of defects (errors) per million opportunities (DPMO). The sigma (σ) value refers to the number of standard deviations (SDs) away from the mean a process can move before it is outside the acceptable limits (Fig. 4-4). For example,

if a sodium test has Six Sigma performance, then the mean could shift by 6 SDs (6σ) and still meet the laboratory requirements for precision and accuracy for sodium measurement. If a test achieves Six Sigma (6σ), it has a narrow process SD (i.e., it is very precise) and produces only three errors for every million tests performed. A test that performs at a three sigma (3σ) has a much wider process SD and produces about 26,674 errors per million tests (Fig. 4-4).

To calculate the sigma, defects must be clearly defined. In the laboratory, any test that does not meet its requirements (i.e., correctly quantified or delivered on time) is considered a defect. The most straightforward method uses the process yield—the percentage of times that a process is defect free. Another method to calculate the process sigma is to calculate the DPMO. For example, in the laboratory, this might be measured by the number of errors that occurs for every 1 million tests. The process sigma can be estimated from a Process Sigma table (Table 4-1) using either the process yield or the DPMO.

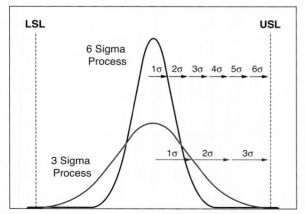

FIGURE 4-4 Comparison of Sigma performance for results distributed between the lower satisfactory limit (LSL) and the upper satisfactory limit (USL).

TABLE 4-1	PROCESS SIGMA TABLE	
YIELD	ERRORS/MILLION RESULTS	PROCESS SIGMA
99.9999%	1	6.27
99.9997%	3	6.04
99.999%	10	5.77
99.99%	100	5.22
99.9%	1,000	4.59
Definition of "Sigma" for a process with a given error rate.		

TABLE 4-2	EXAMPLE OF YIELD AT GIVEN PERFORMANCE (σ): % OF DATA REPORTED CORRECTLY			
NO. OF STEPS	™**3σ**	™**4σ**	™**5σ**	™**6σ**
1	93.3%	99.38%	99.977%	99.9999%
3	82.7%	98.16%	99.931%	99.9953%
4	77.4%	97.56%	99.908%	99.9930%
7	61.6%	95.73%	99.839%	99.9976%
10	50.1%	93.96%	99.768%	99.9966%
20	25.1%	88.29%	99.536%	99.9932%
40	6.3%	77.94%	99.074%	99.9864%
80	1.6%	68.81%	98.614%	99.9796%
100	0.4%	60.75%	98.156%	99.9728%

As stated earlier, eliminating non–value-adding steps and reducing variation have a synergistic positive impact on process performance (Table 4-2). Several examples illustrate this concept. Assume that there are four steps involved in testing a specimen and each step is performed at a 3σ level (each step 93.3% accurate and timely). With this performance, approximately three out of four test results will be accurate and delivered on time (75.8%)! Now imagine that a team improves the quality of the process so that each step is performed correctly and timely at a 4σ level (99.38% accurate and timely). The new level of performance produces 97.5% of the results accurately and delivered on time. Alternatively, if a test has 10 steps, each of which operates at a 3σ level (93.3% accurate and timely) the increase in the number of slightly inaccurate steps, 50% of the tests will be inaccurate and late. Simply by eliminating unnecessary steps and maintaining a high level of performance, the team can drastically reduce the number of total errors. If the improvement team can both eliminate six steps and increase the quality of each step to a 4σ level, the process will improve so that 97.5% of the tests are accurate and on time (Table 4-2). These improvement strategies are designed to be continuous. Once changes have been realized, the improvement process should start again to make the system even better with each cycle.

LEAN SIX SIGMA APPLICATIONS IN THE LABORATORY AND THE GREATER HEALTH-CARE SYSTEM

The popularity of the combination of Lean and Six Sigma principles as an approach to quality management in health care has grown in the last 10 years. In 2004, there were two articles published describing specifically the application of Lean Six Sigma, according to a PubMed search utilizing the phrase "Lean Six Sigma." This number has risen to 29 articles published in 2010/2011. Since 1997, there have been 255 publications on Six Sigma quality improvement strategies alone in the health-care field. Application of Lean and Six Sigma methodology at the Virginia Mason Medical Center showed numerous improvements to patient care.[2] Table 4-3 highlights the major improvements achieved in Lean Six Sigma Quality Management.

Prior to the adoption of Lean Six Sigma strategies, no laboratory result was reported (the time the result was

TABLE 4-3	MAJOR IMPROVEMENTS ACHIEVED FROM LEAN SIX SIGMA QUALITY MANAGEMENT	
	BEFORE LEAN SIX SIGMA	**AFTER LEAN SIX SIGMA**
Results report mailed	100% > 3 d	89% < 3 d
Patient waiting time	[Data not published]	Decreased by 50%
Discharge time	2.5 h	1.5 h
Chemotherapy time	[Data not published]	Decreased by 50%

Source: Bush RW. Reducing waste in US health care systems. *JAMA.* February 2007;297(8):871-874.

available until mailing) within less than 3 days and every physician had an average of 1,800 results waiting to be reported. After application of Lean methodology, 89% of the test results were reported in less than 3 days. Patient waiting time was significantly reduced for chemotherapy infusion time, clinic waiting time decreased by 50%, and discharge time decreased from 2.5 to 1.5 hours. All of these aspects for improvement represent tangible metrics that can be measured and quantified by Lean Six Sigma tools. The results of the improvement process provide superior patient care, improve customer service, and positively impact patient satisfaction, which all contribute toward enhanced customer retention by the individual health-care organization.

A similar application of Lean Six Sigma Methodology was used to develop a new phlebotomy staffing model that better matched demand at Brigham and Women's Hospital in Boston.[3] The project was initiated in response to excessive safety reports filed for missed inpatient collections, thereby delaying laboratory results. Discrepancies between estimated and actual collection demand identified periods of understaffing for the phlebotomy service during peak demand times. After application of the Lean Six Sigma Methodology, new, staggered shifts were implemented to better handle the high-volume times between 5 and 9 am and 7 and 9 pm (Fig. 4-5). Four new shifts were created that increased available personnel during peak hours and decreased available personnel during periods of low collections. The number of full-time equivalents

remained the same between the old and new staffing model. The new staffing model improved collection by 17 minutes, accelerated results for basic chemistry such as potassium by 15 minutes, and reduced by 80% the number of filed safety reports from delayed or missed collections.[3]

PRACTICAL APPLICATION OF SIX SIGMA METRICS

Detecting Laboratory Errors

Recent studies have highlighted that medical errors occur with greater frequency than previously thought.[4-8] As part of the health-care system, the laboratory is a potential source of error. Error rates in laboratory tests have been estimated to occur between 1:164 and 1:8,300 results (Table 4-4).[9-16] Converting these error rates to the standard Six Sigma metric DPMO, laboratory error rates would be expected to occur at a rate of between 120 and 6,098 DPMO; this corresponds to a 4σ to 5σ rating. A 6σ quality level would require less than 3.4 DPMO (Table 4-1).

While an estimated 12.5% of laboratory errors impact patient health, only 37.5 of every 100,000 (0.0375%) errors place patients at risk due to analytical testing mistakes.[8,15,17] Previously, laboratory quality improvement focused on errors that occur in the analytic phase of testing. But currently, analytical testing errors comprise only 4% to 32% of all errors in the laboratory.[18] Most laboratory errors are now attributed to processes occurring either before (pre-analytic) or immediately after (post-analytic) the test. Pre-analytic errors are estimated at between 32% and 75%, and post-analytic errors account for 9% to 55%. As outlined in Figure 4-6, the pre-analytic phase involves steps such as the actual ordering of the tests

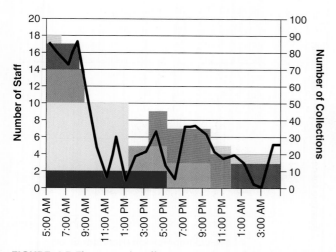

FIGURE 4-5 The revised staffing model that better matches the collection pattern (*black line*) modified through Six Sigma quality improvement strategies. Blocked colors represent different staff shifts. (Reprinted with permission from Morrison AP, Tanasijevic MJ, Torrence-Hill JN, Goonan EM, Gustafson ML, Melanson SEF. A strategy for optimizing staffing to improve the timeliness of inpatient phlebotomy collections. *Arch Pathol Lab Med.* December 2011;135(12):1576-1580.)

TABLE 4-4	RATE OF LABORATORY ERROR DETECTION
ESTIMATED LABORATORY ERROR RATE	**ERRORS/MILLION (DPMO)**
1:164	6,098
1:214	4,672
1:283	3,534
1:8,300	20
Risk of dying in a plane crash	
1:7,000,000 passengers	0.14

Table adapted with permission from Bonini P, Plebani M, Ceriotti F, Rubboli F. Errors in laboratory medicine. *Clin Chem.* May 2002;48(5):691-698.

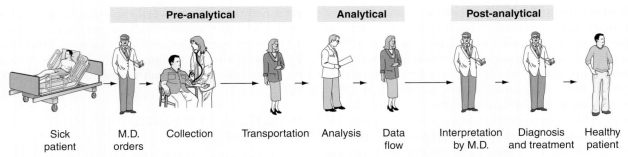

FIGURE 4-6 Schematic representation of the process components involved in clinical laboratory testing.

by physicians, as well as sample collection. Because many of the pre-analytic errors are outside the physical laboratory (i.e., phlebotomy), it is imperative that the process as a whole be considered when reorganizing laboratory processes to improve quality. This often requires collaboration between other departments within the system. With the current emphasis on quality improvement in the health-care setting,[2,19-21] clinical laboratories have been early adopters of Lean Six Sigma methodology to improve the quality of laboratory testing by identifying and reducing pre- and post-analytical sources of error.[3,22-26]

Defining the Sigma Performance of an Assay

From a quality management perspective, Six Sigma metrics can determine how well an analytic process performs and assist in choosing appropriate QC rules based on test performance. For example, if a given test has excellent performance (very precise and accurate over time), then fewer errors will occur. It would take a large shift in the mean for the test to fail the quality requirements. Accordingly, fewer QC rules would be needed to identify errors. These rules are designed to maximize the chance of detecting a problem, while simultaneously minimizing the risk of rejecting a result when it is actually correct (false rejection).

Six Sigma metrics can be plotted graphically using an operational process specification "OPSpecs" chart. This chart incorporates many of the measures described in the Method Evaluation chapter into one graph, including (1) total allowable error, (2) systematic error (inaccuracy), and (3) random error (imprecision) (Fig. 4-7). From the QC section, total allowable error is defined by CLIA (Clinical Laboratory Improvement Amendments) regulations (see Table 3-12). Systematic and random errors are derived from method comparison experiments, described in Chapter 3 (see Fig. 3-16). Consider the following hypothetical example for total calcium.

The performance of the assay is defined by the following linear regression equation:

$$y = 0.91x + 0.2$$

The total allowable error for calcium is 1 mg/dL

The assay has an imprecision of 2%

What is the systemic error for the assay at 10 mg/dL?

$$y = (0.91 \times 10) + 0.2$$

$$y = 9.3 \text{ mg/dL}$$

10 mg/dL – 9.3 mg/dL = 0.7 mg/dL

0.7 mg/dL represents 70% of the total allowable error for calcium (1 mg/dL)

What is the random error of the assay at 10 mg/dL?

Imprecision = 10 mg/dL × 0.02

Imprecision = 0.2 mg/dL

0.2 mg/dL represents 20% of the total allowable error for calcium (1 mg/dL)   **(Eq. 4-1)**

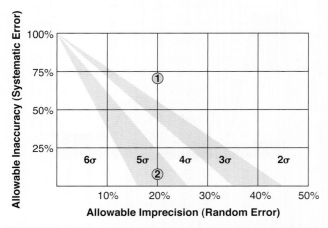

FIGURE 4-7 OPSpecs chart used to determine process performance. The allowable imprecision is plotted against the allowable inaccuracy as percentage of the total allowable error. Assay performance changing from point 1 to point 2 by reducing inaccuracy improves the performance from a 2σ process to a 5σ process.

Plotting the random error of 20% on the *x*-axis and the systemic error of 70% on the *y*-axis using the OPSpecs chart (Fig. 4-7) reveals that the assay has a 2σ performance; this is considered poor performance and would require extensive QC measurements to detect the high number of errors. Many rules are needed because only a small shift in the mean would result in a failure (this principle is evident in Fig. 4-4). If the systemic error (bias) could be eliminated (as demonstrated with point 2, Fig. 4-7), the performance would fall into the 5σ range, which is considered to be very good; only a few QC measurements would be necessary with a minimal use of control rules to detect the low number of errors.

Choosing the Appropriate Westgard Rules

Recently, a straightforward methodology has been published detailing how Six Sigma metrics can be used to choose appropriate Westgard QC rules for any assay.[27] A sigma value for every Westgard rule or set of rules can be deduced from the slope of the line it generates in an OPSpecs chart (Fig. 4-7). In short, the slope of the line is equal to the − (negative) sigma value. Furthermore, the sigma value for an assay can be calculated by the following equation:

$$\text{Sigma} = (\text{Total Allowable Error} - \text{Bias})/ \text{Coefficient of Variation} \qquad \textbf{(Eq. 4-2)}$$

Total allowable error represents the error budget based on the biological variation of the specific analyte. Bias refers to the systematic error of the assay and the coefficient of variation is the analytical SD of the assay. If the calculated sigma for an assay is greater than the sigma of the Westgard rule, that rule is suitable for monitoring the error of the test. Values for total allowable error for specific analytes have been published and are readily available (Table 3-12) so the laboratory must simply calculate bias and coefficient of variation (CV) for the assay in question. Consider the following hypothetical example using potassium:

The total allowable error for potassium = 5.8%

The bias for your laboratory's assay for potassium = 0.7%

The CV for your laboratory's assay for potassium = 1%

$$\text{Sigma}_{\text{potassium}} = (5.8 - 0.7)/1$$
$$\text{Sigma}_{\text{potassium}} = 5.1$$

Using Table 4-5, the Westgard rule with the sigma value closest, but below 5.1 is the 1 2.5s rule. Therefore, a QC rule of 1 2.5s would provide the optimum control to detect error in the laboratory's potassium assay while minimizing false rejection of accurate results.

TABLE 4-5	HYPOTHETICAL SIGMA VALUES FOR WESTGARD RULES
WESTGARD RULE	**SIGMA VALUE**
1 3.5s	6
1 3s	5.6
1 2.5s	5.0
1 3s/2 2s/R 4s/4 1s	4.0

Source: Schoenmakers CHH, Naus AJM, Vermeer HJ, van Loon D, Steen G. Practical application of Sigma Metrics QC procedures in clinical chemistry. *Clin Chem Lab Med.* November 2011;49(11):1837-1843.

CONCLUSIONS

Lean Six Sigma Methodology has emerged as a powerful technique to effectively improve the quality and efficiency of the clinical laboratory. It provides a framework to define, measure, and reduce waste and variation associated with the total testing process. Furthermore, it supplies mathematically sound metrics to assess laboratory processes and assay performance, define QC rules, and develop quality improvement strategies. Lean Six Sigma's role in clinical chemistry will continue to grow in importance and scope as the need for improved quality and reduced cost becomes paramount in the healthcare system. Knowledge of Lean Six Sigma methodology will be critical for laboratorians going forward to achieve the mission of delivering quality health care to patients. Major hospitals have made institutional-wide commitments to quality improvement using Lean Six Sigma. Yellow belt training is currently offered at certain institutions to all laboratory personnel with the goal of having the entire laboratory staff trained. Supervisors and lead technologists are also trained at the blue, purple, and black belt level to participate in quality improvement projects across departments within the institution. For medical technologists, this training provides an unprecedented opportunity to be an agent for change in the health-care system and allows the laboratorian to take a greater ownership in improving patient care and enhancing customer service.

ACKNOWLEDGMENTS

The authors wish to acknowledge Glen Spivak, Vice President of Business Development and Operational Efficiency, and more broadly the University of North Carolina Hospitals for its support and training in Lean Six Sigma Methodologies utilized in writing this chapter and used in our clinical laboratories.

For additional student resources please visit thePoint at **http://thepoint.lww.com.** **thePoint** ☀

QUESTIONS

1. To evaluate a moderately complex laboratory test, all of the following must be done except:
   a. Analytical sensitivity and specificity
   b. Verification of the reference interval
   c. Accuracy and precision
   d. Reportable range

2. An ROC includes all of the following except:
   a. Perfect test = an area under the curve <1.0
   b. Equals receiver operator characteristic
   c. Plots sensitivity and 1 – specificity
   d. Can be used to compare two different tests

3. For method development studies, which analytical performance test should be done first?
   a. Imprecision studies
   b. Comparison of methods (COM)
   c. Recovery
   d. Interference studies
   e. Does not matter, they all need to be done

4. For the following series of laboratory values, the vendor has indicated that a true value is 6.0. Series = 5, 4, 5, 6, 7, 5, 3, 8, 5, 9, 5, 4, 5, 6. The SDI (standard deviation index) is:
   a. −0.3
   b. +0.3
   c. +1.0
   d. −0.7

5. Comparison of method studies:
   a. Estimate systematic error.
   b. Use primary QC material and standards that span the reportable range.
   c. Are usually completed within 4 working days.
   d. Are not required for non-waived tests.

6. Interference studies typically use _____ as an interferent.
   a. All of these

   b. Hemolyzed red cells
   c. Highly icteric samples
   d. Highly lipemic samples

7. Allowable analytical error is:
   a. A combination of random and systematic error.
   b. Best if it is greater than the total error.
   c. Used only for research and initial evaluation studies.
   d. Published by the CDC for an array of clinical tests.

8. The methodology for a Lean Six Sigma quality improvement team will include consideration of all of the following factors EXCEPT:
   a. Define
   b. Measure
   c. Analyze
   d. Improve
   e. Communicate

9. It is reported that the greatest percentage of laboratory errors occur during the _____ phase.
   a. Preanalytical
   b. Analytical
   c. Postanalytical
   d. Proficiency
   e. Phlebotomy

10. Calculate the Sigma value for sodium given that the total allowable error is 8%, the bias is 0.9%, and the CV is 2%.
   a. 3.6
   b. 2.7
   c. 7.1
   d. 4.5
   e. 6.7

REFERENCES

1. Juran JM. *Juran on Leadership for Quality.* 1st ed. New York, NY: Free Press; 1989.
2. Bush RW. Reducing waste in US health care systems. *JAMA.* February 2007;297(8):871-874.
3. Morrison AP, Tanasijevic MJ, Torrence-Hill JN, Goonan EM, Gustafson ML, Melanson SEF. A strategy for optimizing staffing to improve the timeliness of inpatient phlebotomy collections. *Arch Pathol Lab Med.* December 2011;135(12):1576-1580.
4. Institute of Medicine (U.S.). Committee on Crossing the Quality Chasm: Adaptation to Mental Health and Addictive Disorders. *Improving the Quality of Health Care for Mental and Substance-Use Conditions.* Washington, DC: National Academies Press; 2006.
5. Committee on Quality of Health Care in America, Institute of Medicine. *Crossing the Quality Chasm: A New Health System for the 21st Century.* 1st ed. Washington, DC: National Academies Press; 2001.
6. IOM report: patient safety—achieving a new standard for care. *Acad Emerg Med.* October 2005;12(10):1011-1012.

7. Committee on Quality of Health Care in America. Institute of Medicine. *To Err Is Human: Building a Safer Health System*. 1st ed. Washington, DC: National Academies Press; 2000.

8. Committee on Identifying Priority Areas for Quality Improvement. *Priority Areas for National Action: Transforming Health Care Quality*. 1st ed. Washington, DC: National Academies Press; 2003.

9. Siebers R. Laboratory blunders revisited. *Ann Clin Biochem*. July 1994;31(pt 4):390-391.

10. Chambers AM, Johnston J, O'Reilly DS. Laboratory blunders revisited. *Ann Clin Biochem*. July 1994;31(pt 4):390; author reply 391.

11. Lapworth R, Teal TK. Laboratory blunders revisited. *Ann Clin Biochem*. January 1994;31(pt 1):78-84.

12. Stankovic AK. The laboratory is a key partner in assuring patient safety. *Clin Lab Med*. December 2004;24(4):1023-1035.

13. Kalra J. Medical errors: impact on clinical laboratories and other critical areas. *Clin Biochem*. December 2004;37(12):1052-1062.

14. Hollensead SC, Lockwood WB, Elin RJ. Errors in pathology and laboratory medicine: consequences and prevention. *J Surg Oncol*. December 2004;88(3):161-181.

15. Plebani M. Errors in clinical laboratories or errors in laboratory medicine? *Clin Chem Lab Med*. 2006;44(6):750-759.

16. Singla P, Parkash AA, Bhattacharjee J. Preanalytical error occurrence rate in clinical chemistry laboratory of a public hospital in India. *Clin Lab*. 2011;57(9-10):749-752.

17. Plebani M. Exploring the iceberg of errors in laboratory medicine. *Clin Chim Acta*. June 2009;404(1):16-23.

18. Bonini P, Plebani M, Ceriotti F, Rubboli F. Errors in laboratory medicine. *Clin Chem*. May 2002;48(5):691-698.

19. Nicolay CR, Purkayastha S, Greenhalgh A, et al. Systematic review of the application of quality improvement methodologies from the manufacturing industry to surgical healthcare. *Br J Surg* [Internet]. November 2011 [cited Dec 6, 2011]. http://www.ncbi.nlm.nih.gov/pubmed/22101509

20. Sciacovelli L, Sonntag O, Padoan A, Zambon CF, Carraro P, Plebani M. Monitoring quality indicators in laboratory medicine does not automatically result in quality improvement. *Clin Chem Lab Med* [Internet]. December 2011 [cited Dec 22, 2011]. http://www.ncbi.nlm.nih.gov/pubmed/22149744

21. Signori C, Ceriotti F, Sanna A, et al. Process and risk analysis to reduce errors in clinical laboratories. *Clin Chem Lab Med*. 2007;45(6):742-748.

22. DelliFraine JL, Langabeer JR 2nd, Nembhard IM. Assessing the evidence of Six Sigma and Lean in the health care industry. *Qual Manag Health Care*. September 2010;19(3):211-225.

23. Gras JM, Philippe M. Application of the Six Sigma concept in clinical laboratories: a review. *Clin Chem Lab Med*. 2007;45(6):789-796.

24. Kuo AM-H, Borycki E, Kushniruk A, Lee T-S. A healthcare Lean Six Sigma System for postanesthesia care unit workflow improvement. *Qual Manag Health Care*. March 2011;20(1):4-14.

25. Pocha C. Lean Six Sigma in health care and the challenge of implementation of Six Sigma methodologies at a Veterans Affairs Medical Center. *Qual Manag Health Care*. December 2010;19(4):312-318.

26. Vanker N, van Wyk J, Zemlin AE, Erasmus RT. A Six Sigma approach to the rate and clinical effect of registration errors in a laboratory. *J Clin Pathol*. May 2010;63(5):434-437.

27. Schoenmakers CHH, Naus AJM, Vermeer HJ, van Loon D, Steen G. Practical application of Sigma Metrics QC procedures in clinical chemistry. *Clin Chem Lab Med*. November 2011;49(11):1837-1843.

Analytic Techniques

JULIA C. DREES, MATTHEW S. PETRIE, ALAN H.B. WU

CHAPTER 5

CHAPTER OUTLINE

◆ **SPECTROPHOTOMETRY**
   Beer's Law
   Spectrophotometric Instruments
   Components of a Spectrophotometer
   Spectrophotometer Quality Assurance
   Atomic Absorption Spectrophotometer
   Flame Photometry
   Fluorometry
   Basic Instrumentation
   Chemiluminescence
   Turbidity and Nephelometry
   Laser Applications

◆ **ELECTROCHEMISTRY**
   Galvanic and Electrolytic Cells
   Half-Cells
   Ion-Selective Electrodes
   pH Electrodes
   Gas-Sensing Electrodes
   Enzyme Electrodes
   Coulometric Chloridometers and Anodic Stripping
   Voltammetry

◆ **ELECTROPHORESIS**
   Procedure
   Support Materials
   Treatment and Application of Sample
   Detection and Quantitation
   Electroendosmosis
   Isoelectric Focusing
   Capillary Electrophoresis
   Two-Dimensional Electrophoresis
◆ **OSMOMETRY**
   Freezing Point Osmometer
◆ **QUESTIONS**
◆ **REFERENCES**

Chapter Objectives

Upon completion of this chapter, the clinical laboratorian should be able to do the following:

• Explain the general principles of each analytic method.
• Discuss the limitations of each analytic technique.
• Compare and contrast the various analytic techniques.
• Discuss existing clinical applications for each analytic technique.

• Describe the operation and component parts of the following instruments: spectrophotometer, atomic absorption spectrometer, fluorometer, osmometer, ion-selective electrode, and pH electrode.
• Outline the quality assurance and preventive maintenance procedures involved with the following instruments: spectrophotometer, fluorometer, osmometer, ion-selective electrode, and pH electrode.

KEY TERMS

Atomic absorption
Chemiluminescence
Electrochemistry

Electrophoresis
Fluorometry
Ion-selective electrodes
Spectrophotometry

Analytic techniques and instrumentation provide the foundation for all measurements made in a modern clinical chemistry laboratory. The majority of techniques fall into one of four basic disciplines within the field of analytic chemistry: spectrometry (including spectro-photometry, atomic absorption, and mass spectrometry [MS]); luminescence (including fluorescence and chemiluminescence); electroanalytic methods (including electrophoresis, potentiometry, and amperometry); and chromatography (including gas, liquid, and thin layer). Due to the rapid growth and increased utilization in clinical laboratories, chromatography and MS will be covered separately in Chapter 6.

SPECTROPHOTOMETRY

The instruments that measure electromagnetic radiation have several concepts and components in common. Shared instrumental components are discussed in some detail in a later section. Photometric instruments measure light intensity without consideration of wavelength. Most instruments today use filters (photometers), prisms, or gratings (spectrometers) to select (isolate) a narrow range of the incident wavelength. Radiant energy that passes through an object will be partially reflected, absorbed, and transmitted.

Electromagnetic radiation is described as photons of energy traveling in waves. The relationship between wavelength and energy E is described by Planck's formula:

$$E = h\nu \qquad \text{(Eq. 5-1)}$$

where h is a constant (6.62×10^{-27} erg sec), known as Planck's constant, and ν is frequency. Because the frequency of a wave is inversely proportional to the wavelength, it follows that the energy of electromagnetic radiation is inversely proportional to wavelength. Figure 5-1A shows this relationship. Electromagnetic

radiation includes a spectrum of energy from short-wavelength, highly energetic gamma rays and x-rays on the left in Figure 5-1B to long-wavelength radio-frequencies on the right. Visible light falls in between, with the color violet at 400 nm and red at 700 nm wavelengths being the approximate limits of the visible spectrum.

The instruments discussed in this section measure either absorption or emission of radiant energy to determine the concentration of atoms or molecules. The two phenomena, absorption and emission, are closely related. For a ray of electromagnetic radiation to be absorbed, it must have the same frequency as a rotational or vibrational frequency in the atom or molecule that it strikes. Levels of energy that are absorbed move in discrete steps, and any particular type of molecule or atom will absorb only certain energies and not others. When energy is absorbed, valence electrons move to an orbital with a higher energy level. Following energy absorption, the excited electron will fall back to the ground state by emitting a discrete amount of energy in the form of a characteristic wavelength of radiant energy.

Absorption or emission of energy by atoms results in a line spectrum. Because of the relative complexity of molecules, they absorb or emit a bank of energy over a large region. Light emitted by incandescent solids (tungsten or deuterium) is in a continuum. The three types of spectra are shown in Figure 5-2.[1-3]

Beer's Law

The relationship between absorption of light by a solution and the concentration of that solution has been described by Beer and others. Beer's law states that the concentration of a substance is directly proportional to the amount of light absorbed or inversely proportional to the logarithm of the transmitted light. Percent transmittance (%T) and absorbance (A) are related photometric terms that are explained in this section.

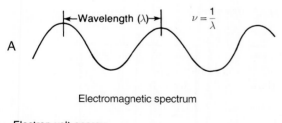
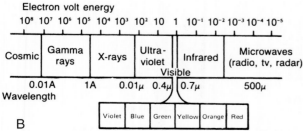

FIGURE 5-1 Electromagnetic radiation—relationship of energy and wavelength.

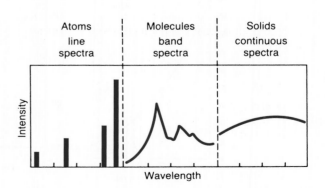

FIGURE 5-2 Characteristic absorption or emission spectra. (Adapted from Coiner D. *Basic Concepts in Laboratory Instrumentation.* Bethesda, MD: ASMT Education and Research Fund; 1975-1979.)

A

$$\% \text{ Transmittance} = \frac{T}{I} \times 100$$

Blank — Defined as 100% T

B

$$\% T = \frac{\text{Sample beam signal}}{\text{Blank beam signal}} \times 100$$

Sample

FIGURE 5-3 Percent transmittance (%T) defined.

Figure 5-3A shows a beam of monochromatic light entering a solution. Some of the light is absorbed. The remainder passes through, strikes a light detector, and is converted to an electric signal. Percent transmittance is the ratio of the radiant energy transmitted (T) divided by the radiant energy incident on the sample (I). All light absorbed or blocked results in 0% T. A level of

100% T is obtained if no light is absorbed. In practice, the solvent without the constituent of interest is placed in the light path, as in Figure 5-3B. Most of the light is transmitted, but a small amount is absorbed by the solvent and cuvette or is reflected away from the detector. The electrical readout of the instrument is set arbitrarily at 100% T, while the light is passing through a "blank" or reference. The sample containing absorbing molecules to be measured is placed in the light path. The difference in amount of light transmitted by the blank and that transmitted by the sample is due only to the presence of the compound being measured. The %T measured by commercial spectrophotometers is the ratio of the sample transmitted beam divided by the blank transmitted beam.

Equal thicknesses of an absorbing material will absorb a constant fraction of the energy incident upon the layers. For example, in a tube containing layers of solution (Fig. 5-4A), the first layer transmits 70% of the light incident upon it. The second layer will, in turn, transmit 70% of the light incident upon it. Thus, 70% of 70% (49%) is transmitted by the second layer. The third layer transmits 70% of 49%, or 34% of the original light. Continuing on, successive layers transmit 24% and 17%, respectively. The %T values, when plotted on linear graph paper, yield the curve shown in Figure 5-4B. Considering each equal layer as many monomolecular layers, we can translate layers of material to concentration. If semilog graph paper is used to plot the same

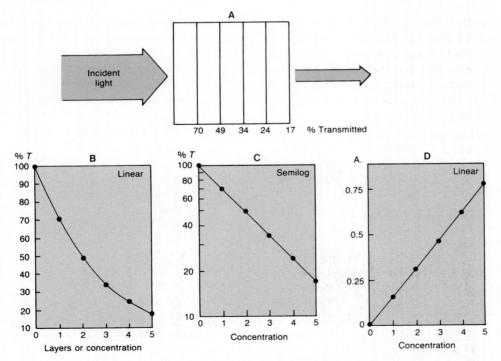

FIGURE 5-4 (**A**) Percent of original incident light transmitted by equal layers of light-absorbing solution. (**B**) Percent T vs. concentration on linear graph paper. (**C**) Percent T vs. concentration on semilog graph paper. (**D**) A versus concentration on linear graph paper.

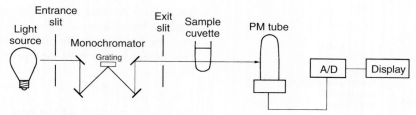

FIGURE 5-5 Single-beam spectrophotometer.

figures, a straight line is obtained (Fig. 5-4C), indicating that, as concentration increases, %T decreases in a logarithmic manner.

Absorbance A is the amount of light absorbed. It cannot be measured directly by a spectrophotometer but rather is mathematically derived from %T as follows:

$$\%T = \frac{I}{I_0} \times 100 \qquad \text{(Eq. 5-2)}$$

where I_0 is the incident light and I is the transmitted light.

Absorbance is defined as follows:

$$A = -\log(I/I_0) = \log(100\%) - \log \%T$$
$$= 2 - \log \%T \qquad \text{(Eq. 5-3)}$$

According to Beer's law, absorbance is directly proportional to concentration (Fig. 5-4D):

$$A = \varepsilon \times b \times c \qquad \text{(Eq. 5-4)}$$

where ε = molar absorptivity, the fraction of a specific wavelength of light absorbed by a given type of molecule; b is the length of light path through the solution; and c is the concentration of absorbing molecules.

Absorptivity depends on the molecular structure and the way in which the absorbing molecules react with different energies. For any particular molecular type, absorptivity changes as wavelength of radiation changes. The amount of light absorbed at a particular wavelength depends on the molecular and ion types present and may vary with concentration, pH, or temperature.

Because the path length and molar absorptivity are constant for a given wavelength,

$$A \sim c \qquad \text{(Eq. 5-5)}$$

Unknown concentrations are determined from a calibration curve that plots absorbance at a specific wavelength versus concentration for standards of known concentration. For calibration curves that are linear and have a zero y-intercept, unknown concentrations can be determined from a single calibrator. Not all calibration curves result in straight lines. Deviations from linearity are typically observed at high absorbances. The stray light within an instrument will ultimately limit

the maximum absorbance that a spectrophotometer can achieve, typically 2.0 absorbance units.

Spectrophotometric Instruments

A spectrophotometer is used to measure the light transmitted by a solution to determine the concentration of the light-absorbing substance in the solution. Figure 5-5 illustrates the basic components of a single-beam spectrophotometer, which are described in subsequent sections.

Components of a Spectrophotometer

Light Source
The most common source of light for work in the visible and near-infrared regions is the incandescent tungsten or tungsten-iodide lamp. Only about 15% of radiant energy emitted falls in the visible region, with most emitted as near-infrared.[1-3] Often, a heat-absorbing filter is inserted between the lamp and the sample to absorb the infrared radiation.

The lamps most commonly used for ultraviolet (UV) work are the deuterium discharge lamp and the mercury arc lamp. Deuterium provides continuous emission down to 165 nm. Low-pressure mercury lamps emit a sharp line spectrum, with both UV and visible lines. Medium and high-pressure mercury lamps emit a continuum from UV to the mid-visible region. The most important factors for a light source are range, spectral distribution within the range, the source of radiant production, stability of the radiant energy, and temperature.

Monochromators
Isolation of individual wavelengths of light is an important and necessary function of a monochromator. The degree of wavelength isolation is a function of the type of device used and the width of entrance and exit slits. The bandpass of a monochromator defines the range of wavelengths transmitted and is calculated as width at more than half the maximum transmittance (Fig. 5-6).

Numerous devices are used for obtaining monochromatic light. The least expensive are colored glass filters. These filters usually pass a relatively wide band of radiant energy and have a low transmittance of the selected

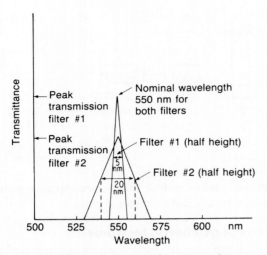

FIGURE 5-6 Spectral transmittance of two monochromators with band pass at half height of 5 and 20 nm.

wavelength. Although not precise, they are simple, inexpensive, and useful.

Interference filters produce monochromatic light based on the principle of constructive interference of waves. Two pieces of glass, each mirrored on one side, are separated by a transparent spacer that is precisely one-half the desired wavelength. Light waves enter one side of the filter and are reflected at the second surface. Wavelengths that are twice the space between the two glass surfaces will reflect back and forth, reinforcing others of the same wavelengths and finally passing on through. Other wavelengths will cancel out because of phase differences (destructive interference). Because interference filters also transmit multiples of the desired wavelengths, they require accessory filters to eliminate these harmonic wavelengths. Interference filters can be constructed to pass a very narrow range of wavelengths with good efficiency.

The prism is another type of monochromator. A narrow beam of light focused on a prism is refracted as it enters the more dense glass. Short wavelengths are refracted more than long wavelengths, resulting in dispersion of white light into a continuous spectrum. The prism can be rotated, allowing only the desired wavelength to pass through an exit slit.

Diffraction gratings are most commonly used as monochromators. A diffraction grating consists of many parallel grooves (15,000 or 30,000 per inch) etched onto a polished surface. Diffraction, the separation of light into component wavelengths, is based on the principle that wavelengths bend as they pass a sharp corner. The degree of bending depends on the wavelength. As the wavelengths move past the corners, wave fronts are formed. Those that are in phase reinforce one another, whereas those not in phase cancel out and disappear. This results in complete spectra. Gratings with very fine line rulings produce a widely dispersed spectrum. They produce linear spectra, called orders, in both directions from the entrance slit. Because the multiple spectra have a tendency to cause stray light problems, accessory filters are used.

Sample Cell

The next component of the basic spectrophotometer is the sample cell or cuvette, which may be round or square. The light path must be kept constant to have absorbance proportional to concentration. This is easily checked by preparing a colored solution to read midscale when using the wavelength of maximum absorption. Fill each cuvette to be tested, take readings, and save those that match within an acceptable tolerance (e.g., ±0.25% T). Because it is difficult to manufacture round tubes with uniform diameters, they should be etched to indicate the position for use. Cuvettes are sold in matched sets. Square cuvettes have plane-parallel optical surfaces and a constant light path. They have an advantage over round cuvettes in that there is less error from the lens effect, orientation in the spectrophotometer, and refraction. Cuvettes with scratched optical surfaces scatter light and should be discarded. Inexpensive glass cuvettes can be used for applications in the visible range, but they absorb light in the UV region. Quartz cuvettes must, therefore, be used for applications requiring UV radiation.

Photodetectors

The purpose of the detector is to convert the transmitted radiant energy into an equivalent amount of electrical energy. The least expensive of the devices is known as a barrier-layer cell, or photocell. The photocell is composed of a film of light-sensitive material, frequently selenium, on a plate of iron. Over the light-sensitive material is a thin, transparent layer of silver. When exposed to light, electrons in the light-sensitive material are excited and released to flow to the highly conductive silver. In comparison with the silver, a moderate resistance opposes the electron flow toward the iron, forming a hypothetical barrier to flow in that direction. Consequently, this cell generates its own electromotive force, which can be measured. The produced current is proportional to the incident radiation. Photocells require no external voltage source but rely on internal electron transfer to produce a current in an external circuit. Because of their low internal resistance, the output of electrical energy is not easily amplified. Consequently, this type of detector is used mainly in filter photometers with a wide bandpass, producing a fairly high level of illumination so that there is no need to amplify the signal. The photocell is inexpensive and durable; however, it is temperature sensitive and nonlinear at very low and very high levels of illumination.

A phototube (Fig. 5-7) is similar to a barrier-layer cell in that it has photosensitive material that gives off

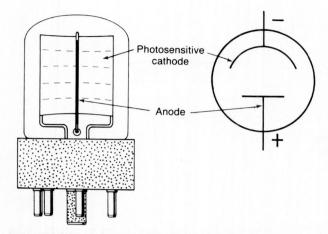

FIGURE 5-7 Phototube drawing and schematic.

are attracted to a series of anodes, known as dynodes, each having a successively higher positive voltage. These dynodes are of a material that gives off many secondary electrons when hit by single electrons. Initial electron emission at the cathode triggers a multiple cascade of electrons within the PM tube itself. Because of this amplification, the PM tube is 200 times more sensitive than the phototube. PM tubes are used in instruments designed to be extremely sensitive to very low light levels and light flashes of very short duration. The accumulation of electrons striking the anode produces a current signal, measured in amperes, that is proportional to the initial intensity of the light. The analog signal is converted first to a voltage and then to a digital signal through the use of an analog-to-digital converter. Digital signals are processed electronically to produce absorbance readings.

In a photodiode, absorption of radiant energy by a reverse-biased pn-junction diode (pn, positive–negative) produces a photocurrent that is proportional to the incident radiant power. Although photodiodes are not as sensitive as PM tubes because of the lack of internal amplification, their excellent linearity (6 to 7 decades of radiant power), speed, and small size make them useful in applications where light levels are adequate.[4] Photodiode array (PDA) detectors are available in integrated circuits containing 256 to 2,048 photodiodes in a linear arrangement. A linear array is shown in Figure 5-9. Each photodiode responds to a specific wavelength, and as a result, a complete UV/visible spectrum can be obtained in less than 1 second. Resolution is 1 to 2 nm and depends on the number of discrete elements. In spectrophotometers using PDA detectors, the grating is positioned after the

electrons when light energy strikes it. It differs in that an outside voltage is required for operation. Phototubes contain a negatively charged cathode and a positively charged anode enclosed in a glass case. The cathode is composed of a material (e.g., rubidium or lithium) that acts as a resistor in the dark but emits electrons when exposed to light. The emitted electrons jump over to the positively charged anode, where they are collected and return through an external, measurable circuit. The cathode usually has a large surface area. Varying the cathode material changes the wavelength at which the phototube gives its highest response. The photocurrent is linear, with the intensity of the light striking the cathode as long as the voltage between the cathode and the anode remains constant. A vacuum within the tubes avoids scattering of the photoelectrons by collision with gas molecules.

The third major type of light detector is the photomultiplier (PM) tube, which detects and amplifies radiant energy. As shown in Figure 5-8, incident light strikes the coated cathode, emitting electrons. The electrons

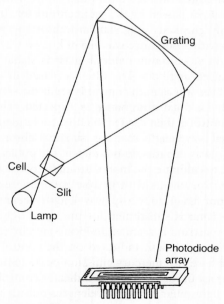

FIGURE 5-9 Photodiode array spectrophotometer illustrating the placement of the sample cuvette before the monochromator.

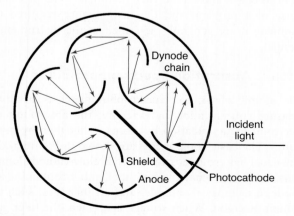

FIGURE 5-8 Dynode chain in a photomultiplier.

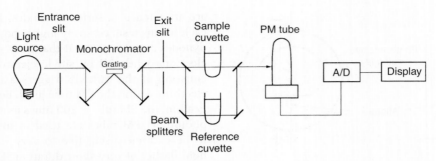

FIGURE 5-10 Double-beam spectrophotometer.

sample cuvette and disperses the transmitted radiation onto the PDA detector (Fig. 5-9).

For single-beam spectrophotometers, the absorbance reading from the sample must be blanked using an appropriate reference solution that does not contain the compound of interest. Double-beam spectrophotometers permit automatic correction of sample and reference absorbance, as shown in Figure 5-10. Because the intensities of light sources vary as a function of wavelength, double-beam spectrophotometers are necessary when the absorption spectrum for a sample is to be obtained. Computerized, continuous zeroing, single-beam spectrophotometers have replaced most double-beam spectrophotometers.

Spectrophotometer Quality Assurance

Performing at least the following checks should validate instrument function: wavelength accuracy, stray light, and linearity. Wavelength accuracy means that the wavelength indicated on the control dial is the actual wavelength of light passed by the monochromator. It is most commonly checked using standard absorbing solutions or filters with absorbance maxima of known wavelength. Didymium or holmium oxide in glass is stable and frequently used as filters. The filter is placed in the light path and the wavelength control is set at the wavelength at which maximal absorbance is expected. The wavelength control is then rotated in either direction to locate the actual wavelength that has maximal absorbance. If these two wavelengths do not match, the optics must be adjusted to calibrate the monochromator correctly.

Some instruments with narrow bandpass use a mercury vapor lamp to verify wavelength accuracy. The mercury lamp is substituted for the usual light source, and the spectrum is scanned to locate mercury emission lines. The wavelength indicated on the control is compared with known mercury emission peaks to determine the accuracy of the wavelength indicator control.

Stray light refers to any wavelengths outside the band transmitted by the monochromator. The most common causes of stray light are reflection of light from scratches

on optical surfaces or from dust particles anywhere in the light path and higher order spectra produced by diffraction gratings. The major effect is absorbance error, especially in the high absorbance range. Stray light is detected by using cutoff filters, which eliminate all radiation at wavelengths beyond the one of interest. To check for stray light in the near-UV region, for example, insert a filter that does not transmit in the region of 200 to 400 nm. If the instrument reading is greater than 0% T, stray light is present. Certain liquids, such as $NiSO_4$, $NaNO_2$, and acetone, absorb strongly at short wavelengths and can be used in the same way to detect stray light in the UV range.

Linearity is demonstrated when a change in concentration results in a straight line calibration curve, as discussed under Beer's law. Colored solutions may be carefully diluted and used to check linearity, using the wavelength of maximal absorbance for that color. Sealed sets of different colors and concentrations are available commercially. They should be labeled with expected absorbance for a given bandpass instrument. Less than expected absorbance is an indication of stray light or of a bandpass that is wider than specified. Sets of neutral-density filters to check linearity over a range of wavelengths are also commercially available.

A routine system should be devised for each instrument to check and record each parameter. The probable cause of a problem and the maintenance required to eliminate it are generally described in the instrument's manual.

Atomic Absorption Spectrophotometer

The atomic absorption spectrophotometer is used to measure concentration by detecting the absorption of electromagnetic radiation by atoms rather than by molecules. The basic components are shown in Figure 5-11. The usual light source, known as a hollow-cathode lamp, consists of an evacuated gas-tight chamber containing an anode, a cylindrical cathode, and an inert gas, such as helium or argon. When voltage is applied, the filler gas is ionized. Ions attracted to the cathode collide with the

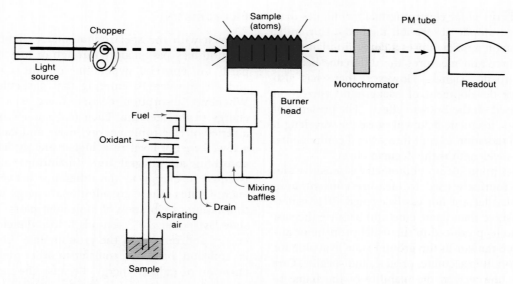

FIGURE 5-11 Single-beam atomic absorption spectrophotometer—basic components.

metal, knock atoms off, and cause the metal atoms to be excited. When they return to the ground state, light energy is emitted that is characteristic of the metal in the cathode. Generally, a separate lamp is required for each metal (e.g., a copper hollow-cathode lamp is used to measure Cu).

Electrodeless discharge lamps are a relatively new light source for atomic absorption spectrophotometers. A bulb is filled with argon and the element to be tested. A radiofrequency generator around the bulb supplies the energy to excite the element, causing a characteristic emission spectrum of the element.

The analyzed sample must contain the reduced metal in the atomic vaporized state. Commonly, this is done by using the heat of a flame to break the chemical bonds and form free, unexcited atoms. The flame is the sample cell in this instrument, rather than a cuvette. There are various designs; however, the most common burner is the premix long-path burner. The sample, in solution, is aspirated as a spray into a chamber, where it is mixed with air and fuel. This mixture passes through baffles, where large drops fall and are drained off. Only fine droplets reach the flame. The burner is a long, narrow slit, to permit a longer path length for absorption of incident radiation. Light from the hollow-cathode lamp passes through the sample of ground state atoms in the flame. The amount of light absorbed is proportional to the concentration. When a ground state atom absorbs light energy, an excited atom is produced. The excited atom then returns to the ground state, emitting light of the same energy as it absorbed. The flame sample thus contains a dynamic population of ground state and excited atoms, both absorbing and emitting radiant energy. The emitted energy from the flame will go in all directions,

and it will be a steady emission. Because the purpose of the instrument is to measure the amount of light absorbed, the light detector must be able to distinguish between the light beam emitted by the hollow-cathode lamp and that emitted by excited atoms in the flame. To do this, the hollow-cathode light beam is modulated by inserting a mechanical rotating chopper between the light and the flame or by pulsing the electric supply to the lamp. Because the light beam being absorbed enters the sample in pulses, the transmitted light will also be in pulses. There will be less light in the transmitted pulses because part of it will be absorbed. There are, therefore, two light signals from the flame—an alternating signal from the hollow-cathode lamp and a direct signal from the flame emission. The measuring circuit is tuned to the modulated frequency. Interference from the constant flame emission is electronically eliminated by accepting only the pulsed signal from the hollow cathode.

The monochromator is used to isolate the desired emission line from other lamp emission lines. In addition, it serves to protect the photodetector from excessive light emanating from flame emissions. A PM tube is the usual light detector.

Flameless atomic absorption requires an instrument modification that uses an electric furnace to break chemical bonds (electrothermal atomization). A tiny graphite cylinder holds the sample, either liquid or solid. An electric current passes through the cylinder walls, evaporates the solvent, ashes the sample, and, finally, heats the unit to incandescence to atomize the sample. This instrument, like the spectrophotometer, is used to determine the amount of light absorbed. Again, Beer's law is used for calculating concentration. A major problem is that background correction is considerably more necessary and critical for electrothermal techniques than for flame-based atomic absorption methods. Currently, the most common approach uses a deuterium lamp as a secondary source and measures the difference between the two absorbance signals. However, there has also been extensive development of background correction techniques based on the Zeeman effect.[1] The presence of an intense static magnetic field will cause the wavelength of the emitted radiation to split into several components. This shift in wavelength is the Zeeman effect.

Atomic absorption spectrophotometry is sensitive and precise. It is routinely used to measure concentration of trace metals that are not easily excited. It is generally more sensitive than flame emission because the vast majority of atoms produced in the usual propane or air-acetylene flame remain in the ground state available for light absorption. It is accurate, precise, and specific. One disadvantage, however, is the inability of the flame to dissociate samples into free atoms. For example, phosphate may interfere with calcium analysis by formation of calcium phosphate. This may be overcome by adding cations that compete with calcium for phosphate. Routinely, lanthanum or strontium is added to samples to form stable complexes with phosphate. Another possible problem is the ionization of atoms following dissociation by the flame, which can be decreased by reducing the flame temperature. Matrix interference, due to the enhancement of light absorption by atoms in organic solvents or formation of solid droplets as the solvent evaporates in the flame, can be another source of error. This interference may be overcome by pretreatment of the sample by extraction.[5]

Recently, inductively coupled plasma (ICP) has been used to increase sensitivity for atomic emission. The torch, an argon plasma maintained by the interaction of a radiofrequency field and an ionized argon gas, is reported to have used temperatures between 5,500 and 8,000 K. Complete atomization of elements is thought to occur at these temperatures. Use of ICP as a source is recommended for determinations involving refractory elements such as uranium, zirconium, and boron. ICP with MS detection is the most sensitive and specific assay technique for all elements on the periodic chart. Atomic absorption spectrophotometry is used less frequently because of this newer technology.

Flame Photometry

The flame emission photometer, which measures light emitted by excited atoms, was widely used to determine concentration of Na^+, K^+, or Li^+. With the development of ion-selective electrodes for these analytes, flame photometers are no longer routinely used in clinical chemistry laboratories. Discussion of this technique, therefore, is no longer included in this edition; the reader should refer to previous editions of this book.

Fluorometry

As seen with the spectrophotometer, light entering a solution may pass mainly through or may be absorbed partly or entirely, depending on the concentration and the wavelength entering that particular solution. Whenever absorption occurs, there is a transfer of energy to the medium. Each molecular type possesses a series of electronic energy levels and can pass from a lower energy level to a higher energy level only by absorbing an integral unit (quantum) of light that is equal in energy to the difference between the two energy states. There are additional energy levels owing to rotation or vibration of molecular parts. The excited state lasts about 10^{-5} seconds before the electron loses energy and returns to the ground state. Energy is lost by collision, heat loss, transfer to other molecules, and emission of radiant energy. Because the molecules are excited by absorption of radiant energy and lose energy by multiple interactions, the radiant energy emitted is less than the absorbed energy. The difference between the maximum wavelengths, excitation, and emitted fluorescence is called Stokes shift. Both excitation (absorption) and fluorescence (emission) energies are characteristic for a given molecular type; for example, Figure 5-12 shows the absorption and fluorescence spectra of quinine in 0.1 N sulfuric acid. The dashed line on the left shows the short-wavelength excitation energy that is maximally absorbed, whereas the solid line on the right is the longer wavelength (less energy) fluorescent spectrum.

Basic Instrumentation

Filter fluorometers measure the concentrations of solutions that contain fluorescing molecules. A basic instrument is shown in Figure 5-13. The source emits short-wavelength high-energy excitation light. A

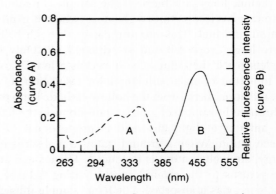

FIGURE 5-12 Absorption and fluorescence spectra of quinine in 0.1 N sulfuric acid. (Adapted from Coiner D. *Basic Concepts in Laboratory Instrumentation.* Bethesda, MD: ASMT Education and Research Fund; 1975-1979.)

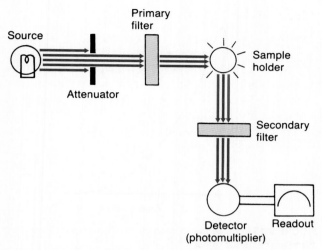

FIGURE 5-13 Basic filter fluorometer. (Adapted from Coiner D. *Basic Concepts in Laboratory Instrumentation.* Bethesda, MD: ASMT Education and Research Fund; 1975-1979.)

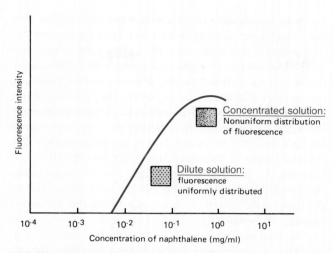

FIGURE 5-14 Dependence of fluorescence on the concentration of fluorophore. (Adapted from Guilbault GG. *Practical Fluorescence, Theory, Methods and Techniques.* New York, NY: Marcel Dekker; 1973.)

mechanical attenuator controls light intensity. The primary filter, placed between the radiation source and the sample, selects the wavelength that is best absorbed by the solution to be measured. The fluorescing sample in the cuvette emits radiant energy in all directions. The detector (placed at right angles to the sample cell) and a secondary filter that passes the longer wavelengths of fluorescent light prevent incident light from striking the photodetector. The electrical output of the photodetector is proportional to the intensity of fluorescent energy. In spectrofluorometers, the filters are replaced by prisms or grating monochromators.

Gas discharge lamps (mercury and xenon arc) are the most frequently used sources of excitation radiant energy. Incandescent tungsten lamps are seldom used because they release little energy in the UV region. Mercury vapor lamps are commonly used in filter fluorometers. Mercury emits a characteristic line spectrum. Resonance lines at 365 to 366 nm are commonly used. Energy at wavelengths other than the resonance lines is provided by coating the inner surface of the lamp with a material that absorbs the 254-nm mercury radiation and emits a broad band of longer wavelengths. Most spectrofluorometers use a high-pressure xenon lamp. Xenon has a good continuum, which is necessary for determining the excitation spectra.

Monochromator fluorometers use grating, prisms, or filters for isolation of incident radiation. Light detectors are almost exclusively PM tubes because of their higher sensitivity to low light intensities. Double-beam instruments are used to compensate for instability due to electric power fluctuation.

Fluorescence concentration measurements are related to molar absorptivity of the compound, intensity of the incident radiation, quantum efficiency of the energy emitted per quantum absorbed, and length of the light path. In dilute solutions with instrument parameters held constant, fluorescence is directly proportional to concentration. Generally, a linear response will be obtained until the concentration of the fluorescent species is so high that the sample begins to absorb significant amounts of excitation light. A curve demonstrating nonlinearity as concentration increases is shown in Figure 5-14. The solution must absorb less than 5% of the exciting radiation for a linear response to occur.[6] As with all quantitative measurements, a standard curve must be prepared to demonstrate that the concentration used falls in a linear range.

In fluorescence polarization, radiant energy is polarized in a single plane. When the sample (fluorophore) is excited, it emits polarized light along the same plane as the incident light if the fluorophore does not rotate in solution (i.e., it is attached or bound to a large molecule). In contrast, a small molecule emits depolarized light because it will rotate out of the plane of polarization during its excitation lifetime. This technique is widely used for the detection of therapeutic and abused drugs. In the procedure, the sample analyte is allowed to compete with a fluorophore-labeled analyte for a limited antibody to the analyte. The lower the concentration of the sample analyte, the higher the macromolecular antibody–analyte–fluorophore formed and the lower the depolarization of the radiant light.

Advantages and Disadvantages of Fluorometry
Fluorometry has two advantages over conventional spectrophotometry: specificity and sensitivity. Fluorometry increases specificity by selecting the optimal wavelength

for both absorption and fluorescence, rather than just the absorption wavelength seen with spectrophotometry.

Fluorometry is approximately 1,000 times more sensitive than most spectrophotometric methods.[6] One reason is because the emitted radiation is measured directly; it can be increased simply by increasing the intensity of the exciting radiant energy. In addition, fluorescence measures the amount of light intensity present over a zero background. In absorbance, however, the quantity of the absorbed light is measured indirectly as the difference between the transmitted beams. At low concentrations, the small difference between 100% *T* and the transmitted beam is difficult to measure accurately and precisely, limiting the sensitivity.

The biggest disadvantage is that fluorescence is very sensitive to environmental changes. Changes in pH affect availability of electrons, and temperature changes the probability of loss of energy by collision rather than fluorescence. Contaminating chemicals or a change of solvents may change the structure. UV light used for excitation can cause photochemical changes. Any decrease in fluorescence resulting from any of these possibilities is known as quenching. Because so many factors may change the intensity or spectra of fluorescence, extreme care is mandatory in analytic technique and instrument maintenance.

Chemiluminescence

In chemiluminescence reactions, part of the chemical energy generated produces excited intermediates that decay to a ground state with the emission of photons.[7] The emitted radiation is measured with a PM tube, and the signal is related to analyte concentration. Chemiluminescence is different from fluorescence in that no excitation radiation is required and no monochromators are needed because the chemiluminescence arises from one species. Most importantly, chemiluminescence reactions are oxidation reactions of luminol, acridinium esters, and dioxetanes characterized by a rapid increase in intensity of emitted light followed by a gradual decay. Usually, the signal is taken as the integral of the entire peak. Enhanced chemiluminescence techniques increase the chemiluminescence efficiency by including an enhancer system in the reaction of a chemiluminescent agent with an enzyme. The time course for the light intensity is much longer (60 minutes) than that for conventional chemiluminescent reactions, which last for about 30 seconds (Fig. 5-15).

Advantages of chemiluminescence assays include subpicomolar detection limits, speed (with flash-type reactions, light is only measured for 10 seconds), ease of use (most assays are one-step procedures), and simple instrumentation.[7] The main disadvantage is that impurities can cause a background signal that degrades the sensitivity and specificity.

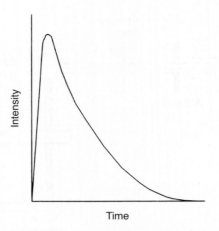

FIGURE 5-15 Representative intensity-vs.-time curve for a transient chemiluminescence signal.

Turbidity and Nephelometry

Turbidimetric measurements are made with a spectrophotometer to determine the concentration of particulate matter in a sample. The amount of light blocked by a suspension of particles depends not only on concentration but also on size. Because particles tend to aggregate and settle out of suspension, sample handling becomes critical. Instrument operation is the same as for any spectrophotometer.

Nephelometry is similar, except that light scattered by the small particles is measured at an angle to the beam incident on the cuvette. Figure 5-16 demonstrates two possible optical arrangements for a nephelometer. Light scattering depends on wavelength and particle size. For macromolecules with a size close to or larger than the wavelength of incident light, sensitivity is increased by measuring the forward light scatter.[8] Instruments are available with detectors placed at various forward angles, as well as at 90° to the incident light. Monochromatic light obtains uniform scatter and minimizes sample heating. Certain instruments use light amplification by stimulated emission of radiation (laser) as a source of monochromatic light; however, any monochromator may be used.

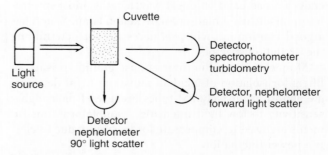

FIGURE 5-16 Nephelometer vs. spectrophotometer—optical arrangements.

Measuring light scatter at an angle other than at 180° in turbidimetry minimizes error from colored solutions and increases sensitivity. Because both methods depend on particle size, some instruments quantitate initial change in light scatter rather than total scatter. Reagents must be free of any particles, and cuvettes must be free of any scratches.

Laser Applications

Laser is based on the interaction of radiant energy with suitably excited atoms or molecules. The interaction leads to stimulated emission of radiation. The wavelength, direction of propagation, phase, and plane of polarization of the emitted light are the same as those of the incident radiation. Laser light is polarized and coherent and has narrow spectral width and small cross-sectional area with low divergence. The radiant emission can be very powerful and either continuous or pulsating.

Laser light can serve as the source of incident energy in a spectrometer or nephelometer. Some lasers produce bandwidths of a few kilohertz in both the visible and infrared regions, making these applications about three to six orders more sensitive than conventional spectrometers.[9]

Laser spectrometry can also be used for the determination of structure and identification of samples, as well as for diagnosis. Quantitation of samples depends on the spectrometer used. An example of the clinical application of laser is the Coulter counter, which is used for differential analysis of white blood cells.[10]

ELECTROCHEMISTRY

Many types of electrochemical analyses are used in the clinical laboratory, including potentiometry, amperometry, coulometry, and polarography. The two basic electrochemical cells involved in these analyses are galvanic and electrolytic cells.

Galvanic and Electrolytic Cells

An electrochemical cell can be set up as shown in Figure 5-17. It consists of two half-cells and a salt bridge, which can be a piece of filter paper saturated with electrolytes. Instead of two beakers as shown, the electrodes can be immersed in a single, large beaker containing a salt solution. In such a setup, the solution serves as the salt bridge.

In a galvanic cell, as the electrodes are connected, there is spontaneous flow of electrons from the electrode with the lower electron affinity (oxidation; e.g., silver). These electrons pass through the external meter to the cathode (reduction), where OH^- ions are liberated. This reaction continues until one of the chemical components is depleted, at which point, the cell is "dead" and cannot produce electrical energy to the external meter.

Current may be forced to flow through the dead cell only by applying an external electromotive force E. This is called an electrolytic cell. In short, a galvanic cell can be built from an electrolytic cell. When the external E is turned off, accumulated products at the electrodes will spontaneously produce current in the opposite direction of the electrolytic cell.

Half-Cells

It is impossible to measure the electrochemical activity of one half-cell; two reactions must be coupled and one reaction compared with the other. To rate half-cell reactions, a specific electrode reaction is arbitrarily assigned 0.00 V. Every other reaction coupled with this arbitrary zero reaction is either positive or negative, depending on the relative affinity for electrons. The electrode defined as 0.00 V is the standard hydrogen electrode: H_2 gas at 1 atmosphere (atm). The hydrogen gas in contact with H^+ in solution develops a potential. The hydrogen electrode coupled with a zinc half-cell is cathodic, with the reaction $2H^+ + 2e^- \rightarrow H_2$, because H_2 has a greater affinity than Zn for electrons. Cu, however, has a greater affinity than H_2 for electrons, and thus the anodic reaction $H_2 \rightarrow 2H^+ + 2e^-$ occurs when coupled to the Cu-electrode half-cell.

The potential generated by the hydrogen-gas electrode is used to rate the electrode potential of metals in 1 mol/L solution. Reduction potentials for certain metals are shown in Table 5-1.[11] A hydrogen electrode is used

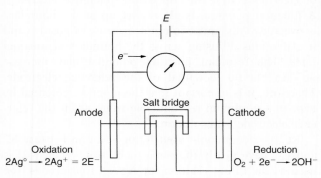

FIGURE 5-17 Electrochemical cell.

TABLE 5-1	STANDARD REDUCTION POTENTIALS	
		POTENTIAL, V
$Zn^{2+} + 2e \leftrightarrow Z$		−0.7628
$Cr^{2+} + 2e \leftrightarrow Cr$		−0.913
$Ni^{2+} + 2e \leftrightarrow Ni$		−0.257
$2H^+ + 2e \leftrightarrow H_2$		0.000
$Cu^{2+} + 2e \leftrightarrow Cu$		0.3419
$Ag^+ + e \leftrightarrow Ag$		0.7996

Data presented are examples from Lide DR. *CRC Handbook of Chemistry and Physics.* 93rd ed. Boca Raton, FL: CRC Press; 2012-2013.

to determine the accuracy of reference and indicator electrodes, the stability of standard solutions, and the potentials of liquid junctions.

Ion-Selective Electrodes

Potentiometric methods of analysis involve the direct measurement of electrical potential due to the activity of free ions. Ion-selective electrodes (ISEs) are designed to be sensitive toward individual ions.

pH Electrodes

An ISE universally used in the clinical laboratory is the pH electrode. The basic components of a pH meter are shown in Figure 5-18.

Indicator Electrode
The pH electrode consists of a silver wire coated with AgCl, immersed into an internal solution of 0.1 mmol/L HCl, and placed into a tube containing a special glass membrane tip. This membrane is only sensitive to hydrogen ions (H^+). Glass membranes that are selectively sensitive to H^+ consist of specific quantities of lithium, cesium, lanthanum, barium, or aluminum oxides in silicate. When the pH electrode is placed into the test solution, movement of H^+ near the tip of the electrode produces a potential difference between the internal solution and the test solution, which is measured as pH and read by a voltmeter. The combination pH electrode also contains a built-in reference electrode, either Ag/AgCl or calomel (Hg/Hg_2Cl_2) immersed in a solution of saturated KCl.

The specially formulated glass continually dissolves from the surface. The present concept of the selective mechanism that causes the formation of electromotive force at the glass surface is that an ion-exchange process is involved. Cationic exchange occurs only in the gel layer—there is no penetration of H^+ through the glass. Although the glass is constantly dissolving, the process is slow, and the glass tip generally lasts for several years. pH electrodes are highly selective for H^+; however, other cations in high concentration interfere, the most common of which is sodium. Electrode manufacturers should list the concentration of interfering cations that may cause error in pH determinations.

Reference Electrode
The reference electrode commonly used is the calomel electrode. Calomel, a paste of predominantly mercurous chloride, is in direct contact with metallic mercury in an electrolyte solution of potassium chloride. As long as the electrolyte concentration and the temperature remain constant, a stable voltage is generated at the interface of the mercury and its salt. A cable connected to the mercury leads to the voltmeter. The filling hole is needed for adding potassium chloride solution. A tiny opening at the bottom is required for completion of electric contact between the reference and indicator electrodes. The liquid junction consists of a fiber or ceramic plug that allows a small flow of electrolyte filling solution.

Construction varies, but all reference electrodes must generate a stable electrical potential. Reference electrodes generally consist of a metal and its salt in contact with a solution containing the same anion. Mercury/mercurous chloride, as in this example, is a frequently used reference electrode; the disadvantage is that it is slow to reach a new stable voltage following temperature change and it is unstable above 80°C.[1,2] Ag/AgCl is another common reference electrode. It can be used at high temperatures, up to 275°C, and the AgCl-coated Ag wire makes a more compact electrode than that of mercury. In measurements in which chloride contamination must be avoided, a mercury sulfate and potassium sulfate reference electrode may be used.

Liquid Junctions
Electrical connection between the indicator and reference electrodes is achieved by allowing a slow flow of electrolyte from the tip of the reference electrode. A junction potential is always set up at the boundary between two dissimilar solutions because of positive and negative ions diffusing across the boundary at unequal rates. The resultant junction potential may increase or decrease the potential of the reference electrode. Therefore, it is important that the junction potential be kept to a minimum reproducible value when the reference electrode is in solution.

KCl is a commonly used filling solution because K^+ and Cl^- have nearly the same mobilities. When KCl is used as the filling solution for Ag/AgCl electrodes, the addition of AgCl is required to prevent dissolution of

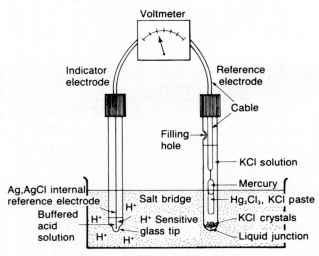

FIGURE 5-18 Necessary components of a pH meter.

the AgCl salt. One way of producing a lower junction potential is to mix K^+, Na^+, NO_3^-, and Cl^- in appropriate ratios.

Readout Meter

Electromotive force produced by the reference and indicator electrodes is in the millivolt range. Zero potential for the cell indicates that each electrode half-cell is generating the same voltage, assuming there is no liquid junction potential. The isopotential is that potential at which a temperature change has no effect on the response of the electrical cell. Manufacturers generally achieve this by making the midscale (pH 7.0) correspond to 0 V at all temperatures. They use an internal buffer whose pH changes due to temperature compensate for the changes in the internal and external reference electrodes.

Nernst Equation

The electromotive force generated because of H^+ at the glass tip is described by Nernst equation, which is shown in a simplified form:

$$\varepsilon = \Delta pH \times \frac{RT \ln 10}{F} = \Delta pH \times 0.059 \text{ V} \qquad \text{(Eq. 5-6)}$$

where ε is the electromotive force of the cell, F is the Faraday constant (96,500C/mol), R is the molar gas constant, and T is temperature, in Kelvin.

As the temperature increases, H^+ activity increases and the potential generated increases. Most pH meters have a temperature compensation knob that amplifies the millivolt response when the meter is on pH function. pH units on the meter scale are usually printed for use at room temperature. On the voltmeter, 59.16 is read as 1 pH unit change. The temperature compensation changes the millivolt response to compensate for changes due to temperature from 54.2 at 0°C to 66.10 at 60°C. However, most pH meters are manufactured for greatest accuracy in the 10°C to 60°C range.

Calibration

The steps necessary to standardize a pH meter are fairly straightforward. First, balance the system with the electrodes in a buffer with a 7.0 pH. The balance or intercept control shifts the entire slope, as shown in Figure 5-19. Next, replace the buffer with one of a different pH. If the meter does not register the correct pH, amplification of the response changes the slope to match that predicted by Nernst equation. If the instrument does not have a slope control, the temperature compensator performs the same function.

pH Combination Electrode

The most commonly used pH electrode has both the indicator and reference electrodes combined in one small probe, which is convenient when small samples are tested. It consists of an Ag/AgCl internal reference electrode sealed in a narrow glass cylinder with a pH-sensitive

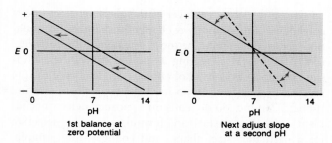

FIGURE 5-19 pH meter calibration. (Adapted from Willard HH, Merritt LL, Dean JA, et al. *Instrumental Methods of Analysis.* Belmont, CA: Wadsworth; 1981.)

glass tip. The reference electrode is an Ag/AgCl wire wrapped around the indicator electrode. The outer glass envelope is filled with KCl and has a tiny pore near the tip of the liquid junction. The solution to be measured must completely cover the glass tip. Examples of other ISEs are shown in Figure 5-20. The reference electrode, electrometer, and calibration system described for pH measurements are applicable to all ISEs.

There are three major ISE types: inert metal electrodes in contact with a redox couple, metal electrodes that participate in a redox reaction, and membrane electrodes. The membrane can be solid material (e.g., glass), liquid (e.g., ion-exchange electrodes), or special membrane (e.g., compound electrodes), such as gas-sensing and enzyme electrodes.

The standard hydrogen electrode is an example of an inert metal electrode. The Ag/AgCl electrode is an example of the second type. The electrode process $AgCl + e^- \rightarrow Ag^+ + Cl^-$ produces an electrical potential proportional to chloride ion (Cl^-) activity. When Cl^- is held constant, the electrode is used as a reference electrode. The electrode in contact with varying Cl^- concentrations is used as an indicator electrode to measure Cl^- concentration.

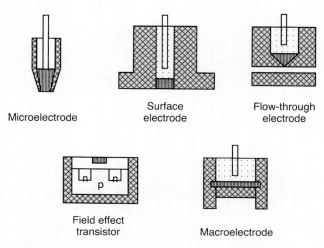

FIGURE 5-20 Other examples of ion-selective electrodes.

The H^+-sensitive gel layer of the glass pH electrode is considered a membrane. A change in the glass formulation makes the membrane more sensitive to sodium ions (Na^+) than to H^+, creating a sodium ISE. Other solid-state membranes consist of either a single crystal or fine crystals immobilized in an inert matrix such as silicone rubber. Conduction depends on a vacancy defect mechanism, and the crystals are formulated to be selective for a particular size, shape, and change—for example, F^--selective electrodes of LaF_3, Cl^--sensitive electrodes with AgCl crystals, and AgBr electrodes for the detection of Br^-.

The calcium ISE is a liquid membrane electrode. An ion-selective carrier, such as dioctylphenyl phosphonate dissolved in an inert water-insoluble solvent, diffuses through a porous membrane. Because the solvent is insoluble in water, the test sample cannot cross the membrane, but calcium ions (Ca^{2+}) are exchanged. The Ag/AgCl internal reference in a filling solution of $CaCl_2$ is in contact with the carrier by means of the membrane.

Potassium-selective liquid membranes use the antibiotic valinomycin as the ion-selective carrier. Valinomycin membranes show great selectivity for K^+. Liquid membrane electrodes are recharged every few months to replace the liquid ion exchanger membrane and the porous membrane.

Gas-Sensing Electrodes

Gas electrodes are similar to pH glass electrodes but are designed to detect specific gases (e.g., CO_2 and NH_3) in solutions and are usually separated from the solution by a thin, gas-permeable hydrophobic membrane. Figure 5-21 shows a schematic illustration of the pCO_2 electrode. The membrane in contact with the solution is permeable only to CO_2, which diffuses into a thin film of sodium bicarbonate solution. The pH of the bicarbonate solution is changed as follows:

$$CO_2 + H_2O \leftrightarrow H_2CO_3 \leftrightarrow H^+ + HCO_3^- \qquad \text{(Eq. 5-7)}$$

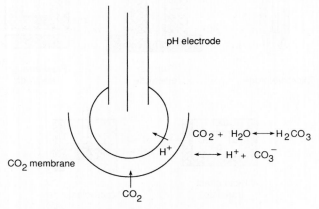

FIGURE 5-21 The pCO_2 electrode.

The change in pH of the HCO_3^- is detected by a pH electrode. The pCO_2 electrode is widely used in clinical laboratories as a component of instruments for measuring serum electrolytes and blood gases.

In the NH_3 gas electrode, the bicarbonate solution is replaced by ammonium chloride solution, and the membrane is permeable only to NH_3 gas. As in the pCO_2 electrode, NH_3 changes the pH of NH_4Cl as follows:

$$NH_3 + H_2O \leftrightarrow NH_4^+ + OH^- \qquad \text{(Eq. 5-8)}$$

The amount of OH^- produced varies linearly with the log of the partial pressure of NH_3 in the sample.

Other gas-sensing electrodes function on the basis of an amperometric principle—that is, measurement of the current flowing through an electrochemical cell at a constant applied electrical potential to the electrodes. Examples are the determination of pO_2, glucose, and peroxidase.

The chemical reactions of the pO_2 electrode (Clark electrode), an electrochemical cell with a platinum cathode and an Ag/AgCl anode, are illustrated in Figure 5-17. The electrical potential at the cathode is set to -0.65 V and will not conduct current without oxygen in the sample. The membrane is permeable to oxygen, which diffuses through to the platinum cathode. Current passes through the cell and is proportional to the pO_2 in the test sample.

Glucose determination is based on the reduction in pO_2 during glucose oxidase reaction with glucose and oxygen. Unlike the pCO_2 electrode, the peroxidase electrode has a polarized platinum anode and its potential is set to $+0.6$ V. Current flows through the system when peroxide is oxidized at the anode as follows:

$$H_2O_2 \rightarrow 2H^+ + 2e^- + O_2 \qquad \text{(Eq. 5-9)}$$

Enzyme Electrodes

The various ISEs may be covered by immobilized enzymes that can catalyze a specific chemical reaction. Selection of the ISE is determined by the reaction product of the immobilized enzyme. Examples include urease, which is used for the detection of urea, and glucose oxidase, which is used for glucose detection. A urea electrode must have an ISE that is selective for NH_4^+ or NH_3, whereas glucose oxidase is used in combination with a pH electrode.

Coulometric Chloridometers and Anodic Stripping Voltammetry

Chloride ISEs have largely replaced coulometric titrations for the determination of chloride in body fluids. Anodic stripping voltammetry was widely used for the analysis of lead and is best measured by electrothermal (graphite furnace) atomic absorption spectroscopy or, preferably, ICP-MS.

ELECTROPHORESIS

Electrophoresis is the migration of charged solutes or particles in an electrical field. Iontophoresis refers to the migration of small ions, whereas zone electrophoresis is the migration of charged macromolecules in a porous support medium such as paper, cellulose acetate, or agarose gel film. An electrophoretogram is the result of zone electrophoresis and consists of sharply separated zones of a macromolecule. In a clinical laboratory, the macromolecules of interest are proteins in serum, urine, cerebrospinal fluid (CSF), and other biologic body fluids and erythrocytes and tissue.

Electrophoresis consists of five components: the driving force (electrical power), the support medium, the buffer, the sample, and the detecting system. A typical electrophoretic apparatus is illustrated in Figure 5-22.

Charged particles migrate toward the opposite charged electrode. The velocity of migration is controlled by the net charge of the particle, the size and shape of the particle, the strength of the electric field, chemical and physical properties of the supporting medium, and the electrophoretic temperature. The rate of mobility[12] of the molecule (μ) is given by

$$\mu = \frac{Q}{K} \leftrightarrow r \leftrightarrow n \qquad \text{(Eq. 5-10)}$$

where Q is net charge of the particle, k is a constant, r is the ionic radius of the particle, and n is the viscosity of the buffer.

From the equation, the rate of migration is directly proportional to the net charge of the particle and inversely proportional to its size and the viscosity of the buffer.

Procedure

The sample is soaked in hydrated support for approximately 5 minutes. The support is put into the electrophoresis chamber, which was previously filled with the buffer. Sufficient buffer must be added to the chamber to maintain contact with the support. Electrophoresis is carried out by applying a constant voltage or constant current for a specific time. The support is then removed and placed in a fixative or rapidly dried to prevent diffusion of the sample. This is followed by staining the zones with an appropriate dye. The uptake of dye by the sample is proportional to sample concentration. After excess dye is washed away, the supporting medium may need to be placed in a clearing agent. Otherwise, it is completely dried.

Power Supply
Power supplies operating at either constant current or constant voltage are available commercially. In electrophoresis, heat is produced when current flows through a medium that has resistance, resulting in an increase in thermal agitation of the dissolved solute (ions) and leading to a decrease in resistance and an increase in current. The increase leads to increases in heat and evaporation of water from the buffer, increasing the ionic concentration of the buffer and subsequent further increases in the current. The migration rate can be kept constant by using a power supply with constant current. This is true because, as electrophoresis progresses, a decrease in resistance as a result of heat produced also decreases the voltage.

Buffers
Two buffer properties that affect the charge of ampholytes are pH and ionic strength. The ions carry the applied electric current and allow the buffer to maintain constant pH during electrophoresis. An ampholyte is a molecule, such as protein, whose net charge can be either positive or negative. If the buffer is more acidic than the isoelectric point (pI) of the ampholyte, it binds H^+, becomes positively charged, and migrates toward the cathode. If the buffer is more basic than the pI, the ampholyte loses H^+, becomes negatively charged, and migrates toward the anode. A particle without a net charge will not migrate, remaining at the point of application. During electrophoresis, ions cluster around a migrating particle. The higher the ionic concentration, the higher the size of the ionic cloud and the lower the mobility of the particle. Greater ionic strength produces sharper protein-band separation but leads to increased heat production. This may cause denaturation of heat-labile proteins. Consequently, the optimal buffer concentration should be determined for any electrophoretic system. Generally, the most widely used buffers are made of monovalent ions because their ionic strength and molality are equal.

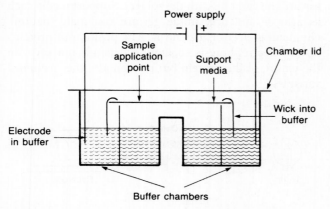

FIGURE 5-22 Electrophoresis apparatus—basic components.

Support Materials

Cellulose Acetate

Paper electrophoresis use has been replaced by cellulose acetate or agarose gel in clinical laboratories. Cellulose is acetylated to form cellulose acetate by treating it with acetic anhydride. Cellulose acetate, a dry, brittle film composed of about 80% air space, is produced commercially. When the film is soaked in buffer, the air spaces fill with electrolyte and the film becomes pliable. After electrophoresis and staining, cellulose acetate can be made transparent for densitometer quantitation. The dried transparent film can be stored for long periods. Cellulose acetate prepared to reduce electroendosmosis is available commercially. Cellulose acetate is also used in isoelectric focusing.

Agarose Gel

Agarose gel is another widely used supporting medium. Used as a purified fraction of agar, it is neutral and, therefore, does not produce electroendosmosis. After electrophoresis and staining, it is detained (cleared), dried, and scanned with a densitometer. The dried gel can be stored indefinitely. Agarose gel electrophoresis requires small amounts of sample (approximately 2 mL); it does not bind protein and, therefore, migration is not affected.

Polyacrylamide Gel

Polyacrylamide gel electrophoresis involves separation of protein on the basis of charge and molecular size. Layers of gel with different pore sizes are used. The gel is prepared before electrophoresis in a tube-shaped electrophoresis cell. The small-pore separation gel is at the bottom, followed by a large-pore spacer gel and, finally, another large-pore gel containing the sample. Each layer of gel is allowed to form a gelatin before the next gel is poured over it. At the start of electrophoresis, the protein molecules move freely through the spacer gel to its boundary with the separation gel, which slows their movement. This allows for concentration of the sample before separation by the small-pore gel. Polyacrylamide gel electrophoresis separates serum proteins into 20 or more fractions rather than the usual 5 fractions separated by cellulose acetate or agarose. It is widely used to study individual proteins (e.g., isoenzymes).

Starch Gel

Starch gel electrophoresis separates proteins on the basis of surface charge and molecular size, as does polyacrylamide gel. The procedure is not widely used because of technical difficulty in preparing the gel.

Treatment and Application of Sample

Serum contains a high concentration of protein, especially albumin, and therefore, serum specimens are routinely diluted with buffer before electrophoresis. In contrast, urine and CSF are usually concentrated. Hemoglobin hemolysate is used without further concentration. Generally, preparation of a sample is done according to the suggestion of the manufacturer of the electrophoretic supplies.

Cellulose acetate and agarose gel electrophoresis require approximately 2 to 5 mL of sample. These are the most common routine electrophoreses performed in clinical laboratories. Because most commercially manufactured plates come with a thin plastic template that has small slots through which samples are applied, overloading of agarose gel with sample is not a frequent problem. After serum is allowed to diffuse into the gel for approximately 5 minutes, the template is blotted to remove excess serum before being removed from the gel surface. Sample is applied to cellulose acetate with a twin-wire applicator designed to transfer a small amount.

Detection and Quantitation

Separated protein fractions are stained to reveal their locations. Different stains come with different plates from different manufacturers. The simplest way to accomplish detection is visualization under UV light, whereas densitometry is the most common and reliable way for quantitation. Most densitometers will automatically integrate the area under a peak, and the result is printed as percentage of the total. A schematic illustration of a densitometer is shown in Figure 5-23.

Electroendosmosis

The movement of buffer ions and solvent relative to the fixed support is called endosmosis or electroendosmosis. Support media, such as paper, cellulose acetate, and agar gel, take on a negative charge from adsorption of hydroxyl ions. When current is applied to the electrophoresis system, the hydroxyl ions remain fixed while the free positive ions move toward the cathode. The ions are highly hydrated, resulting in net cathodic movement of solvent. Molecules that are nearly neutral are swept toward the cathode with the solvent. Support media such as agarose and acrylamide gel are essentially neutral, eliminating electroendosmosis. The position of proteins in any electrophoresis separation depends not only on the nature of the protein but also on all other technical variables.

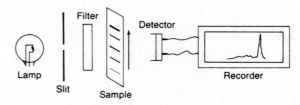

FIGURE 5-23 Densitometer—basic components.

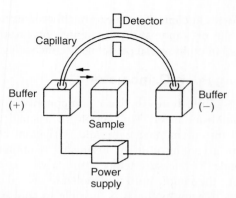

FIGURE 5-24 Schematic of capillary electrophoresis instrumentation. Sample is loaded on the capillary by replacing the anode buffer reservoir with the sample reservoir. (Adapted from Heiger DN. *High-Performance Capillary Electrophoresis*. Waldbronn, Germany: Hewlett-Packard; 1992.)

Isoelectric Focusing

Isoelectric focusing is a modification of electrophoresis. An apparatus is used similar to that shown in Figure 5-24. Charged proteins migrate through a support medium that has a continuous pH gradient. Individual proteins move in the electric field until they reach a pH equal to their isoelectric point, at which point they have no charge and cease to move.

Capillary Electrophoresis

In capillary electrophoresis (CE), separation is performed in narrow-bore fused silica capillaries (inner diameter 25 to 75 μm). Usually, the capillaries are only filled with buffer, although gel media can also be used. A CE instrumentation schematic is shown in Figure 5-24. Initially, the capillary is filled with buffer and then the sample is loaded; applying an electric field performs the separation. Detection can be made near the other end of the capillary directly through the capillary wall.[13]

A fundamental CE concept is the electro-osmotic flow (EOF). EOF is the bulk flow of liquid toward the cathode upon application of an electric field and it is superimposed on electrophoretic migration. EOF controls the amount of time solutes remain in the capillary. Cations migrate fastest because both EOF and electrophoretic attraction are toward the cathode; neutral molecules are all carried by the EOF but are not separated from each other; and anions move slowest because, although they are carried to the cathode by the EOF, they are attracted to the anode and repelled by the cathode (Fig. 5-25). Widely used for monitoring separated analytes, UV-visible detection is performed directly on the capillary; however, sensitivity is poor because of the small dimensions of the capillary, resulting in a short path length. Fluorescence, laser-induced fluorescence, and chemiluminescence detection can be used for higher sensitivity.

CE has been used for the separation, quantitation, and determination of molecular weights of proteins and peptides; for the analysis of polymerase chain reaction products; and for the analysis of inorganic ions, organic acids, pharmaceuticals, optical isomers, and drugs of abuse in serum and urine.[14] While traditionally serum protein electrophoresis (Chapter 11) for the diagnosis of plasma cell dyscrasias has been performed using polyacrylamide gel electrophoresis, CE has now become widely used for this analysis due to its faster run time and its relative automation.

Two-Dimensional Electrophoresis

This electrophoresis assay combines two different electrophoresis dimensions to separate proteins from complex matrices such as serum or tissue. In the first dimension, proteins are resolved according to their isoelectric points (pIs), using immobilized pH gradients. Commercial gradients are available in a variety of pH ranges. In the second dimension, proteins are separated according to their relative size (molecular weight), using sodium dodecyl sulfate–polyacrylamide gel electrophoresis. A schematic of this is shown in Figure 5-26. Gels

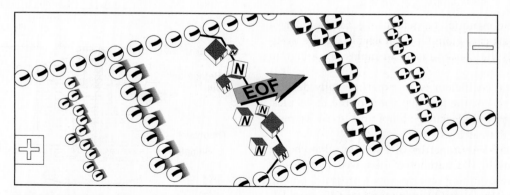

FIGURE 5-25 Differential solute migration superimposed on electro-osmotic flow in capillary zone electrophoresis. (Adapted from Heiger DN. *High-Performance Capillary Electrophoresis*. Waldbronn, Germany: Hewlett-Packard; 1992.)

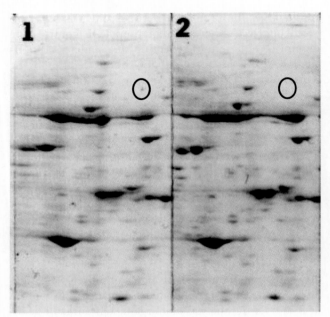

FIGURE 5-26 Hypothetical example of a two-dimensional electrophoretogram from a patient with a disease (*panel 1*) compared with a normal subject (*panel 2*). The patient exhibits a protein (*oval*) that is not expressed in the normal subject. This protein might be a potential marker for this disease. (Gels courtesy of Kendrick Laboratories, Madison, WI.)

can be run under denaturing or nondenaturing conditions (e.g., for the maintenance of enzyme activity) and visualized by a variety of techniques, including the use of colorimetric dyes (e.g., Coomassie blue or silver stain) and radiographic, fluorometric, or chemiluminescence of appropriately labeled polypeptides. These latter techniques are considerably more sensitive than the colorimetric dyes.

OSMOMETRY

An osmometer is used to measure the concentration of solute particles in a solution. The mathematic definition is

$$\text{Osmolality} = \varphi \times n \times C \qquad \text{(Eq. 5-11)}$$

where φ is the osmotic coefficient, n is the number of dissociable particles (ions) per molecule in the solution, and C is the concentration in moles per kilogram of solvent.

The osmotic coefficient is an experimentally derived factor to correct for the fact that some of the molecules, even in a highly dissociated compound, exist as molecules rather than as ions.

The four physical properties of a solution that change with variations in the number of dissolved particles in the solvent are osmotic pressure, vapor pressure, boiling point, and freezing point. Osmometers measure osmolality indirectly by measuring one of these colligative properties, which change proportionally with osmotic pressure.

Osmometers in clinical use measure either freezing point depression or vapor pressure depression; results are expressed in milliosmolal per kilogram (mOsm/kg) units.

Freezing Point Osmometer

Figure 5-27 illustrates the basic components of a freezing point osmometer. The sample in a small tube is lowered into a chamber with cold refrigerant circulating from a cooling unit. A thermistor is immersed in the sample. To measure temperature, a wire is used to gently stir the sample until it is cooled to several degrees below its freezing point. It is possible to cool water to as low as −40°C and still have liquid water, provided no crystals or particulate matter is present. This is referred to as a supercooled solution. Vigorous agitation when the sample is supercooled results in rapid freezing. Freezing can also be started by "seeding" a supercooled solution with crystals. When the supercooled solution starts to freeze as a result of the rapid stirring, a slush is formed and the solution actually warms to its freezing point temperature. The slush, an equilibrium of liquid and ice crystals, will remain at the freezing point temperature until the sample freezes solid and drops below its freezing point.

Impurities in a solvent will lower the temperature at which freezing or melting occurs by reducing the bonding forces between solvent molecules so that the molecules break away from each other and exist as a fluid at a lower temperature. The decrease in the freezing point temperature is proportional to the number of dissolved particles present.

The thermistor is a material that has less resistance when the temperature increases. The readout uses a Wheatstone bridge circuit that detects temperature change as proportional to change in thermistor resistance. Freezing point depression is proportional to the number of solute particles. Standards of known concentration are used to calibrate the instruments in mOsm/kg.

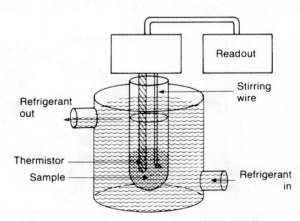

FIGURE 5-27 Freezing point osmometer. (Adapted from Coiner D. *Basic Concepts in Laboratory Instrumentation.* Bethesda, MD: ASMT Education and Research Fund; 1975-1979.)

For additional student resources please visit thePoint at http://thepoint.lww.com.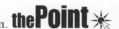

1. Which of the following is *not* necessary for obtaining the spectrum of a compound from 190 to 500 nm?
   a. Tungsten light source
   b. Deuterium light source
   c. Double-beam spectrophotometer
   d. Quartz cuvettes
   e. Photomultiplier

2. Stray light in a spectrophotometer places limits on
   a. Upper range of linearity
   b. Sensitivity
   c. Photometric accuracy below 0.1 absorbance units
   d. Ability to measure in the UV range
   e. Use of a grating monochromator

3. Which of the following light sources is used in atomic absorption spectrophotometry?
   a. Hollow-cathode lamp
   b. Xenon arc lamp
   c. Tungsten light
   d. Deuterium lamp
   e. Laser

4. Which of the following is true concerning fluorometry?
   a. Fluorescence is an inherently more sensitive technique than absorption.
   b. Emission wavelengths are always set at lower wavelengths than excitation.
   c. The detector is always placed at right angles to the excitation beam.
   d. All compounds undergo fluorescence.
   e. Fluorometers require special detectors.

5. Which of the following techniques has the highest potential sensitivity?
   a. Chemiluminescence
   b. Fluorescence
   c. Turbidimetry
   d. Nephelometry
   e. Phosphorescence

6. Which electrochemical assay measures current at fixed potential?
   a. Amperometry
   b. Anodic stripping voltammetry
   c. Coulometry
   d. Analysis with ISEs
   e. Electrophoresis

7. Which of the following refers to the movement of buffer ions and solvent relative to the fixed support?
   a. Electroendosmosis
   b. Isoelectric focusing
   c. Iontophoresis
   d. Zone electrophoresis
   e. Plasmapheresis

8. Reverse-phase liquid chromatography refers to
   a. A polar mobile phase and nonpolar stationary phase
   b. A nonpolar mobile phase and polar stationary phase
   c. Distribution between two liquid phases
   d. Size used to separate solutes instead of charge
   e. Charge used to separate solutes instead of size

9. Which of the following is *not* an advantage of CE?
   a. Multiple samples can be assayed simultaneously on one injection
   b. Very small sample size
   c. Rapid analysis
   d. Use of traditional detectors
   e. Cations, neutrals, and anions move in the same direction at different rates

10. Tandem mass spectrometers
    a. Are two mass spectrometers placed in series with each other
    b. Are two mass spectrometers placed in parallel with each other
    c. Require use of a gas chromatograph
    d. Require use of an electrospray interface
    e. Do not require an ionization source

11. Which of the following is *false* concerning the principles of point-of-care testing devices?
    a. Devices do not require quality control testing.
    b. They use principles that are identical to laboratory-based instrumentation.
    c. Biosensors have enabled miniaturization particularly amendable for point-of-care testing.
    d. Onboard microcomputers control instrument functions and data reduction.
    e. Whole blood analysis is the preferred specimen.

12. Which is the most sensitive detector for spectrophotometry?
    a. Photomultiplier
    b. Phototube
    c. Electron multiplier

d. Photodiode array

e. All are equally sensitive

13. Which of the following is Beer's law?
    a. $A = \varepsilon \times b \times c$
    b. $\%T = I/I_0 \times 100$
    c. $E = h\nu$
    d. $\varepsilon = \Delta pH \times 0.59\ V$
    e. Osmolality $= \varphi \times n \times C$

14. Which of the following correctly ranks electromagnetic radiation from low energy to high energy?
    a. Microwaves, infrared, visible, UV, x-rays, gamma, cosmic
    b. Cosmic, gamma, x-rays, UV, visible, infrared, microwaves
    c. UV, visible, infrared, microwaves, x-rays, cosmic, gamma
    d. UV, visible, infrared, cosmic, gamma, microwaves, x-rays
    e. Visible, UV, infrared, cosmic, gamma, microwaves, x-rays

15. What is the purpose of the chopper in an atomic absorption spectrophotometer?
    a. Correct for the amount of light emitted by the flame
    b. Correct for the fluctuating intensity of the light source
    c. Correct for the fluctuating sensitivity of the detector
    d. Correct for differences in the aspiration rate of the sample
    e. Correct for the presence of stray light

16. Which of the following best describes the process of fluorescence?
    a. Molecules emit a photon at lower energy when excited electrons return to the ground state.
    b. Atoms emit a photon when the electrons are excited.
    c. Molecules emit a photon when the electrons are excited.
    d. Molecules emit a photon at the same energy when excited electrons return to the ground state.

    e. Molecules emit a photon at higher energy when excited electrons return to the ground state.

17. Which is most accurate concerning ISEs?
    a. Gas-specific membranes are necessary for oxygen and carbon dioxide electrodes.
    b. The pH electrode uses a solid-state membrane.
    c. The calcium electrode does not require a reference electrode.
    d. The sodium electrode uses an ion-selective carrier (valinomycin).
    e. The ISE for urea uses immobilized urease.

18. Which of the following regarding MS is *false*?
    a. Mass spectrometers can be used to sequence DNA.
    b. Ions are formed by the bombardment of electrons.
    c. Quadrupole and ion trap sectors separate ions according to their mass-to-charge ratio.
    d. Each chemical compound has a unique mass spectrum.
    e. MS detects for gas and liquid chromatography.

19. Which of the following is not an objective of proteomics research?
    a. Identifying specific gene mutations
    b. Identifying novel proteins as potential new biomarkers for disease
    c. Identifying posttranslational modifications of proteins
    d. Understanding the mechanism of diseases
    e. Determining which genes are expressed and which genes are dormant

20. Which of the following procedures is not currently or routinely used for point-of-care testing devices?
    a. Polymerase chain reaction
    b. Immunochromatography
    c. Biosensors
    d. Colorimetric detection
    e. Electrochemical detection

REFERENCES

1. Christian GD, O'Reilly JE. *Instrumental Analysis.* 2nd ed. Boston, MA: Allyn and Bacon; 1986.
2. Willard HH, Merritt LL, Dean JA, et al. *Instrumental Methods of Analysis.* Belmont, CA: Wadsworth; 1981.
3. Coiner D. *Basic Concepts in Laboratory Instrumentation.* Bethesda, MD: ASMT Education and Research Fund; 1975-1979.
4. Ingle JD, Crouch SR. *Spectrochemical Analysis.* Upper Saddle River, NJ: Prentice-Hall; 1988.
5. Holland JF, Enke CG, Allison J, et al. Mass spectrometry on the chromatographic time scale: realistic expectations. *Anal Chem.* 1983;55:997A.
6. Guilbault GG. *Practical Fluorescence, Theory, Methods and Techniques.* New York, NY: Marcel Dekker; 1973.

7. Kricka LJ. Chemiluminescent and bioluminescent techniques. *Clin Chem*. 1991;37:1472.

8. Wild D. *The Immunoassay Handbook*. London: Macmillan Press; 1994.

9. Svelto O. *Principles of Lasers*. 2nd ed. New York, NY: Plenum Press; 1982.

10. *Coulter Hematology Analyzer: Multidimensional Leukocyte Differential Analysis*. Vol 11(1). Miami, FL: Beckman Coulter; 1989.

11. Weast RC. *CRC Handbook of Chemistry and Physics*. 61st ed. Cleveland, OH: CRC Press; 1981.

12. Burtis CA. *Tietz Textbook of Clinical Chemistry*. 2nd ed. Philadelphia, PA: WB Saunders; 1993.

13. Heiger DN. *High-Performance Capillary Electrophoresis: An Introduction*. 2nd ed. Waldbronn, Germany: Hewlett-Packard; 1992.

14. Monnig CA, Kennedy RT. Capillary electrophoresis. *Anal Chem*. 1994;66:280R.

Chromatography and Mass Spectrometry

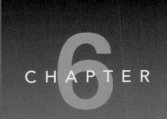

CHAPTER 6

JULIA C. DREES, MATTHEW S. PETRIE, ALAN H.B. WU

CHAPTER OUTLINE

- ◆ **CHROMATOGRAPHY**
  Modes of Separation
  Chromatographic Procedures
  High-Performance Liquid Chromatography
  Gas Chromatography
- ◆ **MASS SPECTROMETRY**
  Sample Introduction and Ionization
  Mass Analyzer
  Detector

- ◆ **APPLICATIONS OF MS IN THE CLINICAL LABORATORY**
  Small Molecule Analysis
  Mass Spectrometry in Proteomics and Pathogen Identification
- ◆ **QUESTIONS**
- ◆ **REFERENCES**

Chapter Objectives

Upon completion of this chapter, the clinical laboratorian should be able to do the following:

- Explain the general principles of each analytic method.
- Discuss the limitations of each analytic technique.
- Compare and contrast the various analytic techniques.
- Discuss existing clinical applications for each analytic technique.

- Describe the operation and component parts of the following instruments: mass spectrometer and gas chromatograph.
- Outline the quality assurance and preventive maintenance procedures involved with the following instruments: mass spectrometer and gas chromatograph.

KEY TERMS

Chromatography
Gas chromatography

High-performance liquid chromatography
Mass spectrometry

Over the past several decades, the number of analytes measured in clinical laboratories has increased dramatically. This has been accompanied by an equally high demand for technologies that can accurately measure a large variety of compounds. Liquid or gas chromatography (GC) coupled to mass spectrometry (MS) has long been considered the gold standard for most testing due to its high sensitivity and specificity. In this chapter, we will discuss how these high-complexity instruments operate and, in turn, how they are utilized in the modern clinical laboratory.

CHROMATOGRAPHY

Chromatography refers to the group of techniques used to separate complex mixtures on the basis of different physical interactions between the individual compounds and the stationary phase of the system. The

basic components in any chromatographic technique are the mobile phase (gas or liquid), which carries the complex mixture (sample); the stationary phase (solid or liquid), through which the mobile phase flows; the column holding the stationary phase; and the separated components (eluate).

Modes of Separation

Adsorption

Adsorption chromatography, also known as liquid–solid chromatography, is based on the competition between the sample and the mobile phase for adsorptive sites on the solid stationary phase. There is an equilibrium of solute molecules being adsorbed to the solid surface and desorbed and dissolved in the mobile phase. The molecules that are most soluble in the mobile phase move fastest; the least soluble move slowest. Thus, a mixture is typically separated into classes according to polar functional groups. The stationary phase can be acidic polar (e.g., silica gel), basic polar (e.g., alumina), or nonpolar (e.g., charcoal). The mobile phase can be a single solvent or a mixture of two or more solvents, depending on the analytes to be desorbed. Liquid–solid chromatography is not widely used in clinical laboratories because of technical problems with the preparation of a stationary phase that has homogeneous distribution of absorption sites.

Partition

Partition chromatography is also referred to as liquid–liquid chromatography. Separation of solute is based on relative solubility in an organic (nonpolar) solvent and an aqueous (polar) solvent. In its simplest form, partition (extraction) is performed in a separatory funnel. Molecules containing polar and nonpolar groups in an aqueous solution are added to an immiscible organic solvent. After vigorous shaking, the two phases are allowed to separate. Polar molecules remain in the aqueous solvent; nonpolar molecules are extracted in the organic solvent. This results in the partitioning of the solute molecules into two separate phases.

The ratio of the concentration of the solute in the two liquids is known as the partition coefficient:

$$K = \frac{\text{solute in stationary phase}}{\text{solute in mobile phase}} \quad \text{(Eq. 6-1)}$$

Modern partition chromatography uses pseudo-liquid stationary phases that are chemically bonded to the support or high-molecular-weight polymers that are insoluble in the mobile phase.[1] Partition systems are considered normal phase when the mobile solvent is less polar than the stationary solvent and reverse phase when the mobile solvent is more polar.

Partition chromatography is applicable to any substance that may be distributed between two liquid phases. Because ionic compounds are generally soluble only in water, partition chromatography works best with nonionic compounds.

Steric Exclusion

Steric exclusion, a variation of liquid–solid chromatography, is used to separate solute molecules on the basis of size and shape. The chromatographic column is packed with porous material, as shown in Figure 6-1. A sample containing different-sized molecules moves down the column dissolved in the mobile solvent. Small molecules enter the pores in the packing and are momentarily trapped. Large molecules are excluded from the small pores and so move quickly between the particles. Intermediate-sized molecules are partially restricted from entering the pores and, therefore, move through the column at an intermediate rate that is between those of the large and small molecules.

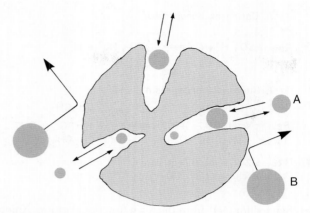

FIGURE 6-1 Pictorial concept of steric exclusion chromatography. Separation of sample components by their ability to permeate pore structure of column-packing material. Smaller molecules (**A**) permeating the interstitial pores; large excluded molecules (**B**). (Adapted from Parris NA. *Instrumental Liquid Chromatography: A Practical Manual on High Performance Liquid Chromatographic Methods.* New York, NY: Elsevier; 1976.)

Early methods used hydrophilic beads of cross-linked dextran, polyacrylamide, or agarose, which formed a gel when soaked in water. This method was termed gel filtration. A similar separation process using hydrophobic gel beads of polystyrene with a nonaqueous mobile phase was called gel permeation chromatography. Current porous packing uses rigid inorganic materials such as silica or glass. The term steric exclusion includes all these variations. Pore size is controlled by the manufacturer, and packing materials can be purchased with different pore sizes, depending on the size of the molecules being separated.

Ion-Exchange Chromatography

In ion-exchange chromatography, solute mixtures are separated by virtue of the magnitude and charge of ionic species. The stationary phase is a resin, consisting of large polymers of substituted benzene, silicates, or cellulose derivatives, with charged functional groups. The resin is insoluble in water, and the functional groups are immobilized as side chains on resin beads that are used to fill the chromatographic column. Figure 6-2A shows a resin with sulfonate functional groups. Hydrogen$^+$ ions are loosely held and free to react. This is an example of a cation-exchange resin. When a cation such as Na^+ comes in contact with these functional groups, an equilibrium is formed, following the law of mass action. Because there are many sulfonate groups, Na^+ is effectively and completely removed from solution. The Na^+ concentrated on the resin column can be eluted from the resin by pouring acid through the column, driving the equilibrium to the left.

Anion-exchange resins are made with exchangeable hydroxyl ions such as the diethylamine functional group illustrated in Figure 6-2B. They are used like cation-exchange resins, except that hydroxyl ions are exchanged for anions. The example shows Cl^- in sample solution

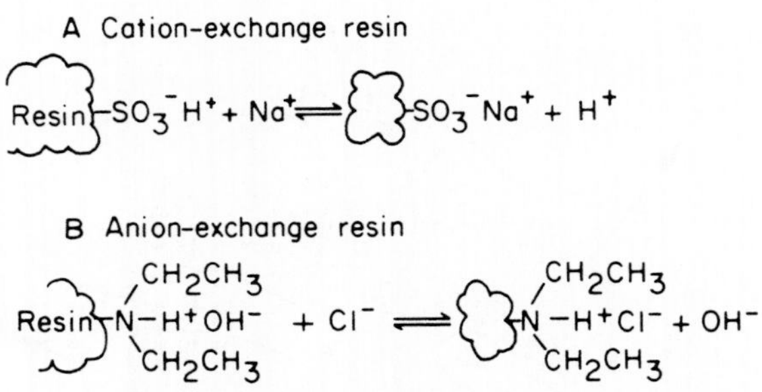

A Cation-exchange resin

Resin─SO$_3^-$H$^+$ + Na$^+$ ⇌ SO$_3^-$Na$^+$ + H$^+$

B Anion-exchange resin

Resin─N─H$^+$OH$^-$ + Cl$^-$ ⇌ N─H$^+$Cl$^-$ + OH$^-$

FIGURE 6-2 Chemical equilibrium of ion-exchange resins. (**A**) Cation-exchange resin. (**B**) Anion-exchange resin.

exchanged for OH$^-$ from the resin functional group. Anion and cation resins mixed together (mixed-bed resin) are used to deionize water. The displaced protons and hydroxyl ions combine to form water. Ionic functional groups other than the illustrated examples are used for specific analytic applications. Ion-exchange chromatography is used to remove interfering substances from a solution, to concentrate dilute ion solutions, and to separate mixtures of charged molecules, such as amino acids. Changing pH and ionic concentration of the mobile phase allows separation of mixtures of organic and inorganic ions.

Chromatographic Procedures

Thin-Layer Chromatography

Thin-layer chromatography (TLC) is a variant of column chromatography. A thin layer of sorbent, such as alumina, silica gel, cellulose, or cross-linked dextran, is uniformly coated on a glass or plastic plate. Each sample to be analyzed is applied as a spot near one edge of the plate, as shown in Figure 6-3. The mobile phase (solvent) is usually placed in a closed container until the atmosphere is saturated with solvent vapor. One edge of the plate is placed in the solvent, as shown. The solvent migrates up the thin layer by capillary action, dissolving and carrying sample molecules. Separation can be achieved by any of the four processes previously described, depending on the sorbent (thin layer) and

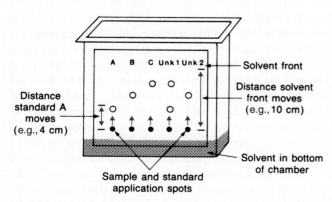

FIGURE 6-3 Thin-layer chromatography plate in chromatographic chamber.

solvent chosen. After the solvent reaches a predetermined height, the plate is removed and dried. Sample components are identified by comparison with standards on the same plate. The distance a component migrates, compared with the distance the solvent front moves, is called the retention factor, R_f:

$$R_f = \frac{\text{distance leading edge of component moves}}{\text{total distance solvent front moves}} \quad \text{(Eq. 6-2)}$$

Each sample component R_f is compared with the R_f of standards. Using Figure 6-3 as an example, standard A has an R_f value of 0.4, standard B has an R_f value of 0.6, and standard C has an R_f value of 0.8. The first unknown contains A and C, because the R_f values are the same. This ratio is valid only for separations run under identical conditions. Because R_f values may overlap for some components, further identifying information is obtained by spraying different stains on the dried plate and comparing colors of the standards.

TLC is most commonly used as a semiquantitative screening test. Technique refinement has resulted in the development of semiautomated equipment and the ability to quantitate separated compounds. For example, sample applicators apply precise amounts of sample extracts in concise areas. Plates prepared with uniform sorbent thickness, finer particles, and new solvent systems have resulted in the technique of high-performance thin-layer chromatography (HPTLC).[2] Absorbance of each developed spot is measured using a densitometer, and the concentration is calculated by comparison with a reference standard chromatographed under identical conditions.

High-Performance Liquid Chromatography

Modern high-performance liquid chromatography (HPLC) uses pressure for fast separations, controlled temperature, in-line detectors, and gradient elution techniques.[3,4] Figure 6-4 illustrates the basic components.

Pumps

A pump forces the mobile phase through the column at a much greater velocity than that accomplished by gravity flow columns and includes pneumatic, syringe, reciprocating, or hydraulic amplifier pumps. The most widely used pump today is the mechanical reciprocating pump, which is used as a multihead pump with two or more reciprocating pistons. During pumping, the pistons operate out of phase (180° for two heads, 120° for three heads) to provide constant flow. Pneumatic pumps are used for preoperative purposes; hydraulic amplifier pumps are no longer commonly used.

Columns

The stationary phase is packed into long stainless steel columns. HPLC is usually run at ambient temperatures, although columns can be put in an oven and heated

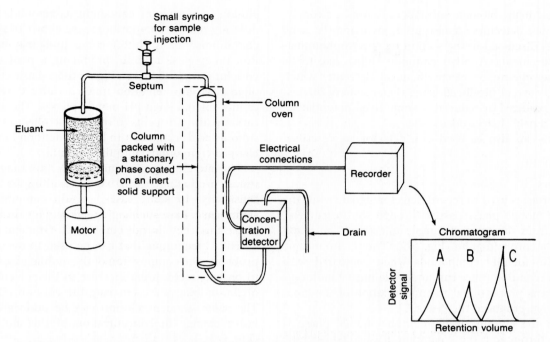

FIGURE 6-4 High-performance liquid chromatography basic components. (Adapted from Bender GT. *Chemical Instrumentation: A Laboratory Manual Based on Clinical Chemistry.* Philadelphia, PA: WB Saunders; 1972.)

to enhance the rate of partition. Fine, uniform column packing results in much less band broadening but requires pressure to force the mobile phase through. The packing can also be pellicular (an inert core with a porous layer), inert and small particles, or macroporous particles. The most common material used for column packing is silica gel. It is very stable and can be used in different ways. It can be used as solid packing in liquid–solid chromatography or coated with a solvent, which serves as the stationary phase (liquid–liquid). As a result of the short lifetime of coated particles, molecules of the mobile-phase liquid are now bonded to the surface of silica particles.

Reversed-phase HPLC is now popular; the stationary phase is nonpolar molecules (e.g., octadecyl C-18 hydrocarbon) bonded to silica gel particles. For this type of column packing, the mobile phase commonly used is acetonitrile, methanol, water, or any combination of solvents. A reversed-phase column can be used to separate ionic, nonionic, and ionizable samples. A buffer is used to produce the desired ionic characteristics and pH for separation of the analyte. Column packings vary in size (3 to 20 mm), using smaller particles mostly for analytic separations and larger ones for preparative separations.

Sample Injectors
A small syringe can be used to introduce the sample into the path of the mobile phase that carries it into the column (Fig. 6-4). The best and most widely used method, however, is the loop injector. The sample is introduced into a fixed-volume loop. When the loop is switched, the sample is placed in the path of the flowing mobile phase and flushed onto the column. Loop injectors have high reproducibility and are used at high pressures. Many HPLC instruments have loop injectors that can be programmed for automatic injection of samples. When the sample size is less than the volume of the loop, the syringe containing the sample is often filled with the mobile phase to the volume of the loop before filling the loop. This prevents the possibility of air being forced through the column because such a practice may reduce the lifetime of the column-packing material.

Detectors
Modern HPLC detectors monitor the eluate as it leaves the column and, ideally, produce an electronic signal proportional to the concentration of each separated component. Spectrophotometers that detect absorbances of visible or UV light are most commonly used. Photodiode array (PDA) and other rapid scanning detectors are also used for spectral comparisons and compound identification and purity. These detectors have been used for drug analyses in urine. Obtaining a UV scan of a compound as it elutes from a column can provide important information as to its identity. Unknowns can be compared against library spectra in a similar manner to MS. Unlike gas chromatography/MS, which requires volatilization of targeted compounds, liquid chromatography (LC)/PDA enables direct injection of aqueous urine samples.

Because many biologic substances fluoresce strongly, fluorescence detectors are also used, involving the same principles discussed in the section on spectrophotometric measurements. Another common HPLC detector is the amperometric or electrochemical detector, which measures current produced when the analyte of interest is either oxidized or reduced at some fixed potential set between a pair of electrodes.

An MS can also be used as a detector, as described later.

Recorders

The recorder is used to record detector signal versus the time the mobile phase passed through the instrument, starting from the time of sample injection. The graph is called a chromatogram (Fig. 6-5). The retention time is used to identify compounds when compared with standard retention times run under identical conditions. Peak area is proportional to concentration of the compounds that produced the peaks.

When the elution strength of the mobile phase is constant throughout the separation, it is called isocratic elution. For samples containing compounds of widely differing relative compositions, the choice of solvent is a compromise. Early eluting compounds may have retention times close to zero, producing a poor separation (resolution), as shown in Figure 6-5A. Basic compounds often have low retention times because C-18 columns cannot tolerate high pH mobile phases. The addition of cation-pairing reagents to the mobile phase (e.g., octane sulfonic acid) can result in better retention of negatively charged compounds onto the column.

The late-eluting compounds may have long retention times, producing broad bands resulting in decreased sensitivity. In some cases, certain components of a sample may have such a great affinity for the stationary phase that they do not elute at all. Gradient elution is an HPLC technique that can be used to overcome this problem. The composition of the mobile phase is varied to provide a continual increase in the solvent strength of the mobile phase entering the column (Fig. 6-5B). The same gradient elution can be performed with a faster change in concentration of the mobile phase (Fig. 6-5C).

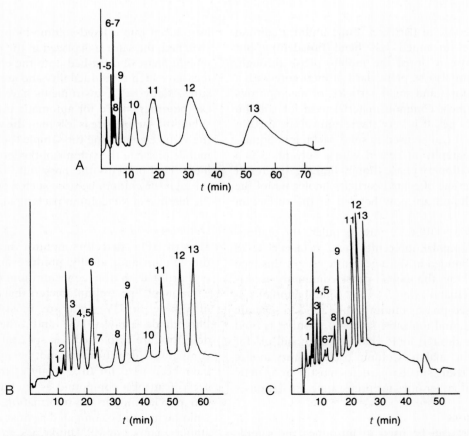

FIGURE 6-5 Chromatograms. (**A**) Isocratic ion-exchange separation mobile phase contains 0.055 mol/L NaNO3. (**B**) Gradient elution mobile phase gradient from 0.01 to 0.1 mol/L NaNO3 at 2% per min. (**C**) Gradient elution—5% per minute. (Adapted from Horváth C. *High Performance Liquid Chromatography, Advances and Perspectives*. New York, NY: Academic Press; 1980.)

Gas Chromatography

Gas chromatography is used to separate mixtures of compounds that are volatile or can be made volatile.[5] GC may be gas–solid chromatography, with a solid stationary phase, or gas–liquid chromatography (GLC), with a nonvolatile liquid stationary phase. GLC is commonly used in clinical laboratories. Figure 6-6 illustrates the basic components of a GC system. The setup is similar to HPLC, except that the mobile phase is a gas and samples are partitioned between a gaseous mobile phase and a liquid stationary phase. The carrier gas can be nitrogen, helium, or argon. The selection of a carrier gas is determined by the detector used in the instrument. The instrument can be operated at a constant temperature or programmed to run at different temperatures if a sample has components with different volatilities. This is analogous to gradient elution described for HPLC.

The sample, which is injected through a septum, must be injected as a gas or the temperature of the injection port must be above the boiling point of the components so that they vaporize upon injection. Sample vapor is swept through the column partially as a gas and partially dissolved in the liquid phase. Volatile compounds that are present mainly in the gas phase will have a low partition coefficient and will move quickly through the column. Compounds with higher boiling points will move slowly through the column. The effluent passes through a detector that produces an electric signal proportional to the concentration of the volatile components. As in HPLC, the chromatogram is used both to identify the compounds by the retention time and to determine their concentration by the area under the peak.

Columns

GLC columns are generally made of glass or stainless steel and are available in a variety of coil configurations and sizes. Packed columns are filled with inert particles such as diatomaceous earth or porous polymer or glass beads coated with a nonvolatile liquid (stationary) phase. These columns are usually 1/8 to 1/4 inch wide and 3 to 12 feet long. Capillary wall–coated open tubular columns have inside diameters in the range of 0.25 to 0.50 mm and are up to 60 m long. The liquid layer is coated on the walls of the column. A solid support coated with a liquid stationary phase may in turn be coated on column walls. The liquid stationary phase must be nonvolatile at the temperatures used, must be thermally stable, and must not react chemically with the solutes to be separated. The stationary phase is termed nonselective when separation is primarily based on relative volatility of the compounds. Selective liquid phases are used to separate polar compounds based on relative polarity (as in liquid–liquid chromatography).

Detectors

Although there are many types of detectors, only thermal conductivity (TC) and flame ionization detectors are discussed because they are the most stable (Fig. 6-7).

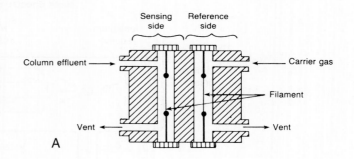

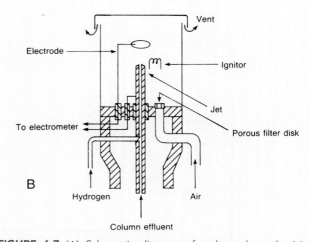

FIGURE 6-7 (**A**) Schematic diagram of a thermal conductivity detector. (**B**) Schematic diagram of a flame ionization detector. (Adapted from Tietz NW, ed. *Fundamentals of Clinical Chemistry*. Philadelphia, PA: WB Saunders, 1987.)

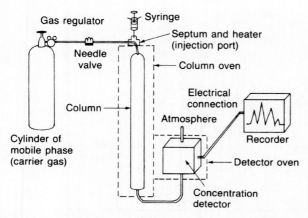

FIGURE 6-6 Gas–liquid chromatography basic components. (Adapted from Bender GT. *Chemical Instrumentation: A Laboratory Manual Based on Clinical Chemistry*. Philadelphia, PA: WB Saunders; 1972.)

TC detectors contain wires (filaments) that change electrical resistance with change in temperature. The filaments form opposite arms of a Wheatstone bridge and are heated electrically to raise their temperature. Helium, which has a high TC, is usually the carrier gas. Carrier gas from the reference column flows steadily across one filament, cooling it slightly. Carrier gas and separated compounds from the sample column flow across the other filament. The sample components usually have a lower TC, increasing the temperature and resistance of the sample filament. The change in resistance results in an unbalanced bridge circuit. The electrical change is amplified and fed to the recorder. The electrical change is proportional to the concentration of the analyte. Flame ionization detectors are widely used in the clinical laboratory. They are more sensitive than TC detectors. The column effluent is fed into a small hydrogen flame burning in excess air or atmospheric oxygen. The flame jet and a collector electrode around the flame have opposite potentials. As the sample burns, ions form and move to the charged collector. Thus, a current proportional to the concentration of the ions is formed and fed to the recorder.

MASS SPECTROMETRY

Definitive identification of samples eluting from GC or HPLC columns is possible when an MS is used as a detector.[6] The coupled techniques, GC/MS and LC/MS, have powerful analytic capabilities with widespread clinical applications. The sample in an MS is first volatilized and then ionized to form charged molecular ions and fragments that are separated according to their mass-to-charge (m/z) ratio; the sample is then measured by a detector, which gives the intensity of the ion current for each species. These steps take place in the four basic components that are standard in all MSs: the sample inlet, ionization source, mass analyzer, and ion detector (Fig. 6-8). Ultimately, molecule identification is based on the formation of characteristic fragments. Figure 6-9 illustrates the mass spectrum of Δ9-carboxytetrahydrocannabinol, a metabolite of marijuana.

Mass Spectrometer Components

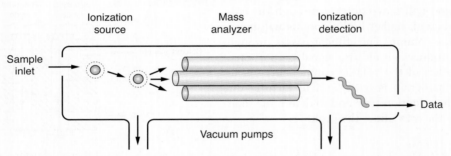

FIGURE 6-8 The components of a mass spectrometer. In this case, the ionization source pictured is electrospray ionization and the mass analyzer is a quadrupole.

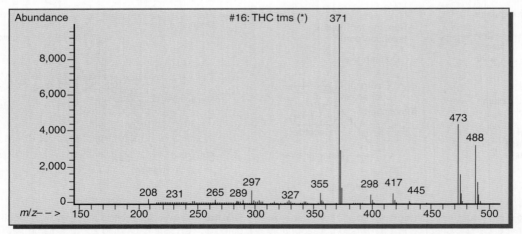

FIGURE 6-9 Mass spectrum of the trimethylsilane derivative of Δ9-carboxytetrahydrocannabinol (marijuana metabolite).

Sample Introduction and Ionization

Direct infusion is commonly used to interface a GC or LC with an MS; however, the challenge of introducing a liquid sample from an LC column into an MS was a significant barrier until recent technological advances in ionization techniques.

Electron Ionization

The most common form of ionization used in GC/MS is electron ionization (EI). This method requires a source of electrons in the form of a filament to which an electric potential is applied, typically at 70 eV.[7] The molecules in the source are bombarded with high-energy electrons, resulting in the formation of charged molecular ions and fragments. Molecules break down into characteristic fragments according to their molecular structure (Fig. 6-10). The ions formed and their relative proportions are reproducible and can be used for qualitative identification of the compound. Since most instruments use the same 70 eV potential, the fragmentation of molecules on different days and different instruments is remarkably similar, allowing the comparison of unknown spectra to spectra in a published reference library.[7]

Atmospheric Pressure Ionization

Unlike EI in GC/MS, most LC/MS ionization techniques are conducted at atmospheric pressure. As such, the ion source of this type of instrument is not included in the high-vacuum region of the instrument. Two types of ionization for LC/MS will be discussed here: electrospray ionization (ESI) and atmospheric pressure chemical ionization (APCI), while matrix-assisted laser desorption ionization (MALDI) and surface-enhanced laser desorption ionization (SELDI) will be discussed later in the section on proteomics. ESI and APCI also differ from EI in that they are "soft" ionization techniques that leave the molecular ion largely intact in the source. Many LC/MS techniques employ technologies after the source, in the mass analyzer, to fragment molecules and generate the daughter or fragment ions used in identification. However, ionization techniques used in LC/MS produce fragments and therefore mass spectra that are somewhat less reproducible between instruments than EI used in GC/MS. This may prove to limit the utility of reference library spectra produced in other instruments.

Electrospray Ionization

Thanks to its wide mass range and high sensitivity, ESI can be applied to a wide range of biological macromolecules in addition to small molecules and has become the most common ionization source for LC/MS. ESI involves passing the LC effluent through a capillary to which a voltage has been applied. The energy is transferred to the solvent droplets, which become charged.[7] Evaporation of the solvent through heat and gas causes the droplets to decrease in size, which increases the charge density on the surface. Eventually, the Coulombic repulsion of like charges leads to the ejection of ions from the droplet (Fig. 6-11).[8] The individually charged molecules are drawn into the MS for mass analysis. ESI is adept at forming singly charged small molecules, but larger molecules can also be ionized using this method. Larger molecules such as proteins become multiply charged in ESI, and since MSs measure the *m/z*, even these large molecules can be observed in an instrument with a relatively small mass range (Fig. 6-12).[8]

Atmospheric Pressure Chemical Ionization

Another important ionization source is APCI, which is similar to ESI in that the liquid from LC is introduced directly into the ionization source. However, the droplets are not charged and the source contains a heated vaporizer to allow rapid desolvation of the drops.[8] A high voltage is applied to a corona discharge needle, which emits a cloud of electrons to ionize compounds after they are converted to the gas phase.

Mass Analyzer

The actual measuring of the *m/z* occurs when the gas phase ions pass into the mass analyzer. Mass analyzers

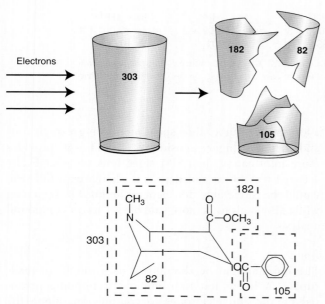

FIGURE 6-10 Electron bombardment breaks cocaine into fragments, with number and size quantified. Unlike the illustrative glass tumbler, the result of mass fragmentation of cocaine or other chemical compounds is both predictable and reproducible, especially with electron ionization.

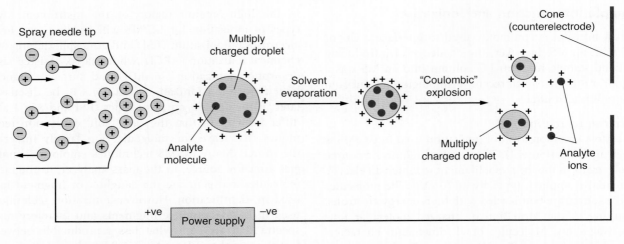

FIGURE 6-11 Diagram of electrospray ionization, the most common ionization source for liquid chromatography/mass spectrometry.

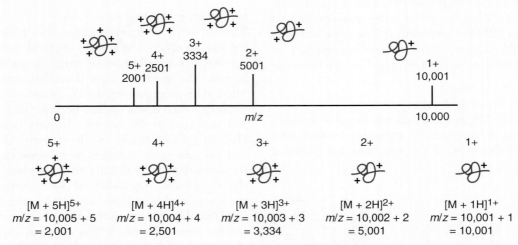

FIGURE 6-12 A theoretical protein with a molecular weight of 10,000 can be multiply charged, which will generate numerous peaks. A mass spectrometer with a relatively small mass range can still detect the multiply charged ions since the m/z is reduced.

generate electric fields that can manipulate the charged molecules to sort them according to their m/z.

Quadrupole

A diagram of a quadrupole MS is shown in Figure 6-13. The quadrupole is the most common mass analyzer in use today. The electric field on the two sets of diagonally opposed rods allows only ions of a single selected m/z value to pass through the analyzer to the detector. All other ions are deflected into the rods. The rods can be scanned from low to high mass to allow ions of increasing mass to form stable sinusoidal orbits and traverse the filtering sector. This technique will generate a full scan mass spectrum. Alternatively, specific masses can be selected to monitor a few target analytes. This technique is called selected ion monitoring (SIM) and it allows for

a longer dwell time (time spent monitoring a single ion) and therefore higher sensitivity.[7] A full scan provides more information than SIM since ions not specifically selected in SIM are not detected. Therefore, a full scan would be preferable for general unknown screening while SIM analysis is more suitable for target compound analysis.

Ion Trap

The ion trap can be thought of as a modified quadrupole. A linear ion trap employs a stopping potential on the end electrodes to confine ions along the two-dimensional axis of the quadrupoles. In a three-dimensional ion trap, the four rods, instead of being arranged parallel to each other, form a three-dimensional sphere in which ions are "trapped." In all ion traps,

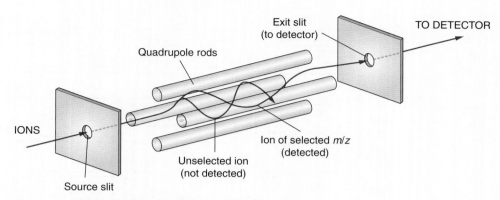

FIGURE 6-13 Single quadrupole mass spectrometer.

after a period of accumulation, the electric field adjusts to selectively destabilize the trapped ions, which are mass-selectively ejected from the cavity to the detector based on their m/z.[7] The unique feature of ion trap MSs is that they trap and store ions generated over time, effectively concentrating the ions of interest and yielding a greater sensitivity.

Tandem Mass Spectrometry

Tandem MSs (GC/MS/MS and LC/MS/MS) can be used for greater selectivity and lower detection limits. A common form of MS/MS is to link three quadrupoles in series; such an instrument is referred to as a triple quad (Fig. 6-14). Generally, each quadrupole has a separate function.[8] Following an appropriate ionization method, the first quadrupole (Q1) is used to scan across a preset m/z range and select an ion of interest. The second quadrupole

(Q2) functions as a collision cell. In a process called collision-induced dissociation, the ions are accelerated to high kinetic energy and allowed to collide with neutral gas molecules (usually nitrogen, helium, or argon) to fragment the ions. The single ion that passed through the first analyzer is called the precursor (or parent) ion while the ions formed during fragmentation of the precursor ions are called product (or daughter) ions. The third quadrupole (Q3) serves to analyze the product ions generated in Q2. This last quadrupole can be set to scan all of the product ions to produce a full product ion scan or to selectively allow one or more of these product ions through to the detector in a process called selected reaction monitoring. Various scanning modes commonly used in a triple quad are shown in Figure 6-15. In some triple quad instruments, the third quadrupole can also function as a linear ion trap to add further sensitivity to MS/MS.

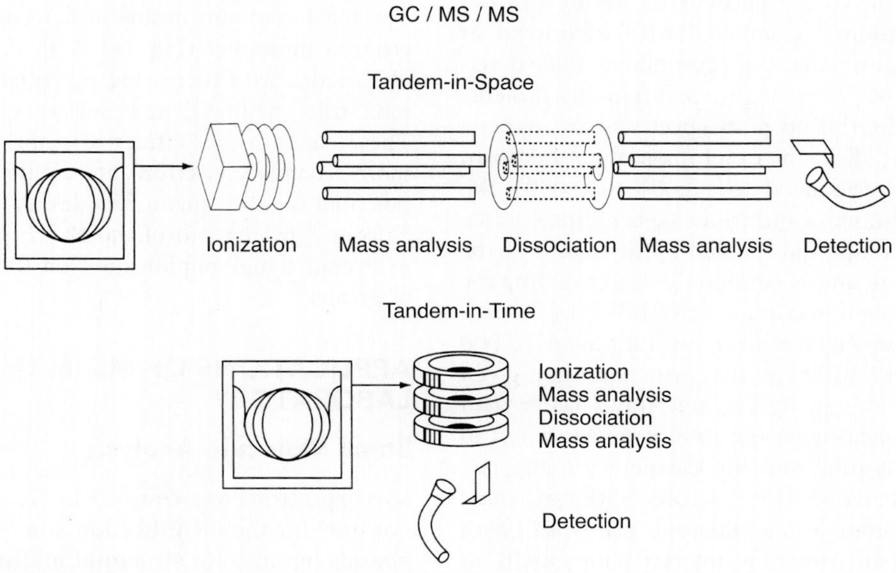

GC / MS / MS

Tandem-in-Space

Ionization   Mass analysis   Dissociation   Mass analysis   Detection

Tandem-in-Time

Ionization
Mass analysis
Dissociation
Mass analysis

Detection

FIGURE 6-14 Triple quadrupole mass spectrometer.

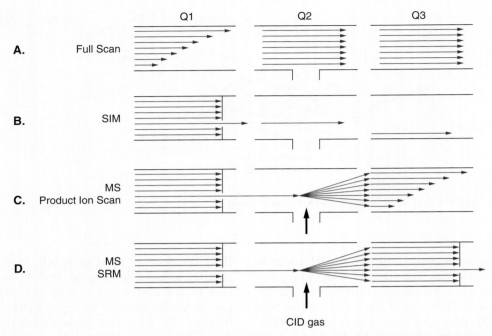

FIGURE 6-15 Scanning modes used in a triple quadrupole mass spectrometer. **(A)** Full scan mass spectrometry (MS) detects all ions. **(B)** Selected ion monitoring (SIM) detects ions of one selected *m/z*. **(C)** Product ion scans select ions of one *m/z* in Q1 to pass on to Q2, the collision cell, where the ion is fragmented. All ion fragments are allowed to pass through to the detector. **(D)** Selected reaction monitoring (SRM) is similar to the product ion scan, but only fragments of one selected *m/z* are allowed to pass on to the detector. Both **(C)** and **(D)** are examples of tandem mass spectrometry (MS/MS). CID, collision-induced dissociation.

High-Resolution MS

Newer technologies utilizing high-resolution mass spectrometers based on time-of-flight (TOF) or Orbitrap (Thermo Fisher) technologies have gained popularity in recent years. These instruments can measure large numbers of analytes simultaneously in complex biological matrices and have been particularly useful for drug screening applications.[9] Compared with traditional or "nominal resolution" mass spectrometers that determine masses to ~0.5 Da, high-resolution instruments such as TOF and Orbitrap mass spectrometers operate at resolutions that allow the exact mass of an unknown compound to be calculated to ~0.001 to 0.0001 Da. The resolution of a mass spectrometer is defined as the mass of a given compound divided by the width of the corresponding peak and is commonly designated by the term full width at half maximum (FWHM) (Fig 6-16A). TOF mass spectrometers achieve resolutions of 10,000 to 50,000 FWHM utilizing the principle that given the same kinetic energy, lighter ions travel faster than heavier ions. By measuring the time it takes an ion to traverse the flight tube and hit the detector, the *m/z* ratio can be calculated (Fig. 6-16B). Orbitrap mass spectrometers operate on a different principle. With Orbitrap instruments, ions are injected tangentially to the electric field between the outer barrel-like electrode

and the inner spindle-like electrode and the stable orbit achieved is proportional to the *m/z* value (Fig. 6-16C). Orbitrap mass spectrometers can achieve 100,000 to 250,000 FWHM.

Detector

The most common means of detecting ions employs an electron multiplier (Fig. 6-17). In this detector, a series of dynodes with increasing potentials are linked. When ions strike the first dynode surface, electrons are emitted. These electrons are attracted to the next dynode where more secondary electrons are emitted due to the higher potential of subsequent dynodes. A cascade of electrons is formed by the end of the chain of dynodes, resulting in overall signal amplification on the order of 1 million or greater.[8]

APPLICATIONS OF MS IN THE CLINICAL LABORATORY

Small Molecule Analysis

Mass spectrometers coupled to GC or LC can be used not only for the identification and quantitation of compounds but also for structural information and molecular weight determination (high-resolution MS).[10] GC/MS

A FWHM Definition

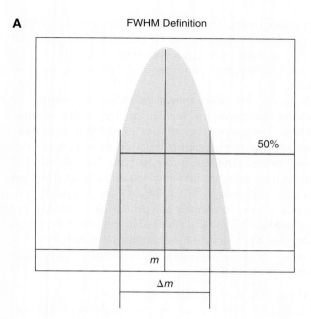

50%

m

Δm

B Linear TOF Mass Spectrometer

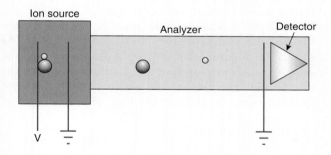

Ion source

Analyzer

Detector

V

C

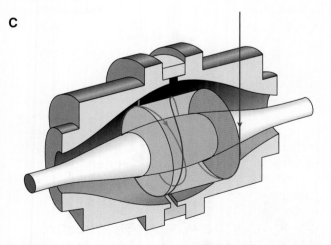

FIGURE 6-16 (**A**) Pictorial representation of the full width at half maximum (FWHM) definition of mass resolution. Reprinted with permission from Thermo Fisher Scientific. (**B**) Diagram of the principle of time-of-flight (TOF) mass spectrometers. Reprinted with permission. (http://msr.dom.wustl.edu/Research/MALDI_TOF_Mass_Spec_and_Proteomics/Time-of-Flight_Mass_Spectrometry_Fundamentals.htm) (**C**) Diagram of Orbitrap mass spectrometry. Reprinted with permission from Thermo Fisher Scientific.

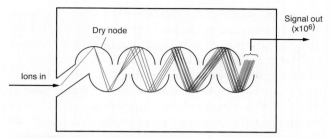

Dry node

Signal out (x10⁶)

Ions in

FIGURE 6-17 Diagram of an electron multiplier detector in a mass spectrometer.

systems are widely used for measuring drugs of abuse in urine toxicology confirmations. Drugs and metabolites must be extracted from body fluids and typically reacted with derivatizing reagents to form compounds that are more volatile for the GC process. Computerized libraries and matching algorithms are available within the instrument to compare mass spectral results of an unknown substance obtained from a sample to the reference library.

Increasingly, LC/MS (including LC/MS/MS) technology is taking its place alongside GC/MS in clinical laboratories. LC offers a number of advantages over GC. Typically, LC requires less extensive extraction procedures and derivatization is rarely used, saving time and expense. In addition, polar and heat-labile compounds fare better in LC.[7] However; the chromatography itself in LC can be somewhat less robust than in GC, resulting in wider peaks and more variable retention times and potentially requiring maintenance that is more frequent. Another disadvantage of LC/MS is the less reproducible mass spectra, as mentioned earlier. One drawback to implementing LC or GC/MS in clinical laboratories is the long run times associated with the chromatographic separation. For low-volume testing, this is not an issue; however, for medium- or high-volume testing, it remains a significant challenge. To overcome this, laboratories can utilize technologies such as ultra-performance liquid chromatography (UPLC) or multiplexing. With UPLC, both the column and the pumps are robust enough to handle very high pressures (>600 bar), allowing faster flow rates which in turn dramatically reduces the run time.

For very high volume testing, several HPLC (or UPLC) pumps can be connected to a single mass spectrometer, which is referred to as multiplexing. This technology works because analyte peaks are only typically ~5 to 30 seconds in width and in theory that is the only time the LC flow needs to be in-line with the mass spectrometer. LC separations typically require much longer gradients for good resolution and additionally the column must be equilibrated before the next run, which takes several minutes. In multiplexing, the LC pumps are staggered so that once the peak of interest has been analyzed by the mass spectrometer, the flow is diverted to waste. At that point, the flow from the next LC pump is placed in-line with the mass spectrometer and the cycle repeats. Multiplexing can reduce the run time by a factor of the number of LC pumps and is well suited for high-volume targeted analysis but not for untargeted screening. For example, if the total run time with a single LC pump takes 8 minutes, then a system with four multiplexed LC pumps would take only 2 minutes to measure the same analyte. Utilizing technologies such as UPLC and multiplexing has allowed clinical laboratories to measure very high volume analytes using MS.

Besides its use in toxicology, LC/MS also has great potential for measuring low-level and mixed-polarity analytes such as vitamin D, testosterone, and immunosuppressant drugs due to its superior sensitivity and specificity over immunoassays. In addition, LC/MS has the advantage of being able to detect multiple analytes (such as a panel of drugs or a series of metabolites) in one run. LC/MS is free from the antibody interferences seen in immunoassays, although LC/MS has its own type of interference in the form of ion suppression. This effect is seen when a co-eluting chemical in the sample prevents a compound of interest from being ionized, thereby reducing or eliminating its signal. LC/MS also requires highly skilled operators and is not nearly as automated as immunoassay instruments.

Mass Spectrometry in Proteomics and Pathogen Identification

The next generation of biomarkers for human diseases will be discovered using techniques found within the research fields of genomics and proteomics. Genomics uses the known sequences of the entire human genome for determining the role of genetics in certain human diseases. Proteomics is the investigation of the protein products encoded by these genes. Protein expression is equal to and, in many cases, more important for disease detection than genomics because these products determine what is currently occurring within a cell, rather than the genes, which indicate what a cell might be capable of performing. Moreover, many (posttranslational) changes can occur to the protein, as influenced by other proteins and enzymes that cannot be easily predicted by knowledge at the genomic level. A "shotgun" approach is often used in the discovery of new biochemical markers. The proteins from samples (e.g., serum, urine, and tissue extract) from normal individuals are compared with those derived from patients with the disease being studied. Before being analyzed on the mass spectrometer, the complex mixture of proteins must first be separated using chromatographic techniques. Proteins can be trypsin digested and separated by HPLC or techniques such as two-dimensional electrophoresis (Chapter 5) can be used to separate proteins into individual spots or bands.

Proteins that only appear in either the normal or diseased specimens are further studied. For proteomic analysis, computer programs are available that digitally compare gels to determine spots or areas that are different. When candidate proteins have been found, the spots can be isolated and subjected to traditional trypsin digestion followed by HPLC-MS/MS or to MALDI-TOF MS (see below) to identify the protein and possibly any posttranslational modifications that may have occurred. Using this approach, the researcher does not have any preconceptions or biases as to what directions or particular proteins to look for.

MALDI-TOF and SELDI-TOF MS

MALDI-TOF MS is used for the analysis of biomolecules, such as peptides and proteins. Protein samples, such as those isolated from a two-dimensional electrophoretogram, are mixed with an appropriate matrix solvent and spotted onto a stainless steel plate. The solvent is dried and the plate is introduced into the vacuum system of the MALDI-TOF analyzer. As shown in Figure 6-18, a laser pulse irradiates the sample, causing desorption and ionization of both the matrix and the sample. Because the monitored mass spectral range is high (>500 Da), the ionization of

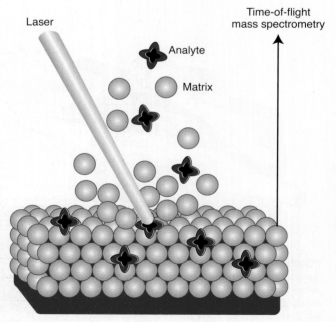

FIGURE 6-18 Sample desorption process prior to matrix-assisted laser desorption ionization time-of-flight (MALDI-TOF) analysis. (Diagram courtesy of Stanford Research Systems, Sunnyvale, CA)

the low-molecular-weight matrix can be readily distinguished from high-molecular-weight peptides and proteins and does not interfere with the assay of the protein. Ions from the sample are focused into the mass spectrometer. The time required for an ion with a given mass to reach the detector is a nonlinear function of the mass, with larger ions requiring more time than smaller ions. The molecular weight of the proteins acquired by mass spectrum is used to determine the identity of the sample and is helpful in determining posttranslational modifications that may have occurred. For very large proteins, samples can be pretreated with trypsin, which cleaves peptide bonds after lysine and arginine, to produce lower-molecular-weight fragments that can then be measured. The detection limit of this assay is about 10^{-15} to 10^{-18} mol. A modification of MALDI-TOF MS is SELDI-TOF MS, in which proteins are directly captured on a chromatographic biochip without the need of sample preparation. Figure 6-19 illustrates the SELDI-TOF process.

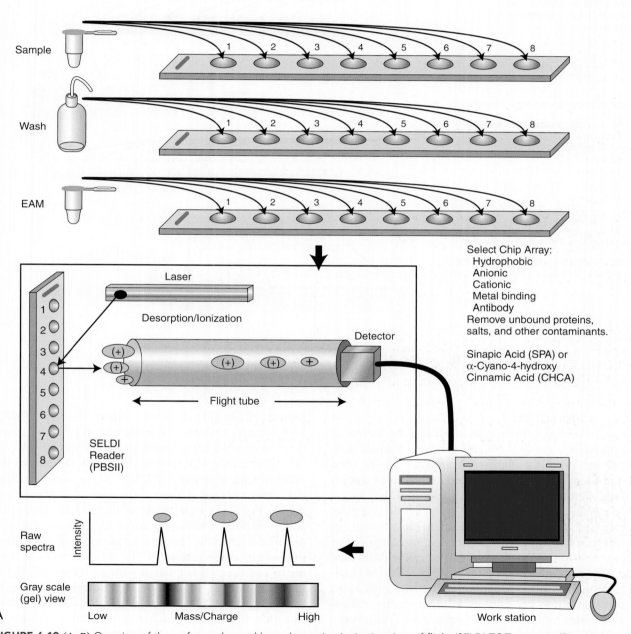

FIGURE 6-19 (**A, B**) Overview of the surface-enhanced laser desorption ionization time-of-flight (SELDI-TOF) process. (Diagram courtesy of Ciphergen Biosystems, Fremont, CA)

1. Apply supernatant from CD8$^+$ cells

Supernatant from stimulated and unstimulated CD8$^+$ cell cultures from Normal, LTPN, and Progressors is added to a Protein Chip Array. Proteins bind to chemical or biological "docking" sites on the array surface through an affinity interaction.

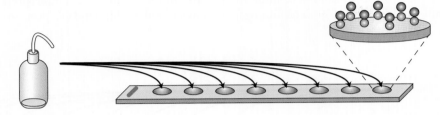

2. Wash Protein Chip Array

Proteins that bind nonspecifically and buffer contaminants are washed away, eliminating sample noise.

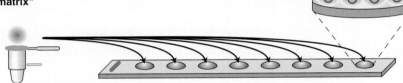

3. Add energy-absorbing molecules or "matrix"

After sample processing, the array is dried and EAM is applied to each spot to facilitate desorption and ionization.

4. Analyze in a Protein Chip Reader

The proteins that are retained on the array are detected on the Protein Chip Reader.

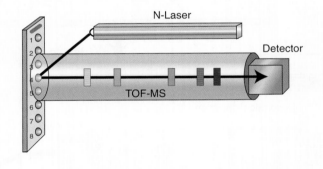

B

FIGURE 6-19 *(Continued)*

Pathogen Identification

Although MS has primarily been utilized in chemistry and toxicology sections for the analysis of small molecules and proteins, high-resolution MS can be used for the identification of pathogens in modern microbiology laboratories.[11] Isolated bacterial or fungal colonies can be directly spotted onto the MALDI plate and ionized, which results in a protein "fingerprint" of the species. This protein "fingerprint" is composed of mainly ribosomal proteins and can be compared with a digital database of species (Fig. 6-20). Because MALDI-TOF MS requires inexpensive reagents and only takes 5 to 10 minutes per run, it is significantly cheaper and faster than traditional automated biochemical identification techniques. Another application of high-resolution MS for pathogen identification is the Abbott PLEX-ID polymerase chain reaction (PCR)/TOF, which combines the sensitivity of PCR and specificity and rapid turnaround time of ESI-TOF MS. In this application, PCR is used to amplify DNA from the unknown pathogen and ESI-TOF MS is used to calculate exact masses of these PCR-generated DNA fragments. From the exact masses, the number of purine and pyrimidine nucleotide bases (As, Ts, Gs, and Cs) can be determined. The unique purine and pyrimidine nucleotide composition of the PCR-generated fragments can then be compared with a preexisting digital library in order to identify the unknown pathogen. Unlike MALDI-TOF and traditional automated identification platforms, which required the organism to be cultured, PCR/ESI-TOF can be used directly from patient specimens.

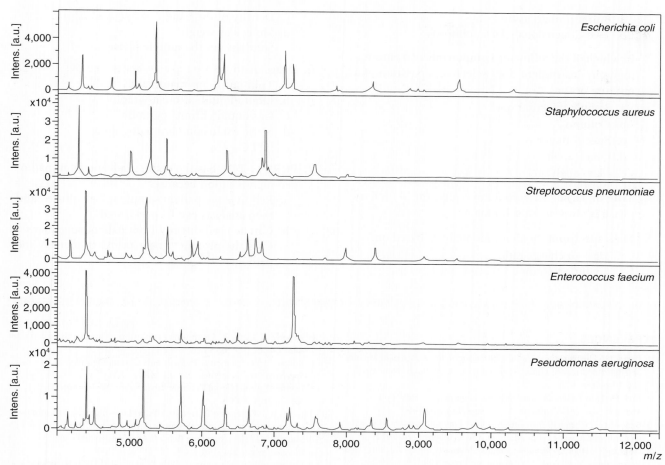

FIGURE 6-20 Matrix-assisted laser desorption ionization time-of-flight (MALDI-TOF) spectral fingerprints of five different bacterial species. (Adapted from Carbonnelle E, Mesquita C, Bille E, et al. *Clin Biochem*. 2011;44:104-109).

For additional student resources please visit thePoint at **http://thepoint.lww.com.** **thePoint**

QUESTIONS

1. Which of the following statements is TRUE?
   a. Partition chromatography is most appropriate to identifying analytes that may be distributed between two liquid phases.
   b. Steric exclusion chromatography is best suited for separating analytes based on their solubility in the mobile solvent.
   c. In liquid–solid chromatography, the stationary phase separates analytes based on size, shape, and polarity.
   d. Ion-exchange chromatography has a resin phase that is soluble to water and separation of the mixture is based on magnitude and charge of ionic species.
   e. The partition coefficient is measured and compared with standards in thin layer chromatography.

2. In high-performance thin-layer chromatography (HPTLC), developed bands are compared with reference standard concentrations. Each band is measured by:
   a. Mass spectrometer
   b. Densitometer
   c. Ruler

d. Buiret protein assay
e. Two-dimensional electrophoresis

3. In which of the following components of a chromatography instrument does selective separation of a mixture occur?
   a. Sample injection port
   b. Column
   c. Spectrometer
   d. Quadrupole
   e. Mass analyzer

4. True or False? In chromatography, the stationary phase is always of a solid matrix.

5. Mass spectrometry identifies analytes based on:
   a. Mass to charge ratio
   b. Retention factor

c. Density of the band
d. Molecular weight
e. Solubility in the mobile phase

6. Drugs of abuse are typically measured by:
   a. Thin-layer chromatography
   b. Liquid/liquid chromatography
   c. Gas/liquid chromatography
   d. Steric exclusion chromatography
   e. HPLC

7. PCR/ESI-TOF has the distinct advantage in pathogen identification because:
   a. Requires the patient sample to be cultured and then analysis can be performed.
   b. Can be used directly from patient specimens.
   c. Uses the protein "finger print" to identify the pathogen.

REFERENCES

1. Parris NA. *Instrumental Liquid Chromatography: A Practical Manual on High Performance Liquid Chromatographic Methods.* New York, NY: Elsevier; 1976.
2. Jurk H. *Thin-Layer Chromatography. Reagents and Detection Methods, Vol. 1a.* Weinheim: Verlagsgesellschaft; 1990.
3. Bender GT. *Chemical Instrumentation: A Laboratory Manual Based on Clinical Chemistry.* Philadelphia, PA: WB Saunders; 1972.
4. Horváth C. *High Performance Liquid Chromatography, Advances and Perspectives.* New York, NY: Academic Press; 1980.
5. Constantin E, Schnell A. *Mass Spectrometry.* New York, NY: Ellis Horwood; 1990.
6. Kebarle E, Liang T. From ions in solution to ions in the gas phase. *Anal Chem.* 1993;65:972A.
7. Karasek FW, Clement RE. *Basic Gas Chromatography: Mass Spectrometry.* New York, NY: Elsevier; 1988.
8. Levine B. *Principles of Forensic Toxicology.* Washington, DC: AACC Press; 2006.
9. Jiwan JL, Wallemacq P, Hérent MF. HPLC—high resolution mass spectrometry in clinical laboratory? *Clin Biochem.* 2011;44:136-147.
10. Siuzdak, G. *The Expanding Role of Mass Spectrometry in Biotechnology.* San Diego, CA: MCC Press; 2006.
11. Carbonnelle E, Mesquita C, Bille E, et al. MALDI-TOF mass spectrometry tools for bacterial identification in clinical microbiology laboratory. *Clin Biochem.* 2011;44:104-109.

Principles of Clinical Chemistry Automation

RYAN W. GREER, JOELY A. STRASESKI,
WILLIAM L. ROBERTS

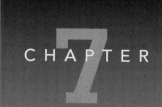

CHAPTER

7

CHAPTER OUTLINE

Chapter Objectives

Upon completion of this chapter, the clinical laboratorian should be able to do the following:

- Define the following terms: automation, channel, continuous flow, discrete analysis, dwell time, flag, random access, and throughput.
- Discuss the history of the development of automated analyzers in the clinical chemistry laboratory.
- List four driving forces behind the development of new automated analyzers.
- Name three basic approaches to sample analysis used by automated analyzers.
- Explain the major steps in automated analysis.
- Provide examples of commercially available discrete chemistry analyzers and modular systems.
- Compare the different approaches to automated analysis used by instrument manufacturers.
- Discriminate between an open versus a closed reagent system.
- Relate three considerations in the selection of an automated analyzer.
- Explain the concept of total laboratory automation.
- Differentiate the three phases of the laboratory testing process.
- Discuss future trends in automated analyzer development.

KEY TERMS

Automation
Bar code
Centrifugal analysis
Channel
Closed tube sampling
Continuous flow
Discrete analysis

Dry chemistry slide
Flag
Modular analyzer
Probe
Random access
Robotics
Rotor
Total laboratory automation

The modern clinical chemistry laboratory uses a high degree of automation. Many steps in the analytic process that were previously performed manually can now be performed automatically, permitting the operator to focus on manual processes and increasing both efficiency and capacity. The analytic process can be divided into three major phases—preanalytic, analytic, and postanalytic—corresponding to sample processing, chemical analysis, and data management, respectively. Substantial improvements have occurred in all three areas during the past decade. Five major diagnostic vendors sell automated analyzers and reagents. These vendors are continually refining their products to make them more functional and user-friendly. The analytic phase is the most automated, and more research and development efforts are focusing on increasing automation of the preanalytic and postanalytic processes.

HISTORY OF AUTOMATED ANALYZERS

Following the introduction of the first automated analyzer by Technicon in 1957, automated instruments proliferated from many manufacturers.[1] This first "AutoAnalyzer" (AA) was a continuous-flow, single-channel, sequential batch analyzer capable of providing a single test result on approximately 40 samples per hour. The next generation of Technicon instruments to be developed was the Simultaneous Multiple Analyzer (SMA) series. SMA-6 and SMA-12 were analyzers with multiple channels (for different tests), working synchronously to produce 6 or 12 test results simultaneously at the rate of 360 or 720 tests per hour. It was not until the mid-1960s that these continuous-flow analyzers had any significant competition in the marketplace.

In 1970, the first commercial centrifugal analyzer was introduced as a spin-off technology from NASA outer space research. Dr. Norman Anderson developed a prototype in 1967 at the Oak Ridge National Laboratory as an alternative to continuous-flow technology, which had significant carryover problems and costly reagent waste. He wanted to perform analyses in parallel and also take advantage of advances in computer technology. The second generation of these instruments (1975) was more successful as a result of miniaturization of computers and advances in the polymer industry for high-grade, optical plastic cuvettes.

The next major development that revolutionized clinical chemistry instrumentation occurred in 1970 with the introduction of the Automatic Clinical Analyzer (ACA) (DuPont [now Siemens]). It was the first non-continuous flow, discrete analyzer as well as the first instrument to have random-access capabilities, whereby stat specimens could be analyzed out of sequence on an as-needed basis. Plastic test packs, positive patient identification, and infrequent calibration were among the unique features of the ACA. Other major milestones were the introduction of thin film analysis technology in 1976 and the production of the Kodak Ektachem (now Vitros) Analyzer (now Ortho-Clinical Diagnostics) in 1978. This instrument was the first to use microsample volumes and reagents on slides for dry chemistry analysis and to incorporate computer technology extensively into its design and use.

Since 1980, several primarily discrete analyzers have been developed that incorporate such characteristics as ion-selective electrodes (ISEs), fiber optics, polychromatic analysis, continually more sophisticated computer hardware and software for data handling, and larger test menus. The popular and more successful analyzers using

these and other technologies since 1980 are Astra (now Synchron) analyzers (Beckman Coulter), which extensively used ISEs; Paramax (no longer available), which introduced primary tube sampling; and the Hitachi analyzers (Boehringer-Mannheim, now Roche Diagnostics), with reusable reaction disks and fixed diode arrays for spectral mapping. Automated systems that are commonly used in clinical chemistry laboratories today are Aeroset and ARCHITECT analyzers (Abbott Diagnostics), Advia analyzers (Siemens), Synchron analyzers (Beckman Coulter), Dimension analyzers (Siemens), Vitros analyzers (Ortho-Clinical Diagnostics), and several Roche analyzer lines.

Many manufacturers of these instrument systems have adopted the more successful features and technologies of other instruments, where possible, to make each generation of their product more competitive in the marketplace. The differences among the manufacturers' instruments, operating principles, and technologies are less distinct now than they were in the beginning years of laboratory automation (TLA).

DRIVING FORCES TOWARD MORE AUTOMATION

Since 1995, the pace of changes with current routine chemistry analyzers and the introduction of new ones has slowed considerably, compared with the first half of the 1990s. Certainly, analyzers are faster and easier to use as a result of continual re-engineering and electronic refinements. Methods are more precise, sensitive, and specific, although some of the same principles are found in today's instruments as in earlier models. Manufacturers have worked successfully toward automation with "walk-away" capabilities and minimal operator intervention.[2] Manufacturers have also responded to the physicians' desire to bring laboratory testing closer to the patient. The introduction of small, portable, easy-to-operate benchtop analyzers in physician office laboratories, as well as in surgical and critical care units that demand immediate laboratory results, has resulted in a hugely successful domain of point-of-care (POC) analyzers.[3] Another specialty area with a rapidly developing arsenal of analyzers is immunochemistry. Immunologic techniques for assaying drugs, specific proteins, tumor markers, and hormones have evolved to an increased level of automation. Instruments that use techniques such as fluorescence polarization immunoassay, nephelometry, and competitive and noncompetitive immunoassay with chemiluminescent detection have become popular in laboratories.

The most recent milestone in chemistry analyzer development has been the combination of chemistry and immunoassay into a single modular analyzer.

The Dimension RxL analyzer with a heterogeneous immunoassay module was introduced in 1997. This design permits further workstation consolidation with consequent improvements in operational efficiency and further reductions in turnaround time. Modular analyzers combining chemistry and immunoassay capabilities are now available from several vendors that meet the needs of mid- and high-volume laboratories (Fig. 7-1).

Other forces are also driving the market toward more focused automation. Higher volume of testing and faster turnaround time have resulted in fewer and more centralized core laboratories performing more comprehensive testing.[4] The use of laboratory panels or profiles has declined, with more diagnostically directed individual tests as dictated by recent policy changes from Medicare and Medicaid. Researchers have known for many years that chemistry panels only occasionally lead to new diagnoses in patients who appear healthy.[5] The expectation of quality results with higher accuracy and precision is ever present with the regulatory standards set by the Clinical Laboratory Improvement Amendments, the Joint Commission (formerly the Joint Commission on Accreditation of Healthcare Organizations), the College of American Pathologists, and others. Intense competition among instrument manufacturers has driven automation into more sophisticated analyzers with creative technologies and unique features. Furthermore, escalating costs have spurred healthcare reform and, more specifically, managed care

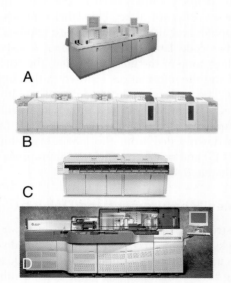

FIGURE 7-1 Modular chemistry/immunoassay analyzers. (**A**) Siemens Dimension Vista 3000T. (Photograph courtesy of Siemens.) (**B**) Roche MODULAR *ANALYTICS*. (Photograph courtesy of Roche Diagnostics.) (**C**) Abbott ARCHITECT ci8200. (Photograph courtesy of Abbott Diagnostics.) (**D**) Beckman Coulter Synchron LXi 725. (Photograph courtesy of Beckman Coulter.)

and capitation environments within which laboratories are forced to operate.

BASIC APPROACHES TO AUTOMATION

There are many advantages to automating procedures. One purpose is to increase the number of tests performed by one laboratorian in a given period. Labor is an expensive commodity in clinical laboratories. Through mechanization, the labor component devoted to any single test is minimized and this effectively lowers the cost per test. A second purpose is to minimize the variation in results from one laboratorian to another. By reproducing the components in a procedure as identically as possible, the coefficient of variation is lowered and reproducibility is increased. Accuracy is then not dependent on the skill or workload of a particular operator on a particular day. This allows better comparison of results from day to day and week to week. Automation, however, cannot correct for deficiencies inherent in methodology. A third advantage is gained because automation eliminates the potential errors of manual analyses such as volumetric pipetting steps, calculation of results, and transcription of results. A fourth advantage accrues because instruments can use very small amounts of samples and reagents. This allows less blood to be drawn from each patient. In addition, the use of small amounts of reagents decreases the cost of consumables.

There are three basic approaches with instruments: continuous flow, centrifugal analysis, and discrete analysis. All three can use batch analysis (i.e., large number of specimens in one run), but only discrete analyzers offer random-access, or stat, capabilities.

In continuous flow, liquids (reagents, diluents, and samples) are pumped through a system of continuous tubing. Samples are introduced in a sequential manner, following each other through the same network. A series of air bubbles at regular intervals serve as separating and cleaning media. Continuous flow, therefore, resolves the major consideration of uniformity in the performance of tests because each sample follows the same reaction path. Continuous flow also assists the laboratory that needs to run many samples requiring the same procedure. The more sophisticated continuous-flow analyzers used parallel single channels to run multiple tests on each sample—for example, SMA. The major drawbacks that contributed to the eventual demise of traditional continuous-flow analyzers (i.e., AA and SMA) in the marketplace were significant carryover problems and wasteful use of continuously flowing reagents. Technicon's (now Siemens) answer to these problems was a non–continuous-flow discrete analyzer (the RA1000), using random-access fluid (a hydrofluorocarbon liquid to reduce surface tension between samples/reagents and their tubing) and, thereby, reducing carryover. Later, the Chem 1 was developed by Technicon to use Teflon tubing and Teflon oil, virtually eliminating carryover problems. The Chem 1 was a continuous-flow analyzer but only remotely comparable to the original continuous-flow principle.

Centrifugal analysis uses the force generated by centrifugation to transfer and then contain liquids in separate cuvettes for measurement at the perimeter of a spinning rotor. Centrifugal analyzers are most capable of running multiple samples, one test at a time, in a batch. Batch analysis is their major advantage because reactions in all cuvettes are read virtually simultaneously, taking no longer to run a full rotor of about 30 samples than it would take to run a few. Laboratories with a high workload of individual tests for routine batch analysis may use these instruments. Again, each cuvette must be uniformly matched to each other to maintain quality handling of each sample. The Cobas-Bio (Roche Diagnostics), with a xenon flash lamp and longitudinal cuvettes,[6] and the IL Monarch, with a fully integrated walk-away design, are two of the more successful centrifugal analyzers.

Discrete analysis is the separation of each sample and accompanying reagents in a separate container. Discrete analyzers have the capability of running multiple tests one sample at a time or multiple samples one test at a time. They are the most popular and versatile analyzers and have almost completely replaced continuous-flow and centrifugal analyzers. However, because each sample is in a separate reaction container, uniformity of quality must be maintained in each cuvette so that a particular sample's quality is not affected by the particular space that it occupies. The analyzers listed in Table 7-1 are examples of current discrete analyzers with random-access capabilities.

STEPS IN AUTOMATED ANALYSIS

In clinical chemistry, automation is the mechanization of the steps in a procedure. Manufacturers design their instruments to mimic manual techniques. The major processes performed by an automated analyzer can be divided into specimen identification and preparation, chemical reaction, and data collection and analysis. An overview of these processes is provided in Table 7-2.

Each step of automated analysis is explained in this section, and several different applications are discussed. Several instruments have been chosen because they have components that represent either common features used in chemistry instrumentation or a unique method of automating a step in a procedure. None of the representative instruments is completely described, but rather the important components are described in the text as examples.

Specimen Preparation and Identification

Preparation of the sample for analysis has been and remains a manual process in most laboratories. The clotting time (if using serum), centrifugation, and the transferring of the sample to an analyzer cup (unless using primary tube sampling) cause delay and expense in the testing process. One alternative to manual preparation is to automate this process by using robotics, or front-end automation, to "handle" the specimen through these steps and load the specimen onto the analyzer. Another option is to bypass the specimen preparation altogether by using whole blood for analysis—for example, Abbott-Vision. Robotics for specimen preparation has already become a reality in some clinical laboratories in the United States and other countries. Another approach is to use a plasma separator tube and perform primary tube sampling with heparin plasma. This eliminates the need both to wait for the sample to clot and to aliquot the sample. More discussion about preanalytic specimen processing, or front-end automation, appears later in this chapter.

The sample must be properly identified and its location in the analyzer must be monitored throughout the test. The simplest means of identifying a sample is by placing a manually labeled sample cup in a numbered analysis position on the analyzer, in accordance with a manually prepared worksheet or a computer-generated load list. The most sophisticated approach that is commonly used today employs a bar code label affixed to the primary collection tube. This label contains patient demographics and also may include test requests.

The bar code–labeled tubes are then transferred to the loading zone of the analyzer, where the bar code is scanned and the information is stored in the computer's memory. The analyzer is then capable of monitoring all functions of identification, test orders and parameters, and sample position. Certain analyzers may take test requests downloaded from the laboratory information system (LIS) and run them when the appropriate sample is identified and ready to be pipetted.

Specimen Measurement and Delivery

Most instruments use either circular carousels or rectangular racks as specimen containers for holding disposable sample cups or primary sample tubes in the loading or pipetting zone of the analyzer. These cups or tubes hold standards, controls, and patient specimens to be pipetted into the reaction chambers of the analyzers. The slots in the trays or racks are usually numbered to aid in sample identification. The trays or racks move automatically in one-position steps at preselected speeds. The speed

TABLE 7-1 SUMMARY OF FEATURES FOR SELECTED MID- AND HIGH-VOLUME CLINICAL CHEMISTRY ANALYZERS

	MID VOLUME					HIGH VOLUME				
	ABBOTT DIAGNOSTICS ARCHITECT C8000	BECKMAN COULTER INC. UNICEL DXC 600I	ORTHO-CLINICAL DIAGNOSTICS VITROS 350	ROCHE DIAGNOSTICS COBAS 6000	SIEMENS HEALTHCARE DIAGNOSTICS INC. DIMENSION VISTA 500	ABBOTT DIAGNOSTICS ARCHITECT C16000	BECKMAN COULTER, INC. UNICEL DXC 680I	ORTHO-CLINICAL DIAGNOSTICS VITROS 5,1 FS	ROCHE DIAGNOSTICS COBAS 8000	SIEMENS HEALTHCARE DIAGNOSTICS INC. DIMENSION VISTA 1500
First year sold in the United States	2003	2006	2005	2006	2009	2007	2009	2004	2010	2006
Throughput (tests per hour, depends on test mix)	133–200	900	40–60	85–300	83–166	1,800	1400	600–700	8,400	1500
No. of assays onboard simultaneously	58	89	60	88	>100	68	115	125	88	>100
No. of open channels	220	100	–	40	10	220	100	20	40	10
No. of ion-selective electrode channels	3	5	3	3	3	3	5	3	3	3
Minimum sample volume aspirated (µL)	2	3	6	1.5	50	2	3	2	1.5	50µL
Dedicated pediatric sample cup/dead volume (µL)	Yes/50	Yes/–	No/35	Yes/50	No/10	Yes/50	Yes/20	No/35	Yes/50	No/10-20µL
Short sample/clot detection	Yes/Yes	Yes/Yes	Yes/Yes	Yes/Yes	Yes/Yes	Yes/Yes	Yes/Yes	Yes/Yes	Yes/Yes	Yes/Yes
Index measurements	Yes	Yes	No	Yes	Yes	Yes	Yes	Yes	Yes	Yes
Onboard test automatic inventory	Yes	Yes	Yes	Yes	Yes	Yes	Yes	Yes	Yes	Yes
Remote troubleshooting by modem	Yes	Yes	No	Yes	Yes	Yes	Yes	Yes	Yes	Yes

Information obtained from Dabkowski B. Vendors toil and tinker to refine chemistry analyzers. CAP Today 2011;July:56–71 and directly from vendors.

TABLE 7-2	SUMMARY OF CHEMISTRY ANALYZER OPERATIONS
IDENTIFICATION AND PREPARATION	
1. Sample identification	This is usually done by reading the bar code. This information can also be entered manually
2. Determine test(s) to perform	The LIS communicates to the analyzer which test(s) have been ordered
CHEMICAL REACTION	
3. Reagent systems and delivery	One or more reagents can be dispensed into the reaction cuvette
4. Specimen measurement and delivery	A small aliquot of the sample is introduced into the reaction cuvette
5. Chemical reaction phase	The sample and reagents are mixed and incubated
DATA COLLECTION AND ANALYSIS	
6. Measurement phase	Optical readings may be initiated before or after all reagents have been added
7. Signal processing and data handling	The analyte concentration is estimated from a calibration curve that is stored in the analyzer
8. Send result(s) to LIS	The analyzer communicates results for the ordered tests to the LIS

Operations generally occur in the order listed from 1 to 8. However, there may be slight variations in the order. Some steps may be deleted or duplicated. Most analyzers have the capability to dilute the sample and repeat the testing process if the analyte concentration exceeds the linear range of the assay.

determines the number of specimens to be analyzed per hour. As a convenience, the instrument can determine the slot number containing the last sample and terminate the analysis after that sample. The instrument's microprocessor holds the number of samples in memory and aspirates only in positions containing samples.

On the Vitros analyzer, sample cup trays are quadrants that hold 10 samples each in cups with conical bottoms. The four quadrants fit on a tray carrier (Fig. 7-2). Although the tray carrier accommodates only 40 samples, more trays of samples can be programmed and then loaded in place of completed trays while tests on other trays are in progress. A disposable sample tip

is hand-loaded adjacent to each sample cup on the tray. Roche/Hitachi analyzers can use five-position racks to hold samples (Fig. 7-3). A modular analyzer can accommodate as many as 60 of these racks at one time.

Nearly all contemporary chemistry analyzers sample from primary collection tubes, or for limited volume samples, there are microsample tubes. The tubes are placed in either racks or carousels. Bar code labels for each sample, which include the patient name and identification number, can be printed on demand by the operator (Fig. 7-4). This allows samples to be loaded in any order. The Dimension analyzers make use of a continuous belt of flexible, disposable plastic cuvettes

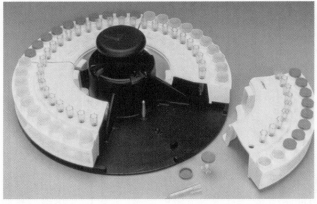

FIGURE 7-2 Vitros. The four quadrant trays, each holding ten samples, fit on a tray carrier. (Photograph courtesy of Ortho-Clinical Diagnostics.)

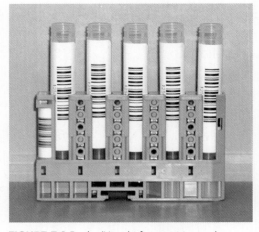

FIGURE 7-3 Roche/Hitachi five-position rack.

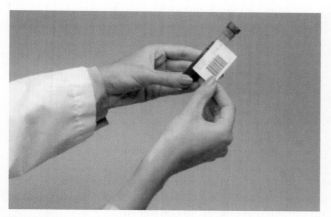

FIGURE 7-4 Sample collection tubes are identified with bar code labels. (Photograph courtesy of Siemens.)

carried through the analyzer's water bath on a main drive track. The cuvettes are loaded onto the analyzer from a continuous spool. These cuvettes index through the instrument at the rate of one every 5 seconds and are cut into sections or groups as required. A schematic of the Dimension RxL cuvette production and reading system is shown in Figure 7-5. Exposure of the sample to air can lead to sample evaporation and produce errors in analysis. Evaporation of the sample may be significant and may cause the concentration of the constituents being analyzed to rise 50% in 4 hours.[7] With instruments measuring electrolytes, the carbon dioxide present in the samples will be lost to the atmosphere, resulting in low carbon dioxide values. Manufacturers have devised a variety of mechanisms to minimize this effect—for

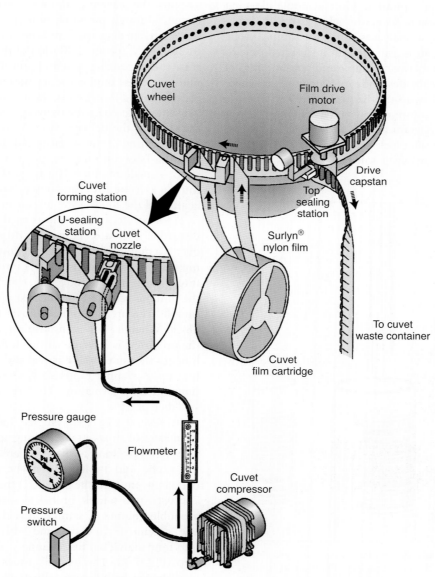

FIGURE 7-5 Analyzer production system for sealed cuvettes. (Photograph courtesy of Siemens.)

example, lid covers for trays and individual caps that can be pierced, which includes closed tube sampling from primary collection tubes.[8]

The actual measurement of each aliquot for each test must be very accurate. This is generally done through aspiration of the sample into a probe. When the discrete instrument is in operation, the probe automatically dips into each sample cup and aspirates a portion of the liquid. After a preset, computer-controlled time interval, the probe quickly rises from the cup. Sampling probes on instruments using specific sampling cups are programmed or adjusted to reach a prescribed depth in those cups to maximize the use of available sample. Those analyzers capable of aspirating sample from primary collection tubes usually have a parallel liquid level–sensing probe that will control entry of the sampling probe to a minimal depth below the surface of the serum, allowing full aliquot aspiration while avoiding clogging of the probe with serum separator gel or clot (Fig. 7-6).

In continuous-flow analyzers, when the sample probe rises from the cup, air is aspirated for a specified time to produce a bubble in between sample and reagent plugs of liquid. Then the probe descends into a container where wash solution is drawn into the probe and through the system. The wash solution is usually deionized water, possibly with a surfactant added. Remembering that all samples follow the same reaction path, the necessity for the wash solution between samples becomes obvious.

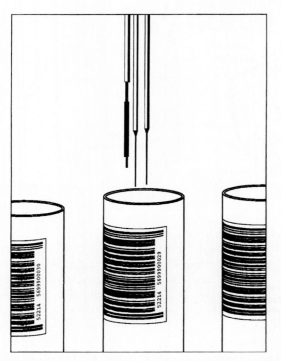

FIGURE 7-6 Dual sample probes of a chemistry analyzer. Note the liquid level sensor to the left of probes. (Photograph courtesy of Roche Diagnostics.)

Immersion of the probe into the wash reservoir cleanses the outside, whereas aspiration of an aliquot of solution cleanses the lumen. The reservoir is continually replenished with an excess of fresh solution. The wash aliquot, plus the previously mentioned air bubble, maintains sample integrity and minimizes sample carryover.

Certain pipetters use a disposable tip and an air-displacement syringe to measure and deliver reagent. When this is used, the pipetter may be reprogrammed to measure sample and reagent for batches of different tests comparatively easily. Besides eliminating the effort of priming the reagent delivery system with the new solution, no reagent is wasted or contaminated because nothing but the pipet tip contacts it.

The cleaning of the probe and tubing after each dispensing to minimize the carryover of one sample into the next is a concern for many instruments. In some systems, the reagent or diluent is also dispersed into the cuvette through the same tubing and probe. Deionized water may be dispensed into the cuvette after the sample to produce a specified dilution of the sample and also to rinse the dispensing system. In the Technicon RA1000, a random-access fluid is the separation medium. The fluorocarbon fluid is a viscous, inert, immiscible, nonwetting substance that coats the delivery system. The coating on the sides of the delivery system prevents carryover due to the wetting of the surfaces and, forming a plug of the solution between samples, prevents carryover by diffusion. A small amount (10 μL) of this fluid is dispensed into the cuvette with the sample. Surface tension leaves a coating of the fluid in the dispensing system.

If a separate probe or tip is used for each sample and discarded after use, as in the Vitros, the issue of carryover is a moot point. Vitros has a unique sample-dispensing system. A proboscis presses into a tip on the sample tray, picks it up, and moves over the specimen to aspirate the volume required for the tests programmed for that sample. The tip is then moved over to the slide-metering block. When a slide is in position to receive an aliquot, the proboscis is lowered so that a dispensed 10-μL drop touches the slide, where it is absorbed from the nonwetting tip. A stepper motor-driven piston controls aspiration and drop formation. The precision of dispensing is specified at ±5%.

In several discrete systems, the probe is attached by means of nonwettable tubing to precision syringes. The syringes draw a specified amount of sample into the probe and tubing. Then the probe is positioned over a cuvette and the sample is dispensed. The Hitachi 736 used two sample probes to simultaneously aspirate a double volume of sample in each probe immersed in one specimen container and, thereby, deliver sample into four individual test channels, all in one operational step (Fig. 7-7). The loaded probes pass through a fine mist shower bath before delivery to wash off any sample

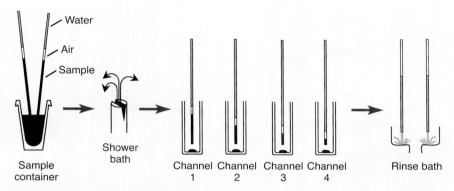

FIGURE 7-7 Sampling operation of the Hitachi 736 analyzer. (Courtesy of Roche Diagnostics.)

residue adhering to the outer surface of the probes. After delivery, the probes move to a rinse bath station for cleaning the inside and outside surfaces of the probes.

Many chemistry analyzers use computer-controlled stepping motors to drive both the sampling and washout syringes. Every few seconds, the sampling probe enters a specimen container, withdraws the required volume, moves to the cuvette, and dispenses the aliquot with a volume of water to wash the probe. The washout volume is adjusted to yield the final reaction volume. If a procedure's range of linearity is exceeded, the system will retrieve the original sample tube, repeat the test using one-fourth the original sample volume for the repeat test, and calculate a new result, taking the dilution into consideration.

Economy of sample size is a major consideration in developing automated procedures, but methodologies have limitations to maintain proper levels of sensitivity and specificity. The factors governing sample and reagent measurement are interdependent. Generally, if sample size is reduced, then either the size of the reaction cuvette and final reaction volume must be decreased or the reagent concentration must be increased to ensure sufficient color development for accurate photometric readings.

Reagent Systems and Delivery

Reagents may be classified as liquid or dry systems for use with automated analyzers. Liquid reagents may be purchased in bulk volume containers or in unit dose packaging as a convenience for stat testing on some analyzers. Dry reagents are packaged in various forms. They may be bottled as lyophilized powder, which requires reconstitution with water or a buffer. Unless the manufacturer provides the diluent, the water quality available in the laboratory is important. A second and unique type of dry reagent is the multilayered **dry chemistry slide** for the Vitros analyzer (rebranded in 2001 as the VITROS Microslide technology). These slides have microscopically thin layers of dry reagents mounted on a plastic support. The slides are approximately the size and thickness of a postage stamp.

Reagent handling varies according to instrument capabilities and methodologies. Many test procedures use sensitive, short-lived working reagents; so contemporary analyzers use a variety of techniques to preserve them. One technique is to keep all reagents refrigerated until the moment of need and then quickly preincubate them to reaction temperature or store them in a refrigerated compartment on the analyzer that feeds directly to the dispensing area. Another means of preservation is to provide reagents in a dried, tablet form and reconstitute them when the test is to be run. A third is to manufacture the reagent in two stable components that will be combined at the moment of reaction. If this approach is used, the first component also may be used as a diluent for the sample. The various manufacturers often use combinations of these reagent-handling techniques.

Reagents also must be dispensed and measured accurately. Many instruments use bulk reagents to decrease the preparation and changing of reagents. Instruments that do not use bulk reagents have unique reagent packaging. In continuous-flow analyzers, reagents and diluents are supplied from bulk containers into which tubing is suspended. The inside diameter, or bore, of the tubing governs the amount of fluid that will be dispensed. A proportioning pump, along with a manifold, continuously and precisely introduces, proportions, and pumps liquids and air bubbles throughout the continuous-flow system.

To deliver reagents, many discrete analyzers use techniques similar to those used to measure and deliver the samples. Syringes, driven by a stepping motor, pipet the reagents into reaction containers. Piston-driven pumps, connected by tubing, may also dispense reagents. Another technique for delivering reagents to reaction containers uses pressurized reagent bottles connected by tubing to dispensing valves. The computer controls the opening and closing of the valves. The fill volume of reagent into the reaction container is determined by the precise amount of time the valve remains open.

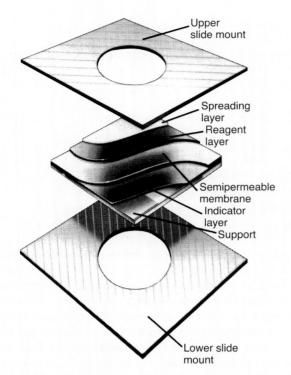

FIGURE 7-8 Vitros slide with multiple layers contains the entire reagent chemistry system. (Courtesy of Ortho-Clinical Diagnostics.)

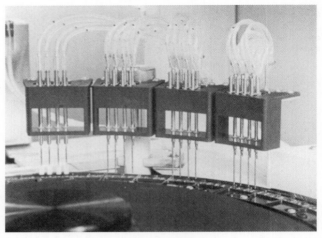

FIGURE 7-9 Wash stations on a chemistry analyzer perform the following: (1) aspirate reaction waste and dispense water; (2) aspirate and dispense rinse water; (3) aspirate rinse water and dispense water for measurement of cell blank; and (4) aspirate cell blank water to dryness. (Photograph courtesy of Roche Diagnostics.)

The Vitros analyzers use slides to contain their entire reagent chemistry system. Multiple layers on the slide are backed by a clear polyester support. The coating itself is sandwiched in a plastic mount. There are three or more layers: (1) a spreading layer, which accepts the sample; (2) one or more central layers, which can alter the aliquot; and (3) an indicator layer, where the analyte of interest may be quantified (Fig. 7-8). The number of layers varies depending on the assay to be performed. The color developed in the indicator layer varies with the concentration of the analyte in the sample. Physical or chemical reactions can occur in one layer, with the product of these reactions proceeding to another layer, where subsequent reactions can occur. Each layer may offer a unique environment and the possibility to carry out a reaction comparable to that offered in a chemistry assay or it may promote an entirely different activity that does not occur in the liquid phase. The ability to create multiple reaction sites allows the possibility of manipulating and detecting compounds in ways not possible in solution chemistries. Interfering materials can be left behind or altered in upper layers.

Chemical Reaction Phase

This phase consists of mixing, separation, incubation, and reaction time. In most discrete analyzers, the chemical reactants are held in individual moving containers that are either disposable or reusable. These reaction containers also function as the cuvettes for optical analysis. If the cuvettes are reusable, then wash stations are set up immediately after the read stations to clean and dry these containers (Fig. 7-9). This arrangement allows the analyzer to operate continuously without replacing cuvettes. Examples of this approach include ADVIA Centaur (Siemens), ARCHITECT (Abbott Diagnostics), Cobas (Roche Diagnostics), and UniCel DxC Synchron (Beckman Coulter) analyzers. Alternatively, the reactants may be placed in a stationary reaction chamber in which a flow-through process of the reaction mixture occurs before and after the optical reading.

Mixing

A vital component of each procedure is the adequate mixing of the reagents and sample. Instrument manufacturers go to great lengths to ensure complete mixing. Nonuniform mixtures can result in noise in continuous-flow analysis and in poor precision in discrete analysis.

Mixing was accomplished in continuous-flow analyzers (e.g., the Chem 1) through the use of coiled tubing. When the reagent and sample stream go through coiled loops, the liquid rotates and tumbles in each loop. The differential rate of liquids falling through one another produces mixing in the coil.

RA1000 used a rapid start–stop action of the reaction tray. This causes a sloshing action against the walls of the cuvettes, which mixes the components. Centrifugal analyzers may use a start–stop sequence of rotation or bubbling of air through the sample and reagent to mix them while these solutions are moving from transfer disk to rotor. This process of transferring and mixing occurs in just a few seconds. The centrifugal force is responsible for the mixing as it pushes sample from its compartment,

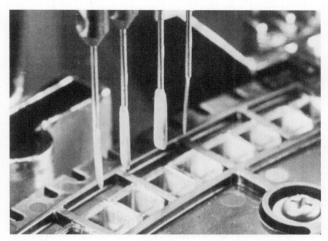

FIGURE 7-10 Stirring paddles on a chemistry analyzer. (Photograph courtesy of Roche Diagnostics.)

over a partition into a reagent-filled compartment and, finally, into the cuvette space at the perimeter of the rotor.

In the VITROS Microslide technology, the spreading layer provides a structure that permits a rapid and uniform spreading of the sample over the reagent layer(s) for even color development.

Most automated wet chemistry analyzers use stirring paddles that dip into the reaction container for a few seconds to stir sample and reagents, after which they return to a wash reservoir (Fig. 7-10). Other instruments use forceful dispensing to accomplish mixing.

Separation

In chemical reactions, undesirable constituents that will interfere with an analysis may need to be separated from the sample before the other reagents are introduced into the system. Protein causes major interference in many analyses. One approach without separating protein is to use a very high reagent-to-sample ratio (the sample is highly diluted) so that any turbidity caused by precipitated protein is not sensed by the spectrophotometer. Another approach is to shorten the reaction time to eliminate slower-reacting interferents.

In the older continuous-flow systems, a dialyzer was the separation or filtering module. It performed the equivalent of the manual procedures of precipitation, centrifugation, and filtration, using a fine-pore cellophane membrane. In the VITROS Microslide technology, the spreading layer of the slide not only traps cells, crystals, and other small particulate matter but also retains large molecules, such as protein. In essence, what passes through the spreading layer is a protein-free filtrate.

Most contemporary discrete analyzers have no automated methodology by which to separate interfering substances from the reaction mixture. Therefore, methods have been chosen that have few interferences or that have known interferences that can be compensated for by the instrument (e.g., using correction formulas).

Incubation

A heating bath in discrete or continuous-flow systems maintains the required temperature of the reaction mixture and provides the delay necessary to allow complete color development. The principal components of the heating bath are the heat-transfer medium (i.e., water or air), the heating element, and the thermoregulator. A thermometer is located in the heating compartment of an analyzer and is monitored by the system's computer. On many discrete analyzer systems, the multicuvettes incubate in a water bath maintained at a constant temperature of usually 37°C.

Slide technology incubates colorimetric slides at 37°C. There is a precondition station to bring the temperature of each slide close to 37°C before it enters the incubator. The incubator moves the slides at 12-second intervals in such a manner that each slide is at the incubator exit four times during the 5-minute incubation time. This feature is used for two-point rate methods and enables the first point reading to be taken part way through the incubation time. Potentiometric slides are held at 25°C. The slides are kept at this temperature for 3 minutes to ensure stability before reading.

Reaction Time

Before the optical reading by the spectrophotometer, the reaction time may depend on the rate of transport through the system to the "read" station, timed reagent additions with moving or stationary reaction chambers, or a combination of both processes. An environment conducive to the completion of the reaction must be maintained for a sufficient length of time before spectrophotometric analysis of the product is made. Time is a definite limitation. To sustain the advantage of speedy multiple analyses, the instrument must produce results as quickly as possible.

It is possible to monitor not only completion of a reaction but also the rate at which the reaction is proceeding. The instrument may delay the measurement for a predetermined time or may present the reaction mixtures for measurement at constant intervals of time. Use of rate reactions may have two advantages: the total analysis time is shortened and interfering chromogens that react slowly may be negated. Reaction rate is controlled by temperature; therefore, the reagent, timing, and spectrophotometric functions must be coordinated to work in harmony with the chosen temperature. The environment of the cuvettes is maintained at a constant temperature by a liquid bath, containing water or some other fluid with good heat-transfer properties, in which the cuvettes move.

Measurement Phase

After the reaction is completed, the formed products must be quantified. Almost all available systems for measurement have been used, such as ultraviolet, fluorescent, and flame photometry; ion-specific electrodes; gamma counters; and luminometers. Still, the most common is visible and ultraviolet light spectrophotometry, although adaptations of traditional fluorescence measurement, such as fluorescence polarization, chemiluminescence, and bioluminescence, have become popular. The Abbott AxSYM, for example, is a popular instrument for drug analysis that uses fluorescence polarization to measure immunoassay reactions.

Analyzers that measure light require a monochromator to achieve the desired component wavelength. Traditionally, analyzers have used filters or filter wheels to separate light. The old AAs used filters that were manually placed in position in the light path. Many instruments still use rotating filter wheels that are microprocessor controlled so that the appropriate filter is positioned in the light path. However, newer and more sophisticated systems offer the higher resolution afforded by diffraction gratings to achieve light separation into its component colors. Many instruments now use such monochromators with either a mechanically rotating grating or a fixed grating that spreads its component wavelengths onto a fixed array of photo diodes—for example, Hitachi analyzers (Fig. 7-11). This latter grating arrangement, as well as rotating filter wheels, easily accommodates polychromatic light analysis, which offers improved sensitivity and specificity over monochromatic measurement. By recording optical readings at different wavelengths, the instrument's computer can then use these data to correct for reaction mixture interferences that may occur at adjacent, as well as desired, wavelengths.

Many newer instruments use fiber optics as a medium to transport light signals from remote read stations back to a central monochromator detector box for analysis of these signals. The fiber-optic cables, or "light pipes" as they are sometimes called, are attached from multiple remote stations where the reaction mixtures reside to a centralized filter wheel/detector unit that, in conjunction with the computer, sequences and analyzes a large volume of light signals from multiple reactions (Fig. 7-12).

The containers holding the reaction mixture also play a vital role in the measurement phase. In most discrete wet chemistry analyzers, the cuvette used for analysis is also the reaction vessel in which the entire procedure has occurred. The reagent volume and, therefore, sample size, speed of analysis, and sensitivity of measurement are some aspects influenced by the method of analysis. A beam of light is focused through the container holding the reaction mixture. The amount of light that exits from the container is dictated primarily by the absorbance of light by the reaction mixture. The exiting light strikes a photodetector, which converts the light into electrical energy. Filters and light-focusing components permit the desired light wavelength to reach the photodetector. The photometer continuously senses the sample photodetector output voltage and, as is the process in most analyzers, compares it with a reference output voltage. The electrical impulses are sent to a readout device, such as a printer or computer, for storage and retrieval.

Centrifugal analysis measurement occurs while the rotor is rotating at a constant speed of approximately 1,000 rpm. Consecutive readings are taken of the sample, the dark current (readings between cuvettes), and the reference cuvette. Each cuvette passes through the light source every few milliseconds. After all the data points have been determined, centrifugation stops and the results are printed. The rotor is removed from the analyzer and discarded. For endpoint analyses, an initial absorbance is measured before the constituents have had time to react, usually a few seconds, and is considered a blank measurement. After enough time has elapsed for the reaction to be completed, another absorbance reading is taken. For rate analyses, the initial absorbance

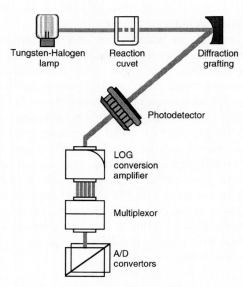

FIGURE 7-11 Photometer for a chemistry analyzer. Fixed diffraction grating separates light into specific wavelengths and reflects them onto a fixed array of 11 specific photodetectors. Photometer has no moving parts. (Courtesy of Roche Diagnostics.)

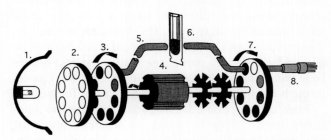

FIGURE 7-12 Photo-optical system for a chemistry analyzer: (**1**) source with reflector, (**2**) fixed focusing lens, (**3**) filter wheel, (**4**) double-shafted motor, (**5**) fiber-optic bundle, (**6**) cuvette, (**7**) filter wheel, and (**8**) photomultiplier tube. (Courtesy of Siemens.)

is measured, and then a lag time is allowed (preset into the instrument for each analysis). For each assay, several data points are determined at a programmed time interval. The instrument monitors the absorbance measurements at each data point and calculates a result.

Slide technology depends on reflectance spectrophotometry, as opposed to traditional transmittance photometry, to provide a quantitative result. The amount of chromogen in the indicator layer is read after light passes through the indicator layer, is reflected from the bottom of a pigment-containing layer (usually the spreading layer), and is returned through the indicator layer to a light detector. For colorimetric determinations, the light source is a tungsten–halogen lamp. The beam focuses on a filter wheel holding up to eight interference filters, which are separated by a dark space. The beam is focused at a 45° angle to the bottom surface of the slide, and a silicon photodiode detects the portion of the beam that reflects down. Three readings are taken for the computer to derive reflectance density. The three recorded signals taken are (1) the filter wheel blocking the beam, (2) reflectance of a reference white surface with the programmed filter in the beam, and (3) reflectance of the slide with the selected filter in the beam (Fig. 7-13).

After a slide is read, it is shuttled back in the direction from which it came, where a trap door allows it to drop into a waste bin. If the reading was the first for a two-point rate test, the trap door remains closed, and the slide reenters the incubator.

There are a number of fully automated, random-access immunoassay systems, which use chemiluminescence or electrochemiluminescence technology for reaction analysis. In chemiluminescence assays, quantification of an analyte is based on emission of light resulting from a chemical reaction.[9] The principles of chemiluminescent immunoassays are similar to those of radioimmunoassay and immunoradiometric assay, except that an acridinium ester is used as the tracer and paramagnetic particles are used as the solid phase. Sample, tracer, and paramagnetic particle reagent are added and incubated in disposable plastic cuvettes, depending on the assay protocol. After incubation, magnetic separation and washing of the particles are performed automatically. The cuvettes are then transported into a light-sealed luminometer chamber, where appropriate reagents are added to initiate the chemiluminescent reaction. On injection of the reagents into the sample cuvette, the system luminometer detects the chemiluminescent signal. Luminometers are similar to gamma counters in that they use a photomultiplier tube detector; however, unlike gamma counters, luminometers do not require a crystal to convert gamma rays to light photons. Light photons from the sample are detected directly, converted to electrical pulses, and then counted.

Signal Processing and Data Handling

Because most automated instruments print the results in reportable form, accurate calibration is essential to obtaining accurate information. There are many variables that may enter into the use of calibration standards. The matrices of the standards and unknowns may be different. Depending on the methodology, this may or may not present problems. If secondary standards are used to calibrate an instrument, the methods used to derive the standard's constituent values should be known. Standards containing more than one analyte per vial may cause interference problems. Because there are no

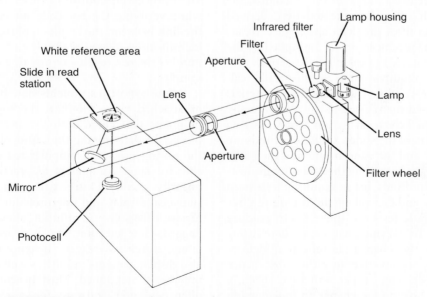

FIGURE 7-13 Components of the system for making colorimetric determinations with slide technology. (Courtesy of Ortho-Clinical Diagnostics.)

primary standards available for enzymes, either secondary standards or calibration factors based on the molar extinction coefficients of the products of the reactions may be used.

Many times, a laboratory will have more than one instrument capable of measuring a constituent. Unless there are different normal ranges published for each method, the instruments should be calibrated so that the results are comparable. The advantage of calibrating an automated instrument is the long-term stability of the standard curve, which requires only monitoring with controls on a daily basis. Some analyzers use low- and high-concentration standards at the beginning of each run and then use the absorbances of the reactions produced by the standards to produce a standard curve electronically for each run. Other instruments are self-calibrating after analyzing standard solutions.

The original continuous-flow analyzers used six standards assayed at the beginning of each run to produce a calibration curve for that particular batch. Now, continuous-flow analyzers use a single-level calibrator to calibrate each run with water used to establish the baseline.

The centrifugal analyzer uses standards pipetted into designated cuvettes in each run for endpoint analyses. After the delta absorbance for each sample has been obtained, the computer calculates the results by determining a constant for each standard. The constants are derived by dividing the concentration of the standard (pre-entered into the computer) by the delta absorbance and averaging the constants for each of the standards to obtain a factor. The concentration of each control and unknown is determined by multiplying the delta absorbance of the unknown by the factor. If the concentration of an unknown exceeds the range of the standards, the result is printed with a flag. Enzyme activity is derived by a linear regression fit of the delta absorbance versus time. The slope of the produced line is multiplied by the enzyme factor (pre-entered) to calculate the activity.

Slide technology requires more sophisticated calculations to produce results. The calibration materials require a protein-based matrix because of the necessity for the calibrators to behave as serum when reacting with the various layers of the slides. Calibrator fluids are bovine serum–based, and the concentration of each analyte is determined by reference methods. Endpoint tests require three calibrator fluids, blank-requiring tests need four calibrator fluids, and enzyme methods require three calibrators. Colorimetric tests use spline fits to produce the standardization. In enzyme analysis, a curve-fitting algorithm estimates the change in reflection density per unit time. This is converted to either absorbance or transmission-density change per unit time. Then, a quadratic equation converts the change in transmission density to volume activity (U/L) for each assay.

Most automated analyzers retain the calibrations for each lot of a particular method until the laboratorian programs the instrument for recalibration. Instrument calibration is initiated or verified by assaying a minimum of three levels of primary standards or, in the case of enzymes, reference samples. The values obtained are compared with the known concentrations by using linear regression, with the x-axis representing the expected values and the y-axis representing the mean of the values obtained. The slope (scale factor) and y-intercept (offset) are the adjustable parameters. On earlier models of this instrument, the parameters were determined and entered manually into the instrument computer by the operator; however, on later, more automated models, the instrument performs calibration automatically on operator's request. After calibration has been performed and the chemical or electrical analysis of the specimen is either in progress or completed, the instrument's computer goes into data acquisition and calculation mode. The process may involve signal averaging, which may entail hundreds of data pulses per second, as with a centrifugal analyzer, and blanking and correction formulas for interferents that are programmed into the computer for calculation of results.

All advanced automated instruments have some method of reporting printed results with a link to sample identification. In sophisticated systems, the demographic-sample information is entered in the instrument's computer together with the tests required. Then the sample identification is printed with the test results. Most laboratories use bar code labels printed by the LIS to identify sample. Bar code–labeled samples can be loaded directly on the analyzer without the need to enter identifying information manually. Microprocessors control the tests, reagents, and timing, while verifying the bar code for each sample. This is the link between the results reported and the specimen identification. Even the simplest of systems sequentially number the test results to provide a connection with the samples.

Because most instruments now have either a built-in or attached video monitor, the sophisticated software programs that come with the instrument can be displayed for determining the status of different aspects of the testing process. Computerized monitoring is available for such parameters as reaction and instrument linearity, quality control data with various options for statistical display and interpretation, short sample sensing with flags on the printout, abnormal patient results flagged, clot detection, reaction vessel or test chamber temperature, and reagent inventories. The printer can also display patients' results as well as various warnings previously mentioned. Most instrument manufacturers offer computer software for preventive maintenance schedules and algorithms for diagnostic troubleshooting.

Some manufacturers also install phone modems on the analyzer for a direct communication link between the instrument and their service center for instant trouble-shooting and diagnosis of problems.

SELECTION OF AUTOMATED ANALYZERS

Each manufacturer's approach to automation is unique. The instruments being evaluated should be rated according to previously identified needs. One laboratory may need a stat analyzer, whereas another's need may be a batch analyzer for high-test volumes. When considering cost, the price of the instrument and, even more importantly, the total cost of consumables are significant. The high capital cost of an instrument may actually be small when divided by the large number of samples to be processed. It is also important to calculate the total cost per test for each instrument that is considered. Moreover, a break-even analysis to study the relationship of fixed costs, variable costs, and profits can be helpful in analyzing the financial justification and economic impact on a laboratory. Of course, the mode of acquisition, that is, purchase, lease, rental, and so on, must also be factored into this analysis. The variable cost of consumables will increase as more tests are performed or samples are analyzed. The ability to use reagents produced by more than one supplier (open versus closed reagent systems) can provide a laboratory with the ability to customize testing and, possibly, save money. The labor component also should be evaluated. With the large number of instruments available on the market, the goal is to find the right instrument for each situation.[10]

Another major concern toward the selection of an instrument is its analytic capabilities. What are the instrument's performance characteristics for accuracy, precision, linearity, specificity and sensitivity (which may be method dependent), calibration stability, and stability of reagents (both shelf-life and onboard or reconstituted)? The best way to verify these performance characteristics of an analyzer before making a decision on an instrument is to see it in operation. Ideally, if a manufacturer will place an instrument in the prospective buyer's laboratory on a trial basis, then its analytic performance can be evaluated to the customer's satisfaction with studies to verify accuracy, precision, and linearity. At the same time, laboratory personnel can observe such design features as its test menus, true walk-away capability, user friendliness, and the space that the instrument and its consumables occupies in their laboratory.

Clinical chemistry instrumentation provides speed and precision for assays that would otherwise be performed manually. The chosen methodologies and adherence to the requirements of the assay provide accuracy. No one may assume that the result produced is the correct value.

Automated methods must be evaluated completely before being accepted as routine. It is important to understand how each instrument actually works.

TOTAL LABORATORY AUTOMATION

The pressures of healthcare reform and managed care have caused increasing interest in improving productivity of the preanalytic and postanalytic phases of laboratory testing.[11] As for the analytic process itself, routine analyzers in clinical chemistry today have nearly all the mechanization they need. The next generation of automation will replicate the Japanese practice of "black box" labs, in which the sample goes in at one end and the printed result comes out the other end.[12] Much effort has been expended during the past decade on the development of automated "front-end" feeding of the sample into the analytic "box" and computerized/automated management of the data that come out the back end of the box. There have been many developments in the three phases of the laboratory testing process—that is, preanalytic (sample processing), analytic (chemical analyses), and postanalytic (data management) as they merge closer into an integrated TLA system. Automation equipment vendors are developing open architecture components that provide more flexibility in automation implementation.[13] An example of a commercial TLA system is shown in Figure 7-14.

Preanalytic Phase (Sample Processing)

The sample-handling protocol currently available on all major chemistry analyzers is to use the original specimen collection tube (primary tube sampling) of any size (after plasma or serum separation) as the sample cup on the analyzer and to use bar code readers, also on the analyzer, to identify the specimen. An automated process is gradually replacing manual handling and presentation of the sample to the analyzer. Increasing efficiency while decreasing costs has been a major impetus for laboratories to start integrating some aspects of TLA into their operations. Conceptually, TLA refers to automated devices and robots integrated with existing analyzers to perform all phases of laboratory testing. Most attention to date has been devoted to development of the front-end systems that can identify and label specimens, centrifuge the specimen and prepare aliquots, and sort and deliver samples to the analyzer or to storage.[14] Back-end systems may include removal of specimens from the analyzer and transport to storage, retrieval from storage for retesting, re-aliquoting, or disposal, as well as comprehensive management of the data from the analyzer and interfacing with the LIS.

Dr. Sasaki[15] installed the first fully automated clinical laboratory in the world at Koshi Medical School in Japan; since then, the concept has gradually, but steadily, become a reality in the United States. The University of Nebraska and the University of Virginia have been

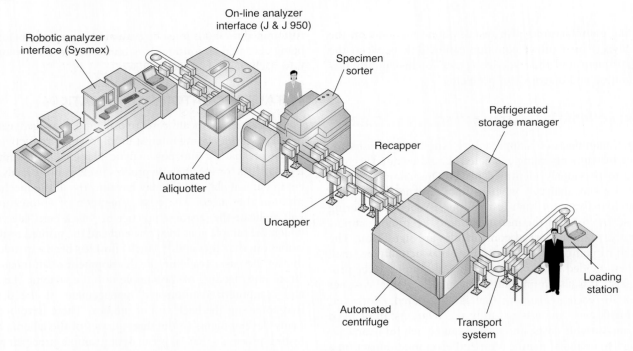

FIGURE 7-14 Schematic of total laboratory automation system. (Courtesy of Labotix Automation.)

pioneers for TLA system development. In 1992, a prototype of a laboratory automation platform was developed at the University of Nebraska, the key components being a conveyance system, bar-coded specimens, a computer software package to control specimen movement and tracking, and coordination of robots with the instruments as work cells.[16] Some of the first automated laboratories in the United States have reported their experiences with front-end automation with a wealth of information for others interested in the technology.[17,18] The first hospital laboratory to install an automated system was the University of Virginia Hospital in Charlottesville in 1995. Their Medical Automation Research Center cooperated with Johnson & Johnson and Coulter Corporation to use a Vitros 950 attached to a Coulter/IDS "U" lane for direct sampling from a specimen conveyor without using intervening robotics.[19] The first commercially available turnkey system was the Hitachi Clinical Laboratory Automation System (Boehringer-Mannheim Diagnostics; now Roche Diagnostics). It couples the Hitachi line of analyzers to a conveyor belt system to provide a completely operational system with all interfaces.[20]

Robotics and front-end automation are changing the face of the clinical laboratory.[21] Much of the benefit derivable from TLA can be realized merely by automating the front end. The planning, implementation, and performance evaluation of an automated transport and sorting system by a large reference laboratory have been described in detail.[22,23] Several instrument manufacturers are currently working on or are already marketing interfacing front-end devices together with software for their own chemistry analyzers. Johnson & Johnson introduced the Vitros 950 AT (Automation Technology) system in 1995 with an open architecture design to allow laboratories to select from many front-end automation systems rather than being locked into a proprietary interface. A Lab-Track interface is now available on the Dimension RxL (Siemens) that is compatible with major laboratory automation vendors and allows for direct sampling from a track system. Also, the technology now exists for microcentrifugal separators to be integrated into clinical chemistry analyzers.[24] Several other systems are now on the market, including the Advia LabCell system (Siemens), which uses a modular approach to automation. The Power Processor Core System (Beckman Coulter) performs sorting, centrifugation, and cap removal. The enGen Series Automation System (Ortho-Clinical Diagnostics) provides sorting, centrifugation, uncapping, and sample archiving functions and interface directly with a Vitros 950 AT analyzer. The instruments listed in Table 7-3 are examples of current TLA solutions offered commercially. Much of the benefit of TLA is derived from automation of the front-end processing steps. Therefore, several manufacturers have developed stand-alone automated front-end processing systems. The Genesis FE500 (Tecan) is an example of a stand-alone front-end system that can centrifuge, uncap, aliquot into a labeled pour-off tube, and sort into analyzer racks. Systems with similar functionality are available from Labotix, Motoman, and PVT. An example of one such system is shown in Figure 7-15. Stand-alone automated sample uncappers and recappers are available from PVT and Sarstedt. These latter devices

TABLE 7-3	SUMMARY OF FEATURES FOR SELECTED LABORATORY AUTOMATION SYSTEMS AND WORKCELLS			
	ABBOTT DIAGNOSTICS "ACCELERATOR APS"	BECKMAN COULTER "POWER PROCESSOR"	ROCHE DIAGNOSTICS CORP. "MODULAR PRE-ANALYTICS"	SIEMENS HEALTHCARE DIAGNOSTICS "ADVIA WORKCELL"
First year sold in the United States	2005	1998	2003	2002
Pre-analytical processor/ total laboratory automation	Yes/Yes	Yes/Yes	Yes/Yes	Yes/Yes
Automated centrifugation available	Yes	Yes	Yes	Yes
Automated input/ accessioning available	Yes	Yes	Yes	Yes
Automated decapping available	Yes	Yes	Yes	Yes
Automated sorting available	Yes	Yes	Yes	Yes
Automated aliquotting available	No	Yes	Yes	No
Automated recapper or sealer available	Sealer	Sealer	Recapper	No
Automated storage and retrieval available	Yes	Yes	Yes	Yes

Information obtained from Aller R. *CAP Today* 2011;September:20–40.

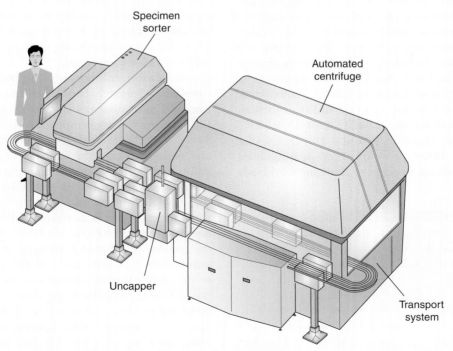

FIGURE 7-15 Schematic of preanalytic automation system. (Courtesy of Labotix Automation.)

are less flexible than the complete stand-alone front-end systems and require samples to be presented to them in racks that will work with a single analyzer. Some laboratories have taken a modular approach with devices for only certain automated functions. Ciba-Corning Clinical Laboratories installed Coulter/IDS robotic systems in several regional laboratories.[19] Recently, a thawing–mixing work cell that is compatible with a track system in a referral laboratory has been described.[25] The bottom line is that robotics and front-end automation are here to stay. As more and more clinical laboratories reengineer for TLA, they are building core laboratories containing all of their automated analyzers as the necessary first step to more easily link the different instruments into one TLA system.[26]

Analytic Phase (Chemical Analyses)

There have been changes and improvements that are now common to many general chemistry analyzers. They include ever smaller microsampling and reagent dispensing with multiple additions possible from randomly replaced reagents; expanded onboard and total test menus, especially drugs and hormones; accelerated reaction times with chemistries for faster throughput and lower dwell time; higher resolution optics with grating monochromators and diode arrays for polychromatic analysis; improved flow-through electrodes; enhanced user-friendly interactive software for quality control, maintenance, and diagnostics; integrated modems for online troubleshooting; LIS-interfacing data management systems; reduced frequencies of calibration and controls; automated modes for calibration, dilution, rerun, and maintenance; as well as ergonomic and physical design improvements for operator ease, serviceability, and maintenance reduction. The features and specifications of five mid- and five high-volume systems are summarized in Table 7-1. One main advantage of modular chemistry analyzers is scalability. As workload increases, additional modules can be added to increase throughput. A schematic of the MODULAR *ANALYTICS* system (Roche) is shown in Figure 7-16. This system can accommodate from one to four D, P, or E modules. This provides flexibility to adapt to changing workloads.

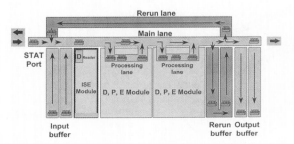

FIGURE 7-16 Schematic drawing of Roche MODULAR *ANALYTICS* system. (Courtesy of Roche Diagnostics.)

Chemistry and immunoassay testing can be combined, obviating the need to split samples. Repeat testing can be accomplished automatically using the rerun buffer, which holds the samples until all testing is completed.

Postanalytic Phase (Data Management)

Although most of the attention in recent years in TLA concept has been devoted to front-end systems for sample handling, several manufacturers have been developing and enhancing back-end handling of data. Bidirectional communication between the analyzer(s) and the host computer or LIS has become an absolutely essential link to request tests and enter patient demographics, automatically transfer this customized information to the analyzer(s), as well as post the results in the patient's record. Evaluation and management of data from the time of analysis until posting have become more sophisticated and automated with the integration of work station managers into the entire communication system.[27] Most data management devices are personal computer–based modules with manufacturers' proprietary software that interfaces with one or more of their analyzers and the host LIS. They offer automated management of quality control data with storage and evaluation of quality control results against the laboratory's predefined quality control perimeters with multiple plotting, displaying, and reporting capabilities. Review and editing of patient results before verification and transmission to the host are enhanced by user-defined perimeters for reportable range limits, panic value limits, delta checks, and quality control comparisons for clinical change, repeat testing, and algorithm analysis. Reagent inventory and quality control, along with monitoring of instrument functions, are also managed by the workstation's software. Most LIS vendors have interfacing software available for all the major chemistry analyzers.

Some data-handling needs associated with automation cannot be adequately handled by most current LISs. For example, most current analyzers are capable of assessing the degree of sample hemolysis, icterus, and lipemia (see Table 7-1). However, making this information available and useful to either the clinician or laboratorian in an automated fashion requires additional manipulation of the data. Ideally, the tests ordered on the sample, the threshold for interference of each test by each of the three agents, and whether the interference is positive or negative needs to be determined. In the case of lipemia, the results for affected tests need to be held until the sample can be clarified and the tests rerun. It is difficult or impossible for the current LISs to perform this latter task. There is a need for a "gap-filler" between the instrument and the LIS. One company, Data Innovations, has developed a system called Instrument Manager, which links the analyzer to the LIS and provides the ability for the user to define rules for release of information to the LIS. In addition, flags can be displayed to the instrument operator to perform additional operations, such as sample clarification and reanalysis. The ability to fully automate data review using rules-based analysis is a key factor in moving toward TLA. The use of "auto-verification" capabilities found with many post-analytic LISs has contributed to a significant reduction in result turnaround time.

FUTURE TRENDS IN AUTOMATION

Clinical chemistry automation continues to evolve at a rapid pace in the 21st century. With most of the same forces driving the automation market as those discussed in this chapter, analyzers will continue to perform more cost effectively and efficiently. More integration and miniaturization of components and systems will persist to accommodate more sophisticated portable analyzers for the successful POC testing market. Effective communications among all automation stakeholders for a given project are key to successful implementation.[28]

More new tests for expanded menus will be developed, with a mixture of measurement techniques used on the analyzers to include more immunoassays and polymerase chain reaction–based assays. Spectral mapping, or multiple wavelength monitoring, with high-resolution photometers in analyzers will be routine for all specimens and tests as more instruments are designed with the monochromator device in the light path after the cuvette, not before. Spectral mapping capabilities will allow simultaneous analysis of multiple chemistry analytes in the same reaction vessel. This will have a tremendous impact on throughput and turnaround time of test results. Mass spectrometry and capillary electrophoresis will be used more extensively in clinical laboratories for identification and quantification of elements and compounds in extremely small concentrations. In the coming years, more system and workflow integration will occur with robotics and data management for more inclusive TLA.[29] To accomplish this, more companies will form alliances to place their instrumentation products in the laboratories. The incorporation of artificial intelligence into analytic systems will evolve, using both experts systems and neural networks.[30,31] This will greatly advance the technologies of robotics, digital processing of data, computer-assisted diagnosis, and data integration with electronic patient records.

Finally, technologic advances in chip technology and biosensors will accelerate the development of noninvasive, in vivo testing.[32-34] Transcutaneous monitoring is already available with some blood gases. "True" or dynamic values from in vivo monitoring of constituents in blood and other body fluids will revolutionize laboratory medicine as we know it today.

For additional student resources please visit thePoint at http://thepoint.lww.com. **thePoint**

QUESTIONS

1. Which of the following is NOT a driving force for more automation?
   a. Increased use of chemistry panels
   b. High-volume testing
   c. Fast turnaround time
   d. Expectation of high-quality, accurate results

2. Which of the following approaches to analyzer automation can use mixing paddles to stir?
   a. Discrete analysis
   b. Centrifugal analysis
   c. Continuous flow
   d. Dry chemistry slide analysis

3. Which of the following types of analyzers offers random-access capabilities?
   a. Discrete analyzers
   b. Continuous-flow analyzers
   c. Centrifugal analyzers
   d. None of these

4. All of the following are primary considerations in the selection of an automated chemistry analyzer EXCEPT
   a. How reagents are added or mixed
   b. The cost of consumables
   c. Total instrument cost
   d. The labor component

5. An example of a modular integrated chemistry/immunoassay analyzer would be the
   a. Aeroset
   b. Dimension Vista 3000T
   c. Paramax
   d. Vitros

6. *Dwell time* refers to the
   a. Time between initiation of a test and the completion of the analysis
   b. Number of tests an instrument can handle in a specified time

c. Ability of an instrument to perform a defined workload in a specified time

d. None of these

7. The first commercial centrifugal analyzer was introduced in what year?

a. 1970
b. 1957
c. 1967
d. 1976

8. All of the following are advantages to automation EXCEPT

a. Correction for deficiencies inherent in methodologies
b. Increased number of tests performed
c. Minimized labor component
d. Use of small amounts of samples and reagents in comparison to manual procedures

9. Which of the following steps in automation generally remains a manual process in most laboratories?

a. Preparation of the sample
b. Specimen measurement and delivery
c. Reagent delivery
d. Chemical reaction phase

10. Which of the following chemistry analyzers uses slides to contain the entire reagent system?

a. Vitros analyzers
b. ACA analyzers
c. Synchron analyzers
d. None of these

11. Reflectance spectrometry uses which of the following?

a. Luminometer
b. Tungsten–halogen lamp
c. Photomultiplier tube
d. UV lamp
e. Thermometer to monitor temperature in reaction vessel

12. Modifications in microsampling and reagent dispensing improve which of the following phases in clinical testing?

a. Physician ordering phase
b. Preanalytical phase
c. Analytical phase
d. Postanalytical phase
e. All of the above phases

13. Bidirectional communication between the chemistry analyzer and the laboratory information system has had the greatest impact on which of the following phases of clinical testing?

a. Preanalytical
b. Analytical
c. Postanalytical
d. All of the above
e. None of the above

REFERENCES

1. Hodnett J. Automated analyzers have surpassed the test of time. *Adv Med Lab.* 1994;6:8.
2. Schoeff LE, Williams RH. *Principles of Laboratory Instruments.* St. Louis, MO: Mosby–Year Book; 1993.
3. Jacobs E, Simson E. Point of care testing and laboratory automation: the total picture of diagnostic testing at the beginning of the next century. *Clin Lab News.* December 1999;25(12):12-14.
4. Boyce N. Why hospitals are moving to core labs. *Clin Lab News.* 1996;22:1-2.
5. Boyce N. Why labs should discourage routine testing. *Clin Lab News.* 1996;22:1, 9.
6. Eisenwiener H, Keller M. Absorbance measurement in cuvets lying longitudinal to the light beam. *Clin Chem.* 1979;25:117-121.
7. Burtis CA. Factors influencing evaporation from sample cups, and assessment of their effect on analytic error. *Clin Chem.* 1975;21:1907-1917.
8. Burtis CA, Watson JS. Design and evaluation of an anti-evaporative cover for use with liquid containers. *Clin Chem.* 1992;38:768-775.
9. Dudley RF. Chemiluminescence immunoassay: an alternative to RIA. *Lab Med.* 1990;21:216.
10. Haboush L. Lab equipment management strategies: balancing costs and quality. *Clin Lab News.* 1997;23:20-21.
11. Schoeff L. Clinical instrumentation (general chemistry analyzers). *Anal Chem.* 1997;69:200R-203R.
12. Ringel M. National survey results: automation is everywhere. *MLO Med Lab Obs.* 1996;28:38-43.
13. Douglas L. Redefining automation: perspectives on today's clinical laboratory. *Clin Lab News.* 1997;23:48-49.
14. Felder R. Front-end automation. In: Kost G, ed. *Handbook of Clinical Laboratory Automation and Robotics.* New York, NY: Wiley; 1995.
15. Sasaki M. A fully automated clinical laboratory. *Lab Inform Mgmt.* 1993;21:159-168.
16. Markin R, Sasaki M. A laboratory automation platform: the next robotic step. *MLO Med Lab Obs.* 1992;24:24-29.
17. Bauer S, Teplitz C. Total laboratory automation: a view of the 21st century. *MLO Med Lab Obs.* 1995;27:22-25.
18. Bauer S, Teplitz C. Laboratory automation, part 2. Total lab automation: system design. *MLO Med Lab Obs.* 1995;27:44-50.
19. Felder R. Cost justifying laboratory automation. *Clin Lab News.* 1996;22:10-11, 17.
20. Felder R. Laboratory automation: strategies and possibilities. *Clin Lab News.* 1996;22:10-11.
21. Boyd J, Felder R, Savory J. Robotics and the changing face of the clinical laboratory. *Clin Chem.* 1996;42:1901-1910.
22. Hawker CD, Garr SB, Hamilton LT, et al. Automated transport and sorting system in a large reference laboratory: part 1. Evaluation of needs and alternatives and development of a plan. *Clin Chem.* 2002;48:1751-1760.
23. Hawker CD, Roberts WL, Garr SB, et al. Automated transport and sorting system in a large reference laboratory: part 2. Implementation of the system and performance measures over three years. *Clin Chem.* 2002;48:1761-1767.

24. Richardson P, Molloy J, Ravenhall R, et al. High speed centrifugal separator for rapid online sample clarification in biotechnology. *J Biotechnol*. 1996;49:111-118.

25. Hawker CD, Roberts WL, DaSilva A, et al. Development and validation of an automated thawing and mixing workcell. *Clin Chem*. 2007;53:2209-2211.

26. Zenie F. Re-engineering the laboratory. *J Automat Chem*. 1996;18:135-141.

27. Saboe T. Managing laboratory automation. *J Automat Chem*. 1995;17:83-88.

28. Fisher JA. Laboratory automation: communicating with all stakeholders is the key to success. *Clin Lab News*. July 2000; 26(7):38-40.

29. Brzezicki L. Workflow integration: does it make sense for your lab? *Adv Lab*. 1996;23:57-62.

30. Place J, Truchaud A, Ozawa K, et al. Use of artificial intelligence in analytical systems for the clinical laboratory. *J Automat Chem*. 1995;17:1-15.

31. Boyce N. Neural networks in the lab: new hope or just hype? *Clin Lab News*. 1997;23:2-3.

32. Boyce N. Tiny "lab chips" with huge potential? *Clin Lab News*. 1996;22:21.

33. Rosen S. Biosensors: where do we go from here? *MLO Med Lab Obs*. 1995;27:24-29.

34. Aller RD. Chemistry analyzers branching out. *CAP Today*. July 2002;16(7):84-106.

Immunochemical Techniques

ALAN H. B. WU

CHAPTER 8

CHAPTER OUTLINE

Chapter Objectives

Upon completion of this chapter, the clinical laboratorian should be able to do the following:

State the principle of each of the following methods:

- Double diffusion
- Radial immunodiffusion
- Immunoelectrophoresis
- Immunofixation electrophoresis
- Nephelometry
- Turbidimetry
- Competitive immunoassay
- Noncompetitive immunoassay
- Immunoblot
- Direct immunocytochemistry
- Indirect immunocytochemistry
- Immunophenotyping by flow cytometry

- Compare and contrast the general types of labels used in immunoassays.
- Classify an immunoassay, given its format, as homogeneous or heterogeneous, competitive or noncompetitive, and by its label.
- Explain how the concentration of the analyte in the test sample is related to the amount of bound labeled reagent for competitive and noncompetitive immunoassays.
- Describe the three methods used to separate unbound labeled reagent from bound labeled reagent.
- Describe the data reduction in the classic competitive radioimmunoassay.
- Compare and contrast EMIT, DELFIA, MEIA, RIA, FPIA, ELISA, CEDIA, ICON, and OIA methodologies.

KEY TERMS

Affinity
Antibody
Antigen
Avidity
Competitive immunoassay
Counterimmunoelectrophoresis
Cross-reactivity
Direct immunofluorescence (DIF)
Enzyme-linked immunosorbent assays (ELISAs)
Epitope
Flow cytometry
Hapten (Hp)
Heterogeneous immunoassay
Homogeneous immunoassay
Immunoblot

Immunocytochemistry
Immunoelectrophoresis (IEP)
Immunofixation electrophoresis (IFE)
Immunohistochemistry
Monoclonal
Nephelometry
Noncompetitive immunoassay
Polyclonal
Postzone
Prozone
Radial immunodiffusion (RID)
Rocket technique
Solid phase
Tracer
Turbidimetry
Western blot

Immunoassays were first developed by Dr. Rosalyn Yallow and colleagues in 1959, who developed a radioimmunoassay (RIA) for the measurement of insulin.[1] Dr. Yallow went on to share the Nobel Prize in physiology or medicine for this discovery in 1977. Today, immunoassays are one of the essential analytical techniques used in clinical chemistry laboratories for the measurement of proteins, hormones, metabolites, therapeutic drugs, drugs of abuse, cells, and even nucleic acids from serum, plasma, whole blood, tissues, and organs. Instrumentation has undergone tremendous advancement from manual RIA to totally automated analyzers capable of random access, high throughput, and wide menu options. Despite these advancement, the basic principle of how immunoassays work remains largely unchanged, a half century later.

This chapter introduces the generic analytic methods used in many areas of the clinical laboratory—the binding of antibody (Ab) to antigen (Ag) for the specific and sensitive detection of an analyte. In immunoassays, an Ag binds to an Ab. The Ag–Ab interactions may involve unlabeled reactants in less analytically sensitive techniques or a labeled reactant in more sensitive techniques. The design, label, and detection system combine to create many different assays, which enable the measurement of a wide range of molecules. This chapter reviews the concepts of binding, describes the nature of the reagents used, and discusses basic assay design of selected techniques used in the clinical laboratory; as such, it is intended to be an overview rather than an exhaustive review.

IMMUNOASSAYS

General Considerations

In an immunoassay, an Ab molecule recognizes and binds to an *Ag*. The molecule of interest may be either an Ag or an Ab. This binding is related to the concentration of each reactant, the specificity of the Ab for the Ag, the affinity and avidity for the pair, and the environmental conditions. Although this chapter focuses on immunoassays that use an Ab molecule as the binding reagent, other assays such as receptor assays and competitive binding protein assays use receptor proteins or transport proteins as the binding reagent, respectively. The same principles apply to these assays. An Ab molecule is an immunoglobulin (Ig) with a functional domain known as F(ab); this area of the Ig protein binds to a site on the Ag. An Ag is relatively large and complex and usually has multiple sites that can bind to antibodies (Abs) with different specificities; each site on the Ag is referred to as an antigenic determinant or epitope. Some confusion exists in the terminology used: some immunologists refer to an *immunogen* as the molecule that induces the biologic response and synthesis of Ab, and some use *Ag* to refer

to that which binds to Ab. However, all agree that the antigenic site to which an F(ab) can bind is the epitope.

The degree of binding is an important consideration in an immunoassay. The binding of an Ab to an Ag is directly related to the affinity and avidity of the Ab for the epitope, as well as the concentration of the Ab and epitope. Under standard conditions, the **affinity** of an Ab is measured using a **hapten** (Hp) because the Hp is a low-molecular-weight Ag considered to have only one epitope. The affinity for the Hp is related to the likelihood to bind or to the degree of complementary nature of each. The reversible reaction is summarized in Equation 8-1:

$$\text{Hapten} + \text{antibody} \rightleftharpoons$$
$$\text{hapten} - \text{antibody complex} \qquad \text{(Eq. 8-1)}$$

The binding between an Hp and the Ab obeys the law of mass action and is expressed mathematically in Equation 8-2:

$$K_a = \frac{k_1}{k_2} = \frac{[\text{Hp} - \text{Ab}]}{[\text{Hp}][\text{Ab}]} \qquad \text{(Eq. 8-2)}$$

K_a is the affinity or equilibrium constant and represents the reciprocal of the concentration of free Hp when 50% of the binding sites are occupied. The greater the affinity of the Hp for the Ab, the smaller is the concentration of Hp needed to saturate 50% of the binding sites of the Ab. For example, if the affinity constant of a monoclonal antibody (MAb) is 3×10^{11} L/mol, it means that an Hp concentration of 3×10^{-11} mol/L is needed to occupy half of the binding sites. Typically, the affinity constant of Abs used in immunoassay procedures ranges from 10^9 to 10^{11} L/mol, whereas the affinity constant for transport proteins ranges from 10^7 to 10^8 L/mol and the affinity for receptors ranges from 10^8 to 10^{11} L/mol.

As with all chemical (molecular) reactions, the initial concentrations of the reactants and the products affect the extent of complex binding. In immunoassays, the reaction moves forward (to the right) (Eq. 8-1) when the concentration of reactants (Ag and Ab) exceeds the concentration of the product (Ag–Ab complex) and when there is a favorable affinity constant.

The forces that bring an antigenic determinant and an Ab together are noncovalent, reversible bonds that result from the cumulative effects of hydrophobic, hydrophilic, and hydrogen bonding and van der Waals forces. The most important factor that affects the cumulative strength of bonding is the goodness (or closeness) of fit between the Ab and the Ag. The strength of most of these interactive forces is inversely related to the distance between the interactive sites. The closer the Ab and Ag can physically approach one another, the greater are the attractive forces.

After the Ag–Ab complex is formed, the likelihood of separation (which is inversely related to the tightness of bonding) is referred to as *avidity*. The avidity represents a value-added phenomenon in which the strength of binding of all Ab–epitope pairs exceeds the sum of single Ab–epitope binding. In general, the stronger the affinity and avidity, the greater is the possibility of cross-reactivity.

The specificity of an Ab is most often described by the Ag that induced the Ab production, the homologous Ag. Ideally, this Ab would react only with that Ag. However, an Ab can react with an Ag that is structurally similar to the homologous Ag; this is referred to as *cross-reactivity*. Considering that an antigenic determinant can be five or six amino acids or one immunodominant sugar, it is not surprising that Ag similarity is common. The greater the similarity between the cross-reacting Ag and the homologous Ag, the stronger is the bond with the Ab.[2] Reagent Ab production is achieved by polyclonal or monoclonal techniques. In polyclonal Ab production, the stimulating Ag is injected in an animal responsive to the Ag; the animal detects this foreign Ag and mounts an immune response to eliminate the Ag. If part of this immune response includes strong Ab production, then blood is collected and Ab is harvested, characterized, and purified to yield the commercial antiserum reagent. This polyclonal Ab reagent is a mixture of Ab specificities. Some Abs react with the stimulating epitopes and some are endogenous to the host. Multiple Abs directed against the multiple epitopes on the Ag are present and can cross-link the multivalent Ag. Polyclonal Abs are often used as "capture" Abs in sandwich or indirect immunoassays.

In contrast, an immortal cell line produces *monoclonal* Abs; each line produces one specific Ab. This method developed as an extension of the hybridoma work published by Kohler and Milstein in 1975.[3] The process begins by selecting cells with the qualities that will allow the synthesis of a homogeneous Ab. First, a host (commonly, a mouse) is immunized with an Ag (the one to which an Ab is desired); later, the sensitized lymphocytes of the spleen are harvested. Second, an immortal cell line (usually a nonsecretory mouse myeloma cell line that is hypoxanthine guanine phosphoribosyltransferase deficient) is required to ensure that continuous propagation in vitro is viable. These cells are then mixed in the presence of a fusion agent, such as polyethylene glycol, that promotes the fusion of two cells to form a hybridoma. In a selective growth medium, only the hybrid cells will survive. B cells have a limited natural life span in vitro and cannot survive, and the unfused myeloma cells cannot survive due to their enzyme deficiency. If the viable fused cells synthesize Ab, then the specificity and isotype of the Ab are evaluated. MAb reagent is commercially produced by growing the hybridoma in tissue culture or in compatible animals. An important feature of MAb reagent is that the Ab is homogeneous (a single Ab, not a mixture of Abs). Therefore, it recognizes only one epitope on a multivalent Ag and cannot cross-link a multivalent Ag.

Unlabeled Immunoassays

Immune Precipitation in Gel

In one of the simplest unlabeled immunoassays introduced into the clinical laboratory, unlabeled Ab was layered on top of unlabeled Ag (both in the fluid phase); during the incubation period, the Ab and Ag diffused and the presence of precipitation was recorded. The precipitation occurred because each Ab recognized an epitope and the multivalent Ags were cross-linked by multiple Abs. When the Ag–Ab complex is of sufficient size, the interaction with water is limited so that the complex becomes insoluble and precipitates.

It has been observed that if the concentration of Ag is increased while the concentration of Ab remains constant, the amount of precipitate formed is related to the ratio of Ab to Ag. As shown in Figure 8-1, there is an optimal ratio of the concentration of Ab to the concentration of Ag that results in the maximal precipitation; this is the zone of equivalence. If the amount of Ag exceeds the amount of Abs supplied by the test kit, cross-linking is decreased (Fig. 8-2), no precipitation is formed, and the assay is in prozone. Although originally described with precipitation reactions, this concept applies in particular to immunonephelometry for the measurement of specific proteins, in which the ratio of Ab to Ag is critical. For these types of calibration curves, a single signal from the reaction can be produced by two different Ag concentrations (see arrows of Fig. 8-1). Therefore, accurate results require dilution of the sample to move the result out of the prozone area and into the area of assay linearity.

Precipitation reactions in gel are not as commonly performed in the clinical laboratory today. Gel is dilute agarose (typically less than 1%) dissolved in an aque-

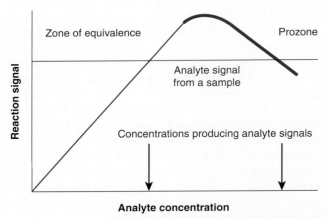

FIGURE 8-1 Precipitin curve showing the amount of precipitate vs. antigen concentration. The concentration of the antibody (from the assay kit) is constant. Note that one signal can be produced by two different analyte concentrations (*arrows*). A similar curve is observed for the hook effect seen in two-site sandwich immunoassays.

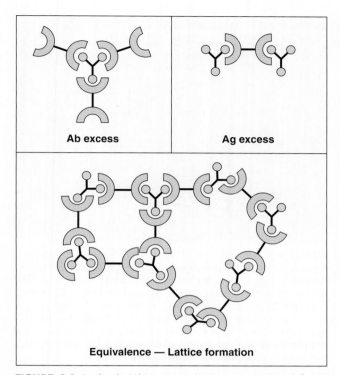

FIGURE 8-2 Antibody (Ab)–antigen (Ag) reactions. Top left: Ab excess condition. Top right: Ag excess condition. Both of these conditions lead to the formation of soluble complexes. Bottom: Bioequivalence leading to the formation of an insoluble "lattice" complex, detectable by immunonephelometry. Used with permission from Immunology, Chapter 7, Immunoglobulins-antigen-Antibody Reactions. Microbiology and Immunology On-Line, University of South Carolina School of Medicine.

TABLE 8-1	IMMUNE PRECIPITATION METHODS
Gel	
Passive	
Double diffusion (Ouchterlony technique)	
Single diffusion (radial immunodiffusion)	
Electrophoresis	
Counterimmunoelectrophoresis	
Immunoelectrophoresis	
Immunofixation electrophoresis	
Rocket electrophoresis	
Soluble Phase	
Turbidimetry	
Nephelometry	

detected using enzyme-linked immunoassays or multiplex bead array systems (e.g., Luminex Corp).

The single-diffusion technique, radial immunodiffusion (RID), is an immune precipitation method used to quantitate protein (the Ag). In this method, monospecific antiserum is added to the liquefied agarose; then the agarose is poured into a plate and cooled. Wells are cut into the solidified agarose. Multiple standards, one or more quality control samples, and patient samples are added to the wells. The Ag diffuses from the well in all directions, binds to the soluble Ab in the agarose, and forms a complex seen as a concentric precipitin ring (Fig. 8-4). The diameter of the ring is related to the concentration

ous buffer. This provides a semisolid medium through which soluble Ag and Ab can easily pass. Precipitated immune complexes are easier to discern in gel versus a liquid suspension. Immune precipitation methods in gel can be classified as passive methods or those using electrophoresis and are summarized in Table 8-1. The simplest and least sensitive method is double diffusion (the Ouchterlony technique).[4] Agarose is placed on a solid surface and allowed to solidify. Wells are cut into the agarose. A common template is six Ab wells, surrounding a single Ag well in the center. Soluble Ag and soluble Ab are added to separate wells and diffusion occurs. The intensity and pattern of the precipitation band are interpreted. As shown in Figure 8-3, the precipitin band of an unknown sample is compared with the precipitin band of a sample known to contain the Ab. A pattern of identity confirms the presence of the Ab in the unknown sample. Patterns of partial identity and nonidentity are ambiguous. This technique can be used to detect Abs associated with autoimmune diseases, such as Sm and ribonucleoprotein detected in systemic lupus erythematosus, SSA and SSB in Sjögren's syndrome, and Scl-70 in progressive systemic sclerosis. However, most of these Abs are also

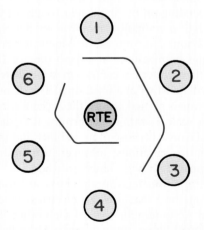

FIGURE 8-3 A schematic demonstrating the pattern of identity. The center well contains the antigen, rabbit thymus extract (RTE). *Well 1* is filled with a serum known to contain Sm antibody. Test sera are in *wells 2* and *3*; the pattern of identity, the smooth continuous line between the three wells, confirms the presence of Sm antibody in the test sera. *Well 4* is filled with a serum known to contain U1-ribonucleoprotein (RNP) antibody. Test sera in *wells 5* and *6* also contain U1-RNP antibody, confirmed by the pattern of identity between the known serum and the test sera.

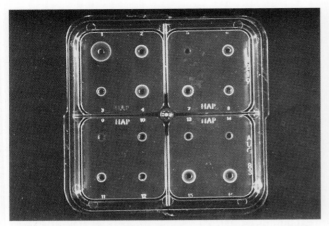

FIGURE 8-4 Radial immunodiffusion plate to detect haptoglobin. The diameter of the precipitin circle is related to the concentration of haptoglobin in the serum.

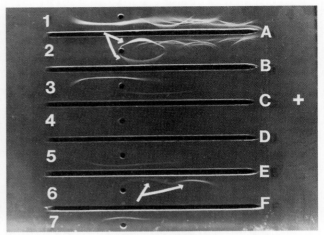

FIGURE 8-5 Immunoelectrophoresis. *Wells 1, 3, 5,* and *7* contain normal human serum, and *wells 2, 4,* and *6* contain the test serum. Antiserum reagent is in the troughs: antihuman whole serum (**A**), antihuman immunoglobulin (Ig)G (**B**), antihuman IgA (**C**), antihuman IgM (**D**), antihuman κ (**E**), and antihuman λ (**F**). The *arrows* at the *top* point to an abnormal γ chain that reacts with the anti-IgG reagent. A similar band is shown at the *bottom* with the anti-κ reagent. There is also a pattern of identity with the anti-κ reagent that shows free κ chains in the test serum.

of the Ag that diffused from the well. A standard curve is constructed to determine the concentration in the quality control and patient samples. The usable analytic range is between the lowest and highest standards. If the ring is greater than the highest standard, the sample should be diluted and retested. If the ring is less than the lowest standard, the sample should be run on a low-level plate. Two variations exist: the endpoint (Mancini) method[5] and the kinetic (Fahey-McKelvey) method.[6] The endpoint method requires that all Ag diffuse from the well and the concentration of the Ag is related to the square of the diameter of the precipitin ring; the standard curve is plotted and a line of the best fit is computed. To ensure that all of the Ag has diffused, the incubation time is 48 to 72 hours, depending on the molecular weight of the Ag; for example, IgG quantitation requires 48 hours, and IgM requires 72 hours. In contrast, the kinetic method requires that all rings be measured at a fixed time of 18 hours; a sample with a greater concentration will diffuse at a faster rate and will be larger at a fixed time. The diameter of the precipitin ring is plotted against the Ag concentration on a logarithmic scale. For those performing RID, the endpoint method is favored because of its stability and indifference to temperature variations; however, turnaround time is longer compared with the kinetic method.

Counterimmunoelectrophoresis is an immune precipitation method that uses an electrical field to cause the Ag and Ab to migrate toward each other. Two parallel lines of wells are cut into agarose; Ab is placed in one line and Ag is placed in the other. Ab will migrate to the cathode and the Ag to the anode; a precipitin line forms where they meet. This qualitative test is useful to detect bacterial Ags in cerebrospinal fluid and other fluids when a rapid laboratory response is needed.

Immunoelectrophoresis (IEP) and immunofixation electrophoresis (IFE) are two methods used in the clinical laboratory to characterize monoclonal proteins in serum and urine. In 1964, Grabar and Burtin[7] published methods for examining serum proteins using electrophoresis coupled with immunochemical reactions in agarose. Serum proteins are electrophoretically separated and then reagent Ab is placed in a trough running parallel to the separated proteins. The Ab reagent and separated serum proteins diffuse; when the reagent Ab recognizes the serum protein and the reaction is in the zone of equivalence, a precipitin arc is seen (Fig. 8-5). The agarose plate is stained (typically, with a protein stain such as Amido black 10), destained, and dried to enhance the readability of precipitin arcs, especially weak arcs. The size, shape, density, and location of the arcs aid in the interpretation of the protein. All interpretation is made by comparing the arcs of the patient sample with the arcs of the quality control sample, a normal human serum. Because IEP is used to evaluate a monoclonal gammopathy, the heavy chain class and light chain type must be determined. To evaluate the most common monoclonal proteins, the following antisera are used: antihuman whole serum (which contains a mixture of Abs against the major serum proteins), antihuman IgG (γ-chain specific), antihuman IgM (μ-chain specific), antihuman IgA (α-chain specific), antihuman λ (λ-chain specific), and antihuman κ (κ-chain specific). The test turnaround time and the subtlety in interpretation have discouraged the use of IEP as the primary method to evaluate MAbs.

IFE has replaced IEP in essentially all clinical laboratories.[8] A serum, urine, or cerebrospinal fluid sample is

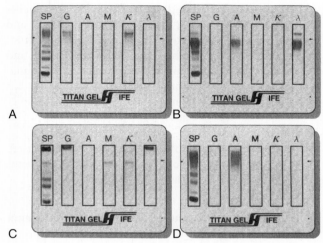

FIGURE 8-6 Immunofixation electrophoresis. **A.** IgG κ monoclonal immunoglobulin. **B.** IgA λ monoclonal immunoglobulin with free λ light chains. **C.** IgG λ and IgM κ biclonal immunoglobulins. **D.** Diffuse IgA heavy chain band without a corresponding light chain.

placed in all six lanes of an agarose gel and electrophoresed to separate the proteins. Cellulose acetate (or some other porous material) is saturated with Ab reagent and then applied to one lane of the separated protein. If the Ab reagent recognizes the protein, an insoluble complex is formed. After staining and drying of the agarose film, interpretation is based on the migration and appearance of bands. As shown in Figure 8-6, the monoclonal protein will appear as a discrete band (with both a heavy and a light chain monospecific antiserum occurring at the same position). Polyclonal proteins will appear as a diffuse band. The concentration of patient sample may need adjustment to ensure the reaction is in the zone of equivalence.

The rocket technique (Laurell technique, or electroimmunoassay) is also an immune precipitation method.[9,10] In this quantitative technique, reagent Ab is mixed with agarose; Ag is placed in the well and electrophoresed. As the Ag moves through the agarose, it reacts with the reagent Ab and forms a "rocket," with stronger precipitation along the edges. The height of the rocket is proportional to the concentration of Ag present; the concentration is determined based on a calibration curve. The narrow range of linearity may require dilution or concentration of the unknown sample.

Detection of Fluid-Phase Ag–Ab Complexes

A different strategy to quantitate Ag–Ab complexes is to use an instrument to detect the soluble Ag–Ab complexes as they interact with light. When Ag and Ab combine, complexes are formed that act as particles in suspension and thus can scatter light. The size of the particles determines the type of scatter that will dominate when the solution interacts with nearly monochromatic light.[11] When the particle, such as albumin or IgG, is relatively

small compared with the wavelength of incident light, the particle will scatter light symmetrically, both forward and backward. A minimum of scattered light is detectable at 90° from the incident light. Larger molecules and Ag–Ab complexes have diameters that approach the wavelength of incident light and scatter light with a greater intensity in the forward direction. The wavelength of light is selected based on its ability to be scattered in a forward direction and the ability of the Ag–Ab complexes to absorb the wavelength of light.

Turbidimetry measures the light transmitted and nephelometry measures the light scattered. Turbidimeters (spectrophotometers or colorimeters) are designed to measure the light passing through a solution so the photodetector is placed at an angle of 180° from the incident light. If light absorbance is insignificant, turbidity can be expressed as the absorbance, which is directly related to the concentration of suspended particles and path length. Nephelometers measure light at an angle other than 180° from the incident light; most measure forward light scattered at less than 90° because the sensitivity is increased (see Chapter 5). The relative concentration of the Ab reagent and Ag is critical to ensure that the size of the complex generated is best detected by the nephelometer or turbidimeter and that the immune reaction is not in prozone. Therefore, it may be important to test more than one concentration of patient sample, to monitor the presence of excess Ab, or to add additional antiserum and monitor the peak rate. Specific protein analyzers that use immunonephelometry as the detection scheme have automated sample dilution protocols in order to find an optimum Ag concentration to produce measurable precipitants.

For both turbidimetry and nephelometry, all reagents and sera must be free of particles that could scatter the light. Pretreatment of serum with polyethylene glycol, a nonionic, hydrophilic polymer, enhances the Ag–Ab interaction. Because the polymer is more hydrophilic than the Ag or Ab, water is attracted from the Ag and Ab to the polyethylene glycol. This results in a faster rate and greater quantity of Ag–Ab complex formation.

Both methods can be performed in an endpoint or a kinetic mode. In the endpoint mode, a measurement is taken at the beginning of the reaction (the background signal) and one is taken at a set time later in the reaction (plateau or endpoint signal); the concentration is determined using a calibration curve. In the kinetic mode, the rate of complex formation is continuously monitored and the peak rate is determined. The peak rate is directly related to the concentration of the Ag, although this is not necessarily linear. Thus, a calibration curve is required to determine concentration in unknown samples.

In general, turbidimetry is less sensitive of an analytical technique than nephelometry. In the former case, the decrease in the amount of light due to scattering is measured relative to the intensity of the reference blank, i.e., no sample, equivalent to 100% transmittance. If the sample concentration of the analyte is high, a large precipitate is formed resulting in a significant decrease in the amount of light that can easily be measured by turbidimetry. If however, the amount of precipitate is small due to a low sample concentration, the amount of light decreased is minimal and the instrument must measure the difference between two high-intensity light signals. Because in turbidimetry the amount of light is measured at an angle of 90°, the reference blank produces no signal (no light scattering). When a microprecipitate is formed, the light-scattered signal is more analytically discernible when measured against a dark reference baseline.

Labeled Immunoassays

General Considerations

In all labeled immunoassays, a reagent (Ag or Ab) is usually labeled by attaching a particle or molecule that will better detect lower concentrations of Ag–Ab complexes. Therefore, the label improves analytic sensitivity. All assays have a binding reagent, which can bind to the Ag or ligand. If the binding reagent is an Ab, the assay is an immunoassay. If the binding agent is a receptor (e.g., estrogen or progesterone receptor), the assay is a receptor assay. If the binding reagent is a transport protein (e.g., thyroxine-binding globulin or transcortin), the assay may be called competitive protein-binding assay. Immunoassays are used today almost exclusively, with two notable exceptions: estrogen and progesterone receptor assays and the thyroid hormone–binding ratio, which uses thyroxine-binding globulin.

Immunoassays may be described based on the label—which reactant is labeled, the relative concentration and source of the Ab, the method used to separate free from bound labeled reagents, the signal that is measured, and the method used to assign the concentration of the analyte in the sample. Immunoassay design, therefore, has many variables to consider, leading to diverse assays.

Labels

The simplest way to identify an assay is by the label used. Table 8-2 lists the commonly used labels and the methods used to detect the label.

Radioactive Labels

Atoms with unstable nuclei that spontaneously emit radiation are radioactive and referred to as radionuclides. The emission is known as radioactive decay and is independent of chemical or physical parameters, such as temperature, pressure, or concentration. Of the three forms of radiation, only beta and gamma are used in the clinical laboratory. In beta emission, the nucleus can emit negatively charged electrons or positively charged particles called positrons. The emitted electrons are also known as beta particles. Tritium (^3H) is the radionuclide commonly used in cellular immunology assays for diagnosis and research.

Gamma emission is electromagnetic radiation with very short wavelengths originating from unstable nuclei. As a radionuclide releases energy and becomes more stable, it disintegrates or decays, releasing energy. A specific spectrum of energy levels is associated with each radionuclide. The standardized unit of radioactivity is the becquerel (Bq), which is equal to one disintegration

TABLE 8-2	LABELS AND DETECTION METHODS	
IMMUNOASSAY	**COMMON LABEL**	**DETECTION METHOD**
RIA	^3H	Liquid scintillation counter
	^{125}I	Gamma counter
EIA	Horseradish peroxidase	Photometer, fluorometer, luminometer
	Alkaline phosphatase	Photometer, fluorometer, luminometer
	β-D-Galactosidase	Fluorometer, luminometer
	Glucose-6-phosphate dehydrogenase	Photometer, luminometer
CLA	Isoluminol derivative	Luminometer
	Acridinium esters	Luminometer
FIA	Fluorescein	Fluorometer
	Europium	Fluorometer
	Phycobiliproteins	Fluorometer
	Rhodamine B	Fluorometer
	Umbelliferone	Fluorometer

CLA, chemiluminescent assay; EIA, enzyme immunoassay; FIA, fluorescent immunoassay; RIA, radioimmunoassay.

per second. The traditional unit is the curie (Ci), which equals 3.7×10^{10} Bq; 1 μCi = 37 kBq. The half-life of the radionuclide is the time needed for 50% of the radionuclide to decay and become more stable. The longer the half-life, the more slowly it decays, increasing the length of time it can be measured. For radioactive substances used in diagnostic tests, it is preferable that the emission have an appropriate energy level and that the long half-life be relatively long; ^{125}I satisfies these requirements and is the most commonly used gamma-emitting radionuclide in the clinical laboratory.

Gamma-emitting nuclides are detected using a crystal scintillation detector (also known as a gamma counter). The energy released during decay excites a fluor, such as thallium-activated sodium iodide. The excited fluor releases a photon of visible light, which is amplified and detected by a photomultiplier tube; the amplified light energy is then translated into electrical energy. Detectable decay of the radionuclide is expressed as counts per minute (CPM).

In immunoassays, one reactant is radiolabeled. In competitive assays, the Ag is labeled and called the tracer. The radiolabel must allow the tracer to be fully functional and to compete equally with the unlabeled Ag for the binding sites. When the detector Ab is radiolabeled, the Ag-combining site must remain biologically active and unhindered.

Enzyme Labels

Enzymes are commonly used to label the Ag/Hp or Ab.[12,13] Horseradish peroxidase (HRP), alkaline phosphatase (ALP), and glucose-7-phosphate dehydrogenase are used most often. Enzymes are biologic catalysts that increase the rate of conversion of substrate to product and are not consumed by the reaction. As such, an enzyme can catalyze many substrate molecules, amplifying the amount of product generated. The enzyme activity may be monitored directly by measuring the product formed or by measuring the effect of the product on a coupled reaction. Depending on the substrate used, the product can be photometric, fluorometric, or chemiluminescent. For example, a typical photometric reaction using HRP-labeled Ab (Ab-HRP) and the substrate (a peroxide) generates the product (oxygen). The oxygen can then oxidize a reduced chromogen (reduced orthophenylenediamine [OPD]) to produce a colored compound (oxidized OPD), which is measured using a photometer:

$$Ab - HRP + peroxide \rightarrow Ab = HRP + O_2$$
$$O_2 + reduced\ OPD \rightarrow oxidized\ OPD + H_2O \quad \textbf{(Eq. 8-3)}$$

Fluorescent Labels

Fluorescent labels (fluorochromes or fluorophores) are compounds that absorb radiant energy of one wavelength and emit radiant energy of a longer wavelength in less than 10^{-4} seconds. Generally, the emitted light is detected at an angle of 90° from the path of excitation light using a fluorometer or a modified spectrophotometer. The difference between the excitation wavelength and emission wavelength (Stokes shift) usually ranges between 20 and 80 nm for most fluorochromes. Some fluorescence immunoassays simply substitute a fluorescent label (such as fluorescein) for an enzyme label and quantitate the fluorescence.[14] Another approach, time-resolved fluorescence immunoassay, uses a highly efficient fluorescent label, such as europium chelate,[15] which fluoresces approximately 1,000 times slower than the natural background fluorescence and has a wide Stokes shift. The delay allows the fluorescent label to be detected with minimal interference from background fluorescence. The long Stokes shift facilitates measurement of emission radiation while excluding the excitation radiation. The resulting assay is highly sensitive and time-resolved, with minimized background fluorescence.

Luminescent Labels

Luminescent labels emit a photon of light as the result of an electrical, biochemical, or chemical reaction.[16,17] Some organic compounds become excited when oxidized and emit light as they revert to the ground state. Oxidants include hydrogen peroxide, hypochlorite, or oxygen. Sometimes a catalyst is needed, such as peroxidase, ALP, or metal ions.

Luminol, the first chemiluminescent label used in immunoassays, is a cyclic diacylhydrazide that emits light energy under alkaline conditions in the presence of peroxide and peroxidase. Because peroxidase can serve as the catalyst, assays may use this enzyme as the label; the chemiluminogenic substrate, luminol, will produce light that is directly proportional to the amount of peroxidase present (Eq. 8-4):

$$Luminol + 2H_2O_2 + OH^- \xrightarrow{Peroxidase}$$
$$3\text{-aminophthalate} + light\ (425\ nm) \quad \textbf{(Eq. 8-4)}$$

A popular chemiluminescent label, acridinium esters, is a triple-ringed organic molecule linked by an ester bond to an organic chain. In the presence of hydrogen peroxide and under alkaline conditions, the ester bond is broken and an unstable molecule (*N*-methylacridone) remains. Light is emitted as the unstable molecule reverts to its more stable ground state:

$$Acridinium\ ester + 2H_2O_2 + OH^- \rightarrow$$

$$N\text{-methylacridone} + CO_2 + H_2O + light\ (430\ nm) \quad \textbf{(Eq. 8-5)}$$

ALP commonly conjugated to an Ab has been used in automated immunoassay analyzers to produce some of the most sensitive chemiluminescent assays. ALP catalyzes adamantyl 1,2-dioxetane aryl phosphate substrates to release light at 477 nm. The detection limit approaches 1 zmol, or approximately 602 enzyme molecules.[18,19]

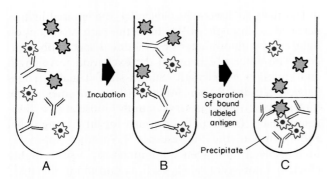

FIGURE 8-7 Competitive labeled immunoassay. During simultaneous incubation, labeled antigen and unlabeled antigen compete for the antibody-binding sites. The bound label in the precipitate is frequently measured.

Assay Design

Competitive Immunoassays

The earliest immunoassay was a competitive immunoassay in which the radiolabeled Ag (A*; also called the tracer) competed with unlabeled Ag for a limited number of binding sites (Ab) (Fig. 8-7). The proportion of Ag and Ag* binding with the Ab is related to the Ag and Ag* concentration and requires limited Ab in the reaction. In the competitive assay, the Ag* concentration is constant and limited. As the concentration of Ag increases, more binds to the Ab, resulting in less binding of Ag*. These limited reagent assays were very sensitive because low

concentrations of unlabeled Ag yielded a large measurable signal from the bound labeled Ag. If the competitive assay is designed to reach equilibrium, the incubation times are often long.

The Ag–Ab reaction can be accomplished in one step when labeled antigen (Ag*), unlabeled antigen (Ag), and reagent antibody (Ab) are simultaneously incubated together to yield bound labeled antigen (Ag*Ab), bound unlabeled antigen (AgAb), and free label (Ag*), as shown in Figure 8-7 and Equation 8-6:

$$\text{Ag* (fixed reagent) + Ag + Ab (limited reagent)}$$
$$\rightarrow \text{Ag* Ab + AgAb + Ag*} \qquad \text{(Eq. 8-6)}$$

A generic, heterogeneous, competitive simultaneous assay begins by pipetting the test sample (quality control, calibrator, or patient) into test tubes. Next, labeled Ag and Ab reagents are added. After incubation and separation of free labeled (unbound) Ag, the bound labeled Ag is measured.

Alternatively, the competitive assay may be accomplished in sequential steps. First, labeled Ag is incubated with the reagent Ab and then labeled Ag is added. After a longer incubation time and a separation step, the bound labeled Ag is measured. This approach increases the analytic sensitivity of the assay.

Consider the example in Table 8-3. A relatively small, yet constant, number of Ab combining sites is available to combine with a relatively large, constant amount of Ag* (tracer) and calibrators with known Ag concentrations.

TABLE 8-3	COMPETITIVE BINDING ASSAY EXAMPLE								
AG	+	**AG***	+	**AB**	→	**AGAB**	+	**AG*AB**	+	**AG***
CONCENTRATION OF REACTANTS						CONCENTRATION OF PRODUCTS			
AG		**AG***		**AB**		**AGAB**		**AG*AB**		**AG***
0		200		100		0		100		100
50		200		100		20		80		120
100		200		100		34		66		134
200		200		100		50		50		150
400		200		100		66		34		166
SAMPLE CALCULATIONS									
Dose of [Ag]		% B		B/F					
0		$\frac{100}{200} = 50$		$\frac{100}{100} = 1$					
50		$\frac{80}{200} = 40$		$\frac{80}{120} = 67$					
100		$\frac{66}{200} = 33$		$\frac{66}{134} = 33$					
200		$\frac{50}{200} = 25$		$\frac{50}{150} = 33$					
400		$\frac{34}{200} = 17$		$\frac{34}{166} = 20$					

Because the amount of tracer and Ab is constant, the only variable in the test system is the amount of unlabeled Ag. As the concentration of unlabeled Ag increases, the concentration (or percentage) of free tracer increases.

By using multiple calibrators, a dose–response curve is established. As the concentration of unlabeled Ag increases, the concentration of tracer that binds to the Ab decreases. In the example presented in Table 8-3, if the amount of unlabeled Ag is zero, maximum tracer will combine with the Ab. When no unlabeled Ag is present, maximum binding by the tracer is possible; this is referred to as B_0, B_{max}, maximum binding, or the zero standard. When the amount of unlabeled Ag is the same as the tracer, each will bind equally to the Ab. As the concentration of Ag increases in a competitive assay, the amount of tracer that complexes with the binding reagent decreases. If the tracer is of low molecular weight, free tracer is often measured. If the tracer is of high molecular weight, the bound tracer is measured. The data may be plotted in one of three ways: bound/free versus the arithmetic dose of unlabeled Ag; percentage bound versus the log dose of unlabeled Ag; and logit bound/B_0 versus the log dose of the unlabeled Ag (Fig. 8-8).

The bound fraction can be expressed in several different formats. Bound/free is CPM of the bound fraction compared with the CPM of the free fraction. Percent bound (% B) is the CPM of the bound fraction compared with the CPM of maximum binding of the tracer (B_0) multiplied by 100. Logit B/B_0 transformation is the natural log of $(B/B_0)/(1 - B/B_0)$. When B/B_0 is plotted on the ordinate and the log dose of the unlabeled Ag is plotted on the abscissa, a straight line with a negative slope is produced using linear regression.

It is important to remember that the best type of curve-fitting technique is determined by experiment and that there is no assurance that a logit-log plot of the data will always generate a straight line. To determine the best method, several different methods of data plotting should be tried when a new assay is introduced. Every time the assay is performed, a dose–response curve should be prepared to check the performance of the assay. The relative error for all RIA dose–response curves is minimal when $B/B_0 = 0.5$ and increases at both high and low concentrations of the plot. As shown in the plot of B/B_0 versus log of the Ag concentration (Fig. 8-8), a relatively large change in the concentration at either end of the curve produces little change in the B/B_0 value. Patient values derived from a B/B_0 value >0.9 or <0.1 should be interpreted with caution. When the same data are displayed using the logit-log plot, it is easy to overlook the error at either end of the straight line.

Noncompetitive Immunoassays
Sometimes known as immunometric assays, noncompetitive immunoassays use a labeled reagent Ab to detect the Ag. Excess labeled Ab is required to ensure that the labeled Ab reagent does not limit the reaction. The concentration of the Ag is directly proportional to the bound labeled Ab as shown in Figure 8-9. The relationship is

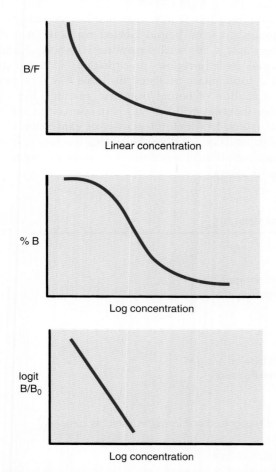

FIGURE 8-8 Dose–response curves in a competitive assay. B, bound labeled antigen; F, free labeled antigen; B_0, maximum binding; % B, $B/B_0 \times 100$.

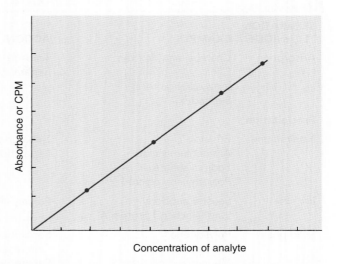

FIGURE 8-9 Dose–response curve in a noncompetitive immunoassay. CPM, counts per minute.

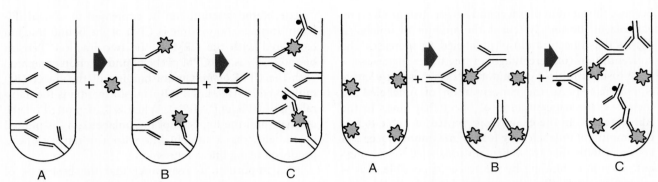

FIGURE 8-10 Two-site noncompetitive sandwich assay to detect antigen. Immobilized antibody captures the antigen. Then labeled antibody is added, binds to the captured antigen, and is detected.

FIGURE 8-11 Two-site noncompetitive sandwich assay to detect antibody. Immobilized antigen captures the antibody. Then labeled antibody is added, binds to the captured antibody, and is detected.

linear up to a limit and then is subject to the high-dose hook effect.

In the sandwich assay to detect Ag (also known as an Ag capture assay), immobilized unlabeled Ab captures the Ag. After washing to remove unreacted molecules, the labeled detector Ab is added. After another washing to remove free labeled detector Ab, the signal from the bound labeled Ab is proportional to the Ag captured. This format relies on the ability of the Ab reagent to react with a single epitope on the Ag. The specificity and quantity of MAbs have allowed the rapid expansion of diverse assays. A schematic is shown in Figure 8-10.

The sandwich assay is another noncompetitive assay used to detect Ab, in which the immobilized Ag captures specific Ab. After washing, the labeled detector Ab is added and binds to the captured Ab. The amount of bound labeled Ab is directly proportional to the amount of specific Ab present (Fig. 8-11). This assay can be modified to determine the Ig class of the specific Ab present in serum. For example, if the detector Ab was labeled and monospecific (e.g., rabbit antihuman IgM [μ-chain specific]), it would detect and quantitate only human IgM captured by the immobilized Ag.

Separation Techniques

All immunoassays require that free labeled reactant be distinguished from bound labeled reactant. In *heterogeneous assays*, physical separation is necessary and is achieved by adsorption, precipitation, or interaction with a solid phase as listed in Table 8-4. The better the separation of bound from free reactant, the more reliable the assay will be. This is in contrast to *homogeneous assays*, in which the activity or expression of the label depends on whether the labeled reactant is free or bound. No physical separation step is needed in homogeneous assays.

TABLE 8-4	CHARACTERISTICS OF SEPARATION TECHNIQUES	
SEPARATION TECHNIQUE	**EXAMPLE**	**ACTION**
Adsorption	Charcoal and dextran Silica Ion exchange resin Sephadex	Traps free labeled antigen Separation by centrifugation
Precipitation		
Nonimmune	Ethanol Ammonium sulfate Sodium sulfate Polyethylene glycol	Denatures bound labeled antigen Separation by centrifugation
Immune	Second antibody Staphylococcal protein A	Primary antibody is recognized and forms an insoluble complex
Solid phase	Polystyrene Membranes Magnetized particles	Separation by centrifugation One reactant is adsorbed or covalently attached to the inert surface Separation by washing

Adsorption

Adsorption techniques use particles to trap small Ags, labeled or unlabeled. A mixture of charcoal and cross-linked dextran is used. Charcoal is porous and readily combines with small molecules to remove them from solution; dextran prevents nonspecific protein binding to the charcoal. The size of the dextran influences the size of the molecule that can be adsorbed; the lower the molecular weight of dextran used, the smaller is the molecular weight of free Ag that can be adsorbed. Other adsorbents include silica, ion exchange resin, and Sephadex. After adsorption and centrifugation, the free labeled Ag is found in the precipitate. The binding of the capture Ab to paramagnetic particles is the most common method used by automated immunoassay analyzers. Separation takes place by applying a powerful magnet, thereby adhering bound analytes to each reaction chamber (Fig. 8-12). Unbound constituents and labels are removed by aspiration. Thereafter, the magnet is removed that enables the pellet to reconstitute and additional reagents added in order to generate the analytical signal (usually a chemiluminescent reaction).

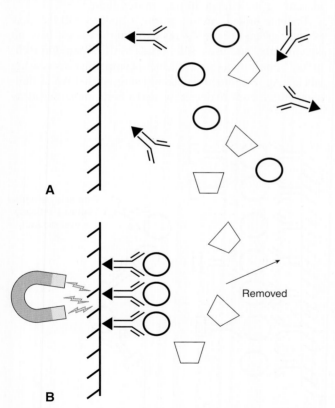

A

B

FIGURE 8-12 Separation by paramagnetic particles. **A.** Addition of sample containing the analyte (circle) and other constituent (rhomboid) to a capture antibody containing a paramagnetic particle (solid triangle). **B.** Application of a magnet to adhere capture antibodies and analyte to the side of the reaction chamber. The unbound constituent is removed by aspiration. Removal of the magnet and addition of signal antibody facilitate measurement (not shown).

Precipitation

Nonimmune precipitation occurs when the environment is altered, affecting the solubility of protein. Compounds such as ammonium sulfate, sodium sulfate, polyethylene glycol, and ethanol precipitate protein nonspecifically; both free Ab and Ag–Ab complexes will precipitate. Ammonium sulfate and sodium sulfate "salt out" free globulins and Ag–Ab complexes. Ethanol denatures protein and Ag–Ab complexes, causing precipitation. Polyethylene glycol precipitates larger protein molecules with or without the Ag attached. Ideally, after centrifugation, all bound labeled Ag will be in the precipitate, leaving free labeled Ag in the supernatant.

Soluble Ag–Ab complexes can be precipitated by a second Ab that recognizes the primary Ab in the soluble complex. The result is a larger complex that becomes insoluble and precipitates. Centrifugation is again used to aid in the separation. This immune precipitation method is also known as the double-Ab or second-Ab method. For example, in a growth hormone assay, the primary or Ag-specific Ab produced in a rabbit recognizes growth hormone. The second Ab, produced in a sheep or goat, would recognize rabbit Ab. Labeled Ag–Ab complexes, unlabeled Ag–Ab complexes, and free primary Abs are precipitated by the second Ab. This separation method is more specific than nonimmune precipitation because only the primary Ab is precipitated. A similar separation occurs when staphylococcal protein A (SPA) replaces the second Ab. SPA binds to human IgG causing precipitation.

Solid Phase

The use of a *solid phase* to immobilize reagent Ab or Ag provides a method to separate free from bound labeled reactant after washing. The solid-phase support is an inert surface to which reagent Ag or Ab is attached. The solid-phase support may be, but is not limited to, polystyrene surfaces, membranes, and magnetic beads. The immobilized Ag or Ab may be adsorbed or covalently bound to the solid-phase support; covalent linkage prevents spontaneous release of the immobilized Ag or Ab. Immunoassays using solid-phase separation are easier to perform and to automate and require less manipulation and time to perform than other immunoassays. However, a relatively large amount of reagent Ab or Ag is required to coat the solid-phase surface, and consistent coverage of the solid phase is difficult to achieve.

Interferences with Sandwich Immunoassays

While an advantage of sandwich-type immunoassays is the production of linear calibration curves (Fig. 8-1), the disadvantage is that these assays are subjected to false-positive and false-negative interferences. Normally, the target analyte is required for the production of a positive analytical signal (Fig. 8-13A). If, however, the sample contains unusual Abs, such as human anti-mouse

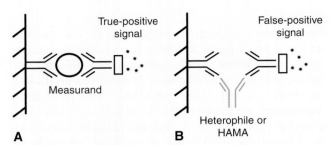

FIGURE 8-13 Heterophile or human anti-mouse interference. **A.** Analytical signal in the presence of the analyte. The capture antibody (left), attached to a solid support binds to the analyte (circle) at one epitope of the analyte. The labeled antibody (right) is added and binds to the analyte at a second analyte epitope. **B.** False-positive signal in the presence of an interfering antibody. The interfering antibody (gray middle) binds to both the capture (left) and label (right) antibodies, forming a "sandwich" in the absence of the analyte causing a false-positive signal.

antibodies (HAMA) or heterophile Abs, they can bind to both the capture and labeled Abs producing an analytical signal in the absence of the analyte (Fig. 8-13B). Individuals who are exposed to mouse Ags can develop HAMA Abs that recognize monoclonal Abs derived from murine cell lines as Ags.[20] Heterophile Abs are formed from patients who have autoimmune disease and other disorders.[21] Although the principle is different, the "hook" effect is similar to the prozone effect in that excess concentrations of the Ag from the sample reduces

the analytical signal.[22] As shown in Figure 8-14, excess Ag binds to free labeled Ab, prohibiting the labeled Ab to bind to the capture Ab (via the analyte), and the resulting signal is reduced after the wash step. Analytes that are present in very low and high concentrations, such as human chorionic gonadotropin (hCG) during the first trimester of pregnancy, are subjected to the hook effect. Commercial assays must be designed to either be immune to the hook effect or produce some warning flag to the analyst that the sample must be diluted in order to obtain an accurate result. In anticipation of the need for sample dilution, some laboratories automatically perform dilutions of a sample from a patient known to have high analyte values (e.g., hCG during pregnancy).

Examples of Labeled Immunoassays

Particle-enhanced turbidimetric inhibition immunoassay is a homogeneous competitive immunoassay in which low-molecular-weight Hps bound to particles compete with unlabeled analyte for the specific Ab. The extent of particle agglutination is inversely proportional to the concentration of unlabeled analyte and is assessed by measuring the change in transmitted light.[23]

Enzyme-linked immunosorbent assays (ELISAs), a popular group of heterogeneous immunoassays, have an enzyme label and use a solid phase as the separation technique. Four formats are available: a competitive assay using labeled Ag, a competitive assay using labeled Ab, a noncompetitive assay to detect Ag, and a noncompetitive assay

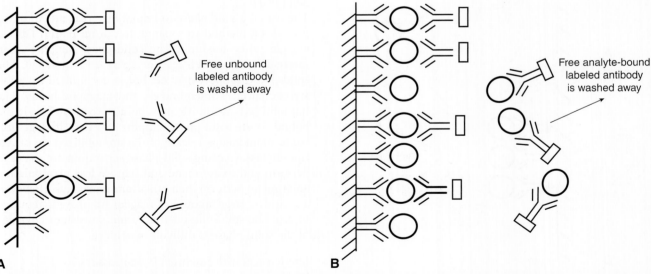

FIGURE 8-14 The hook effect. **A.** Analytical signal in the presence of the analyte at a concentration that is within the dynamic range of the assay. There is an excess amount of capture (left) and labeled (right) antibodies such that all analytes are bound (none are free in solution). Excess free unbound labeled antibody is washed away, and the resulting signal is proportional to the number of captured labeled antibody (4 units in this example). **B.** Analytical signal in the presence of the analyte at a concentration that is above the dynamic range of the assay. All of the capture antibody is bound with the analyte. The excess antigen is found free in solution and binds to excess labeled antibody found free in solution. These labeled antibodies cannot bind to the analyte-bound capture antibody because the site is already occupied with the analyte. The free analyte-bound labeled antibody is washed away. This leaves 4 units remaining, the same number as in example A despite the much higher analyte concentration.

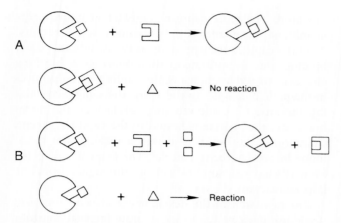

FIGURE 8-15 Enzyme-multiplied immunoassay technique. **A.** When enzyme-labeled antigen is bound to the antibody, the enzyme activity is inhibited. **B.** Free patient antigen binds to the antibody and prevents antibody binding to the labeled antigen. The substrate indicates the amount of free labeled antigen.

to detect Ab. ELISAs are widely used in clinical research as there are commercial assays available to hundreds of analytes. If the analyte has clinical value, an automated version would be made available to the clinical laboratory scientist. If the assay is only used for research purposes, e.g., cytokine analysis, then ELISAs are the technique of choice because they can be easily produced by the manufacturers and most research laboratories have ELISA plate readers. The disadvantage of ELISAs are that they typically use enzyme or fluorescence detection, which is not as sensitive as chemiluminescence or radiodetection. The assays are more labor intensive than modern clinical assays, although some laboratories have automated plate washing and reading stations to improve workflow if there is a high volume of testing needed.

One of the earliest homogeneous assays was enzyme-multiplied immunoassay technique (EMIT), an enzyme immunoassay (Siemens Healthcare Corp).[24] As shown in Figure 8-15, the reactants in most test systems include an enzyme-labeled Ag (commonly, a low-molecular-weight analyte, such as a drug), an Ab directed against the Ag, the substrate, and test Ag. The enzyme is catalytically active when the labeled Ag is free (not bound to the Ab). It is thought that when the Ab combines with the labeled Ag, the Ab sterically hinders the enzyme. The conformational changes that occur during Ag–Ab interaction inhibit the enzyme activity. In this homogeneous assay, the unlabeled Ag in the sample competes with the labeled Ag for the Ab-binding sites; as the concentration of unlabeled Ag increases, less enzyme-labeled Ag can bind to the Ab. Therefore, more labeled Ag is free, and the enzymatic activity is greater.

Cloned enzyme donor immunoassays (CEDIAs) are competitive, homogeneous assays in which the genetically engineered label is β-galactosidase (Microgenics Corp).[25] The enzyme is in two inactive pieces: the enzyme acceptor and the enzyme donor. When these two pieces bind together, enzyme activity is restored. In the assay, the Ag labeled with the enzyme donor and the unlabeled Ag in the sample compete for specific Ab-binding sites. When the Ab binds to the labeled Ag, the enzyme acceptor cannot bind to the enzyme donor; therefore, the enzyme is not restored and the enzyme is inactive. More unlabeled Ag in the sample results in more enzyme activity.

Microparticle capture enzyme immunoassay (MEIA) is an automated assay available on the AxSYM Analyzer (Abbott Laboratories). The microparticles serve as the solid phase, and a glass fiber matrix separates the bound labeled reagent. Both competitive and noncompetitive assays are available. Although the label is an enzyme (ALP), the substrate (4-methylumbelliferyl phosphate) is fluorogenic.

Solid-phase fluorescence immunoassays are analogous to the ELISA methods except that the label fluoresces. Of particular note is FIAX (BioWhittaker). In this assay, fluid-phase unlabeled Ag is captured by Ab on the solid phase; after washing, the detector Ab (with a fluorescent label attached) reacts with the solid-phase captured Ag.

Particle concentration fluorescence immunoassay is a heterogeneous, competitive immunoassay in which particles are used to localize the reaction and concentrate the fluorescence. Labeled Ag and unlabeled Ag in the sample compete for Ab bound to polystyrene particles. The particles are trapped and the fluorescence is measured. The assay can also be designed so that labeled Ab and unlabeled Ab compete for Ag fixed onto particles.

Fluorescence excitation transfer immunoassay is a competitive, homogeneous immunoassay using two fluorophores (such as fluorescein and rhodamine).[26] When the two labels are in close proximity, the emitted light from fluorescein will be absorbed by rhodamine. Thus, the emission from fluorescein is quenched. Fluorescein-labeled Ag and unlabeled Ag compete for rhodamine-labeled Ab. More unlabeled Ag lessens the amount of fluorescein-labeled Ag that binds; therefore, more fluorescence is present (less quenching).

Substrate-level fluorescence immunoassay is another competitive, homogeneous assay. This time, the Hp is labeled with a substrate; when catalyzed by an appropriate enzyme, fluorescent product is generated. Substrate-labeled Hp and unlabeled Hp in the sample compete with Ab; the bound labeled Hp cannot be catalyzed by the enzyme.

Fluorescence polarization immunoassay (FPIA) is another assay that uses a fluorescent label.[27] This homogeneous immunoassay uses polarized light to excite the fluorescent label. Polarized light is created when light passes through special filters and consists of parallel light waves oriented in one plane. When polarized light is used to excite a fluorescent label, the emitted light could be polarized or depolarized. Small molecules, such as free fluorescent-labeled Hp, rotate rapidly and randomly, interrupting the polarized light. Larger molecules, such as those created when the fluorescent-labeled Hp binds to an Ab, rotate more slowly and emit polarized light parallel to the excitation polarized light. The polarized light is measured at a 90° angle compared with the path of the excitation light. In a competitive FPIA, fluorescent-labeled Hp and unlabeled Hp in the sample compete for limited Ab sites. When no unlabeled Hp is present, the labeled Hp binds maximally to the Ab, creating large complexes that rotate slowly and emit a high level of polarized light. When Hp is present, it competes with the labeled Hp for the Ab sites; as the Hp concentration increases, more labeled Hp is displaced and is free. The free labeled Hp rotates rapidly and emits less polarized light. The degree of labeled Hp displacement is inversely related to the amount of unlabeled Hp present.

Dissociation-enhanced lanthanide fluoroimmunoassay (DELFIA) is an automated system (Thermo Fisher Scientific) that measures time-delayed fluorescence from the label europium. The assay can be designed as a competitive, heterogeneous assay or a noncompetitive (sandwich), heterogeneous assay.[28]

The classic RIA is a heterogeneous, competitive assay with a tracer.[1] When bound tracer is measured, the signal from the label (CPM) is inversely related to the concentration of the unlabeled Ag in the sample.

Rapid Immunoassay for Point-of-Care Testing

The sensitivity and specificity of automated labeled assays and the trend for decentralized laboratory testing have led to the development of assays that are easy to use, simple (many classified as waived or moderately complex related to the Clinical Laboratory Improvement Amendments of 1988), fast, and site neutral and require no instrumentation. Those discussed here are representative of currently available commercial kits; however, this discussion is not intended to be exhaustive. Three categories of rapid immunoassays emerge: (1) latex particles for visualization of the reaction, (2) fluid flow and labeled reactant, and (3) changes in a physical or chemical property following Ag–Ab binding.

The earliest rapid tests were those in which a latex particle suspension was added to the sample; if the immunoreactive component attached to the particle recognized its counterpart in the sample, macroscopic agglutination occurred. Colored latex particles are now available to facilitate reading the reaction.

Self-contained devices that use the liquid nature of the specimen have evolved. In flowthrough systems, a capture reagent is immobilized onto a membrane, the solid phase. The porous nature of the membranes increases the surface area to which the capture reagent can bind. The more capture reagent that binds to the membrane, the greater is the potential assay sensitivity. After the capture reagent binds to the membrane, other binding sites are saturated with a nonreactive blocking chemical to reduce nonspecific binding by substances in the patient sample. In the assay, the sample containing the analyte is allowed to pass through the membrane and the analyte is bound to the capture reagent. Commonly, the liquid is attracted through the membrane by an absorbent material. The analyte is detected by a labeled reactant, as well as the signal from the labeled reactant.

The next step in the development of self-contained, single-use devices was to incorporate internal controls. One scheme to detect hCG, the ImmunoConcentration Assay (ICON; Hybritech),[29] creates three zones in which specifically treated particles are deposited. In the assay zone, particles are coated with reagent Ab specific for the assay; in the negative control zone, particles are coated with nonimmune Ab; and, in the positive control zone, particles are coated with an immune complex specific for the assay. The patient sample (serum or urine) passes through the membrane, and the analyte is captured by the specific reagent Ab in the assay zone. Next, a labeled Ab passes through the membrane, which fixes to the specific immune complex formed in the assay zone or the positive control zone. Following color development, a positive reaction is noted when the assay and positive zones are colored.

A second homogeneous immunoassay involves the tangential flow of fluid across a membrane. The fluid dissolves and binds to the dried capture reagent; the complex flows to the detection area, where it is concentrated and viewed.

A third homogeneous immunoassay, enzyme immunochromatography, involves vertical flow of fluid along a membrane.[30] This is quantitative and does not require any instrumentation. A dry paper strip with immobilized Ab is immersed in a solution of unlabeled analyte and an enzyme-labeled analyte; the liquid migrates up the strip by capillary action. As the labeled and unlabeled analyte migrate, they compete and bind to the immobilized Ab. A finite amount of labeled and unlabeled analyte mixture is absorbed. The migration distance of the labeled analyte is visualized when the strip reacts with a substrate reagent and develops a colored reaction product. Comparing the migration distance of the sample with the calibrator allows the concentration of the unlabeled ligand to be assigned.

The next generation of rapid immunoassays involves change in physical or chemical properties after an Ag–Ab interaction occurs. One example is the optical immunoassay (OIA).[31] A silicon wafer is used to support a thin film of optical coating; this is then topped with the capture Ab. Sample is applied directly to the device. If an Ag–Ab complex forms, the thickness of the optical surface increases and changes the optical path of light. The color changes from gold to purple. Some studies suggest that this method has better analytic sensitivity than immunoassays, which rely on the fluid flow.

Immunoblots

Most assays described this far are designed to measure a single analyte. In some circumstances, it is beneficial to separate multiple Ags by electrophoresis so as to be able to simultaneously detect multiple serum Abs. The Western blot is a transfer technique used to detect specific Abs. As shown in Figure 8-16, multiple protein Ags

(such as those associated with the human immunodeficiency virus) are isolated, denatured, and separated by sodium dodecyl sulfate–polyacrylamide gel electrophoresis (SDS-PAGE). SDS denatures the protein and adds an overall negative charge proportional to the molecular weight of the protein. The PAGE of SDS-treated proteins allows the separation of protein based on molecular weight. The separated proteins are then transferred to a new medium (e.g., nylon, nitrocellulose, or polyvinylidene difluoride membrane). The separated proteins will be fixed on the new medium and may be stained to assure separation. Each lane on the membrane is then incubated with patient or control sample. The Ab recognizes and binds to the Ag, forming an insoluble complex. After washing, a labeled Ab reagent detects the complex. Depending on the label, it may yield a photometric, fluorescent, or chemiluminescent product that appears as a band. The bands from the patient sample are compared with those from the control containing Ab that will react with known Ags. Molecular weight markers are also separated and stained to provide a guide for interpretation of molecular weight.

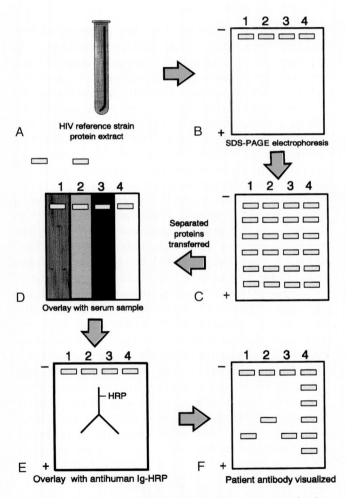

FIGURE 8-16 Immunoblot (Western blot) to detect antibodies to human immunodeficiency virus (HIV) antigens. **A.** The HIV is disrupted and extracted to generate its antigens. **B.** The HIV antigens are separated by sodium dodecyl sulfate–polyacrylamide gel electrophoresis (SDS-PAGE). **C.** The separated antigens are visualized and then transferred to a membrane. **D.** Each lane of the membrane is overlaid with a patient or control serum. **E.** After incubation and washing, a labeled antibody reagent is overlaid onto all lanes. **F.** The bound labeled antibody is detected. Ig, immunoglobulin; HRP, horseradish peroxidase.

Immunocytochemistry and Immunohistochemistry

When Ab reagents are used to detect Ags in cells or tissue, the methods are known as immunocytochemistry and immunohistochemistry, respectively. When the Ag is an integral part of the cell or tissue, this is direct testing. A second strategy, indirect testing, uses cells or tissue as a substrate (the source of Ag) to capture serum Ab; this complex is then detected using a labeled Ab reagent.

Fluorescent labels are most commonly used in immunocytochemistry and immunohistochemistry. When used to microscopically identify bacteria or constituents in tissue (e.g., immune complexes deposited in vivo), the method is called direct immunofluorescence (DIF) or direct fluorescence assay (DFA). A specially configured fluorescence microscope is necessary. Appropriate wavelengths of light are selected by a filter monochromator to excite the fluorescent label; the fluorescent label emits light of a second wavelength that is selected for viewing by a second filter monochromator. Examples of DFA include detection of *Treponema pallidum* in lesional fluid or detection of immune complexes in glomerulonephritis associated with Goodpasture's syndrome and lupus nephritis.

When a fluorescent label is used in indirect testing, this is *indirect immunofluorescence (IIF)* or an indirect immunofluorescence assay (IFA). The substrate is placed on a microscopic slide, serum is overlaid and allowed to react with the Ag, and the bound Ab is detected by the labeled antihuman globulin reagent. The slide is viewed using a fluorescence microscope. The most common IFA performed in the clinical laboratory detects Abs to nuclear Ags. Both the titer and pattern of fluorescence provide useful information to diagnose connective tissue disease. Other autoantibodies and Abs to infectious disease can be detected by IFA.

Immunophenotyping

An important and more recent advance in immunocytochemistry is the use of a flow cytometer to detect intracellular and cell surface Ags. This technique, *immunophenotyping*, is used to classify cell lineage and identify the stage of cell maturation. In particular, immunophenotyping aids in the diagnosis of leukemias and lymphomas. Differentiating between acute myelogenous leukemia and acute lymphoblastic leukemia is difficult morphologically and requires additional information to identify the phenotypically expressed molecules. In lymphoid leukemias and lymphomas, identification of tumor cells as either T- or B-lymphocytes can be an important predictor of clinical outcome. Another application is to determine the CD4/CD8 ratio (the ratio of the number of helper T-lymphocytes to cytotoxic T-lymphocytes) and, more recently, the absolute number of CD4 positive (CD4+) cells. This is the standard method to diagnose infection and to initiate and monitor treatment, although viral load quantitation is considered by many to be a better marker.

Immunophenotyping begins with a living cell suspension. The cells may come from peripheral blood, bone marrow, or solid tissue. Leukocytes or mononuclear cells can be isolated using density gradient separation (centrifugation through Ficoll-Hypaque) or by red blood cell lysis. Tissue, such as lymph node and bone marrow, requires mechanical removal of cells from the tissue to collect a cell suspension. Based on patient history and type of specimen, a panel of fluorochrome-labeled MAbs is used. Fluorochromes commonly used in immunophenotyping include fluorescein isothiocyanate, phycoerythrin, peridinin chlorophyll, CY-5, allophycocyanin, and tetramethyl rhodamine isothiocyanate. An aliquot of the cell suspension is incubated with one or more MAbs, depending on the design of the flow cytometer. If the cell expresses the Ag, then the labeled MAb binds and the fluorescent label can be detected. Flow cytometry is based on cells transported under fluidic pressure passing one by one through a laser beam. The forward light scatter, side light scatter, and light emitted from fluorescent labels are detected by photomultiplier tubes. Forward light scatter is related to the size of the cell, and side light scatter is related to the granularity of the cell. When these two parameters are used together in a scattergram (two-parameter histogram), the desired cell population can be electronically selected. This cell population is also evaluated for emission from the labeled MAb. For a single parameter, the frequency of cells versus the intensity of fluorescence (the channel number) is recorded and displayed as a single-parameter histogram. Alternatively, if two parameters are evaluated on the same cell, then a scattergram is generated that diagrams the expression of two Ags simultaneously. By using a panel of MAbs, the cell can be identified and the relative or absolute number of the cell can be determined.

Future Directions for Immunoassays

For many years, immunoassays have occupied an irreplaceable space within the clinical laboratory due to the attributes of this technology. Automated immunoassay analyzers are prevalent and will continue to have a major role in clinical testing. Newer instrumentation has focused on the integration of chemistry and immunochemistry within a single testing platform (e.g., Dimension Vista, Siemens Healthcare Corp.). These instruments have advantages to "stand-alone" chemistry analyzers for testing analytes that require spectrophotometry, electrochemistry, and immunoassays on a single sample.

Aptamers are oligonucleotides that have been designed and engineered to bind to specific analytes and offer an alternative to Abs used in immunoassays.[32] Aptamers may be easier to develop than Abs and may offer some advantages regarding analyte specificity. However, aptamers have not yet been adopted into routine clinical practice.

Advancements in mass spectrometry have begun to challenge immunoassays in a few areas for the measurement of low-molecular-weight analytes including hormones, therapeutic drug monitoring (i.e., immunosuppressants), inborn errors of metabolism, and vitamin D.[33] Liquid chromatography/mass spectrometry (LC-MS) offers the advantages of high analytical sensitivity, freedom from matrix effects, and multi-analyte analysis. However, LC-MS instruments are expensive and require a high degree of operator expertise; therefore, implementation has been limited to larger academic hospitals.

For additional student resources please visit thePoint at **http://thepoint.lww.com.** **thePoint**✷

QUESTIONS

1. The strength of binding between an antigen and antibody is related to the:
   a. Goodness of fit between the epitope and the F(ab)

   b. Concentration of antigen and antibody
   c. Source of antibody production, because monoclonal antibodies bind better
   d. Specificity of the antibody

2. In monoclonal antibody production, the specificity of the antibody is determined by the:
   a. Sensitized B lymphocytes
   b. Myeloma cell line
   c. Sensitized T lymphocytes
   d. Selective growth medium

3. Which unlabeled immune precipitation method in gel is used to quantitate a serum protein?
   a. Radial immunodiffusion
   b. Double diffusion
   c. Counterimmunoelectrophoresis
   d. Immunofixation electrophoresis

4. In immunofixation electrophoresis, discrete bands appear at the same electrophoretic location, one reacted with antihuman IgA (α chain specific) reagent and the other reacted with antihuman λ reagent. This is best described as:
   a. An IgA λ monoclonal protein
   b. An IgA λ polyclonal protein
   c. IgA biclonal proteins
   d. Cross-reactivity

5. In nephelometry, the antigen–antibody complex formation is enhanced in the presence of:
   a. Polyethylene glycol
   b. High-ionic-strength saline solution
   c. Normal saline
   d. Complement

6. Which homogeneous immunoassay relies on inhibiting the activity of the enzyme label when bound to antibody reagent to eliminate separating free-labeled from bound-labeled reagent?
   a. EMIT
   b. CEDIA
   c. MEIA
   d. ELISA

7. In flow cytometry, the side scatter is related to the:
   a. Granularity of the cell
   b. DNA content of the cell
   c. Size of the cell
   d. Number of cells in G_0 and G_1

8. You analyze the DNA content on a sample of breast tissue for suspected malignancy using flow cytometry and get the following results: DI = 2.5 and % cells in S phase = 29%. Based on these results you can conclude:
   a. These results are likely indicative of a malignant breast tumor
   b. This is normal breast tissue
   c. These results are consistent with a mostly diploid population
   d. The results are not consistent with one another; no information is gained

9. The nucleic acid technique in which RNA is converted to cDNA, which is then amplified, is known as:
   a. RT-PCR
   b. PCR
   c. RFLP
   d. In situ hybridization

REFERENCES

1. Berson SA, Yalow RS. Assay of plasma insulin in human subjects by immunological methods. *Nature.* 1959;184:1648-1649.
2. Sheehan C. An overview of antigen–antibody interaction and its detection. In: Sheehan C, ed. *Clinical Immunology: Principles and Laboratory Diagnosis.* 2nd ed. Philadelphia, PA: Lippincott-Raven Publishers; 1997:109.
3. Kohler G, Milstein C. Continuous cultures of fused cells secreting antibody of predefined specificity. *Nature.* 1975;256:495.
4. Ouchterlony O. Antigen–antibody reactions in gel. *Acta Pathol Microbiol Scand.* 1949;26:507.
5. Mancini G, Carbonara AO, Heremans JF. Immunochemical quantitation of antigens by single radial immunodiffusion. *Immunochemistry.* 1965;2:235.
6. Fahey JL, McKelvey EM. Quantitative determination of serum immunoglobulins in antibody-agar plates. *J Immunol.* 1965;98:84.
7. Grabar P, Burtin P. *Immunoelectrophoresis.* Amsterdam: Elsevier; 1964.
8. Alper CC, Johnson AM. Immunofixation electrophoresis: a technique for the study of protein polymorphism. *Vox Sang.* 1969;17:445.
9. Laurell CB. Quantitative estimation of proteins by electrophoresis in agarose gel containing antibodies. *Anal Biochem.* 1966;15:45.
10. Laurell CB. Electroimmunoassay. *Scand J Clin Lab Invest.* 1972;29(Suppl 124):21.
11. Kusnetz J, Mansberg HP. Optical considerations: nephelometry. In: Ritchie RF, ed. *Automated Immunoanalysis. Part 1.* New York, NY: Marcel Dekker; 1978.
12. Engvall E, Perlmann P. Enzyme-linked immunosorbent assay (ELISA). Quantitative assay of immunoglobulin G. Immunochemistry 1971;8:871.
13. Van Weemen BK, Schuurs AHWM. Immunoassay using antigen-enzyme conjugates. *FEBS Lett.* 1971;15:232.
14. Nakamura RM, Bylund DJ. Fluorescence immunoassays. In: Rose NR, deMarcario EC, Folds JD, Lane HC, Nakamura RM, eds. *Manual of Clinical Laboratory Immunology.* 5th ed. Washington, DC: ASM Press; 1997:39.
15. Diamandis EP, Evangelista A, Pollack A, et al. Time-resolved fluoroimmunoassays with europium chelates as labels. *Am Clin Lab.* 1989;8(8):26.
16. Kricka LJ. Chemiluminescent and bioluminescent techniques. *Clin Chem.* 1991;37:1472.
17. Kricka LJ. Selected strategies for improving sensitivity and reliability of immunoassays. *Clin Chem.* 1994;40:347.
18. Bronstein I, Juo RR, Voyta JC. Novel chemiluminescent adamantyl 1,2-dioxetane enzyme substrates. In: Stanley PE, Kricka LJ, eds. *Bioluminescence and Chemiluminescence: Current Status.* Chichester: Wiley; 1991:73.
19. Edwards B, Sparks A, Voyta JC, et al. New chemiluminescent dioxetane enzyme substrates. In: Campbell AK, Kricka LJ,

Stanley PE, eds. *Bioluminescence and Chemiluminescence: Fundamentals and Applied Aspects.* Chichester: Wiley; 1994: 56-59.

20. Kricka L. Human anti-animal antibody interferences in immunological assays. *Clin Chem.* 1999;45:942.

21. Kaplan IV, Levinson SS. When is a heterophile antibody not a heterophile antibody? When it is an antibody against a specific immunogen. *Clin Chem.* 1999;45:616.

22. Butch AW. Dilution protocols for detection of hook effects/prozone phenomenon. *Clin Chem.* 2000;46:1719.

23. Litchfield WJ. Shell-core particles for the turbidimetric immunoassays. In: Ngo TT, ed. *Nonisotopic Immunoassay.* New York, NY: Plenum Press; 1988.

24. Rubenstein KE, Schneider RS, Ullman EF. "Homogeneous" enzyme immunoassay. A new immunochemical technique. *Biochem Biophys Res Commun.* 1972;47:846.

25. Henderson DR, Freidman SB, Harris JD, et al. CEDIA, a new homogeneous immunoassay system. *Clin Chem.* 1986;32:1637.

26. Ullman EF, Schwartzberg M, Rubinstein KD. Fluorescent excitation transfer assay: a general method for determination of antigen. *J Biol Chem.* 1976;251:4172.

27. Dandliker WB, Kelly RJ, Dandiker BJ, et al. Fluorescence polarization immunoassay: theory and experimental methods. *Immunochemistry.* 1973;10:219.

28. Diamandis EP. Immunoassays with time-resolved fluorescence spectroscopy: principles and applications. *Clin Biochem.* 1988; 21:139.

29. Valkirs GE, Barton R. ImmunoConcentration: a new format for solid-phase immunoassays. *Clin Chem.* 1985;31:1427.

30. Rubenstein AS, Hostler RD, White CC, et al. Particle entrapment: application to ICON immunoassay. *Clin Chem.* 1986;32:1072.

31. Harbeck RJ, Teague J, Crossen GR, et al. Novel, rapid optical immunoassay technique for detection of group A streptococci from pharyngeal specimens: comparison with standard culture methods. *J Clin Microbiol.* 1993;31:839.

32. Min K, Cho M, Han S, Shim Y, Ku J, Ban C. A simple and direct electrochemical detection of interferon-gamma using its RNA and DNA aptamers. *Biosens Bioelectron.* 2008;23: 1819.

33. Grebe SKG, Singh RJ. LC-MS/MS in the clinical laboratory—where to from here? *Clin Biochem Rev.* 2011;32:5-31.

Molecular Theory and Techniques

SHASHI MEHTA

CHAPTER 9

CHAPTER OUTLINE

- ◆ NUCLEIC ACID–BASED TECHNIQUES
  Nucleic Acid Chemistry
  Nucleic Acid Extraction
  Hybridization Techniques
  DNA Sequencing
  DNA Chip Technology

  Target Amplification
  Probe Amplification
  Signal Amplification
  Nucleic Acid Probe Applications
- ◆ QUESTIONS
- ◆ REFERENCES

Chapter Objectives

Upon completion of this chapter, the clinical laboratorian should be able to do the following:

- Explain the principles of hybridization.
- State the principle of each of the following methods:
  - DNA sequencing
  - Polymerase chain reaction
  - Transcription-based amplification system

- Southern blot
- In situ hybridization
- Restriction fragment length polymorphism
- Describe the three types of amplification assays and list examples of each type of assay.
- Describe the process of dideoxy sequencing.
- Describe the principle of fluorescence resonance energy transfer as it is used in a real-time polymerase chain reaction assay.

KEY TERMS

Amplicon
Anneal
Branched chain DNA (bDNA)
Deoxyribonucleic acid (DNA)
Dideoxynucleotides
DNA sequencing
Hybridization
In situ hybridization
Ligase chain reaction (LCR)
Messenger RNA (mRNA)

Northern blot
Nucleic acid probe
Nucleic acid sequence–based amplification (NASBA)
Polymerase chain reaction (PCR)
Restriction fragment length polymorphism
Reverse transcriptase–polymerase chain reaction (RT-PCR)
Ribonucleic acid (RNA)
Self-sustained sequence replication
Southern blot
Strand displacement amplification (SDA)
Transcription-mediated amplification (TMA)

Molecular techniques, assays that target nucleic acid instead of protein, are the latest development in clinical laboratory testing. This chapter introduces molecular techniques that at their core consist of the binding of a nucleic acid to its complementary target nucleic acid sequence. The target nucleic acid may or may not be amplified prior to detection and/or quantitation. Thus, nucleic acid–based methods are designed to detect changes at the deoxyribonucleic acid (DNA) or ribonucleic acid (RNA) level rather than to detect a synthesized gene product, such as a protein detected in immunoassays. Molecular techniques used in the clinical laboratory to identify unique nucleic acid sequences include enzymatic cleavage of nucleic acids, gel electrophoresis, enzymatic amplification of target sequences, and hybridization with nucleic acid probes. This chapter reviews the concepts of binding, describes the nature of the reagents used, discusses basic assay design of selected techniques used in the clinical laboratory, and illustrates the importance of single nucleotide polymorphism (SNP) and DNA sequence; as such, it is intended to be an overview rather than an exhaustive review.

NUCLEIC ACID–BASED TECHNIQUES

Molecular testing is a rapidly expanding area in the clinical laboratory. Research laboratories have used these techniques for many years; however, U.S. Food and Drug Administration (FDA)–approved assays for the detection and quantitation of DNA and RNA in clinical samples have only developed within the past 10 to 15 years. Key quality issues to be addressed in any clinical DNA-based assays include sample quality and preparation, sensitivity of reagents to inactivating contaminants, amplification bias and variability, selection of appropriate controls, restriction enzyme efficiency, and reproducibility and cross-contamination of amplification reactions. Nucleic acids store all genetic information and direct the synthesis of specific proteins. By evaluating nucleic acids, insight into cellular changes may be recognized before specific protein products are detectable. Genetically based diseases, presence of infectious organisms, differences between individuals for forensic and transplantation purposes, and altered cell growth regulation are areas that have been investigated using nucleic acid hybridization. The most recent development is the use of molecular arrays (up to 10^5 to 10^6 probes per single array) for high-speed analysis of multiple ligands, analysis of gene expression, and determination of mutations with possible therapeutic implications.

Nucleic Acid Chemistry

DNA stores human genetic information and directs the amino acid sequence of peptides and proteins. It is composed of two strands of nucleotides; each strand is a polymer of deoxyribose molecules linked by strong 3′–5′ phosphodiester bonds that join the 3′ hydroxyl group of one sugar to the 5′ phosphate group of a second sugar. A purine or pyrimidine base is also attached to each sugar. The two strands are arranged in a double helix, with the bases pointing toward the center. The strands are antiparallel, so that the 3′–5′ end of one strand bonds with a strand in the 5′ → 3′ direction. Because the phosphate esters are strong acids and dissociated at neutral pH, the strand has a negative charge that is proportional to its length. The purine bases (adenine [A] and thymine [T]) and the pyrimidine bases (cytosine [C] and guanine [G]) maintain the double helix by forming hydrogen bonds between base pairs as shown in Figure 9-1. Adenine pairs with thymine with two hydrogen bonds and cytosine pairs with guanine with three hydrogen bonds. The strands are complementary due to the fixed manner in which the base pairs bond.

Under physiologic conditions, the helical structure of double-stranded DNA (dsDNA) is stable due to the numerous, although weak, hydrogen bonds between base pairs and the hydrophobic interaction between the bases in the center of the helix. However, the weak

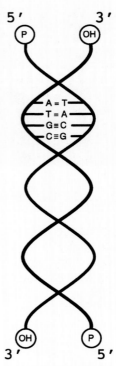

FIGURE 9-1 DNA molecule. The double helix of the DNA is shown along with details of how the bases, sugars, and phosphates connect to form the structure of the molecule. DNA is a double-stranded molecule twisted into a helix (think of a spiral staircase). Each spiraling strand, composed of a sugar–phosphate backbone and attached bases, is connected to a complementary strand by noncovalent hydrogen bonding between paired bases. The bases are adenine (A), thymine (T), cytosine (C), and guanine (G). A and T are connected by two hydrogen bonds. G and C are connected by three hydrogen bonds.

bonds can be broken in vitro by changing environmental conditions; the strands are denatured and separate from each other. Once denatured, the negative charge of each strand causes the strands to repel each other. The two complementary strands can be reassociated or reannealed if the conditions change and favor this process. The renaturation will follow the rules of base pairing so the original DNA molecule is recovered.

RNA is also present in human cells and is chemically similar to DNA. RNA differs from DNA in three ways: (1) ribose replaces deoxyribose as the sugar; (2) uracil replaces thymine as a purine base; and (3) RNA is single stranded. DNA and RNA work together to synthesize proteins. Genomic dsDNA is enzymatically split into its two strands, one of which serves as the template for the synthesis of complementary messenger RNA (mRNA). As mRNA is released from the template DNA, the DNA strands reanneal. The mRNA specifies the amino acid to be added to the peptide chain by transfer RNA, which transports the amino acid to the ribosome, where peptide chain elongates.

This discussion of protein synthesis highlights that physiologically DNA is routinely denatured, binds to RNA, and reanneals to reestablish the original DNA, always following base pair rules. These processes form the foundation of nucleic acid hybridization assays in which complementary strands of nucleic acid from unrelated sources bind together to form a hybrid or *duplex.* Molecular testing in the clinical laboratory consists of two major areas: (1) the use of DNA probes to directly detect or characterize a specific target and (2) the use of nucleic acid amplification technologies to detect or characterize a specific target DNA or RNA. Procedures that use probes include solid-phase assays (capture hybridization and Southern and Northern blotting), solution-based assays (protection assays and hybrid capture assays), and in situ hybridization assays. Amplification procedures include nucleic acid amplification (polymerase chain reaction [PCR], nucleic acid–based sequence amplification, transcription-mediated amplification [TMA], and strand displacement amplification [SDA]), probe amplification (ligase chain reaction [LCR]), and signal amplification (branched chain DNA assay).

Nucleic Acid Extraction

Nucleic acid extraction requires the release of DNA or RNA from the cell followed by its purification and quantitation. Nucleic acid can be extracted from a variety of specimens that include whole blood, serum, plasma, bone marrow, cerebrospinal fluid, urine, cultured cells, amniotic fluid, and paraffin-embedded tissue.[1,2] The extracted DNA or RNA needs to be free of each other and also proteins, lipids, carbohydrates, and other contaminants. A commercial kit–based liquid and solid phase as well as automated methods have been utilized to obtain nucleic acids for hybridization techniques described in this chapter.

In liquid phase, DNA extraction detergent such as sodium dodecyl sulfate liberates DNA and proteins, which are digested by protease or salt precipitated and removed. The lipids and protein remnants can also be removed by organic extraction with phenol and chloroform. The isolated nucleic acid from free nucleus and other cellular contents is then purified by precipitation with cold ethanol. In solid-phase nucleic acid extraction method, DNA is reversibly absorbed onto coated silica either onto filters or magnetic beads at higher ionic strength solutions. The contaminants are washed away in the presence of chaotropic salts and alcohol. The DNA is then eluted by changing to low ionic strength buffer solutions and re-precipitated with cold ethanol. The purpose of these extraction methods is to isolate target nucleic acid, remove inhibitors, and concentrate nucleic acids.

There are commercial QIAamp/DNeasy kits available for extractions of genomic DNA. The buffer formulation is altered in these kits to favor genomic DNA rather than RNA binding (however, some RNA will co-purify unless RNase is added during the procedure). These kits may be directed to samples that have a matrix (e.g., collagen, plant cell wall, and Gram-positive bacterial cell wall), samples that have a membrane but are not embedded within a matrix (cell culture, blood, and *Escherichia coli*), and samples that have neither a matrix nor cell membrane (viruses, extracellular DNA in urine, or cell culture). These kits differ by the proteases included or by the addition of carrier nucleic acid to compensate for low concentrations.

The factors to consider for the nucleic acid extractions are usually the specimen, sample volume needed for hybridization procedures, purity, size of the nucleic acid to be isolated, ease of operation, and potential for high throughput in clinical laboratories. A number of automated workstations for nucleic acid extractions are commercially available. Many of these automated workstations can work with anticoagulated blood, which is fresh or frozen or tissue specimens and isolate DNA or RNA in less than 1 hour. The automated isolation procedures for total RNA in some instances require the addition of genomic DNA binding agent prior to sample loading in the automated workstation.

Hybridization Techniques

A nucleic acid probe is a short strand of DNA or RNA of a known sequence that is well characterized and complementary for the base sequence on the test target. Probes may be fragments of genomic nucleic acids, cloned DNA (or RNA), or synthetic DNA. The genomic nucleic acids are isolated from purified organisms. Some probes are molecularly cloned in a bacterial host. First, the sequence of DNA to be used as the probe must be isolated using bacterial restriction endonucleases to cut the DNA at a specific base sequence. The desired base sequence (the probe) is inserted into a plasmid vector, circular dsDNA. The vector with the insert is incorporated into a host cell, such as *E. coli*, where the vector replicates. The replicated desired base sequence is then isolated and purified. For short DNA segments, an oligonucleotide probe can be synthesized using an automated process; if the amino acid sequence of the protein is known, it is possible to determine the base sequence based on amino acid sequence.

In a hybridization reaction, the probe must be detected. The probe can be labeled directly with a radionuclide (such as ^{32}P), enzyme, or biotin. ^{32}P is detected by autoradiography when the radioactive label exposes x-ray film wherever the probe is located. If the probe is directly labeled with an enzyme, an appropriate substrate must be added to generate a colorimetric, fluorescent, or chemiluminescent product. Biotin-labeled probes can bind to avidin, which is complexed to an enzyme

TABLE 9-1	PROBE TECHNIQUES

UNAMPLIFIED

Southern blot

Northern blot

In situ hybridization

Restriction fragment length polymorphism

TARGET AMPLIFICATION

Polymerase chain reaction

Reverse transcriptase–polymerase chain reaction

Transcription-based amplification systems

   Transcription-mediated amplification

   Nucleic acid sequence–based amplification

   Strand displacement assay

PROBE AMPLIFICATION

Ligase chain reaction

SIGNAL AMPLIFICATION

Branched DNA assay

(e.g., alkaline phosphatase and horseradish peroxidase); the enzyme activity can then be detected. Alternatively, the biotinylated probe can be detected by a labeled avidin antibody reagent.

The probe techniques to be discussed are listed in Table 9-1. Hybridization can take place either in a solid support medium or in solution.

Solid Support Hybridization

Dot-blot and sandwich hybridization assays are the simplest types of solid support hybridization assays.[3] In the dot-blot assay, clinical samples are applied directly to a membrane surface. The membrane is heated to denature or separate DNA strands, and then labeled probes are added. After careful washing to remove any unhybridized probe, the presence of the remaining probe is detected by autoradiography or enzyme assays. A positive result indicates the presence of a specific sequence of interest. This permits qualitative testing of a clinical specimen because it only indicates the presence or absence of a particular genetic sequence. It is much easier to handle multiple samples in this manner.[4] However, there may be difficulty with the interpretation of weak positive reactions because there can be background interference.[3]

Sandwich hybridization is a modification of the dot-blot procedure. It was designed to overcome some of the background problems associated with the use of unpurified samples.[5] The technique uses two probes, one of which is bound to the membrane and serves to capture target sample DNA. The second probe anneals to a different site on the target DNA, and it has a label for detection. The sample nucleic acid is thus sandwiched in between the capture probe on the membrane and the signal-generating probe.[5] Because of the fact that two hybridization events must take place, specificity is increased. Sandwich hybridization assays have been developed using microtiter plates instead of membranes, which has made the procedure more adaptable to automation.[5]

A classic method for DNA analysis, attributed to E. M. Southern, is the Southern blot.[6] In this method, DNA is extracted from a sample using a phenolic reagent and then enzymatically digested using restriction endonucleases to produce DNA fragments. These fragments are then separated by agarose gel electrophoresis. The separated DNA fragments are denatured and transferred to a solid support medium—most commonly, nitrocellulose or a charged nylon membrane. The transfer occurs by the capillary action of a salt solution, transferring DNA to the membrane, or using an electric current to transfer the DNA. When the DNA is on the membrane, a labeled probe is added that binds to the complementary base sequence and appears as a band. In a similar method, the Northern blot, RNA is extracted, digested, electrophoresed, blotted, and finally probed.

Restriction fragment length polymorphism (RFLP) is a technique that evaluates differences in genomic DNA sequences.[7] This technique can help establish identity or nonidentity in forensic or paternity testing or to identify a gene associated with a disease. Genomic DNA is extracted from a sample (e.g., peripheral blood leukocytes) and is purified and quantitated. A restriction endonuclease, which cleaves DNA sequences at a specific site, is added. If there is a mutation or change in the DNA sequence, this may cause the length of the DNA fragment to be different from usual. Southern blotting can be used to identify the different lengths of the DNA fragments. A labeled specific probe could be used to identify a specific aberration. PCR can be used to amplify the target DNA sequence before RFLP analysis.

Solution Hybridization

Hybridization assays can also be performed in a solution phase. In this type of setting, both the target nucleic acid and the probe are free to interact in a reaction mixture, resulting in increased sensitivity compared with that of solid support hybridization. It also requires a smaller amount of sample, although the sensitivity is improved when target DNA is extracted and purified.[8]

For solution hybridizations, the probe must be single stranded and incapable of self-annealing.[4] Several unique detection methods exist. In one of these, an S1 nuclease is added to the reaction mix. This will only digest unannealed or single-stranded DNA, leaving the hybrids intact. dsDNA can then be recovered by precipitation with trichloroacetic acid or by binding it to hydroxyapatite columns.[4,9]

A second and less technically difficult means of solution hybridization is the hybridization protection assay. For this assay, a chemiluminescent acridinium ester is attached to a probe. After the hybridization reaction takes place, the solution is subjected to alkaline hydrolysis, which hydrolyzes the chemiluminescent ester if the probe is not attached to the target molecule. If the probe is attached to the target DNA, the ester is protected from hydrolysis. Probes that remain bound to a specific target sequence give off light when exposed to a chemical trigger such as hydrogen peroxide at the end of the assay.

Digene's Hybrid Capture 2 (Digene Corp., Gaithersburg, MD) assay for the detection of human papilloma virus (HPV) is a solution phase hybridization assay that uses an antibody specific for DNA/RNA hybrids to "capture" and detect the hybrids that are formed during the solution hybridization of HPV DNA in the sample with an unlabeled RNA probe.

Solution phase hybridization assays are fairly adaptable to automation, especially those using chemiluminescent labels. Assays can be performed in a few hours.[4] However, low positive reactions are difficult to interpret because of the possibility of cross-reacting target molecules.[10]

In situ hybridization is performed on cells, tissue, or chromosomes that are fixed on a microscope slide.[11] After the DNA is heat denatured, a labeled probe is added and will hybridize the target sequence after the slide is cooled. Colorimetric or fluorescent products are generally used. One strength of this method is the morphologic context in which the localization of target DNA is viewed.

DNA Sequencing

DNA sequencing is considered the "gold standard" for many molecular applications from mutation detection to genotyping, but it requires proper methodology and interpretation to prevent misinterpretation. The sequence should be analyzed on both DNA strands to provide even greater accuracy. Patient sequences are compared with known reference sequences to detect mutations. Most sequencing strategies include PCR amplification as the first step to amplify the region of interest to be sequenced. The sequencing reaction itself is based on the dideoxy chain termination reaction developed by Sanger and colleagues in 1977.[12] This reaction generates fragments of newly synthesized DNA, which upon incorporation of one of four dideoxynucleotides halts synthesis of the new DNA. The fragments are of varying lengths due to incorporation of the dideoxynucleotides. These nucleotides lack the 3'- and 2'-hydroxyl (OH) group on the pentose ring, and because DNA chain elongation requires the addition of deoxynucleotides to the 3'-OH group, incorporation of the dideoxynucleotide terminates chain length. Varying lengths of DNA

are synthesized, all with a dideoxynucleotide at the end. The reaction mixture is then run on a gel, separating the various DNA fragments by size, and the sequence is read directly from the gel. The most commonly used form of this sequencing method in the clinical laboratory uses "cycle sequencing," which is similar to a PCR in that the steps involved include denaturation, annealing of a primer, chain extension, and termination by varying the temperature of the reaction. The newly generated fragments are tagged with a fluorescent dye and separated, based upon size, by denaturing gel or capillary electrophoresis and detected by fluorescence detectors as the fragments pass through the detector. Using this automated method with capillary electrophoresis, about 600 base pairs can be sequenced in a 2½-hour period (Fig. 9-2). DNA sequencing is most commonly used to detect mutations. For example, in infectious disease, testing such as sequencing of the human immunodeficiency virus (HIV) for drug resistance and of the hepatitis C virus (HCV) is used to establish appropriate therapy and treatment decisions.

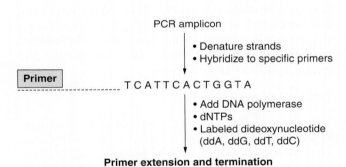

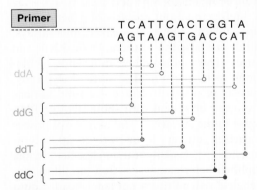

FIGURE 9-2 Sanger dideoxy DNA sequencing. The region of interest is first amplified using polymerase chain reaction. Sequence-specific primers then hybridize with the denatured amplicons, followed by extension of the new strand by DNA polymerase. At various points in the DNA extension, a dideoxy base (ddA, ddG, ddT, or ddC) is incorporated, which stops further extension of DNA. This results in a mixture of newly synthesized products of various lengths. Each dideoxy terminator base is labeled with a specific fluorescent tag, which can be detected with a fluorescent detector. The fragments are separated based upon their size, and fluorescence is read on each strand, resulting in the sequence of the DNA.

Pyrosequencing[1,2] is a relatively new technique for a short to moderate sequence analysis that is based on the release of pyrophosphate during DNA synthesis as each dNTP (deoxyribonucleotide triphosphate) is incorporated with elongation of DNA. In this method, after primer annealing to template strand and with subsequent addition of the complementary dNTPs toward the 3′-end by DNA polymerase, PPi (pyrophosphate) is released as the nucleotide forms a phosphodiester bond with the primer. Sulfurylase and its substrate adenosine 5′-phosphosulfate then convert PPi to ATP, which subsequently transforms luciferin to oxyluciferin by luciferase. This conversion of oxyluciferin generates a luminescent signal proportional to the amount of ATP. The light signal is detected by a charge-coupled device and seen as a peak in a pyrogram. The number of nucleotides incorporated is proportional to the height of each peak observed. Apyrase degrades unincorporated nucleotides and ATP. When degradation is completed, another nucleotide is added. As the complementary DNA (cDNA) is synthesized, the nucleotide sequence is determined from the signal peaks in real time by built-in computer software. The technique does not require gel electrophoretic separation of ddNTPs (dideoxyribonucleoside triphosphate), DNA fragments, and radioactive or fluorescent labels. The pyrosequencing technique is useful for the detection of SNP and has been applied in the diagnosis of infectious diseases and human leukocyte antigen typing.

DNA Chip Technology

Previously, genetic studies examined individual gene expression by Northern blotting or polymorphisms by gel-based restriction digests and sequence analysis, but with advances in microchips and bead-based array technologies, high-throughput analysis of genetic variation is now possible. Biochips, also called microarrays, are very small devices used to examine DNA, RNA, and other substances. These chips allow thousands of biological reactions to be performed at once.[13] Typically, a biochip consists of a small rectangular solid surface that is made of glass or silicon with short DNA or RNA probes anchored to the surface.[14] The number of probes on a biochip surface can vary from 10 to 20 up to hundreds of thousands.[13,14] Usually, the nucleic acid in the sample is amplified before analysis. After amplification, the sample, labeled with a fluorescent tag, is loaded onto the chip. Hybridization occurs on the surface of the chip, allowing thousands of hybridization reactions to occur at one time. Unbound strands of the target sample are then washed away. The fluorescent tagged hybridized samples are detected using a fluorescent detector.[13] The intensity of the fluorescent signal at a particular location is proportional to the sequence homology at a particular locus. Complete sequence matches result in bright fluorescence, while single-base mismatches result in a dimmer signal,

indicative of a point mutation. Because most SNPs are silent and have no apparent functional consequence, the challenge is to identify the set of SNPs that are directly related to or cause disease. Detection of point mutations can be used for classification of leukemias, molecular staging of tumors, and characterization of microbial agents.[15] One prime example is the determination of genes associated with drug resistance in HIV testing. Identification of such genes guides the physician in selecting a proper drug regimen for a particular patient.

Currently, Affymetrix, Inc. has developed GeneChips, proprietary, high-density microarrays that contain 10,000 to 400,000 different short DNA probes on a 1.2 cm × 1.2 cm glass wafer. GeneChips are available for HIV-1 genotyping,[15] human p53 tumor suppressor gene mutation analysis, and human cytochrome p450 gene mutation analysis, with other GeneChips currently under development.

Target Amplification

Target amplification systems are in vitro methods for the enzymatic replication of a target molecule to levels at which it can be readily detected.[8] This allows the target sequence to be identified and further characterized. There are numerous different types of target amplification. Examples include PCR, TMA, SDA, and nucleic acid sequence–based amplification (NASBA). Of these, PCR (Table 9-1) is by far the best known and most widely used technique in clinical laboratories.[16] However, the other non-PCR methods have become more popular in recent years.

The PCR, developed by K. B. Mullis of Cetus Company,[17,18] is an amplified hybridization technique that enzymatically synthesizes millions of identical copies of the target DNA to increase the analytic sensitivity. The test reaction mixture (Table 9-2) includes the test DNA sample (lysed cells or tissue enzymatically digested with RNase and proteinase and then extracted),

TABLE 9-2	REAL-TIME POLYMERASE CHAIN REACTION COMPONENTS
Taq POLYMERASE	
Primers	
Probe are used in real-time PCR master mix solutions	
Magnesium salts	
Nucleic acid bases	
Buffers, other salts, additives, water	
DNA or RNA template	
Reverse transcriptase if RNA template is used	

PCR, polymerase chain reaction.

TABLE 9-3	**PRIMERS**

A single-stranded DNA or RNA that can hybridize to a single-stranded template DNA and provide a free 3′-hydroxyl end to which DNA polymerase can add deoxynucleotides to synthesize a chain of DNA complementary to the template DNA

They are short nucleic acid sequences, one forward, one reverse that functions as a starting point for addition of nucleotides

Sequences are complementary to target regions

Target regions are typically 60–200 bases apart

T_m of the primers are 58–60°C (lower than the probe so they anneal after the probe anneals)

They "prime" DNA synthesis by *Taq* polymerase during polymerase chain reaction

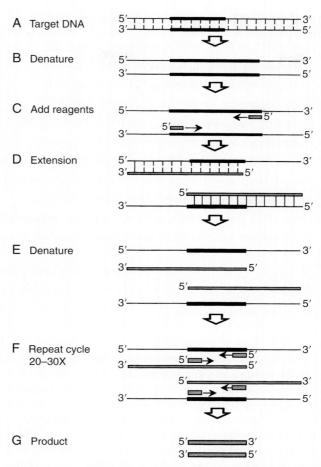

FIGURE 9-3 Polymerase chain reaction. **(A)** Target DNA sequence is indicated by the *bold line*. **(B)** Double-stranded DNA is denatured (separated) by heating. **(C)** Reagents are added, and the primer binds to the target DNA sequence. **(D)** Polymerase extends the primers. **(E–G)** Heating, annealing of the primer, and extension are repeated.

oligonucleotide primers (Table 9-3), thermostable DNA polymerase (e.g., *Taq* polymerase, from *Thermus aquaticus*), and nucleotide triphosphates (ATP, GTP, CTP, and TTP) in a buffer. The process, shown in Figure 9-3, begins by heating the target DNA to denature it and then separating the strands. Two oligonucleotide primers (probes) that recognize the edges of the target DNA are added and anneal to the target DNA. Thermostable DNA polymerase and nucleotide triphosphates extend the primer. The process of heat denaturation, cooling to allow the primers to anneal and heating again to extend the primers, is repeated manyfold (15 to 30 times or more). PCR is an exponential amplification reaction in which after n cycles, there is $(1 + x)^n$ times as much target as was present initially, where x is the mean efficiency of the reaction for each cycle. Theoretically, as few as 20 cycles would yield approximately 1 million times the amount of target DNA initially present. However, in reality, the theoretical maxima are never reached and more cycles are necessary to achieve such levels of amplification. The amplified target DNA sequences, known as amplicons, can be analyzed by gel electrophoresis, Southern blot, sequencing, or directly labeled probes.

When the target is microbial RNA or mRNA, the RNA must be enzymatically converted to DNA by reverse transcriptase; the product, cDNA, can then be analyzed by PCR. This method is referred to a reverse transcriptase–polymerase chain reaction (RT-PCR). Initially, PCR was a qualitative assay, but assays have been developed that allowed for quantitation of amplicons. Quantitative RT-PCR is used to measure viral loads in HIV- and HCV-infected patients. These numbers allow physicians to determine disease status and evaluate efficacy of antiviral treatments.

The latest PCR innovation is the development of "real-time" RT-PCR, which allows for direct measurement of amplicon accumulation during the exponential phase of the reaction. Two important findings led to the discovery of real-time PCR: (1) finding that the *Taq* polymerase (Table 9-4) possesses 5′ → 3′-exonuclease activity[19,20] and (2) the construction of dual-labeled oligonucleotide probes that emit a fluorescence signal only on cleavage, based on the

TABLE 9-4	***Taq* POLYMERASE**

Is a thermostable enzyme

5′–3′ polymerase activity

Some modified versions must be heat activated (usually 5–10 min) to eliminate false priming at start of PCR

Magnesium salts are needed for polymerase and nuclease activities of *Taq* polymerase. Higher Mg concentrations increase nuclease activity (5–9 mM) and must be optimized in real-time PCRs

PCR, polymerase chain reaction.

TABLE 9-5	PROBES
It is a defined RNA or DNA fragment, usually 20–35 bases long	
Reporter dye at 5′-end, e.g., FAM™, TET™, TAMRA™	
Quencher dye is at 3′-end, e.g., TAMRA™, QSY7™	
3′-End blocked to prevent extension during PCR	
T_m is 10°C above the primers, so the probe anneals first	
Reporter dye and quencher dye are in close proximity in the intact probe	
Energy from the reporter dye is transferred to quencher dye	
There is suppression of reporter fluorescence with an intact probe	
Probe sequence is complementary to target sequence	
During PCR, if the target is present, the probe specifically anneals before the primers anneal	
5′–3′ nuclease activity of *Taq* polymerase cleaves the annealed probe into fragments, which are displaced from the target	
The reporter dye is no longer in close proximity to quencher dye; fluorescence not suppressed	
Fluorescence is then emitted by reporter dye and increases with each PCR cycle	

PCR, polymerase chain reaction.

principle of *fluorescence resonance energy transfer (FRET)*.[21] FRET involves the nonradioactive transfer of energy from a donor molecule to an acceptor molecule. Probe-based (Table 9-5) systems, such as TaqMan probes,[22] molecular beacons,[23] and scorpion primers,[24] rely on the close proximity of donor fluorophores and nonfluorophore acceptor molecules (quenchers) in the unhybridized probe, so that little or no signal is generated as the fluorescence of the donor is quenched by the acceptor. Upon hybridization to the target, the fluorophore and quencher become separated through either conformational changes (molecular beacons

and scorpion primers) or enzymatic cleavage of the fluorophore from the quencher as a result of the 5′ to 3′-nuclease activity of *Taq* polymerase. Real-time detection occurs when the fluorescence emission of the reporter probe (driven by the accumulation of amplicons) is monitored cycle by cycle. The results are available immediately and, more importantly, there is no manipulation of the postamplification sample, reducing the chance of contaminating other samples with amplified products. A typical post RT-PCR sigmoidal curve is demonstrated in Figure 9-4. The threshold cycle (C_T) is defined as the value at which

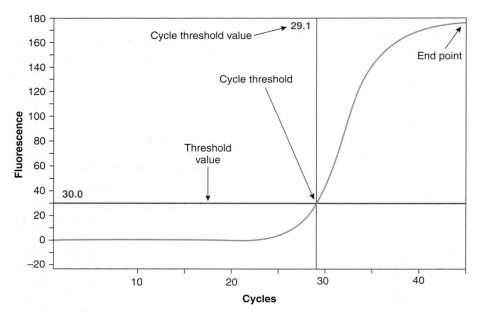

FIGURE 9-4 The plot of fluorescence observed in real time (*x*-axis) and numbers of cycles completed (*y*-axis). The graph demonstrates a typical polymerase chain reaction run analysis.

the sample fluorescence crosses the threshold. A standard chart of the target copy number against C_T can provide a reference plot for quantitation of the unknown target in samples.

PCR is limited by expense, the need for special thermocyclers, potential aerosol contamination from one sample to another, nonspecific annealing, and degree of stringency. Stringency is related to the stability of the bonding between target DNA or RNA and the probe and is based on the degree of match and the length of the probe. Stability of the duplex is strongly influenced by temperature, pH, and ionic strength of the hybridization solution. Under low stringency conditions (low temperature or increased ionic strength), imperfect binding occurs.

Additionally, DNA melt curve analysis has been extremely useful. DNA melting temperature (T_m) is defined as the temperature at which 50% of the DNA is double stranded and 50% is single stranded. Each PCR product or amplicon has its own specific melting temperature and is determined by its G-C content, the number of base pair mismatches, and the ionic strength of the solution. T_m can be used (1) to determine the purity of amplification product, (2) to identify amplification products, and (3) to optimize the assay annealing temperature. The melting curve analysis is accomplished by slowly raising the temperature at the end of the PCR run followed by the continuous fluorescence measurements at 2°C increments.[1,25]

Transcription-Based Amplification

Other techniques have evolved to overcome some of these shortcomings, to standardize methods for use in clinical laboratories, or to provide new proprietary approaches. Amplification of the target, probe, and signal has been described. The classic target amplification method, PCR, increases the number of target nucleic acids so that simple signal detection systems can be used. Another target amplification method is self-sustained sequence replication or *transcription-based amplification system (TAS)*, which detects target RNA and involves continuous isothermic cycles of reverse transcription.[26,27] The first non-PCR nucleic acid amplification method developed was a TAS by Kwoh et al. in 1989 that amplified an RNA target.[28] The principle of the reaction was a two-step process that involved generation of cDNA from the target RNA followed by reverse transcription of the cDNA template into multiple copies of RNA. Multiple cycles result in amplification of the target (Fig. 9-5). From this

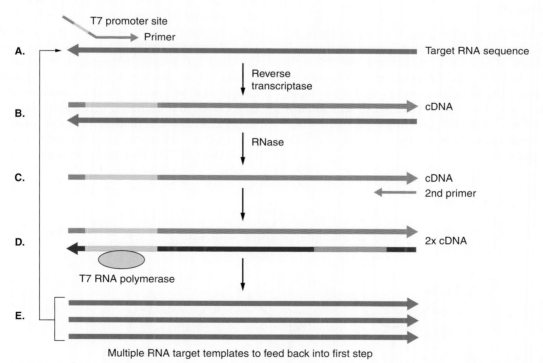

FIGURE 9-5 Transcription-based amplification systems. Non–polymerase chain reaction (PCR) method of amplifying RNA targets. Nucleic acid sequence–based amplification (NASBA) and transcription-mediated amplification (TMA) are based upon this methodology; NASBA uses three enzymes (reverse transcriptase, RNase H, and T7 DNA-dependent RNA polymerase), while TMA only uses RNA polymerase and a reverse transcriptase with inherent RNase H activity. Initial steps in the procedure involve generation of complementary DNAs (cDNAs) from the target RNA using primers (which incorporate a T7 RNA polymerase binding site) **(A and B)**. RNase H then destroys the initial strands of target RNA from the RNA cDNA hybrids **(C)**. The cDNA then serves as template for the generation of double-stranded cDNA, with one strand (containing the T7 binding site) serving as the template for reverse transcription and synthesis of multiple copies of RNA using the T7 RNA polymerase **(D)**. The RNAs then serve as templates for more cDNA templates to be made, and the cycles continue **(E)**.

system, two other non-PCR target amplification methods have been developed that are currently used in clinical assays: NASBA and TMA. The advantages of these two methods are that they are both isothermal reactions that do not require the use of a thermal cycler.

SDA was originally developed and patented by Becton Dickinson, Inc. (Franklin Lakes, NJ) in 1991.[29,30] One set of primers incorporates a specific restriction enzyme site that is later attacked by an endonuclease. The resulting "nick" created in only one strand by the restriction enzyme allows for displacement of the amplified strands that then, in turn, serve as targets for further amplification and nick digestion. A modified deoxynucleotide (dATPαS; one of the oxygen molecules in the triphosphate moiety has been replaced with sulfur) is used to synthesize a double-stranded, hemiphosphorothioated DNA recognition site for the restriction enzyme cleavage that allows only single-strand nicking of the unmodified strand instead of cutting through both strands. Becton Dickinson currently markets this methodology under the label BD ProbeTec, and it is FDA approved for the detection of *Legionella pneumophila*, with a combination kit for *Chlamydia trachomatis* and *Neisseria gonorrhoeae*.[31]

Probe Amplification

Rather than directly amplifying the target, there are several techniques that amplify the detection molecule or probe itself. The LCR is an example of this technique. The LCR is a probe amplification technique that uses two pairs of labeled probes that are complementary for two, short-target DNA sequences in close proximity.[32] After hybridization, the DNA ligase interprets the break between the ends as a nick and links the probe pairs.

Signal Amplification

Signal amplification methods are designed to increase the signal strength by increasing the concentration of the label. This technique uses multiple probes and several simultaneous hybridization steps. It has been compared to decorating a Christmas tree, and it involves several sandwich hybridizations. In the first step, target-specific oligonucleotide probes capture the target sequence to a solid support. Then a second set of target-specific probes called extenders hybridize to adjoining sequences and act as binding sites for a large piece called the branched amplification multimer. Each branch of the amplification multimer has multiple side branches capable of binding numerous (up to 10,000) enzyme-labeled oligonucleotides onto each target molecule (Fig. 9-6). Perhaps the best known of the signal amplification systems is the branched chain signal amplification (bDNA) system originally developed by Chiron Corporation and now sold through Siemens Healthcare Diagnostics (Tarrytown, NJ).[33] The most recent bDNA system has high specificity and can provide quantitative detection over a range of several orders of magnitude (10^2 to 10^5 copies/mL).[34,5] Branched chain systems are well suited for the detection of nucleic acid target with sequence heterogeneity, such as HCV and HIV, because if one or two of the capture or extender probes fail to hybridize, the signal-generating capacity is not lost as a result of the presence of several remaining probe complexes. Additionally, the need for several independent probe-target hybridization events provides a great deal of specificity. The danger of false-positive results caused by carryover of target material is decreased because the target itself is not amplified. However, nonspecific localization of reagents can result in background amplification.[5] Assays for hepatitis B virus, HCV, HIV-1, and cytomegalovirus have been

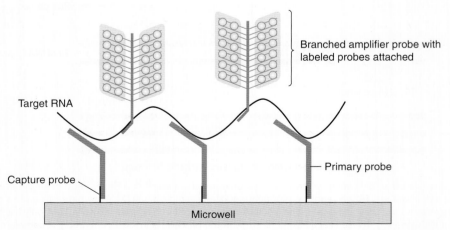

FIGURE 9-6 Branched chain amplification. Several different probes are used to amplify the signal rather than the target DNA itself. The first probe captures the target. Amplifier 1 binds in a different place and forms the base for amplifier 2, the branched chain. Amplifier 3 contains the signal.

developed using this method.[34] This system is also used to quantitate HIV-1 with a lower limit of detection at 75 copies/mL.[31] It has been validated for the quantitation of viral load testing of all the subtypes. Therefore, this technique can be used for quantitation and to help monitor the therapeutic response.

Nucleic Acid Probe Applications

Nucleic acid probes are used to detect infectious organisms; to detect gene rearrangements, chromosomal translocations, or chromosomal breakage; to detect changes in oncogenes and tumor suppressor factors; to aid in prenatal diagnosis of an inherited disease or carrier status; to identify polymorphic markers used to establish identity or nonidentity; and to aid in donor selection. Nucleic acid probes are useful in identifying microorganisms in a patient specimen or confirming an organism isolated in culture. Probes are currently available to confirm *Mycobacterium* sp., *Legionella* sp., *Salmonella*, diarrheogenic *E. coli* strains, *Shigella,* and *Campylobacter* sp. Probes also are available to identify fungi such as *Blastomyces dermatitidis, Coccidioides immitis, Cryptococcus neoformans,* and *Histoplasma capsulatum.* Direct identification of microorganisms in patient specimens includes *Chlamydia trachomatis, N. gonorrhoeae,* cytomegalovirus, Epstein-Barr virus, and herpes simplex virus. In addition, viral load testing for HIV and HCV is detected using probe technology. Detection of multidrug-resistant strains of *Mycobacterium tuberculosis* may lead to more timely public health control measures. Identification of genes for antimicrobial resistance in other organisms will help in more effective treatment for severe infections.[35] HCV genotyping and pretreatment viral load testing in newly diagnosed infections provide the physician with valuable information to determine therapy regimens.[36] HIV viral load testing can play a role in the diagnosis of HIV in neonates born to HIV-infected mothers as well as in the diagnosis of acute HIV infections, which are defined as the period after exposure to the virus but before seroconversion.[37]

Gene rearrangement studies by Southern blot are helpful to distinguish between T- and B-lymphocyte lineage.[38] Also, the chromosome translocation associated with most follicular, non-Hodgkin's lymphomas and certain diffuse, large-cell lymphomas has been detected and monitored. The Philadelphia chromosome in chronic myelogenous leukemia is associated with the translocation that results in the detection of the *bcr/abl* fusion gene.[39] Other mutations associated with hematologic and solid tumors are being described daily.

Prenatal diagnosis of genetic diseases such as sickle cell anemia, cystic fibrosis,[40] Huntington's chorea,[41] Duchenne-type muscular dystrophy,[42] and von Willebrand's disease[43] has been made possible using probe technology. In addition, the carrier status in Duchenne-type muscular dystrophy and von Willebrand's disease can be determined.

PCR has been used to detect major histocompatibility complex class I and class II polymorphism.[44] The increased accuracy of detecting differences in the genes, rather than the gene product, has been used to improve transplant compatibility.

For additional student resources please visit thePoint at **http://thepoint.lww.com.** **thePoint** ⁎

QUESTIONS

1. True or False? Molecular arrays typically contain a single probe for high-throughput analysis of gene expression or determination of mutations in patient samples.

2. Which of the following is LEAST likely to affect the purification of genomic DNA for analysis in molecular methods?
   a. Sample volume required for hybridization
   b. Size of the nucleic acid to be isolated
   c. Presence of RNA in the sample
   d. Presence of protein in the sample
   e. Presence of deoxyribose

3. Why is it important to add RNase to the patient sample when isolating genomic DNA?

   a. RNase serves as an enzymatic tag on DNA probes.
   b. RNase will remove excess collagen from the patient sample.
   c. RNase will transport the amino acid to the ribosome, where the peptide chain elongates.
   d. RNase clones DNA to RNA.
   e. RNase digests RNA in the patient sample that could co-purify with genomic DNA.

4. All of the following describe a nucleic acid probe except:
   a. Short strand of DNA of a known sequence
   b. Short strand of RNA of a known sequence
   c. Can be cloned in bacteria

   d. Can be inserted into a plasmid vector

   e. Can be labeled with avidin

5. Of the following, which is a common example of solid support hybridization?
   a. Southern blot
   b. Chemiluminescence
   c. Hybridization protection assay
   d. Digene's Hybrid Capture 2
   e. In situ hybridization

6. When sequencing DNA, _____ stops DNA synthesis in polymerase chain reaction amplification.
   a. Dideoxynucleotides
   b. DNA polymerase
   c. Insertion of thymine
   d. 3′-OH group
   e. Pyrophosphates

7. One of the most common clinical applications for identifying SNPs in patients is:
   a. SNPs have been useful in optimizing the treatment of HIV.
   b. SNPs have been useful in diagnosing metabolic syndrome.
   c. SNPs have been used to facilitate transcription-mediated amplification.
   d. Currently, there are no clinical applications for the identification of SNPs as these are silent and have no apparent function.
   e. SNPs are added to the patient sample during polymerase amplification reactions to create the complimentary nucleic acid sequence.

8. The development of "real-time" PCR was driven by:
   a. Learning that Taq polymerase that has 5′- to 3′-exonuclease activity.
   b. The development of a dot-blot hybridization methods.
   c. The development of chain ligase reaction.
   d. The ability to volatilize a sample in a nebulizer.
   e. The development of scorpion primers.

REFERENCES

1. Buckingham L. *Molecular Diagnostics: Fundamentals, Methods and Clinical Applications.* 2nd ed. Philadelphia, PA: F. A. Davis and Company; 2012.
2. Ronaghi M. Pyrosequencing sheds light on DNA sequencing. *Genome Res.* 2001;11:3-11.
3. Parslow TG. Molecular genetic techniques for clinical analysis of the immune system. In: Stites DP, Terr AI, Parslow TG, eds. *Medical Immunology.* 9th ed. Stamford, CT: Appleton & Lange; 1997:309-318.
4. Podzorski RP. Molecular methods. In: Detrick B, Hamilton RG, Folds JD, et al., eds. *Manual of Molecular and Clinical Laboratory Immunology.* 7th ed. Washington, DC: American Society for Microbiology; 2006:26-52.
5. Lo DYM, Chiu RWK. Principles of molecular biology. In: Burtis CA, Ashwood ER, Bruns DE, eds. *Tietz Textbook of Clinical Chemistry and Molecular Diagnostics.* 4th ed. St. Louis, MO: Elsevier Saunders; 2006:1393-1406.
6. Southern EM. Detection of specific sequences among DNA fragments separated by gel electrophoresis. *J Mol Biol.* 1975;98:503.
7. Saiki RK, Scharf S, Faloona F, et al. Enzymatic amplification of beta-globulin genomic sequences and restriction site analysis for diagnosis of sickle cell anemia. *Science.* 1985;230:1350-1354.
8. Tenover FC, Unger ER. Nucleic acid probes for detection and identification of infectious agents. In: Persing DH, Smith TF, Tenover FC, et al., eds. *Diagnostic Molecular Microbiology: Principles and Applications.* Washington, DC: American Society for Microbiology; 1993:3-25.
9. Hansen CA. Clinical applications of molecular biology in diagnostic hematology. *Lab Med.* 1993;24:562.
10. Unger ER, Piper MA. Molecular diagnostics: basic principles and techniques. In: Henry JB, ed. *Clinical Diagnosis and Management by Laboratory Methods.* 20th ed. Philadelphia, PA: WB Saunders; 2001:1275-1295.
11. Hankin RC. In situ hybridization: principles and applications. *Lab Med.* 1992;23:764.
12. Sanger F, Nicklen S, Coulson AR. DNA sequencing with chain terminating inhibitors. *Proc Natl Acad Sci U S A.* 1977;74:5463.
13. Friedrich MJ. New chip on the block. *Lab Med.* 1996;30:180.
14. Check W. Clinical microbiology eyes nucleic acid-based technologies. *ASM News.* 1998;64:84.
15. Vahey M, Nau ME, Barrick S, et al. Performance of the Affymetrix GeneChip HIV PRT 440 platform for antiretroviral drug resistance genotyping of human immunodeficiency virus type 1 clades and viral isolates with length polymorphisms. *J Clin Microbiol.* 1999; 37:2533.
16. Forbes BA, Sahm DF, Weissfeld AS. *Bailey and Scott's Diagnostic Microbiology.* 10th ed. St. Louis, MO: Mosby; 1998:188-207.
17. Mullis KB, Faloona FA. Specific synthesis of DNA in vitro via a polymerase-catalyzed chain reaction. *Methods Enzymol.* 1987;155:335.
18. Mullis KB. The unusual origin of the polymerase chain reaction. *Sci Am.* 1990;262:56.
19. Foy CA, Parkes HC. Emerging homogenous DNA-based technologies in the clinical laboratory. *Clin Chem.* 2001;47:990.
20. Holland PA, Abramson RD, Watson R, Gelfand DH. Detection of specific polymerase chain reaction by utilizing the 5′ to 3′ exonuclease activity of *Thermus aquaticus* DNA polymerase. *Proc Natl Acad Sci U S A.* 1991;88:7276.
21. Szollosi J, Damjanovich S, Matyus L. Application of fluorescence resonance energy transfer in the clinical laboratory: routine and research. *Cytometry.* 1998;15:159.
22. Livak K, Flood S, Marmaro J, et al. Oligonucleotides with fluorescent dyes at opposite ends provide a quenched probe system useful for detecting PCR product and nucleic acid hybridization. *PCR Methods Appl.* 1995;4:357.
23. Tyagi S, Kramer F. Molecular beacons: probes that fluoresce upon hybridization. *Nat Biotechnol.* 1996;14:303.
24. Whicombe D, Theaker J, Guy S, et al. Detection of PCR products using self-probing amplicons and fluorescence. *Nat Biotechnol.* 1999;17:804.
25. Coleman WB, Tsongalis GJ. *Molecular Diagnostics for the Clinical Laboratorian.* 2nd ed. Totowa, NJ: Humana Press; 2006.

26. Guatelli JC, Whitfield KM, Kwoh DY, et al. Isothermal in vitro amplification of nucleic acids by a multienzyme reaction modeled after retroviral replication. *Proc Natl Acad Sci U S A.* 1990;87:1874.

27. Fahy E, Kwoh DY, Gingeras TR. Self-sustained sequence replication (3SR): an isothermal transcription-based amplification system alternative to PCR. *PCR Methods Appl.* 1991;1:25.

28. Kwoh DY, Davis GR, Whitfield KM, et al. Transcription-based amplification system and detection of amplified human immunodeficiency virus type 1 with a bead-based sandwich hybridization format. *Proc Natl Acad Sci U S A.* 1989;86:1173-1177.

29. Little MC, Andrews J, Moore R, et al. Strand displacement amplification and homogenous real-time detection incorporated in a second-generation DNA probe system, BDProbe TecET. *Clin Chem.* 1999;45:777-784.

30. Walker G, Fraiser M, Schram J, et al. Strand displacement amplification: an isothermal in vitro DNA amplification technique. *Nucleic Acid Res.* 1992;20:1691-1696.

31. BD ProbeTec™ ET System. http://www.bd.com/ds/productCenter/MD-ProbetecEt.asp. Accessed July 31, 2012.

32. Barany F. Genetic disease detection and DNA amplification using cloned thermostable ligase. *Proc Natl Acad Sci U S A.* 1991;88:189.

33. Wiedbrauk DL. Molecular methods for virus detection. *Lab Med.* 1992;23:737.

34. Persing DH. In vitro nucleic acid amplification techniques. In: Persing DH, Smith TF, Tenover FC, et al., eds. *Diagnostic Molecular Microbiology: Principles and Applications.* Washington, DC: American Society for Microbiology; 1993:51-87.

35. Mitchell PS, Persing DH. Current trends in molecular microbiology. *Lab Med.* 1999;30:263.

36. Zein NN. Clinical significance of hepatitis C virus genotypes. *Clin Microbiol Rev.* 2000;13:223-235.

37. Ferreira-Gonzalez A, Versalovic J, Habecbu S, Caliendo AM. Molecular methods in diagnosis and monitoring of infectious diseases. In: Bruns DE, Ashwood ER, Burtis CA, eds. *Fundamentals of Molecular Diagnostics.* St. Louis, MO: Saunders Elsevier; 2007:171-196.

38. Farkas DH. The Southern blot: application to the B- and T-cell gene rearrangement test. *Lab Med.* 1992;23:723.

39. Ni H, Blajchman MA. Understanding the polymerase chain reaction. *Transfus Med Rev.* 1994;8:242.

40. Gasparini P, Novelli G, Savoia A, et al. First-trimester prenatal diagnosis of cystic fibrosis using the polymerase chain reaction: report of eight cases. *Prenat Diagn.* 1989;9:349.

41. Thies U, Zuhlke C, Bockel B, et al. Prenatal diagnosis of Huntington's disease (HD): experience with six cases and PCR. *Prenat Diagn.* 1992;12:1055.

42. Clemens PR, Fenwick RG, Chamberlain JS, et al. Carrier detection and prenatal diagnosis in Duchenne and Becker muscular dystrophy families, using dinucleotide repeat polymorphism. *Am J Hum Genet.* 1991;49:951.

43. Peake IR, Bowen D, Bignell P. Family studies and prenatal diagnosis in severe von Willebrand disease by polymerase chain reaction amplification of variable number tandem repeat region of the von Willebrand factor gene. *Blood.* 1990;76:555.

44. Erlich H, Tugawan T, Begovich AB, et al. HLA-DR, DQ, and DP typing using PCR amplification and immobilized probes. *Eur J Immunogenet.* 1991;18:33.

Point-of-Care Testing

JANETTA BRYKSIN, CORINNE R. FANTZ

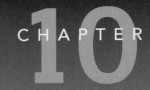

CHAPTER 10

CHAPTER OUTLINE

Chapter Objectives

Upon completion of this chapter, the clinical laboratorian should be able to do the following:

• Define point-of-care testing (POCT).
• Explain what basic structure is required to manage a POCT program.

• Explain the nuts and bolts process of implementing a POC test.
• State the basic principles behind common POC applications.

KEY TERMS

Connectivity
High-complexity test
Moderately complex test

Point-of-care testing (POCT)
Standardization
Waived tests

INTRODUCTION

Point-of-care testing (POCT) is defined as "those analytical patient-testing activities provided within the institution, but performed outside the physical facilities of the clinical laboratories."[1] POCT is also known by many names including "near-patient testing,"[2] "extra-laboratory analyses,"[3] "ancillary testing," "bedside testing,"[4] "physician's office testing,"[5] and "alternative site testing." A convenience for the patient and physician, POCT brings the laboratory to the patient. POCT is increasingly being used not only in the emergency department, operating rooms, and intensive care units (ICUs) but also in the clinics, physician offices, nursing homes, pediatric units, pharmacies, counseling centers, and ambulances. Advances in medical, analytical, and engineering technologies in the last two decades led to the appearance of a large number of portable measurement devices for a variety of the different analytes. These include tests for electrolytes,

glucose, hemoglobin A1c, urinalysis, pregnancy, drugs of abuse, therapeutic drug monitoring, occult blood, blood gases, coagulation tests, enzymes, and cardiac markers. POCT is also available for infectious diseases such as HIV, gonorrhea, syphilis, streptococcus, influenza, fungal infections, and tuberculosis.

POCT offers several advantages compared with central laboratory testing (Table 10-1). The major advantage of POCT is faster delivery of results. POCT is designed to work with the flow of patient management and care—physicians can order and perform the test and immediately make a medical decision.

Smaller sample volume allows POCT use in neonatal and pediatric population and is ideal for those patients requiring frequent testing. The overall cost of patient care is arguably smaller due to improved patient workflows. Testing near the patient requires fewer steps than transporting a specimen to the laboratory, processing, aliquoting, testing, and communicating results back to

TABLE 10-1	POTENTIAL ADVANTAGES AND DISADVANTAGES OF POCT*

ADVANTAGES	DISADVANTAGES
Convenience for both the attending physician/nurse and patient	POCT is significantly more expensive than the cost of central laboratory testing due to the higher disposable and reagent costs of the POCT analyzers
Reduced turnaround time for test results to expedite medical decision-making in operating rooms, emergency department, and intensive care units	Maintenance of quality control and quality assurance is difficult as anyone can run the analysis
Reduction in clinic visits, hospital admissions, and length of hospital stay due to faster laboratory services	Management of POCT is challenging—there are numerous operators to train, multiple sites to manage, and hundreds of POC tests to validate
Better patient management due to improved visibility and interaction with a patient	Preanalytic, analytic, and postanalytic issues are not recognized easily if tests are performed by untrained staff
Decreased manpower needs associated with test requesting and reporting, especially for patients necessitating tests several times a day (e.g., glucose determination)	Inter-individual variability in POCT results may be greater when compared with central laboratory testing
Fingerstick POCT is less traumatic for a patient as smaller sample volume is required	Difficulties with documentation of test results, billing, and regulatory compliance
Reduced risk of preanalytical errors due to absence of transporting a specimen to a core laboratory, processing, aliquoting, testing, and communicating results back to clinical staff. Reduced risk of sample deterioration	Proper integration of test result into the patient's electronic medical record may be more difficult
Improved patient outcome	Managing reagent supply and storage at multiple sites is problematic
Improved cost of overall patient care	Central laboratory test results and POCT results are not always comparable due to differences in specimen types, technology, interfering substances, etc.
Wide menu of POC analytes for specimens that do not require processing	
Availability to a wider variety of sites (e.g., rural areas, areas with limited infrastructure/personnel, and sites with underserved populations)	

*POCT, point-of-care testing.

clinical staff, all of which may reduce preanalytical and postanalytical laboratory-related errors. Portability of POCT allows for increased access to testing in a wider variety of sites, e.g., rural areas, accident sites, areas with limited infrastructure and personnel, and locations with underserved populations. One example of the latter is the use of a portable POCT to test for tuberculosis in the risk populations in low-income countries.[6]

Although POCT offers many advantages, there are some negative aspects of POCT (Table 10-1). On a cost per test basis, POCT is more expensive than the cost of central laboratory testing as a result of the higher disposable and reagent costs of the POCT analyzers. End-users may be able to counterbalance these increased costs by gaining efficiencies in improved patient workflows. Additionally, quality of results is a concern because POCT is usually performed by non-laboratory personnel

who may include nurses, physicians, emergency medical technicians, pharmacists, medics, patients, and medical office assistants. End-users with multiple responsibilities and limited laboratory training may not appreciate the value of laboratory quality control (QC) in ensuring quality test results.

LABORATORY REGULATIONS

Accreditation

In the United States, laboratory testing for patient care (with limited exceptions) requires a Clinical Laboratory Improvement Amendments (CLIA) certificate. CLIA was enacted by Congress and established quality standards for all laboratory testing, thereby ensuring the accuracy, reliability, and timeliness of patient test results regardless of where the test was performed.[7] The requirements are based

TABLE 10-2	TYPES OF CLIA CERTIFICATES[a]
Certificate of Waiver	Issued to a laboratory to perform only waived tests
Certificate of Registration	Issued to a laboratory that enables the entity to conduct moderate- or high-complexity laboratory testing or both until the entity is determined by survey to be in compliance with CLIA regulations
Certificate for PPMPs	Issued to a laboratory in which a physician, midlevel practitioner, or dentist performs no tests other than the microscopy procedures
	Permits the laboratory to also perform waived tests
Certificate of Compliance	Issued to a laboratory after an inspection that finds the laboratory to be in compliance with all applicable CLIA requirements
Certificate of Accreditation	Issued to a laboratory on the basis of the laboratory's accreditation by an accreditation organization approved by the Health Care Finance Administration

CLIA, Clinical Laboratory Improvement Amendments; POCT, point-of-care testing; PPMP, provider-performed microscopy procedure.
[a]Clinical Laboratory Improvement Act. How to Obtain a CLIA Certificate of Waiver, http://www.cms.gov/Regulations-and-Guidance/Legislation/CLIA/downloads//howobtaincertificateofwaiver.pdf

on the complexity of the test and not the type of laboratory where the testing is performed (POC or central laboratory). All laboratories performing POCT must be certified under one of the five types of CLIA certificates listed in Table 10-2. The CLIA certificate must be appropriate for the testing that is performed in the laboratory (i.e., appropriate complexity). In addition to the federal program, state departments of public health or public organizations may apply for "deemed" status, which allows these organizations to perform laboratory accreditation and inspections.

POCT Complexity

Tests are classified based on their complexity. The Food and Drug Administration (FDA) uses several criteria to assign complexity to any test, and the three categories are "waived" tests, moderate-complexity tests, and high-complexity tests. Waived tests are a category of tests defined by CLIA, such as dipstick tests, urine pregnancy tests, and blood glucose monitoring devices, which are subject to the lowest level of regulation and are cleared by the FDA for home uses. They employ methodologies that are so simple and accurate as to render the likelihood of erroneous results negligible and pose almost no risk of harm to the patient if the test is performed incorrectly. A full list of currently waived tests can be found on the FDA web site (http://www.accessdata.fda.gov/scripts/cdrh/cfdocs/cfClia/testswaived.cfm). Laboratories performing non-waived tests (moderate-complexity tests and high-complexity tests) must fulfill all the requirements for personnel qualifications, proficiency testing and inspections, quality assurance and QCs, and patient test management. The majority of POCT is moderate complexity.

The fourth category of POCT is *provider-performed microscopy procedures*, or *PPMPs*, which is a subcategory of moderate-complexity testing. These tests involve the use of a microscope, limited to bright-field or phase-contrast microscopy. Generally, the specimens are labile and cannot survive transport to a clinical laboratory. Only licensed physicians, dentists, and midlevel practitioners may perform PPMP. There are usually no QC materials available for PPMP.

To determine to which category POC test or procedure belongs, refer to the following searchable and continuously renewable FDA-approved test menu: http://www.accessdata.fda.gov/scripts/cdrh/cfdocs/cfClia/search.cfm.

IMPLEMENTATION

Establishing Need

When establishing a POCT site, the approach and steps in the implementation will be different in nearly every case insofar as organizational characteristics, personnel competency, and financial situation of any given institution may vary greatly. However, there are some common guidelines to implementation that apply to nearly every case. Support of the organization must be present to evaluate the requests for POCT. Typically, a multidisciplinary committee consisting of laboratory staff, physician, nursing representatives, and hospital/laboratory administration is formed to create a structure for receiving and establishing criteria for approving requests for POCT. Before implementing a POCT service, an interdisciplinary committee should address the questions similar to those listed in Box 10-1. The decision to establish POCT program is made after justifying the clinical need, cost, and the analytic performance requirements. Other factors should also be considered, including space, any previous track record of regulatory compliance, personnel who will be performing the testing, and metrics to determine if the POCT implementation is successful.

BOX 10-1 QUESTIONS TO ASK WHEN IMPLEMENTING POCT

- Which test is required and in which specific area? How is the service currently provided and what are the problems?
- What is the expected annual test volume?
- What clinical question is being asked when requesting this test?
- What clinical decision is likely to be made and action to be taken upon receipt of the result?
- How will POCT increase patient satisfaction?
- Are personnel competent to perform the POCT? Are facilities available to perform the test and store equipment, reagents, and documentation?

- Will a change in practice be required?
- Can central laboratory deliver the required service? How do POCT cost, reference ranges, accuracy, and precision compare to similar tests in a laboratory?
- Are available POCT analyzers user-friendly? Can POCT analyzers interface with an LIS and a patient electronic medical record?
- Are both internal and external QC materials available?
- Does the company providing POCT analyzers and reagents offer a reliable support service?

POCT Implementation Protocol

After making the decision to implement POCT, the responsible party selects the method of choice and begins validation. Desirable characteristics of POCT analyzers include ease of use, method accuracy and comparability to main laboratory method, portability, durability, low maintenance, simple QC, QC lockout features, simple sample handling requirements, bar code patient and operator identification capabilities, and the ability to interface with a laboratory information system (LIS). The manufacturer should aid in providing minimum acceptability requirements, instrument manuals, package inserts for reagents and QCs, materials safety data sheet, and training materials. Method validation should confirm the manufacturer's specifications and a *procedure/policy* should be written for each test. This should not be simply a collection of materials obtained from a manufacturer; rather, these documents should aid in the development of an easy-to-follow, simple, and concise procedure. The procedure should include information on the principle of the method; personnel qualifications; specimen, reagents, supplies, and equipment requirements; QC and calibrations; patient testing procedure; reference ranges; reporting limits; and interfering substances if applicable. All required regulatory or certifying standards should be in place prior to initiating patient testing (Box 10-2).

BOX 10-2 POINT-OF-CARE CHECKLIST

1. *Quality Management*
   The POC program has a written QM program as well as organizational system setting forth levels of authority, responsibility, and accountability. There is a documented system to address unusual patient results or instrument troubleshooting. There is a written procedure for each POCT.
2. *Specimen Handling*
   There is a documented procedure describing methods for patient identification and preparation, as well as for specimen collection, accessioning, and preservation before testing. There is a procedure for entering POCT results into the permanent medical record of a patient. Reference intervals should be established.
3. *Reagents*
   All reagents should be stored and labeled as recommended by the manufacturer.
4. *Instruments and Equipment*
   Equipment must be evaluated and scheduled for a regular maintenance.

5. *Personnel*
   The director of the POCT program is a physician or a doctoral scientist. The testing personnel have adequate, specific training to ensure competence and this must be documented.
6. *Quality Control and Calibration*
   Calibrations and quality controls are run at regular intervals (at least daily). Acceptable limits are defined for control procedures, and there are documented corrective actions when control results exceed defined acceptability limits. Upper and lower limits of the analytical measurement range (AMR) for each analyte are defined.
7. *Safety*
   There is a program to assure that the safety of patients and health-care personnel is not compromised by POCT.

Adapted from the College of American Pathologists Point-of-Care-Testing Checklist 01.04.2012 (http://www.cap.org).

Personnel Requirements

For a POC program with moderate-complexity tests, unlike for those POC with Certificate of Waiver or certificate for PPMP, institutions are required to have a certain organizational and administrative structure where staff has established qualifications, competency, and experience. The *director of laboratory* is usually a Ph.D. scientist, or a physician with at least 1 year of experience directing a laboratory with 20 continuing medical education credits,[8] or a person with a bachelor's degree with 2 years' laboratory experience plus 2 years of supervising experience. Responsibilities of a director are very broad and include policy making, ensuring compliance with regulatory standards, and administrative duties. Importantly, the director is responsible for the analytic performance of all tests. The director must make technical decisions based on a constant monitoring of ongoing proficiency, accuracy, and precision. Such individuals should be a liaison between the clinicians, hospital administration, and laboratory personnel.

Each laboratory performing moderate-complexity tests must have a technical and a clinical consultant. The *technical consultant* is responsible for scientific oversight of the POCT, while the *clinical consultant* is required to provide clinical and medical advice. The director of a POCT program, the technical consultant, and the clinical consultant may be the same person.

Even though the implementation of the POCT program may be done differently depending on an institution, the entity responsible for quality management of the POCT program is always the laboratory. It is useful, therefore, for a laboratory to have a person supervising the POCT program, so a *POCT coordinator (POCC)* fulfills this role. Even though a POCC does not monitor day-to-day activities of *testing personnel*, it is the responsibility of the POCC to coordinate POC patient testing and facilitate compliance with procedures and policies and regulatory requirements. The POCC develops a training program for testing personnel and ensures documentation of competency training. The POCC also oversees completion of proficiency testing programs, performs on-site review of patient testing, QC, and maintenance logs and reports problems and regulatory noncompliance to appropriate management personnel.

Even though the laboratory is responsible for the POCT policies and procedures, it is the clinical staff that does the actual testing. Fostering a partnership between the operators and laboratory will help solve problems that may arise during the testing process. In this decentralized testing model, the specifics of how training is performed, how competency records are maintained, and how reagents are ordered may be different for each institution. The laboratory should monitor POC areas and ensure consistent feedback is provided regarding compliance with any applicable regulations. However, before any testing is initiated, clarifying individual roles and expectations is key to the success of the program.

QUALITY MANAGEMENT

Accuracy Requirements

Understanding how accurate the results need to be in the context of how the test will be used clinically is important before any patient testing is initiated. Ideally, a POC test will provide equivalent results with those from the central laboratory. If this were the case, depending on a clinical situation, physicians would have an option to choose either test and achieve the same clinical outcome. Unfortunately, despite the ongoing harmonization and standardization efforts, currently, there are still accuracy and imprecision concerns with some POCT. One example is the ongoing accuracy and precision problems with glucose meters. Authors of one study applied simulation modeling to relate performance characteristics of glucose analyzers to error rates in insulin dosage.[9] Interestingly, glucose meters that met existing POCT quality specifications allowed a large fraction of administrated insulin doses to differ from the intended doses. In addition, two landmark studies on tight glycemic controls gave completely different outcomes.[10,11] While one study showed that tight glycemic controls and the following intensive insulin therapy reduce morbidity and mortality among critically ill patients in the surgical ICU,[10] authors of another study found that intensive glucose control increased mortality among adults in the ICU.[11] There has been a considerable debate in the laboratory medicine literature that the difference in these two studies' outcome was due to the test method.[12-14] Due to complaints about glucose meter inaccuracy, the FDA is currently developing new standards for glucose meter accuracy.

QC and Proficiency Testing

The purpose of a quality management program is to ensure quality test results. A thorough validation should verify the analytical performance and any applicable limitations with the assay. Ongoing daily QC will alert the operator to any reagent or instrument issues. Some devices have both internal and external QC, both of which have distinctly different roles. Internal QC, which is also referred to as onboard QC, internal checks, electronic QC, or intelligent QC,[15] is performed at specific time intervals or at least daily. Internal QC ensures the electronics of the device are performing as expected or, if a manual test, the integrity of the device unit. Some instruments automate QC and/or calibration, which is helpful for regulatory compliance, but also ensures the instrument is ready to perform quality testing at all times. Another important feature is to tie QC performance requirements to test availability. If QC has not been performed as required and is unsatisfactory, the instrument does not allow patient testing until corrective action has taken place. This is known as QC lockout.

The entire testing process should be checked periodically according to the manufacturer and regulatory requirements by running an external QC. Here, a control sample is introduced to the test system in the same manner as a patient sample. Another form of external QC is proficiency testing where blind samples are sent to participating laboratories to perform testing. In the United States, results from one laboratory are compared with the results from the laboratories using the same method (peer group). Laboratories performing non-waived testing are not required to participate.

Quality management programs also need to ensure that the operators are competent to perform testing. After initial training, ongoing assessment of their performance is required. Careful control of personnel records is an important part of the quality management program and may be managed at the POCT site or directly by the laboratory. Some instruments will allow "super-users" (supervisors, managers, or POCC) to track training renewal dates and to lockout operators whose training has expired.

The greatest source of error in POCT is the preanalytical error. While the above features are necessary for any POCT program, it is more difficult to identify errors arising from poor specimen, e.g., sample contamination, dilution, circulating interference (lipemia, icterus, and hemolysis), and proper specimen source (arterial, venous, and fingerstick). For this reason, careful assessment of an area's compliance in proper specimen collection and handling is needed prior to implementing testing.

Preventing postanalytic errors in reporting can be achieved more reliably with connectivity. With the aid of bar codes, modern technology has improved patient identification and decreased transcription errors in many health-care applications. However, linear bar code identification methods are not fail-safe.[16] Hospitals should work with laboratories, pharmacy, radiology, and admissions to standardize scanning and printing specifications across a system. Careful control of bar code scanning and printing equipment specifications will minimize the misidentification threat to patient safety.

Total-system POCT quality assurance is thus the combination of several QC mechanisms:

- A mechanism to perform a thorough systems validation
- Reliable, user-friendly POCT device
- Training of POCT operators
- Competency assessment of all individuals involved in POCT
- QC testing and monitoring
- Proficiency testing
- Connectivity and bar coding technologies

POC APPLICATIONS

POCT makes up nearly 30% of the total in vitro diagnostics market in United States.[17] A wide variety of POCT devices can be loosely classified into the single-use, hand-held devices, the bench top devices, and the wearable devices (Box 10-3). POCT devices are designed with a consideration for the operators who may have little to no laboratory training. Hand-held devices are getting smaller and more ergonomic with every generation. A variety of analytical principles used in a laboratory have also been implemented in POCT devices, including the following:

- Reflectance
- Electrochemistry, electrical impedance
- Light scattering/optical motion
- Immunoturbidimetry
- Lateral flow, flow-through, or solid phase immunoassays
- Spectrophotometry, multiwavelength spectrophotometry
- Fluorescence, time-resolved fluorescence
- Polymerase chain reaction

BOX 10-3 TYPES OF POCT ANALYZERS

1. Single-use, qualitative, or semiquantitative cartridge/strip tests
   - Urine and blood chemistry
   - Infectious disease agents, cardiac markers, hCG
2. Single-use quantitative cartridge/strip tests with a reader device
   - Glucose
   - Blood chemistry
   - Coagulation
   - Cardiac markers, drugs, C-reactive protein (CRP), allergy, fertility tests
   - *Chlamydia*

   - HbA1c, urine albumin
   - Blood chemistry
   - pH, blood gases, electrolytes, metabolites
3. Multiple-use quantitative cartridge/benchtop devices
   - Hemoglobin species, bilirubin
   - pH, blood gases, electrolytes, metabolites
   - Cardiac markers, drugs, CRP
   - Complete blood count

Modified from the *Tietz Textbook of Clinical Chemistry and Molecular Diagnostics.* 5th ed., table 20-1.

Contemporary POCT analyzers are capable of delivering test results in less than a minute using a single-step protocol on a variety of unprocessed specimens such as whole blood, cerebrospinal fluid, urine, and stool specimens. Ideally, the results of POCT should meet the analytical specifications that are "fit-for-purpose" and should be comparable to those of the central laboratory.

Glucose testing is the highest volume POCT. These are devices with single-use cartridges or strips that use the reflectance or electrochemistry analytical principles for glucose measurement. Hemoglobin A1c testing is also rapidly increasing, although we are yet to see a device that measures both glucose and hemoglobin A1c. Both of these tests should not be used for a tight glucose control at bedside but rather employed as monitoring procedures because of the cases of hypoglycemia as well as cases of erroneous POCT measurements due to interfering substances.[18,19]

Mature POCT areas are measurements of urine and blood chemistry, coagulation testing, pH and blood gases, hemoglobin and bilirubin, and complete blood count. Other areas of POCT that are rapidly evolving are intraoperative immunoassay of parathyroid hormone, creatinine and cardiac markers in emergency departments, and infectious diseases (HIV).

INFORMATICS AND POCT

Capturing patient ID, operator ID, reference range, and the result documentation in the permanent record can be challenging without connectivity. Due to the number of interfaces that would be required, POCT analyzers are usually connected with LIS via a docking station and/or data management (DM) system that can connect to multiple POCT devices from different manufacturers through a single interface connection to the LIS/hospital information system (HIS) for all data transmissions. This creates an additional step to entering test result into LIS and later to the patient medical record.

With a multitude of POCT devices, it is not practical to have a separate device–LIS interfacing system for each device. Accordingly, the Connectivity Industry Consortium (CIC) represented by more than 30 instrument manufacturers, information technology companies, and end-users has developed a set of standards to ensure POCT devices bidirectionality, device connection commonality, commercial software intraoperability and security, and regulatory compliance. The developed standards govern the communication between the POCT devices and the DM as well as the actual interface between the DM and the LIS. The standards have been adopted by the National Committee for Clinical Laboratory Standards (now the Clinical and Laboratory Standards Institute, or CLSI).[20,21] Prior to the CIC, each vendor developed its own proprietary means of communicating data from POCT devices, with different physical connections, the wiring, and even the language and communication format or protocol. Nowadays, the CIS standards are becoming widely accepted by vendors and by users who necessitate a more universal POCT connectivity.

According to the CLSI guidelines,[21] certain patient information should always accompany the patient test result across the POCT device, the DM, the LIS, and the medical records. These include:

- Patient, sample, operator, and device identifiers
- Date and time of specimen collection and analysis
- Type of specimen
- Test requested and test result with appropriate units
- Error messages and action messages

These obligatory information items might also be accompanied by additional information such as reference intervals, calibrator/reagent/QC detail (e.g., lot number and expiration date), and specific comments and alerts.

In the course of selecting a POCT device, consideration must be given to the type of data output a POCT device provides. These include visual readings, printers, display screens, Ethernet and RS232 ports, modems, infrared beams, and radio signals. Preference is usually given to a device that is suitable for an already developed POCT connectivity system of an institution, which also makes the training of operators easier. Additionally, the connectivity communication system between a device and the DM can be unidirectional (one-way) or bidirectional (two-way). One-way connectivity allows the DM to only read information from the POCT device, while the two-way connectivity also lets the DM to upload data to the POCT devices. This is especially helpful in the POC system with multiple devices insofar as the DM can update information (e.g., lists of valid operators, reagent lot information, and patient information) for all POCT devices simultaneously.

Integration of POCT results with LIS and medical records allows for better management of such diseases as diabetes mellitus and hyperlipidemia and also in critical situations such as glycemic control in intensive care, management of heart failure, and assistance with dosing of anticoagulants. In these particular instances, the wireless connectivity of POCT devices in conjunction with docking stations is in great demand.

For additional student resources please visit thePoint at http://thepoint.lww.com.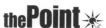

QUESTIONS

1. A CLIA waived test requires that operators
   a. must follow manufacturer's instructions.
   b. must have annual competence assessment.
   c. must perform proficiency testing.
   d. must perform QC daily.

2. Quality control lockout
   a. prevents quality control from being recorded when outside 2 standard deviations.
   b. prevents testing when quality control has not been performed.
   c. prevents operators from changing quality control records.
   d. prevents the wrong quality control material to be used for a particular test.

3. EQC per CLIA means
   a. equivalent.
   b. electronic.
   c. external.
   d. essential.

4. For laboratories with a provider-performed microscopy procedure CLIA certificate, which of the following would NOT be approved?
   a. Urinalysis
   b. Semen analysis

   c. Hematology differential
   d. Wet prep

5. Connectivity for POCT provides the ability to
   a. charge meters at docking stations on the hospital units.
   b. accept barcode patient identification.
   c. perform electronic quality control.
   d. transmit patient results to the medical record.
   e. prevent password sharing for operator identification.

6. Which of the following specimens is NOT used for a waived POC test?
   a. Urine
   b. Whole blood
   c. Plasma
   d. Eye fluid

7. Competency for non-waived testing
   a. is required for the CLIA director.
   b. is NOT required for physicians in their specialty.
   c. should be performed and documented annually for all operators.
   d. should be performed and documented initially after 6 months, then annually thereafter.

REFERENCES

1. CAP Commission on Laboratory Accreditation, Laboratory Accreditation Program. *Point-of-Care Testing Checklist.* Northfield, IL: CAP; April 2012.
2. Crook M. *Handbook of Near-Patient Testing.* London: Greenwich Medical Media Limited; 1999:1-116.
3. Price CP. Quality assurance of extra-laboratory analyses. In: Marks V, Alberti KG, eds. *Clinical Biochemistry Nearer the Patient II.* London: Bailliere Tindall; 1987:166-178.
4. Oliver G. *On Bedside Testing.* London: HK Lewis; 1884:1-128.
5. Mass D. Consulting to physician office laboratories. In: Snyder JR, Wilkinson DS, eds. *Management in Laboratory Medicine.* 3rd ed. New York, NY: Lippincott; 1998:443-450.
6. Boehme CC, Nabeta P, Hillemann D, et al. Rapid molecular detection of tuberculosis and rifampin resistance. *N Engl J Med.* 2010;363:1005-1015.
7. U.S. Department of Health and Human Services. Medicare, Medicaid and CLIA Programs. Regulations implementing the Clinical Laboratory Improvement Amendments of 1988 (CLIA): final rule. *Fed Regist.* 1992;57:7002-7186.
8. A List of CME Courses for Laboratory Directors of Moderate Complexity Laboratories: http://www.cms.gov/Regulations-and-Guidance/Legislation/CLIA/CME_Courses_for_Laboratory_

Directors_of_Moderate_Complexity_Laboratories.html. Accessed July 30, 2012.
9. Boyd JC, Bruns DE. Quality specifications for glucose meters: assessment by simulation modeling of errors in insulin dose. *Clin Chem.* February 2001;47(2):209-214.
10. van den Berghe G, Wouters P, Weekers F, et al. Intensive insulin therapy in critically ill patients. *N Engl J Med.* November 2001;345(19):1359-1367.
11. NICE-SUGAR Study Investigators, Finfer S, Chittock DR, et al. Intensive versus conventional glucose control in critically ill patients. *N Engl J Med.* 2009;360:1283-1297.
12. Cembrowski GS, Tran DV, Slater-MacLean L, Chin D, Gibney RT, Jacka M. Could susceptibility to low hematocrit interference have compromised the results of the NICE-SUGAR trial? *Clin Chem.* July 2010;56(7):1193-1195.
13. Mahoney JJ, Maguire P, Ellison JM, Cariski AT. Response to Cembrowski et al. regarding "Could susceptibility to low hematocrit interference have compromised the results of the NICE-SUGAR trial?". *Clin Chem.* October 2010;56(10):1643; author reply 1643-1644.
14. Hoedemaekers CW, Klein Gunnewiek JM, Van der Hoeven JG. Point-of-care glucose measurement systems should be used with great caution in critically ill intensive care unit patients. *Crit Care Med.* January 2010;38(1):339; author reply 339-340.

15. Gill JP, Shephard M. The conduct of quality control and quality assurance testing for POCT outside the laboratory. *Clin Biochem Rev.* August 2010;31(3):85-88.

16. Snyder ML, Carter A, Jenkins K, Fantz CR. Patient mis-identification caused by errors in standard barcode technology. *Clin Chem.* October 2010;56(10):1554-1560.

17. Kalorama Information Worldwide Point of Care Diagnostics. http://www.kaloramainformation.com/. Accessed July 30, 2012.

18. Hoedemaekers CW, Klein Gunnewiek JM, Prinsen MA, et al. Accuracy of bedside glucose measurement from three glucometers in critically ill patients. *Crit Care Med.* 2008;36: 3062-3066.

19. Eastham JH, Mason D, Barnes DL, et al. Prevalence of interfering substances with point-of-care glucose testing in a community hospital. *Am J Health Syst Pharm.* 2009;66:167-170.

20. Clinical Laboratory Standards Institute. *Point-of-Care Connectivity: Approved Standard.* 2nd ed. CLSI Document POCT01-A2. Wayne, PA: CLSI; 2006.

21. Clinical Laboratory Standards Institute. *Implementation Guide of POCT01 for Healthcare Providers: Approved Guideline.* CLSI Document POCT02-A. Wayne, PA: CLSI; 2008.

Clinical Correlations and Analytic Procedures

Amino Acids and Proteins

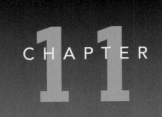

DEBORAH E. KEIL

CHAPTER

11

CHAPTER OUTLINE

- ◆ **AMINO ACIDS**
  Overview
  Basic Structure
  Metabolism
  Essential Amino Acids
  Nonessential Amino Acids
  Two New Amino Acids
  Aminoacidopathies
  Amino Acid Analysis
- ◆ **PROTEINS**
  Importance
  Molecular Size
  Synthesis
  Catabolism and Nitrogen Balance
  Structure
  Nitrogen Content
  Charge and Isoelectric Point
  Solubility
  Classification
- ◆ **PLASMA PROTEINS**
  Prealbumin (Transthyretin)
  Albumin
  Globulins
- ◆ **OTHER PROTEINS OF IMPORTANCE**
  Myoglobin
  Cardiac Troponin

- Brain Natriuretic Peptide and N-Terminal–Brain
  Natriuretic Peptide
  Fibronectin
  Adiponectin
  β-Trace Protein
  Cross-Linked C-Telopeptides
  Cystatin C
  Amyloid
- ◆ **TOTAL PROTEIN ABNORMALITIES**
  Hypoproteinemia
  Hyperproteinemia
- ◆ **METHODS OF ANALYSIS**
  Total Nitrogen
  Total Proteins
  Fractionation, Identification, and Quantitation of
  Specific Proteins
  Serum Protein Electrophoresis
  High-Resolution Protein Electrophoresis
  Capillary Electrophoresis
  Isoelectric Focusing
  Immunochemical Methods
- ◆ **PROTEINS IN OTHER BODY FLUIDS**
  Urinary Protein
  CSF Proteins
- ◆ **QUESTIONS**
- ◆ **REFERENCES**

Chapter Objectives

Upon completion of this chapter, the clinical laboratorian should be able to do the following:

- Describe the structures and general properties of amino acids and proteins, including both conjugated and simple proteins.
- Outline protein synthesis and catabolism.
- Discuss the general characteristics of the aminoacidopathies, including the metabolic defect in each and the procedure used for detection.
- Briefly discuss the function and clinical significance of the following proteins:
  - Prealbumin
  - Albumin
  - α_1-antitrypsin

- α_1-fetoprotein
- Haptoglobin
- Ceruloplasmin
- Transferrin
- Fibrinogen
- C-reactive protein
- Immunoglobulin
- Troponin
- Discuss at least five general causes of abnormal serum protein concentrations.
- List the reference intervals for total protein and albumin and discuss any nonpathologic factors that influence their levels.
- Describe and compare methodologies used in the analysis of total protein, albumin, and protein fractionation. Include the structural characteristics or chemical

- properties that are relevant to each measurement and the clinical usage of each.
- Recognize and name the fractions, interpret any abnormality in the pattern, and associate these patterns with common disease states given a densitometric scan of a serum protein electrophoresis using the routine method (five zones).

- Differentiate the types of proteinuria on the basis of etiology and type of protein found in the urine, and describe the principle of the methods used for both qualitative and quantitative determination and identification of urine proteins.
- Describe the diseases associated with alterations in cerebrospinal fluid proteins.

KEY TERMS

Albumin
Aminoacidopathies
Amino acid
Ampholytes
Conjugated protein
Denaturation
Globulins
Hyperproteinemia
Hypoproteinemia

Isoelectric point (pI)
Monoclonal immunoglobulin
Nitrogen balance
Opsonization
Peptide bond
Phenylketonuria (PKU)
Principal fetal protein
Proteinuria
Quaternary structure
Simple protein

AMINO ACIDS

Overview

Amino acids are the building blocks of proteins. The precise amino acid content, and the sequence of those amino acids, of a specific protein is determined by the sequence of the bases in the gene that encodes that protein. The chemical properties of the amino acids of proteins determine the biologic activity of the protein.[1] Growth, repair, and maintenance of all cells are dependent on amino acids. The chemical properties of the amino acids of proteins determine the biologic activity of the protein. Proteins catalyze almost all of the reactions in living cells, controlling virtually all cellular processes.

Basic Structure

An amino acid contains at least one of both amino and carboxylic acid functional groups. The basic structure of an amino acid is depicted in Figure 11-1. The N-terminal end amino group ($-NH_2$) and the C-terminal end carboxyl group ($-COOH$) bond to the α-carbon, with the amino group of one amino acid linking with the carboxyl group of another, forming a peptide bond (Fig. 11-2).

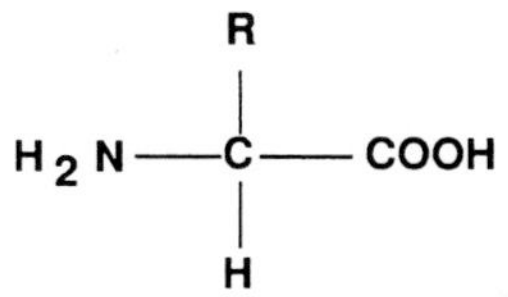

FIGURE 11-1 General structure of an α-amino acid.

A chain of amino acids is known as a *polypeptide*, and a large polypeptide constitutes a *protein*. In human serum, proteins average about 100 to 150 amino acids in the polypeptide chains. Amino acids differ from one another by the chemical composition of their R group (side chains). The R groups found on the 20 different amino acids used in building proteins are shown in Table 11-1.

Metabolism

About half of the 20 amino acids needed by humans cannot be synthesized at a rapid enough rate to support growth; they must be supplied in food. These nutritionally essential amino acids must be supplied by the diet in the form of proteins. The essential amino acids are arginine (often called semiessential as it is required for

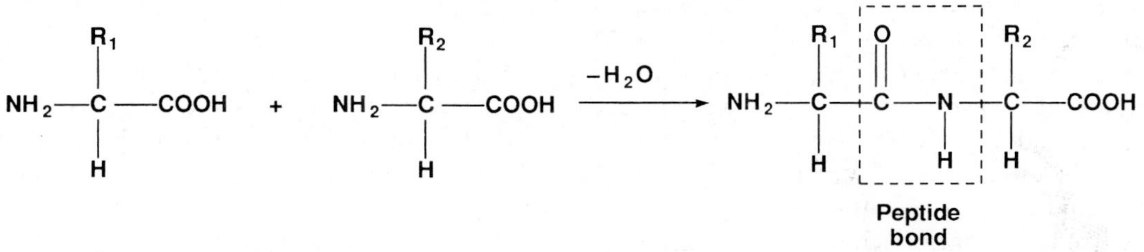

FIGURE 11-2 Formation of a dipeptide.

TABLE 11-1	AMINO ACIDS REQUIRED IN THE SYNTHESIS OF PROTEINS		
AMINO ACID	**R**	**AMINO ACID**	**R**
Glycine (Gly)	—H	Glutamine (Gln)	$-CH_2-CH_2-\overset{\overset{\displaystyle O}{\|\|}}{C}-NH_2$
Alanine (Ala)	$-CH_3$	Serine (Ser)	$\overset{\overset{\displaystyle OH}{\|}}{-CH_2}$
Valine (Val)[a]	$-CH\overset{-CH_3}{\underset{-CH_3}{}}$	Threonine (Thr)[a]	$\overset{\overset{\displaystyle OH}{\|}}{-CH}-CH_3$
Leucine (Leu)[a]	$-CH_2-CH\overset{CH_3}{\underset{CH_3}{}}$	Tyrosine (Tyr)	$-CH_2-\bigcirc-OH$
Isoleucine (Ile)[a]	$-CH\overset{CH_3}{\underset{-CH_2-CH_3}{}}$	Lysine (Lys)[a]	$-CH_2-CH_2-CH_2-CH_2-NH_2$
Cysteine (Cys)	$-CH_2-SH$	Arginine (Arg)	$-CH_2-CH_2-CH_2-\overset{}{\underset{H}{N}}-\overset{\overset{\displaystyle NH_2}{\|\|}}{C}-NH_2$
Methionine (Met)[a]	$-CH_2-CH_2-S-CH_3$	Histidine (His)	$-CH_2-\text{(imidazole ring)}$
Tryptophan (Trp)[a]	$-CH_2-\text{(indole ring)}$	Aspartate (Asp)	$-CH_2-COOH$
Phenylalanine (Phe)[a]	$-CH_2-\text{(benzene ring)}$	Glutamate (Glu)	$-CH_2-CH_2-COOH$
Asparagine (Asn)	$-CH_2-\overset{\overset{\displaystyle O}{\|\|}}{C}-NH_2$	Proline (Pro)[a,b]	$\text{(pyrrolidine ring)}-COOH$

The R group is the group attached to the α carbon.

[a]Nutritionally essential

[b]Exception to attachment of R group is proline.

the young but not for adults and can be synthesized in high enough amounts than what the body needs), histidine, isoleucine, leucine, lysine, methionine, phenylalanine, threonine, tryptophan, and valine. The 10 amino acids that the body can produce are alanine, asparagine, aspartic acid, cysteine, glutamic acid, glutamine, glycine, proline, serine, and tyrosine. Tyrosine is produced from phenylalanine, so if the diet is deficient in phenylalanine, tyrosine will be required as well. Humans do not have all the enzymes required for the biosynthesis of all of the amino acids. Under normal circumstances, proteolytic enzymes, such as pepsin and trypsin, completely digest dietary proteins into their constituent amino acids. Amino acids are then rapidly absorbed from the intestine into the blood and subsequently become part of the body's pool of amino acids. Amino acids are also released by the normal breakdown of body proteins.

The primary purpose of amino acids is for the synthesis of body proteins, including plasma, intracellular, and structural proteins. Amino acids are also used for the synthesis of nonprotein nitrogen-containing compounds such as purines, pyrimidines, porphyrins, creatine, histamine, thyroxine, epinephrine, and the coenzyme NAD. In addition, protein provides 12% to 20% of the total daily body energy requirement. The amino group is removed from amino acids by either deamination or transamination. The resultant ketoacid can enter into a common metabolic pathway with carbohydrates and fats. Glucogenic amino acids generate precursors of glucose, such as pyruvate or a citric acid cycle intermediate. Examples include alanine, which can be deaminated to pyruvate; arginine, which is converted to α-ketoglutarate; and aspartate, which is converted to oxaloacetate. Ketogenic amino acids generate ketone bodies. They are degraded to acetyl-CoA or acetoacetyl-CoA (e.g., leucine or lysine), with some amino acids being both ketogenic and glucogenic. The ammonium ion that is produced during deamination of the amino acids is converted into urea via the urea cycle in the liver.[2]

Essential Amino Acids

Arginine (Arg)

Arginine is a complex amino acid that is often found at the catalytic (active) site in proteins and enzymes due to its amine-containing side chain. Arginine plays an important role in cell division, the healing of wounds, stimulation of protein synthesis, immune function, and the release of hormones. Arginine is required for the generation of urea, which is necessary for the removal of toxic ammonia from the body, and is also required for the synthesis of creatine, which degrades to creatinine, a waste product that is cleared from the body by the kidney.

Histidine (His)

Histidine is one of the basic (by pH) amino acids due to its imidazole side chain. It is the direct precursor of histamine, one of the proteins involved in immune response. Histidine is also an important source of carbon atoms in the synthesis of purines, one of the two groups of nitrogen bases that make up DNA and RNA. Histidine is needed to help grow and repair body tissues and to maintain the myelin sheaths that protect nerve cells. It also helps manufacture red and white blood cells and helps to protect the body from heavy metal toxicity. Histamine stimulates the secretion of the digestive enzyme gastrin and acts as a catalytic site in certain enzymes.

Isoleucine (Ile)

Isoleucine is in the group of branched-chain amino acids that are needed to help maintain, heal, and repair muscle tissue, skin, and bones. Isoleucine is needed for hemoglobin formation, and it helps to regulate blood glucose levels and maintain energy levels.

Leucine (Leu)

Leucine is also in the group of branched-chain amino acids, along with valine and isoleucine. Leucine is the second most common amino acid found in protein besides glycine. Leucine, in conjunction with valine and isoleucine, boosts the healing of muscle, skin, and bones; aids in recovery from surgery; and lowers blood glucose levels. Leucine is necessary for the optimal growth of infants and for nitrogen balance in adults.

Lysine (Lys)

Lysine has a net positive charge, which makes it one of the three basic (by charge) amino acids. Lysine plays a role in the production of antibodies and lowers triglyceride levels. Lysine is needed for proper growth and bone development in children and to maintain a proper nitrogen balance in adults. Lysine helps in the absorption and conservation of calcium and plays an important role in the formation of collagen, a component of cartilage and connective tissue.

Methionine (Met)

Methionine is an important amino acid that helps to initiate translation of messenger RNA (mRNA) by being the first amino acid incorporated into the N-terminal position of all proteins.[3] Methionine is a source of sulfur, required by the body for normal metabolism and growth. Methionine assists the breakdown of fats, helps to detoxify lead and other heavy metals, helps diminish muscle weakness, and prevents brittle hair. Methionine reacts with adenosine triphosphate (ATP) to contribute to the synthesis of many important substances, including epinephrine and choline.

Phenylalanine (Phe)

Phenylalanine is classified as a nonpolar amino acid because of the hydrophobic nature of its benzyl side chain. It promotes alertness and vitality, elevates mood, decreases pain, aids memory and learning, and is used to treat arthritis and depression. Phenylalanine is used by the brain to produce norepinephrine, a neurotransmitter that transmits signals between nerve cells. Phenylalanine uses an active transport channel to cross the blood–brain barrier and, in large quantities, interferes with the production of serotonin, another neurotransmitter. Phenylalanine is part of the composition of aspartame, a common sweetener used in prepared foods as a sugar replacement. Phenylalanine plays a key role in the biosynthesis of other amino acids.

Threonine (Thr)

Threonine is an alcohol-containing amino acid that is an important component in the formation of protein, collagen, elastin (a connective tissue protein), and tooth enamel. It is also important in the production of neurotransmitters and health of the nervous system. Threonine helps maintain proper protein balance in the body and aids liver function, metabolism, and assimilation.

Tryptophan (Trp)

Tryptophan is formed from proteins during digestion by the action of proteolytic enzymes. Tryptophan is also a precursor for serotonin and melatonin, a neurohormone and powerful antioxidant. Tryptophan is a natural relaxant; it helps alleviate insomnia by inducing sleep, soothes anxiety, and reduces depression. It is used in the treatment of migraine headaches, aids in weight control by reducing appetite, and helps control hyperactivity in children.

Valine (Val)

Valine is another branched-chain amino acid that is a constituent of fibrous protein in the body. Valine is needed for muscle metabolism and coordination, tissue repair, and maintenance of nitrogen balance. It is used by muscle tissue as an energy source. Valine is used in treatments for muscle, mental, and emotional problems; insomnia; anxiety; and liver and gallbladder disease.

Nonessential Amino Acids

Alanine (Ala)

Alanine is one of the simplest of the amino acids and is involved in the energy-producing breakdown of glucose. Alanine itself is a product of the breakdown of DNA or the dipeptides, anserine and carnosine, and the conversion of pyruvate, a pivotal compound in carbohydrate metabolism.[4] Alanine plays a major role in the transfer of nitrogen from peripheral tissue to the liver, helps in reducing the buildup of toxic substances that are released into muscle cells when muscle protein is broken down quickly to meet energy needs, and strengthens the immune system through production of antibodies.

Asparagine (Asn)

Asparagine was first isolated in 1806 from asparagus juice, becoming the first amino acid to be isolated. Asparagine is one of the principal and frequently the most abundant of the amino acids involved in the transport of nitrogen. Asparagine is the β-amide of aspartic acid synthesized from aspartic acid and ATP.[4] The main function of asparagine is converting one amino acid into another via amination, the process by which an amine group is introduced into an organic molecule, and transamination, the reaction when an amino acid is transferred to an α-ketoacid. Asparagine is required by the nervous system and plays an important role in the synthesis of ammonia.

Aspartic Acid (Asp)

Aspartic acid is alanine with one of the β-hydrogens replaced by a carboxylic acid group. Aspartic acid plays a vital role in metabolism during construction of other amino acids and metabolites in the citric acid cycle. Among the amino acids that are synthesized from aspartic acid are asparagine, arginine, lysine, methionine, threonine, isoleucine, and several nucleotides. Aspartic acid is also a metabolite in the urea cycle and participates in gluconeogenesis, the generation of glucose from nonsugar carbon substrates.

Cysteine (Cys)

Cysteine is classified as a nonessential amino acid, but it may be essential for infants, the elderly, and individuals with certain metabolic diseases or malabsorption syndromes. Cysteine is an important structural and functional component of many proteins and enzymes. Cysteine is named after cystine, its oxidized dimer.[5] Cysteine is potentially toxic and is catabolized in the gastrointestinal tract and blood. In opposition, cysteine is absorbed during digestion as cystine, which is more stable in the gastrointestinal tract. It is cystine that travels to cells, where it is reduced to two cysteine molecules upon cell entry. Cysteine is used as a constituent in the food, pharmaceutical, and personal care industries. One of its largest applications is in the production of flavors.

Glutamic Acid (Glu)

Glutamic acid is synthesized from a number of amino acids, and when an amino group is added to glutamic acid, it forms the important amino acid glutamine. Glutamic acid is one of the two amino acids that have a net negative charge (by pH), making it a very polar molecule. Glutamic acid serves as a neurotransmitter and its dysregulation has been linked to epileptic seizures. It is also important in the metabolism of sugars and fats and aids transporting potassium into the spinal fluid. Glutamic acid is present in a wide variety of foods and is responsible for one of the five basic tastes of the human sense of taste (umami). Glutamic acid is often used as a food additive and flavor enhancer in the form of its sodium salt, monosodium glutamate.

Glutamine (Gln)

Glutamine is the most abundant amino acid in the body, being involved in more metabolic processes than any other amino acid. Over 61% of skeletal muscle tissue is glutamine. Glutamine is converted to glucose when more glucose is required for energy and aids in immune function. Glutamine assists in maintaining the proper acid/alkaline balance in the body, provides fuel for a healthy digestive tract,[6] and is the basis of the building blocks for the synthesis of RNA and DNA. Studies have shown glutamine to be useful in the treatment of serious illnesses, injury, trauma, burns, and cancer treatment–related side effects and in wound healing for postoperative patients.[7] Glutamine is also marketed as a supplement used for muscle growth in weightlifting and bodybuilding. Glutamine transports ammonia, the toxic metabolic by-product of protein breakdown, to the liver, where it is converted into less toxic urea and then excreted by the kidneys.

Glycine (Gly)

Glycine is the simplest amino acid synthesized in the body and is the only amino acid that is not optically active because it has no stereoisomers (any of a group of isomers [compounds with the same molecular formula but a different structural formula] in which atoms are linked in the same order but differ in their spatial arrangement). Glycine is essential for the synthesis of nucleic acids, bile acids, proteins, peptides, purines, ATP, porphyrins, hemoglobin, glutathione, creatine, bile salts, glucose, glycogen, and other amino acids. The liver uses glycine to help in the detoxification of compounds and to help in the synthesis of bile acids. Glycine has a sweet taste and is used as a sweetener/taste enhancer. Glycine is an inhibitory neurotransmitter in the central nervous system (CNS), is a metal complexing agent, retards muscle degeneration, improves glycogen storage, and promotes healing.

Proline (Pro)
Proline is the precursor of hydroxyproline, which is manufactured into collagen, tendons, ligaments, and heart muscle by the body. Proline is involved in wound healing, plays important roles in molecular recognition, and is an important component in certain medical wound dressings that use collagen to stimulate wound healing. Proline helps in the healing of cartilage and in the strengthening of joints, tendons, and heart muscle, and it works with vitamin C to promote healthy connective tissues.

Serine (Ser)
Serine is the second amino acid that is also an alcohol because of its methyl side chain, which contains a hydroxy group. Serine is needed for the proper metabolism of fats and fatty acids and plays an important role in the body's synthetic pathways for pyrimidines, purines (making it important for DNA and RNA function), creatine, and porphyrins. It is highly concentrated in all cell membranes, is a component of the protective myelin sheaths surrounding nerve fibers, and aids in the production of immunoglobulins and antibodies for the maintenance of a healthy immune system.

Tyrosine (Tyr)
Tyrosine is metabolically synthesized from the important amino acid phenylalanine to become the para-hydroxy derivative of phenylalanine. Tyrosine is a precursor of the adrenal hormones epinephrine, norepinephrine, and dopamine and the thyroid hormones, including thyroxine. It is important in overall metabolism, aiding in the functions of the adrenal, thyroid, and pituitary glands. Tyrosine stimulates metabolism and the nervous system, acts as a mood elevator, suppresses appetite, and helps reduce body fat, making it useful in the treatment of chronic fatigue, narcolepsy, anxiety, depression, low sex drive, allergies, and headaches.

Two New Amino Acids

Selenocysteine (Sec)
Selenocysteine is recognized as the 21st amino acid but, unlike other amino acids present in proteins, it is not coded for directly in the genetic code. Selenocysteine is encoded by a UGA codon, which is normally a stop codon; however, like the other amino acids used by cells, selenocysteine has a specialized transfer RNA (tRNA). Selenocysteine was named as an amino acid in 2002 and found to be the selenium analogue of cysteine, in which a selenium atom replaces sulfur. Selenocysteine is present in several enzymes, such as formate dehydrogenases, glycine reductases, and some hydrogenases. It has been discovered that HIV-1 encodes a functional selenoprotein, and patients with HIV infection have been shown to have a lower-than-average blood plasma selenium level.[8,9]

Pyrrolysine (Pyl)
Pyrrolysine is the 22nd naturally occurring genetically encoded amino acid used by some Archaea (prokaryotic [lacking a membrane-bound nucleus] and single-celled microorganisms) in enzymes that are part of their methane-producing metabolism. This lysine derivative is encoded by the UAG codon, normally a stop codon, possibly modified by the presence of a specific downstream sequence forcing the incorporation of pyrrolysine instead of terminating translation.[10]

Aminoacidopathies

Aminoacidopathies are a class of inherited errors of metabolism in which there is an enzyme defect that inhibits the body's ability to metabolize certain amino acids. The abnormalities exist either in the activity of a specific enzyme in the metabolic pathway or in the membrane transport system for amino acids. Phenylketonuria (PKU), an aminoacidopathy, was the first newborn screening test introduced in the early 1960s. Now, some states require screening tests for up to 26 amino acids.[11] More than 100 diseases have been identified that result from inherited errors of amino acid metabolism. The aminoacidopathy disorders cause severe medical complications due to the buildup of toxic amino acids and/or by-products of amino acid metabolism in the blood.

Phenylketonuria
PKU is inherited as an autosomal recessive trait and occurs in about 1 in 15,000 births. The metabolic defect in the classic form of PKU is an absence of activity of the enzyme phenylalanine hydroxylase (PAH), which catalyzes the conversion of phenylalanine to tyrosine (Fig. 11-3). In the absence of the enzyme, phenylalanine levels are usually greater than 1,200 μmol/L. In the newborn, the upper limit of normal for a phenylalanine level is 120 μmol/L (2 mg/dL).[12] In untreated classic PKU, blood levels as high as 2.4 mM/L can be found. Chronically high levels of phenylalanine and some of its metabolites—e.g., phenylpyruvic acid, phenylpyruvate (also known as phenylketone), and phenyllactic acid—can cause significant brain problems.

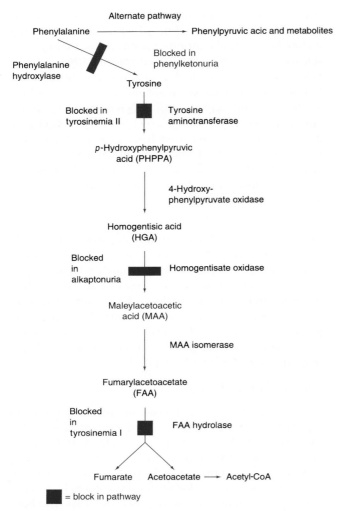

FIGURE 11-3 Metabolism of phenylalanine and tyrosine.

All of these compounds are found in both the blood and the urine of a PKU patient, giving the urine a characteristic musty odor. Partial deficiencies of PAH activity are typically classified as mild PKU if phenylalanine levels are between 600 and 1,200 μmol/L or as non-PKU mild hyperphenylalaninemia if phenylalanine levels are in the range of 180 to 600 μmol/L and there is no accompanying accumulation of phenylketones.

In infants and children with this inherited defect, retarded mental development and microcephaly occur as a result of the toxic effects of phenylalanine or its metabolic by-products on the brain. Brain damage can be avoided if the disease is detected at birth and the infant is maintained on a diet containing very low levels of phenylalanine. Also, women with PKU who are untreated during pregnancy almost always have babies who are microcephalic and mentally retarded. The fetal effects of maternal PKU are preventable if the mother is maintained on a phenylalanine-restricted diet from before conception through term.

Hyperphenylalaninemia cases that are not the result of the lack of the PAH enzyme also occur. The defect in these cases is a deficiency in the enzymes needed for the regeneration and synthesis of tetrahydrobiopterin (BH_4). BH_4 is a cofactor required for the enzymatic hydroxylation of the aromatic amino acids phenylalanine, tyrosine, and tryptophan. Deficiency of BH_4 results in elevated blood levels of phenylalanine and deficient production of neurotransmitters from tyrosine and tryptophan. Although cofactor defects account for only 1% to 5% of all cases of elevated phenylalanine levels, they must be identified so that appropriate treatment of the active cofactor along with the neurotransmitter precursors ʟ-DOPA and 5-OH tryptophan can be initiated.[13]

Every state now screens the blood phenylalanine level of all newborns at about 3 days of age. If the screening test is abnormal, other tests are needed to confirm or exclude PKU. Newborn screening allows early identification and implementation of treatment. The goal of PKU treatment is to maintain the blood level of phenylalanine between 2 and 10 mg/dL (120 to 600 μmol/L). Some phenylalanine is needed for normal growth, therefore a diet that has some phenylalanine but in much lower amounts than normal is the recommended treatment. High-protein foods, such as meat, fish, poultry, eggs, cheese, and milk, are avoided. Instead, calculated amounts of cereals, starches, fruits, and vegetables, along with a milk substitute, are usually recommended.

In December 2007, the U.S. Food and Drug Administration (FDA) approved Kuvan® (sapropterin dihydrochloride), the first drug to help manage PKU.[14] The drug helps reduce phenylalanine levels by increasing the activity of the PAH enzyme. Kuvan is effective only in patients who have some PAH activity and who continue to follow a phenylalanine-restricted diet and have their phenylalanine levels monitored.

Tests for PKU
The Guthrie test is a semiquantitative, bacterial inhibition assay for phenylalanine that uses the ability of phenylalanine to facilitate bacterial growth in a culture medium with an inhibitor. Newborn infant blood is collected on a piece of filter paper, and a small disk of the filter paper is punched out and placed on an agar gel plate containing *Bacillus subtilis* and β-2-thienylalanine. The agar gel is able to support bacterial growth, but the β-2-thienylalanine inhibits bacterial growth. In the presence of extra phenylalanine leached from the impregnated filter paper disk, the inhibition is overcome and the bacteria grow. The Guthrie assay is sensitive enough to detect serum phenylalanine levels of 180 to 240 μmol/L (3 to 4 mg/dL). The test has been widely used throughout North America and Europe as one of the core

newborn screening tests since the late 1960s. In recent years, it is gradually being replaced in many areas by newer techniques, such as tandem mass spectrometry (MS/MS), the gold standard for detecting a variety of congenital diseases.

Another approach to the screening for PKU involves a microfluorometric assay for the direct measurement of phenylalanine in dried blood filter disks. This method yields quantitative results, is more adaptable to automation, and is not affected by the presence of antibiotics. The procedure is based on the fluorescence of a complex formed of phenylalanine–ninhydrin–copper in the presence of a dipeptide. The test requires pretreatment of the filter paper specimen with trichloroacetic acid (TCA). The extract is then reacted in a microtiter plate with a mixture of ninhydrin, succinate, and leucylalanine in the presence of copper tartrate. The fluorescence of the complex is measured using excitation/emission wavelengths of 360 and 530 nm, respectively.[15]

Any positive results found in screening tests must be verified. The reference method for quantitative serum phenylalanine is high-performance liquid chromatography (HPLC); however, both fluorometric and enzymatic methods are available. Now, MS/MS is being used in screening for inherited disorders in newborns. Mass spectrometry is an analytical technique that measures the mass-to-charge ratio of charged particles.[16] It is most generally used to find the composition of a physical sample by generating a mass spectrum representing the masses of the sample's components. Because both the increase in phenylalanine and the decrease in tyrosine levels seen in PKU can be identified, the ratio of phenylalanine to tyrosine (Phe/Try) can be calculated. Using the ratio between metabolites rather than an individual level increases the specificity of the measurement and lowers the false-positive rate for PKU to less than 0.01%. The MS/MS method has a greater sensitivity, detecting lower levels of phenylalanine and allowing for diagnosis of PKU as early as the first day of life. Because MS/MS has the ability to detect more than 25 different genetic disorders with a single specimen, this method is replacing the multiple procedures currently used in newborn screening programs.

Another fast diagnostic procedure for neonatal PKU was developed in 2005 using microwave-assisted silylation followed by gas chromatography–mass spectrometry (GC/MS). Amino acids are extracted from neonatal blood samples and rapidly derived with *N,O-bis*(trimethylsilyl)-trifluoroacetamide under microwave irradiation. The derivatives are then analyzed by GC/MS.

Prenatal diagnosis and detection of carrier status in families with PKU are now available using DNA analysis. PKU results from multiple independent mutations (more than 400 identified) at the PAH locus.

Tyrosinemia

The inborn metabolic disorders of tyrosine catabolism are characterized by the excretion of tyrosine and tyrosine catabolites in urine. There are three types of tyrosinemia, each with distinctive symptoms and caused by the deficiency of a different enzyme.

Type I tyrosinemia is the most severe form of this aminoacidopathy and is found in about 1 in 100,000 births. It is caused by low levels of the enzyme fumarylacetoacetate hydrolase, the fifth of five enzymes needed to break down tyrosine. Symptoms of type I tyrosinemia include failure to thrive, diarrhea, vomiting, jaundice, cabbage-like odor, distended abdomen, swelling of legs, and increased predisposition for bleeding. Type I tyrosinemia can lead to liver and kidney failure, problems affecting the nervous system, and an increased risk of cirrhosis or liver cancer later in life.

Type II tyrosinemia is caused by a deficiency of the enzyme tyrosine aminotransferase. It occurs in fewer than 1 in 250,000 births. Tyrosine aminotransferase is the first in a series of five enzymes that converts tyrosine to smaller molecules, which are excreted by the kidneys or used in energy-producing reactions. About half of the individuals with type II tyrosinemia are mentally retarded and have symptoms of excessive tearing, photophobia (abnormal sensitivity to light), eye pain and redness, and painful skin lesions on the palms and soles of the feet.

Type III tyrosinemia is a rare disorder (only a few cases have been reported) caused by a deficiency of the enzyme 4-hydroxyphenylpyruvate dioxygenase. This enzyme is found mainly in the liver, with lesser amounts found in the kidneys. It, too, is one of the series of enzymes needed to break down tyrosine. The clinical picture of type III tyrosinemia patients includes mild mental retardation, seizures, and periodic loss of balance and coordination.

Diagnostic criteria include an elevated tyrosine level using tandem MS/MS coupled with a confirmatory test for an elevated level of the abnormal metabolite succinylacetone.[17] Treatment for tyrosinemia is a low-protein diet; the drug nitisinone (NTBC), which prevents the formation of maleylacetoacetic acid and fumarylacetoacetic acid, which can be converted to succinylacetone, a toxin that damages the liver and kidneys; or full or partial liver transplant. Since nitisinone's first use for tyrosinemia in 1991, it has replaced liver transplantation as the first-line treatment for this rare condition.

Alkaptonuria

Alkaptonuria is an inborn metabolic disease transmitted as an autosomal recessive gene, the *HGD* gene, which causes the lack of the enzyme homogentisate oxidase, which is needed in the metabolism of tyrosine and phenylalanine. This disorder occurs in about 1 of 250,000 births. A predominant clinical manifestation of alkaptonuria is that the patient's urine turns brownish-black when it mixes with air. This phenomenon is due to an accumulation of homogentisic acid (HGA) in the urine, which oxidizes to produce this dark pigment. Alkaptonuric patients have no immediate problems; however, late in the disease, the high level of HGA gradually accumulates in connective tissue, causing ochronosis (pigmentation of these tissues), an arthritis-like degeneration from the buildup of HGA in the cartilage, dark spots on the sclera (white of the eye), and deposition of pigment in the cartilage of the ears, nose, and tendons of the extremities.

Urinalysis is done to test for alkaptonuria. When ferric chloride is added to the urine, it will turn the urine black in patients with alkaptonuria. Treatment for alkaptonuria is high-dose vitamin C, which has been shown to decrease the buildup of brown pigment in the cartilage and may slow the development of arthritis.

Maple Syrup Urine Disease

Maple syrup urine disease (MSUD) results from an absence or greatly reduced activity of the enzyme branched-chain α-ketoacid decarboxylase, blocking the normal metabolism of the three essential branched-chain amino acids leucine, isoleucine, and valine. MSUD is an autosomal recessive genetic inherited disorder. Newborn screening for MSUD has been part of several state screening programs since the mid-1970s, with a reported prevalence of 1 in 150,000 births in the general population. The most striking feature of this hereditary disease is the characteristic maple syrup or burnt sugar odor of the urine, breath, and skin. The result of this enzyme defect is an accumulation of the branched-chain amino acids and their corresponding ketoacids in the blood, urine, and cerebrospinal fluid (CSF).

Infants with MSUD seem normal at birth but, within a week, develop lethargy, vomiting, lack of appetite, and signs of failure to thrive. CNS symptoms follow, including muscle rigidity, stupor, and respiratory irregularities. The disease progresses to cause severe mental retardation, seizures, acidosis, and hypoglycemia. If treatment is not given, the disease can lead to death. Intermediate forms of MSUD have been reported where the activity of the decarboxylase is approximately 25% of normal. Although this still results in a persistent elevation of the branched-chain amino acids, the levels frequently can be controlled by restricting the diet of leucine, isoleucine, and valine.

A modified Guthrie test is commonly used for neonatal screening. The metabolic inhibitor to *B. subtilis,* included in the growth media, is 4-azaleucine. A microfluorometric assay for the three branched-chain amino acids uses a filter paper specimen treated with a solvent mixture of methanol and acetone to denature the hemoglobin. Leucine dehydrogenase is added to an aliquot of the extract, and the fluorescence of the NADH produced in the subsequent reaction is measured at 450 nm, with an excitation wavelength of 360 nm.[18] A leucine level above 4 mg/dL is indicative of MSUD. MS/MS is also being used in testing for MSUD. Prenatal diagnosis of MSUD is made by testing the decarboxylase enzyme concentration in cells cultured from amniotic fluid.

Isovaleric Acidemia

Isovaleric acidemia is an autosomal recessive metabolic disorder from a deficiency of the enzyme isovaleryl-CoA dehydrogenase, preventing normal metabolism of the branched-chain amino acid leucine. The prevalence of isovaleric acidemia is approximately 1 in 250,000 births in the United States, caused by mutations in the isovaleryl-CoA dehydrogenase (*IVD*) gene.

A characteristic feature of isovaleric acidemia is a distinctive odor of sweaty feet caused by the buildup of isovaleric acid. Health problems related to isovaleric acidemia range from very mild to life threatening, but when severe, it can damage the brain and nervous system. Clinical manifestations of this disorder become apparent a few days after birth and include failure to thrive, vomiting, and lethargy that can progress to seizures, coma, and possibly death. Some people with gene mutations that cause isovaleric acidemia are asymptomatic and never experience any signs and symptoms of the condition.

Treatment includes a protein-restrictive diet to lower the levels of accumulating isovaleric acid, which is toxic to the CNS. Oral administration of glycine and carnitine supplementation may be prescribed because they interact with isovaleric acid to form nontoxic, readily excreted products.

The urine of newborns can be screened for isovaleric acidemia using MS/MS or chromatography. Laboratory results reveal metabolic acidosis, mild-to-moderate ketonuria, hyperammonemia, thrombocytopenia, and neutropenia.

Homocystinuria

Homocystinuria is yet another inherited autosomal recessive disorder of amino acid metabolism. In homocystinuria, it is the lack of the enzyme cystathionine β-synthase necessary for the metabolism of the amino acid methionine, that results in elevated plasma and urine levels of methionine and of the precursor homocysteine. The incidence of this disease is about 1 in 200,000 births. Infants seem to be healthy, and early symptoms, if any, are indistinct. Associated clinical findings in late childhood include osteoporosis, dislocated lenses in the eye resulting from the lack of cysteine synthesis essential for collagen formation, and, frequently, mental retardation.[19] This defect leads to a multisystemic disorder of the connective tissue, muscles, CNS, thinning and weakening of bones, and thrombosis resulting from the toxicity of homocysteine to the vascular endothelium if it goes untreated.

Treatment is a dietary restriction of methionine (low protein) as well as high doses of vitamin B_6. Slightly less than 50% of patients respond to this treatment and need an intake of supplemental vitamin B_6 for the rest of their lives. Those who do not respond to this usual treatment need trimethylglycine, and a normal dose of folic acid supplement and sometimes cysteine added in the diet is helpful.

Neonatal screening consists of the Guthrie test using L-methionine sulfoximine as the metabolic inhibitor. Increased plasma methionine levels from affected infants will result in bacterial growth. HPLC is the test used as the confirmatory method, with a methionine level greater than 2 mg/dL confirming positive results from the screening test. MS/MS is also used in screening programs to test for methionine levels. Alternatively, elevations in urinary total homocysteine can be measured in high testing volumes and provide a rapid turnaround by using liquid chromatography–electrospray tandem mass spectrometry (LC-MS/MS). This method is based on the analysis of 100 μL of either plasma or urine with homocysteine (2 nmol) added as the internal standard. After sample reduction and deproteinization, the analysis is performed in the multiple reaction monitoring mode, with detection through the transition from the precursor to the production. A batch of 40 specimens can be completed in less than 1 hour and can be automated.[20]

Elevations of homocysteine are also of interest in the investigation of cardiovascular risk. Approximately 50% of individuals with untreated homocystinuria and significantly elevated levels of plasma homocysteine (200 to 300 mmol/L) experience a thromboembolic event before the age of 30. Furthermore, mild homocysteine elevation (>15 mmol/L) occurs in 20% to 30% of patients with atherosclerotic disease. In addition to the cystathionine β-synthase deficiency described earlier, hyperhomocysteinemia can be caused by low folate concentrations, vitamin B_{12} deficiency, decline in renal function, and a genetic alteration in the enzyme methylenetetrahydrofolate reductase, which converts homocysteine back to methionine.

Citrullinemia
Citrullinemia belongs to a class of genetic diseases called urea cycle disorders. The urea cycle is a metabolic sequence that takes place in liver cells to process excess nitrogen that is generated when protein is used by the body. The excess nitrogen is used in urea formation, which is then excreted in urine.

Citrullinemia is inherited in an autosomal recessive pattern. Type I citrullinemia is the most common form of the disorder, affecting about 1 in 57,000 births. Type II

citrullinemia is found primarily in the Japanese population, where it occurs in an estimated 1 in 100,000 to 230,000 people.

Type I citrullinemia is the metabolic defect caused by the lack of the enzyme argininosuccinic acid synthetase, which causes a buildup of the amino acid citrulline as well as ammonia in the blood. In affected infants, clinical symptoms include lack of appetite, failure to thrive, vomiting, lethargy, seizures, and coma, as ammonia builds up in the body. If not treated promptly, the result is severe brain damage or death. Less commonly, a milder form of type I citrullinemia can develop later in childhood or adulthood.

Type II citrullinemia is caused by a mutation of the gene that would otherwise provide instructions for making the protein citrin. Citrin helps transport molecules inside cells that are used in the production and breakdown of simple sugars, the production of proteins, and the urea cycle. Molecules transported by citrin are also involved in the production of nucleotides, the building blocks of DNA and RNA. In type II citrullinemia, cells are prevented from making citrin, which inhibits the urea cycle and disrupts the production of proteins and nucleotides. The resulting buildup of ammonia and other toxic substances leads to clinical symptoms affecting the nervous system. These symptoms can be life threatening and are known to be triggered by certain medications, infections, surgery, and alcohol intake in people with adult-onset type II citrullinemia.

Treatment of citrullinemia includes a high-caloric, protein-restrictive diet; arginine supplementation; and administration of sodium benzoate and sodium phenylacetate.

Argininosuccinic Aciduria
Argininosuccinic aciduria (ASA) is inherited in an autosomal recessive pattern that also belongs to a class of genetic diseases, the urea cycle disorders. ASA occurs in approximately 1 in 70,000 newborns. Babies born with argininosuccinic acidemia lack the enzyme argininosuccinic acid lyase, which prevents the conversion of argininosuccinic acid into arginine. Elevated levels of argininosuccinic acid also cause buildup of the amino acid citrulline in the blood. Due to mutation of the *ASL* gene, the cause of ASA, the urea cycle cannot proceed normally and nitrogen accumulates in the blood in the form of ammonia. Ammonia is especially damaging to the nervous system, as well as causing eventual damage to the liver. ASA usually becomes evident while the newborn is still in the hospital. Clinical symptoms of ASA may begin with lethargy and unwillingness to eat.

Treatment of ASA includes a high-calorie, protein-restrictive diet; arginine supplementation; and administration of sodium benzoate and sodium phenylacetate.

CASE STUDY 11-1

Victoria and Rusty were worried about their infant Bailey since his first trip to the hospital at 3 weeks of age. That time he had a temperature of 103°F and a runny nose. The emergency physician checked Bailey over but sent him home saying it was only a common cold, probably brought home by his older siblings, and that all would be fine. But Bailey's health has not been fine as he has been having an unusual number of bacterial infections and he is not yet quite 1 year old. The antibiotics that Bailey's physician prescribed have cleared up his bacterial respiratory infections but another infection always follows.

Now that Bailey is back at the hospital with pneumonia, his physician has ordered a number of other laboratory tests as he is now worried about Bailey's immune system. The studies showed that Bailey had normal levels of B cells and T cells, with his immunoglobulin levels and hematology results listed in CASE STUDY TABLE 11-1.1.

CASE STUDY TABLE 11-1.1
LABORATORY RESULTS

TEST	BAILEY'S VALUE	REFERENCE RANGE
Hct	35%	6 mo–2 y: 30.9–37.0%
Hgb	11.9 g/dL	6 mo–2 y: 10.3–12.4 g/dL
WBC	$14.0 \times 10^3/\mu L$	6 mo–2 y: $6.2–14.5 \times 10^3/\mu L$
IgG	153 mg/dL	1–3 y: 507–1,407 mg/dL
IgM	576 mg/dL	1–3 y: 18–171 mg/dL
IgA	11 mg/dL	1–3 y: 63–298 mg/dL
IgD	0 mg/dL	Newborn to adult: 0–8 mg/dL
IgE	1 kIU/L	1–3 y: <90 kIU/L
Total protein	8.7 g/dL	1 y: 5.4–7.5 g/dL
Albumin	3.8 g/dL	1–3 y: 3.4–4.2 g/dL

Questions

1. List the immunoglobulin types, Bailey's level as normal or abnormal, and the function(s) of each type.

2. Why do Bailey's recurring bacterial infections correlate with these laboratory results?

3. What is immunoglobulin isotype switching? How does isotype switching explain the lack of IgG, IgA, and IgE in Bailey's blood?

4. List the immunoglobulin type and the age it appears in the blood of a baby from birth to 18 months.

5. What treatment can be given to Bailey? Immediately? In the future?

It should be noted that the newborn screening test cannot differentiate citrullinemia from argininosuccinic acidemia.[21]

Cystinuria

Cystinuria is an inherited autosomal recessive defect that is caused by a defect in the amino acid transport system rather than a metabolic enzyme deficiency. Cystinuria is characterized by the inadequate reabsorption of cystine during the filtering process in the kidneys, resulting in an excessive concentration of this amino acid. Cystine precipitates out of the urine and forms stones in the kidneys, ureters, or bladder. The kidney stones often recur throughout a patient's lifetime and are directly or indirectly responsible for all of the signs and symptoms of the disease, including hematuria, pain in the side due to kidney pain, and urinary tract infections.

Treatment for cystinuria is to prevent the formation of cystine stones. This is mainly accomplished by increasing the volume of urine to reduce the concentration of cystine in the urine and reduce its precipitating from the urine and forming stones. High fluid intake means an absolute minimum of 4 L of water per day. When a consistent high fluid intake does not stop the formation of stones, the drug penicillamine is prescribed. Penicillamine forms a more soluble complex with cystine, because cystine, itself, is relatively insoluble. Percutaneous nephrolithotripsy has been performed as an alternative to surgery to remove the kidney stones.

Cystinuria can be diagnosed by testing the urine for cystine using cyanide nitroprusside, which produces a red-purple color on reaction with sulfhydryl groups. False-positive results as a result of homocysteine must be ruled out. Another laboratory finding is a large amount of urinary levels of three other amino acids with a similar structure to cystine—lysine, arginine, and ornithine. Ion exchange chromatography can be used for quantitative analysis of amino acids in urine or plasma.

Amino Acid Analysis

Blood samples for amino acid analysis should be drawn after at least a 6- to 8-hour fast to avoid the effect of absorbed amino acids originating from dietary proteins. The sample is collected in a heparin tube with the plasma promptly removed from the cells, taking care not to aspirate the platelet and white cell layer to prevent contamination with platelet or leukocyte amino acids. White blood cell levels of aspartic acid and glutamic acid, for example, are about 100 times higher than those in plasma. Hemolysis is unacceptable for the same reason. Deproteinization should be performed within 30 minutes of sample collection, and analysis should be performed immediately or the sample frozen at −20°C to −40°C.

Urinary amino acid analysis can be performed on a random specimen for screening purposes. For quantitation, a

24-hour urine sample preserved with thymol or organic solvents is required. Amniotic fluid also may be analyzed.

For a screening test, the method of choice is thin-layer chromatography. The application of either one- or two-dimensional separations depends on the purpose of the analysis. If searching for a particular category of amino acids, such as branched-chain amino acids or even a single amino acid, usually one-dimensional separations are sufficient. For more general screening, two-dimensional chromatography is essential. The amino acids migrate along one solvent front and then the chromatogram is rotated 90° and a second solvent migration occurs. A variety of solvents have been used, including butanol, acetic acid, water and ethanol, and ammonia and water mixtures. The chromatogram is viewed by staining with ninhydrin, which gives most amino acids a blue color. Amino acids can be separated and quantitated by ion exchange chromatography, an HPLC reversed-phase system equipped with fluorescence detection,[22] or capillary electrophoresis. Another technique that provides a highly specific and sensitive method for the measurement of amino acids is MS/MS.[23]

PROTEINS

Importance

Every function in the living cell depends on proteins. From the few examples of the functions of proteins given next, it is easy to see that proteins are truly the physical basis of life.[24] Motion and locomotion depend on contractile proteins—muscle movement, for example.

- All biochemical reactions are catalyzed by enzymes, which contain protein.
- The structure of cells and the extracellular matrix that surrounds all cells is largely made of the protein group collagens. Collagens are the most abundant protein in the human body.
- The transport of materials in body fluids depends on proteins such as transferrin, receptors for hormones are transmembrane proteins, and transcription factors, needed to initiate the transcription of a gene, are proteins.
- Proteins make up antibodies, which are a major component of the immune system.

Molecular Size

Proteins are macromolecules (a molecule with a molecular mass of several thousand or more). They are polymers built from one or more unbranched chains of amino acids. A typical protein contains 200 to 300 amino acids, but some are much smaller (peptides) and some are much larger (titin, in muscle) and range in molecular mass from approximately 6,000 for insulin to several millions for some structural proteins.

Synthesis

Most plasma proteins are synthesized in the liver and secreted by the hepatocyte into the circulation. The immunoglobulins are exceptions because they are synthesized in plasma cells. It is the information encoded in genes, specified by the nucleotide sequence, that provides each protein with its own unique amino acid sequence. This amino acid sequence of a polypeptide chain is determined by a corresponding sequence of bases (guanine, cytosine, adenine, and thymine) in the DNA contained in the specific gene. This genetic code is a set of three nucleotides known as codons, with each three-nucleotide combination standing for a specific amino acid. Because DNA contains four nucleotides, the total number of possible codons is 64; therefore, some redundancy in the genetic code allows for some amino acids to be specified by more than one codon. The double-stranded DNA unfolds in the nucleus, and one strand is used as a template for the formation of a complementary strand of mRNA. This first process is known as *transcription*, when genes encoded in DNA are first used to produce a mature mRNA. The mRNA is then used as a template for protein synthesis by the ribosome. The mRNA is manufactured in the cell nucleus and then translocated across the nuclear membrane into the cytoplasm where it attaches to ribosomes, for protein synthesis to take place.

The process of synthesizing a protein from an mRNA template is known as translation. The mRNA is loaded onto the ribosome and is read three nucleotides at a time by matching each codon to its base pairing anticodon located on a tRNA molecule, which carries the amino acid corresponding to the codon it recognizes to the ribosome. This process continues until the mRNA message is read and all amino acids are in the specific sequence to form the polypeptide chain. The code on the mRNA also contains initiation and termination codons for the peptide chain.

The next step in protein synthesis is getting the amino acid to the ribosomes. First, the amino acid is activated in a reaction that requires energy and a specific enzyme for each amino acid. This activated amino acid complex is then attached to another kind of RNA, tRNA, with the subsequent release of the activating enzyme and adenosine monophosphate. The tRNA is a short chain of RNA that occurs free in the cytoplasm. Each amino acid has a specific tRNA that contains three bases that correspond to the three bases in the mRNA. The tRNA carries its particular amino acid to the ribosome and attaches to the mRNA in accordance with the matching codon. In this manner, the amino acids are aligned in sequence. As each new tRNA brings in the next amino acid, the preceding amino acid is transferred onto the amino group of the new amino acid and enzymes located in the ribosomes form a peptide bond. The tRNA is released

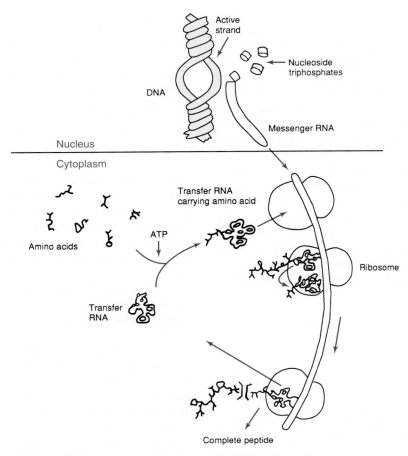

FIGURE 11-4 Schematic summary of protein synthesis.

into the cytoplasm, where it can pick up another amino acid, and the cycle repeats. When the terminal codon is reached, the peptide chain is detached and the ribosome and mRNA dissociate. Figure 11-4 illustrates protein synthesis. Intracellular proteins are generally synthesized on free ribosomes, whereas proteins made by the liver for secretion are made on ribosomes attached to the rough endoplasmic reticulum. Protein synthesis occurs at the rate of approximately two to six peptide bonds per second. The hormones that assist in controlling protein synthesis are thyroxine, growth hormone, insulin, and testosterone. The hormones that assist in controlling protein catabolism are glucagon and cortisol.

Catabolism and Nitrogen Balance

Unlike fats and carbohydrates, nitrogen has no designated storage depots in the body. The biologic value of dietary proteins is related to the extent to which they provide all the necessary amino acids.

Insufficient dietary quantities of even one amino acid can quickly limit the synthesis and lower the body levels of many essential proteins.[25] Most proteins in the body are constantly being repetitively synthesized and then degraded. Ordinarily, a balance exists between protein anabolism (synthesis) and catabolism (breakdown). Normally, this turnover totals about 125 to 220 g of protein each day, with the rate of individual proteins widely varying. For example, the plasma proteins and most intracellular proteins are rapidly degraded, having half-lives of hours or days; some of the structural proteins, such as collagen, are metabolically stable and have half-lives of years. Normal, healthy adults are generally in nitrogen balance, with intake and excretion being equal. Pregnant women, growing children, and adults recovering from major illness are often in positive nitrogen balance. Their intake of nitrogen exceeds their loss as net protein synthesis proceeds. When more nitrogen is excreted than is incorporated into the body, an individual is in negative nitrogen balance, and this occurs in conditions in which there is excessive tissue destruction, such as burns, wasting diseases, continual high fevers, or starvation.

The disintegration of protein occurs in the digestive tract, kidneys, and, particularly, the liver. Nitrogen elimination begins intracellularly with protein degradation.

There are two main routes for converting intracellular proteins to free amino acids: a lysosomal pathway, which degrades extracellular and some intracellular proteins, and cytosolic pathways, which are important in degrading intracellular proteins.

The central reactions that remove amino acid nitrogen from the body are known as transaminations. Transaminations involve moving an α-amino group from a donor α-amino acid to the keto carbon of an acceptor α-ketoacid. These reversible reactions are catalyzed by a group of intracellular enzymes known as *transaminases*. These reactions remove nitrogen from free amino acids, ultimately producing ammonia and ketoacids. The ammonia is converted to urea by the urea cycle in hepatocytes and excreted in the urine, and the ketoacids are oxidized by means of the citric acid cycle and converted to glucose or fat.

Structure

There are four distinct levels of a protein's structure: primary, secondary, tertiary, and quaternary. *Primary structure* represents the number and types of amino acids in the specific amino acid sequence. In order to function properly, proteins must have the correct sequence of amino acids. For example, when the amino acid valine is substituted for glutamic acid in the α-chain of hemoglobin A, hemoglobin S is formed, which results in sickle cell disease.

Secondary structure is regularly repeating structures stabilized by hydrogen bonds between the amino acids within the protein. Common secondary structures are the α-helix, β-pleated sheet, and turns, with most serum proteins forming a helix.[26] Secondary structures add new properties to a protein such as strength and flexibility (Fig. 11-5).

Tertiary structure refers to the overall shape, or conformation, of the protein molecule. The conformation is known as the *fold*, or the spatial relationship of the secondary structures to one another. Tertiary structures are three-dimensional. Tertiary structure results from the interaction of side chains and is stabilized through the hydrophobic effect, ionic attraction, hydrogen bonds, and disulfide bonds. The function and physical and chemical properties of a protein depend on its tertiary structure.[27]

Quaternary structure is defined as the shape or structure that results from the interaction of more than one protein molecule, or protein subunits, held together by noncovalent forces such as hydrogen bonds and electrostatic interactions, which are part of the larger protein complex with a precise three-dimensional configuration.

When the secondary, tertiary, or quaternary structure of a protein is disturbed, the protein may lose its functional and chemical characteristics. This loss of its native, or naturally occurring, folded structure is called denaturation. Denaturation can be caused by heat, hydrolysis by strong acid or alkali, enzymatic action, exposure to urea or other substances, or exposure to ultraviolet light.

Nitrogen Content

Proteins consist of the elements carbon, oxygen, hydrogen, nitrogen, and sulfur. It is the fact that proteins contain nitrogen that sets them apart from pure carbohydrates and lipids, which do not contain nitrogen atoms. The nitrogen content of serum protein is, on average, approximately 16%. This measurement of nitrogen content is used in one method for total protein.

Charge and Isoelectric Point

Proteins contain many ionizable groups on the side chains of their amino acids as well as on their N- and C-terminal ends. Because of this, proteins can be positively and negatively charged. The acid or basic groups that are not involved in the peptide bond can exist in different charged forms, depending on the pH of the surrounding environment (Fig. 11-6).

The side chains of lysine, arginine, and histidine include basic groups, and acidic groups are found on the side chains of glutamate, aspartate, cysteine, and tyrosine. The pH of the solution, the pK_a of the side chain, and the side chain's environment influence the charge on each side chain. The relationship between pH, pK_a, and charge for individual amino acids can be described by the Henderson-Hasselbalch equation:

$$pH = pK_a + \log \frac{[\text{conjugate base}]}{[\text{conjugate acid}]} \quad \text{(Eq. 11-1)}$$

In general terms, as the pH of a solution increases, deprotonation of the acidic and basic groups on proteins occurs, so that carboxyl groups are converted to carboxylate anions (R–COOH to R–COO⁻) and ammonium

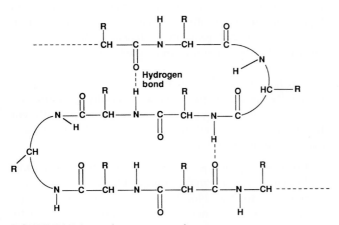

FIGURE 11-5 Secondary structure of proteins.

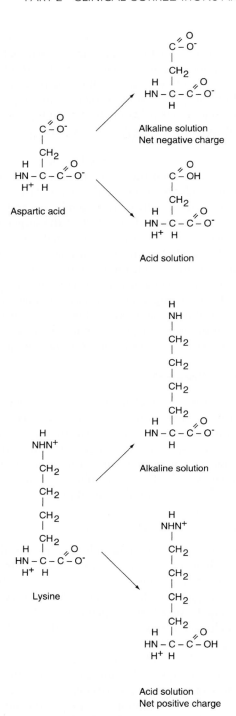

FIGURE 11-6 Charged states of amino acids.

positively charged groups equals the number of negatively charged groups in a protein. If a protein is placed in a solution that has a pH greater than the pI, the protein will be negatively charged; at a pH less than the pI, the protein will be positively charged. Proteins differ in their pI values, but for most proteins it occurs in the pH range of 5.5 to 8. Because proteins carry different net charges at any given pH, this difference in size of the charge is the basis for several procedures for separating and quantifying proteins.

Solubility

Soluble proteins have a charge on their surfaces. The surface of a protein has a net charge that depends on the number and type of its amino acids and on pH. A protein has its lowest solubility at its pI. If there is a charge at the protein surface, the protein is hydrophilic (prefers to interact with water, rather than with other protein molecules). This charge makes it more soluble. Without a net charge, protein–protein interactions and precipitation are more likely. The solubility of proteins in blood requires a pH in the range of 7.35 to 7.45. Methods have been developed to separate proteins based on their solubility.

Classification

From 2003 to 2005, the Human Plasma Proteome Project directed by the Human Plasma Proteome Organization (HUPO) prepared and distributed reference specimens of human serum and plasma to 55 participating laboratories worldwide. Some of the long-term goals of this project are the comprehensive analysis of plasma and serum protein constituents in people and their physiologic, pathologic, and pharmacologic applications. Protocols used combinations of depletion, fractionation, mass spectrometry, and immunoassay methods linked via search engines and annotation groups to gene and protein databases. A new human plasma proteome database was created with, obviously, much work yet to be done.[28] The findings from the collaborative project and from laboratory-specific ancillary projects were published in a special issue of *Proteomics*, "Exploring the Human Plasma Proteome" in August 2005.

Classification by Protein Functions
Generally speaking, proteins do everything in the living cells.[29] Proteins are responsible for many different functions in a cell, making function one of the common classifications of proteins.

- **Enzymes**—proteins that catalyze chemical reactions. Enzymes are normally found inside cells but are released to the blood in tissue damage, making enzyme measurement a very important diagnostic tool. Examples of groups of enzymes tested in the

groups are converted to amino groups ($R-NH_3^+$ to $R-NH_2$).

The pH at which an amino acid or protein has no net charge is known as its isoelectric point (pI). When the pH > pI, a protein has a net negative charge, and when the pH < pI, a protein has a net positive charge. Therefore, the pI is the point at which the number of clinical laboratory are the transaminases, dehydrogenases, and phosphatases.

- **Hormones**—proteins that are chemical messengers that control the actions of specific cells or organs. Hormones affect growth and development, metabolism, sexual function, reproduction, and behavior. Examples of hormones that are tested in the clinical laboratory in blood, urine, or saliva are insulin, testosterone, growth hormone, follicle-stimulating hormone, and cortisol.
- **Transport proteins**—proteins that transport movement of ions, small molecules, or macromolecules, such as hormones, vitamins, minerals, and lipids, across a biologic membrane. Examples of commonly measured transport proteins are hemoglobin, albumin, and transferrin.
- **Immunoglobulins (antibodies)**—proteins produced by B cells (lymphocytes) in the bone marrow that mediate the humoral immune response to identify and neutralize foreign objects. Examples of immunoglobulins are IgG, IgM, and IgA.
- **Structural proteins**—fibrous proteins that are the structures of cells and tissues such as muscle, tendons, and bone matrix. Collagen, elastin, and keratin are examples of structural proteins.
- **Storage proteins**—proteins that serve as reserves of metal ions and amino acids that can be released and used later without harm occurring to cells during the time of storage. The most widely studied and tested storage protein is ferritin, which stores iron to be later used in the manufacture of hemoglobin.
- **Energy source**—plasma proteins that serve as a reserve source of energy for tissues and muscle.
- **Osmotic force**—plasma proteins that function in the distribution of water throughout the compartments of the body. Their colloid osmotic force, due to their size, does not allow proteins to cross the capillary membranes. As a result, water is absorbed from the tissue into the venous portion of the capillary.

When the concentration of plasma proteins is significantly decreased, the concomitant decrease in the plasma colloidal osmotic (oncotic) pressure results in increased levels of interstitial fluid and edema. This is often seen in renal disease when proteinuria occurs due to loss of plasma proteins into urine.

Protein functions are summarized in Table 11-2.

Classification by Protein Structure

- **Database (manual)**—The Structural Classification of Proteins (SCOP) database was created by manual inspection and is aided by a battery of automated methods. The goal of SCOP is to provide a detailed and comprehensive description of the structural domains based on similarities of their amino acid sequences and three-dimensional structures. SCOP utilizes four levels of structural classification: class, fold, superfamily, and family. Originally published in 1995, SCOP is usually updated at least once yearly by Alexei G. Murzin et al., upon whose expertise the classification rests.[30]
- **Database (automated)**—The Families of Structurally Similar Proteins (FSSP) is also known as Fold classification based on the structure–structure alignment of proteins. The FSSP protein classification is based on a three-dimensional structure comparison of protein structures in the Protein Data Bank. Alignments and classification are done automatically and are updated continuously by the Dali (Distance matrix ALIgnment) server, which is an automatic server that makes a three-dimensional comparison of protein structures.[31]
- **Simple proteins**—Simple proteins contain peptide chains composed of only amino acids. Simple proteins may be globular or fibrous in shape. Globular proteins are globe-like, symmetrical proteins that are soluble in water. Globular proteins are transporters, enzymes, and messengers. Examples of globular proteins are

TABLE 11-2	FUNCTIONS OF PROTEINS
Energy—tissue nutrition	
Osmotic force—maintenance of water distribution between cells and tissue, interstitial compartments, and the vascular system of the body	
Acid–base balance—participation as buffers to maintain pH	
Transport—metabolic substances	
Antibodies—part of immune defense system	
Hormones—hormones and receptors	
Structure—connective tissue	
Enzymes—catalysts	
Hemostasis—participation in coagulation of blood	

albumin, hemoglobin, and the immunoglobulins IgG, IgA, and IgM. Fibrous proteins form long protein filaments or subunits, are asymmetrical and usually inert, and are generally water insoluble due to their hydrophobic R groups. Fibrous proteins are structural, such as connective tissues, tendons, bone, and muscle. Examples of fibrous proteins include troponin and collagen.

- **Conjugated Proteins**—Conjugated proteins consist of a protein and a nonprotein (prosthetic) group. The prosthetic group is the nonamino part of a conjugated protein. The prosthetic group may be lipids, carbohydrates, porphyrins, metals, and others. It is the prosthetic groups that define the characteristics of these proteins. Examples of conjugated proteins are the metalloproteins, glycoproteins, lipoproteins, and nucleoproteins. Metalloproteins have a metal ion attached to the protein, either directly, as in ferritin (which contains iron) and ceruloplasmin (which contains copper), or as complex metals (metal plus another prosthetic group), such as hemoglobin and flavoproteins. Lipoproteins have lipids such as cholesterol and triglyceride linked to proteins, such as high-density lipoproteins (HDLs) and very low density lipoproteins (VLDLs). Several protein groups are used to describe carbohydrates joined to proteins. Generally, those molecules with 10% to 40% carbohydrate are called glycoproteins. Examples of glycoproteins are haptoglobin and α_1-antitrypsin. When the percentage of carbohydrate linked to protein is higher, the proteins are called mucoproteins or proteoglycans. An example of a mucoprotein is mucin, a lubricant that protects body surfaces from friction or erosion. Increased mucin production occurs in many adenocarcinomas, including cancer of the pancreas, lung, breast, ovary, and colon. Moreover, mucins are also being investigated for their potential as diagnostic markers.[32] Nucleoproteins are those proteins that are combined with nucleic acids, DNA or RNA. Chromatin is an example of a nucleoprotein that is the complex of DNA and protein that makes up chromosomes.

PLASMA PROTEINS

The plasma proteins are the most frequently analyzed of all the proteins. The major measured plasma proteins are divided into two groups: albumin and globulins. There are four major types of globulins, each with specific properties and actions. A typical blood panel will provide four different measurements—total protein, albumin, globulins, and the albumin/globulin (A/G) ratio. Some of the more significant plasma proteins and their functions, structures, and relation to disease states are discussed later. Characteristics of selected plasma proteins are listed in Table 11-3.

TABLE 11-3	CHARACTERISTICS OF SELECTED PLASMA PROTEINS				
	REFERENCE VALUE (ADULT, G/L)	**MOLECULAR MASS (Da)**	**ISOELECTRIC POINT, pI**	**ELECTROPHORETIC MOBILITY pH 8.6**	
Prealbumin	0.1–0.4	55,000	4.7	7.6	Indicator of nutrition; binds thyroid hormones and retinol-binding protein
Albumin	35–55	66,300	4.9	5.9	Binds bilirubin, steroids, fatty acids; major contributor to oncotic pressure
α_1-Globulins					
α_1-Antitrypsin	2–4	53,000	4.0	5.4	Acute-phase reactant; protease inhibitor
α_1-Fetoprotein	1×10^5	76,000	2.7	6.1	Principal fetal protein. Elevated levels indicate risk for spina bifida
α_1-Acid glycoprotein (orosomucoid)	0.55–1.4	44,000		5.2	Acute-phase reactant, may be related to immune response
α_1-Lipoprotein	2.5–3.9	200,000		4.4–5.4	Transports lipids (HDL)

TABLE 11-3	CHARACTERISTICS OF SELECTED PLASMA PROTEINS (CONTINUED)				
	REFERENCE VALUE (ADULT, G/L)	MOLECULAR MASS (Da)	ISOELECTRIC POINT, pI	ELECTROPHORETIC MOBILITY pH 8.6	
α_1-Antichymotrypsin	0.3–0.6	68,000		Inter α	Inhibits serine proteinases
Inter-α–trypsin inhibitor	0.2–0.7	160,000		Inter α	Inhibits serine proteinases
Gc-globulin	0.2–0.55	59,000		Inter α	Transports vitamin D and binds actin
α_2-GLOBULINS					
HAPTOGLOBINS					
Type 1-1	1.0–2.2	100,000		4.5	Acute-phase reactant; binds hemoglobin
Type 2-1	1.6–3.0	200,000	4.1	3.5–4.0	Binds hemoglobin
Type 2-2	1.2–1.6	400,000		3.5–4.0	Binds hemoglobin
Ceruloplasmin	0.15–0.60	134,000	4.4	4.6	Acute-phase reactant, oxidase activity; contains copper
α_2-Macroglobulin	1.5–4.2	725,000	5.4	4.2	Inhibits proteases
β-GLOBULINS					
Pre-β lipoprotein	1.5–2.3	250,000		3.4–4.3	Transports lipids (primarily VLDL triglyceride)
Transferrin	2.04–3.60	76,000	5.9	3.1	Transports iron
Hemopexin	0.5–1.0	57,000–80,000		3.1	Binds heme
β-Lipoprotein	2.5–4.4	3,000,000		3.1	Transports lipids (primarily LDL cholesterol)
β_2-Microglobulin (B2M)	0.001–0.002	11,800		β_2	Component of leukocyte antigen (HLA) molecules
C4 complement	0.20–0.65	206,000		0.8–1.4	Immune response
C3 complement	0.55–1.80	180,000		0.8–1.4	Immune response
C1q complement	0.15	400,000			Immune response
Fibrinogen	2.0–4.5	341,000	5.8	2.1	Precursor of fibrin clot
CRP	0.01	118,000	6.2		Acute-phase reactant, motivates phagocytosis in inflammatory disease
g-GLOBULINS					
Immunoglobulin G	8.0–12.0	150,000	5.8–7.3	0.5–2.6	Antibodies
Immunoglobulin A	0.7–3.12	180,000		2.1	Antibodies (in secretions)
Immunoglobulin M	0.5–2.80	900,000		2.1	Antibodies (early response)
Immunoglobulin D	0.005–0.2	170,000		1.9	Antibodies
Immunoglobulin E	6×10^4	190,000		2.3	Antibodies (reagins, allergy)

HDL, high-density lipoproteins; VLDL, very low density lipoprotein; HLA, human leukocyte antigen; CRP, C-reactive protein.

Prealbumin (Transthyretin)

Prealbumin is so named because it migrates before albumin in the classic electrophoresis of serum or plasma proteins. It can also be separated by high-resolution electrophoresis (HRE) or immunoelectrophoresis techniques. Prealbumin is the transport protein for thyroxine and triiodothyronine (thyroid hormones); it also binds with retinol-binding protein to form a complex that transports retinol (vitamin A) and is rich in tryptophan. Prealbumin is decreased in hepatic damage, acute-phase inflammatory response, and tissue necrosis. A low prealbumin level is a sensitive marker of poor nutritional status. When a diet is deficient in protein, hepatic synthesis of proteins is reduced, with the resulting decrease in the level of the proteins originating in the liver, including prealbumin, albumin, and β-globulins. Because prealbumin has a short half-life of approximately 2 days, it decreases more rapidly than do other proteins. Prealbumin is increased in patients receiving steroids, in alcoholism, and in chronic renal failure.

Albumin

Albumin is synthesized in the liver from 585 amino acids at the rate of 9 to 12 g/d with no reserve or storage. It is the protein present in highest concentration in the plasma. Albumin also exists in the extravascular (interstitial) space. In fact, the total extravascular albumin exceeds the total intravascular amount by 30%, but the concentration of albumin (plasma albumin concentration = intravascular albumin mass/plasma volume) in the blood is much greater than its concentration in the interstitial space. Albumin leaves the circulation at a rate of 4% to 5% of total intravascular albumin per hour. This rate of movement is known as the transcapillary escape rate, which measures systemic capillary efflux of albumin. Albumin is responsible for nearly 80% of the colloid osmotic pressure (COP) of the intravascular fluid, which maintains the appropriate fluid balance in the tissue. Albumin also buffers pH and is a negative acute-phase reactant protein.

Another prime function of albumin is its capacity to bind various substances in the blood. There are four binding sites on albumin, and these have varying specificities for different substances. Albumin transports thyroid hormones; other hormones, particularly fat-soluble ones; iron; and fatty acids. For example, albumin binds unconjugated bilirubin, salicylic acid (aspirin), fatty acids, calcium (Ca^{2+}) and magnesium (Mg^{2+}) ions, and many drugs, and serum albumin levels can affect the half-life of drugs. This binding characteristic is also exhibited with certain dyes, providing a method for the quantitation of albumin.

Several recent studies have focused the clinical applications of glycated (or glycosylated) albumin as a more sensitive indicator of short-term hyperglycemic control. Glycated hemoglobin represents trends in serum glucose over a period of 3 months or approximately 120 days (the life span of red blood cells [RBCs]). As the half-life of serum albumin is 20 days, glycated albumin represents serum glucose patterns approximating 1 month. Affinity chromatographic methods based on specific interaction of boronic acids with glycated proteins have also been applied to determine serum concentrations of glycated albumin.[33]

Decreased concentrations of serum albumin may be caused by the following:

- An inadequate source of amino acids that occurs in malnutrition and malabsorption
- Liver disease, resulting in decreased synthesis by the hepatocytes. Note that the increase in globulins that occurs in early cirrhosis, however, balances the loss in albumin to give a total protein concentration within acceptable limits
- Protein-losing enteropathy or gastrointestinal loss as interstitial fluid leaks out in inflammation and disease of the intestinal tract as in diarrhea
- Kidney loss of albumin via urine in renal disease. Albumin is normally excreted in very small amounts. This excess excretion occurs when the glomerulus no longer functions to restrict the passage of proteins from the blood as in nephrotic syndrome
- Skin loss in the absence of the skin barrier such as in burns or exfoliative dermatitis
- Hypothyroidism
- Dilution by excess: polydipsia (drinking too much water) or excess administration of intravenous fluids
- Acute disease states
- Mutation resulting from an autosomal recessive trait causing analbuminemia (absence of albumin) or bisalbuminemia (the presence of albumin that has unusual molecular characteristics) demonstrated by the presence of two albumin bands instead of the single band usually seen by electrophoresis. Both are rare.
- Redistribution by hemodilution, increased capillary permeability (increased interstitial albumin), or decreased lymph clearance. In sepsis, there is a profound reduction in plasma albumin associated with marked fluid shifts.

Abnormally high albumin levels are seldom clinically important. Increased serum albumin levels are seen only with dehydration or after excessive albumin infusion.[34]

Globulins

The globulin group of proteins consists of α_1, α_2, β, and γ fractions. Each fraction consists of a number of different proteins with different functions. The following subsections describe selected examples of the globulins.

α_1-Antitrypsin

α_1-Antitrypsin, a glycoprotein mainly synthesized in the liver, has as its most important function the inhibition of the protease neutrophil elastase. Mutations in the *SERPINA1* gene cause α_1-antitrypsin deficiency. Neutrophil elastase is released from leukocytes to fight infection, but it can destroy alveoli, which can lead to emphysema if not controlled by α_1-antitrypsin. Mutations in the *SERPINA1* gene can lead to a deficiency of α_1-antitrypsin protein or an abnormal form of the protein that cannot control neutrophil elastase. The abnormal form of α_1-antitrypsin can also accumulate in the liver and can cause cirrhosis. α_1-Antitrypsin is an acute-phase reactant. Increased levels of α_1-antitrypsin are seen in inflammatory reactions, pregnancy, and contraceptive use. Several phenotypes of α_1-antitrypsin deficiency have been identified. The most common phenotype is MM (allele *Pi*^{M}) and is associated with normal antitrypsin activity. Other alleles are *Pi*^{S}, Pi^Z, Pi^F, and *Pi*$^-$ (null). The homozygous phenotype ZZ individual is most at risk for liver and lung disease from a deficiency of α_1-antitrypsin. Protein replacement therapy, using purified α_1-antitrypsin protein from pooled plasma samples, and smoking cessation can dramatically slow disease progression.

Abnormal α_1-antitrypsin levels are most often found in the laboratory by the lack of an α_1-globulin band on protein electrophoresis because it is the major component (approximately 90%) of the fraction of serum proteins that migrates immediately following albumin. Quantitative methods used to confirm electrophoresis findings are radial immunodiffusion and automated immunonephelometric assays. Phenotyping is done using immunofixation.[35]

α_1-Fetoprotein

α_1-Fetoprotein (AFP) is synthesized in the developing embryo and fetus and then by the parenchymal cells of the liver. AFP levels decrease gradually after birth, reaching adult levels by 8 to 12 months; however, AFP has no known function in normal adults. In normal fetuses, AFP binds the hormone estradiol. It has an electrophoretic mobility between that of albumin and α_1-globulin.

The physiologic function of AFP has not been completely identified, but it has been proposed that the protein protects the fetus from immunologic attack by the mother. Conditions associated with an elevated AFP level include spina bifida, neural tube defects, abdominal wall defects, anencephaly (absence of the major portion of the brain), and general fetal distress. Low levels of maternal AFP indicate an increased risk for Down syndrome and trisomy 18, while it is increased in the presence of twins and neural tube defects.

AFP screening is done between 15 and 20 weeks' gestational age when the maternal AFP increases gradually; therefore, interpretation requires accurate dating of the pregnancy. Measurements of AFP can be affected by laboratory technique, resulting in difficulty comparing absolute results between centers. AFP levels are also affected by maternal weight, race, and diabetes; therefore, test results need to be adjusted for these variables. Because multiples of the median (MoM) is a reflection of an individual patient's value compared with the median, it is used to compensate for these issues. MoM is calculated by dividing the patient's AFP value by the median reference value for that gestational age. Most screening laboratories use 2.0 MoM as the upper limit and 0.5 MoM as the lower limit of normal for maternal serum. The methods commonly used for AFP determinations are radioimmunoassay (RIA) and enzyme-labeled immunoassay (EIA). Maternal screening tests have been established as a triple or quadruple test group using a mathematical calculation involving the levels of these three or four substances (AFP, hCG, unconjugated estriol, and inhibin A) to determine a numeric risk for chromosomal abnormalities in the fetus. This risk is compared with an established cutoff. The interpretation of a test result should be provided by a genetic counselor or clinician to help women and their physicians make decisions about the management of their pregnancies. AFP may also serve as a tumor marker (see Chapter 32).

AFP can be fractionated by affinity electrophoresis into three isoforms—L1, L2, and L3—based on their reactivity with the lectin *Lens culinaris* agglutinin (LCA). AFP-L3 is now being considered as a tumor marker for the North American population for screening chronic liver disease patients for hepatocellular carcinoma (HCC). Results for AFP-L3 are reported as a ratio of LCA-reactive AFP to total AFP (AFP-L3%). Studies have shown that AFP-L3% test results of greater than 10% are associated with a sevenfold increase in the risk of developing HCC within the next 21 months.[36]

α_1-Acid Glycoprotein (Orosomucoid)

α_1-Acid glycoprotein (AAG), a major plasma glycoprotein, is negatively charged even in acid solutions, a fact that gave it its name. This protein is produced by the liver and is an acute-phase reactant. The possibility that AAG regulates immune responses has been suggested by several findings.[37] There is a strong similarity in the amino acid sequences between AAG and immunoglobulin. It is elevated following stress, inflammation and tissue damage, acute myocardial infarction (AMI), trauma, pregnancy, cancer, pneumonia, rheumatoid arthritis, and surgery. Serum AAG levels also provide a useful diagnostic tool in neonates with bacterial infections. In the past decade, the binding of drugs to this plasma protein has become increasingly important in regard to drug action, distribution, and disposition. The analytic methods used

CASE STUDY 11-2

Immediately following the birth of a baby girl, the attending physician requested a protein electrophoretic examination of the mother's serum. This was done on a sample that was obtained on the mother's admission to the hospital the previous day. An electrophoretic examination was also performed on the cord-blood specimen. Laboratory reports are shown in CASE STUDY TABLE 11-2.1.

The appearance of the mother's electrophoretic pattern was within that expected for a healthy person. The electrophoretic pattern of the cord-blood serum resembled the one shown in Figure 11-9C.

**CASE STUDY TABLE 11-2.1
ELECTROPHORESIS VALUES (g/dL)**

	ADULT REFERENCE VALUES	MOTHER'S SERUM	CORD BLOOD
Albumin	3.5–5.0	4.2	3.3
α_1-Globulins	0.1–0.4	0.3	0.0
α_2-Globulins	0.3–0.8	1.2	0.4
β-Globulins	0.6–1.1	1.3	0.7
γ-Globulins	0.5–1.7	1.3	1.0

Questions

1. What protein fraction(s) is/are abnormal in the mother's serum and the cord-blood serum?

2. An abnormality in this/these fraction(s) is/are most often associated with what disease?

3. What other test(s) may be done to confirm this abnormality?

most commonly for the determination of AAG are radial immunodiffusion, immunoturbidity, and nephelometry. Immunofixation has been used to study inherited variants. The normal range for healthy individuals is 50 to 120 mg/dL.

α_1-Antichymotrypsin

α_1-Antichymotrypsin is an α-globulin glycoprotein that is a member of the serine proteinase inhibitor (serpin) family. It inhibits the activity of the enzymes cathepsin G, pancreatic elastase, mast cell chymase, and chymotrypsin by cleaving them into a different shape (conformation). α_1-Antichymotrypsin is produced in the liver and is an acute-phase protein that is increased during inflammation.

Deficiency of this protein has been associated with liver disease. Mutations have been identified in patients with Parkinson disease and chronic obstructive pulmonary disease. α_1-Antichymotrypsin is also associated with the pathogenesis of Alzheimer disease as it is an integral component of the amyloid deposits in Alzheimer disease.[38]

Inter-α-Trypsin Inhibitor

Inter-α-trypsin inhibitors (ITIs) are a family of serine protease inhibitors, assembled from two precursor proteins: a light chain (bikunin) and either one or two heavy chains. While there is only one type of light chain, there are five different homologous heavy chains (ITIHs). ITIH molecules have been shown to play a particularly important role in inflammation and carcinogenesis.[39] Elevations are seen in inflammatory disorders.

Gc-Globulin (Group-Specific Component; Vitamin D–Binding Protein)

Gc-globulin (Gc), synthesized mainly by hepatocytes, is the major carrier protein of vitamin D and its metabolites in the circulation and also transports components such as fatty acids and endotoxin. Due to genetic polymorphism in the Gc gene (codominant alleles), three major electrophoretic variants of Gc exist (Gc2, Gc1s, and Gc1f). Elevations of Gc-globulin are seen in the third trimester of pregnancy and in patients taking estrogen oral contraceptives. Severe liver disease and protein-losing syndromes are associated with low levels.

Gc binds actin released from cells upon injury, and the Gc–actin complexes are rapidly cleared from the circulation, thereby preventing the harmful effects of actin filaments in blood vessels. The resulting decrease in Gc concentration makes Gc usable as a prognostic indicator of survival of patients with significant tissue injury after trauma and among patients with hepatic failure.[40]

Gc may be of importance for bone formation and in the immune system. Gc may act as a co-chemotactic factor in facilitating chemotaxis of neutrophils and monocytes in inflammation. Immunonephelometry, which can be automated, is the method of choice for measurement in the laboratory.

Haptoglobin

Haptoglobin (Hp), an α_2-glycoprotein, is synthesized in the hepatocytes. The mature haptoglobin molecule is a tetramer, consisting of two α and two β chains. Haptoglobin is considered an acute-phase protein that is elevated in many inflammatory diseases, such as ulcerative colitis, acute rheumatic disease, heart attack, and severe infection. It is one of the proteins used to evaluate the rheumatic diseases. Increases are also seen in conditions such as burns and nephrotic syndrome when large amounts of fluid and lower-molecular-weight proteins have been lost. (Haptoglobin testing is not generally used to help diagnose or monitor these conditions.) Haptoglobin phenotype has also been reported as an independent risk factor for cardiovascular disease (CVD) in individuals with type 2 diabetes mellitus.[41]

Three phenotypes of haptoglobin are found in humans: Hp1-1, Hp2-1, and Hp2-2. Homozygous Hp1-1 gives one band. The peptide chains form polymers with each other and with haptoglobin 1 chains to provide the other two electrophoretic patterns, which have been designated as Hp2-1 and Hp2-2 phenotypes. The function of haptoglobin is to bind free hemoglobin to prevent the loss of hemoglobin and its constituent, iron, into the urine. Free hemoglobin is not contained within RBCs. When the haptoglobin and hemoglobin attach, the reticuloendothelial cells (mainly in the spleen) remove the haptoglobin–hemoglobin complex from circulation within minutes of its formation, with iron and amino acids being recycled. The haptoglobin is destroyed.

Haptoglobin testing is used primarily to help detect and evaluate hemolytic anemia and to distinguish it from anemia due to other causes. When haptoglobin levels are decreased, along with an increased reticulocyte count and usually also a decreased RBC count, hemoglobin, and hematocrit, then it is likely that the patient has hemolytic anemia. Haptoglobin has been used to evaluate the degree of intravascular hemolysis that has occurred in transfusion reactions or hemolytic disease of the newborn. If the haptoglobin is normal and the reticulocyte count is increased, then RBC destruction may be occurring in organs such as the spleen and liver. Since the freed hemoglobin is not released into the bloodstream, the haptoglobin is not consumed and therefore will be within the normal reference range. If the haptoglobin concentrations are normal and the reticulocyte count is not increased, then it is likely that any anemia present is not due to RBC breakdown. If haptoglobin levels are decreased without any signs of hemolytic anemia, then it is possible that the liver is not producing adequate amounts of haptoglobin. Radial immunodiffusion and immunonephelometric methods have been used for the quantitative determination of haptoglobin.

Ceruloplasmin

Ceruloplasmin is a copper-containing, α_2-glycoprotein enzyme that is synthesized in the liver. Ceruloplasmin is an acute-phase reactant. It is frequently elevated in inflammation, severe infection, and tissue damage and may be increased with some cancers. It may be increased during pregnancy and with the use of estrogen, oral contraceptives, and medications such as carbamazepine, phenobarbital, and valproic acid. Ninety percent or more of total serum copper is found in ceruloplasmin; the other 10% is bound to albumin.

Ceruloplasmin is primarily ordered along with blood and/or urine copper tests to help diagnose Wilson's disease, an autosomal recessive inherited disorder associated with decreased levels (typically 0.1 g/L) of ceruloplasmin and excess storage of copper in the liver, brain, and other organs resulting in hepatic cirrhosis and neurologic damage. Total serum copper is decreased, but the direct reacting fraction is elevated and the urinary excretion of copper is increased. Copper also deposits in the cornea, producing the characteristic Kayser-Fleischer rings. Low ceruloplasmin is also seen in malnutrition; malabsorption; severe liver disease; nephrotic syndrome; and Menkes syndrome (kinky hair disease), in which a decreased absorption of copper results in a decrease in ceruloplasmin.

The early analytic method of ceruloplasmin determination was based on its copper oxidase activity. Most assays today use immunochemical methods, including radial immunodiffusion and nephelometry.

α_2-Macroglobulin

α_2-Macroglobulin, a large protein, is synthesized by the liver and is a major component of the α_2 band in protein electrophoresis. It is a tetramer of four identical subunits that inhibits proteases such as trypsin, thrombin, kallikrein, and plasmin by means of a bait region that can entrap proteinases, reducing the accessibility of the proteinase functional sites, particularly to large molecules, but not completely inactivating them. After binding with and inhibiting proteases, it is removed by the reticuloendothelial tissues.

In nephrosis, the levels of serum α_2-macroglobulin may increase as much as 10 times because its large size aids in its retention. The protein is also increased in diabetes and liver disease. Use of contraceptive medications and pregnancy increase the serum levels by 20%. The analytic methods that have been used for the assay of this protein are radial immunodiffusion, immunonephelometry, enzyme-linked immunosorbent assay (ELISA), and latex agglutination immunoassay.

Transferrin (Siderophilin)

Transferrin, a glycoprotein, is a negative acute-phase protein synthesized primarily by the liver. Two molecules of ferric iron can bind to each molecule of transferrin, which binds iron very tightly but reversibly. Although iron bound to transferrin is less than 0.1% (4 mg) of the total body iron, dynamically it is the most important iron pool. Normally, only about 20% to 50% of the iron-binding sites on transferrin are occupied. Transferrin is the major component of the β-globulin fraction and appears as a distinct band on HRE.

The major functions of transferrin are the transport of iron and the prevention of loss of iron through the kidney. Its binding of iron prevents iron deposition in the tissue during temporary increases in absorbed iron or free iron. Transferrin transports iron to its storage sites, where it is incorporated into apoferritin, another protein, to form ferritin. Transferrin also carries iron to cells, such as bone marrow, that synthesize hemoglobin and other iron-containing compounds.

Transferrin levels are tested to determine the cause of anemia, to gauge iron metabolism, and to determine the iron-carrying capacity of the blood. Low transferrin can impair hemoglobin production and lead to anemia. A decreased transferrin level can be due to poor production of transferrin as seen in liver disease, malnutrition, or excessive loss of transferrin through the kidneys into the urine in protein-losing disorders such as nephrotic syndrome. Many conditions, including infection and malignancy, can depress transferrin levels.

Transferrin is abnormally high in iron deficiency anemia. A deficiency of plasma transferrin may result in the accumulation of iron in apoferritin or in histiocytes, or it may precipitate in tissue as hemosiderin. Transferrin is also decreased in inflammation. An increase of iron bound to transferrin is found in a hereditary disorder of iron metabolism, hemochromatosis, in which excess iron is deposited in the tissue, especially the liver and the pancreas. This disorder is associated with bronze skin, cirrhosis, diabetes mellitus, and low plasma transferrin levels.

Atransferrinemia is inherited as an autosomal recessive trait due to mutation of both transferrin genes, with a resulting absence of transferrin. It is characterized by anemia and hemosiderosis (iron deposition) in the heart and liver. The iron damage to the heart can lead to heart failure. This disease can be effectively treated by plasma infusions of transferrin.

The analytic methods used for the quantitation of transferrin are immunodiffusion and immunonephelometry. Total iron-binding capacity (TIBC) is typically measured along with serum iron to evaluate either iron deficiency or iron overload. The iron concentration divided by TIBC gives the transferrin saturation, which is a more useful indicator of iron status than iron or TIBC alone. In iron deficiency, iron is low, but TIBC is increased, and transferrin saturation becomes very low. In iron overload, iron is high and TIBC is low or normal, causing the transferrin saturation to increase. It is customary to test for transferrin (rather than TIBC) when evaluating nutritional status or liver function. Because it is made in the liver, transferrin is low in liver disease or when there is not enough protein in the diet.[42]

Hemopexin

The parenchymal cells of the liver synthesize hemopexin, which migrates electrophoretically in the β-globulin region and is an acute-phase reactant. The function of hemopexin is to scavenge the heme released or lost by the turnover of heme proteins such as hemoglobin, which protects the body from the oxidative damage that free heme can cause. Hemopexin binds heme with the highest affinity of any known protein. When free heme (ferroprotoporphyrin IX) is formed during the breakdown of hemoglobin, myoglobin, or catalase, it binds to hemopexin in a 1:1 ratio. The heme–hemopexin complex is carried to the liver, where the complex is destroyed. In this manner, hemopexin preserves the body's iron. Hemopexin also induces intracellular antioxidant activities. Increased concentrations are also found in inflammation, diabetes mellitus, Duchenne-type muscular dystrophy, and some malignancies, especially melanomas. Low hemopexin levels are diagnostic of a hemolytic anemia. Hemopexin can be determined by radial immunodiffusion.[43]

Lipoproteins

Lipoproteins are complexes of proteins and lipids whose function is to transport cholesterol, triglycerides, and phospholipids in the blood. Lipoproteins are subclassified according to the apoprotein and specific lipid content into chylomicrons, VLDL, intermediate-density lipoproteins, low-density lipoproteins (LDLs) and lipoprotein(a), and HDL. On HRE, HDL migrates between the albumin and α_1-globulin zone; VLDL migrates at the beginning of the β-globulin fraction (pre-β); and LDL appears as a separate band in the β-globulin region. For a more detailed discussion of structure, function, and laboratory methods, refer Chapter 15.

β₂-Microglobulin

β_2-Microglobulin (B2M) is the light chain component of the major histocompatibility complex (human leukocyte antigen [HLA]). This protein is found on the surface of most nucleated cells and is present in high concentrations on lymphocytes. Because of its small size (molecular weight, 11,800 kDa), B2M is filtered by the renal glomerulus, but most (>99%) is reabsorbed and catabolized in the proximal tubules. Elevated serum levels are the result of impaired clearance by the kidney or overproduction of the protein that occurs in a number of inflammatory diseases, such as rheumatoid arthritis and systemic lupus erythematosus (SLE). In patients with human immunodeficiency virus, a high B2M level in the absence of renal failure indicates a large lymphocyte turnover rate, which suggests the virus is killing lymphocytes. B2M may sometimes be seen on HRE but, because of its low concentration, it is usually measured by immunoassay.

Complement

The complement system is one of the natural defense mechanisms that protects the human body from infections. These proteins are synthesized in the liver as single polypeptide chains and circulate in the blood as nonfunctional precursors. Complement C3 is the most abundant complement protein in the human serum, with complement C4 being the second. In the classic pathway, activation of these proteins begins when the first complement factor, C1q, binds to an antigen–antibody complex. Each complement protein (C2–C9) is then activated sequentially and can bind to the membrane of the cell to which the antigen–antibody complex is bound, leading to the final result—lysis of the cell. An alternate pathway (properdin pathway) for complement activation exists in which the early components are bypassed and the process begins with C3. This pathway is triggered by different substances (does not require the presence of an antibody); however, the lytic attack on membranes is the same (sequence C5–C9).

Complement is increased in inflammatory states and decreased in malnutrition and hemolytic anemia. Inherited deficiencies of individual complement proteins have also been described. Complements C3 and C4 are the components most frequently measured. Complement C3 is used as a screening test because of its pivotal position in the complement cascade; C3 is consumed by activation of either the classic or alternative pathway. However, C3 levels are not the most sensitive indicators of classic pathway activation, and a decreased complement C4 level is frequently found to be a more sensitive measure of mild classic pathway activation.

Decreased levels of C3 are associated with autoimmune disease, neonatal respiratory distress syndrome, bacteremia, tissue injury, and chronic hepatitis. Complement C3 is important in the pathogenesis of age-related macular degeneration. This finding further underscores the influence of the complement pathway in the pathogenesis of this disease.[44]

Decreased levels of C4 may indicate disseminated intravascular coagulation, acute glomerulonephritis, chronic hepatitis, and SLE. Increased levels of both C3 and C4 are linked to acute inflammatory disease and tissue inflammation. Methods for measuring C3 and C4 include nephelometric immunoassay and turbidimetry.

Fibrinogen

Fibrinogen is one of the largest proteins in blood plasma. It is synthesized in the liver, and it is classified as a glycoprotein because it has considerable carbohydrate content. On plasma electrophoresis, fibrinogen is seen as a distinct band between the β- and γ-globulins. The function of fibrinogen is to form a fibrin clot when activated by thrombin; therefore, all fibrinogen is virtually removed in the clotting process and is not seen in serum.

Fibrinogen customarily has been determined as clottable protein. Fibrinogen concentration is proportional to the time required to form a clot after the addition of thrombin to citrated plasma. Fibrin split products (degradation products of fibrinogen and fibrin) are determined by immunoassay methods such as radial immunodiffusion, nephelometry, and RIA.

Fibrinogen is one of the acute-phase reactants, a term that refers to proteins that are significantly increased in plasma during the acute phase of the inflammatory process. Fibrinogen levels also rise with pregnancy and the use of oral contraceptives. Decreased values generally reflect extensive coagulation, during which the fibrinogen is consumed.

C-Reactive Protein

C-reactive protein (CRP) is synthesized in the liver and is one of the first acute-phase proteins to rise in response to inflammatory disease. CRP received its name because it precipitates with the C substance, a polysaccharide of pneumococci. CRP rises sharply whenever there is tissue necrosis, whether the damage originates from a pneumococcal infection or some other source. CRP bound to bacteria and fungi promotes the binding of complement, which facilitates their uptake by phagocytes. This protein-coating process to enhance phagocytosis is known as opsonization. Inflammation, the process by which the body responds to injury or an infection, has been demonstrated through many studies to be important in atherosclerosis (the fatty deposits that build up in the inner lining of arteries). Atherosclerosis, in addition to being a disease of lipid accumulation, also represents a chronic inflammatory process. Elevated levels of CRP stimulate the production of tissue factor that initiates coagulation, activates complement, and binds to LDL in the atherosclerotic plaque—evidence that points to a causal relationship between CRP levels and CVD. Furthermore, interventions such as weight loss, diet, exercise, and smoking cessation and administration of pharmacologic agents such as statins all lead to both reduced CRP levels and reduced vascular risk. The major factors that promote atherosclerosis—cigarette smoking, hypertension, plaque-causing lipoproteins, and hyperglycemia—are well established.[45] These risk factors contribute to the release of chemicals and the activation of cells involved in the inflammatory process and contribute to the formation of plaque but may also contribute to plaque breaking off the artery wall, resulting in the formation of a blood clot.

The American Heart Association and the Centers for Disease Control and Prevention published a joint scientific statement in 2003 on the use of inflammatory markers in clinical and public health practice. This statement was developed after systematically reviewing the evidence of association between inflammatory markers (mainly CRP) and coronary heart disease and stroke.[46] Most studies to date have focused on heart disease, but new research shows that having CRP in the high-normal range may also be associated with other diseases such as colon cancer, complications of diabetes, obesity, and the risk of developing type 2 diabetes.[47] Individuals with CRP levels greater than 3 mg/L have a risk of the development of diabetes four to six times higher than that of individuals with lower levels of CRP. Part of the link between heart disease and diabetes is due to inflammation.

CRP is not specific but does have value as a general indicator. Normally, there are minimal levels of CRP in blood. A high or increasing amount of CRP suggests an acute infection or inflammation. Although a result above 1 mg/dL is usually considered high for CRP, most infections and inflammations result in CRP levels above 10 mg/dL. In cases of inflammatory rheumatic diseases, such as rheumatoid arthritis and SLE, the CRP test is used to assess the effectiveness of a specific arthritis treatment and monitor periods of disease eruption. However, even in known cases of inflammatory disease, a low CRP level is possible and is not indicative of absence of inflammation. It is significantly elevated in acute rheumatic fever, bacterial infections, myocardial infarctions, rheumatoid arthritis, carcinomatosis, gout, and viral infections. CRP is generally measured by immunologic methods, including nephelometry and EIA. The traditional methods have a sensitivity of approximately 3 to 5 mg/L.

High-Sensitivity CRP

High-sensitivity CRP (hsCRP) is the same protein but is named for the newer, monoclonal antibody–based test methodologies that can detect CRP at levels below 1 mg/L. The hsCRP test determines risk of CVD. Using the hsCRP assay, levels of less than 1, 1 to 3, and greater than 3 mg/L correspond to low-, moderate-, and high-risk groups for future cardiovascular events.[48] High levels of hsCRP consistently predict recurrent coronary events in patients with unstable angina and AMI. Higher hsCRP levels are also associated with lower survival rates in these patients. Studies also suggest that higher levels of hsCRP may increase the risk that an artery will reclose after it has been opened with balloon angioplasty. A more detailed discussion of cardiac risk factors is found in Chapter 26.

Immunoglobulins

The immunoglobulins (antibodies or Igs) are glycoproteins composed of 82% to 96% protein and 4% to 18% carbohydrate produced by white blood cells, known as B cells, that confer humoral immunity. These proteins consist of two identical heavy (H) and two identical light (L) chains linked by two disulfide bonds that can be in the form of monomers with one unit, dimers with two units, or pentamers with five units. There are five classes of immunoglobulins (IgG, IgA, IgM, IgD, and IgE) or isotypes based on the type of heavy chain they possess. The heavy chains are γ, α, μ, δ, and ε, respectively. Each heavy chain has two regions—the constant region and the variable region. The constant region is identical in all antibodies of the same isotype but differs in antibodies of different isotypes. The variable region of the heavy chain differs in antibodies produced by different B cells but is the same for all antibodies produced by a single B cell or B-cell clone. There are two types of light chains—kappa (κ) and lambda (λ) chains. The ratio of κ to λ chains is 2:1, which is sometimes used as a marker of immune abnormalities. Four distinct heavy chain subgroups (subclasses 1, 2, 3, and 4) of IgG were first demonstrated in the 1960s based on their relative concentration in normal serum.

The N-terminal regions of the heavy and light chains exhibit highly variable amino acid composition referred to as VH and VL, respectively. This variable region is involved in antigen binding. In contrast to the variable region, the constant domains of light and heavy chains are referred to as CL and CH, respectively. The constant regions are involved in complement binding, placental passage, and binding to cell membrane. For example, IgG has two γ-type H chains and two identical L chains (either κ or λ).

Multiple genes for the variable regions contain three distinct types of segments encoded in the human genome. For example, the immunoglobulin heavy chain region contains 65 *Variable* (V) genes plus 27 *Diversity* (D) genes and six functional *Joining* (J) genes.[49] The light chains also possess numerous V and J genes but do not have D genes. By the mechanism of DNA rearrangement of these regional genes, it is possible to generate an antibody repertoire of more than 10^7 possible combinations. V(D)J recombination is a mechanism of genetic recombination that randomly selects and assembles segments of genes encoding specific proteins, which generates a diverse repertoire of T-cell receptor and immunoglobulin (Ig) molecules that are necessary for the recognition of diverse antigens from bacterial, viral, and parasitic invaders and from dysfunctional cells such as tumor cells.[50]

Immunoglobulin class switching (or isotype switching) is a biologic mechanism that changes an antibody from one class to another, for example, from an isotype IgM to an isotype IgG. This process occurs after activation of the B cell, which allows the cell to produce different classes of antibody. Only the constant region of the antibody heavy chain changes during class switching. Because the variable region does not change, class switching does not affect the antigens that are bound by the antibody. Instead, the antibody retains affinity for the same antigens but can interact with different effector molecules (any regulatory molecule that binds to a protein and alters the activity of that protein).[51]

The antibody molecule has a "Y" shape, with the tip being the site that binds antigen, and, therefore, recognizes specific foreign objects. This region of the antibody is called the Fab (fragment, antigen binding) region. It is composed of one constant and one variable domain from each heavy and light chain of the antibody. The base of the Y is called the Fc (fragment, crystallizable) region and is composed of two heavy chains that contribute two or three constant domains depending on the class of the antibody.[52] By binding to specific proteins, the Fc region ensures that each antibody generates an appropriate immune response for a given antigen. The Fc region also binds to various cell receptors, such as Fc receptors, and other immune molecules, such as complement proteins. By doing this, it mediates different physiologic effects including opsonization, cell lysis, and degranulation of mast cells, basophils, and eosinophils.[53]

The immunoglobulins are not synthesized to any extent by the neonate. IgG crosses the placenta; the IgG present in the newborn's serum is that synthesized by the mother. IgM does not cross the placenta but rather is the only immunoglobulin synthesized by the neonate. IgA is generally higher in males than in females; IgM and IgG levels are somewhat higher in females. IgE levels vary with the allergic condition of the individual.

The immunoglobulins have been determined using radial immunodiffusion, nephelometry, turbidimetry, electrochemiluminescent immunoassay (ECLIA), and RIA. Fluorescent immunoassay techniques and immunonephelometric assays have also been used. The automated immunonephelometric method is available for IgG, IgA, and IgM. Monoclonal increases are seen on serum protein electrophoresis (SPE) patterns as spikes.

IgG is the most abundant class of antibodies found in blood plasma and lymph. Immunoglobulin G antibodies act on bacteria, fungi, viruses, and foreign particles by agglutination, by opsonization (the process by which a pathogen is marked for ingestion and destruction by a phagocyte), by activating complement, and by neutralizing toxins. IgG is increased in liver disease, infections, IgG myeloma, parasitic disease, and many rheumatic diseases. Decreased IgG levels are associated with acquired immunodeficiency, an increased susceptibility to infections, hereditary deficiency, protein-losing states, and non-IgG myeloma.

IgA is the main immunoglobulin found in mucous secretions, including tears, saliva, colostrum, vaginal fluid, and secretions from the respiratory and gastrointestinal mucosa. It is also found in small amounts in blood. It exists in two isotypes, IgA1 (90%) and IgA2 (10%). IgA1 is found in serum and made by bone marrow B cells, while IgA2 is made by B cells located in the mucosae. IgA is also classified based upon location— serum IgA and secretory IgA. IgA found in secretions is a specific form known as secretory IgA, polymers of two to four IgA monomers linked by two additional chains, one being the J chain (Joining chain), which is a polypeptide-containing cysteine and completely different structurally from other immunoglobulin chains. Secretory IgA is resistant to enzyme degradation and remains active in the digestive and respiratory tracts to provide antibody protection in body secretions. Increases in the serum IgA are found in liver disease, infections, and autoimmune diseases. Decreased serum concentrations are found in depressed protein synthesis and immunodeficiency.

IgM is the first antibody that appears in response to antigenic stimulation. IgM is present in B cells. Because the J chain is found in pentameric IgM, it is also important as a secretory immunoglobulin. IgM is the naturally occurring antibody, anti-A and anti-B, to red cell antigens, in rheumatoid factors, and are heterophile antibodies. Increased IgM concentration is found in toxoplasmosis, primary biliary cirrhosis, cytomegalovirus, rubella, herpes, syphilis, and various bacterial and fungal diseases. A monoclonal increase is seen in Waldenström's macroglobulinemia as a spike in the vicinity of the late β zone on protein electrophoresis. Decreases are seen in protein-losing conditions and hereditary immunodeficiency.

IgD molecules are present on the surface of most, but not all, B cells early in their development, but little IgD is ever released into the circulation. IgD may help regulate B-cell function; however, the function of circulating IgD is largely unknown. Its concentration is increased in infections, liver disease, and connective tissue disorders.[54]

IgE is produced by B cells and plasma cells and is the immunoglobulin associated with allergic and anaphylactic reactions. In contrast to other immunoglobulins, the concentration of IgE in the circulation is very low. An elevated IgE concentration is not diagnostic of any single condition. Elevated IgE levels are observed in many inflammatory and infectious diseases, including asthma and hay fever. Monoclonal increases are seen in IgE myeloma, a rare disease. Solid-phase displacement RIAs, double-antibody RIAs, solid-phase sandwich RIAs, and nephelometry are all used to measure IgE.[55]

OTHER PROTEINS OF IMPORTANCE

Myoglobin

Myoglobin is a single-chain globular protein of 153 amino acids, containing a heme (iron-containing) prosthetic group. Myoglobin is the primary oxygen-carrying protein (approximately 2% of total muscle protein) found in striated skeletal and cardiac muscle. It can reversibly bind oxygen similarly to the hemoglobin molecule, but myoglobin requires a very low oxygen tension to release the bound oxygen. Most of the myoglobin found in cells is dissolved in the cytoplasm.

As a cardiac biomarker, myoglobin has been used in conjunction with troponin to help diagnose or rule out a heart attack. When striated muscle is damaged, myoglobin is released, elevating the blood levels. In an AMI, this increase is seen within 2 to 3 hours of onset and reaches peak concentration in 8 to 12 hours. Myoglobin is a small molecule freely filtered by the kidneys, allowing levels to return to normal in 18 to 30 hours after the AMI. Because of the speed of appearance and clearance of myoglobin, it is also a useful marker for monitoring the success or failure of reperfusion. Although the diagnostic sensitivity

TABLE 11-4	CAUSES OF MYOGLOBIN ELEVATIONS
Acute myocardial infarction	
Angina without infarction	
Rhabdomyolysis	
Muscle trauma	
Renal failure	
Myopathies	
Vigorous exercise	
Intramuscular injections	
Open heart surgery	
Seizures (tonic–clonic)	
Electric shock	
Arterial thrombosis	
Certain toxins	

of myoglobin elevations following an AMI has been reported to be between 75% and 100%, myoglobin is not cardiac specific. Elevations are also seen in conditions such as progressive muscular dystrophy and crushing injury in which skeletal muscle is damaged. Myoglobin is toxic to the kidneys and in severe muscle injury, levels of myoglobin may rise very quickly and the kidneys may be damaged by the increased amounts. Renal failure can also elevate the level of serum myoglobin. Table 11-4 lists some of the causes of myoglobin elevation.

Latex agglutination, ELISA, immunonephelometry, ECLIA, and fluoroimmunoassays for myoglobin are used in the clinical laboratory for myoglobin measurement. A qualitative spot test using immunochromatography is also available.

Cardiac Troponin

Cardiac troponin (cTn) represents a complex of regulatory proteins that include troponin I (cTnI) and troponin T (cTnT) that are specific to heart muscle. cTnI and cTnT are the "gold standard" in the diagnosis of acute coronary syndrome (ACS). cTn should be measured in all patients presenting with symptoms suggestive of ACS, in conjunction with physical examination and ECG.[57] Because of the specificity of cTn for myocardial damage, a single cTn above the decision limit, along with clinical evidence, is indicative of myocardial injury.

The American College of Cardiology and the European Society of Cardiology in conjunction with the National Academy of Clinical Biochemistry recommend the use of a decision limit for myocardial injury at the 99th percentile of the reference population for cTnT and cTnI.[56] Although it is acceptable to use the manufacturer's

decision limits, each laboratory should, if possible, define its own cutoff value based on its reference population. Furthermore, assays should ideally not exceed a total imprecision of 10% at the diagnostic cutoff. cTnI or cTnT testing can be performed by itself or along with other cardiac biomarkers, such as creatine kinase (CK), CK-MB, and myoglobin. cTnI and cTnT tests have begun to replace CK and CK-MB tests because they are more specific for heart injury (vs. skeletal muscle injury) and are elevated for a longer period of time.[57] If CK, CK-MB, and myoglobin concentrations are normal but troponin levels are increased, then it is likely that either a lesser degree of heart injury is present or that the injury took place more than 24 hours in the past. If the first troponin performed is normal but subsequent (6- and 12-hour samples) troponin tests are increased, then the heart injury likely occurred within a couple of hours prior to the first test and had not had time to increase. When a CK test is elevated but CK-MB (which is more heart specific than CK) and troponin tests are normal, then it is likely that whatever symptoms are present are due to another cause, such as skeletal muscle injury.

Cardiac troponins can be measured on serum or heparinized plasma by ELISA or immunoenzymometric assays using two monoclonal antibodies directed against different epitopes (antigenic determinants) on the protein. The reference interval for cTnT is <0.1 ng/mL (mg/L). The cutoff concentration for cTnI immunoassays varies from 0.1 to 3.1 ng/mL (mg/L) (see Chapter 26 for a detailed discussion of cardiac markers).

Brain Natriuretic Peptide and N-Terminal–Brain Natriuretic Peptide

The natriuretic peptides are a family of structurally related hormones that include atrial natriuretic peptide, B-type (or brain) natriuretic peptide (BNP), C-type natriuretic peptide, and dendroaspis natriuretic peptide. B-type natriuretic peptides are produced initially as a 134–amino acid pre pro peptide, which is cleaved into proBNP108, a precursor molecule stored in myocytes. Upon release, proBNP108 is cleaved by the protease, furin, into N-terminal (NT)-proBNP (a 76–amino acid biologically inert portion) and BNP (which is biologically active). NT-proBNP and BNP are found in largest concentration in the left ventricular myocardium but are also detectable in atrial tissue as well as in the myocardium of the right ventricle.

In the past few years, BNP has become a popular marker for congestive heart failure.[58] The natriuretic peptides are neurohormones that affect body fluid homeostasis (through natriuresis and diuresis) and blood pressure (through decreased angiotensin II and norepinephrine synthesis), both major components in the pathology of congestive heart failure.

Methods for BNP and NT-proBNP include immunoradiometric assay, microparticle enzyme immunoassay, and ECLIA.

Fibronectin

Fibronectin is a glycoprotein composed of two nearly identical subunits. Although fibronectin is the product of a single gene, the resulting protein can exist in multiple forms due to splicing of a single pre-mRNA. The variants demonstrate a wide variety of cellular interactions, including roles in cell adhesion, tissue differentiation, growth, and wound healing. These proteins are found in plasma and on cell surfaces and can be synthesized by the liver hepatocytes, endothelial cells, peritoneal macrophages, and fibroblasts. Plasma fibronectin has been used as a nutritional marker.

Fetal fibronectin (fFN) is a glycoprotein used to help predict the short-term risk of premature delivery. fFN is produced at the boundary between the amniotic sac and the decidua (the lining of the uterus) and functions to maintain the adherence of the placenta to the uterus. fFN is thought to help maintain the integrity of this boundary. fFN is normally detectable in amniotic fluid and placental tissue during early pregnancy, and in a normal pregnancy it is no longer detectable after 24 weeks. fFN should not be detectable between 22 and 36 weeks of pregnancy. Elevated levels during this period reflect a disturbance at the uteroplacental junction and have been associated with an increased risk of preterm labor and delivery.

Adiponectin

Adiponectin is a 247–amino acid fat hormone composed of an N-terminal collagen-like domain and a C-terminal globular domain produced by adipocytes. Adiponectin exists in trimers, hexamers, and multimers in the blood. Recent studies have shown an inverse correlation between body mass index and adiponectin values. Lower levels of adiponectin correlate with an increased risk of heart disease, type 2 diabetes, metabolic syndrome, and obesity.[59]

β-Trace Protein

β-Trace protein (BTP; synonym prostaglandin D synthase) is a 168–amino acid, low-molecular-mass protein in the lipocalin protein family. Recently, it was verified that BTP was established as an accurate marker of CSF leakage. It has also been reported recently as a potential marker in detecting impaired renal function, although no more sensitive than cystatin C.[60] BTP serum values correlate significantly with serum cystatin C, glomerular filtration rate, and urine microproteins, but BTP is not a diagnostic efficient test for glomerular filtration rate. The benefit of BTP measurement could be findings that BTP concentrations, in contrast to cystatin C concentrations, are not influenced by glucocorticoid therapy. BTP might be a promising marker in the diagnosis of perilymphatic fluid fistulas.

Cross-Linked C-Telopeptides

Cross-linked C-telopeptides (CTXs) are proteolytic fragments of collagen I formed during bone resorption (turnover). CTX is a biochemical marker of bone resorption that can be detected in serum and urine. The bone turnover rate increases at menopause. After an effective 3 to 6 months of antiresorptive therapy, CTX concentrations drop 35% to 55% from baseline levels. Limitations of measuring CTX values are as follows: (1) the need to establish a baseline level; (2) CTX levels may vary due to a patient's diet, exercise, time of day, etc.; and (3) it cannot replace bone mineral density to diagnose osteoporosis. The CTX test is most useful for monitoring the response to antiresorptive therapy; it is noninvasive and can be repeated often. ECLIA technology is used to measure CTX in the laboratory. It can also be automated.

Cystatin C

Cystatin C, a low-molecular-mass protein with 120 amino acids, is a cysteine proteinase inhibitor. It is produced and destroyed at a constant rate, making it a recently proposed new marker for the early assessment of changes to the glomerular filtration rate. Cystatin C is freely filtered by the glomerulus and almost completely reabsorbed and catabolized by the proximal tubular cells. Cystatin C has been recently proposed as a new sensitive endogenous serum marker for the glomerular filtration rate. When the rate at which the fluid filtrate is formed is reduced, indicating decreased kidney function, blood levels of substances removed by them (such as cystatin C) increase and are an indication of kidney function. Cystatin C levels are not affected by muscle mass, gender, age, or race unlike creatinine, nor are they generally affected by most drugs, infections, diet, or inflammation. Cystatin C may be used as an alternative to creatinine and creatinine clearance to screen for and monitor kidney dysfunction. While there are growing data and literature supporting the use of cystatin C, there is still a degree of uncertainty about when and how it should be used.[61] It may be especially useful in those cases where creatinine measurement is not appropriate, such as in patients with cirrhosis, obesity, or malnutrition or who have a reduced muscle mass. In addition to kidney dysfunction, it has been associated with an increased risk of CVD and heart failure in the elderly.[72] Cystatin C levels require particle-enhanced immunoturbidimetry or immunonephelometric laboratory methods for their measurement. These methods have been FDA approved and can also be automated.

Amyloid

Amyloids are insoluble fibrous protein aggregates formed due to an alteration in their secondary structure known as β-pleated sheets. Amyloid characteristically stains with Congo red. Amyloidosis refers to a variety of conditions in which amyloid proteins are abnormally deposited in organs and/or tissues. Amyloid fibrils may infiltrate many organs, including the heart and blood vessels, brain and peripheral nerves, kidneys, liver, spleen, and intestines, causing localized or widespread organ failure. Amyloidosis can be inherited due to different diseases, for example, chronic infections, malignancies, and rheumatologic disorders, which cause overabundant or abnormal protein production.

Amyloid β42 (Aβ42) and Tau protein tests are not currently part of a typical patient assessment but can be used as supplemental tests to help differentiate a diagnosis of Alzheimer disease from other forms of dementia. Abnormal forms of Tau, a brain phosphoprotein, make up part of the structure of neurofibrillary tangles (twisted protein fragments that clog nerve cells), while Aβ42, which is formed from β amyloid precursor protein, is associated with the creation of senile plaques. Tau protein and Aβ42 tests are performed primarily in research settings (the specimen used is CSF). In a symptomatic patient, low Aβ42 along with high Tau reflects an increased likelihood of Alzheimer disease, but it does not mean that the person definitely has Alzheimer disease. If a patient does not have abnormal levels of these proteins, then the dementia is more likely due to a cause other than Alzheimer disease.

TOTAL PROTEIN ABNORMALITIES

The total protein test is a rough measure of all of the proteins in the plasma. Total protein measurements can reflect nutritional status, kidney disease, liver disease, and many other conditions. If total protein is abnormal, further tests must be performed to identify which protein fraction is abnormal, so that a specific diagnosis can be made.

Hypoproteinemia

Hypoproteinemia, a total protein level less than the reference interval, occurs in any condition where a negative nitrogen balance exists. One cause of a low level of plasma proteins is excessive loss. Plasma proteins can be lost by excretion in the urine in renal disease; leakage into the gastrointestinal tract in inflammation of the digestive system; and the loss of blood in open wounds, internal bleeding, or extensive burns. Another circumstance producing hypoproteinemia is decreased intake either because of malnutrition or through intestinal malabsorption as seen in sprue. Without adequate dietary intake of proteins, there is a deficiency of certain essential amino acids and protein synthesis is impaired. A decrease in serum proteins as a result of decreased synthesis is also seen in liver disease (site of all nonimmune protein synthesis) or in inherited immunodeficiency disorders, in which antibody production is diminished. Additionally, hypoproteinemia may result from accelerated catabolism of proteins, such as occurs in burns, trauma, or other injuries.

Hyperproteinemia

Hyperproteinemia, an increase in total plasma proteins, is not an actual disease state but is the result of the underlying cause, dehydration. When excess water is lost from the vascular system, the proteins, because of their size, remain within the blood vessels. Although the absolute quantity of proteins remains unchanged, the concentration is elevated due to a decreased volume of solvent water. Dehydration results from a variety of conditions, including vomiting, diarrhea, excessive sweating, diabetic acidosis, and hypoaldosteronism.

In addition to dehydration, hyperproteinemia may be the result of excessive production, primarily of the γ-globulins. Some disorders are characterized by the appearance of a monoclonal protein or paraprotein in the serum and often in the urine as well. This protein is an intact immunoglobulin molecule or, occasionally, κ or λ light chains only. The most common disorder is multiple myeloma, in which the neoplastic plasma cells proliferate in the bone marrow. The paraprotein in this case is usually IgG, IgA, or κ or λ light chains. IgD and IgE paraproteins rarely occur. Paraproteins in multiple myeloma may reach a serum concentration of several grams per deciliter. IgM paraprotein is found in patients with Waldenström's macroglobulinemia, a rare type of slow-growing, non-Hodgkin lymphoma. Many disorders, including chronic inflammatory states, collagen vascular disorders, and other neoplasms, may be associated with paraproteins. Polyclonal increases in immunoglobulins, which would be represented by increases in both κ and λ chains, are seen in the serum and urine in many chronic diseases.

CASE STUDY 11-3

A 76-year-old woman was admitted to the hospital with gangrene of her right toe. She was disoriented and had difficulty finding the right words to express herself. On evaluation, it was revealed she lived alone and was responsible for her own cooking. A daughter who lived in the area said her mother was a poor eater, even with much encouragement. An ECG, performed on admission, showed possible ectopic rhythm with occasional premature supraventricular contractions. The cardiologist suspected

CASE STUDY 11-3 (continued)

a possible inferior myocardial infarction of undetermined age. Laboratory results are shown in CASE STUDY TABLE 11-3.1.

CASE STUDY TABLE 11-3.1 LABORATORY RESULTS

DAY 1	RESULTS	REFERENCE RANGE
CK total	187 U/L	40–325 U/L
CK-MB mass	6 µg/L	<8 µg/L
Troponin I	16.3 µg/L	0–2 µg/L
NT-proBNP	60 pmol/L	2–50 pmol/L (generic cutoff)
Prealbumin	15 mg/dL	17–42 mg/dL
Albumin	2.7 g/dL	3.7–4.9 g/dL
REPEAT (5 H LATER)		
CK total	180 U/L	
CK-MB mass	5.4 µg/L	
Troponin I	17.5 µg/L	
NT-proBNP	100.5 pmol/L	
DAY 2		
CK total	177 U/L	
CK-MB mass	4.5 µg/L	
Troponin I	13.7 µg/L	
NT-proBNP	143 pmol/L	
Myoglobin	>500 µg/L	(<76)

Questions

1. In this patient, what is the clinical value of the troponin I measurements?

2. What is a possible explanation for the elevated myoglobin?

3. What condition is indicated by the low prealbumin value?

Table 11-5 summarizes the disease states affecting total protein levels with the relative changes in the albumin and globulin fractions.

METHODS OF ANALYSIS

Total Nitrogen

A total nitrogen determination measures all chemically bound nitrogen in the sample. The method can be applied to various biologic samples, including plasma and urine. In plasma, both the total protein and nonprotein nitrogenous compounds, such as urea and creatinine, are measured. The analysis of total nitrogen level is useful in assessing nitrogen balance. Monitoring the nitrogen nutritional status is particularly important in patients receiving total parenteral nutrition, such as individuals with neurologic injuries who are sustained on intravenous fluids for an extended period.

The method for total nitrogen analysis uses chemiluminescence.[62] The sample, in the presence of oxygen, is heated to a high temperature $(1,100 \pm 20°C)$. Any chemically bound nitrogen is oxidized to nitric oxide. The nitric oxide is then mixed with ozone (O_3) to form an excited nitrogen dioxide molecule (NO_2). When this molecule decays to the ground state, it emits chemiluminescent light, which is detected, amplified, and converted to an electronic signal, proportional to the total nitrogen content in the sample. This chemiluminescence signal is compared with that of a standard for quantitation.

Total Proteins

The specimen most often used to determine the total protein is serum rather than plasma. A fasting specimen is not needed. Interferences in some of the methods occur in the presence of lipemia; hemolysis falsely elevates the total protein result because of the release of RBC proteins into the serum.

The reference interval for serum total protein is 6.5 to 8.3 g/dL (65 to 83 g/L) for ambulatory adults. In the recumbent position, the serum total protein concentration is 6.0 to 7.8 g/dL (60 to 78 g/L). The reduction in serum albumin reduces blood COP. Therefore, the distribution of fluid shifts toward extracellular compartments. At birth, the total protein concentration is lower, reaching adult levels by age 3. As a person ages, there is a slight decrease in albumin levels. Lower total protein levels are also seen in pregnancy. Methods for the determination of total protein are described below and summarized in Table 11-6.

Kjeldahl

The classic method for quantitation of total protein is the Kjeldahl method, which determines nitrogen. This method is not used in the clinical laboratory because it is time consuming and too tedious for routine use. In this method, an average of 16% nitrogen mass in protein is assumed to calculate the protein concentration. The actual nitrogen content of serum proteins varies from 15.1% to 16.8%. Therefore, error is introduced if a protein standard (calibrated with the Kjeldahl method) is used that differs in composition from the serum specimen to be analyzed, because the percentage of nitrogen will not be the same. The method also requires the assumption that no proteins of significant concentration in the unknown specimen are lost in the precipitation step.

The serum proteins are precipitated with an organic acid such as TCA or tungstic acid. The nonprotein

TABLE 11-5	PROTEIN LEVELS IN SELECTED DISEASE STATES		
TOTAL PROTEIN	**ALBUMIN**	**GLOBULIN**	**DISEASE**
N, ↓	↓	↑	Hepatic damage
			• Cirrhosis β-γ bridging
			• Hepatitis ↑ γ-globulins
			• Obstructive jaundice ↑ α_2-, β-globulins
			Burns, trauma
			Infections
			• Acute ↑ α_1-, α_2-globulins
			• Chronic ↑ α_1-, α_2-, γ-globulins
↓	↓	N	Malabsorption
			Inadequate diet
			Nephrotic syndrome ↑ α_2-, β-globulins; ↓ γ-globulins
↓	N	↓	Immunodeficiency syndromes
↓	↓	↓	Salt retention syndrome
↑	↑	↑	Dehydration
↑	N	↑	Multiple myeloma
			Monoclonal and polyclonal gammopathies

↑, increased; ↓, decreased; N, normal levels.

nitrogen is removed with the supernatant. The protein pellet is digested in H_2SO_4 with heat (340°C to 360°C) and a catalyst, such as cupric sulfate, to speed the reaction. Potassium sulfate is also introduced to increase the boiling point to improve the efficiency of digestion. The H_2SO_4 oxidizes the C, H, and S in protein to CO_2, CO, H_2O, and SO_2. The nitrogen in the protein is converted to ammonium bisulfite (NH_4HSO_4), which is then measured by adding alkali and distilling the ammonia into a standard boric acid solution. The ammonium borate ($NH_4H_2BO_3$) formed is then titrated with a standard solution of HCl to determine the amount of nitrogen in the original protein solution.

Biuret

The biuret procedure is the most widely used method and the one recommended by the International Federation of Clinical Chemistry expert panel for the determination of total protein. In this reaction, cupric ions (Cu^{2+}) complex with the groups involved in the peptide bond. In an alkaline medium and in the presence of at least two peptide bonds, a violet-colored chelate (a bound metal in complex) is formed. The reagent also contains sodium potassium tartrate, to complex cupric ions to prevent their precipitation in the alkaline solution, and potassium iodide, which acts as an antioxidant. The absorbance of the colored chelate formed is measured at 540 nm. When small peptides react, the color of the chelate produced has a different shade than that seen with larger peptides. The color varies from a pink to a reddish violet. The color that is formed is proportional to the number of peptide bonds present and reflects the total protein level. However, in the presence of abnormally small proteins, such as those

TABLE 11-6	TOTAL PROTEIN METHODS	
METHOD	**PRINCIPLE**	**COMMENT**
Kjeldahl	Digestion of protein; measurement of nitrogen content	Reference method; assume average nitrogen content of 16%
Biuret	Formation of violet-colored chelate between Cu^{2+} ions and peptide bonds	Routine method; requires at least two peptide bonds and an alkaline medium
Dye binding	Protein binds to dye and causes a spectral shift in the absorbance maximum of the dye	Research use

Refractometry is a rapid, simple method, but is not commonly used for total protein analysis.[63]

seen in multiple myeloma, the C-protein concentration is underestimated due to the lighter shade of color produced. Lipemia in the sample is an interferent.[64]

In addition to the NHCO group that occurs in the peptide bond, cupric ions will react with any compound that has two or more of the following groups: $NHCH_2$ and NHCS. The method was named because a substance called biuret ($NH_2CONHCONH_2$) reacted with cupric ions in the same manner. There must be a minimum of two of the reactive groups; therefore, amino acids and dipeptides will not react.

Dye Binding

The dye-binding methods are based on the ability of most proteins in serum to bind dyes, although the affinity with which they bind may vary. Bromophenol blue, Ponceau S, amido black 10B, lissamine green, and Coomassie brilliant blue have been used to stain protein bands after electrophoresis. A dye-binding method, Coomassie brilliant blue 250, relies on the binding of Coomassie brilliant blue 250 to protein, causing a shift in the absorbance maximum of the dye from 465 to 595 nm. The increase in absorbance at 595 is used to determine the protein concentration. Although the method is simple and fast, the unequal dye-binding responses of individual proteins require caution when applying this test to the complex mixture of protein found in serum.

Fractionation, Identification, and Quantitation of Specific Proteins

In the assay of total serum proteins, useful diagnostic information can be obtained by determining the albumin fraction and the globulins. A reversal or significant change in the ratio of albumin and total globulin, the A/G ratio, is found in diseases of the kidney and liver. To determine the A/G ratio, total protein and albumin are measured and globulins are calculated by subtracting the albumin from the total protein (total protein − albumin = globulins). The following are methods for measuring protein fractions.

Salt Fractionation

Fractionation of proteins is done using precipitation. Globulins are separated from albumin by salting out, using sodium salt to cause precipitation of the globulins. The albumin that remains in solution in the supernatant is then measured by any of the routine total protein methods. Salting out is not used today because direct methods are available that react specifically with albumin in a mixture of proteins.

Albumin

The most widely used methods for determining albumin are dye-binding procedures. The pH of the solution is adjusted so that albumin is positively charged. The albumin is attracted to and binds to an anionic dye by electrostatic forces. When bound to albumin, the dye has a different absorption maximum than the free dye. The amount of albumin is calculated by measurement of the absorbance of the albumin–dye complex. A variety of dyes have been used, including methyl orange, 2,4′-hydroxyazobenzene-benzoic acid (HABA), bromocresol green (BCG), and bromocresol purple (BCP). Methyl orange is nonspecific for albumin; β-lipoproteins and some α_1- and α_2-globulins also will bind to this dye. HABA has a low sensitivity but is more specific for albumin. In addition, several compounds, such as salicylates, penicillin, conjugated bilirubin, and sulfonamides, interfere with the binding of albumin to HABA. BCG is not affected by interfering substances such as bilirubin and salicylates; however, hemoglobin binds to BCG. For every 100 mg/dL of hemoglobin, albumin is increased by 0.1 g/dL.[65] BCG has been reported to overestimate low albumin values in patients when the low albumin level was accompanied by an elevated α-globulin fraction, such as occurs in nephrotic syndrome or end-stage renal disease.[66] It was found that the α-globulins react with BCG, giving a color intensity that is approximately one-third of the reaction seen with albumin. The specificity of the reaction for albumin can be improved by taking absorbance readings within a standardized short interval (<5 minutes due to α-globulins contributing significantly to the absorbance at long incubation) after mixing.[67]

BCP is an alternate dye used for albumin determinations, binding specifically to albumin. BCP is not subject to most interferences, is precise, and exhibits excellent correlation with immunodiffusion reference methods. The BCP method, however, is not without its disadvantages. In patients with renal insufficiency, the BCP method underestimates the serum albumin.[68] The serum of these patients appears to contain either a substance tightly bound to albumin or a structurally altered albumin that affects the binding of BCP. Bilirubin interferes with BCP binding to albumin while BCG binding is unaffected. Today, both the BCG and BCP methods are used to quantitate albumin, with BCP commonly preferred. Albumin methods are summarized in Table 11-7.

Total Globulins

Another approach to fractionation of proteins is the measurement of total globulins. Albumin can then be calculated by subtraction of the globulin from total protein. The total globulin level in serum is determined by a direct colorimetric method using glyoxylic acid. Glyoxylic acid, in the presence of Cu^{2+} and in an acid medium (acetic acid and H_2SO_4), condenses with tryptophan found in globulins to produce a purple color. Albumin has approximately 0.2% tryptophan, compared with 2% to 3% for the serum globulins. When calibrated using a serum of known albumin and globulin concentrations, the total globulins can be determined. The measurement of globulins based on their tryptophan content

TABLE 11-7	ALBUMIN METHODS	
METHOD	**PRINCIPLE**	**COMMENT**
Salt precipitation	Globulins are precipitated in high salt concentrations; albumin in supernatant is quantitated by biuret reaction	Labor intensive
DYE BINDING		
Methyl orange	Albumin binds to dye; causes shift in absorption maximum	Nonspecific for albumin
HABA [2,4'-hydroxyazobenzene-benzoic acid]	Albumin binds to dye; causes shift in absorption maximum	Many interference (salicylates, bilirubin)
BCG (bromocresol green)	Albumin binds to dye; causes shift in absorption maximum	Sensitive; overestimates low albumin levels; most commonly used dye
BCP (bromocresol purple)	Albumin binds to dye; causes shift in absorption maximum	Specific, sensitive, precise
Electrophoresis	Proteins separated based on electric charge	Accurate; gives overview of relative changes in different protein fractions

has never come into common use because of the ease and simplicity of the dye-binding methods for albumin.

Electrophoresis

When an abnormality is found in the total protein or albumin, an electrophoresis is usually performed. If an abnormality is seen on the electrophoretic pattern, an analysis of the individual proteins within the area of abnormality is made.

Electrophoresis separates proteins on the basis of their electric charge densities. Protein, when placed in an electric current, will move according to their charge density, which is determined by the pH of a surrounding buffer. At a pH greater than the pI, the protein is negatively charged (AA~COO⁻) and vice versa (AA~NH₃⁺). The direction of movement depends on whether the charge is positive or negative; cations (positive net charge) migrate to the cathode (negative terminal), whereas anions (negative net charge) migrate to the anode (positive terminal). The speed of the migration can be estimated from the difference between the pI of the protein and the pH of the buffer. The more the pH of the buffer differs from the pI, the greater is the magnitude of the net charge of that protein and the faster it will move in the electric field. In addition to the charge density, the velocity of the movement also depends on the electric field strength, size, and shape of the molecule; temperature; and the characteristics of the buffer such as pH, qualitative composition, and ionic strength. The specific electrophoretic mobility (μ of a protein) is calculated by

$$\mu = \frac{(s/t)}{F}$$ (Eq. 11-2)

where s is the distance traveled in cm, t is time of migration in seconds, and F is field strength in V/cm.

Cellulose acetate or agarose gel is the support media used in today's laboratories. Historically, electrophoresis using an aqueous medium was called *moving boundary electrophoresis*. Later, paper was used as a solid medium in the process known as *zone electrophoresis*.

CASE STUDY 11-4

A 60-year-old woman with a history of rheumatoid arthritis, smoking of 60 packs/y, chronic obstructive pulmonary disease, and treated hypertension underwent a screening colonoscopy and then felt poorly for a week. She saw her family physician, who referred her to the local hospital clinic, where they did the tests listed in CASE STUDY TABLE 11-4.1. Her creatinine and BUN levels 2 weeks after the colonoscopy were 4.6 and 46 mg/dL, respectively; a baseline (from previous physician's office testing) serum creatinine was 0.9 mg/dL. Laboratory results are shown in the chart.

Questions

1. What disease state is the most likely explanation for the patient's laboratory results?

2. What is the significance of the polyclonal hypergammaglobulinemia with no monoclonal immunoglobulin spike identified on SPE?

3. Is the patient's urine protein normal?

4. Describe the immunofixation electrophoresis method.

CASE STUDY 11-4 (continued)

CASE STUDY TABLE 11-4.1 LABORATORY RESULTS

TEST	RESULTS	REFERENCE RANGE
Creatinine	3.7 mg/dL	Women <1.2 mg/dL
BUN	35 mg/dL	5–20 mg/dL
Creatinine clearance	12.5 mL/min	75–115 mL/min
C3	148 mg/dL	80–200 mg/dL
C4	19 mg/dL	15–80 mg/dL
Albumin	4.1 g/dL	3.5–5.0 g/dL
Calcium	9 mg/dL	8–10 mg/dL
Phosphorous	4.6 mg/dL	2.5–4.5 mg/dL
Cryoglobulin screen	Negative	

Serum protein electrophoresis—polyclonal hypergammaglobulinemia with no monoclonal immunoglobulin spike identified

Urine protein electrophoresis—protein 15.9 mg/dL with normal immunofixation electrophoresis

Urine sediment—no RBCs, 4–8 WBCs/hpf, granular and hyaline casts

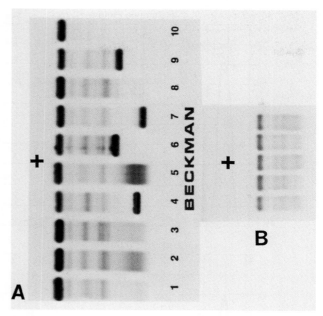

FIGURE 11-7 Serum protein electrophoretic patterns on agarose and cellulose acetate. **(A)** Agarose gel—note the monoclonal γ-globulin. **(B)** Cellulose acetate. (Courtesy of Department of Laboratory Medicine, The University of Texas M.D. Anderson Hospital, Drs. Liu, Fritsche, and Trujillo and Ms. McClure, Supervisor.)

Serum Protein Electrophoresis

In the standard method for SPE, serum samples are applied close to the cathode end of a support medium that is saturated with an alkaline buffer (pH 8.6). The support medium is connected to two electrodes and a current is passed through the medium to separate the proteins. All major serum proteins carry a net negative charge at pH 8.6 and migrate toward the anode. Using standard SPE methods, serum proteins appear in five bands: albumin travels farthest to the anode, followed by α_1-globulins, α_2-globulins, β-globulins, and γ-globulins, in that order. The width of the band of proteins in a fraction depends on the number of proteins present in that fraction. Homogeneous protein gives a narrow band.

After separation, the protein fractions are fixed by immersing the support medium in an acid solution (e.g., acetic acid) to denature the proteins and immobilize them on the support medium. In the next step, the proteins are stained. A variety of dyes have been used, including Ponceau S, amido black, and Coomassie blue. The proteins appear as bands on the support medium. Typical cellulose acetate electrophoretic patterns are shown in Figure 11-7A, and Figure 11-7B shows the patterns obtained using agarose gel as the support medium.

Visual inspection of the membrane can be done, but usually the cleared transparent medium is placed in a scanning densitometer for reading. Reflectance measurements also may be made on the uncleared membranes. The pattern on the membrane moves past a slit through which light is transmitted to a phototube to record the absorbance of the dye that is bound to each protein fraction. This absorbance is normally recorded on a strip-chart recorder to obtain a pattern of the fractions (Fig. 11-8).

Many scanning densitometers compute the area under the absorbance curve for each band and the percentage of total dye that appears in each fraction. The concentration is then calculated as a percentage of the total protein that was determined by one of the protein methods, such as the biuret procedure.

The computation also may be made by cutting out the small bands from the membrane and eluting the dye from each band in 0.1 mol/L NaOH. The absorbances are added to obtain the total absorbance, and the percentage of the total absorbance found in each fraction is then calculated.

A reference serum control is processed with each electrophoretic run (Fig. 11-8A). Reference values for each fraction are as follows:

Albumin, 53% to 65% of the total protein (3.5 to 5.0 g/dL)
α_1-Globulin, 2.5% to 5% (0.1 to 0.3 g/dL)
α_2-Globulin, 7% to 13% (0.6 to 1.0 g/dL)
β-Globulin, 8% to 14% (0.7 to 1.1 g/dL)
γ-Globulin, 12% to 22% (0.8 to 1.6 g/dL)

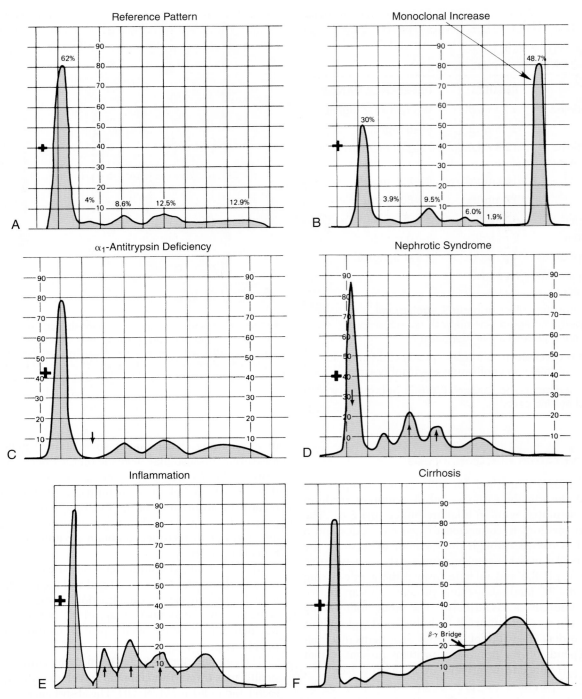

FIGURE 11-8 Selected densitometric patterns of protein electrophoresis. Albumin is at the anodal (+) end followed by α₁-, α₂-, β-, and γ-globulin fractions. *Arrows* indicate decrease or increase in fractions. **(A)** Reference pattern (agarose). **(B)** Monoclonal increase in γ area (agarose). **(C)** α₁-Antitrypsin deficiency (cellulose acetate). **(D)** Nephrotic syndrome (cellulose acetate). **(E)** Inflammation (cellulose acetate). **(F)** Cirrhosis (cellulose acetate). (**A** and **B** are courtesy of Drs. Liu and Fritsche and Jose Trujillo, Director, and Ms. McClure of the Department of Laboratory Medicine, The University of Texas M.D. Anderson Hospital. Others are courtesy of Dr. Wu of the Hermann Hospital Laboratory/The University of Texas Medical School.)

Inadvertent use of plasma will result in a narrow band in the β_2-globulin region because of the presence of fibrinogen. The presence of free hemoglobin will cause a blip in the pattern in the late α_2 or early β zone, and the presence of hemoglobin–haptoglobin complexes will cause a small blip in the α_2 zone. The great advantage of electrophoresis compared with the quantitation of specific proteins is the overview it provides. The electrophoretic pattern can give information about the relative increases and decreases within the protein population, as well as information about the homogeneity of a fraction.

Probably the most significant finding from an electrophoretic pattern is **monoclonal immunoglobulin disease.** The densitometric scan shows a sharp peak if the increase in immunoglobulins is a result of a monoclonal increase (Fig. 11-8B). A spike in the γ, β, or, sometimes, α_2 region signals the need for examination of the immunoglobulins and observation for clinical signs of myelomatosis. A deficiency of the predominant immunoglobulin, IgG, is seen as a much paler stain in the γ area. Another significant finding is a decrease in α_1-antitrypsin (Fig. 11-8C).

In nephrotic syndrome, the patient loses serum albumin and low-molecular-weight proteins in the urine. Some IgG is also lost. At the same time, an increase occurs in α_2-macroglobulin, β-lipoprotein, complement components, and haptoglobin. These two events lead to a dramatic decrease in the relative amount of albumin and a significant increase in the relative amounts of α_2-globulin and β-globulin fractions (Fig. 11-8D).

An inflammatory pattern indicating an inflammatory condition is seen when there is a decrease in albumin and an increase in the α_1-globulins (AAG and α_1-antitrypsin), α_2-globulins (ceruloplasmin and haptoglobin), and β-globulin band (CRP) (Fig. 11-8E). This pattern, also called an acute-phase reactant pattern, is seen in trauma, burns, infarction, malignancy, and liver disease. Acute-phase reactants are so named because they are increased in the serum within days following trauma or exposure to inflammatory agents. Fibrinogen, haptoglobin, ceruloplasmin, and serum amyloid A increase severalfold, whereas CRP and α_2-macroglobulin are increased several hundredfold. Chronic infections also produce a decrease in the albumin, but the globulin increase is found in the γ fraction as well as the α_1, α_2, and β fractions.

The electrophoretic pattern of serum proteins in liver disease shows the decrease in serum albumin concentration and the increase in γ-globulin. In the pattern in cirrhosis of the liver, there are some fast-moving γ-globulins that prevent resolution of the β- and γ-globulin bands. This is known as the β–γ bridge of cirrhosis (Fig. 11-8F). In infectious hepatitis, the γ-globulin fraction rises with increasing hepatocellular damage. In obstructive jaundice, there is an increase in the α_2- and β-globulins. Also noted in obstructive jaundice is an increased concentration of lipoproteins, which is an indicator of its biliary origin. This is especially the case when there is little or no decrease of the serum albumin.

High-Resolution Protein Electrophoresis

Standard SPE separates the protein into 5 distinct bands but, by modifying the electrophoretic parameters, proteins can be further separated into as many as 12 bands. The modification, known as HRE, uses a higher voltage coupled with a cooling system in the electrophoretic apparatus and a more concentrated buffer. The support medium most commonly used is agarose gel. To obtain the HRE patterns, samples are applied on the agarose gel, electrophoresed in a chamber cooled by a gel block, stained, and then visually inspected. Each band is compared with the same band on a reference pattern for color density, appearance, migration rates, and appearance of abnormal bands or regions of density. A normal serum HRE pattern is shown in Figure 11-9. As with SPE, the

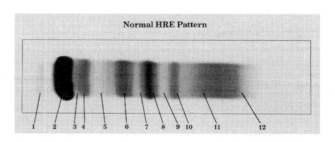

Normal HRE Pattern

Zones	Serum proteins found in zones
1. PREALBUMIN ZONE	-Prealbumin
2. ALBUMIN ZONE	-Albumin
3. ALBUMIN-α_1 INTERZONE	-α-Lipoprotein (α-Fetoprotein)
4. α_1 ZONE	-α_1-Antitrypsin, α_1-Acid glycoprotein
5. α_1-α_2 INTERZONE	-Gc-globulin, inter-α-trypsin inhibitor, α_1-antichymotrypsin
6. α_2 ZONE	-α_2-Macroglobulin, Haptoglobin
7. α_2-β_1 INTERZONE	-Cold insoluble globulin, (Hemoglobin)
8. β_1 ZONE	-Transferrin
9. β_1-β_2 INTERZONE	-β-Lipoprotein
10. β_2 ZONE	-C3
11. γ_1 ZONE	-IgA (Fibrinogen), IgM (Monoclonal Igs, light chains)
12. γ_2 ZONE	-IgC (C-reactive protein) (Monoclonal Igs, light chains)

Proteins listed in ( ) are normally found in too low a concentration to be visible in a normal pattern.

FIGURE 11-9 High-resolution electrophoretic (HRE) pattern of serum. (Courtesy of Helena Laboratories, Beaumont, TX.)

patterns may be scanned with a densitometer to obtain semiquantitative estimates of the protein found in each band. HRE is particularly useful in detecting small monoclonal bands and differentiating unusual bands or prominent increases of normal bands that can be confused with a monoclonal gammopathy.[69]

Capillary Electrophoresis

Capillary electrophoresis is a collection of techniques in which the separation of molecules takes place in silica capillaries. The capillaries are typically 30 to 50 cm long, with an internal diameter between 25 and 100 μm. In capillary zone electrophoresis, the capillaries are filled with a conducting solution, usually an aqueous buffer. The detection end of the capillary is grounded and the sample injection end is connected to a high-voltage power supply. When a positive voltage is applied, the positively charged buffer molecules flow to the detection end, which is negative relative to the injection end. The net flow of buffer is called electroosmotic flow (EOF). When a sample is injected, all molecules have a tendency to move toward the detector (negative) end of the capillary due to EOF; however, the negatively charged molecules in the specimen also have a tendency to migrate back toward the injector (positive) end. This is referred to as *electrophoretic mobility*. EOF is usually stronger than electrophoretic mobility, and all ions (positively charged, neutral, and negatively charged) migrate to the detector end but with different net mobilities based on size and charge differences. The separated molecules are detected by their absorbance as they pass through a small window near the detection end of the capillary. Use of the capillaries allows heat to be effectively dissipated, which means that higher operating voltages can be used and, therefore, analysis times are faster. Additionally, the sample size required is small (nanoliters).

Isoelectric Focusing

Isoelectric focusing (IEF) is zone electrophoresis that separates proteins on the basis of pI. IEF uses constant power and polyacrylamide or agarose gel mediums, which contain a pH gradient. The pH gradient is established by the incorporation of small polyanions and polycations (**ampholytes**, or molecules that contain both acidic and basic groups) in the gel. The varying pIs of the polyions cause them, in the presence of an electric field, to seek their place in the gradient and to remain there. The pH gradient may range from 3.5 to 10.

When a protein is electrophoresed in the gel, it migrates to a place on the gel where the pH is the same as its pI. The protein becomes focused there because, if it should diffuse in either direction, it leaves its pI and gains

a net charge. When this occurs, the electric current once again carries it back to its point of no charge, or its pI.

The clinical applications of IEF include phenotyping of α₁-antitrypsin deficiencies, determination of genetic variants of enzymes and hemoglobins, detection of paraproteins in serum and oligoclonal bands in CSF, and isoenzyme determinations.

Immunochemical Methods

Specific proteins may be identified by immunochemical assays in which the reaction of the protein (antigen) and its antibody is measured. Methods using various modifications of this principle include radial immunodiffusion, immunoelectrophoresis, immunofixation electrophoresis (Fig. 11-10), electroimmunodiffusion, immunoturbidimetry, and immunonephelometry. These techniques are discussed in Chapter 8.

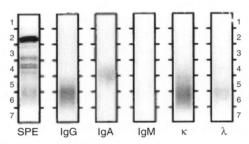

Normal IFE electrophoresis

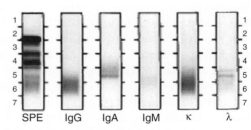

IFE electrophoresis showing IgA λmonoclonal band

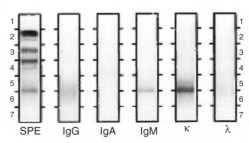

IFE electrophoresis showing IgM κmonoclonal band

FIGURE 11-10 Patterns of immunofixation electrophoresis (IFE).

PROTEINS IN OTHER BODY FLUIDS

The development of a disease-oriented relational database for proteins found in body fluids has been stimulated by the development of computers capable of handling large amounts of data and the development of high-resolution methods for the quantitative analysis of proteins in body fluids.[70]

Body fluids now being studied for their protein content include peritoneal, pleural, seminal, and vaginal fluids and tears. This section includes a discussion of the two fluids whose protein contents are studied most often—urine and CSF.

CASE STUDY 11-5

A male patient aged 47 years came to the clinic after a minor work accident. He worked as a painter, and he had fallen off a 12-foot scaffold and hurt his ankle. He had a complicated medical history that included severe diabetes, diagnosed a decade earlier, with peripheral neuropathy and retinopathy; chronic renal insufficiency; hypertension for the past 20 years; and hyperlipidemia. At this clinic visit, the patient was noted to have mild hepatomegaly. The patient's blood showed a normochromic normocytic anemia. An SPE with immunofixation demonstrated a monoclonal IgGκ of less than 100 mg/dL. An urine protein electrophoresis (UPE) with immunofixation was negative for light chains (Bence Jones protein). Although his ankle was not sprained, the patient continued to have breathing problems over the next several months and returned to the clinic often. Among many other tests, a follow-up SPE and an UPE with immunofixation were performed. The results are shown below.

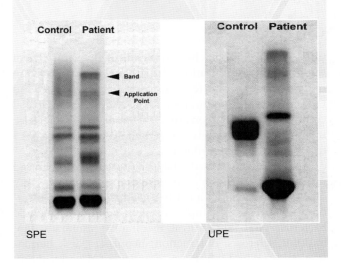

SPE   UPE

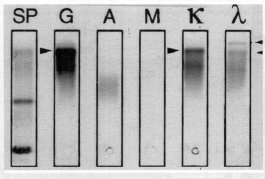

UPE Immunofixation

Questions

1. What does the presence of the monoclonal IgGκ band indicate?

2. What further information is obtained from the UPE?

3. Was this patient's SPE finding consistent with his complicated medical history?

4. What is MGUS?

Urinary Protein

Proteins found in the urine are from the blood; however, urinary proteins can originate from the kidney and urinary tract and from extraneous sources such as the vagina and prostate. Plasma proteins appear in the urine because they have passed through the renal glomerulus and have not been reabsorbed by the renal tubules. The qualitative tests for proteinuria are commonly performed using a reagent test strip. These methods are based on the change of an indicator dye in the presence of protein, known as protein error of indicators (ability of protein to alter the color of some acid–base indicators without altering the pH). In an acid pH, the indicator that is yellow in the absence of protein progresses through various shades of green and finally to blue as the concentration of protein increases. A protein concentration of 6 mg/dL or greater produces a color change.

Most quantitative assays are performed on urine specimens for 12 or 24 hours. The 24-hour timing allows for circadian rhythmic changes in excretion at certain times of day. The patient should void, completely emptying the bladder, and discard this urine. Urine is collected from that time for the next 24 hours. At the end of the 24-hour period, the bladder is completely emptied and that urine included in the sample. The volume of the timed specimen is measured accurately and recorded. The results are reported generally in terms of weight of protein per

TABLE 11-8	URINE PROTEIN METHODS	
METHOD	**PRINCIPLE**	**COMMENT**
Turbidimetric methods (sulfosalicylic acid, trichloroacetic acid, or benzethonium chloride)	Proteins are precipitated as fine particles, turbidity is measured spectrophotometrically	Rapid, easy to use; unequal sensitivity for individual protein
Biuret	Proteins are concentrated by precipitation, redissolved in alkali, then reacted with Cu^{2+}; Cu^{2+} forms colored complex with peptide bonds	Accurate
Folin-Lowry	Initial biuret reaction; oxidation of tyrosine, tryptophan, and histidine residues by Folin phenol reagent (mixture of phosphotungstic and phosphomolybdic acids): measurement of resultant blue color	Very sensitive
Dye binding (Coomassie blue, Ponceau S)	Protein binds to dye, causes shift in absorption maximum	Limited linearity; unequal sensitivity for individual proteins

24 hours by calculating the amount of protein present in the total volume of urine collected during that time.

There are several precipitation methods for the determination of total protein in urine and other body fluids, including the measurement of turbidity when urinary proteins are mixed with an anionic organic acid such as sulfosalicylic acid, TCA, or benzethonium chloride. These methods are sensitive, but the reagent does not react equally with each protein fraction. This is particularly true of sulfosalicylic acid, which produces four times more turbidity with albumin than with α-globulin.

A quantitative method consists of precipitation of the urine proteins, dissolution of the protein precipitate, and color formation with biuret reagent. Another chemical procedure for urinary protein uses the Folin-Ciocalteu reagent, which is a phosphotungstomolybdic acid solution, frequently called phenol reagent because it oxidizes phenolic compounds. The reagent changes color from yellow to blue during reaction with tyrosine, tryptophan, and histidine residues in protein. This method is about 10 times more sensitive than the biuret method. Lowry et al. increased the sensitivity of the Folin-Ciocalteu reaction by incorporating a biuret reaction as the initial step. After the binding of the Cu^{2+} to the peptide bonds, the Folin-Ciocalteu reagent is added. As the Cu^{2+}–protein complex is oxidized, the reagent is reduced, forming the chromogens tungsten blue and molybdenum blue. This increased the sensitivity to 100 times greater than that of the biuret method alone. Another modification uses a pyrogallol red–molybdate complex that reacts with protein to produce a blue-purple complex. This procedure is easily automated.

Dye-binding methods using Coomassie blue and Ponceau S have also been used to determine the quantitative total protein content of urine. However, dye-binding assays are too insensitive for urine microalbumin (MAU) testing, making immunochemical assays the most widely used MAU methods.[71] These immunoassays include immunoturbidimetry, immunofluorescence, ELISA, RIA, and zone immunoelectrophoresis. Table 11-8 summarizes the various methods for measurement of urinary total protein.

The reference values or intervals for urinary proteins are highly method dependent, ranging from 100 to 250 mg every 24 hours. Because of ease of use, speed, and sensitivity, the techniques used most frequently today are turbidimetric procedures. Immunochemical, chromatographic, and liquid chromatography–mass spectrometry methods for quantifying urine albumin are being used. Even a fluorescence resonance energy transfer assay for point-of-care testing of urinary albumin has been developed.[72]

CSF Proteins

CSF is formed in the choroid plexus of the ventricles of the brain by ultrafiltration of the blood plasma. Protein measurement is one test that is usually requested on CSF, in addition to glucose level and differential cell count, culture, and sensitivity. The accepted reference interval for patients between 10 and 40 years of age is 15 to 45 mg/dL of CSF protein.

Abnormally increased total CSF proteins may be found in conditions in which there is an increased permeability of the capillary endothelial barrier through which ultrafiltration occurs. Examples of such conditions include bacterial, viral, and fungal meningitis; traumatic tap; multiple sclerosis; obstruction; neoplasm; disk herniation; and cerebral infarction. The degree of permeability

CASE STUDY 11-6

A 55-year-old man with no history of illness suffered a blow to the head. He was unconscious when admitted to the hospital and remained in that state until his death 15 days later. A nasogastric tube was inserted to administer the required nutrients (protein, carbohydrates, fat, minerals, and vitamins). The total water intake was 1,500 mL/d. Starting on day 5, his blood pressure gradually fell. The 24-hour urine volumes recorded from an indwelling catheter were as follows:

DAY AFTER ADMISSION	URINE VOLUME (mL/24 h)
6	1,500
8	1,300
10	1,200
12	1,100
14	900

The patient's hemoglobin and hematocrit were elevated.

Blood chemistry analysis on day 13 revealed the following:

TOTAL PROTEIN	9.4 g/dL
Albumin	6.0 g/dL
BUN	80 mg/dL
Na^+	175 mmol/L
K^+	4.0 mmol/L
Cl^-	134 mmol/L

Questions

1. What is the probable cause of the elevated proteins?

2. What other results support this conclusion?

3. Why is the BUN elevated?

can be evaluated by measuring the CSF albumin and comparing it with the serum albumin. Albumin is usually used as the reference protein for permeability because it is not synthesized to any degree in the CNS. The reference value for the CSF albumin–serum albumin ratio is less than 2.7 to 7.3; a value greater than this indicates that the increase in the CSF albumin came from plasma due to a damaged blood–brain barrier. Low CSF protein values are found in hyperthyroidism and when fluid is leaking from the CNS.

The total CSF protein may be determined by several of the more sensitive chemical or spectrophotometric methods referred to earlier in the discussion on urinary proteins. The most frequently used procedures are turbidimetric using TCA, sulfosalicylic acid with sodium sulfate, or benzethonium chloride. Also available are dye-binding methods (e.g., Coomassie brilliant blue), a kinetic biuret reaction, and the Lowry method using a Folin phenol reagent.

Although total protein levels in the CSF are informative, diagnosis of specific disorders often requires measurement of individual protein fractions. The pattern of types of proteins present can be seen by electrophoresis of CSF that has been concentrated. This may be performed on cellulose acetate or agarose gel. The normal CSF pattern shows prealbumin, a prominent albumin band, α_1-globulin composed predominantly of α_1-antitrypsin, an α_2 band consisting primarily of haptoglobin and ceruloplasmin, a β_1 band composed principally of transferrin, and a CSF-specific transferrin that is deficient in carbohydrate, referred to as τ protein, in the β_2 zone. The globulin present in the γ band is typically IgG with a small amount of IgA.

CASE STUDY 11-7

An 84-year-old woman resident of a nursing home was admitted to the hospital for treatment of lower back pain resulting from a fall. Radiologic examination revealed a vertebral compression fracture. Because she demonstrated signs of general deterioration, further medical evaluation was performed. A neurologic examination and CT scan were normal. Serologic examinations for collagen vascular disease were also negative, although the CRP showed a modest increase. Serum protein electrophoresis was done to rule out multiple myeloma. The serum protein fractions were as follows: albumin, 3.2 g/dL; α_1-globulins, 0.31 g/dL; α_2-globulins, 1.59 g/dL (elevated in a tight band); β-globulins, 0.72 g/dL; and γ-globulins, 0.96 g/dL.

Questions

1. What would the next step be in the evaluation of this patient?

2. Given the following additional result (haptoglobin: 416 mg/dL), what condition would explain her abnormal protein electrophoresis pattern?

3. What other proteins would you expect to be abnormal?

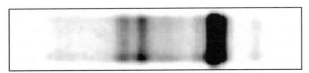

Normal CSF protein electrophoresis

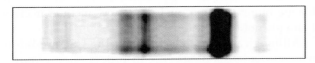

3 X Oligoclonal bands in CSF protein electrophoresis

FIGURE 11-11 Patterns of cerebrospinal fluid (CSF) protein electrophoresis.

Electrophoretic patterns of CSF from patients who have multiple sclerosis have multiple, distinct oligoclonal bands in the γ zone (Fig. 11-11). The identification of discrete bands in the γ region that are present in the CSF but not in the serum is consistent with production of IgG in the CSF. These bands cannot be seen on routine cellulose acetate electrophoresis but require a high-resolution technique in which agarose is usually used. More than 90% of patients with multiple sclerosis have oligoclonal bands, although the bands also have been found in inflammatory conditions and infectious neurologic diseases such as Guillain-Barre syndrome, bacterial meningitis, viral encephalitis, subacute sclerosing panencephalitis, and neurosyphilis.[73]

To distinguish raised CSF IgG due to local CNS production from leakage of plasma into the CSF, the laboratory can compare CSF and serum IgG levels with reference to albumin, a value known as the IgG index. A CSF IgG:albumin ratio higher than that of serum (raised IgG index) is indicative of local CNS production of IgG. A serum IgG:albumin ratio much higher than that of CSF (low IgG index) is suggestive of hypergammaglobulinemia or low serum albumin. The reference range for IgG index is 0.26 to 0.70. To identify the source of the elevated CSF IgG levels, the IgG-albumin index can be calculated as follows:

CSF IgG index =

$$\frac{CSF\ IgG\ (mg/dL) \times serum\ albumin\ (g/dL)}{serum\ IgG\ (g/dL) \times CSF\ albumin\ (mg/dL)} \quad \text{(Eq. 11-3)}$$

The CSF albumin concentration corrects for increased permeability. Another index to aid in discriminating the source of the IgG in the CSF is the IgG synthesis rate calculation using the formula of Tourtellotte et al.[74]

The reference interval for the synthesis rate is −9.9 to +3.3 mg/d.

In the investigation of multiple sclerosis, myelin basic proteins present in the CSF are also assayed because these proteins can provide an index of active demyelination. Myelin basic proteins are constituents of myelin, the sheath that surrounds many of the CNS axons. In very active demyelination, concentrations of myelin basic proteins of 17 to 100 ng/mL are found on RIA. In slow demyelination, values of 6 to 16 ng/mL occur and, in remission, the values are less than 4 ng/mL. In addition to multiple sclerosis, other conditions that induce CNS demyelination and therefore elevated levels of myelin basic protein include meningoencephalitis, SLE of CNS, diabetes mellitus, and chronic renal failure.

CASE STUDY 11-8

A 36-year-old woman complained of intermittent blurred vision and numbness and weakness in her left leg that had persisted for longer than 3 weeks. On examination, vertical nystagmus (involuntary back-and-forth or circular movements of eyes) was noted on upward gaze. CSF was drawn and the specimen was clear and colorless with normal cell count. The CSF total protein level was 49 mg/dL with an IgG of 8.1 mg/dL. Electrophoresis of the patient's serum and CSF revealed the following pattern: more than two oligoclonal bands in CSF (seen in Fig. 11-7) and a polyclonal pattern on SPE.

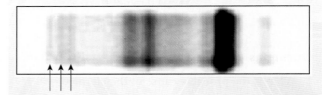

Questions

1. What is the significance of the CSF protein bands indicated by the arrows?

2. What conditions would produce this type of CSF protein electrophoresis pattern?

3. What other tests would be helpful in the investigation of this patient's diagnosis?

4. What laboratory test can be useful for monitoring the course of this patient's condition?

For additional student resources please visit thePoint at http://thepoint.lww.com.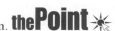

QUESTIONS

1. The acute-phase reactant proteins include all of the following EXCEPT
   a. Transferrin
   b. α_1-antitrypsin
   c. Haptoglobin
   d. Fibrinogen

2. The three-dimensional spatial configuration of a single polypeptide chain as determined by disulfide linkages, hydrogen bonds, electrostatic attractions, and van der Waals forces is referred to as the
   a. Tertiary structure
   b. Primary structure
   c. Secondary structure
   d. Quaternary structure

3. The plasma protein mainly responsible for maintaining colloidal osmotic pressure in vivo is
   a. Albumin
   b. Hemoglobin
   c. Fibrinogen
   d. α_2-macroglobulin

4. A peptide bond is
   a. Amino group and carboxyl group bonded to the alpha-carbon
   b. A double carbon bond
   c. A tertiary ring of amino group and carboxyl group bonded to the alpha-carbon
   d. Two amino groups bonded to the alpha-carbon

5. Nutritional assessment with poor protein-caloric status is associated with
   a. A decreased level of prealbumin
   b. A low level of γ-globulins
   c. An elevated ceruloplasmin concentration
   d. An increased level of α_1-fetoprotein

6. In which of the following conditions would a normal level of myoglobin be expected?
   a. Multiple myeloma
   b. Acute myocardial infarction
   c. Renal failure
   d. Crushing trauma received in a car accident

7. An immunofixation protein electrophoresis is performed on serum from a patient with the most common type of multiple myeloma. The resulting pattern revealed
   a. Monoclonal bands of the IgG type
   b. Oligoclonal bands

   c. β-γ bridging
   d. Monoclonal bands of the IgM type

8. The protein electrophoretic pattern of plasma, as compared with serum, reveals a
   a. Fibrinogen peak between the β- and γ-globulins
   b. Broad increase in the γ-globulins
   c. Fibrinogen peak with the α_2-globulins
   d. Decreased albumin peak

9. The following pattern of serum protein electrophoresis is obtained:
   albumin: decreased
   α_1- and α_2-globulins: increased
   γ-globulins: normal
   This pattern is characteristic of which of the following conditions?
   a. Acute inflammation (primary response)
   b. Cirrhosis
   c. Nephrotic syndrome
   d. Gammopathy

10. Distinct oligoclonal bands in the γ zone on CSF protein electrophoresis are diagnostic of
    a. Multiple sclerosis
    b. Multiple myeloma
    c. Waldenström's macroglobulinemia
    d. Myoglobinemia

11. When a protein is dissolved in a buffer solution, the pH of which is more alkaline than the pI, and an electric current is passed through the solution, the protein will act as
    a. An anion and migrate to the anode
    b. A cation and migrate to the cathode
    c. An anion and migrate to the cathode
    d. An uncharged particle and will not move

12. High serum total protein with high levels of both albumin and globulins is usually seen in
    a. Dehydration
    b. Waldenström's macroglobulinemia
    c. Glomerulonephritis
    d. Cirrhosis

13. In a patient with nephrotic syndrome, the total protein levels in urine would be:
    a. Normal.
    b. Lower than normal.
    c. Higher than normal.
    d. Similar to levels in CSF total protein levels.
    e. Lower albumin levels and higher levels of IgG.

14. Isoelectric focusing is the type of electrophoresis used to phenotype for α_1-antitrypsin deficiencies. When the protein is electrophoresed, it migrates to:
   a. The site where the pH is the same as its pI.
   b. The site where the molecular weight of the protein correlates with the pI.
   c. The site where the protein's net charge exceeds the pI.
   d. The site where the protein's net charge is less than the pI.
   e. The site where the gel pore size inhibits further migration.

15. A CSF albumin–serum albumin ratio was reported at 9.8 in a patient. How is this best interpreted?
   a. This ratio is in the normal range for the patient.
   b. The blood–brain barrier may be compromised leading to increased plasma albumin present in the CSF.
   c. There is an analytical error as it is biologically unlikely to achieve this value.
   d. This is diagnostic of fungal meningitis.
   e. This is diagnostic of multiple sclerosis.

16. Which of the following CSF proteins would be measured when investigating active demyelination in multiple sclerosis?
   a. CSF albumin to serum albumin ratio
   b. α_1-Antitrypsin
   c. Myelin basic protein
   d. Ceruloplasmin
   e. IgG

REFERENCES

1. Baldwin A, Lapointe M. The chemistry of amino acids. The Biology Project. 2004. www.biology.arizona.edu/biochemistry/problem_sets/aa/aa.html. Accessed August 21, 2012.
2. Brosnan J. Interorgan amino acid transport and its regulation. *J Nutr.* 2003;133(6 suppl 1):2068S-2072S.
3. Nelson DL, Cox MM. *Lehninger's Principles of Biochemistry.* 3rd ed. New York: Worth Publishing; 2000.
4. IUPAC-IUBMB Joint Commission on Biochemical Nomenclature. Nomenclature and symbolism for amino acids and peptides. Recommendations on organic & biochemical nomenclature, symbols & terminology etc. www.iupac.org/publications/pac/1984/pdf/5605x0595.pdf. Accessed May 17, 2007.
5. Wear JE, Keevil BG. Measurement of cystine in urine by liquid chromatography–tandem mass spectrometry. *Clin Chem.* 2005;51:787-789.
6. Boza JJ, Dangin M, Moennoz D, et al. Free and protein-bound glutamine have identical splanchnic extraction in healthy human volunteers. *Am J Physiol Gastrointest Liver Physiol.* 2001;281:267-274.
7. Morlion BJ, Stehle P, Wachtler P, et al. Total parenteral nutrition with glutamine dipeptide after major abdominal surgery: a randomized, double-blind, controlled study. *Ann Surg.* 1998;227:302-308.
8. Francesconi KA, Pannier F. Selenium metabolites in urine: a critical overview of past work and current status. *Clin Chem.* 2004;50:2240-2253.
9. Gill M, Gupta S, Zichittella L. Selenocysteine: the 21st amino acid. www.albany.edu/faculty/cs812/bio366/selenocysteine_ppt.pdf. Accessed October 4, 2008.
10. Atkins JF, Gesteland R. Biochemistry. The 22nd amino acid. *Science.* 2002;296:1409-1410.
11. National Newborn Screening and Genetics Resource Center. Current newborn conditions by state. http://genes-r-us.uthscsa.edu. Accessed August 21, 2012.
12. Chace DH, Millington DS, Terada N, et al. Rapid diagnosis of phenylketonuria by quantitative analysis for phenylalanine and tyrosine in neonatal blood spots by tandem mass spectrometry. *Clin Chem.* 1993;39:66-71.
13. Williams RA, Mamotte CDS, Burnett JR. Phenylketonuria: An Inborn Error of Phenylalanine Metabolism. *Clin Biochem Rev.* February 2008;29(1):31-41. PMCID: PMC2423317.
14. Food and Drug Administration (FDA). FDA approves Kuvan for treatment of phenylketonuria (PKU http://www.fda.gov/bbs/topics/news/2007/new01761.html. Accessed December 13, 2007.
15. Yamaguchi A, Mizushima Y, Fukushi M, et al. Microassay system for newborn screening for phenylketonuria, maple syrup urine disease, homocystinuria, histidinemia and galactosemia with use of a fluorometric microplate reader. *Screening.* 1992;1:49.
16. Sparkman OD. *Mass Spectrometry Desk Reference.* Pittsburgh, PA: Global View; 2000.
17. Pass KA, Morrissey M. Enhancing newborn screening for tyrosinemia type I. *Clin Chem.* 2008;54:627-629.
18. Oglesbee D, Sanders KA, Lacey JM, et al. Second-tier test for quantification of alloisoleucine and branched-chain amino acids in dried blood spots to improve newborn screening for maple syrup urine disease (MSUD). *Clin Chem.* 2008;54:542-549.
19. Picker JD, Levy HL. Homocystinuria caused by cystathionine beta-synthase deficiency. In: GeneReviews at GeneTests: medical genetics information resource (database online) (updated March 29, 2006). Copyright University of Washington, Seattle. 1997–2008. http://www.genetests.org. Accessed April 2, 2008.
20. Magera MJ, Lacey JM, Casetta B, Rinaldo P. Method for the determination of total homocysteine in plasma and urine by stable isotope dilution and electrospray tandem mass spectrometry. *Clin Chem.* 1999;45:1517-1522.
21. Thoene JG. Citrullinemia type I. In: GeneReviews at GeneTests: medical genetics information resource (database online) (updated December 22, 2006). Copyright University of Washington, Seattle. 1997–2008. http://www.genetests.org. Accessed April 2, 2008.
22. Turnell DC, Cooper JD. Rapid assay for amino acids in serum or urine by pre-column derivatization and reversed-phase liquid chromatography. *Clin Chem.* 1982;28:527-531.
23. Chace DH. Use of tandem mass spectrometry for multianalyte screening of dried blood specimens from newborns. *Clin Chem.* 2003;49:1797-1817.
24. Kimball J. *Biology.* 6th ed. Dubuque, IA: William C. Brown; 1995.
25. Branden C, Tooze J. *Introduction to Protein Structure.* 2nd ed. New York, NY: Garland Publishing; 1999.
26. Proteins: introduction. http://www.elmhurst.edu/~chm/vchembook/565proteins.html. Accessed October 2, 2008.
27. Proteins, peptides, and amino acids. http://www.cem.msu.edu/~reusch/VirtualText/proteins.htm. Accessed October 2, 2008.
28. Omenn GS, States DJ, Adamski M, et al. Overview of the HUPO Plasma Proteome Project: results from the pilot phase with 35 collaborating laboratories and multiple analytical groups, generating a core dataset of 3020 proteins and a publicly-available database. *Proteomics.* 2005;5:3226-3245.

29. Petsko GA, Ringe D. *Protein Structure and Function*. London: New Science Press in association with Sinauer Associates and Blackwell Science; 2003:180.

30. Lo Conte L, Brenner SE, Hubbard TJ, et al. SCOP database in 2002: refinements accommodate structural genomics. *Nucleic Acids Res*. 2002;30:264-267.

31. Holm L, Ouzounis C, Sander C, et al. A database of protein structure families with common folding motifs. *Protein Sci*. 1992;1:1691-1698.

32. Singh AP, Moniaux N, Chauhan SC, et al. Inhibition of MUC4 expression suppresses pancreatic tumor cell growth and metastasis. *Cancer Res*. 2004;64:622-630.

33. Kazuyoshi I, Yuichiro S, Yukie K, et al. Determination of glycated albumin by enzyme-linked boronate immunoassay (ELBIA). *Clin Chem*. 1998;44:256-263.

34. Albumin: the test sample. http://labtestsonline.org/understanding/analytes/albumin/sample.html. Accessed October 2, 2008.

35. Technical Bulletin. *Alpha-1-Antitrypsin Deficiency, Genotyping: DNA Test for the S and Z Alleles and Protein Measurement*. Salt Lake City, UT: ARUP Laboratories; 2007.

36. Technical Bulletin. *AFP-L3% in Serum (Includes Total Alpha Fetoprotein): For Risk Assessment of Hepatocellular Carcinoma in Patients with Chronic Liver Disease*. Salt Lake City, UT: ARUP Laboratories; 2007.

37. Israili ZH, Dayton PG. Human alpha-1-glycoprotein and its interactions with drugs. *Drug Metab Rev*. 2001;3:161-235.

38. Nilsson LNG, Bales KR, DiCarlo G, et al. α-1-Antichymotrypsin promotes β-sheet amyloid plaque deposition in a transgenic mouse model of Alzheimer's disease. *J Neurosci*. 2001;21:1444-1451.

39. Hamm A, Veeck J, Bektas N, et al. Frequent expression loss of Inter-alpha-trypsin inhibitor heavy chain (ITIH) genes in multiple human solid tumors: a systematic expression analysis. *BMC Cancer*. 2008;8:25.

40. Lis Lauridsen A, Vestergaard P, Nexo E. Mean serum concentration of vitamin D-binding protein (Gc globulin) is related to the Gc phenotype in women. *Clin Chem*. 2001;47:753-756.

41. Levy A. Haptoglobin phenotype and prevalent coronary heart disease in the Framingham offspring cohort. *Atherosclerosis*. 2003;172:361-365.

42. TIBC and transferrin. http://labtestsonline.org/understanding/analytes/tibc/glance.html. Accessed October 2, 2008.

43. Tolosano E, Altruda F. Hemopexin: structure, function, and regulation. *DNA Cell Biol*. 2002;21:297-306.

44. Yates JR, Sepp T, Matharu BK, et al. Complement C3 variant and the risk of age-related macular degeneration. *N Engl J Med*. 2007;357:553-561.

45. Wong SS. Strategic utilization of cardiac markers for the diagnosis of acute myocardial infarction. *Ann Clin Lab Sci*. 1996;26:301.

46. Ridker PM. Clinical application of C-reactive protein for cardiovascular disease detection and prevention. *Circulation*. 2003;107:363-369.

47. King DE, Mainous AG, Buchanan TA, Pearson WS. C-reactive protein and glycemic control in adults with diabetes. *Diabetes Care*. 2003;26:1535-1539.

48. Ridker PM. C-reactive protein: a simple test to help predict risk of heart attack and stroke. *Circulation*. 2003;108:e81.

49. Matsuda F, Ishii K, Bourvagnet P, et al. The complete nucleotide sequence of the human immunoglobulin heavy chain variable region locus. *J Exp Med*. 1998;188:2151-2162.

50. Abbas AK, Lichtman AH. *Cellular and Molecular Immunology*. 5th ed. Philadelphia, PA: WB Saunders; 2003.

51. Tangye SG, Ferguson A, Avery DT, et al. Isotype switching by human B cells is division-associated and regulated by cytokines. *J Immunol*. 2002;169:4298-4306.

52. Janeway CA Jr, Travers P, Walport M, et al. *Immunobiology*. 5th ed. New York, NY: Garland Publishing; 2001.

53. Woof J, Burton D. Human antibody-Fc receptor interactions illuminated by crystal structures. *Nat Rev Immunol*. 2004;4:89-99.

54. Preud'homme JL, Petit I, Barra A, et al. Structural and functional properties of membrane and secreted IgD. *Mol Immunol*. 2000;37:871-887.

55. Winter WE, Hardt MS, Fuhrman S. Immunoglobulin E: importance in parasitic infections and hypersensitivity responses. *Arch Pathol Lab Med*. 2000;124:1382-1385.

56. Morrow DA, Cannon CP, Jesse RL, et al. National Academy of Clinical Biochemistry Laboratory Medicine Practice Guidelines: clinical characteristics and utilization of biochemical markers in acute coronary syndromes. *Clin Chem*. 2007;53:552-574.

57. Chiu A, Chan W-K, Cheng S-H, et al. Troponin-I, myoglobin, and mass concentration of creatine kinase-MB in acute myocardial infarction. *QJM: Int J Med*. 1999;92:711-718.

58. Sakhuja R, Januzzi JL. NT-proBNP: a new test for diagnosis, prognosis and management of congestive heart failure. *Cardiology*. August 2004:1-5.

59. Nakamura Y, Shimada K, Fukuda D, et al. Implications of plasma concentrations of adiponectin in patients with coronary artery disease. *Heart*. 2004;90:528-533.

60. Huber AR, Risch L. Recent developments in the evaluation of glomerular filtration rate: is there a place for beta-trace? *Clin Chem*. 2005;51:1329-1330.

61. Shlipak MG, Sarnak MJ, Katz R, et al. Cystatin C and the risk of death and cardiovascular events among elderly persons. *N Engl J Med*. 2005;352:2049-2060.

62. Peters T Jr, Biamonte ET, Doumas BT. Protein (total) in serum, urine, cerebrospinal fluid, albumin in serum. In: Faulkner WR, Meites S, eds. *Selected Methods in Clinical Chemistry*. Vol 9. Washington, DC: American Association for Clinical Chemistry; 1982:317.

63. Reichert TS-METER. *Total Solids Refractometer Model 1310400A Instruction Manual 2003*. Depew, NY: Reichert, Inc. (publication 10400A-101 Rev. D).

64. Chromy V, Fischer J. Photometric determination of total protein in lipemic serum. *Clin Chem*. 1977;23:754.

65. Doumas BT, Watson WA, Biggs HG. *Albumin Standards and the Measurement of Serum Albumin with Bromcresol Green. Clin Chem Acta*. 1971;31:87.

66. Speicher CE, Widish JR, Gaudot FJ, et al. An evaluation of the overestimation of serum albumin by bromcresol green. *Am J Clin Pathol*. 1978;69:347.

67. Gustafsson JEC. Improved specificity of serum albumin determination and estimation of acute phase reactants by use of the bromocresol green reaction. *Clin Chem*. 1976;22:616.

68. Clase CM, St Pierre MW, Churchill DN. Conversion between bromcresol green- and bromcresol purple-measured albumin in renal disease. *Nephrol Dial Transplant*. 2001;16:1925-1929.

69. Keren D. High resolution electrophoresis aids detection of gammopathies. *Clin Chem News*. 1989;14:26-29.

70. Merril CR, Goldstein MP, Myrick JE, et al. The Protein Disease Database of human body fluids: I. Rationale for the development of this database. *Appl Theor Electrophor*. 1995;5:49-54.

71. Choi S, Choi EY, Kim HS, Sang WO. On-site quantification of human urinary albumin by a fluorescence immunoassay. *Clin Chem*. 2004;50:1052-1055.

72. Qin Q-P, Peltola O, Pettersson K. Time-resolved fluorescence resonance energy transfer assay for point-of-care testing of urinary albumin. *Clin Chem*. 2003;49:1105-1113.

73. Fact Sheet Immunopathology. CSF electrophoresis and the detection of oligoclonal bands. *Inst Clin Pathol Med Res*. 2002 (9/02 0119).

74. Tourtellotte WW, Staugaitis SM, Walsh MJ, et al. The basis of intra-blood-brain-barrier IgG synthesis. *Ann Neurol*. 1985;17:21-27.

Nonprotein Nitrogen Compounds

ELIZABETH L. FRANK

CHAPTER 12

CHAPTER OUTLINE

Chapter Objectives

Upon completion of this chapter, the clinical laboratorian should be able to do the following:

- List the nonprotein nitrogen components of the blood and recognize their chemical structures and relative physiologic concentrations.
- Describe the biosynthesis and excretion of urea, uric acid, creatinine, creatine, and ammonia.
- Describe the major pathological conditions associated with increased and decreased plasma concentrations of urea, uric acid, creatinine, creatine, and ammonia.
- State the specimen collection, transport, and storage requirements necessary for determinations of urea, uric acid, creatinine, creatine, and ammonia.
- Discuss commonly used methods for the determination of urea, uric acid, creatinine, creatine, and ammonia in

plasma and urine. Identify sources of error and variability in these methods and describe the effects on the clinical utility of the laboratory measurements.
- Recognize the reference intervals for urea, uric acid, creatinine, and ammonia in plasma and urine. State the effects of age and gender on these values.
- Describe the use of the urea nitrogen/creatinine ratio to distinguish prerenal, renal, and postrenal causes of uremia.
- Relate the solubility of uric acid to the pathologic consequences of increased plasma uric acid.
- Explain the use and limitations of serum creatinine for calculations of estimated glomerular filtration rate.
- Describe the toxic effects related to an increased plasma ammonia concentration.
- Suggest possible clinical conditions associated with test results, given patient values for urea, uric acid, creatinine, and ammonia and supporting clinical history.

KEY TERMS

Ammonia
Azotemia
Coupled enzymatic method
Creatine
Creatinine
Creatinine clearance
Estimated glomerular filtration rate
Glomerular filtration rate
Gout

Hyperuricemia
Hypouricemia
Postrenal
Prerenal
Protein-free filtrate
Reabsorption
Secretion
Urea
Urea nitrogen/creatinine ratio
Uremia or uremic syndrome
Uric acid

The term nonprotein nitrogen (NPN) originated in the early days of clinical chemistry when analytic methodology required removal of protein from a specimen before analysis. The concentration of nitrogen-containing compounds in this protein-free filtrate was quantified spectrophotometrically by converting nitrogen to ammonia and subsequent reaction with Nessler's reagent ($K_2[HgI_4]$) to produce a yellow color.[1] The method was technically difficult but provided an accurate determination of total NPN concentration. Although determination of total urinary nitrogen is of value in the assessment of nitrogen balance for nutritional management,[2] more useful clinical information is obtained by analyzing a patient's specimen for individual nitrogen-containing compounds.

Numerous compounds of clinical interest are included in the NPN fraction of plasma and urine. The most abundant of these are listed in Table 12-1.[3] The majority of these compounds arise from the catabolism of proteins and nucleic acids. The biochemistry, clinical utility, and analytical methods for measurement of the NPN compounds urea, uric acid, creatinine, creatine, and ammonia are presented in this chapter.

UREA

The NPN compound present in highest concentration in the blood is urea (Fig. 12-1). Urea is the major excretory product of protein metabolism.[4] It is formed in the liver from amino groups ($-NH_2$) and free ammonia generated during protein catabolism.[5] This enzymatically catalyzed process is termed the urea cycle. Since historic assays for urea were based on the measurement of nitrogen, the term blood urea nitrogen (BUN) has been used to refer to urea determination. Urea nitrogen (urea N) is a more appropriate term.[6]

Biochemistry

Protein metabolism produces amino acids that can be oxidized to produce energy or stored as fat and glycogen. These processes release nitrogen which is converted to urea and excreted as a waste product. Following

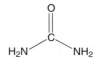

FIGURE 12-1 Structure of urea.

synthesis in the liver, urea is carried in the blood to the kidney, where it is readily filtered from the plasma by the glomerulus. Most of the urea in the glomerular filtrate is excreted in the urine, although some urea is reabsorbed by passive diffusion during passage of the filtrate through the renal tubules. The amount reabsorbed depends on the urine flow rate and extent of hydration. Small quantities of urea (<10% of the total) are excreted through the gastrointestinal (GI) tract and skin. The concentration of urea in the plasma is determined by the protein content of the diet, the rate of protein catabolism, and renal function and perfusion.[7]

Clinical Application

Measurement of urea is used to evaluate renal function, to assess hydration status, to determine nitrogen balance, to aid in the diagnosis of renal disease, and to verify adequacy of dialysis.[4]

Measurements of urea were originally performed on a protein-free filtrate of whole blood and based on measuring the amount of nitrogen. Current analytic methods have retained this custom and urea is often reported in terms of nitrogen concentration rather than urea concentration. Urea N concentration can be converted to urea concentration by multiplying by 2.14, as follows:

$$\frac{1 \text{ mg urea N}}{dL} \times \frac{1 \text{ mmol N}}{14 \text{ mg N}} \times \frac{1 \text{ mmol urea}}{2 \text{ mmol N}} \times$$
$$\frac{60 \text{ mg urea}}{1 \text{ mmol urea}} = \frac{2.14 \text{ mg urea}}{dL} \qquad \text{(Eq. 12-1)}$$

In the International System of Units (SI), urea is reported in units of millimoles per liter. Urea N concentration in milligrams per deciliter may be converted to urea concentration in millimoles per liter by multiplying by 0.36.[8]

	TABLE 12-1	**CLINICALLY SIGNIFICANT NONPROTEIN NITROGEN COMPOUNDS**	

COMPOUND	APPROXIMATE PLASMA CONCENTRATION (% OF TOTAL NPN)	APPROXIMATE URINE CONCENTRATION (% OF EXCRETED NITROGEN)
Urea	45–50	86.0
Amino acids	25	—
Uric acid	10	1.7
Creatinine	5	4.5
Creatine	1–2	—
Ammonia	0.2	2.8

Analytical Methods

Several analytic approaches have been used to assay urea. Enzymatic methods are used most frequently in clinical laboratories.[9] The enzyme urease (urea amidohydrolase, EC 3.5.1.5) hydrolyzes urea in the sample and the ammonium ion (NH_4^+) produced in the reaction is quantified.[10] The most common method couples the urease reaction with glutamate dehydrogenase (GLDH, EC 1.4.1.3), and the rate of disappearance of nicotinamide adenine dinucleotide (reduced, NADH) at 340 nm is measured (Fig. 12-2).[11]

Ammonium from the urease reaction can also be measured by the color change associated with a pH indicator. This approach has been incorporated into instruments using liquid reagents, a multilayer film format, and reagent strips.[12-14] A method that uses an electrode to measure the rate of increase in conductivity as ammonium ions are produced from urea is in use in approximately 15% of laboratories in the United States.[9,15] Because the rate of change in conductivity is measured, ammonia contamination is not a problem as it is in other methods.

A reference method using isotope dilution mass spectrometry (IDMS) has been developed.[16] Analytic methods are summarized in Table 12-2.

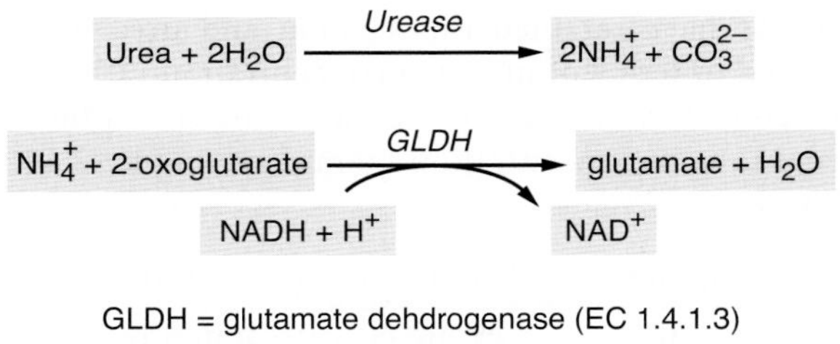

$$\text{Urea} + 2H_2O \xrightarrow{\text{Urease}} 2NH_4^+ + CO_3^{2-}$$

$$NH_4^+ + \text{2-oxoglutarate} \xrightarrow[\text{NADH} + H^+]{\text{GLDH}} \text{glutamate} + H_2O \quad NAD^+$$

GLDH = glutamate dehdrogenase (EC 1.4.1.3)

FIGURE 12-2 Enzymatic assay for urea.

Specimen Requirements

Urea concentration may be measured in plasma, serum, or urine. If plasma is collected, ammonium ions and high concentrations of sodium citrate and sodium fluoride must be avoided; citrate and fluoride inhibit urease.[8] Although the protein content of the diet influences urea concentration, the effect of a single protein-containing meal is minimal and a fasting sample is not required usually. A nonhemolyzed sample is recommended. Urea is susceptible to bacterial decomposition, so specimens (particularly urine) that cannot be analyzed within a few hours should be refrigerated. Timed urine specimens should be refrigerated during the collection period. Methods for plasma or serum may require modification for use with urine specimens because of high urea concentration and the presence of endogenous ammonia.[8]

Reference Intervals

UREA NITROGEN[8]		
Adult		
Plasma or serum	6–20 mg/dL	2.1–7.1 mmol/L
Urine, 24 h	12–20 g/d	0.43–0.71 mol urea/d

Pathophysiology

An elevated concentration of urea in the blood is called azotemia. Very high plasma urea concentration accompanied by renal failure is called uremia or the uremic syndrome. This condition is eventually fatal if not treated by dialysis or transplantation. Conditions causing increased plasma urea are classified according to the cause into three main categories: prerenal, renal, and postrenal.[7]

TABLE 12-2	SUMMARY OF ANALYTIC METHODS—UREA	
ENZYMATIC METHODS		
Methods use a similar first step—catalyzed by urease	Enzymatic production of ammonium ion (NH_4^+) from urea	See Figure 12-2
GLDH coupled enzymatic	Enzymatic reaction of NH_4^+, 2-oxoglutarate and NADH to form glutamate and NAD^+	Used on many automated instruments; best as a kinetic measurement
Indicator dye	NH_4^+ + pH indicator → color change	Used in automated systems, multilayer film reagents, and dry reagent strips
Conductimetric	Conversion of unionized urea to NH_4^+ and CO_3^{2-} results in increased conductivity	Specific and rapid
OTHER METHODS		
Isotope dilution mass spectrometry	Detection of characteristic fragments following ionization; quantification using isotopically labeled compound	Proposed reference method

Prerenal azotemia is a result of reduced renal blood flow. Less blood is delivered to the kidney; consequently, less urea is filtered. Causative factors include congestive heart failure, shock, hemorrhage, dehydration, and other factors resulting in a significant decrease in blood volume. The amount of protein metabolism also induces prerenal changes in blood urea concentration. A high-protein diet or increased protein catabolism, such as occurs in stress, fever, major illness, corticosteroid therapy, and GI hemorrhage, may increase the urea concentration.[7]

Decreased renal function causes an increase in plasma urea concentration as a result of compromised urea excretion. Renal causes of elevated urea include acute and chronic renal failure, glomerular nephritis, tubular necrosis, and other intrinsic renal disease (see Chapter 27). Postrenal azotemia can be due to obstruction of urine flow anywhere in the urinary tract by renal calculi, tumors of the bladder or prostate, or severe infection.

The major causes of decreased plasma urea concentration include low protein intake and severe liver disease. Plasma urea concentration is decreased during late pregnancy and in infancy as a result of increased protein synthesis. The conditions affecting plasma urea concentration are summarized in Table 12-3.

Differentiation of the cause of abnormal urea concentration is aided by calculation of the urea N/creatinine ratio, which is normally 10:1 to 20:1. Prerenal conditions tend to elevate plasma urea, whereas plasma creatinine remains normal, causing a high urea N/creatinine ratio. A high urea N/creatinine ratio with an elevated creatinine is usually seen in postrenal conditions. A low urea N/creatinine ratio is observed in conditions associated with decreased urea production, such as low protein intake, acute tubular necrosis, and severe liver disease.[17]

TABLE 12-3 CAUSES OF ABNORMAL PLASMA UREA CONCENTRATION

INCREASED CONCENTRATION

Prerenal	Congestive heart failure
	Shock, hemorrhage
	Dehydration
	Increased protein catabolism
	High-protein diet
Renal	Acute and chronic renal failure
	Renal disease, including glomerular nephritis and tubular necrosis
Postrenal	Urinary tract obstruction

DECREASED CONCENTRATION

	Low protein intake
	Severe vomiting and diarrhea
	Liver disease
	Pregnancy

CASE STUDY 12-1

A 65-year-old man was first admitted for treatment of chronic obstructive lung disease, renal insufficiency, and significant cardiomegaly. Pertinent laboratory data on admission (5/31) are shown in Case Study Table 12-1.1.

CASE STUDY TABLE 12-1.1 LABORATORY RESULTS—FIRST ADMISSION

Test	5/31	6/3	6/7
Urea N (mg/dL)	45	24	11
Creatinine (mg/dL)	1.8	1.3	0.9
Urea N/creatinine	25	18.5	12.2
pH	7.22	7.50	
pCO_2 (mm Hg)	74.4	48.7	
pO_2 (mm Hg)	32.8	57.6	
O_2 sat (%)	51.3	91.0	

Because of severe respiratory distress, the patient was transferred to the intensive care unit, placed on a respirator, and given diuretics and intravenous (IV) fluids to promote diuresis. This treatment brought about a significant improvement in both cardiac output and renal function, as shown by laboratory results several days later (6/3). After two additional days on a respirator with IV therapy, the patient's renal function had returned to normal and, at discharge, his laboratory results were within normal limits (6/7).

The patient was readmitted 6 months later because of the increasing inability of his family to arouse him. On admission, he was shown to have a tremendously enlarged heart with severe pulmonary disease, heart failure, and probable renal failure. Laboratory studies on admission were as shown in Case Study Table 12-1.2. Numerous attempts were made to improve the patient's cardiac and pulmonary function, all to no avail, and the patient died 4 days later.

CASE STUDY TABLE 12-1.2
LABORATORY RESULTS—SECOND ADMISSION

Urea N (mg/dL)	90
Creatinine (mg/dL)	3.9
Uric acid (mg/dL)	12.0
Urea N/creatinine	23
pH	7.35
pCO_2 (mm Hg)	59.9
pO_2 (mm Hg)	34.6
O_2 sat (%)	63.7

Question

1. What is the most likely cause of the patient's elevated urea nitrogen? Which data support your conclusion?

URIC ACID

Uric acid is the product of catabolism of the purine nucleic acids.[18] Although it is filtered by the glomerulus and secreted by the distal tubules into the urine, most uric acid is reabsorbed in the proximal tubules and reused.[7] Uric acid is relatively insoluble in plasma and, at high concentrations, can be deposited in the joints and tissue, causing painful inflammation.

Biochemistry

Purines, such as adenine and guanine from the breakdown of ingested nucleic acids or from tissue destruction, are converted into uric acid, primarily in the liver. Uric acid is transported in the plasma from the liver to the kidney, where it is filtered by the glomerulus. Reabsorption of 98% to 100% of the uric acid from the glomerular filtrate occurs in the proximal tubules. Small amounts of uric acid are secreted by the distal tubules

into the urine. Renal excretion accounts for about 70% of uric acid elimination; the remainder passes into the GI tract and is degraded by bacterial enzymes.[7]

Nearly, all of the uric acid in plasma is present as monosodium urate. At the pH of plasma (pH ~7), urate is relatively insoluble; at concentrations > 6.8 mg/dL, the plasma is saturated. As a result, urate crystals may form and precipitate in the tissues. In acidic urine (pH <5.75), uric acid is the predominant species and uric acid crystals may form.[7]

Clinical Application

Uric acid is measured to confirm diagnosis and monitor treatment of gout, to prevent uric acid nephropathy during chemotherapeutic treatment, to assess inherited disorders of purine metabolism, to detect kidney dysfunction, and to assist in the diagnosis of renal calculi.[19]

Analytical Methods

In higher primates, such as humans and apes, uric acid is the final breakdown product of purine metabolism.[4] Most other mammals have the ability to catabolize purines to allantoin, a more water-soluble end product. This reaction is shown in Figure 12-3. Uric acid is readily oxidized to allantoin and, therefore, can function as a reducing agent in chemical reactions. This property was exploited in early analytic procedures for the determination of uric acid. The most common method of this type is the Caraway method, which is based on the oxidation of uric acid in a protein-free filtrate, with subsequent reduction of phosphotungstic acid in alkaline solution to tungsten blue.[20] The method lacks specificity.

Methods using uricase (urate oxidase, EC 1.7.3.3), the enzyme that catalyzes the oxidation of uric acid to allantoin, are more specific and are used almost exclusively in clinical laboratories. The simplest of these methods measures the differential absorption of uric acid and allantoin at 293 nm.[21] The difference in absorbance before and after incubation with uricase is proportional to the uric acid concentration. Proteins can cause high

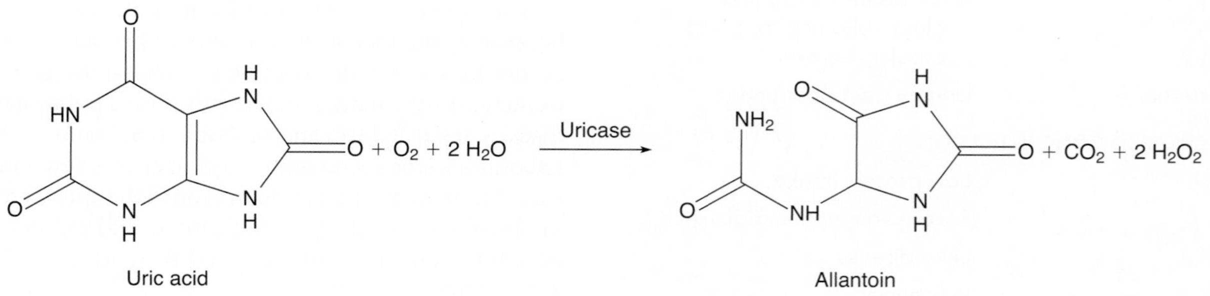

FIGURE 12-3 Conversion of uric acid to allantoin.

background absorbance, reducing sensitivity; hemoglobin and xanthine can cause negative interference.[22]

Coupled enzyme methods measure the hydrogen peroxide produced as uric acid is converted to allantoin.[23,24] Peroxidase or catalase (EC 1.11.1.6) is used to catalyze a chemical indicator reaction. The color produced is proportional to the quantity of uric acid in the specimen. Enzymatic methods of this kind have been adapted for use on traditional wet chemistry analyzers and for dry chemistry slide analyzers. Bilirubin and ascorbic acid, which destroy peroxide, if present in sufficient quantity, can interfere. Commercial reagent preparations often include potassium ferricyanide and ascorbate oxidase to minimize these interferences.

IDMS has been proposed as a candidate reference method.[25] Analytic methods are summarized in Table 12-4.

Specimen Requirements

Uric acid may be measured in heparinized plasma, serum, or urine. Serum should be removed from cells as quickly as possible to prevent dilution by intracellular contents. Diet may affect uric acid concentration overall, but a recent meal has no significant effect and a fasting specimen is unnecessary. Gross lipemia should be avoided. High bilirubin concentration may falsely decrease results obtained by peroxidase methods. Significant hemolysis, with concomitant glutathione release, may result in low values. Drugs such as salicylates and thiazides have been shown to increase values for uric acid.[26]

Uric acid is stable in plasma or serum after red blood cells have been removed. Serum samples may be stored refrigerated for 3 to 5 days. Ethylenediaminetetraacetic acid (EDTA) or fluoride additives should not be used for specimens that will be tested by an uricase method. Urine collections must be alkaline (pH 8).[8]

Reference Intervals

URIC ACID (URICASE METHOD)[8]

Adult	Plasma or Serum		
Male		3.5–7.2 mg/dL	0.21–0.43 mmol/L
Female		2.6–6.0 mg/dL	0.16–0.36 mmol/L
Child		2.0–5.5 mg/dL	0.12–0.33 mmol/L
Adult	Urine, 24 h	250–750 mg/d	1.5–4.4 mmol/d

Results expressed in conventional units of milligrams per deciliter can be converted to SI units using the molecular mass of uric acid (168 g/mol).

Pathophysiology

Abnormally increased plasma uric acid concentration is found in gout, increased catabolism of nucleic acids, and renal disease.[7] Gout is a disease found primarily in men and is usually first diagnosed between 30 and 50 years of age. Affected individuals have pain and inflammation of the joints caused by precipitation of sodium urates. In 25% to 30% of these patients, hyperuricemia is a result of overproduction of uric acid, although hyperuricemia may be exacerbated by a purine-rich diet, drugs,

TABLE 12-4	SUMMARY OF ANALYTIC METHODS—URIC ACID	
CHEMICAL METHODS		
Phosphotungstic acid	In carbonate solution (Na_2CO_3/OH^-), uric acid + $H_3PW_{12}O_{40}$ + O_2 → allantoin + tungsten blue + CO_2	Nonspecific; requires protein removal
ENZYMATIC METHODS		
Similar first step—Catalyzed by uricase	Enzymatic production of allantoin from uric acid	See Figure 12-3 Very specific
Coupled enzymatic—Peroxidase	H_2O_2 + indicator dye → colored compound	Readily automated; reducing agents interfere
Spectrophotometric	Decrease in absorbance at 293 nm measured	Hemoglobin and xanthine interfere
OTHER METHODS		
Isotope dilution mass spectrometry	Detection of characteristic fragments following ionization; quantification using isotopically labeled compound	Proposed reference method

and alcohol. Plasma uric acid concentration in affected individuals is usually greater than 6.0 mg/dL. Patients with gout are susceptible to the formation of renal calculi, although not all persons with abnormally high serum urate concentrations develop this complication. In women, urate concentration rises after menopause. Postmenopausal women may develop hyperuricemia and gout. In severe cases, deposits of crystalline uric acid and urates called tophi form in tissue, causing deformities.[7]

Another common cause of elevated plasma uric acid concentration is increased metabolism of cell nuclei, as occurs in patients on chemotherapy for such proliferative diseases as leukemia, lymphoma, multiple myeloma, and polycythemia. Monitoring uric acid concentration in these patients is important to avoid nephrotoxicity. Allopurinol, which inhibits xanthine oxidase (EC 1.1.3.22), an enzyme in the uric acid synthesis pathway, is used for treatment.

Patients with hemolytic or megaloblastic anemia may exhibit elevated uric acid concentration. Increased urate concentrations may be found following ingestion of a diet rich in purines (e.g., liver, kidney, sweetbreads, and shellfish) or as a result of increased tissue catabolism due to inadequate dietary intake (starvation).[7]

Inherited disorders of purine metabolism are associated with significant increases in physiological uric acid concentrations. Lesch-Nyhan syndrome is an X-linked genetic disorder (seen only in males) caused by the complete deficiency of hypoxanthine-guanine phosphoribosyltransferase (EC 2.4.2.8), an important enzyme in the biosynthesis of purines. Lack of this enzyme prevents the reutilization of purine bases in the nucleotide salvage pathway and results in increased de novo synthesis of purine nucleotides and high plasma and urine concentrations of uric acid.[7] Neurologic symptoms, mental retardation, and self-mutilation characterize this extremely rare disease. Mutations in the first enzyme in the purine synthesis pathway, phosphoribosylpyrophosphate synthetase (EC 2.7.6.1), also cause elevated uric acid concentration.[6] Increased uric acid is found secondary to glycogen storage disease (deficiency of glucose-6-phosphatase, EC 3.1.3.9) and fructose intolerance (deficiency of fructose-1-phosphate aldolase, EC 2.1.2.13).[7] Metabolites such as lactate and triglycerides are produced in excess and compete with urate for renal excretion in these diseases.

Hyperuricemia as a result of decreased uric acid excretion is a common feature of toxemia of pregnancy (preeclampsia) and lactic acidosis presumably as a result of competition for binding sites in the renal tubules. Chronic renal disease causes elevated uric acid concentration because filtration and secretion are impaired.

Uric acid nephrolithiasis, the formation of kidney stones (renal calculi), may occur due to a variety of predisposing factors and conditions. In acidic urine, the

TABLE 12-5	CAUSES OF ABNORMAL PLASMA URIC ACID CONCENTRATION

INCREASED CONCENTRATION

Gout

Treatment of myeloproliferative disease with cytotoxic drugs

Hemolytic and proliferative processes

Purine-rich diet

Increased tissue catabolism or starvation

Enzyme deficiencies

    Lesch-Nyhan syndrome (hypoxanthine guanine phosphoribosyltransferase deficiency)

    Phosphoribosylpyrophosphate synthetase deficiency

    Glycogen storage disease type I (glucose-6-phosphatase deficiency)

    Fructose intolerance (fructose-1-phosphate aldolase deficiency)

Toxemia of pregnancy

Lactic acidosis

Chronic renal disease

Drugs and poisons

DECREASED CONCENTRATION

Liver disease

Defective tubular reabsorption (Fanconi syndrome)

Chemotherapy with azathioprine or 6-mercaptopurine

Overtreatment with allopurinol

relatively insoluble uric acid precipitates to form calculi, which can cause intense flank pain. The stones may be dissolved by alkalinization of the urine, or treated by increased fluid intake and administration of xanthine oxidase inhibitors to reduce uric acid production.[27]

Hypouricemia is less common than hyperuricemia and is usually secondary to severe liver disease or defective tubular reabsorption, as in Fanconi syndrome (a disorder of reabsorption in the proximal convoluted tubules of the kidney).[28] Decreased plasma uric acid can be caused by chemotherapy with 6-mercaptopurine or azathioprine, inhibitors of de novo purine synthesis, and as a result of overtreatment with allopurinol. The conditions affecting plasma urate concentrations are shown in Table 12-5.[7]

CREATININE/CREATINE

Creatinine is formed from creatine and creatine phosphate in muscle and is excreted into the plasma at a constant rate related to muscle mass. Plasma creatinine is inversely related to glomerular filtration rate (GFR) and, although an imperfect measure, it is commonly used to assess renal filtration function.[29]

Biochemistry

Creatine is synthesized primarily in the liver from arginine, glycine, and methionine.[4] It is then transported to other tissues, such as muscle, where it is converted to creatine phosphate, which serves as a high-energy source. Creatine phosphate loses phosphoric acid and creatine loses water to form the cyclic compound, creatinine, which diffuses into the plasma and is excreted in the urine.[29] The structures and relationship of these compounds are shown in Figure 12-4.

Creatinine is released into the circulation at a relatively constant rate that has been shown to be proportional to an individual's muscle mass. It is removed from the circulation by glomerular filtration and excreted in the urine.[29] Small amounts of creatinine are secreted by the proximal tubule and reabsorbed by the renal tubules.[6] Daily creatinine excretion is reasonably stable.

Clinical Application

Measurement of creatinine concentration is used to determine the sufficiency of kidney function, to determine the severity of kidney damage, and to monitor the progression of kidney disease.[30]

Plasma creatinine concentration is a function of relative muscle mass, the rate of creatine turnover, and renal function. The amount of creatinine in the bloodstream is reasonably stable, although the protein content of the diet does influence the plasma concentration. Because of the constancy of endogenous production, urinary creatinine excretion has been used as a measure of the completeness of 24-hour urine collections in a given individual, although the uncertainty associated with this practice may exceed that introduced by use of the urine volume and collection time for standardization.[31] Urinary constituents may be expressed as a ratio to creatinine quantity rather than as mass excreted per day.

Creatinine clearance (CrCl), a measure of the amount of creatinine eliminated from the blood by the kidneys, and GFR are used to gauge renal function.[30] The GFR is the volume of plasma filtered (V) by the glomerulus per unit of time (t):

$$GFR = \frac{V}{t} \qquad \text{(Eq. 12-2)}$$

Assuming a substance, S, can be measured and is freely filtered at the glomerulus and neither secreted nor reabsorbed by the tubules, the volume of plasma filtered would be equal to the mass of S filtered (M_S) divided by its plasma concentration (P_S):

$$V = \frac{M_S}{P_S} \qquad \text{(Eq. 12-3)}$$

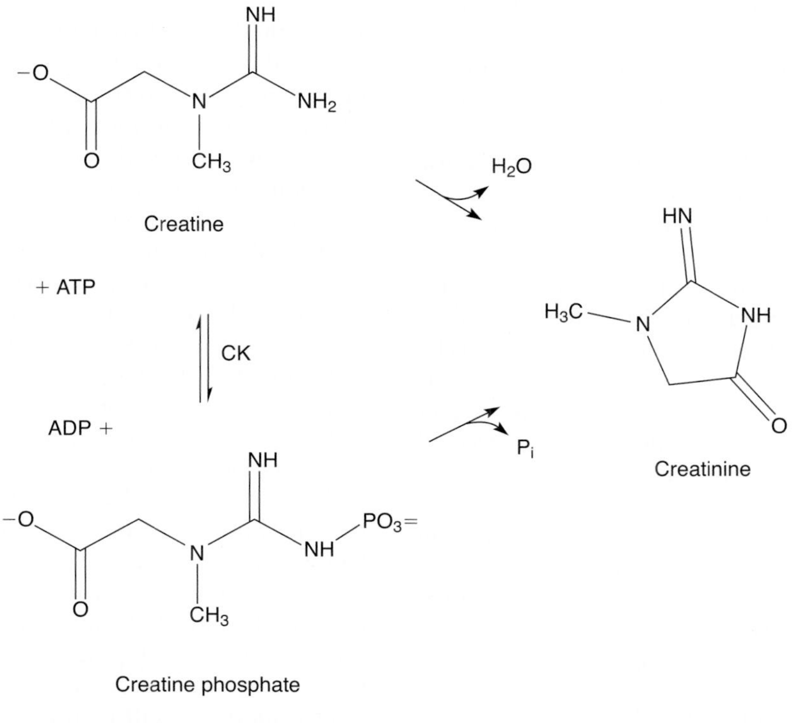

CK = creatine kinase (EC 2.7.3.2)

FIGURE 12-4 Interconversion of creatine, creatine phosphate, and creatinine.

The mass of S filtered is equal to the product of its urine concentration (U_S) and the urine volume (V_U):

$$M_S = U_S V_S \quad \text{(Eq. 12-4)}$$

If the urine and plasma concentrations of S, the volume of urine collected, and the time over which the sample was collected are known, the GFR can be calculated:

$$GFR = \frac{U_S V_U}{P_S t} \quad \text{(Eq. 12-5)}$$

The clearance of a substance is the volume of plasma from which that substance is removed per unit time. The formula for CrCl is given as follows, where U_{Cr} is urine creatinine concentration and P_{Cr} is plasma creatinine concentration:

$$CrCl = \frac{U_{Cr} V_U}{P_{Cr} t} \quad \text{(Eq. 12-6)}$$

CrCl is usually reported in units of mL/min and can be corrected for body surface area (see Chapter 27). CrCl overestimates GFR because a small amount of creatinine is reabsorbed by the renal tubules and up to 10% of urine creatinine is secreted by the tubules. However, CrCl provides a reasonable approximation of GFR.[30]

The observed relationship between plasma creatinine and GFR and relatively constant plasma creatinine concentrations should make the analyte a good endogenous filtration marker. However, measurement of plasma creatinine does not provide sufficient sensitivity for the detection of mild renal dysfunction. Measured creatinine concentration used in combination with other variables in one of several empirically determined equations provides a better assessment of renal disease, in part because the equations estimate GFR, not CrCl.

Clinical laboratories have been strongly encouraged to report an estimated GFR when serum creatinine is ordered as a means to increase identification of kidney disease and improve patient care.[32] Initially, the abbreviated Modification of Diet in Renal Disease (MDRD) equation was advocated.[33] The equation includes four variables—serum creatinine concentration, age, gender (sex), and ethnicity—and makes the assumption that all filtered creatinine is excreted.[32] The MDRD equation is most useful when serum creatinine results are produced in an assay that has been calibrated to be traceable to an IDMS method.[34]

When serum creatinine is measured using an IDMS-traceable method, the MDRD equation for estimated glomerular filtration rate (eGFR) is

$$eGFR(mL/min/1.73\ m^2) = 175 \times (S_{Cr})^{-1.154} \times$$
$$(Age)^{-0.203} \times (0.742\ \text{if female}) \times$$
$$(1.210\ \text{if African-American}) \quad \text{(Eq. 12-7)}$$

where S_{cr} is serum (plasma) creatinine concentration in mg/dL and age is in years.[35] Results are normalized to a standard body surface area (1.73 m^2). The equation is valid for individuals older than 18 years and younger than 70 years.[34] The formula was developed with data from non-hospitalized patients known to have chronic kidney disease and is reasonably accurate for this population, although eGFR values > 60 mL/min/1.73 m^2 calculated using this equation are negatively biased and should not be reported.

Effectiveness of the equation in other populations is being investigated and alternate equations have been proposed.[36] The Chronic Kidney Disease Epidemiology (CKD-EPI) Collaboration published an equation developed using results from healthy adults and adults with chronic kidney disease.[37] The CKD-EPI equation is used to report higher values (>60 mL/min/1.73 m^2) for adults 18 years and older. A modified Schwartz equation has been developed to calculate eGFR in the pediatric population.[38] The equation is

$$eGFR(mL/min/1.73\ m^2) = (0.41 \times height)/S_{Cr} \quad \text{(Eq. 12-8)}$$

Height is measured in cm and S_{cr} is serum (plasma) creatinine concentration in mg/dL. The equation can be used to calculate eGFR for children <18 years old.

Analytical Methods

Creatinine

The methods most frequently used to measure creatinine are based on the Jaffe reaction first described in 1886.[39] In this reaction, creatinine reacts with picric acid in alkaline solution to form a red-orange chromogen. The reaction was adopted for the measurement of blood creatinine by Folin and Wu in 1919.[40] The reaction is nonspecific and subject to positive interference by a large number of compounds, including acetoacetate, acetone, ascorbate, glucose, and pyruvate. More accurate results are obtained when creatinine in a protein-free filtrate is adsorbed onto Fuller's earth (aluminum magnesium silicate) or Lloyd's reagent (sodium aluminum silicate), then eluted and reacted with alkaline picrate.[41] Because this method is time consuming and not readily automated, it is not routinely used.

Two approaches have been used to increase the specificity of assay methods for creatinine: a kinetic Jaffe method and reaction with various enzymes. In the kinetic Jaffe method, serum is mixed with alkaline picrate and the rate of change in absorbance is measured.[42] Although this method eliminates some of the nonspecific reactants, it is subject to interference by α-keto acids and cephalosporins.[43] Bilirubin and hemoglobin may cause a negative bias, probably a result of their destruction in the strong base used. The kinetic Jaffe method is used routinely despite these problems because it is inexpensive, rapid, and easy to perform.

In an effort to enhance the specificity of the Jaffe reaction, several coupled enzymatic methods have been developed.[44,45] The method using creatininase (creatinine amidohydrolase, EC 3.5.2.10), creatinase (creatine amidinohydrolase, EC 3.5.3.3), sarcosine oxidase (EC 1.5.3.1), and peroxidase (EC 1.11.1.7) was adapted for use on a dry slide analyzer.[46]

IDMS is used as a reference method.[34] Assays used on automated analyzers are designated as "traceable" (calibrated) to an IDMS method. Analytic methods for creatinine are summarized in Table 12-6.

Specimen Requirements

Creatinine may be measured in plasma, serum, or urine. Hemolyzed and icteric samples should be avoided, particularly if a Jaffe method is used. Lipemic samples may produce erroneous results in some methods. A fasting sample is not required, although high-protein ingestion may transiently elevate serum concentrations. Urine should be refrigerated after collection or frozen if longer storage than 4 days is required.[8]

Sources of Error

Ascorbate, glucose, α-keto acids, and uric acid may increase creatinine concentration measured by the Jaffe reaction, especially at temperatures above 30°C. This interference is significantly decreased when kinetic measurement is applied. Depending on the concentration of reactants and measuring time, interference from α-keto acids may persist in kinetic Jaffe methods. Some of these substances interfere in enzymatic methods for creatinine measurement. Bilirubin causes a negative bias in both Jaffe and enzymatic methods. Ascorbate will interfere in enzymatic methods that use peroxidase as a reagent.[8]

Patients taking cephalosporin antibiotics may have falsely elevated results when the Jaffe reaction is used. Other drugs have been shown to increase creatinine results. Dopamine, in particular, is known to affect both

TABLE 12-6	SUMMARY OF ANALYTIC METHODS—CREATININE	
CHEMICAL METHODS BASED ON JAFFE REACTION		
Jaffe reaction	In alkaline solution, creatinine + picrate → red-orange complex	
Jaffe-kinetic	Jaffe reaction performed directly on sample; detection of color formation timed to avoid interference of non-creatinine chromogens	Positive bias from α-keto acids and cephalosporins; requires automated equipment for precision
Jaffe with adsorbent	Creatinine in protein-free filtrate adsorbed onto Fuller's earth (aluminum magnesium silicate), then reacted with alkaline picrate to form colored complex	Adsorbent improves specificity; previously considered reference method
Jaffe without adsorbent	Creatinine in protein-free filtrate reacts with alkaline picrate to form colored complex	Positive bias from ascorbic acid, glucose, glutathione, α-keto acids, uric acid, and cephalosporins
ENZYMATIC METHODS		
Creatininase-H_2O_2	In a series of enzymatically catalyzed reactions, creatinine is hydrolyzed to creatine, which is converted to sarcosine and urea. Sarcosine is oxidized to glycine, CH_2O, and H_2O_2. Peroxidase-catalyzed oxidation of a colorless substrate produces a colored product + H_2O	Adapted for use as dry slide method; potential to replace Jaffe; no interference from acetoacetate or cephalosporins; some positive bias due to lidocaine
Creatininase-CK	In a series of reactions catalyzed by the enzymes creatininase, creatine kinase, pyruvate kinase, and lactate dehydrogenase, NAD^+ is produced and measured as a decrease in absorbance	Lacks sensitivity; not used widely
OTHER METHODS		
Isotope dilution mass spectrometry	Detection of characteristic fragments following ionization; quantification using isotopically labeled compound	Highly specific; accepted reference method

enzymatic and Jaffe methods. Lidocaine causes a positive bias in some enzymatic methods.[26]

Creatine

The traditional method for creatine measurement relies on the analysis of the sample using an end point Jaffe method for creatinine before and after it is heated in acid solution. Heating converts creatine to creatinine and the

difference between the two sample measurements is the creatine concentration. High temperatures may result in the formation of additional chromogens and the precision of this method is poor. Several enzymatic methods have been developed; one is the creatininase assay. The initial enzyme is omitted and creatine kinase (EC 2.7.3.2), pyruvate kinase (EC 2.1.7.40), and lactate dehydrogenase (EC 1.1.1.27) are coupled to produce a measurable colored product.[47] Creatine can be measured by HPLC (high performance liquid chromatography).[48,49]

Reference Intervals

Reference intervals vary with assay type, age, and gender.[8] Creatinine concentration decreases with age beginning in the 5th decade of life.

CASE STUDY 12-2

A 3-year-old girl was admitted with a diagnosis of acute lymphocytic leukemia. Her admitting laboratory data are shown in Case Study Table 12-2.1. After admission, she was treated by administration of packed red cells, 2 units of platelets, IV fluids, and allopurinol. On the second hospital day, chemotherapy was begun, using IV vincristine and prednisone and intrathecal injections of methotrexate, prednisone, and cytosine arabinoside. She was discharged for home care 5 days later. She was continued on prednisone and allopurinol at home. She received additional chemotherapy 1 month later (11/1) and again on 11/14. On 12/6, she was readmitted because she had painful sores in her mouth and was unable to eat.

Questions

1. How would you explain the significant elevations of uric acid on admission?

2. Which two factors are responsible for the normal concentrations of uric acid seen in subsequent admissions?

3. Which is the most likely cause of the abnormally low concentration of urea nitrogen observed on 12/6? Which other laboratory test would confirm your suspicions?

CASE STUDY TABLE 12-2.1 LABORATORY RESULTS

	10/1	10/2	10/3	10/4	11/14	12/6	6/20
Urea N (mg/dL)	12.0	a	a	15	4.0	2.0	a
Creatinine (mg/dL)	0.7	a	a	1.0	0.7	a	0.7
Uric acid (mg/dL)	12.0	9.2	4.0	1.9	2.3	a	3.1
WBC (mm³)	56,300	a	a	3,700	2,800	3,700	a

[a]Indicates test not performed.

CREATININE

Adult	Plasma or serum	Jaffe method	Enzymatic method
Male		0.9–1.3 mg/dL (80–115 μmol/L)	0.6–1.1 mg/dL (53–97 μmol/L)
Female		0.6–1.1 mg/dL (53–97 μmol/L)	0.5–0.8 mg/dL (44–71 μmol/L)
Child		0.3–0.7 mg/dL (27–62 μmol/L)	0.0–0.6 mg/dL (0–53 μmol/L)
Adult	Urine, 24 h		
Male		800–2,000 mg/d (7.1–17.7 mmol/d)	
Female		600–1,800 mg/d (5.3–15.9 mmol/d)	

Pathophysiology

Creatinine

Elevated creatinine concentration is associated with abnormal renal function, especially as it relates to glomerular function. Plasma concentration of creatinine is inversely proportional to the clearance of creatinine. Therefore, when plasma creatinine concentration is elevated, GFR is decreased, indicating renal damage. Plasma creatinine is a relatively insensitive marker and may not be measurably increased until renal function has deteriorated more than 50%.[4]

Creatine

In muscle disease such as muscular dystrophy, poliomyelitis, hyperthyroidism, and trauma, both plasma creatine and urinary creatinine are often elevated. Plasma creatinine concentrations are usually normal in these patients. Measurement of creatine kinase is used typically for the diagnosis of muscle disease because analytic

CASE STUDY 12-3

An 80-year-old woman was admitted with a diagnosis of hypertension, congestive heart failure, anemia, possible diabetes, and chronic renal failure. She was treated with diuretics and IV fluids and released 4 days later. Her laboratory results are shown in Case Study Table 12-3.1.

Five months later, she was readmitted for treatment of repeated bouts of dyspnea. She was placed on a special diet and medication to control her hypertension and was discharged. Medical staff believed that she had not been taking her medication as prescribed, and she was counseled regarding the importance of regular doses.

Questions

1. What is the most probable cause of the patient's elevated urea nitrogen? Which data support your conclusion?

2. Note that this patient's admitting diagnosis is "possible diabetes." If the patient had truly been diabetic, with an elevated blood glucose and a positive acetone, what effect would this have had on the measured values of creatinine? Explain.

CASE STUDY TABLE 12-3.1
LABORATORY RESULTS

	FIRST ADMISSION		SECOND ADMISSION	
	2/11	2/15	7/26	7/28
Urea N (mg/dL)	58	a	a	61
Creatinine (mg/dL)	6.2	6.2	6.4	6.0
Uric acid (mg/dL)	10.0	a	a	9.2
Urea N/creatinine	9.4	a	a	10.1
Glucose (mg/dL)	86	80	113	a

aIndicates test not performed.

methods for creatine are not readily available in most clinical laboratories. Plasma creatine concentration is not elevated in renal disease.[6]

AMMONIA

Ammonia is produced in the deamination of amino acids during protein metabolism.[5] It is removed from the circulation and converted to urea in the liver. Free ammonia is toxic; however, ammonia is present in the plasma in low concentrations.

Biochemistry

Ammonia (NH_3) is produced in the catabolism of amino acids and by bacterial metabolism in the lumen of the intestine.[7] Some endogenous ammonia results from anaerobic metabolic reactions that occur in skeletal muscle during exercise. Ammonia is consumed by the parenchymal cells of the liver in the production of urea. At normal physiologic pH, most ammonia in the blood exists as ammonium ion (NH_4^+). Figure 12-5 shows the pH-dependent equilibrium between NH_3 and NH_4^+. Ammonia is excreted as ammonium ion by the kidney and acts to buffer urine.[29]

Clinical Application

Clinical conditions in which blood ammonia concentration provides useful information are hepatic failure, Reye's syndrome, and inherited deficiencies of urea cycle enzymes. Severe liver disease is the most common cause of disturbed ammonia metabolism. The monitoring of blood ammonia may be used to determine prognosis, although correlation between the extent of hepatic encephalopathy and plasma ammonia concentration is not always consistent. Arterial ammonia concentration is a better indicator of the severity of disease.[50]

Reye's syndrome, occurring most commonly in children, is a serious disease that can be fatal. Frequently, the disease is preceded by a viral infection and the administration of aspirin. Reye's syndrome is an acute metabolic disorder of the liver, and autopsy findings show severe fatty infiltration of that organ.[7] Blood ammonia concentration can be correlated with both the severity of the disease and prognosis. Survival reaches 100% if plasma NH_3 concentration remains below five times normal.[51]

Ammonia is of use in the diagnosis of inherited deficiency of urea cycle enzymes. Testing should be considered for any neonate with unexplained nausea, vomiting, or neurological deterioration associated with feeding.[19]

Assay of blood ammonia can be used to monitor hyperalimentation therapy and measurement of urine ammonia can be used to confirm the ability of the kidneys to produce ammonia.[8]

Analytical Methods

The accurate laboratory measurement of ammonia in plasma is complicated by its low concentration, instability, and pervasive contamination. Two approaches have been used for the measurement of plasma ammonia. One is a two-step approach in which ammonia is isolated from the sample and then assayed. The second involves

$$NH_4^+ + H_2O \rightleftharpoons NH_3 + H_3O^+$$

FIGURE 12-5 Interconversion of ammonium ion and ammonia.

direct measurement of ammonia by an enzymatic method or ion-selective electrode. Assays detect NH_3 or NH_4^+.

One of the first analytic methods for ammonia, developed by Conway in 1935, exploited the volatility of ammonia to separate the compound in a microdiffusion chamber.[52] Ammonia gas from the sample diffuses into a separate compartment and is absorbed in a solution containing a pH indicator. The amount of ammonia is determined by titration.

Ammonia can be measured by an enzymatic method using GLDH. This method is convenient and the most common technique used currently.[53] The decrease in absorbance at 340 nm as nicotinamide adenine dinucleotide phosphate (reduced, NADPH) is consumed in the reaction is proportional to the ammonia concentration in the specimen. NADPH is the preferred coenzyme because it is used specifically by GLDH; NADH will participate in reactions of other endogenous substrates, such as pyruvate. Adenosine diphosphate is added to the reaction mixture to increase the rate of the reaction and to stabilize GLDH.[54] This method is used on many automated systems and is available as a prepared kit from numerous manufacturers.

A dry slide automated system uses a thin film colorimetric assay.[55] In this method, ammonia reacts with an indicator to produce a colored compound that is detected spectrophotometrically. Direct measurement using an ion-selective electrode has been developed.[56] The electrode measures the change in pH of a solution of ammonium chloride as ammonia diffuses across a semipermeable membrane. Analytic methods for ammonia are summarized in Table 12-7.

Specimen Requirements
Careful specimen handling is extremely important for plasma ammonia assays. Whole blood ammonia concentration increases rapidly following specimen collection because of in vitro amino acid deamination. Venous blood should be obtained without trauma and placed on ice immediately. Heparin and EDTA are suitable anticoagulants. Commercial collection containers should be evaluated for ammonia interference before a new lot is put into use. Samples should be centrifuged at 0 to 4°C within 20 minutes of collection and the plasma or serum removed. Specimens should be assayed as soon as possible or frozen. Frozen plasma is stable for several days at −20°C. Erythrocytes contain two to three times as much ammonia as plasma; hemolysis should be avoided.

Cigarette smoking by the patient is a significant source of ammonia contamination. It is recommended that patients do not smoke for several hours before a specimen is collected.[8]

Many substances influence the *in vivo* ammonia concentration.[8,22] Ammonium salts, asparaginase, barbiturates, diuretics, ethanol, hyperalimentation, narcotic analgesics, and some other drugs may increase ammonia in plasma. Diphenhydramine, *Lactobacillus acidophilus*, lactulose, levodopa, and several antibiotics decrease concentrations. Glucose at concentrations > 600 mg/dL (33 mmol/L) interferes in dry slide methods.

Sources of Error
Ammonia contamination is a potential problem in the laboratory measurement of ammonia.[19] Precautions must be taken to minimize contamination in the laboratory in which the assay is performed. Elimination of sources of ammonia contamination can significantly improve the accuracy of ammonia assay results. Sources of contamination include tobacco smoke, urine, and ammonia in detergents, glassware, reagents, and water.

The ammonia content of serum-based control material is unstable. Frozen aliquots of human serum albumin containing known amounts of ammonium chloride or ammonium sulfate may be used. Solutions containing known amounts of ammonium sulfate are commercially available.

TABLE 12-7	SUMMARY OF ANALYTIC METHODS—AMMONIA	
CHEMICAL METHODS		
Ion-selective electrode	Diffusion of NH_3 through selective membrane into NH_4Cl causes a pH change, which is measured potentiometrically	Good accuracy and precision; membrane stability may be a problem
Spectrophotometric	NH_3 + bromophenol blue → blue color	
ENZYMATIC METHODS		
Catalyzed by GLDH	Enzymatic reaction of NH_4^+, 2-oxoglutarate, and NADPH to form glutamate and $NADP^+$, which is detected spectrophotometrically	Most common on automated instruments; accurate and precise

Reference Interval

Values obtained vary somewhat with the method used.[8] Higher concentrations are seen in newborns.

AMMONIA			
Adult	Plasma	19–60 µg/dL	11–35 µmol/L
	Urine, 24 h	140–1,500 mg N/d	10–107 mmol N/d
Child (10 d to 2 y)	Plasma	68–136 µg/dL	40–80 µmol/L

Pathophysiology

In severe liver disease in which there is significant collateral circulation or if parenchymal liver cell function is severely impaired, ammonia is not removed from the circulation and blood concentration increases. High concentrations of NH_3 are neurotoxic and often associated with encephalopathy. Toxicity may be partly a result of increased extracellular glutamate concentration and subsequent depletion of adenosine triphosphate in the brain.[57]

Hyperammonemia is associated with inherited deficiency of urea cycle enzymes.[58] Measurement of plasma ammonia is important in the diagnosis and monitoring of these inherited metabolic disorders (see Chapter 35).

For additional student resources please visit thePoint at http://thepoint.lww.com. **thePoint** ✳

QUESTIONS

1. Which one of the following is not an NPN substance?
   a. Allantoin
   b. Ammonia
   c. Creatinine
   d. Urea

2. Which compound constitutes nearly half of the NPN substances in the blood?
   a. Ammonia
   b. Creatine
   c. Urea
   d. Uric acid

3. An urea N result of 9 mg/dL is obtained by a technologist. What is the urea concentration?
   a. 3.2 mg/dL
   b. 4.2 mg/dL
   c. 18.0 mg/dL
   d. 19.3 mg/dL

4. Prerenal azotemia is caused by
   a. Acute renal failure
   b. Chronic renal failure
   c. Congestive heart failure
   d. Urinary tract obstruction

5. A technologist obtains a urea N value of 61 mg/dL and a serum creatinine value of 2.5 mg/dL on a patient. These results indicate
   a. Congestive heart failure
   b. Dehydration
   c. Glomerular nephritis
   d. Urinary tract obstruction

6. Uric acid is the final product of
   a. Allantoin metabolism
   b. Amino acid metabolism
   c. Purine metabolism
   d. The urea cycle

7. Which one of the listed conditions is not associated with elevated plasma uric acid concentration?
   a. Allopurinol overtreatment
   b. Gout
   c. Lesch-Nyhan syndrome
   d. Renal disease

8. In the Jaffe reaction, a red-orange chromogen is formed when creatinine reacts with
   a. Aluminum magnesium silicate
   b. Creatininase
   c. Phosphocreatine
   d. Picric acid

9. Substances known to increase results when measuring creatinine by the Jaffe reaction include all of the following EXCEPT
   a. Ascorbic acid
   b. Bilirubin
   c. Glucose
   d. α-Keto acids

10. Ammonia concentrations are usually measured to evaluate
    a. Acid–base status
    b. Glomerular filtration
    c. Hepatic encephalopathy
    d. Renal failure

11. A complete deficiency of hypoxanthine guanine phosphoribosyltransferase results in which disease?
    a. Lesch-Nyhan syndrome
    b. Modification of diet in renal disease
    c. Maple syrup urine disease
    d. Reye's syndrome
    e. Megaloblastic anemia

12. When calculating creatinine clearance using the MDRD equation, which of the following factors are considered?
    a. Verification that the patient has been fasting
    b. Identification of ethnicity
    c. Body mass
    d. Time of day of blood collection
    e. Physical workout schedule of the patient

13. True or False? Serum creatinine levels may be falsely elevated when a patient is taking cephalosporin.

14. When measuring ammonia blood levels, which of the following might cause a false increase in this analyte?
    a. The patient had two cigarettes 15 minutes prior to blood draw.
    b. The patient was fasting for hours prior to blood collection.
    c. Immediately after phlebotomy, the blood sample was maintained on ice.
    d. The patient had a steak dinner the night before the blood draw.
    e. None of the above will falsely increase the blood ammonia levels.

REFERENCES

1. Gentzkow CJ. An accurate method for determination of blood urea nitrogen by direct nesslerization. *J Biol Chem.* 1942;143:531-544.
2. Matthews DE. Proteins and amino acids. In: Shils ME, ed. *Modern Nutrition in Health and Disease.* 10th ed. Philadelphia, PA: Lippincott Williams & Wilkins; 2006:23-61.
3. Montgomery R, Conway TW, Spector AA, Chappell D. *Biochemistry: A Case-Oriented Approach.* 6th ed. St. Louis, MO: Mosby; 1996.
4. Oh MS. Evaluation of renal function, water, electrolytes and acid-base balance. In: McPherson RA, Pincus MR, eds. *Henry's Clinical Diagnosis and Management by Laboratory Methods.* 21st ed. Philadelphia, PA: Saunders Elsevier; 2007:147-169.
5. Coomes MW. Amino acid metabolism. In: Devlin TM, ed. *Textbook of Biochemistry with Clinical Correlations.* 6th ed. Hoboken, NJ: Wiley-Liss; 2006;743-787.
6. Lamb EJ, Price CP. Kidney function tests. In: Burtis CA, Ashwood ER, Bruns DE, eds. *Tietz Textbook of Clinical Chemistry and Molecular Diagnostics.* 5th ed. St. Louis, MO: Elsevier Saunders; 2012;669-707.
7. Harrison's Online. www.harrisonsonline.com. Accessed February 2012.
8. Wu AHB. *Tietz Clinical Guide to Laboratory Tests.* 4th ed. St. Louis, MO: WB Saunders; 2006.
9. SURVEYS 2011: C-B Chemistry/Therapeutic Drug Monitoring and U-B Urine Chemistry. Northfield, IL: College of American Pathologists; 2011.
10. Berthelot MPE. Violet d'aniline. *Repert Chim Appl.* 1859;1:284.
11. Talke H, Schubert GE. Enzymatic urea determination in the blood and serum in the warburg optical test. *Klin Wochenschr.* 1965;43:174-175.
12. Orsonneau J, Massoubre C, Cabanes M, et al. Simple and sensitive determination of urea in serum and urine. *Clin Chem.* 1992;38:619-623.
13. Ohkubo A, Kamei S, Yamanaka M, et al. Multilayer-film analysis for urea nitrogen in blood, serum, or plasma. *Clin Chem.* 1984;30:1222-1225.
14. Akai T, Naka K, Yoshikawa C, et al. Salivary urea nitrogen as an index to renal function: a test-strip method. *Clin Chem.* 1983;29:1825-1827.
15. Paulson G, Ray R, Sternberg J. A rate sensing approach to urea measurement. *Clin Chem.* 1971;17:644.
16. Kessler A, Siekmann L. Measurement of urea in human serum by isotope dilution mass spectrometry: a reference procedure. *Clin Chem.* 1999;45:1523-1529.
17. Dufour DR. *Clinical Use of Laboratory Data: A Practical Guide.* Baltimore, MD: Williams & Wilkins; 1998.
18. Cory JG. Purine and pyrimidine nucleotide metabolism. In: Devlin TM, ed. *Textbook of Biochemistry with Clinical Correlations,* 6th ed. Hoboken, NJ: Wiley-Liss, 2006;789-822.
19. Jacobs DS, DeMott WR, Oxley DK. *Jacobs & DeMott Laboratory Test Handbook.* Hudson, OH: Lexi-Comp, Inc.; 2001.
20. Caraway WT, Hald PM. Uric acid. In: Seligson D, ed. *Standard Methods of Clinical Chemistry,* Vol. 4. New York, NY: Academic Press; 1963:239-247.
21. Feichtmeier TV, Wrenn HT. Direct determination of uric acid using uricase. *Am J Clin Pathol.* 1955;25:833-839.
22. Young DS. *Effects of Preanalytical Variables on Clinical Laboratory Tests.* 3rd ed. Washington, DC: American Association for Clinical Chemistry Press; 2007.
23. Gochman N, Schmitz JM. Automated determination of uric acid with use of a uricase-peroxidase system. *Clin Chem.* 1971;17:1154-1159.
24. Kageyama N. A direct colorimetric determination of uric acid in serum and urine with uricase-catalase system. *Clin Chim Acta.* 1971;31:421-426.
25. Ellerbe P, Cohen A, Welch MJ, et al. Determination of serum uric acid by isotope dilution mass spectrometry as a new candidate reference method. *Anal Chem.* 1990;62:2173-2177.
26. Young DS. *Effects of Drugs on Clinical Laboratory Tests.* 5th ed. Washington, DC: American Association for Clinical Chemistry Press; 2000.
27. Uric acid nephrolithiasis. http://www.uptodate.com. Accessed February 2012.
28. Webster's Medical Dictionary. www.merriam-webster.com/medical. Accessed February 2012.
29. Apps DK, Cohen BB, Steel CM. *Biochemistry: A Concise Text for Medical Students.* 5th ed. London: WB Saunders; 1992.
30. Assessment of Kidney Function: Serum Creatinine, BUN, and GFR. http://www.uptodate.com. Accessed Spring 2012.
31. Garde AH, Hansen AM, Kristiansen J, Knudsen LE. Comparison of uncertainties related to standardization of urine samples with volume and creatinine concentration. *Ann Occup Hyg.* 2004;48:171-179.

32. National Kidney Disease Education Program. www.nkdep.nih.gov. Accessed February 2012.

33. Levey AS, Coresh J, Balk E, et al. National kidney foundation practice guidelines for chronic kidney disease: evaluation, classification, and stratification. *Ann Intern Med.* 2003;139:137-147.

34. Myers GL, Miller WG, Coresh J, et al. Recommendations for improving serum creatinine measurement: a report from the Laboratory Working Group of the National Kidney Disease Education Program. *Clin Chem.* 2006;52:5-18.

35. Levey AS, Coresh J, Greene T, et al. Expressing the modification of diet in renal disease study equation for estimating glomerular filtration rate with standardized serum creatinine vales. *Clin Chem.* 2007;53:766-772.

36. Miller WG. Glomerular filtration rate: the importance of standardized serum creatinine in detecting kidney disease. *Clin Lab News.* December 2011;37:10-12.

37. Levey AS, Stevens LA, Schmid CH, et al. A new equation to estimate glomerular filtration rate. *Ann Intern Med.* 2009;150:604-612.

38. Schwartz GJ, Munoz A, Schneider MF, et al. New equations to estimate GFR in children with CKD. *J Am Soc Nephrol.* 2009;20:629-637.

39. Jaffe M. Uber den niederschlag welchen pikrinsaure in normalen harn erzeugt und uber eine neue reaktion des kreatinins. *Z Physiol Chem.* 1886;10:391.

40. Folin O, Wu H. System of blood analysis. *J Biol Chem.* 1919;31:81.

41. Haeckel R. Assay of creatinine in serum with use of Fuller's earth to remove interferents. *Clin Chem.* 1981;27:179-183.

42. Larsen K. Creatinine assay by a reaction kinetic principle. *Clin Chim Acta.* 1972;41:209-217.

43. Bowers LD, Wong ET. Kinetic serum creatinine assays. II. A critical evaluation and review. *Clin Chem.* 1980;26:555-561.

44. Moss GA, Bondar RJL, Buzzelli DM. Kinetic enzymatic method for determining serum creatinine. *Clin Chem.* 1975;21:1422-1426.

45. Fossati P, Prencipe L, Berti G. Enzymic creatinine assay: a new colorimetric method based on hydrogen peroxide measurement. *Clin Chem.* 1983;29:1494-1496.

46. *Creatinine Test Methodology. Kodak Ektachem Clinical Chemistry Products.* Rochester, NY: Eastman Kodak Company; 1992:Pub No MP2-49.

47. Beyer, C. Creatine measurement in serum and urine with an automated enzymatic method. *Clin Chem.* 1993;39:1613-1619.

48. Murakita H. Simultaneous determination of creatine and creatinine in serum by high-performance liquid chromatography. *J Chromatogr.* 1988;431:471-473.

49. Yang YD. Simultaneous determination of creatine, uric acid, creatinine and hippuric acid in urine by high performance liquid chromatography. *Biomed Chromatogr.* 1998;12:47-49.

50. Pincus MR, Tierno P, Dufour DR. Evaluation of liver function. In: McPherson RA, Pincus MR, eds. *Henry's Clinical Diagnosis and Management by Laboratory Methods.* 21st ed. Philadelphia, PA: Saunders Elsevier; 2007:263-278.

51. Fitzgerald JF, Clark JH, Angelides AG, et al. The prognostic significance of peak ammonia levels in Reye's syndrome. *Pediatrics.* 1982;70:997-1000.

52. Conway EJ, O'Malley E. Microdiffusion methods: ammonia and urea using buffered absorbents (revised methods for ranges greater than 10 μg N). *Biochem J.* 1942;36:655-661.

53. Mondzac A, Ehrlich GE, Seegmiller JE. An enzymatic determination of ammonia in biological fluids. *J Lab Clin Med.* 1965;66:526-531.

54. *Ammonia Test Methodology. Roche/Hitachi Products.* Indianapolis, IN: Roche Diagnostics Corporation; 2001.

55. *VITROS AMON Slides. Instructions for Use. VITROS Chemistry Products.* Rochester, NY: Ortho-Clinical Diagnostics; 2002:Pub No MP2–90.

56. Willems D, Steenssens W. Ammonia determined in plasma with a selective electrode. *Clin Chem.* 1988;34:2372.

57. Monfort P, Kosenko E, Erceg S, et al. Molecular mechanism of acute ammonia toxicity: role of NMDA receptors. *Neurochem Int.* 2002;41:95-102.

58. Pasquali M, Longo N. Newborn screening and inborn errors of metabolism. In: Burtis CA, Ashwood ER, Bruns DE, eds. *Tietz Textbook of Clinical Chemistry and Molecular Diagnostics.* 5th ed. St. Louis, MO: Elsevier Saunders; 2012:2045-2082.

Enzymes

KAMISHA L. JOHNSON-DAVIS

CHAPTER OUTLINE

Chapter Objectives

Upon completion of this chapter, the clinical laboratorian should be able to do the following:

- Define the term enzyme, including physical composition and structure.
- Classify enzymes according to the International Union of Biochemistry.
- Discuss the different factors affecting the rate of an enzymatic reaction.
- Explain enzyme kinetics including zero-order and first-order kinetics.
- Explain why the measurement of serum enzyme levels is clinically useful.
- Discuss which enzymes are useful in the diagnosis of various disorders, including cardiac, hepatic, bone, and muscle, malignancies, and acute pancreatitis.
- Discuss the tissue sources, diagnostic significance, and assays, including sources of error, for the following enzymes: creatine kinase, lactate dehydrogenase, aspartate aminotransferase, alanine aminotransferase, alkaline phosphatase, acid phosphatase, γ-glutamyltransferase, amylase, lipase, cholinesterase, and glucose-6-phosphate dehydrogenase.
- Evaluate patient serum enzyme levels in relation to disease states.
- Discuss the clinical importance for detecting macroenzymes.
- Discuss the role of enzymes in drug metabolism.

KEY TERMS

Activation energy
Activators
Apoenzyme
Coenzyme
Cofactor
Enzyme
Enzyme–substrate (ES) complex
First-order kinetics
Holoenzyme

Hydrolase
International unit (IU)
Isoenzyme
Isoform
Kinetic assay
LD flipped pattern
Michaelis-Menten constant
Oxidoreductase
Transferase
Zero-order kinetics
Zymogen

Enzymes are specific biologic proteins that catalyze biochemical reactions without altering the equilibrium point of the reaction or being consumed or changed in composition. The other substances in the reaction are converted to products. The catalyzed reactions are frequently specific and essential to physiologic functions, such as the hydration of carbon dioxide, nerve conduction, muscle contraction, nutrient degradation, and energy use. Found in all body tissues, enzymes frequently appear in the serum following cellular injury or, sometimes, in smaller amounts, from degraded cells. Certain enzymes, such as those that facilitate coagulation, are specific to plasma and, therefore, are present in significant concentrations in plasma. Plasma or serum enzyme levels are often useful in the diagnosis of particular diseases or physiologic abnormalities. This chapter discusses the general properties and principles of enzymes, aspects relating to the clinical diagnostic significance of specific physiologic enzymes, and assay methods for those enzymes.

GENERAL PROPERTIES AND DEFINITIONS

Enzymes catalyze many specific physiologic reactions. These reactions are facilitated by the enzyme structure and several other factors. As a protein, each enzyme contains a specific amino acid sequence (*primary structure*), with the resultant polypeptide chains twisting (*secondary structure*), which then folds (*tertiary structure*) and results in structural cavities. If an enzyme contains more than one polypeptide unit, the *quaternary structure* refers to the spatial relationships between the subunits. Each enzyme contains an *active site*, often a water-free cavity, where the substance on which the enzyme acts (the *substrate*) interacts with particular charged amino acid residues. An *allosteric site*—a cavity other than the active site—may bind regulator molecules and, thereby, be significant to the basic enzyme structure.

Even though a particular enzyme maintains the same catalytic function throughout the body, that enzyme may exist in different forms within the same individual. The different forms may be differentiated from each other based on certain physical properties, such as electrophoretic mobility, solubility, or resistance to inactivation. The term isoenzyme is generally used when discussing such enzymes; however, the International Union of Biochemistry (IUB) suggests restricting this term to multiple forms of genetic origin. An isoform results when an enzyme is subject to posttranslational modifications. Isoenzymes and isoforms contribute to heterogeneity in properties and function of enzymes.

In addition to the basic enzyme structure, a nonprotein molecule, called a cofactor, may be necessary for enzyme activity. Inorganic cofactors, such as chloride or magnesium ions, are called activators. A coenzyme is an organic cofactor, such as nicotinamide adenine dinucleotide (NAD). When bound tightly to the enzyme, the coenzyme is called a *prosthetic group*. The enzyme portion (apoenzyme), with its respective coenzyme, forms a complete and active system, a holoenzyme.

Some enzymes, mostly digestive enzymes, are originally secreted from the organ of production in a structurally inactive form, called a *proenzyme* or zymogen. Other enzymes later alter the structure of the proenzyme to make active sites available by hydrolyzing specific amino acid residues. This mechanism prevents digestive enzymes from digesting their place of synthesis.

ENZYME CLASSIFICATION AND NOMENCLATURE

To standardize enzyme nomenclature, the Enzyme Commission (EC) of the IUB adopted a classification system in 1961; the standards were revised in 1972 and 1978. The IUB system assigns a *systematic name* to each enzyme, defining the substrate acted on, the reaction catalyzed, and, possibly, the name of any coenzyme involved in the reaction. Because many systematic names are lengthy, a more usable, trivial, *recommended name* is also assigned by the IUB system.[1]

In addition to naming enzymes, the IUB system identifies each enzyme by an EC numerical code containing four digits separated by decimal points. The first digit places the enzyme in one of the following six classes:

1. **Oxidoreductases.** Catalyze an oxidation–reduction reaction between two substrates
2. **Transferases.** Catalyze the transfer of a group other than hydrogen from one substrate to another
3. **Hydrolases.** Catalyze hydrolysis of various bonds
4. **Lyases.** Catalyze removal of groups from substrates without hydrolysis; the product contains double bonds
5. **Isomerases.** Catalyze the interconversion of geometric, optical, or positional isomers
6. **Ligases.** Catalyze the joining of two substrate molecules, coupled with breaking of the pyrophosphate bond in adenosine triphosphate (ATP) or a similar compound

The second and third digits of the EC code number represent the subclass and subsubclass of the enzyme, respectively, divisions that are made according to criteria specific to the enzymes in the class. The final number is the serial number specific to each enzyme in a subsubclass. Table 13-1 provides the EC code numbers, as well as the systematic and recommended names, for enzymes frequently measured in the clinical laboratory.

Table 13-1 also lists common and standard abbreviations for commonly analyzed enzymes. Without IUB recommendation, capital letters have been used as a convenience to identify enzymes. The common abbreviations, sometimes developed from previously accepted

TABLE 13-1 CLASSIFICATION OF FREQUENTLY QUANTITATED ENZYMES

CLASS	RECOMMENDED NAME	COMMON ABBREVIATION	STANDARD ABBREVIATION	EC CODE NO.	SYSTEMATIC NAME
Oxidoreductases	Lactate dehydrogenase	LD	LD	1.1.1.27	L-Lactate:NAD$^+$ oxidoreductase
	Glucose-6-phosphate dehydrogenase	G-6-PDH	G-6-PD	1.1.1.49	D-Glucose-6-phosphate:NADP$^+$ 1-oxidoreductase
	Glutamate dehydrogenase	GLD	GLD	1.4.1.3	L-glutamate:NAD(P) oxidoreductase, deaminase
Transferases	Aspartate aminotransferase	GOT (glutamate oxaloacetate transaminase)	AST	2.6.1.1	L-Aspartate:2-oxaglutarate aminotransferase
	Alanine aminotransferase	GPT (glutamate transaminase)	ALT	2.6.1.2	L-Alanine:2-oxaglutarate aminotransferase
	Creatine kinase	CPK (creatine phosphokinase)	CK	2.7.3.2	ATP:creatine N-phosphotransferase
	γ-Glutamyltransferase	GGTP	GGT	2.3.2.2	(5-Glutamyl)peptide: amino acid-5-glutamyl-transferase
	Glutathione-S-transferase	α-GST	GST	2.5.1.18	Glutathione transferase
	Glycogen phosphorylase	GP	GP	2.4.1.1	1,4-D-Glucan: orthophosphate α-D-glucosyltransferase
	Pyruvate kinase	PK	PK	2.7.1.40	Pyruvate kinase
Hydrolases	Alkaline phosphatase	ALP	ALP	3.1.3.1	Orthophosphoric monoester phospho-hydrolase (alkaline optimum)
	Acid phosphatase	ACP	ACP	3.1.3.2	Orthophosphoric monoester phosphohy-drolase (acid optimum)
	α-Amylase	AMS	AMY	3.2.1.1	1,4-D-Glucan glucanohydrolase
	Cholinesterase	PCHE	CHE	3.1.1.8	Acylcholine acylhydrolase
	Chymotrypsin	CHY	CHY	3.4.21.1	Chymotrypsin
	Elastase-1	E1	E1	3.4.21.36	Elastase
	5-Nucleotidase	NTP	NTP	3.1.3.5	5′-Ribonucleotide phosphohydrolase
	Triacylglycerol lipase		LPS	3.1.1.3	Triacylglycerol acylhydrolase
	Trypsin	TRY	TRY	3.4.21.4	Trypsin
Lyases	Aldolase	ALD	ALD	4.1.2.13	D-D-Fructose-1,6-bisdi-phosphateD-glyceral-dehyde-3-phosphate-lyase
Isomerases	Triosephosphate isomerase	TPI	TPI	5.3.1.1	Triose-phosphate isomerase
Ligase	Glutathione synthetase	GSH-S	GSH-S	6.3.2.3	Glutathione synthase

Adapted from Competence Assurance, ASMT. *Enzymology, an Educational Program.* Bethesda, MD: RMI Corporation; 1980.

names for the enzymes, were used until the standard abbreviations listed in the table were developed.[2,3] These standard abbreviations are used in the United States and are used later in this chapter to indicate specific enzymes.

ENZYME KINETICS

Catalytic Mechanism of Enzymes

A chemical reaction may occur spontaneously if the free energy or available kinetic energy is higher for the reactants than for the products. The reaction then proceeds toward the lower energy if a sufficient number of the reactant molecules possess enough excess energy to break their chemical bonds and collide to form new bonds. The excess energy, called activation energy, is the energy required to raise all molecules in 1 mol of a compound at a certain temperature to the transition state at the peak of the energy barrier. At the transition state, each molecule is equally likely to either participate in product formation or remain an unreacted molecule. Reactants possessing enough energy to overcome the energy barrier participate in product formation.

One way to provide more energy for a reaction is to increase the temperature and thus increase intermolecular collisions; however, this does not normally occur physiologically. Enzymes catalyze physiologic reactions by lowering the activation energy level that the reactants (*substrates*) must reach for the reaction to occur (Fig. 13-1). The reaction may then occur more readily to a state of equilibrium in which there is no net forward or reverse reaction, even though the equilibrium constant of the reaction is not altered. The extent to which the reaction progresses depends on the number of substrate molecules that pass the energy barrier.

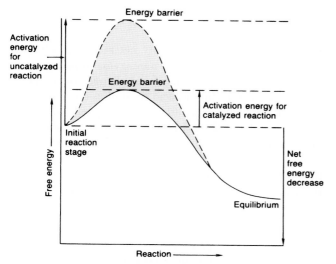

FIGURE 13-1 Energy vs. progression of reaction, indicating the energy barrier that the substrate must surpass to react with and without enzyme catalysis. The enzyme considerably reduces the free energy needed to activate the reaction.

The general relationship among the enzyme, substrate, and product may be represented as follows:

$$E + S \rightarrow ES \rightarrow E + P \qquad \text{(Eq. 13-1)}$$

where E is the enzyme, S is the substrate, ES is the enzyme–substrate complex, and P is the product.

The ES complex is a physical binding of a substrate to the active site of an enzyme. The structural arrangement of amino acid residues within the enzyme makes the three-dimensional active site available. At times, the binding of ligand drives active site rearrangement. The transition state for the ES complex has a lower energy of activation than the transition state of S alone, so that the reaction proceeds after the complex is formed. An actual reaction may involve several substrates and products.

Different enzymes are specific to substrates in different extents or respects. Certain enzymes exhibit *absolute specificity*, meaning that the enzyme combines with only one substrate and catalyzes only the one corresponding reaction. Other enzymes are *group specific* because they combine with all substrates containing a particular chemical group, such as a phosphate ester. Still other enzymes are specific to chemical bonds and thereby exhibit *bond specificity*.

Stereoisometric specificity refers to enzymes that predominantly combine with only one optical isomer of a certain compound. In addition, an enzyme may bind more than one molecule of substrate, and this may occur in a cooperative fashion. Binding of one substrate molecule, therefore, may facilitate binding of additional substrate molecules.

Factors That Influence Enzymatic Reactions

Substrate Concentration

The rate at which an enzymatic reaction proceeds and whether the forward or reverse reaction occurs depend on several reaction conditions. One major influence on enzymatic reactions is substrate concentration. In 1913, Michaelis and Menten hypothesized the role of substrate concentration in the formation of the enzyme–substrate (ES) complex. According to their hypothesis, represented in Figure 13-2, the substrate readily binds to free enzyme at a low substrate concentration. With the amount of enzyme exceeding the amount of substrate, the reaction rate steadily increases as more substrate is added. The reaction is following first-order kinetics because the reaction rate is directly proportional to substrate concentration. Eventually, however, the substrate concentration is high enough to saturate all available enzyme, and the reaction velocity reaches its maximum. When the product is formed, the resultant free enzyme immediately combines with excess free substrate. The reaction is in zero-order kinetics, and the reaction rate depends only on enzyme concentration.

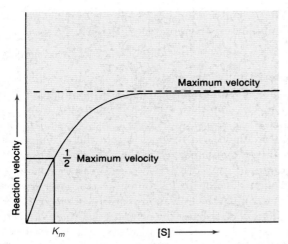

FIGURE 13-2 Michaelis-Menten curve of velocity vs. substrate concentration for enzymatic reaction. K_m is the substrate concentration at which the reaction velocity is half of the maximum level.

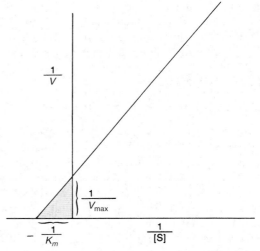

FIGURE 13-3 Lineweaver-Burk transformation of Michaelis-Menten curve. V_{max} is the reciprocal of the x-intercept of the straight line. K_m is the negative reciprocal of the x-intercept of the same line.

The Michaelis-Menten constant (K_m), derived from the theory of Michaelis and Menten, is a constant for a specific enzyme and substrate under defined reaction conditions and is an expression of the relationship between the velocity of an enzymatic reaction and substrate concentration. The assumptions are made that equilibrium among E, S, ES, and P is established rapidly and that the E + P → ES reaction is negligible. The rate-limiting step is the formation of product and enzyme from the ES complex. Then, maximum velocity is fixed, and the reaction rate is a function of only the enzyme concentration. As designated in Figure 13-2, K_m is specifically the substrate concentration at which the enzyme yields half the possible maximum velocity. Therefore, K_m indicates the amount of substrate needed for a particular enzymatic reaction.

The Michaelis-Menten hypothesis of the relationship between reaction velocity and substrate concentration can be represented mathematically as follows:

$$V = \frac{V_{max}[S]}{K_m + [S]} \qquad \text{(Eq. 13-2)}$$

where V is the measured velocity of reaction, V_{max} is the maximum velocity, [S] is the substrate concentration, and K_m is the Michaelis-Menten constant of enzyme for a specific substrate.

Theoretically, V_{max} and then K_m could be determined from the plot in Figure 13-2. However, V_{max} is difficult to determine from the hyperbolic plot and often not actually achieved in enzymatic reactions because enzymes may not function optimally in the presence of excessive substrate. A more accurate and convenient determination of V_{max} and K_m may be made through a Lineweaver-Burk plot, a double-reciprocal plot of the Michaelis-Menten constant, which yields a straight line (Fig. 13-3). The reciprocal is

taken of both the substrate concentration and the velocity of an enzymatic reaction. The equation becomes

$$\frac{1}{V} = \frac{K_m}{V_{max}} \frac{1}{[S]} + \frac{1}{V_{max}} \qquad \text{(Eq. 13-3)}$$

Enzyme Concentration

Because enzymes catalyze physiologic reactions, the enzyme concentration affects the rate of the catalyzed reaction. As long as the substrate concentration exceeds the enzyme concentration, the velocity of the reaction is proportional to the enzyme concentration. The higher the enzyme level, the faster the reaction will proceed because more enzyme is present to bind with the substrate.

pH

Enzymes are proteins that carry net molecular charges. Changes in pH may denature an enzyme or influence its ionic state, resulting in structural changes or a change in the charge of an amino acid residue in the active site. Hence, each enzyme operates within a specific pH range and maximally at a specific pH. Most physiologic enzymatic reactions occur in the pH range of 7.0 to 8.0, but some enzymes are active in wider pH ranges than others. In the laboratory, the pH for a reaction is carefully controlled at the optimal pH by means of appropriate buffer solutions.

Temperature

Increasing the temperature usually increases the rate of a chemical reaction by increasing the movement of molecules, the rate at which intermolecular collisions occur, and the energy available for the reaction. This is the case with enzymatic reactions until the temperature is high enough to denature the protein composition of the enzyme. For each 10° increase in temperature, the rate of the reaction will approximately double until, of course, the protein is denatured.

Each enzyme functions optimally at a particular temperature, which is influenced by other reaction variables, especially the total time for the reaction. The optimal temperature is usually close to that of the physiologic environment of the enzyme; however, some denaturation may occur at the human physiologic temperature of 37°C. The rate of denaturation increases as the temperature increases and is usually significant at 40°C to 50°C.

Because low temperatures render enzymes reversibly inactive, many serum or plasma specimens for enzyme measurement are refrigerated or frozen to prevent activity loss until analysis. Storage procedures may vary from enzyme to enzyme because of individual stability characteristics. Repeated freezing and thawing, however, tends to denature protein and should be avoided.

Because of their temperature sensitivity, enzymes should be analyzed under strictly controlled temperature conditions. Incubation temperatures should be accurate within ±0.1°C. Laboratories usually attempt to establish an analysis temperature for routine enzyme measurement of 25°C, 30°C, or 37°C. Attempts to establish a universal temperature for enzyme analysis have been unsuccessful, and therefore, reference ranges for enzyme levels may vary significantly among laboratories. In the United States, however, 37°C is most commonly used.

Cofactors

Cofactors are nonprotein entities that must bind to particular enzymes before a reaction occurs. Common *activators* (inorganic cofactors) are metallic (Ca^{2+}, Fe^{2+}, Mg^{2+}, Mn^{2+}, Zn^{2+}, and K^+) and nonmetallic (Br^- and Cl^-). The activator may be essential for the reaction or may only enhance the reaction rate in proportion with concentration to the point at which the excess activator begins to inhibit the reaction. Activators function by alternating the spatial configuration of the enzyme for proper substrate binding, linking substrate to the enzyme or coenzyme, or undergoing oxidation or reduction.

Some common coenzymes (organic cofactors) are nucleotide phosphates and vitamins. Coenzymes serve as second substrates for enzymatic reactions. When bound tightly to the enzyme, coenzymes are called *prosthetic groups*. For example, NAD as a cofactor may be reduced to nicotinamide adenine dinucleotide phosphate (NADP) in a reaction in which the primary substrate is oxidized. Increasing coenzyme concentration will increase the velocity of an enzymatic reaction in a manner synonymous with increasing substrate concentration. When quantitating an enzyme that requires a particular cofactor, that cofactor should always be provided in excess so that the extent of the reaction does not depend on the concentration of the cofactor.

Inhibitors

Enzymatic reactions may not progress normally if a particular substance, an *inhibitor*, interferes with the reaction. *Competitive inhibitors* physically bind to the active site of an enzyme and compete with the substrate for the active site. With a substrate concentration significantly higher than the concentration of the inhibitor, the inhibition is reversible because the substrate is more likely than the inhibitor to bind the active site and the enzyme has not been destroyed.

A *noncompetitive inhibitor* binds an enzyme at a place other than the active site and may be reversible in that some naturally present metabolic substances combine reversibly with certain enzymes. Noncompetitive inhibition also may be *irreversible* if the inhibitor destroys part of the enzyme involved in catalytic activity. Because the inhibitor binds the enzyme independently from the substrate, increasing substrate concentration does not reverse the inhibition.

Uncompetitive inhibition is another kind of inhibition in which the inhibitor binds to the ES complex—increasing substrate concentration results in more ES complexes to which the inhibitor binds and, thereby, increases the inhibition. The enzyme–substrate–inhibitor complex does not yield product.

Each of the three kinds of inhibition is unique with respect to effects on the V_{max} and K_m of enzymatic reactions (Fig. 13-4). In competitive inhibition, the effect of the inhibitor can be counteracted by adding excess substrate to bind the enzyme. The amount of the inhibitor is then negligible by comparison, and the reaction will proceed at a slower rate but to the same maximum velocity as an uninhibited reaction. K_m is a constant for each enzyme and cannot be altered. However, because the amount of substrate needed to achieve a particular velocity is higher in the presence of a competing inhibitor, K_m appears to increase when exhibiting the effect of the inhibitor.

The substrate and inhibitor, commonly a metallic ion, may bind an enzyme simultaneously in noncompetitive inhibition. The inhibitor may inactivate either an ES complex or just the enzyme by causing structural changes in the enzyme. Even if the inhibitor binds reversibly and does not inactivate the enzyme, the presence of the inhibitor when it is bound to the enzyme slows the rate of the reaction. Thus, for noncompetitive inhibition, the maximum reaction velocity cannot be achieved. Increasing substrate levels have no influence on the binding of a noncompetitive inhibitor, so that K_m is unchanged.

Because uncompetitive inhibition requires the formation of an ES complex, increasing substrate concentration increases inhibition. Therefore, maximum velocity equal to that of an uninhibited reaction cannot be achieved, and K_m appears to be decreased.

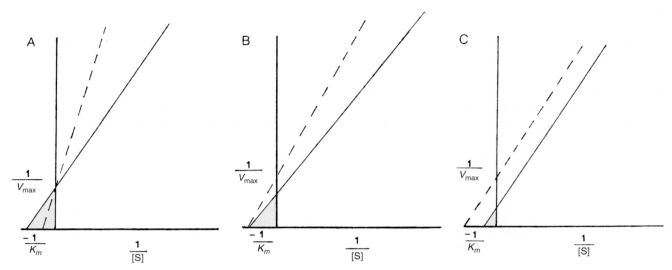

FIGURE 13-4 Normal Lineweaver-Burk plot (*solid line*) compared with each type of enzyme inhibition (*dotted line*). **(A)** Competitive inhibition V_{max} unaltered; K_m appears increased. **(B)** Noncompetitive inhibition V_{max} decreased; K_m unchanged. **(C)** Uncompetitive inhibition V_{max} decreased; K_m appears decreased.

Measurement of Enzyme Activity

Because enzymes are usually present in very small quantities in biologic fluids and often difficult to isolate from similar compounds, a convenient method of enzyme quantitation is measurement of catalytic activity. Activity is then related to concentration. Common methods might photometrically measure an increase in product concentration, a decrease in substrate concentration, a decrease in coenzyme concentration, or an increase in the concentration of an altered coenzyme.

If the amount of substrate and any coenzyme is in excess in an enzymatic reaction, the amount of substrate or coenzyme used, or product or altered coenzyme formed, will depend only on the amount of enzyme present to catalyze the reaction. Enzyme concentrations, therefore, are always performed in zero-order kinetics, with the substrate in sufficient excess to ensure that no more than 20% of the available substrate is converted to product. Any coenzyme also must be in excess. NADH is a coenzyme frequently measured in the laboratory. NADH absorbs light at 340 nm, whereas NAD does not, and a change in absorbance at 340 nm is easily measured.

In specific laboratory methodologies, substances other than substrate or coenzyme are necessary and must be present in excess. NAD or NADH is often convenient as a reagent for a *coupled-enzyme* assay when neither NAD nor NADH is a coenzyme for the reaction. In other coupled-enzyme assays, more than one enzyme is added in excess as a reagent and multiple reactions are catalyzed. After the enzyme under analysis catalyzes its specific reaction, a product of that reaction becomes the substrate on which an intermediate *auxiliary enzyme* acts. A product of the intermediate reaction becomes the substrate for the final reaction, which is catalyzed by an *indicator enzyme* and commonly involves the conversion of NAD to NADH or vice versa.

When performing an enzyme quantitation in zero-order kinetics, inhibitors must be lacking and other variables that may influence the rate of the reaction must be carefully controlled. A constant pH should be maintained by means of an appropriate buffer solution. The temperature should be constant within ±0.1°C throughout the assay at a temperature at which the enzyme is active (usually, 25°C, 30°C, or 37°C).

During the progress of the reaction, the period for the analysis also must be carefully selected. When the enzyme is initially introduced to the reactants and the excess substrate is steadily combining with the available enzyme, the reaction rate rises. After the enzyme is saturated, the rates of product formation, release of the enzyme, and recombination with more substrate proceed linearly. After some time, usually 6 to 8 minutes after reaction initiation, the reaction rate decreases as the substrate is depleted, the reverse reaction occurs appreciably, and the product begins to inhibit the reaction. Hence, enzyme quantitations must be performed during the linear phase of the reaction.

One of two general methods may be used to measure the extent of an enzymatic reaction: (1) fixed-time and (2) continuous-monitoring or kinetic assay. In the *fixed-time method*, the reactants are combined, the reaction proceeds for a designated time, the reaction is stopped (usually by inactivating the enzyme with a weak acid), and a measurement of the amount of reaction that has occurred is made. The reaction is assumed to be linear over the reaction time; the larger the reaction, the more the enzyme present.

In *continuous-monitoring* or kinetic assays, multiple measurements, usually of absorbance change, are made during the reaction, either at specific time intervals (usually every 30 or 60 seconds) or continuously by a continuous-recording spectrophotometer. These assays are advantageous over fixed-time methods because the linearity of the reaction may be more adequately verified. If absorbance is measured at intervals, several data points are necessary to increase the accuracy of linearity assessment. Continuous measurements are preferred because any deviation from linearity is readily observable.

The most common cause of deviation from linearity occurs when the enzyme is so elevated that all substrate is used early in the reaction time. For the remainder of the reaction, the rate change is minimal, with the implication that the coenzyme concentration is very low. With continuous monitoring, the laboratorian may observe a sudden decrease in the reaction rate (deviation from zero-order kinetics) of a particular determination and may repeat the determination using less patient sample. The decrease in the amount of patient sample operates as a dilution, and the answer obtained may be multiplied by the dilution factor to obtain the final answer. The sample itself is not diluted so that the diluent cannot interfere with the reaction. (Sample dilution with saline may be necessary to minimize negative effects in analysis caused by hemolysis or lipemia.) Enzyme activity measurements may not be accurate if storage conditions compromise integrity of the protein, if enzyme inhibitors are present, or if necessary cofactors are not present.

Calculation of Enzyme Activity

When enzymes are quantified relative to their activity rather than a direct measurement of concentration, the units used to report enzyme levels are *activity units*. The definition for the activity unit must consider variables that may alter results (e.g., pH, temperature, and substrate). Historically, specific method developers frequently established their own units for reporting results and often named the units after themselves (i.e., Bodansky and King units). To standardize the system of reporting quantitative results, the EC defined the international unit (IU) as the amount of enzyme that will catalyze the reaction of 1 μmol of substrate per minute under specified conditions of temperature, pH, substrates, and activators. Since specified conditions may vary among laboratories, reference values are still often laboratory specific. Enzyme concentration is usually expressed in units per liter (IU/L). The unit of enzyme activity recognized by the International System

of Units (Système International d'Unités [SI]) is the katal (mol/s). The mole is the unit for substrate concentration, and the unit of time is the second. Enzyme concentration is then expressed as katals per liter (kat/L) (1.0 IU = 17 nkat).

When enzymes are quantitated by measuring the increase or decrease of NADH at 340 nm, the molar absorptivity (6.22×10^3 mol/L) of NADH is used to calculate enzyme activity.

Measurement of Enzyme Mass

Immunoassay methodologies that quantify enzyme concentration by mass are also available and are routinely used for quantification of some enzymes, such as creatine kinase (CK)-MB. Immunoassays may overestimate active enzyme as a result of possible cross-reactivity with inactive enzymes, such as zymogens, inactive isoenzymes, macroenzymes, or partially digested enzyme. The relationship between enzyme activity and enzyme quantity is generally linear but should be determined for each enzyme. Enzymes may also be determined and quantified by electrophoretic techniques, which provide resolution of isoenzymes and isoforms.

Ensuring the accuracy of enzyme measurements has long been a concern of laboratorians. The Clinical Laboratory Improvement Amendment of 1988 (CLIA '88) has established guidelines for quality control and proficiency testing for all laboratories. Problems with quality control materials for enzyme testing have been a significant issue. Differences between clinical specimens and control sera include species of origin of the enzyme, integrity of the molecular species, isoenzyme forms, matrix of the solution, addition of preservatives, and lyophilization processes. Many studies have been conducted to ensure accurate enzyme measurements and good quality control materials.[4]

Enzymes as Reagents

Enzymes may be used as reagents to measure many nonenzymatic constituents in serum. For example, glucose, cholesterol, and uric acid are frequently quantified by means of enzymatic reactions, which measure the concentration of the analyte due to the specificity of the enzyme. Enzymes are also used as reagents for methods to quantify analytes that are substrates for the corresponding enzyme. One example, lactate dehydrogenase (LD), may be a reagent when lactate or pyruvate concentrations are evaluated. For such methods, the enzyme is added in excess in a quantity sufficient to provide a complete reaction in a short period.

Immobilized enzymes are chemically bonded to adsorbents, such as agarose or certain types of cellulose, by azide groups, diazo, and triazine. The enzymes act as recoverable reagents. When substrate is passed through the preparation, the product is retrieved and analyzed, and the enzyme is present and free to react with more substrate. Immobilized enzymes are convenient for batch analyses and are more stable than enzymes in a solution. Enzymes are also commonly used as reagents in competitive and noncompetitive immunoassays, such as those used to measure human immunodeficiency virus antibodies, therapeutic drugs, and cancer antigens. Commonly used enzymes include horseradish peroxidase, alkaline phosphatase (ALP), glucose-6-phosphate dehydrogenase (G-6-PD), and β-galactosidase. The enzyme in these assays functions as an indicator that reflects either the presence or the absence of the analyte.

ENZYMES OF CLINICAL SIGNIFICANCE

Table 13-2 lists the commonly analyzed enzymes, including their systematic names and clinical significance. Each enzyme is discussed in this chapter with respect to tissue

TABLE 13-2	MAJOR ENZYMES OF CLINICAL SIGNIFICANCE
ENZYME	**CLINICAL SIGNIFICANCE**
Acid phosphatase (ACP)	Prostatic carcinoma
Alanine aminotransferase (ALT)	Hepatic disorder
Aldolase (ALD)	Skeletal muscle disorder
Alkaline phosphatase (ALP)	Hepatic disorder
	Bone disorder
Amylase (AMY)	Acute pancreatitis
Angiotensin-converting enzyme (ACE)	Blood pressure regulation
Aspartate aminotransferase (AST)	Myocardial infarction
	Hepatic disorder
	Skeletal muscle disorder
Chymotrypsin (CHY)	Chronic pancreatitis insufficiency
Creatine kinase (CK)	Myocardial infarction
	Skeletal muscle disorder
Elastase-1 (E1)	Chronic pancreatitis insufficiency
Glucose-6-phosphate dehydrogenase (G-6-PD)	Drug-induced hemolytic anemia
Glutamate dehydrogenase (GLD)	Hepatic disorder
γ-Glutamyltransferase (GGT)	Hepatic disorder
Glutathione-S-transferase (GST)	Hepatic disorder
Glycogen phosphorylase (GP)	Acute myocardial infarction
Lactate dehydrogenase (LD)	Myocardial infarction
	Hepatic disorder
	Hemolysis
	Carcinoma
Lipase (LPS)	Acute pancreatitis
5′-Nucleotidase	Hepatic disorder
Pseudocholinesterase (PChE)	Organophosphate poisoning
	Genetic variants
	Hepatic disorder
	Suxamethonium sensitivity
Pyruvate kinase (PK)	Hemolytic anemia
Trypsin (TRY)	Acute pancreatitis

CASE STUDY 13-1

A 51-year-old, overweight white man visits his family physician with a symptom of "indigestion" of 5 days' duration. He has also had bouts of sweating, malaise, and headache. His blood pressure is 140/105 mm Hg; his family history includes a father with diabetes who died at age 62 of AMI secondary to diabetes mellitus. An electrocardiogram revealed changes from one performed 6 months earlier. The results of the patient's blood work are as follows:

CK	129 U/L (30–60)
CK-MB	4% (<6%)
LD	280 U/L (100–225)
LD	Isoenzymes LD-1 > LD-2
AST	35 U/L (5–30)

Questions

1. Can a diagnosis of AMI be ruled out in this patient?

2. What further cardiac markers should be run on this patient?

3. Should this patient be admitted to the hospital?

source, diagnostic significance, assay method, source of error, and reference range.

Creatine Kinase

CK is an enzyme with a molecular weight of approximately 82,000 Da that is generally associated with ATP regeneration in contractile or transport systems. Its predominant physiologic function occurs in muscle cells, where it is involved in the storage of high-energy creatine phosphate. Every contraction cycle of muscle results in creatine phosphate use, with the production of ATP. This results in relatively constant levels of muscle ATP. The reversible reaction catalyzed by CK is shown in Equation 13-4:

$$\text{Creatine} + \text{ATP} \xrightleftharpoons{\text{CK}} \text{Creatine phosphate} + \text{ADP}$$

(Eq. 13-4)

Tissue Source

CK is widely distributed in tissue, with highest activities found in skeletal muscle, heart muscle, and brain tissue. CK is present in much smaller quantities in other tissue sources, including the bladder, placenta, gastrointestinal tract, thyroid, uterus, kidney, lung, prostate, spleen, liver, and pancreas.

Diagnostic Significance

Due to the high concentrations of CK in muscle tissue, CK levels are frequently elevated in disorders of cardiac and skeletal muscle (myocardial infarction [MI], rhabdomyolysis, and muscular dystrophy). The CK level is considered a sensitive indicator of acute myocardial infarction (AMI) and muscular dystrophy, particularly the Duchenne type. Extreme elevations of CK occur in Duchenne-type muscular dystrophy, with values reaching 50 to 100 times the upper limit of normal (ULN). Although total CK levels are sensitive indicators of these disorders, they are not entirely specific indicators as CK elevation is found in various other abnormal cardiac and skeletal muscle conditions. Levels of CK also vary with muscle mass and, therefore, may depend on gender, race, degree of physical conditioning, and age.

Elevated CK levels are also occasionally seen in central nervous system disorders such as strokes, seizures, nerve degeneration, and central nervous system shock. Damage to the blood–brain barrier must occur to allow enzyme release to the peripheral circulation.

Other pathophysiologic conditions in which elevated CK levels occur are hypothyroidism, malignant hyperpyrexia, and Reye's syndrome. Table 13-3 lists the major disorders associated with abnormal CK levels. Serum CK levels and CK/progesterone ratio have been useful in the diagnosis of ectopic pregnancies.[5] Total serum CK levels have also been used as an early diagnostic tool to identify patients with *Vibrio vulnificus* infections.[6]

Because enzyme elevation is found in numerous disorders, the separation of total CK into its various isoenzyme fractions is considered a more specific indicator of various disorders than total levels. Typically, the clinical relevance of CK activity depends more on isoenzyme fractionation than on total levels.

CK occurs as a dimer consisting of two subunits that can be separated readily into three distinct molecular forms. The three isoenzymes have been designated as CK-BB (brain type), CK-MB (hybrid type), and CK-MM (muscle type). On electrophoretic separation, CK-BB will migrate fastest toward the anode and is therefore called *CK-1*. CK-BB is followed by CK-MB (*CK-2*) and, finally, by CK-MM (*CK-3*), exhibiting the slowest mobility (Fig. 13-5). Table 13-3 indicates the tissue localization of the isoenzymes and the major conditions associated with elevated levels. Separation of CK isoforms may also be visualized by high-voltage electrophoretic separation. Isoforms occur following cleavage of the carboxyl-terminal amino acid from the M subunit by serum carboxypeptidase N. Three isoforms have been described for CK-MM and two isoforms for CK-MB; the clinical significance is not well established.

The major isoenzyme in the sera of healthy people is the MM form. Values for the MB isoenzyme range from undetectable to trace (<6% of total CK). It also appears that CK-BB is present in small quantities in the sera of

TABLE 13-3	CREATINE KINASE ISOENZYMES—TISSUE LOCALIZATION AND SOURCES OF ELEVATION	
ISOENZYME	**TISSUE**	**CONDITION**
CK-MM	Heart	Myocardial infarction
	Skeletal muscle	Skeletal muscle disorder
		Muscular dystrophy
		Polymyositis
		Hypothyroidism
		Malignant hyperthermia
		Physical activity
		Intramuscular injection
CK-MB	Heart	Myocardial infarction
	Skeletal muscle	Myocardial injury
		Ischemia
		Angina
		Inflammatory heart disease
		Cardiac surgery
		Duchenne-type muscular dystrophy
		Polymyositis
		Malignant hyperthermia
		Reye's syndrome
		Rocky Mountain spotted fever
		Carbon monoxide poisoning
CK-BB	Brain	Central nervous system shock
	Bladder	Anoxic encephalopathy
	Lung	Cerebrovascular accident
	Prostate	Seizure
	Uterus	Placental or uterine trauma
	Colon	Carcinoma
	Stomach	Reye's syndrome
	Thyroid	Carbon monoxide poisoning
		Malignant hyperthermia
		Acute and chronic renal failure

healthy people; however, the presence of CK-BB in serum depends on the method of detection. Most techniques cannot detect CK-BB in normal serum.

CK-MM is the major isoenzyme fraction found in striated muscle and normal serum. Skeletal muscle contains almost entirely CK-MM, with a small amount of CK-MB. The majority of CK activity in heart muscle is also attributed to CK-MM, with approximately 20% as a result of CK-MB.[7] Normal serum consists of approximately 94% to 100% CK-MM. Injury to both cardiac and skeletal muscle accounts for the majority of cases of CK-MM elevations

(Table 13-3). Hypothyroidism results in CK-MM elevations because of the involvement of muscle tissue (increased membrane permeability), the effect of thyroid hormone on enzyme activity, and, possibly, the slower clearance of CK as a result of slower metabolism.

Mild to strenuous activity may contribute to elevated CK levels, as may intramuscular injections. In physical activity, the extent of elevation is variable. However, the degree of exercise in relation to the exercise capacity of the individual is the most important factor in determining the degree of elevation.[8] Patients who are

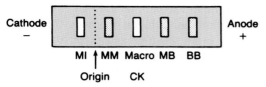

FIGURE 13-5 Electrophoretic migration pattern of normal and atypical creatine kinase (CK) isoenzymes.

physically well conditioned show lesser degrees of elevation than do patients who are less conditioned. Levels may be elevated for as long as 48 hours following exercise. CK elevations are generally less than five times the ULN following intramuscular injections and usually not apparent after 48 hours, although elevations may persist for 1 week. The predominant isoenzyme is CK-MM.

The quantity of CK-BB in the tissue (Table 13-3) is usually small. The small quantity, coupled with its relatively short half-life (1 to 5 hours), results in CK-BB activities that are generally low and transient and not usually measurable when tissue damage occurs. Highest concentrations are found in the central nervous system, the gastrointestinal tract, and the uterus during pregnancy. Although brain tissue has high concentrations of CK, serum rarely contains CK-BB of brain origin. Because of its molecular size (80,000 Da), its passage across the blood–brain barrier is hindered. However, when extensive damage to the brain has occurred, significant amounts of CK-BB can sometimes be detected in the serum. It has been observed that CK-BB may be significantly elevated in patients with carcinoma of various organs. It has been found in association with untreated prostatic carcinoma and other adenocarcinomas. These

findings indicate that CK-BB may be a useful tumor-associated marker.[9] The most common causes of CK-BB elevations are central nervous system damage, tumors, childbirth, and the presence of macro-CK, an enzyme–immunoglobulin complex. In most of these cases, the CK-BB level is greater than 5 U/L, usually in the range of 10 to 50 U/L. Other conditions listed in Table 13-3 usually show CK-BB activity below 10 U/L.[10]

The value of CK isoenzyme separation can be found principally in the detection of myocardial damage. Cardiac tissue contains significant quantities of CK-MB, approximately 20% of all CK-MB. Whereas CK-MB is found in small quantities in other tissue, myocardium is essentially the only tissue from which CK-MB enters the serum in significant quantities. Demonstration of elevated levels of CK-MB, greater than or equal to 6% of the total CK, is considered a good indicator of myocardial damage, particularly AMI. Other nonenzyme proteins, called troponins, have been found to be even more specific and may elevate in the absence of CK-MB elevations. Following MI, the CK-MB levels begin to rise within 4 to 8 hours, peak at 12 to 24 hours, and return to normal levels within 48 to 72 hours. This time frame must be considered when interpreting CK-MB levels.

CK-MB activity has been observed in other cardiac disorders (Table 13-3). Therefore, increased quantities are not entirely specific for AMI but probably reflect some degree of ischemic heart damage. The specificity of CK-MB levels in the diagnosis of AMI can be increased if interpreted in conjunction with LD isoenzymes and/or troponins and if measured sequentially over a 48-hour period to detect the typical rise and fall of enzyme activity seen in AMI (Fig. 13-6). The MB isoenzyme also has

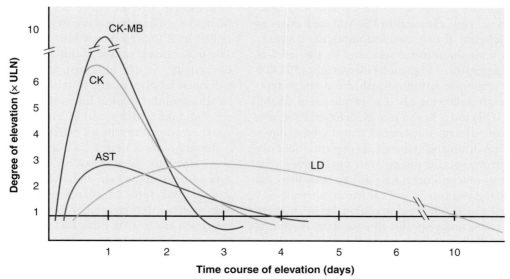

FIGURE 13-6 Time-activity curves of enzymes in myocardial infarction for aspartate aminotransferase (AST), creatine kinase (CK), CK-MB, and lactate dehydrogenase (LD). CK, specifically the MB fraction, increases initially, followed by AST and LD. LD is elevated the longest. All enzymes usually return to normal within 10 d. ULN, upper limit of normal.

been detected in the sera of patients with noncardiac disorders. CK-MB levels found in these conditions probably represent leakage from skeletal muscle, although in Duchenne-type muscular dystrophy, there may be some cardiac involvement as well. CK-MB levels in Reye's syndrome also may reflect myocardial damage. Despite the findings of CK-MB levels in disorders other than MI, its presence still remains a significant indicator of AMI.[11] The typical time course of CK-MB elevation following AMI is not found in other conditions.

Nonenzyme proteins (troponin I and troponin T) have been used as a more sensitive and specific marker of myocardial damage. These proteins are released into the bloodstream earlier and persist longer than CK and its isoenzyme CK-MB. More information on these protein markers of AMI can be found in Chapter 26.

Numerous reports have been made describing the appearance of unusual CK isoenzyme bands displaying electrophoretic properties that differ from the three major isoenzyme fractions (Fig. 13-5).[12-16] These atypical forms are generally of two types and are referred to as macro-CK and mitochondrial CK (CK-Mi).

Macro-CK appears to migrate to a position midway between CK-MM and CK-MB. This type of macro-CK largely comprises CK-BB complexed with immunoglobulin. In most instances, the associated immunoglobulin is IgG, although a complex with IgA also has been described. The term *macro-CK* has also been used to describe complexes of lipoproteins with CK-MM. The incidence of macro-CK in sera ranges from 0.8% to 1.6%. Currently, no specific disorder is associated with its presence, although it appears to be age and sex related, occurring most frequently in women older than age 50.

CK-Mi is bound to the exterior surface of the inner mitochondrial membranes of muscle, brain, and liver. It migrates to a point cathodal to CK-MM and exists as a dimeric molecule of two identical subunits. It occurs in serum in both the dimeric state and in the form of oligomeric aggregates of high molecular weight (350,000 Da). CK-Mi is not present in normal serum and is typically not present following MI. The incidence of CK-Mi ranges from 0.8% to 1.7%. For it to be detected in serum, extensive tissue damage must occur, causing breakdown of the mitochondrion and cell wall. Its presence does not correlate with any specific disease state but appears to be an indicator of severe illness. CK-Mi has been detected in cases of malignant tumor and cardiac abnormalities.

In view of the indefinite correlation between these atypical CK forms and a specific disease state, it appears that their significance relates primarily to the methods used for detecting CK-MB. In certain analytic procedures, these atypical forms may be measured as CK-MB, resulting in erroneously high CK-MB levels.

Methods used for the measurement of CK isoenzymes include electrophoresis, ion-exchange chromatography, and several immunoassays, including radioimmunoassay (RIA) and immunoinhibition methods. Although mass methods are more sensitive and preferred for quantitation of CK-MB, electrophoresis has been the reference method. The electrophoretic properties of the CK isoenzymes are shown in Figure 13-5. Generally, the technique consists of performing electrophoresis on the sample, measuring the reaction using an overlay technique, and then visualizing the bands under ultraviolet light. With electrophoresis, the atypical bands can be separated, allowing their detection apart from the three major bands. Often a strongly fluorescent band appears, which migrates in close proximity to the CK-BB form. The exact nature of this fluorescence is unknown, but it has been attributed to the binding of fluorescent drugs or bilirubin by albumin.

In addition to visualizing atypical CK bands, other advantages of electrophoresis methods include detecting an unsatisfactory separation and allowing visualization of adenylate kinase (AK). AK is an enzyme released from erythrocytes in hemolyzed samples and appearing as a band cathodal to CK-MM. AK may interfere with chemical or immunoinhibition methods, causing a falsely elevated CK or CK-MB value.

Ion-exchange chromatography has the potential for being more sensitive and precise than electrophoretic procedures performed with good technique. On an unsatisfactory column, however, CK-MM may merge into CK-MB and CK-BB may be eluted with CK-MB. Also, macro-CK may elute with CK-MB.

Antibodies against both the M and B subunits have been used to determine CK-MB activity. Anti-M inhibits all M activity but not B activity. CK activity is measured before and after inhibition. Activity remaining after M inhibition is a result of the B subunit of both MB and BB activity. The residual activity after inhibition is multiplied by 2 to account for MB activity (50% inhibited). The major disadvantage of this method is that it detects BB activity, which, although not normally detectable, will cause falsely elevated MB results when BB is present. In addition, the atypical forms of CK-Mi and macro-CK are not inhibited by anti-M antibodies and also may cause erroneous results for MB activity.

Immunoassays detect CK-MB reliably with minimal cross-reactivity. Immunoassays measure the concentration of enzyme protein rather than enzymatic activity and can, therefore, detect enzymatically inactive CK-MB. This leads to the possibility of permitting detection of infarction earlier than other methods. A double-antibody immunoinhibition assay is also available. This technique allows differentiation of MB activity due to AK and the atypical isoenzymes, resulting in a more specific analytic procedure for CK-MB.[17] Point-of-care assay systems for CK-MB are available but not as widely used as those for troponins.

Assay Enzyme Activity

As indicated by Equation 13-4, CK catalyzes both forward and reverse reactions involving phosphorylation of creatine or ADP. Typically, for analysis of CK activity, this reaction is coupled with other enzyme systems and a change in absorbance at 340 nm is determined. The forward reaction is coupled with the pyruvate kinase–LD–NADH system and proceeds according to Equation 13-5:

$$\text{Creatine} + \text{ATP} \xrightleftharpoons{CK} \text{Creatine phosphate} + \text{ADP}$$

$$\text{ADP} + \text{phosphoenolpyruvate} \xrightleftharpoons{PK} \text{Pyruvate} + \text{ATP}$$

$$\text{Pyruvate} + \text{NADH} + \text{H}^+ \xrightleftharpoons{LD} \text{Lactate} + \text{NAD}^+$$

(Eq. 13-5)

The reverse reaction is coupled with the hexokinase–G-6-PD–NADP system, as indicated in Equation 13-6:

$$\text{Creatine phosphate} + \text{ADP} \xrightleftharpoons{CK} \text{Creatine ADP}$$

$$\text{ATP} + \text{glucose} \xrightleftharpoons{KH} \text{ADP} + \text{glucose-6-phosphate}$$

$$\text{Glucose 6-phosphate} + \text{NADPH}^+ \xrightleftharpoons{G\text{-}6\text{-}PD}$$
$$\text{6-phosphogluconate} + \text{NADPH}$$ (Eq. 13-6)

The reverse reaction proposed by Oliver and modified by Rosalki is the most commonly performed method in the clinical laboratory.[13] The reaction proceeds two to six times faster than the forward reaction, depending on the assay conditions and there is less interference from side reactions. The optimal pH for the reverse reaction is 6.8; for the forward reaction, it is 9.0.

CK activity in serum is unstable, being rapidly inactivated because of oxidation of sulfhydryl groups. Inactivation can be partially reversed by the addition of sulfhydryl compounds to the assay reagent. Compounds such as N-acetylcysteine, mercaptoethanol, thioglycerol, and dithiothreitol are among those used.

Source of Error

Hemolysis of serum samples may be a source of elevated CK activity. Erythrocytes are virtually devoid of CK; however, they are rich in AK activity. AK reacts with ADP to produce ATP, which is then available to participate in the assay reaction, causing falsely elevated CK levels. This interference can occur with hemolysis of greater than 320 mg/L hemoglobin, which releases sufficient AK to exhaust the AK inhibitors in the reagent. Trace hemolysis causes little, if any, CK elevation. Serum should be stored in a dark place because CK is inactivated by light. Activity can be restored after storage in the dark at 4°C for 7 days or at −20°C for 1 month when the assay is conducted using a sulfhydryl activator.[18] Because of the effect of muscular activity and muscle mass on CK levels, it should be noted that people who are physically well trained tend to have elevated baseline levels and that patients who are bedridden for prolonged periods may have decreased CK activity.

Reference Range

Total CK:

Males: 46 to 171 U/L (37°C) (0.8 to 2.9 μkat/L)
Females: 34 to 145 U/L (37°C) (0.6 to 2.4 μkat/L)
CK-MB: <5% total CK

The higher values in males are attributed to increased muscle mass. Note that enzyme reference ranges are subject to variation, depending on the method used and the assay conditions.

Lactate Dehydrogenase

LD is an enzyme that catalyzes the interconversion of lactic and pyruvic acids. It is a hydrogen-transfer enzyme that uses the coenzyme NAD$^+$ according to Equation 13-7:

$$\begin{array}{ccc}
\text{CH}_3 & & \text{CH}_3 \\
| & & | \\
\text{HC—OH} + \text{NAD}^+ \xrightleftharpoons{LD} & \text{C}{=}\text{O} + \text{NADH} + \text{H}^+ \\
| & & | \\
\text{COOH} & & \text{COOH} \\
\text{Lactate} & & \text{Pyruvate}
\end{array}$$

(Eq. 13-7)

Tissue Source

LD is widely distributed in the body. High activities are found in the heart, liver, skeletal muscle, kidney, and erythrocytes; lesser amounts are found in the lung, smooth muscle, and brain.

Diagnostic Significance

Because of its widespread activity in numerous body tissue, LD is elevated in a variety of disorders. Increased levels are found in cardiac, hepatic, and skeletal muscle and renal diseases, as well as in several hematologic and neoplastic disorders. The highest levels of total LD are seen in pernicious anemia and hemolytic disorders. Intramedullary destruction of erythroblasts causes elevation as a result of the high concentration of LD in erythrocytes. Liver disorders, such as viral hepatitis and cirrhosis, show slight elevations of two to three times the ULN. AMI and pulmonary infarct also show slight elevations of approximately the same degree (2 to 3× ULN). In AMI, LD levels begin to rise within 12 to 24 hours, reach peak levels within 48 to 72 hours, and may remain elevated for 10 days. Skeletal muscle disorders and some leukemias contribute to increased levels. Marked elevations can be observed in most patients with acute lymphoblastic leukemia in particular.

Because of the many conditions that contribute to increased activity, an elevated total LD value is a rather nonspecific finding. LD assays, therefore, assume more clinical significance when separated into isoenzyme fractions. The enzyme can be separated into five major fractions, each comprising four subunits. It has a molecular

TABLE 13-4	LACTATE DEHYDROGENASE ISOENZYMES—TISSUE LOCALIZATION AND SOURCES OF ELEVATION	
ISOENZYME	**TISSUE**	**DISORDER**
LD-1 (HHHH)	Heart	Myocardial infarction
	Red blood cells	Hemolytic anemia
LD-2 (HHHM)	Heart	Megaloblastic anemia
	Red blood cells	Acute renal infarct
		Hemolyzed specimen
LD-3 (HHMM)	Lung	Pulmonary embolism
	Lymphocytes	Extensive
	Spleen	Pulmonary pneumonia
	Pancreas	Lymphocytosis
		Acute pancreatitis
		Carcinoma
LD-4 (HMMM)	Liver	Hepatic injury or inflammation
LD-5 (MMMM)	Skeletal muscle	Skeletal muscle injury

LD, lactate dehydrogenase.

weight of 128,000 Da. Each isoenzyme comprises four polypeptide chains with a molecular weight of 32,000 Da each. Two different polypeptide chains, designated H (heart) and M (muscle), combine in five arrangements to yield the five major isoenzyme fractions. Table 13-4 indicates the tissue localization of the LD isoenzymes and the major disorders associated with elevated levels. LD-1 migrates most quickly toward the anode, followed in sequence by the other fractions, with LD-5 migrating the slowest.

In the sera of healthy individuals, the major isoenzyme fraction is LD-2, followed by LD-1, LD-3, LD-4, and LD-5 (for the isoenzyme ranges, see Table 13-5). LD-1 and LD-2 are present to approximately the same extent in the tissues listed in Table 13-4. However, cardiac tissue and red blood cells contain a higher concentration of LD-1. Therefore, in conditions involving cardiac necrosis (AMI) and intravascular hemolysis, the serum levels of LD-1 will increase to a point at which they are present in greater concentration than LD-2, resulting in a condition known as the LD flipped pattern (LD-1 > LD-2).[19] This flipped pattern is suggestive of AMI. However, LD is not specific to cardiac tissue and is not a preferred marker of diagnosis of AMI. LD-1/LD-2 ratios greater than 1 also may be observed in hemolyzed serum samples.[20] Elevations of LD-3 occur most frequently with pulmonary involvement and are also observed in patients with various carcinomas. The LD-4 and LD-5 isoenzymes are found primarily in liver and skeletal muscle tissue, with LD-5 being the predominant fraction in these tissues. LD-5 levels have greatest

clinical significance in the detection of hepatic disorders, particularly intrahepatic disorders. Disorders of skeletal muscle will reveal elevated LD-5 levels, as depicted in the muscular dystrophies.

A sixth LD isoenzyme has been identified, which migrates cathodic to LD-5.[21-23] LD-6 is alcohol dehydrogenase. In reporting studies, LD-6 has been present in patients with arteriosclerotic cardiovascular failure. It is believed that its appearance signifies a grave prognosis and impending death. LD-5 is elevated concurrently with the appearance of LD-6, probably representing hepatic congestion due to cardiovascular disease. It is suggested, therefore, that LD-6 may reflect liver injury secondary to severe circulatory insufficiency.

TABLE 13-5	LACTATE DEHYDROGENASE (LD) ISOENZYMES AS A PERCENTAGE OF TOTAL LD
ISOENZYME	**%**
LD-1	14–26
LD-2	29–39
LD-3	20–26
LD-4	8–16
LD-5	6–16

Source: Lott JA, Stang JM. Serum enzymes and isoenzymes in the diagnosis and differential diagnosis of myocardial ischemia and necrosis. *Clin Chem*. 1980;26:1241.

LD has been shown to complex with immunoglobulins and to reveal atypical bands on electrophoresis. LD complexed with IgA and IgG usually migrates between LD-3 and LD-4. This macromolecular complex is not associated with any specific clinical abnormality.

Analysis of LD isoenzymes can be accomplished by electrophoresis, by immunoinhibition or chemical inhibition methods, or by differences in substrate affinity. Because of limited clinical utility, such tests are not commonly used. The electrophoretic procedure has been widely used historically. After electrophoretic separation, the isoenzymes can be detected either fluorometrically or colorimetrically. LD can use other substrates in addition to lactate, such as α-hydroxybutyrate. The H subunits have a greater affinity for α-hydroxybutyrate than to the M subunits. This has led to the use of this substrate in an attempt to measure the LD-1 activity, which consists entirely of H subunits. The chemical assay, known as the measurement of α-hydroxybutyrate dehydrogenase activity (α-HBD), is outlined in Equation 13-8:

$$\underset{\substack{\text{α-Ketobutyrate}}}{\begin{array}{c}CH_3\\|\\CH_2\\|\\HC=O\\|\\COOH\end{array}} + NADH + H^+ \xrightarrow{\text{α-HBD}} \underset{\substack{\text{α-Hydroxybutyrate}}}{\begin{array}{c}CH_3\\|\\CH_2\\|\\HC-OH\\|\\COOH\end{array}} + NAD^+$$

(Eq. 13-8)

α-HBD is not a separate and distinct enzyme but is considered to represent the LD-1 activity of total LD. However, α-HBD activity is not entirely specific for the LD-1 fraction because LD-2, LD-3, and LD-4 also contain varying amounts of the H subunit. HBD activity is increased in those conditions in which the LD-1 and LD-2 fractions are increased.

LD is commonly used to measure lactic and pyruvic acids or as a coupled reaction.

Assay for Enzyme Activity

LD catalyzes the interconversion of lactic and pyruvic acids using the coenzyme NAD^+. The reaction sequence is outlined in Equation 13-9:

$$\text{Lactate} + NAD^+ \rightleftharpoons \text{Pyruavate} + NADH + H^+$$

(Eq. 13-9)

The reaction can proceed in either a forward (lactate [L]) or reverse (pyruvate [P]) direction. Both reactions have been used in clinical assays. The rate of the reverse reaction is approximately three times faster, allowing smaller sample volumes and shorter reaction times.

However, the reverse reaction is more susceptible to substrate exhaustion and loss of linearity. The optimal pH for the forward reaction is 8.3 to 8.9; for the reverse reaction, it is 7.1 to 7.4.

Source of Error

Erythrocytes contain an LD concentration approximately 100 to 150 times that found in serum. Therefore, any degree of hemolysis should render a sample unacceptable for analysis. LD activity is unstable in serum regardless of the temperature at which it is stored. If the sample cannot be analyzed immediately, it should be stored at 25°C and analyzed within 48 hours. LD-5 is the most labile isoenzyme. Loss of activity occurs more quickly at 4°C than at 25°C. Serum samples for LD isoenzyme analysis should be stored at 25°C and analyzed within 24 hours of collection.

Reference Range

LD, 125 to 220 U/L (37°C)

Aspartate Aminotransferase

Aspartate aminotransferase (AST) is an enzyme belonging to the class of transferases. It is commonly referred to as a *transaminase* and is involved in the transfer of an amino group between aspartate and α-keto acids. The older terminology, *serum glutamic oxaloacetic transaminase (SGOT, or GOT)*, may also be used. Pyridoxal phosphate functions as a coenzyme. The reaction proceeds according to Equation 12-10:

$$\underset{\substack{\text{Asparate}}}{\begin{array}{c}COOH\\|\\CH_2\\|\\HC-NH_2\\|\\COOH\end{array}} + \underset{\substack{\text{α-Keto-}\\\text{glutarate}}}{\begin{array}{c}COOH\\|\\CH_2\\|\\CH_2\\|\\C=O\\|\\COOH\end{array}} \rightleftharpoons \underset{\substack{\text{Oxalo-}\\\text{acetate}}}{\begin{array}{c}COOH\\|\\CH_2\\|\\C=O\\|\\COOH\end{array}} + \underset{\substack{\text{Glutamate}}}{\begin{array}{c}COOH\\|\\CH_2\\|\\CH_2\\|\\HC-NH_2\\|\\COOH\end{array}}$$

(Eq. 13-10)

The transamination reaction is important in intermediary metabolism because of its function in the synthesis and degradation of amino acids. The ketoacids formed by the reaction are ultimately oxidized by the tricarboxylic acid cycle to provide a source of energy.

Tissue Source

AST is widely distributed in human tissue. The highest concentrations are found in cardiac tissue, liver, and skeletal muscle, with smaller amounts found in the kidney, pancreas, and erythrocytes.

Diagnostic Significance

The clinical use of AST is limited mainly to the evaluation of hepatocellular disorders and skeletal muscle involvement. In AMI, AST levels begin to rise within 6 to 8 hours, peak at 24 hours, and generally return to normal within 5 days. However, because of the wide tissue distribution, AST levels are not useful in the diagnosis of AMI.

AST elevations are frequently seen in pulmonary embolism. Following congestive heart failure, AST levels also may be increased, probably reflecting liver involvement as a result of inadequate blood supply to that organ. AST levels are highest in acute hepatocellular disorders. In viral hepatitis, levels may reach 100 times the ULN. In cirrhosis, only moderate levels—approximately four times the ULN—are detected (see Chapter 25). Skeletal muscle disorders, such as the muscular dystrophies, and inflammatory conditions also cause increases in AST levels (4 to 8× ULN).

AST exists as two isoenzyme fractions located in the cell cytoplasm and mitochondria. The intracellular concentration of AST may be 7,000 times higher than the extracellular concentration. The cytoplasmic isoenzyme is the predominant form occurring in serum. In disorders producing cellular necrosis, the mitochondrial form may be significantly increased. Isoenzyme analysis of AST is not routinely performed in the clinical laboratory.

Assay for Enzyme Activity

Assay methods for AST are generally based on the principle of the Karmen method, which incorporates a coupled enzymatic reaction using malate dehydrogenase as the indicator reaction and monitors the change in absorbance at 340 nm continuously as NADH is oxidized to NAD^+ (Equation 13-11). The optimal pH is 7.3 to 7.8:

$$\text{Aspartate} + \alpha\text{-ketoglutarate} \underset{}{\overset{\text{AST}}{\rightleftharpoons}}$$
$$\text{Oxaloacetate} + \text{glutamate}$$

$$\text{Oxaloacetate} + \text{NADH} + H^+ \rightleftharpoons \text{Malate} + NAD^+$$

(Eq. 13-11)

Source of Error

Hemolysis should be avoided because it can dramatically increase serum AST concentration. AST activity is stable in serum for 3 to 4 days at refrigerated temperatures.

Reference Range

AST, 5 to 35 U/L (37°C) (0.1 to 0.6 µkat/L)

Alanine Aminotransferase

Alanine aminotransferase (ALT) is a transferase with enzymatic activity similar to that of AST. Specifically, it catalyzes the transfer of an amino group from alanine to α-ketoglutarate with the formation of glutamate and pyruvate. The older terminology was serum *glutamic*

CASE STUDY 13-2

While a 71-year-old woman is walking home from a shopping center, she faints and falls. She is driven home by a friend. When home, she realizes that she is bleeding from her mouth and is slightly disoriented. She appears injured from the fall, but she does not remember tripping or falling. The woman is taken to a local emergency department. The examining physician determines that there was a loss of consciousness; to determine the reason, he orders a head CT and ECG and the following laboratory tests: CBC, PT, aPTT, CK, LD, AST, and troponin T and troponin I. All tests are within normal limits. The woman is sutured for the mouth injuries and admitted to a 24-hour observation unit.

Questions

1. What possible diagnoses is the physician considering?

2. What laboratory tests would be elevated at 6, 12, and 24 hours if this patient had an AMI?

3. What isoenzyme tests would be useful with this patient?

pyruvic transaminase (*SGPT*, or *GPT*). Equation 13-12 indicates the transferase reaction. Pyridoxal phosphate acts as the coenzyme:

(Eq. 13-12)

Tissue Source

ALT is distributed in many tissues, with comparatively high concentrations in the liver. It is considered the more liver-specific enzyme of the transferases.

Diagnostic Significance

Clinical applications of ALT assays are confined mainly to evaluation of hepatic disorders. Higher elevations are found in hepatocellular disorders than in extrahepatic or intrahepatic obstructive disorders. In acute inflammatory conditions of the liver, ALT elevations are frequently higher than those of AST and tend to remain elevated longer as a result of the longer half-life of ALT in serum (16 and 24 hours, respectively).

Cardiac tissue contains a small amount of ALT activity, but the serum level usually remains normal in AMI unless subsequent liver damage has occurred. ALT levels have historically been compared with levels of AST to help determine the source of an elevated AST level and to detect liver involvement concurrent with myocardial injury.

Assay for Enzyme Activity

The typical assay procedure for ALT consists of a coupled enzymatic reaction using LD as the indicator enzyme, which catalyzes the reduction of pyruvate to lactate with the simultaneous oxidation of NADH. The change in absorbance at 340 nm measured continuously is directly proportional to ALT activity. The reaction proceeds according to Equation 13-13. The optimal pH is 7.3 to 7.8:

$$\text{Alanine} + \alpha\text{-ketoglutarate} \xrightleftharpoons{\text{ALT}} \text{Pyruvate} + \text{glutamate}$$

$$\text{Pyruvate} + \text{NADH} + \text{H}^+ \xrightleftharpoons{\text{LD}} \text{Lactate} + \text{NAD}^+$$

$$\text{(Eq. 13-13)}$$

Source of Error

ALT is stable for 3 to 4 days at 4°C. It is relatively unaffected by hemolysis.

Reference Range

ALT, 7 to 45 U/L (37°C) (0.1 to 0.8 μkat/L)

Alkaline Phosphatase

ALP belongs to a group of enzymes that catalyze the hydrolysis of various phosphomonoesters at an alkaline pH. Consequently, ALP is a nonspecific enzyme capable of reacting with many different substrates. Specifically, ALP functions to liberate inorganic phosphate from an organic phosphate ester with the concomitant production of an alcohol. The reaction proceeds according to Equation 13-14:

$$
\underset{\text{Phosophomonoester}}{\text{R}\!-\!\overset{\displaystyle O}{\underset{\displaystyle O^-}{\overset{\|}{\underset{|}{P}}}}\!-\!O^-} + H_2O \underset{\text{pH 9-10}}{\overset{\text{ALP}}{\rightleftharpoons}} \underset{\text{Alcohol}}{\text{R}\!-\!\text{OH}} + \underset{\text{Phosphate ion}}{\text{HO}\!-\!\overset{\displaystyle O}{\underset{\displaystyle O^-}{\overset{\|}{\underset{|}{P}}}}\!-\!O^-}
$$

$$\text{(Eq. 13-14)}$$

The optimal pH for the reaction is 9.0 to 10.0, but optimal pH varies with the substrate used. The enzyme requires Mg^{2+} as an activator.

Tissue Source

ALP activity is present on cell surfaces in most human tissue. The highest concentrations are found in the intestine, liver, bone, spleen, placenta, and kidney. In the liver, the enzyme is located on both sinusoidal and bile canalicular membranes; activity in bone is confined to the osteoblasts, those cells involved in the production of bone matrix. The specific location of the enzyme within this tissue accounts for the more predominant elevations in certain disorders.

Diagnostic Significance

Elevations of ALP are of most diagnostic significance in the evaluation of hepatobiliary and bone disorders. In hepatobiliary disorders, elevations are more predominant in obstructive conditions than in hepatocellular disorders; in bone disorders, elevations are observed when there is involvement of osteoblasts.

In biliary tract obstruction, ALP levels range from 3 to 10 times the ULN. Increases are primarily a result of increased synthesis of the enzyme induced by cholestasis. In contrast, hepatocellular disorders, such as hepatitis and cirrhosis, show only slight increases, usually less than three times the ULN. Because of the degree of overlap of ALP elevations that occurs in the various liver disorders, a single elevated ALP level is difficult to interpret. It assumes more diagnostic significance when evaluated along with other tests of hepatic function (see Chapter 25).

Elevated ALP levels may be observed in various bone disorders. Perhaps the highest elevations of ALP activity occur in Paget's disease (osteitis deformans). Other bone disorders include osteomalacia, rickets, hyperparathyroidism, and osteogenic sarcoma. In addition, increased levels are observed in healing bone fractures and during periods of physiologic bone growth.

In normal pregnancy, increased ALP activity, averaging approximately 1½ times the ULN, can be detected between weeks 16 and 20 and is two to three times the ULN during the third trimester. ALP activity increases and persists until the onset of labor. Activity then returns to normal within 3 to 6 days.[24] Elevations also may be seen in complications of pregnancy such as hypertension, preeclampsia, and eclampsia, as well as in threatened abortion.

ALP levels are significantly decreased in the inherited condition of hypophosphatasia. Subnormal activity is a result of the absence of the bone isoenzyme and results in inadequate bone calcification.

ALP exists as a number of isoenzymes, which have been studied by a variety of techniques. The major isoenzymes, which are found in the serum and have been most extensively studied, are those derived from the liver, bone, intestine, and placenta.[25]

Electrophoresis is considered the most useful single technique for ALP isoenzyme analysis. However, because there may still be some degree of overlap between the fractions, electrophoresis in combination with another separation technique may provide the most reliable information. A direct immunochemical method for the measurement of bone-related ALP is now available; this has made ALP electrophoresis unnecessary in most cases.

The liver fraction migrates the fastest, followed by bone, placental, and intestinal fractions. Because of the similarity between liver and bone phosphatases, there often is not a clear separation between them. Quantitation with use of a densitometer is sometimes difficult because of the overlap between the two peaks. The liver isoenzyme can actually be divided into two fractions—the major liver band and a smaller fraction called *fast liver*, or α_1 liver, which migrates anodal to the major band and corresponds to the α_1 fraction of protein electrophoresis. When total ALP levels are increased, the major liver fraction is the most frequently elevated. Many hepatobiliary conditions cause elevations of this fraction, usually early in the course of the disease. The fast-liver fraction has been reported in metastatic carcinoma of the liver, as well as in other hepatobiliary diseases. Its presence is regarded as a valuable indicator of obstructive liver disease. However, it is occasionally present in the absence of any detectable disease state.

The bone isoenzyme increases due to osteoblastic activity and is normally elevated in children during periods of growth and in adults older than age 50. In these cases, an elevated ALP level may be difficult to interpret.[26]

The presence of intestinal ALP isoenzyme in serum depends on the blood group and secretor status of the individual. Individuals who have B or O blood group and are secretors are more likely to have this fraction. Apparently, intestinal ALP is bound by erythrocytes of group A. Furthermore, in these individuals, increases in intestinal ALP occur after consumption of a fatty meal. Intestinal ALP may increase in several disorders, such as diseases of the digestive tract and cirrhosis. Increased levels are also found in patients undergoing chronic hemodialysis.

Difference in heat stability is the basis of a second approach used to identify the isoenzyme source of an elevated ALP. Typically, ALP activity is measured before and after heating the serum at 56°C for 10 minutes. If the residual activity after heating is less than 20% of the total activity before heating, then the ALP elevation is assumed to be a result of bone phosphatase. If greater than 20% of the activity remains, the elevation is probably a result of liver phosphatase. These results are based on the finding that placental ALP is the most heat stable of the four major fractions, followed by intestinal, liver, and bone fractions in decreasing order of heat stability. Placental ALP will resist heat denaturation at 65°C for 30 minutes.

Heat inactivation is an imprecise method for differentiation because inactivation depends on many factors, such as correct temperature control, timing, and analytic methods sensitive enough to detect small amounts of residual ALP activity. In addition, there is some degree of overlap between heat inactivation of liver and bone fractions in both liver and bone diseases.

A third approach to identification of ALP isoenzymes is based on selective chemical inhibition. Phenylalanine is one of several inhibitors that have been used. Phenylalanine inhibits intestinal and placental ALP to a much greater extent than liver and bone ALP. With phenylalanine use, however, it is impossible to differentiate placental from intestinal ALP or liver from bone ALP.

In addition to the four major ALP isoenzyme fractions, certain abnormal fractions are associated with neoplasms. The most frequently seen are the Regan and Nagao isoenzymes. They have been referred to as *carcinoplacental ALPs* because of their similarities to the placental isoenzyme. The frequency of occurrence ranges from 3% to 15% in cancer patients. The Regan isoenzyme has been characterized as an example of an ectopic production of an enzyme by malignant tissue. It has been detected in various carcinomas, such as lung, breast, ovarian, and colon, with the highest incidences in ovarian and gynecologic cancers. Because of its low incidence in cancer patients, diagnosis of malignancy is rarely based on its presence. It is, however, useful in monitoring the effects of therapy because it will disappear on successful treatment.

The Regan isoenzyme migrates to the same position as the bone fraction and is the most heat stable of all ALP isoenzymes, resisting denaturation at 65°C for 30 minutes. Its activity is inhibited by phenylalanine.

The Nagao isoenzyme may be considered a variant of the Regan isoenzyme. Its electrophoretic, heat stability, and phenylalanine inhibition properties are identical to those of the Regan fraction. However, Nagao also can be inhibited by L-leucine. Its presence has been detected in metastatic carcinoma of pleural surfaces and in adenocarcinoma of the pancreas and bile duct.

Assay for Enzyme Activity

Because of the relative nonspecificity of ALP with regard to substrates, a variety of methodologies for its analysis have been proposed and are still in use today. The major differences between these relate to the concentration and types of substrate and buffer used and the pH of the reaction. A continuous-monitoring technique based on a method devised by Bowers and McComb allows calculation of ALP activity based on the molar absorptivity of *p*-nitrophenol. The reaction proceeds according to Equation 13-15:

p-Nitrophenyl-   *p*-Nitro-   Phosphate ion
phosphate   phenol

(Eq. 13-15)

p-Nitrophenylphosphate (colorless) is hydrolyzed to *p*-nitrophenol (yellow), and the increase in absorbance at 405 nm, which is directly proportional to ALP activity, is measured.

Source of Error

Hemolysis may cause slight elevations because ALP is approximately six times more concentrated in erythrocytes than in serum. ALP assays should be run as soon as possible after collection. Activity in serum increases approximately 3% to 10% on standing at 25°C or 4°C for several hours. Diet may induce elevations in ALP activity of blood group B and O individuals who are secretors. Values may be 25% higher following ingestion of a high-fat meal.

Reference Range
ALP (total) (37°C)

Males/Females	4–15 y	54–369 U/L (0.9–6.3 µkat/L)
Males	20–50 y	53–128 U/L (0.9–2.1 µkat/L)
	≥60 y	56–119 U/L (0.9–2.0 µkat/L)
Females	20–50 y	42–98 U/L (0.7–1.6 µkat/L)
	≥60 y	53–141 U/L (0.9–2.4 µkat/L)

Acid Phosphatase

Acid phosphatase (ACP) belongs to the same group of phosphatase enzymes as ALP and is a hydrolase that catalyzes the same type of reactions. The major difference between ACP and ALP is the pH of the reaction. ACP functions at an optimal pH of approximately 5.0. Equation 13-16 outlines the reaction sequence:

Phosphomonoester   Alcohol   Phosphate ion

(Eq. 13-16)

Tissue Source

ACP activity is found in the prostate, bone, liver, spleen, kidney, erythrocytes, and platelets. The prostate is the richest source, with many times the activity found in other tissue.

Diagnostic Significance

Historically, ACP measurement has been used as an aid in the detection of prostatic carcinoma, particularly metastatic carcinoma of the prostate. Total ACP determinations are relatively insensitive techniques, detecting elevated ACP levels resulting from prostatic carcinoma in the majority of cases only when the tumor has metastasized. Newer markers, such as prostate-specific antigen (PSA), are more useful screening and diagnostic tools (see Chapter 34).

One of the most specific substrates for prostatic ACP is thymolphthalein monophosphate. Chemical inhibition methods used to differentiate the prostatic portion most frequently use tartrate as the inhibitor. The prostatic fraction is inhibited by tartrate. Serum and substrate are incubated both with and without the addition of L-tartrate. ACP activity remaining after inhibition with L-tartrate is subtracted from the total ACP activity determined without inhibition, and the difference represents the prostatic portion:

Total ACP − ACP after tartrate inhibition
    = Prostatic ACP   (Eq. 13-17)

The reaction is not entirely specific for prostatic ACP; lysosomal ACP is also inhibited by tartrate. However, other tissue sources are largely uninhibited.

Neither of these methods of ACP determination is sensitive to prostatic carcinoma that has not metastasized. Values are usually normal in the majority of cases and, in fact, may be elevated only in about 50% of cases of prostatic carcinoma that has metastasized.

One technique with much improved sensitivity over conventional ACP assays is the immunologic approach using antibodies that are specific for the prostatic portion. Immunochemical techniques, however, are not of value as screening tests for prostatic carcinoma.

PSA is more likely than ACP to be elevated at each stage of prostatic carcinoma, even though a normal PSA level may be found in stage D tumors. PSA is particularly useful to monitor the success of treatment; however, PSA is controversial as a screening test for prostatic malignancy because PSA elevation may occur in conditions other than prostatic carcinoma, such as benign prostatic hypertrophy and prostatitis.[27-29]

Other prostatic conditions in which ACP elevations have been reported include hyperplasia of the prostate and prostatic surgery. There are conflicting reports of elevations following rectal examination and prostate massage. Certain studies have reported ACP elevations; others have indicated no detectable change. When elevations are found, levels usually return to normal within 24 hours.[30]

ACP assays have proved useful in forensic clinical chemistry, particularly in the investigation of rape. Vaginal washings are examined for seminal fluid–ACP activity, which can persist for up to 4 days.[31] Elevated activity is presumptive evidence of rape in such cases.

Serum ACP activity may frequently be elevated in bone disease. Activity has been shown to be associated with the osteoclasts.[32] Elevations have been noted in Paget's disease, in breast cancer with bone metastases, and in Gaucher's disease, in which there is an infiltration of bone marrow and other tissue by Gaucher cells rich in ACP activity. Because of ACP activity in platelets, elevations are observed when platelet damage occurs, as in the thrombocytopenia resulting from excessive platelet destruction from idiopathic thrombocytopenic purpura.

Assay for Enzyme Activity

Assay procedures for total ACP use the same techniques as in ALP assays but are performed at an acid pH:

$$p\text{-Nitrophenolphosphate} \xrightleftharpoons[\text{pH 5}]{\text{ACP}}$$
$$p\text{-Nitrophenol} + \text{phosphate ion} \qquad \text{(Eq. 13-18)}$$

The reaction products are colorless at the acid pH of the reaction, but the addition of alkali stops the reaction and transforms the products into chromogens, which can be measured spectrophotometrically.

Some substrate specificities and chemical inhibitors for prostatic ACP measurements have been discussed previously. Thymolphthalein monophosphate is the substrate of choice for quantitative endpoint reactions. For continuous-monitoring methods, α-naphthyl phosphate is preferred.

Immunochemical techniques for prostatic ACP use several approaches, including RIA, counterimmunoelectrophoresis, and immunoprecipitation. Also, an immunoenzymatic assay (Tandem E) includes incubation with an antibody to prostatic ACP followed by washing and incubation with p-nitrophenylphosphate. The p-nitrophenol formed, measured photometrically, is proportional to the prostatic ACP in the sample.

Source of Error

Serum should be separated from the red cells as soon as the blood has clotted to prevent leakage of erythrocyte and platelet ACP. Serum activity decreases within 1 to 2 hours if the sample is left at room temperature without the addition of a preservative. Decreased activity is a result of a loss of carbon dioxide from the serum, with a resultant increase in pH. If not assayed immediately, serum should be frozen or acidified to a pH lower than 6.5. With acidification, ACP is stable for 2 days at room temperature. Hemolysis should be avoided because of contamination from erythrocyte ACP.

RIA procedures for measurement of prostatic ACP require nonacidified serum samples. Activity is stable for 2 days at 4°C.

Reference Range

Prostatic ACP, 0 to 3.5 ng/mL
Tartrate-resistant ACP, adults: 1.5–4.5 U/L (37°C); children: 3.5–9.0 U/L (37°C)

γ-Glutamyltransferase

γ-Glutamyltransferase (GGT) is an enzyme involved in the transfer of the γ-glutamyl residue from γ-glutamyl peptides to amino acids, H_2O, and other small peptides. In most biologic systems, glutathione serves as the γ-glutamyl donor. Equation 13-19 outlines the reaction sequence:

$$\text{Glutathione} + \text{amino acid} \xrightleftharpoons{\text{AST}}$$
$$\text{Glutamyl peptide} + \text{L-cysteinylglycine}$$

$$\text{(Eq. 13-19)}$$

The specific physiologic function of GGT has not been clearly established, but it is suggested that GGT is involved in peptide and protein synthesis, regulation of tissue glutathione levels, and the transport of amino acids across cell membranes.[33]

Tissue Source

GGT activity is found primarily in tissues of the kidney, brain, prostate, pancreas, and liver. Clinical applications of assay, however, are confined mainly to evaluation of liver and biliary system disorders.

Diagnostic Significance

In the liver, GGT is located in the canaliculi of the hepatic cells and particularly in the epithelial cells lining the biliary ductules. Because of these locations, GGT is elevated in virtually all hepatobiliary disorders, making it one of the most sensitive of enzyme assays in these conditions (see Chapter 25). Higher elevations are generally observed in biliary tract obstruction.

Within the hepatic parenchyma, GGT exists to a large extent in the smooth endoplasmic reticulum and is, therefore, subject to hepatic microsomal induction. Therefore, GGT levels will be increased in patients receiving enzyme-inducing drugs such as warfarin, phenobarbital, and phenytoin. Enzyme elevations may reach levels four times the ULN.

Because of the effects of alcohol on GGT activity, elevated GGT levels may indicate alcoholism, particularly chronic alcoholism. Generally, enzyme elevations in persons who are alcoholics or heavy drinkers range from two to three times the ULN, although higher levels have been observed. GGT assays are useful in monitoring the effects of abstention from alcohol and are used as such by alcohol treatment centers. Levels usually return to normal within 2 to 3 weeks after cessation but can rise again if alcohol consumption is resumed. Because of the susceptibility to enzyme induction, any interpretation of GGT levels must be done with consideration of the consequent effects of drugs and alcohol.

GGT levels are also elevated in other conditions, such as acute pancreatitis, diabetes mellitus, and MI. The source of elevation in pancreatitis and diabetes is probably the pancreas, but the source of GGT in MI is unknown. GGT assays are of limited value in the diagnosis of these conditions and are not routinely requested.

GGT activity is useful in differentiating the source of an elevated ALP level because GGT levels are normal in skeletal disorders and during pregnancy. It is particularly useful in evaluating hepatobiliary involvement in adolescents because ALP activity will invariably be elevated as a result of bone growth.

Assay for Enzyme Activity

The most widely accepted substrate for use in GGT analysis is γ-glutamyl-p-nitroanilide. The γ-glutamyl residue is transferred to glycylglycine, releasing p-nitroaniline, a chromogenic product with a strong absorbance at 405 to 420 nm. The reaction, which can be used as a continuous-monitoring or fixed-point method, is outlined in Equation 13-20:

$$HOOC - CHNH_2 - CH_2 - CH_2 - CO$$

HN — ⟨⟩ — NO$_2$

γ-Glutamyl-p-nitroanilide

$$+ H_2N - CH_2 - CONH - CH_2 - COOH$$

Glycylglycine

$$HOOC - CHNH_2 - CH_2 - CH_2 - CO$$

HN — CH$_2$ — CONH — CH$_2$ — COOH

γ-Glutamyl-glycylglycine

+

$$\xrightarrow[\text{pH 8.2}]{\text{GGT}}$$

H$_2$N — ⟨⟩ — NO$_2$

p-Nitroaniline

(Eq. 13-20)

Source of Error

GGT activity is stable, with no loss of activity for 1 week at 4°C. Hemolysis does not interfere with GGT levels because the enzyme is lacking in erythrocytes.

Reference Range

GGT: male, 6 to 55 U/L (37°C) (0.1 to 0.9 μkat/L); female, 5 to 38 U/L (37°C) (0.1 to 0.6 μkat/L)

Values are lower in females, presumably because of suppression of enzyme activity resulting from estrogenic or progestational hormones.

Amylase

Amylase (AMY) is an enzyme belonging to the class of hydrolases that catalyze the breakdown of starch and glycogen. Starch consists of both amylose and amylopectin. Amylose is a long, unbranched chain of glucose molecules, linked by α, 1-4 glycosidic bonds; amylopectin is a branched-chain polysaccharide with α, 1-6 linkages at the branch points. The structure of glycogen is similar to that of amylopectin but is more highly branched. α-AMY attacks only the α, 1-4 glycosidic bonds to produce degradation products consisting of glucose; maltose; and intermediate chains, called *dextrins*, which contain α, 1-6 branching linkages. Cellulose and other structural polysaccharides consisting of linkages are not attacked by α-AMY. AMY is therefore an important enzyme in the physiologic digestion of starches. The reaction proceeds according to Equation 13-21:

$$\xrightarrow{\text{AMS}} \text{glucose, maltose, dextrins}$$

(Eq. 13-21)

AMY requires calcium and chloride ions for its activation.

Tissue Source

The acinar cells of the pancreas and the salivary glands are the major tissue sources of serum AMY. Lesser concentrations are found in skeletal muscle and the small intestine and fallopian tubes. AMY is the smallest enzyme, with a molecular weight of 50,000 to 55,000 Da. Because of its small size, it is readily filtered by the renal glomerulus and also appears in the urine.

Digestion of starches begins in the mouth with the hydrolytic action of salivary AMY. Salivary AMY activity, however, is of short duration because, on swallowing, it is inactivated by the acidity of the gastric contents. Pancreatic AMY then performs the major digestive action of starches once the polysaccharides reach the intestine.

Diagnostic Significance

The diagnostic significance of serum and urine AMY measurements is in the diagnosis of acute pancreatitis.[34] Disorders of tissue other than the pancreas can also produce elevations in AMY levels. Therefore, an elevated AMY level is a nonspecific finding. However, the degree of elevation of AMY is helpful, to some extent, in the differential diagnosis of acute pancreatitis. In addition, other laboratory tests (e.g., measurements of urinary AMY levels, AMY clearance studies, AMY isoenzyme studies, and measurements of serum lipase [LPS] levels), when used in conjunction with serum AMY measurement, increase the specificity of AMY measurements in the diagnosis of acute pancreatitis.

In acute pancreatitis, serum AMY levels begin to rise 5 to 8 hours after the onset of an attack, peak at 24 h, and return to normal levels within 3 to 5 days. Values generally range from 250 to 1,000 Somogyi units per dL (2.55× ULN). Values can reach much higher levels.

Other disorders causing an elevated serum AMY level include salivary gland lesions, such as mumps and parotitis, and other intra-abdominal diseases, such as perforated peptic ulcer, intestinal obstruction, cholecystitis, ruptured ectopic pregnancy, mesenteric infarction, and acute appendicitis. In addition, elevations have been reported in renal insufficiency and diabetic ketoacidosis. Serum AMY levels in intra-abdominal conditions other than acute pancreatitis are usually less than 500 Somogyi units per dL.

An apparently asymptomatic condition of hyperamylasemia has been noted in approximately 1% to 2% of the population. Hyperamylasemia can occur in neoplastic diseases with elevated results as high as 50 times the ULN. *Macroamylasemia* is a condition that results when the AMY molecule combines with immunoglobulins to form a complex that is too large to be filtered across the glomerulus. Serum AMY levels increase because of the reduction in normal renal clearance of the enzyme, and consequently, the urinary excretion of AMY is abnormally low. The diagnostic significance of macroamylasemia lies in the need to differentiate it from other causes of hyperamylasemia.

Much interest has been focused recently on the possible diagnostic use of AMY isoenzyme measurements.[34,35] Serum AMY is a mixture of a number of isoenzymes that can be separated on the basis of differences in physical properties, most notably electrophoresis, although chromatography and isoelectric focusing also have been applied. In normal human serum, two major bands and as many as four minor bands may be seen. The bands are designated as P-type and S-type isoamylase. P isoamylase is derived from pancreatic tissue; S isoamylase is derived from salivary gland tissue, as well as the fallopian tube and lung. The isoenzymes of salivary origin (S1, S2, and S3) migrate most quickly, whereas those of pancreatic origin (P1, P2, and P3) are slower. In normal human serum, the isoamylases migrate in regions corresponding to the β- to α-globulin regions of protein electrophoresis. The most commonly observed fractions are P2, S1, and S2.

In acute pancreatitis, there is typically an increase in P-type activity, with P3 being the most predominant isoenzyme. However, P3 also has been detected in cases of renal failure and, therefore, is not entirely specific for acute pancreatitis. S-type isoamylase represents approximately two-thirds of AMY activity of normal serum, whereas P-type predominates in normal urine.

Assay for Enzyme Activity

AMY can be assayed by a variety of different methods, which are summarized in Table 13-6. The four main approaches are categorized as amyloclast, saccharogenic, chromogenic, and continuous monitoring. Continuous monitoring has replaced previous methods for AMY activity.

In the amyloclastic method, AMY is allowed to act on a starch substrate to which iodine has been attached. As AMY hydrolyzes the starch molecule into smaller units, the iodine is released and a decrease occurs in the initial dark-blue color intensity of the starch–iodine complex. The decrease in color is proportional to the AMY concentration.

The saccharogenic method uses a starch substrate that is hydrolyzed by the action of AMY to its constituent carbohydrate molecules that have reducing properties. The amount of reducing sugars is then measured where the concentration is proportional to AMY activity. The saccharogenic method, the classic reference method for determining AMY activity, is reported in Somogyi units. Somogyi units are an expression of the number of milligrams of glucose released in 30 minutes at 37°C under specific assay conditions.

Chromogenic methods use a starch substrate to which a chromogenic dye has been attached, forming an insoluble dye–substrate complex. As AMY hydrolyzes the starch substrate, smaller dye–substrate fragments are produced, and these are water soluble. The increase in

TABLE 13-6	AMYLASE METHODOLOGIES
Amyloclastic	Measures the disappearance of starch substrate
Saccharogenic	Measures the appearance of the product
Chromogenic	Measures the increasing color from production of product coupled with a chromogenic dye
Continuous monitoring	Coupling of several enzyme systems to monitor amylase activity

color intensity of the soluble dye–substrate solution is proportional to AMY activity.

Recently, coupled-enzyme systems have been used to determine AMY activity by a continuous-monitoring technique in which the change in absorbance of NAD^+ at 340 nm is measured. Equation 13-22 is an example of a continuous-monitoring method. For AMY activity, the optimal pH is 6.9:

$$\text{Maltopentose} \xrightleftharpoons{AMS} \text{Maltrotriose} + \text{maltose}$$

$$\text{Maltrotriose} + \text{maltose} \xrightleftharpoons{\alpha\text{-glucosidase}} \text{5-Glucose}$$

$$\text{5-Glucose} + \text{5 ATP} \xrightarrow{\text{Hexokinase}}$$
$$\text{5-Glucose-6-phosphate} + \text{5 ADP}$$

$$\text{5-Glucose-6-phosphate} + \text{5 NAD} + \xrightleftharpoons{\text{G-6-PD}}$$
$$\text{5,6-Phosphogluconolactone} + \text{5 NADH}$$

(Eq. 13-22)

Because salivary AMY is preferentially inhibited by wheat germ lectin, salivary and pancreatic AMY can be estimated by measuring total AMY in the presence and absence of lectin. Specific immunoassays are also available for measuring isoenzymes of AMY.

Source of Error
AMY in serum and urine is stable. Little loss of activity occurs at room temperature for 1 week or at 4°C for 2 months. Because plasma triglycerides suppress or inhibit serum AMY activity, AMY values may be normal in acute pancreatitis with hyperlipemia.

The administration of morphine and other opiates for pain relief before blood sampling will lead to falsely elevated serum AMY levels. The drugs presumably cause constriction of the sphincter of Oddi and of the pancreatic ducts, with consequent elevation of inarticulate pressure causing regurgitation of AMY into the serum.

Reference Range
AMY: serum, 28 to 100 U/L (37°C) (0.5 to 1.7 μkat/L); urine, 1 to 15 U/h

Because of the various AMY procedures currently in use, activity is expressed according to each procedure. There is no uniform expression of AMY activity, although Somogyi units are frequently used. The approximate conversion factor between Somogyi units and IUs is 1.85.

Lipase

LPS is an enzyme that hydrolyzes the ester linkages of fats to produce alcohols and fatty acids. Specifically, LPS catalyzes the partial hydrolysis of dietary triglycerides in the intestine to the 2-monoglyceride intermediate, with the production of long-chain fatty acids. The reaction proceeds according to Equation 13-23:

$$\begin{array}{c}
CH_2-O-\overset{O}{\overset{\|}{C}}-R_1 \\
CH_2-O-\overset{O}{\overset{\|}{C}}-R_2 + 2H_2O \xrightleftharpoons{LPS} \\
CH_2-O-\overset{O}{\overset{\|}{C}}-R_3
\end{array}
\begin{array}{c}
CH_2OH \\
CH-O-\overset{O}{\overset{\|}{C}}-R_2 + 2\text{ fatty acids} \\
CH_2OH
\end{array}$$

Triacylgycerol   2-Monoglyceride

(Eq. 13-23)

The enzymatic activity of pancreatic LPS is specific for the fatty acid residues at positions 1 and 3 of the triglyceride molecule, but substrate must be an emulsion for activity to occur. The reaction rate is accelerated by the presence of colipase and a bile salt.

Tissue Source
LPS concentration is found primarily in the pancreas, although it is also present in the stomach and small intestine.

Diagnostic Significance
Clinical assays of serum LPS measurements are confined almost exclusively to the diagnosis of acute pancreatitis. Serum LPS activity increases 4 to 8 hours after an attack of acute pancreatitis; concentrations peak at 24 hours and decrease within 8 to 14 days. LPS is similar in this respect to AMY measurements but is considered more specific for pancreatic disorders than AMY measurement. Both AMY and LPS levels rise quickly, but LPS elevations persist for approximately 8 days in acute pancreatitis, whereas AMY elevations persist for only 2 to 3 days. The extent of elevations does not correlate with severity of disease. Elevated LPS levels also may be found in other intra-abdominal conditions but with less frequency than elevations of serum AMY. Elevations have been reported in cases of penetrating duodenal ulcers and perforated peptic ulcers, intestinal obstruction, and acute cholecystitis. In contrast to AMY levels, LPS levels are normal in conditions of salivary gland involvement. Therefore, LPS levels are useful in differentiating serum AMY elevation as a result of pancreatic versus salivary involvement. Of the three LPS isoenzymes, L2 is thought to be the most clinically specific and sensitive.

Assay for Enzyme Activity
Procedures used to measure LPS activity include estimation of liberated fatty acids (titrimetric) and turbidimetric methods. The reaction is outlined in Equation 13-24:

$$\text{Triglyceride} + 2\,H_2O \xrightleftharpoons[(pH = 8.6-9.0)]{LPS}$$
$$\text{2-Monoglyceride} + 2\text{ fatty acids}$$

(Eq. 13-24)

Early methods for LPS were historically poor. The classic Cherry-Crandall method used an olive oil substrate and measured the liberated fatty acids by titration after a 24-hour incubation. Modifications of the Cherry-Crandall method have been complicated by the lack of stable and uniform substrates. However, triolein is one substrate now used as a more pure form of triglyceride.

Turbidimetric methods are simpler and more rapid than titrimetric assays. Fats in solution create a cloudy emulsion. As the fats are hydrolyzed by LPS, the particles disperse, and the rate of clearing can be measured as an estimation of LPS activity. Colorimetric methods are also available and are based on coupled reactions with enzymes such as peroxidase or glycerol kinase.

Source of Error

LPS is stable in serum, with negligible loss in activity at room temperature for 1 week or for 3 weeks at 4°C. Hemolysis should be avoided because hemoglobin inhibits the activity of serum LPS, causing falsely low values.

Reference Range

LPS, <38 U/L (37°C) (<0.6 μkat/L)

Glucose-6-Phosphate Dehydrogenase

G-6-PD is an oxidoreductase that catalyzes the oxidation of glucose-6-phosphate to 6-phosphogluconate or the corresponding lactone. The reaction is important as the first step in the pentose phosphate shunt of glucose metabolism with the ultimate production of NADPH. The reaction is outlined in Equation 13-25:

Glucose-6-phosphate

6-Phosphogluconate

(Eq. 13-25)

Tissue Source

Sources of G-6-PD include the adrenal cortex, spleen, thymus, lymph nodes, lactating mammary gland, and erythrocytes. Little activity is found in normal serum.

Diagnostic Significance

Most of the research interest in G-6-PD focuses on its role in the erythrocyte. Here, it functions to maintain NADPH in reduced form. An adequate concentration of NADPH is required to regenerate sulfhydryl-containing proteins, such as glutathione, from the oxidized to the reduced state. Glutathione in the reduced form, in turn, protects hemoglobin from oxidation by agents that may be present in the cell. A deficiency of G-6-PD results in an inadequate supply of NADPH and, ultimately, in the inability to maintain reduced glutathione levels. When erythrocytes are exposed to oxidizing agents, hemolysis occurs because of oxidation of hemoglobin and damage of the cell membrane.

G-6-PD deficiency is an inherited sex-linked trait. The disorder can result in several different clinical manifestations, one of which is drug-induced hemolytic anemia. When exposed to an oxidant drug such as primaquine, an antimalarial drug, affected individuals experience a hemolytic episode. The severity of the hemolysis is related to the drug concentration. G-6-PD deficiency is most common in African Americans but has been reported in virtually every ethnic group.

Increased levels of G-6-PD in the serum have been reported in MI and megaloblastic anemias. No elevations are seen in hepatic disorders. G-6-PD levels, however, are not routinely performed as diagnostic aids in these conditions.

CASE STUDY 13-3

A 36-year-old woman presents to the emergency department with intense upper abdominal pain radiating to her back, weakness, loss of appetite, and severe indigestion after eating. She had not traveled in recent months. She has not been well for several days.

Questions

1. What laboratory tests should be ordered to help diagnose this patient?

2. What enzyme tests will be useful in diagnosing this patient?

3. What two diagnoses are most likely for this patient?

Assay for Enzyme Activity

The assay procedure for G-6-PD activity is outlined in Equation 13-26:

$$\text{Glucose-6-phosphate} + \text{NADPH}^+ \xrightleftharpoons{\text{G-6-PD}}$$
$$\text{6-Phosphogluconate} + \text{NADPH} + \text{H}^+$$

(Eq. 13-26)

A red cell hemolysate is used to assay for deficiency of the enzyme; serum is used for evaluation of enzyme elevations.

Reference Range

G-6-PD, 7.9 to 16.3 U/g Hgb (0.1 to 0.3 μkat/g Hgb)

Macroenzymes

Macroenzymes are high-molecular-mass forms of the serum enzymes (ACP, ALP, ALT, AMY, AST, CK, GGT, LD, and LPS) that can be bound to either an immunoglobulin (macroenzyme type 1) or a nonimmunoglobulin substance (macroenzyme type 2). Macroenzymes are usually found in patients who have an unexplained persistent increase of enzyme concentrations in serum.[36] The presence of macroenzymes can also increase with increasing age.[37] Enzymes can bind to immunoglobulins in a nonspecific manner, but there is also evidence that the enzyme–immunoglobulin complex can be formed by specific interactions between circulating autoantibodies and serum enzymes.[36] The reason for the formation of antienzyme antibodies is not known, but there are two theories to explain their formation. According to the "antigen-driven theory," the self-antigen becomes immunogenic by being altered or released from a sequestered site and reacts with an antibody that is initially formed against a foreign antigen.[38] The dysregulation of immune tolerance theory explains the formation of enzymes with autoantibodies in patients with autoimmune disorders.[38] To date, there has not been a strong correlation between the presence of antienzyme antibodies and the pathogenesis of disease.[36] However, the presence of macroenzymes should be documented in the patient's medical records because macroenzymes can persist for long periods.[36]

Macroenzymes accumulate in plasma because their high molecular masses prevent them from being filtered out of the plasma by the kidneys. The detection of macroenzymes is clinically significant because the presence of macroenzymes can cause difficulty in the interpretation of diagnostic enzyme results. The formation of high-molecular-weight enzyme complexes can cause false elevations in plasma enzymes or they can falsely decrease the activity of the enzyme by blocking the activity of the bound enzyme.[36]

The principal method to identify enzymes that are bound to immunoglobulins and nonimmunoglobulins is protein electrophoresis. The binding of enzymes to high-molecular-weight complexes can alter the nor-

mal electrophoretic pattern of enzymes (see Fig. 13-5 for an example). Antienzyme antibodies can cause the formation of new enzyme bands on a gel, can alter the intensity of enzyme bands, and can cause band broadening on the gel.[36] Other test methods used to determine the presence of macroenzymes include gel filtration, immunoprecipitation, immunoelectrophoresis, counter-immunoelectrophoresis, and immunofixation. Last, the immunoinhibition test can also be used to determine the presence of macro-CK.

Drug-Metabolizing Enzymes

Drug-metabolizing enzymes function primarily to transform xenobiotics into inactive, water-soluble compounds for excretion through the kidneys. Metabolic enzymes can also transform inactive prodrugs into active drugs, convert xenobiotics into toxic compounds, or prolong the elimination half-life. Drug-metabolizing enzymes catalyze addition or removal of functional groups through hydroxylation, oxidation, dealkylation, dehydrogenation, reduction, deamination, and desulfuration reactions. These transformation reactions are referred to as phase I reactions and are often mediated by cytochrome P450 (CYP 450) enzymes. Xenobiotics can also become transformed into more polar compounds through enzyme-mediated conjugation reactions, also known as phase II reactions, in which xenobiotics are conjugated with glucuronide (UDP-glucuronosyltransferase 1A1 [UGT1A1]), acetate (N-acetyltransferase [NAT]), glutathione (glutathione-S-transferase [GST]), sulfate (sulfotransferase), and methionine groups.[39]

CYP 450 enzymes are a superfamily of isoenzymes that are involved in the metabolism of more than 50% of all drugs. These enzymes contain heme molecules, and they are given the name CYP 450 because they absorb the maximum amount of light at 450 nm. More than 500 CYP 450 enzymes have been identified, and they are classified into families according to their homology to other enzymes.[42] There are at least four CYP 450 (CYP1, 2, 3, and 4) families that are expressed primarily in the liver, but some isoforms are also expressed in extrahepatic tissues such as the lung, kidney, gastrointestinal tract, skin, and placenta.[39] The specific isozyme is classified by not only its family number but also a subfamily letter, a number for an individual isozyme within the subfamily, and, if applicable, an asterisk followed by a number for each genetic (allelic) variant. Genetic variants have been identified that lead to complete enzyme deficiency (e.g., a frame shift, splice variant, stop codon, or a complete gene deletion), reduced enzyme function or expression, or enhanced enzyme function or expression. Recognition of genetic variants can explain interindividual differences in drug response and pharmacokinetics.[40-43] For example, four phenotypes are recognized for CYP2D6: ultra-metabolizers, extensive metabolizers, intermediate metabolizers, and poor metabolizers. Patients who are poor metabolizers for the CYP2D6 enzyme are at risk for therapeutic failure when inactive prodrugs such as tamoxifen require CYP2D6 for drug activation. Tricyclic antidepressants such as nortriptyline require CYP2D6 for inactivation. Thus, CYP2D6 poor metabolizers may require lower dose requirements than will patients with extensive ("normal") metabolism and may be at high risk for adverse drug reactions.[39,41]

In addition to xenobiotic metabolism, CYP 450 enzymes are also involved in the biosynthesis of endogenous compounds. The CYP5 family consists of thromboxane synthases that catalyze the reaction that leads to platelet aggregation. CYP7 and CYP27 families catalyze the hydroxylation of cholesterol for the biosynthesis of bile acids. The CYP24 family catalyzes the hydroxylation and inactivation of vitamin D_3. CYP 450 enzymes are also found in steroid-producing tissues and function to synthesize steroid hormones from cholesterol (CYP11, 17, 19, and 21).[42]

Genetic variants that affect drug-metabolizing enzyme function and expression are recognized for other enzymes such as NAT, UGT1A1, GST, and thiopurine methyltransferase (TPMT). These variants are associated with distinct extensive (fast), intermediate, or poor (slow) metabolizer phenotypes, which could lead to adverse drug reactions or therapeutic failure. For example, two phenotypes—fast or slow acetylators—are recognized for N-acetyltransferase 2 (NAT2). NAT2 is the primary enzyme involved in the acetylation of isoniazid, a drug used to treat tuberculosis. Acetylation is the primary mechanism for the elimination of isoniazid, and therefore, patients with low NAT2 activity will not be able to inactivate isoniazid, putting those patients at increased risk for adverse drug reactions.[39] UGT1A1 has polymorphisms that can lead to a nonfunctioning enzyme. UGT1A1 is responsible for the metabolism of bilirubin;

patients with nonfunctioning UGT1A1 are at risk for hyperbilirubinemia.[43] Last, TPMT is an enzyme that can be found in bone marrow and erythrocytes and functions to inactivate chemotherapeutic thiopurine drugs like azathioprine and 6-mercaptopurine. The TPMT enzyme has genetic polymorphisms, which causes variable responses (normal, intermediate, and low activity) to thiopurine metabolism. Patients with low TPMT activity are at risk for developing severe bone marrow toxicity when the standard dose therapy for thiopurine drugs is administered; thus, genetic testing is essential for identifying patients with metabolizing enzyme polymorphisms.[43]

Pharmacogenetic testing is often used prior to drug therapy to assist clinicians in identifying patients with genetic polymorphisms and to guide drug and dose selection. Pharmacogenetic testing can be performed through phenotype tests that measure metabolic enzyme activity, through administration of a probe drug and subsequent evaluation of metabolic ratios, or through genotype testing that identifies clinically significant genetic variants.

The activity of drug-metabolizing enzymes can also be altered by food, nutritional supplements, or other drugs. Compounds that stimulate an increase in the synthesis of CYP 450 enzymes are called *inducers*. Inducers will increase the metabolism of drugs and reduce the bioavailability of the parent compound. Compounds that reduce the expression or activity of a drug-metabolizing enzyme are referred to as *inhibitors*. For example, inhibitors can compete with substrates for the active site of CYP 450 and thereby decrease the metabolism of drugs and increase the bioavailability of the parent compound, or block activity or expression through noncompetitive means.[39] Table 13-7 lists the common families of CYP 450 enzymes along with some of their substrates and drugs that can induce or inhibit enzyme activity.

TABLE 13-7	COMMON SUBSTRATES FOR DRUG-METABOLIZING ENZYMES		
ENZYME	**SUBSTRATES**	**INDUCERS**	**INHIBITORS**
CYP1A1	(R)-Warfarin	Omeprazole	
		TCDD	
		Benzo[a]pyrene, 3MC	
CYP1A2	Acetaminophen	Insulin	Ciprofloxacin
	Caffeine	Tobacco	Cimetidine
	(R)-Warfarin	Polycyclic aromatic hydrocarbons	Amiodarone
	Estradiol		Fluoroquinolones
	Theophylline		
CYP2A6	Cyclophosphamide	Dexamethasone	Pilocarpine
	Halothane		Coumarin
	Zidovudine		
	Coumarin		

(Continued)

TABLE 13-7	COMMON SUBSTRATES FOR DRUG-METABOLIZING ENZYMES (CONTINUED)		
ENZYME	**SUBSTRATES**	**INDUCERS**	**INHIBITORS**
CYP2B6	Cyclophosphamide	Phenobarbital	Ticlopidine
	Diazepam	Rifampin	
	Bupropion		
CYP2C9	(S)-Warfarin	Rifampin	Fluconazole
	Ibuprofen	Secobarbital	Amiodarone
	Tolbutamide		Isoniazid
	Diclofenac		Probenecid
	Losartan		Sertraline
	Phenytoin		Sulfamethoxazole
CYP2C19	Diazepam	Barbiturate	Omeprazole
	Omeprazole	Phenytoin	Chloramphenicol
	Chloripramine		Cimetidine
	Indomethacin		Ketoconazole
			Indomethacin
CYP2D6	Carvedilol	Dexamethasone	Bupropion
	Amitriptyline	Rifampin	Fluoxetine
	Haloperidol		Quinidine
	Amphetamine		Amiodarone
	Chlorpromazine		Sertraline
	Dextromethorphan		Celecoxib
	Codeine		Chlorpromazine
CYP2E1	Acetaminophen	Ethanol	Disulfiram
	Chlorzoxazone	Isoniazid	Diethyldithiocarbamate
	Halothane		
	Ethanol		
CYP3A4	Erythromycin	HIV antivirals	HIV antivirals
	Quinidine	Barbiturates	Ketoconazole
	Diazepam	Carbamazepine	Erythromycin
	Cortisol	Phenobarbital	Grapefruit juice
	Cyclosporine	Phenytoin	Cimetidine
	Indinavir	Rifampin	Chloramphenicol
	Chlorpheniramine	St. John's wort	
	Nifedipine	Troglitazone	
	Lovastatin		
	Testosterone		
	Cocaine		
	Fentanyl		
	Tamoxifen		
TPMT	Azathioprine		Naproxen
	6-Mercaptopurine		Furosemide

Source: Rendic S, Di Carlo FJ. Human cytochrome P450 enzymes: a status report summarizing their reactions, substrates, inducers, and inhibitors. *Drug Metab Rev.* 1997;29:413-580.

For additional student resources please visit thePoint at http://thepoint.lww.com. **thePoint** ✳

QUESTIONS

1. When a reaction is performed in zero-order kinetics
   a. The rate of the reaction is independent of the substrate concentration
   b. The substrate concentration is very low
   c. The rate of reaction is directly proportional to the substrate concentration
   d. The enzyme level is always high

2. Activation energy is
   a. Decreased by enzymes
   b. The energy needed for an enzyme reaction to stop
   c. Increased by enzymes
   d. Very high in catalyzed reactions

3. Enzyme reaction rates are increased by increasing temperatures until they reach the point of denaturation at
   a. 40–60°C
   b. 25–35°C
   c. 100°C
   d. 37°C

4. An example of using enzymes as reagents in the clinical laboratory is
   a. The hexokinase glucose method
   b. The diacetyl monoxime blood urea nitrogen (BUN) method
   c. The alkaline picrate creatinine method
   d. The biuret total protein method

5. Activity of enzymes in serum may be determined rather than concentration because
   a. The amount of enzyme is too low to measure
   b. The temperature is too high
   c. There is not enough substrate
   d. The amount of enzyme is too high to measure

6. The isoenzymes LD-4 and LD-5 are elevated in
   a. Liver disease
   b. Pulmonary embolism
   c. Renal disease
   d. Myocardial infarction

7. Which CK isoenzyme is elevated in muscle diseases?
   a. CK-MM
   b. CK-BB
   c. CK-MB
   d. CK-NN

8. Elevation of serum amylase and lipase is commonly seen in
   a. Acute pancreatitis
   b. Acute appendicitis
   c. Gallbladder disease
   d. Acid reflux disease

9. The saccharogenic method for amylase determinations measures
   a. The amount of product produced
   b. The amount of substrate consumed
   c. The amount of iodine present
   d. The amount of starch present

10. Elevation of tissue enzymes in serum may be used to detect
    a. Tissue necrosis or damage
    b. Inflammation
    c. Infectious diseases
    d. Diabetes mellitus

11. Which of the following enzyme patterns is MOST diagnostic of Duchenne-type muscular dystrophy?
    a. Total CK level that is 5 to 10 times the ULN
    b. Total CK level that is 25 times the ULN
    c. Total CK level that is 50 to 100 times the ULN
    d. Total CK level that is 1,000 times the ULN

12. Which of the following preanalytical errors most commonly causes false increases in serum enzyme measurements?
    a. The patient was not fasting prior to blood draw.
    b. The blood sample was not maintained on ice upon collection and during transport to the laboratory.
    c. The serum was not separated from red blood cells within 1 hour.
    d. The patient smoked three cigarettes just prior to blood collection.
    e. The blood sample was not protected from light upon collection and during transport to the laboratory.

REFERENCES

1. Enzyme Nomenclature 1978. *Recommendations of the Nomenclature Committee of the International Union of Biochemistry on the Nomenclature and Classification of Enzymes.* New York, NY: Academic Press; 1979.
2. Baron DN, Moss DW, Walker PG, et al. Abbreviations for names of enzymes of diagnostic importance. *J Clin Pathol.* 1971;24:656.
3. Baron DN, Moss DW, Walker PG, et al. Revised list of abbreviations for names of enzymes of diagnostic importance. *J Clin Pathol.* 1975;28:592.
4. Rej R. Accurate enzyme measurements. *Arch Pathol Lab Med.* 1998;117:352.
5. Spitzer M, Pinto A. Early diagnosis of ectopic pregnancy: can we do it accurately using a chemical profile? *J Women's Health Gender Based Med.* 2000;9:537.
6. Nakafusa J, Misago N, Miura Y, Kayaba M, Tanaka T, Narisawa Y. The importance of serum creatine phosphokinase levels in the early diagnosis, and as a prognostic factor, of *Vibrio vulnificus* infection. *Br J Dermatol.* 2001;145:280-284.
7. Galen RS. The enzyme diagnosis of myocardial infarction. *Hum Pathol.* 1975;6:141.
8. Wilkinson JH. *The Principles and Practice of Diagnostic Enzymology.* Chicago, IL: Year Book Medical Publishers; 1976:395.
9. Silverman LM, Dermer GB, Zweig MH, et al. Creatine kinase BB: a new tumor-associated marker. *Clin Chem.* 1979;25:1432.
10. Lang H, ed. *Creatine Kinase Isoenzymes: Pathophysiology and Clinical Application.* Berlin, Germany: Springer-Verlag; 1981.
11. Irvin RG, Cobb FR, Roe CR. Acute myocardial infarction and MB creatine phosphokinase: relationship between onset of symptoms of infarction and appearance and disappearance of enzyme. *Arch Intern Med.* 1980;140:329.
12. Bark CJ. Mitochondrial creatine kinase—a poor prognostic sign. *JAMA.* 1980;243:2058.
13. Batsakis J, Savory J, eds. Creatine kinase. *Crit Rev Clin Lab Sci.* 1982;16:291.
14. Lang H, Wurzburg U. Creatine kinase, an enzyme of many forms. *Clin Chem.* 1982;28:1439.
15. Lott JA. Electrophoretic CK and LDH isoenzyme assays in myocardial infarction. *Lab Manage.* February 1983;2:23.
16. Pesce MA. The CK isoenzymes: findings and their meaning. *Lab Manage.* October 1982;20:25-37.
17. Roche Diagnostics. *Isomune-CK Package Insert.* Nutley, NJ: Hoffman-La Roche; 1979.
18. Faulkner WR, Meites S, eds. *Selected Methods for the Small Clinical Chemistry Laboratory: Selected Methods of Clinical Chemistry.* Vol. 9. Washington, DC: American Association for Clinical Chemistry; 1982:475.
19. Lott JA, Stang JM. Serum enzymes and isoenzymes in the diagnosis and differential diagnosis of myocardial ischemia and necrosis. *Clin Chem.* 1980;26:1241.
20. Leung FY, Henderson AR. Influence of hemolysis on the serum lactate dehydrogenase-1/lactate dehydrogenase-2 ratio as determined by an accurate thin-layer agarose electrophoresis procedure. *Clin Chem.* 1981;27:1708.
21. Bhagavan NV, Darm JR, Scottolini AG. A sixth lactate dehydrogenase isoenzyme (LDH-6) and its significance. *Arch Pathol Lab Med.* 1982;106:521.
22. Cabello B, Lubin J, Rywlin AM, et al. Significance of a sixth lactate dehydrogenase isoenzyme (LDH$_6$). *Am J Clin Pathol.* 1980;73:253.
23. Goldberg DM, Werner M, eds. *LDH-6, A Sign of Impending Death from Heart Failure, Selected Topics in Clinical Enzymology.* New York, NY: Walter de Gruyter; 1983:347.
24. Posen S, Doherty E. The measurement of serum alkaline phosphatase in clinical medicine. *Adv Clin Chem.* 1981;22:165.
25. Warren BM. *The Isoenzymes of Alkaline Phosphatase.* Beaumont, TX: Helena Laboratories; 1981.
26. Fleisher GA, Eickelberg ES, Elveback LR. Alkaline phosphatase activity in the plasma of children and adolescents. *Clin Chem.* 1977;23:469.
27. Gittes RF. Carcinoma of the prostate. *N Engl J Med.* 1991;324:236.
28. Gittes RF. Prostate specific antigen. *N Engl J Med.* 1987;318:954.
29. Oesterling JE. Prostate specific antigen: a critical assessment of the most useful tumor marker for adenocarcinoma of the prostate. *J Urol.* 1991;145:907.
30. Griffiths JC. The laboratory diagnosis of prostatic adenocarcinoma. *Crit Rev Clin Lab Sci.* 1983;19:187.
31. Lantz RK, Berg MJ. From clinic to court: acid phosphatase testing. *Diagn Med.* 1981;March/April:55.
32. Yam LT. Clinical significance of the human acid phosphatases. A review. *Am J Med.* 1974;56:604.
33. Rosalki SB. Gamma-glutamyl transpeptidase. *Adv Clin Chem.* 1975;17:53.
34. Salt WB II, Schenker S. Amylase: its clinical significance. A review of the literature. *Medicine.* 1976;4:269.
35. Murthy UK, DeGregorio F, Oates RP, Blair DC. Hyperamylasemia in patients with acquired immunodeficiency syndrome. *Am J Gastroenterol.* 1992;87:332.
36. Remaley AT, Wilding P. Macroenzymes: biochemical characterization, clinical significance, and laboratory detection. *Clin Chem.* 1989;35:2261-2270.
37. Turecky L. Macroenzymes and their clinical significance. *Bratisl Lek Listy.* 2004;105:260-263.
38. Theofilopoulous AN. Autoimmunity. In: Stites DP, Stobo JD, Wells JV, eds. *Basic and Clinical Immunology.* 6th ed. Norwalk, CT: Appleton & Lange; 1987:128-158.
39. Hardman JG, Limbird LE, eds. *Goodman and Gilman's The Pharmacological Basis of Therapeutics.* 9th ed. New York, NY: McGraw-Hill; 1996:11-16.
40. Wilkinson GR. Drug metabolism and variability among patients in drug response. *N Engl J Med.* 2005;352:2211-2221.
41. Nebert DW, Dieter MZ. The evolution of drug metabolism. *Pharmacology.* 2000;61:124-135.
42. Rendic S, Di Carlo FJ. Human cytochrome P450 enzymes: a status report summarizing their reactions, substrates, inducers, and inhibitors. *Drug Metab Rev.* 1997;29:413-580.
43. McMillin GA. Pharmacogenetics fundamental of molecular diagnostics. St Louis, MO: WB Saunders; 2007:197-215.

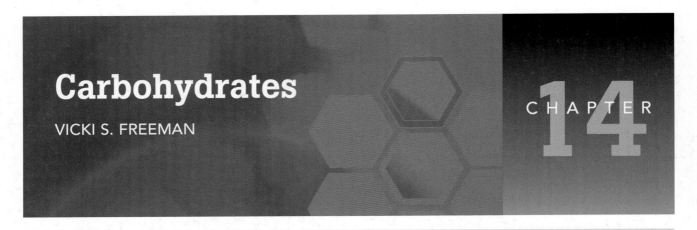

Carbohydrates

VICKI S. FREEMAN

C H A P T E R
14

Chapter Objectives

Upon completion of this chapter, the clinical
laboratorian should be able to do the following:

• Classify carbohydrates into their respective groups.
• Discuss the metabolism of carbohydrates in the body
and the mode of action of hormones in carbohydrate
metabolism.
• Differentiate the types of diabetes by clinical symptoms
and laboratory findings according to the American
Diabetes Association
• Explain the clinical significance of the three ketone
bodies.
• Relate expected laboratory results and clinical symptoms
to the following metabolic complications of diabetes:

• Ketoacidosis
• Hyperosmolar coma
• Distinguish between reactive and spontaneous
hypoglycemia.
• Describe the principle, specimen of choice, and the
advantages and disadvantages of the glucose analysis
methods.
• Describe the three commonly encountered methods of
glycated hemoglobin, specimen of choice, and source
of error.
• Describe the use of glycosylated hemoglobin in the
long-term monitoring of diabetes.
• Discuss the methods of analysis and the advantages and
disadvantages of ketone bodies.

KEY TERMS

Carbohydrates
Diabetes mellitus
Disaccharide
Embden-Meyerhof pathway
Fisher projection
Glucagon
Gluconeogenesis

Glycogen
Glycogenolysis
Glycolysis
Glycosylated hemoglobin
Haworth projection
Hyperglycemic
Hypoglycemic

Insulin
Ketone
Microalbuminuria
Monosaccharide
Oligosaccharide
Polysaccharide
Triose

Organisms rely on the oxidation of complex organic compounds to obtain energy. Three general types of such compounds are carbohydrates, amino acids, and lipids. Although all three are used as a source of energy, carbohydrates are the primary source for brain, erythrocytes, and retinal cells in humans. Carbohydrates are the major food source and energy supply for the body and are stored primarily as liver and muscle glycogen. Disease states involving carbohydrates are split into two groups—hyperglycemia and hypoglycemia. Early detection of diabetes mellitus is the aim of the American Diabetes Association (ADA) guidelines established in 1997. Acute and chronic complications may be avoided with proper diagnosis, monitoring, and treatment. The laboratory plays an important role through periodic measurements of glycosylated hemoglobin and microalbumin.

GENERAL DESCRIPTION OF CARBOHYDRATES

Carbohydrates are compounds containing C, H, and O. The general formula for a carbohydrate is $C_x(H_2O)_y$. All carbohydrates contain C=O and –OH functional groups. There are some derivatives from this basic formula because carbohydrate derivatives can be formed by the addition of other chemical groups, such as phosphates, sulfates, and amines. The classification of carbohydrates is based on four different properties: (1) the size of the base carbon chain, (2) the location of the CO function group, (3) the number of sugar units, and (4) the stereochemistry of the compound.

Classification of Carbohydrates

Carbohydrates can be grouped into generic classifications based on the number of carbons in the molecule. For example, trioses contain three carbons, tetroses contain four, pentoses contain five, and hexoses contain six. In actual practice, the smallest carbohydrate is glyceraldehyde, a three-carbon compound.

Carbohydrates are hydrates of aldehyde or ketone derivatives based on the location of the CO functional group (Fig. 14-1). The two forms of carbohydrates are aldose and ketose (Fig. 14-2). The aldose form has a terminal carbonyl group (O=CH–) called an aldehyde group, whereas the ketose form has a carbonyl group (O=C) in the middle linked to two other carbon atoms (called a ketone group).

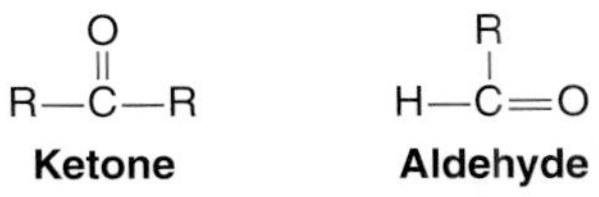

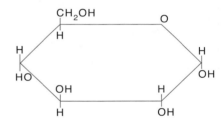

FIGURE 14-1 Pathways in glucose metabolism.

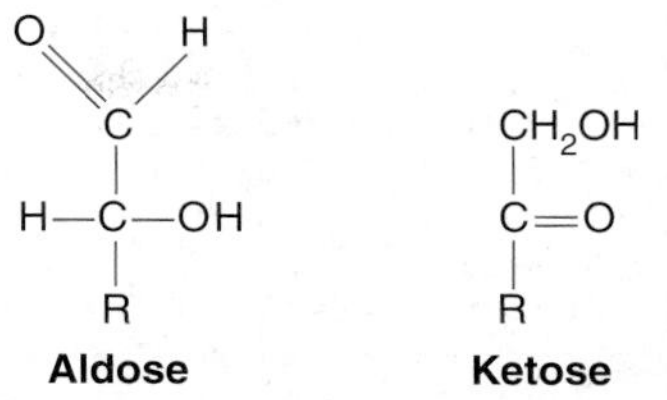

FIGURE 14-2 Two forms of carbohydrates.

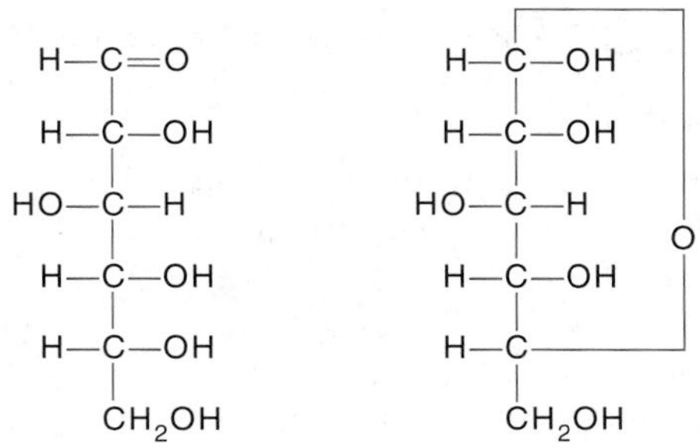

FIGURE 14-3 Fisher projection of glucose. *(Left)* Open-chain Fisher projections. *(Right)* Cyclic Fisher projection.

FIGURE 14-4 Haworth projection of glucose.

Several models are used to represent carbohydrates. The **Fisher** projection of a carbohydrate has the aldehyde or ketone at the top of the drawing. The carbons are numbered starting at the aldehyde or ketone end. The compound can be represented as a straight chain or might be linked to show a representation of the cyclic, hemiacetal form (Fig. 14-3). The **Haworth projection** represents the compound in the cyclic form that is more representative of the actual structure. This structure is formed when the functional (carbonyl) group (ketone or aldehyde) reacts with an alcohol group on the same sugar to form a ring called either a *hemiketal* or a *hemiacetal ring*, respectively (Fig. 14-4).

Stereoisomers

The central carbons of a carbohydrate are asymmetric (chiral)—four different groups are attached to the carbon atoms. This allows for various spatial arrangements around each asymmetric carbon (also called stereogenic centers) forming molecules called *stereoisomers*. Stereoisomers have the same order and types of bonds

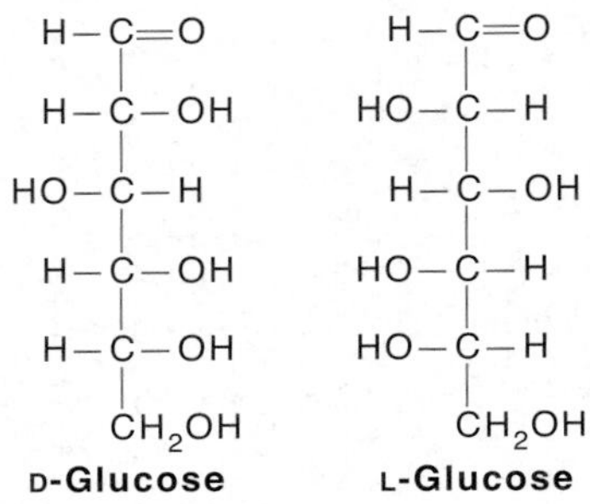

FIGURE 14-5 Stereoisomers of glucose.

but different spatial arrangements and different properties. For each asymmetric carbon, there are 2^n possible isomers; therefore, there are 2^1, or two, forms of glyceraldehyde. Because an aldohexose contains four asymmetric carbons, there are 2^4, or 16, possible isomers. A monosaccharide is assigned to the D or the L series according to the configuration at the highest numbered asymmetric carbon. This asymmetrically substituted carbon atom is called the "configurational atom" or chiral center. Thus, if the hydroxyl group (or the oxygen bridge of the ring form) projects to the right in the Fisher projection, the sugar belongs to the D series and receives the prefix D-, and if it projects to the left, then it belongs to the L series and receives the prefix L-. These stereoisomers, called enantiomers, are images that cannot be overlapped and are nonsuperimposable. In Figure 14-5, D-glucose is represented in the Fisher projection with the hydroxyl group on carbon number 5 positioned on the right. L-Glucose has the hydroxyl group of carbon number 5 positioned on the left. Most sugars in humans are in the D-form.

Monosaccharides, Disaccharides, and Polysaccharides

Another classification of carbohydrates is based on the number of sugar units in the chain: monosaccharides, disaccharides, oligosaccharides, and polysaccharides. This chaining of sugars relies on the formation of glycoside bonds that are bridges of oxygen atoms. When two carbohydrate molecules join, a water molecule is produced. When they split, one molecule of water is used to form the individual compounds. This reaction is called *hydrolysis*. The glycoside linkages of carbohydrate can

involve any number of carbons; however, certain carbons are favored, depending on the carbohydrate.

Monosaccharides are simple sugars that cannot be hydrolyzed to a simpler form. These sugars can contain three, four, five, and six or more carbon atoms (known as trioses, tetroses, pentoses, and hexoses, respectively). The most common include glucose, fructose, and galactose.

Disaccharides are formed when two monosaccharide units are joined by a glycosidic linkage. On hydrolysis, disaccharides will be split into two monosaccharides by disaccharide enzymes (e.g., lactase) located on the microvilli of the intestine. These monosaccharides are then actively absorbed. The most common disaccharides are maltose (comprising two D-glucose molecules in a $1 \rightarrow 4$ linkage), lactose, and sucrose.

Oligosaccharides are the chaining of 2 to 10 sugar units, whereas polysaccharides are formed by the linkage of many monosaccharide units. On hydrolysis, polysaccharides will yield more than 10 monosaccharides. Amylase hydrolyzes starch to disaccharides in the duodenum. The most common polysaccharides are starch (glucose molecules) and glycogen (Fig. 14-6).

Chemical Properties of Carbohydrates

Some carbohydrates are reducing substances; these carbohydrates can reduce other compounds. To be a reducing substance, the carbohydrate must contain a ketone or an aldehyde group. This property was used in many laboratory methods in the past in the determination of carbohydrates.

Carbohydrates can form glycosidic bonds with other carbohydrates and with noncarbohydrates. Two sugar molecules can be joined in tandem forming a glycosidic bond between the hemiacetal group of one molecule and the hydroxyl group on the other molecule. In forming the glycosidic bond, an acetal is generated on one sugar (at carbon 1) in place of the hemiacetal. If the bond forms with one of the other carbons on the carbohydrate other than the anomeric (reducing) carbon, the anomeric carbon is unaltered and the resulting compound remains a reducing substance. Examples of reducing substances include glucose, maltose, fructose, lactose, and galactose. If the bond is formed with the anomeric carbon on the other carbohydrate, the resulting compound is *no longer a reducing substance*. Nonreducing carbohydrates *do not* have an active ketone or aldehyde group. They *will*

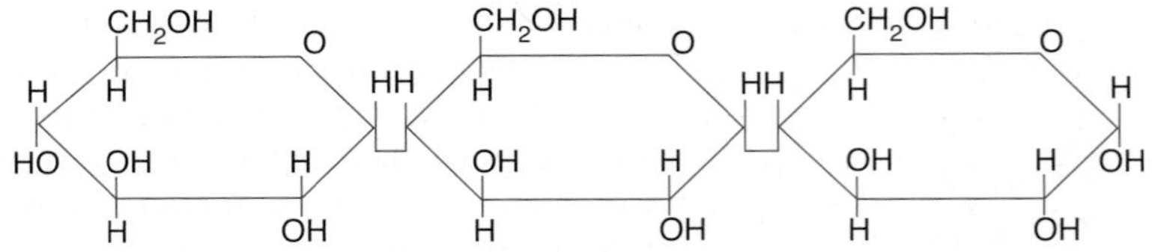

FIGURE 14-6 Linkage of monosaccharides.

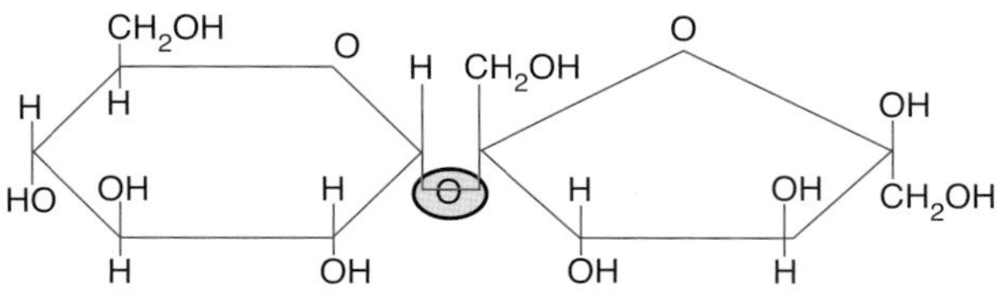

FIGURE 14-7 Haworth projection of sucrose.

not reduce other compounds. The most common nonreducing sugar is sucrose—table sugar (Fig. 14-7).

All monosaccharides and many disaccharides are reducing agents. This is because a free aldehyde or ketone (the open-chain form) can be oxidized under the proper conditions. As dissacharide remains a reducing agent when the hemiacetal or ketal hydroxyl group is not linked to another molecule, both maltose and lactose are reducing agents, whereas sucrose is not.

Glucose Metabolism

Glucose is a primary source of energy for humans. The nervous system, including the brain, totally depends on glucose from the surrounding extracellular fluid (ECF) for energy. Nervous tissue cannot concentrate or store carbohydrates; therefore, it is critical to maintain a steady supply of glucose to the tissue. For this reason, the concentration of glucose in the ECF must be maintained in a narrow range. When the concentration falls below a certain level, the nervous tissue loses the primary energy source and is incapable of maintaining normal function.

Fate of Glucose

Most of our ingested carbohydrates are polymers, such as starch and glycogen. Salivary amylase and pancreatic amylase are responsible for the digestion of these nonabsorbable polymers to dextrins and disaccharides, which are further hydrolyzed to monosaccharides by maltase, an enzyme released by the intestinal mucosa. Sucrase and lactase are two other important gut-derived enzymes that hydrolyze sucrose to glucose and fructose and lactose to glucose and galactose.

When disaccharides are converted to monosaccharides, they are absorbed by the gut and transported to the liver by the hepatic portal venous blood supply. Glucose is the only carbohydrate to be directly used for energy or stored as glycogen. Galactose and fructose must be converted to glucose before they can be used. After glucose enters the cell, it is quickly shunted into one of three possible metabolic pathways, depending on the availability of substrates or the nutritional status of the cell. The ultimate goal of the cell is to convert glucose to carbon dioxide and water. During this process, the cell obtains the high-energy molecule adenosine triphosphate (ATP) from inorganic phosphate and adenosine diphosphate. The cell requires oxygen for the final steps in the electron

transport chain (ETC). Nicotinamide adenine dinucleotide (NAD) in its reduced form (NADH) will act as an intermediate to couple glucose oxidation to the ETC in the mitochondria where much of the ATP is gained.

The first step for all three pathways requires glucose to be converted to glucose-6-phosphate using the high-energy molecule, ATP. This reaction is catalyzed by the enzyme hexokinase (Fig. 14-8). Glucose-6-phosphate can enter the Embden-Meyerhof pathway or the *hexose monophosphate pathway* (HMP) or can be converted to glycogen (Fig. 14-8). The first two pathways are important for the generation of energy from glucose; the conversion to glycogen pathway is important for the storage of glucose.

In the Embden-Meyerhof pathway, glucose is broken down into two- and three-carbon molecules of pyruvic acid that can enter the *tricarboxylic acid* (TCA) *cycle* on conversion to acetyl-coenzyme A (acetyl-CoA). This pathway requires oxygen and is called the *aerobic pathway* (Fig. 14-8). Other substrates have the opportunity to enter the pathway at several points. Glycerol released from the hydrolysis of triglycerides can enter at 3-phosphoglycerate, and fatty acids and ketones and some amino acids are converted or catabolized to acetyl-CoA, which is part of the TCA cycle. Other amino acids enter the pathway as pyruvate or as deaminated α-ketoacids and α-oxoacids. The conversion of amino acids by the liver and other specialized tissue, such as the kidney, to substrates that can be converted to glucose is called gluconeogenesis. Gluconeogenesis also encompasses the conversion of glycerol, lactate, and pyruvate to glucose.

Anaerobic glycolysis is important for tissue such as muscle, which often have important energy requirements without an adequate oxygen supply. These tissues can derive ATP from glucose in an oxygen-deficient environment by converting pyruvic acid into lactic acid. The lactic acid diffuses from the muscle cell, enters the systemic circulation, and is then taken up and used by the liver (Fig. 14-8). For anaerobic glycolysis to occur, 2 mol of ATP must be consumed for each mole of glucose; however, 4 mol of ATP are directly produced, resulting in a net gain of 2 mol of ATP. Further gains of ATP result from the introduction of pyruvate into the TCA cycle and NADH into the ETC.

The second energy pathway is the hexose monophosphate (HMP) *shunt*, which is actually a detour of glucose-6-phosphate from the glycolytic pathway to become 6-phosphogluconic acid. This oxidized product permits the formation of ribose-5-phosphate and NADP in its reduced form (NADPH). NADPH is important to erythrocytes that lack mitochondria and are therefore incapable of the TCA cycle. The reducing power of NADPH is required for the protection of the cell from oxidative and free radical damage. Without NADPH, the lipid bilayer membrane of the cell and critical enzymes

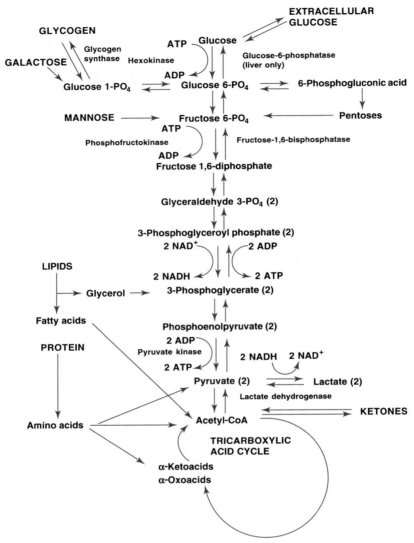

FIGURE 14-8 The Embden-Meyerhof pathway for anaerobic glycolysis.

would eventually be destroyed, resulting in cell death. The HMP shunt also permits pentoses, such as ribose, to enter the glycolytic pathway.

When the cell's energy requirements are being met, glucose can be stored as glycogen. This third pathway, which is called *glycogenesis*, is relatively straightforward. Glucose-6-phosphate is converted to glucose-1-phosphate, which is then converted to uridine diphosphoglucose and then to glycogen by glycogen synthase. Several tissues are capable of the synthesis of glycogen, especially the liver and muscles. Hepatocytes are capable of releasing glucose from glycogen or other sources to maintain the blood glucose concentration. This is because the liver synthesizes the enzyme glucose-6-phosphatase. Without this enzyme, glucose is trapped in the glycolytic pathway. Muscle cells do not synthesize glucose-6-phosphatase and, therefore, they are incapable of dephosphorylating glucose. Once

glucose enters a muscle cell, it remains as glycogen unless it is catabolized. Glycogenolysis is the process by which glycogen is converted back to glucose-6-phosphate for entry into the glycolytic pathway. Table 14-1 outlines the major energy pathways involved either directly or indirectly with glucose metabolism.

Overall, dietary glucose and other carbohydrates either can be used by the liver and other cells for energy or can be stored as glycogen for later use. When the supply of glucose is low, the liver will use glycogen and other substrates to elevate the blood glucose concentration. These substrates include glycerol from triglycerides, lactic acid from skin and muscles, and amino acids. If the lipolysis of triglycerides is unregulated, it results in the formation of ketone bodies, which the brain can use as a source of energy through the TCA cycle. The synthesis of glucose from amino acids is gluconeogenesis.

TABLE 14-1	PATHWAYS IN GLUCOSE METABOLISM
Glycolysis	Metabolism of glucose molecule to pyruvate or lactate for production of energy
Gluconeogenesis	Formation of glucose-6-phosphate from noncarbohydrate sources
Glycogenolysis	Breakdown of glycogen to glucose for use as energy
Glycogenesis	Conversion of glucose to glycogen for storage
Lipogenesis	Conversion of carbohydrates to fatty acids
Lipolysis	Decomposition of fat

This process is used in conjunction with the formation of ketone bodies when glycogen stores are depleted—conditions normally associated with starvation. The principal pathway for glucose oxidation is through the Embden-Meyerhof pathway. NADPH can be synthesized through the HMP shunt, which is a side pathway from the anaerobic glycolytic pathway (Fig. 14-8).

Regulation of Carbohydrate Metabolism

The liver, pancreas, and other endocrine glands are all involved in controlling the blood glucose concentrations within a narrow range. During a brief fast, glucose is supplied to the ECF from the liver through glycogenolysis. When the fasting period is longer than 1 day, glucose is synthesized from other sources through gluconeogenesis. Control of blood glucose is under two major hormones: insulin and glucagon, both produced by the pancreas. Their actions oppose each other. Other hormones and neuroendocrine substances also exert some control over blood glucose concentrations, permitting the body to respond to increased demands for glucose or to survive prolonged fasts. It also permits the conservation of energy as lipids when excess substrates are ingested.

Insulin is the primary hormone responsible for the entry of glucose into the cell. It is synthesized by the β-cells of islets of Langerhans in the pancreas. When these cells detect an increase in body glucose, they release insulin. The release of insulin causes an increased movement of glucose into the cells and increased glucose

metabolism. Insulin is normally released when glucose levels are high and is *not* released when glucose levels are decreased. It decreases plasma glucose levels by increasing the transport entry of glucose in muscle and adipose tissue by way of nonspecific receptors. It also regulates glucose by increasing glycogenesis, lipogenesis, and glycolysis and inhibiting glycogenolysis. Insulin is the only hormone that decreases glucose levels and can be referred to as a hypoglycemic agent (Table 14-2).

Glucagon is the primary hormone responsible for increasing glucose levels. It is synthesized by the α-cells of islets of Langerhans in the pancreas and released during stress and fasting states. When these cells detect a decrease in body glucose, they release glucagon. Glucagon acts by increasing plasma glucose levels by glycogenolysis in the liver and an increase in gluconeogenesis. It can be referred to as a **hyperglycemic** agent (Table 14-2).

Two hormones produced by the adrenal gland affect carbohydrate metabolism. *Epinephrine*, produced by the adrenal medulla, increases plasma glucose by inhibiting insulin secretion, increasing glycogenolysis, and promoting lipolysis. Epinephrine is released during times of stress. *Glucocorticoids*, primarily cortisol, are released from the adrenal cortex on stimulation by adrenocorticotropic hormone (ACTH). Cortisol increases plasma glucose by decreasing intestinal entry into the cell and increasing gluconeogenesis, liver glycogen, and lipolysis.

Two anterior pituitary hormones, growth hormone and ACTH, promote increased plasma glucose. *Growth*

TABLE 14-2	THE ACTION OF HORMONES
ACTION OF INSULIN	
Increases glycogenesis and glycolysis: glucose → glycogen → pyruvate → acetyl-CoA	
Increases lipogenesis	
Decreases glycogenolysis	
ACTION OF GLUCAGON	
Increases glycogenolysis: glycogen → glucose	
Increases gluconeogenesis: fatty acids → acetyl-CoA → ketone, proteins → amino acids	

hormone increases plasma glucose by decreasing the entry of glucose into the cells and increasing glycolysis. Its release from the pituitary is stimulated by decreased glucose levels and inhibited by increased glucose. Decreased levels of cortisol stimulate the anterior pituitary to release ACTH. ACTH, in turn, stimulates the adrenal cortex to release cortisol and increases plasma glucose levels by converting liver glycogen to glucose and promoting gluconeogenesis.

Two other hormones affect glucose levels: thyroxine and somatostatin. The thyroid gland is stimulated by the production of thyroid-stimulating hormone to release *thyroxine* that increases plasma glucose levels by increasing glycogenolysis, gluconeogenesis, and intestinal absorption of glucose. *Somatostatin*, produced by the δ-cells of the islets of Langerhans of the pancreas, increases plasma glucose levels by the inhibition of insulin, glucagon, growth hormone, and other endocrine hormones.

HYPERGLYCEMIA

Hyperglycemia is an increase in plasma glucose levels. In healthy patients, during a hyperglycemia state, insulin is secreted by the β-cells of the pancreatic islets of Langerhans. Insulin enhances membrane permeability to cells in the liver, muscle, and adipose tissue. It also alters the glucose metabolic pathways. Hyperglycemia, or increased plasma glucose levels, is caused by an imbalance of hormones.

Diabetes Mellitus

Diabetes mellitus is actually a group of metabolic diseases characterized by hyperglycemia resulting from defects in insulin secretion, insulin action, or both. In 1979, the National Diabetes Data Group developed a classification and diagnosis scheme for diabetes mellitus.[1] This scheme included dividing diabetes into two broad categories: type 1, insulin-dependent diabetes mellitus (IDDM); and type 2, non–insulin-dependent diabetes mellitus (NIDDM).

Established in 1995, the International Expert Committee on the Diagnosis and Classification of Diabetes Mellitus, working under the sponsorship of the ADA, was given the task of updating the 1979 classification system. The proposed changes included eliminating the older terms of IDDM and NIDDM. The categories of type 1 and type 2 were retained, with the adoption of Arabic numerals instead of Roman numerals (Table 14-3).[2]

Therefore, the ADA/World Health Organization (WHO) guidelines recommend the following categories of diabetes:

- Type 1 diabetes
- Type 2 diabetes
- Other specific types of diabetes
- Gestational diabetes mellitus (GDM)

CASE STUDY 14-1

An 18-year-old male high school student who had a 4-year history of diabetes mellitus was brought to the emergency department because of excessive drowsiness, vomiting, and diarrhea. His diabetes had been well controlled with 40 units of NPH insulin daily until several days ago when he developed excessive thirst and polyuria. For the past 3 days, he has also had headaches, myalgia, and a low-grade fever. Diarrhea and vomiting began 1 day ago.

URINALYSIS RESULTS		CHEMISTRY TEST RESULTS	
Specific gravity	1.012	Sodium	126 mmol/L
pH	5.0	Potassium	6.1 mmol/L
Glucose	4+	Chloride	87 mmol/L
Ketone	Large	Bicarbonate	6 mmol/L
		Plasma glucose	600 mg/dL
		BUN	48 mg/dL
		Creatinine	2.0 mg/dL
		Serum ketones	4+

Questions

1. What is the probable diagnosis of this patient based on the data presented?
2. What laboratory test(s) should be performed to follow this patient and aid in adjusting insulin levels?
3. Why are the urine ketones positive?
4. What methods are used to quantitate urine ketones? Which ketone(s) do they detect?

Type 1 diabetes is characterized by inappropriate hyperglycemia primarily a result of pancreatic islet β-cell destruction and a tendency to ketoacidosis. Type 2 diabetes, in contrast, includes hyperglycemia cases that result from insulin resistance with an insulin secretory defect. An intermediate stage, in which the fasting glucose is increased above-normal limits but not to the level of diabetes, has been named *impaired fasting glucose*. Use of the term *impaired glucose tolerance* to indicate glucose tolerance values above normal but below diabetes levels was retained. Also, the term GDM was retained for women who develop glucose intolerance during pregnancy.

Type 1 diabetes mellitus is a result of cellular-mediated autoimmune destruction of the β-cells of the pancreas, causing an absolute deficiency of insulin secretion. Upper limit of 110 mg/dL on the fasting plasma glucose is designated as the upper limit of normal blood

TABLE 14-3	CLASSIFICATION OF DIABETES MELLITUS
CLASSIFICATION	**PATHOGENESIS**
Type 1	β-Cell destruction
	Absolute insulin deficiency
	Autoantibodies
	• Islet cell autoantibodies
	• Insulin autoantibodies
	• Glutamic acid decarboxylase autoantibodies
	• Tyrosine phosphatase IA-2 and IA-2B autoantibodies
Type 2	Insulin resistance with an insulin secretory defect
	Relative insulin deficiency
Other	Associated with secondary conditions
	• Genetic defects of β-cell function
	• Pancreatic disease
	• Endocrine disease
	• Drug or chemical induced
	• Insulin receptor abnormalities
	• Other genetic syndromes
Gestational	Glucose intolerance during pregnancy
	Due to metabolic and hormonal changes

TABLE 14-4	LABORATORY FINDINGS IN HYPERGLYCEMIA
Increased glucose in plasma and urine	
Increased urine-specific gravity	
Increased serum and urine osmolality	
Ketones in serum and urine (ketonemia and ketonuria)	
Decreased blood and urine pH (acidosis)	
Electrolyte imbalance	

glucose. Type 1 constitutes only 10% to 20% of all cases of diabetes and commonly occurs in childhood and adolescence. This disease is usually initiated by an environmental factor or infection (usually a virus) in individuals with a genetic predisposition and causes the immune destruction of the β-cells of the pancreas and, therefore, a decreased production of insulin. Characteristics of type 1 diabetes include abrupt onset, insulin dependence, and ketosis tendency. This diabetic type is genetically related. One or more of the following markers are found in 85% to 90% of individuals with fasting hyperglycemia: islet cell autoantibodies, insulin autoantibodies, glutamic acid decarboxylase autoantibodies, and tyrosine phosphatase IA-2 and IA-2B autoantibodies.

Signs and symptoms include polydipsia (excessive thirst), polyphagia (increased food intake), polyuria (excessive urine production), rapid weight loss, hyperventilation, mental confusion, and possible loss of consciousness (due to increased glucose to brain). Complications include microvascular problems such as nephropathy, neuropathy, and retinopathy. Increased heart disease is also found in patients with diabetes. Table 14-4 lists the laboratory findings in hyperglycemia. *Idiopathic type 1 diabetes* is a form of type 1 diabetes that has no known etiology, is strongly inherited, and does not have β-cell autoimmunity. Individuals with this form of diabetes have episodic requirements for insulin replacement.

Type 2 diabetes mellitus is characterized by hyperglycemia as a result of an individual's resistance to insulin with an insulin secretory defect. This resistance results in a relative, not an absolute, insulin deficiency. Type 2 constitutes the majority of the diabetes cases. Most patients in this type are obese or have an increased percentage of body fat distribution in the abdominal region. This type of diabetes often goes undiagnosed for many years and is associated with a strong genetic predisposition, with patients at increased risk with an increase in age, obesity, and lack of physical exercise. Characteristics usually include adult onset of the disease and milder symptoms than in type 1, with ketoacidosis seldom occurring. However, these patients are more likely to go into a hyperosmolar coma and are at an increased risk of developing macrovascular and microvascular complications.

Other specific types of diabetes are associated with certain conditions (secondary), including genetic defects of β-cell function or insulin action, pancreatic disease, diseases of endocrine origin, drug- or chemical-induced insulin receptor abnormalities, and certain genetic syndromes. The characteristics and prognosis of this form of diabetes depend on the primary disorder. Maturity-onset diabetes of youth is a rare form of diabetes that is inherited in an autosomal dominant fashion.[3]

GDM has been defined as any degree of glucose intolerance with onset or first recognition during pregnancy. However, the latest recommendations suggest that "high-risk women found to have diabetes at their initial prenatal visit, using standard criteria (Table 14-5), receive a diagnosis of overt, not gestational, diabetes."[4] Women identified through the oral glucose tolerance, listed in Table 14-8, should receive a diagnosis of GDM. Causes of GDM include metabolic and hormonal changes. Patients with GDM frequently return to normal postpartum. However, this disease is associated with

TABLE 14-5	**DIAGNOSTIC CRITERIA FOR DIABETES MELLITUS**
1. HbA$_1$c ≥ 6.5% using a method that is NGSP certified and standardized to the DCCT assay[a]	
2. Fasting plasma glucose ≥ 126 mg/dL (≥7.0 mmol/L)[a]	
3. Two-hour plasma glucose ≥ 200 mg/dL (≥11.1 mmol/L) during an OGTT[a]	
4. Random plasma glucose ≥ 200 mg/dL (≥11.1 mmol/L) plus symptoms of diabetes[a]	

HbA$_1$c, hemoglobin A$_1$c; NGSP, National Glycohemoglobin Standardization Program; OGTT, oral glucose tolerance test.

[a]In the absence of unequivocal hyperglycemia, these criteria should be confirmed by repeat testing on a different day. The fourth measure (OGTT) is not recommended for routine clinical use.

increased perinatal complications and an increased risk for the development of diabetes in later years. Infants born to mothers with diabetes are at increased risk for respiratory distress syndrome, hypocalcemia, and hyperbilirubinemia. Fetal insulin secretion is stimulated in the neonate of a mother with diabetes. However, when the infant is born and the umbilical cord is severed, the infant's oversupply of glucose is abruptly terminated, causing severe hypoglycemia.

Pathophysiology of Diabetes Mellitus

In both type 1 and type 2 diabetes, the individual will be hyperglycemic, which can be severe. Glucosuria can also occur after the renal tubular transporter system for glucose becomes saturated. This happens when the glucose concentration of plasma exceeds roughly 180 mg/dL in an individual with normal renal function and urine output. As hepatic glucose overproduction continues, the plasma glucose concentration reaches a plateau around 300 to 500 mg/dL (17 to 28 mmol/L). Provided renal output is maintained, glucose excretion will match the overproduction, causing the plateau.

The individual with type 1 diabetes has a higher tendency to produce ketones. Patients with type 2 diabetes seldom generate ketones but instead have a greater tendency to develop hyperosmolar nonketotic states. The difference in glucagon and insulin concentrations in these two groups appears to be responsible for the generation of ketones through increased β-oxidation. In type 1, there is an absence of insulin with an excess of glucagon. This permits gluconeogenesis and lipolysis to occur. In type 2, insulin is not absent and may, in fact, present as hyperinsulinemia at times; therefore, glucagon is attenuated. Fatty acid oxidation is inhibited in type 2. This causes fatty acids to be incorporated into triglycerides for release as very low-density lipoproteins.

The laboratory findings of a patient with diabetes with ketoacidosis tend to reflect dehydration, electrolyte disturbances, and acidosis. Acetoacetate, β-hydroxybutyrate, and acetone are produced from the oxidation of fatty acids. The two former ketone bodies contribute to the acidosis. Lactate, fatty acids, and other organic acids can also contribute to a lesser degree. Bicarbonate and total carbon dioxide are usually decreased due to Kussmaul-Kien respiration (deep respirations). This is a compensatory mechanism to blow off carbon dioxide and remove hydrogen ions in the process. The anion gap in this acidosis can exceed 16 mmol/L. Serum osmolality is high as a result of hyperglycemia; sodium concentrations tend to be lower due in part to losses (polyuria) and in part to a shift of water from cells because of the hyperglycemia. The sodium value should not be falsely underestimated because of hypertriglyceridemia. Grossly elevated triglycerides will displace plasma volume and give the appearance of decreased electrolytes when flame photometry or prediluted, ion-specific electrodes are used for sodium determinations. Hyperkalemia is almost always present as a result of the displacement of potassium from cells in acidosis. This is somewhat misleading because the patient's total body potassium is usually decreased.

More typical of the untreated patient with type 2 diabetes is the nonketotic hyperosmolar state. The individual presenting with this syndrome has an overproduction of glucose; however, there appears to be an imbalance between production and elimination in urine. Often, this state is precipitated by heart disease, stroke, or pancreatitis. Glucose concentrations exceed 300 to 500 mg/dL (17 to 28 mmol/L) and severe dehydration is present. The severe dehydration contributes to the inability to excrete glucose in the urine. Mortality is high with this condition. Ketones are not observed because the severe hyperosmolar state inhibits the ability of glucagon to stimulate lipolysis. The laboratory findings of nonketotic hyperosmolar coma include plasma glucose values exceeding 1,000 mg/dL (55 mmol/L), normal or elevated plasma sodium and potassium, slightly decreased bicarbonate, elevated blood urea nitrogen (BUN) and creatinine, and an elevated osmolality (>320 mOsm/dL). The gross elevation in glucose and osmolality, the elevation in BUN, and the absence of ketones distinguish this condition from diabetic ketoacidosis.

Other forms of impaired glucose metabolism that do not meet the criteria for diabetes mellitus include impaired fasting glucose and impaired glucose tolerance. These forms are discussed in the following section.

CASE STUDY 14-2

A 58-year-old obese man with frequent urination was seen by his primary care physician. The following laboratory work was performed, and the following results were obtained:

CASUAL PLASMA GLUCOSE   225 mg/dL

Urinalysis Results

Color and appearance	Pale/clear	Blood	Negative
pH	6.0	Bilirubin	Negative
Specific	1.025	Urobilinogen	Negative
Glucose	2+	Nitrites	Negative
Ketones	Negative	Leukocyte esterase	Negative

Questions

1. What is the probable diagnosis of this patient?

2. What other test(s) should be performed to confirm this? Which is the preferred test?

3. What values from #2 would confirm the diagnosis of diabetes?

3. After diagnosis, what test(s) should be performed to monitor his condition?

Criteria for Testing for Prediabetes and Diabetes

The testing criteria for asymptomatic adults for type 2 diabetes mellitus were modified by the ADA Expert Committee to allow for earlier detection of the disease. According to the ADA recommendations, all adults beginning at the age of 45 years should be tested for diabetes every 3 years using either the hemoglobin A_1c (HbA$_1$c), fasting plasma glucose, or a 2-hour 75 g oral glucose tolerance test (OGTT) unless the individual has otherwise been diagnosed with diabetes.[4] Testing should be carried out at an earlier age or more frequently in individuals who display overweight tendencies, i.e., BMI $\geq$ 25 kg/m^2 (at-risk BMI may be lower in some ethnic groups), and have additional risk factors, as follows:

- Habitually physically inactive
- Family history of diabetes in a first-degree relative
- In a high-risk minority population (e.g., African American, Latino, Native American, Asian American, and Pacific Islander)
- History of GDM or delivering a baby weighing more than 9 lb (4.1 kg)
- Hypertension (blood pressure $\geq$ 140/90 mm Hg)

- Low high-density lipoprotein (HDL) cholesterol concentrations (<35 mg/dL [0.90 mmol/L])
- Elevated triglyceride concentrations > 250 mg/dL (2.82 mmol/L)
- History of impaired fasting glucose/impaired glucose tolerance
- Women with polycystic ovarian syndrome (PCOS)
- Other clinical conditions associated with insulin resistance (e.g., severe obesity and acanthosis nigricans)
- History of cardiovascular disease

In the absence of the above criteria, testing for prediabetes and diabetes should begin at the age of 45 years. If results are normal, testing should be repeated at least at 3-year intervals, with consideration of more frequent testing depending on initial results and risk status.

As the incidence of adolescent type 2 diabetes has risen dramatically in the past few years, criteria for the testing for type 2 diabetes in asymptomatic children have been developed. These criteria include initiation of testing at the age 10 years or at the onset of puberty, if puberty occurs at a younger age, with follow-up testing every 2 years. Testing should be carried out on children who display the following characteristics: Overweight (BMI >85th percentile for age and sex, weight for height

CASE STUDY 14-3

A 14-year-old male student was seen by his physician. His chief complaints were fatigue; weight loss; and increases in appetite, thirst, and frequency of urination. For the past 3 to 4 weeks, he had been excessively thirsty and had to urinate every few hours. He began to get up three to four times a night to urinate. The patient has a family history of diabetes mellitus.

LABORATORY DATA

Fasting plasma glucose	160 mg/dL	
Urinalysis	Specific gravity	1.040
	Glucose	4+
	Ketones	Moderate

Questions

1. Based on the preceding information, can this patient be diagnosed with diabetes?

2. What further tests might be performed to confirm the diagnosis?

3. According to the American Diabetes Association, what criteria are required for the diagnosis of diabetes?

4. Assuming this patient has diabetes, which type would be diagnosed?

>85th percentile, or weight >120% of ideal for height) plus any two of the following risk factors:

- Family history of type 2 diabetes in first- or second-degree relative
- Race/ethnicity (e.g., Native American, African American, Latino, Asian American, and Pacific Islander)
- Signs of insulin resistance or conditions associated with insulin resistance (e.g., acanthosis nigricans, hypertension, dyslipidemia, and PCOS)
- Maternal history of diabetes or GDM

Criteria for the Diagnosis of Diabetes Mellitus

Four methods of diagnosis are suggested: (1) HbA$_1$c ≥6.5% using a National Glycohemoglobin Standardization Program (NGSP)–certified method, (2) a fasting plasma glucose ≥ 126 mg/dL, or (3) an OGTT with a 2-hour postload (75 g glucose load) level ≥ 200 mg/dL, and (4) symptoms of diabetes plus a random plasma glucose level ≥ 200 mg/dL, each of which should be confirmed on a subsequent day by any one of the first three methods (Tables 14-5, 14-6, and 14-7). Any of the first three methods are considered appropriate for the diagnosis of diabetes. The decision on which method to use is the decision of the healthcare provider depending on various patient factors. Point-of-care assay methods for either plasma glucose or HbA$_1$c are not recommended for diagnosis.

TABLE 14-6	CATEGORIES OF FASTING PLASMA GLUCOSE
Normal fasting glucose	FPG 70–99 mg/dL (3.9–5.5 mmol/L)
Impaired fasting glucose	FPG 100–125 mg/dL (5.6–6.9 mmol/L)
Provisional diabetes diagnosis	FPG ≥126 mg/dL (≥7.0 mmol/l)[a]

FPG, fasting plasma glucose.
[a]Must be confirmed.

TABLE 14-7	CATEGORIES OF ORAL GLUCOSE TOLERANCE
Normal glucose tolerance	Two-hour PG ≤140 mg/dL (≤7.8 mmol/L)
Impaired glucose tolerance	Two-hour PG 140–199 mg/dL (7.8–11.1 mmol/l)
Provisional diabetes diagnosis	Two-hour PG ≥ 200 mg/dL (≥11.1 mmol/L)[a]

PG, plasma glucose.
[a]Must be confirmed.

An intermediate group of individuals who did not meet the criteria of diabetes mellitus but who have glucose levels above normal be placed into three categories for the risk of developing diabetes. First, those individuals with fasting glucose levels ≥100 mg/dL but <126 mg/dL are placed in the impaired fasting glucose category. Another set of individuals who have 2-hour OGTT levels ≥140 mg/dL but <200 mg/dL are placed in the impaired glucose tolerance category. Additionally, individuals with a HbA$_1$c of 5.7% to 6.4% are placed in the third at-risk category. Individuals in these three categories are referred to as having "prediabetes" indicating the relatively high risk for the development of diabetes in these patients.

Criteria for the Testing and Diagnosis of GDM

The diagnostic criteria for gestational diabetes were revised by the International Association of the Diabetes and Pregnancy Study Groups. The revised criteria recommend that all nondiabetic pregnant women should be screened for GDM at 24 to 28 weeks of gestation.

CASE STUDY 14-4

A 13-year-old girl collapsed on a playground at school. When her mother was contacted, she mentioned that her daughter had been losing weight and making frequent trips to the bathroom in the night. The emergency squad noticed a fruity breath. On entrance to the emergency department, her vital signs were as follows:

Blood pressure	98/50 mm Hg
Respirations	Rapid
Temperature	99°F

Stat lab results included:

RANDOM URINE		SERUM CHEMISTRIES	
pH	5.5	Glucose	500 mg/dL
Protein	Negative	Ketones	Positive
Glucose	4+	BUN	6 mg/dL
Ketones	Moderate	Creatinine	0.4 mg/dL
Blood	Negative		

Questions

1. Identify this patient's most likely type of diabetes.

2. Based on your identification, circle the common characteristics associated with that type of diabetes in the case study above.

3. What is the cause of the fruity breath?

TABLE 14-8	DIAGNOSTIC CRITERIA FOR GESTATIONAL DIABETES
Fasting plasma glucose	≥92 mg/dL (5.1 mmol/L)
One-hour plasma glucose	≥180 mg/dL (10 mmol/L)
Two-hour plasma glucose	≥153 mg/dL (8.5 mmol/L)

TABLE 14-9	CAUSES OF HYPOGLYCEMIA	
PATIENT APPEARS HEALTHY		
No coexisting disease	Drugs	
	Insulinoma	
	Islet hyperplasia/ nesidioblastosis	
	Factitial hypoglycemia from insulin or sulfonylurea	
	Severe exercise	
	Ketotic hypoglycemia	
Compensated coexistent	Drugs/disease	
PATIENT APPEARS ILL		
Drugs		
Predisposing illness		
Hospitalized patient		

The approach for screening and diagnosis is the performance of a 2-hour OGTT using a 75 g glucose load. Glucose measurements should be taken at fasting, 1 hour, and 2 hours. A fasting plasma glucose value ≥ 92 mg/dL (5.1 mmol/L), a 1-hour value ≥ 180 mg/dL (10 mmol/L), or a 2-hour glucose value ≥ 153 mg/dL (8.5 mmol/L) is diagnostic of GDM if any one of the three criteria are met. This test should be performed in the morning after an overnight fast of at least 8 hours (Table 14-8).

HYPOGLYCEMIA

Hypoglycemia involves decreased plasma glucose levels and can have many causes—some are transient and relatively insignificant, but others can be life threatening. The plasma glucose concentration at which glucagon and other glycemic factors are released is between 65 and 70 mg/dL (3.6 to 3.9 mmol/L); at about 50 to 55 mg/dL (2.8 to 3.1 mmol/L), observable symptoms of hypoglycemia appear. The warning signs and symptoms of hypoglycemia are all related to the central nervous system. The release of epinephrine into the systemic circulation and of norepinephrine at nerve endings of specific neurons acts in unison with glucagon to increase plasma glucose. Glucagon is released from the islet cells of the pancreas and inhibits insulin. Epinephrine is released from the adrenal gland and increases glucose metabolism and inhibits insulin. In addition, cortisol and growth hormone are released and increase glucose metabolism.

Historically, hypoglycemia was classified as postabsorptive (fasting) and postprandial (reactive) hypoglycemia. However, the reactive hypoglycemia only described the timing of hypoglycemia, not the etiology. Current approaches suggest classification based on clinical characteristics. This classification separates patients into those who appear healthy and those who are sick (Table 14-9).[5] Among healthy-appearing patients are those with and without a compensated coexistent disease. This category includes individuals in whom medications may be the cause of hypoglycemia through accidental ingestion by dispensing error. Sick persons may have an illness that predisposes to hypoglycemia or may experience drug and illness interaction leading to hypoglycemia. Hypoglycemia in hospitalized patients can often be ascribed to iatrogenic factors. Symptoms of hypoglycemia are increased hunger, sweating, nausea and vomiting, dizziness, nervousness and shaking, blurring of speech

and sight, and mental confusion. Laboratory findings include decreased plasma glucose levels during hypoglycemic episode and extremely elevated insulin levels in patients with pancreatic β-cell tumors (insulinoma). To investigate an insulinoma, the patient is required to fast under controlled conditions. Men and women have different metabolic patterns in prolonged fasts. The healthy male will maintain plasma glucose of 55 to 60 mg/dL (3.1 to 3.3 mmol/L) for several days. Healthy females will produce ketones more readily and permit plasma glucose to decrease to 40 mg/dL (2.2 mmol/L) or lower. Diagnostic criteria for an insulinoma include a change in glucose level ≥ 25 mg/dL (1.4 mmol/L) coincident with an insulin level ≥ 6 μU/mL (41.7 pmol/L), C-peptide levels ≥ 0.2 nmol/L, proinsulin levels ≥ 5 pmol/L, and/or β-hydroxybutyrate levels ≤ 2.7 mmol/L.[6]

Genetic Defects in Carbohydrate Metabolism

Glycogen storage diseases are the result of the deficiency of a specific enzyme that causes an alternation of glycogen metabolism. The most common congenital form of glycogen storage disease is glucose-6-phosphatase deficiency type 1, which is also called von Gierke disease, an autosomal recessive disease. This disease is characterized by severe hypoglycemia that coincides with metabolic acidosis, ketonemia, and elevated lactate and alanine. Hypoglycemia occurs because glycogen cannot be converted back to glucose by way of hepatic glycogenolysis. A glycogen buildup is found in the liver, causing hepatomegaly. The patients usually have severe hypoglycemia, hyperlipidemia, uricemia, and growth retardation. A liver biopsy will show a positive glycogen stain. Although the

CASE STUDY 14-5

A 28-year-old woman delivered a 9.5-lb infant. The infant was above the 95th percentile for weight and length. The mother's history was incomplete; she claimed to have had no medical care through her pregnancy. Shortly after birth, the infant became lethargic and flaccid. A whole blood glucose and ionized calcium were performed in the nursery with the following results:

Whole blood glucose	25 mg/dL
Ionized calcium	4.9 mg/dL

Plasma glucose was drawn and analyzed in the main laboratory to confirm the whole blood findings

Plasma glucose	33 mg/dL

An intravenous glucose solution was started and whole blood glucose was measured hourly

Questions

1. Give the possible explanation for the infant's large birth weight and size.

2. If the mother was a gestational diabetic, why was her baby hypoglycemic?

3. Why was there a discrepancy between the whole blood glucose concentration and the plasma glucose concentration?

4. If the mother had been monitored during pregnancy, what laboratory tests should have been performed and what criteria would have indicated that she had gestational diabetes?

glycogen accumulation is irreversible, the disease can be kept under control by avoiding the development of hypoglycemia. Liver transplantation corrects the hypoglycemic condition. Other enzyme defects or deficiencies that cause hypoglycemia include glycogen synthase, fructose-1,6-bisphosphatase, phosphoenolpyruvate carboxykinase, and pyruvate carboxylase. Glycogen debrancher enzyme deficiency does not cause hypoglycemia but does cause hepatomegaly.

Galactosemia, a cause of failure to thrive syndrome in infants, is a congenital deficiency of one of three enzymes involved in galactose metabolism, resulting in increased levels of galactose in plasma. The most common enzyme deficiency is galactose-1-phosphate uridyltransferase. Galactosemia occurs because of the inhibition of glycogenolysis and is accompanied by diarrhea and vomiting. Galactose must be removed from the diet to prevent the development of irreversible complications. If left untreated, the patient will develop mental retardation and cataracts. The disorder can be identified by measuring erythrocyte galactose-1-phosphate uridyltransferase activity. Laboratory findings include hypoglycemia, hyperbilirubinemia, and galactose accumulation in the blood, tissue, and urine following milk ingestion. Another enzyme deficiency, fructose-1-phosphate aldolase deficiency, causes nausea and hypoglycemia after fructose ingestion.

Specific inborn errors of amino acid metabolism and long-chain fatty acid oxidation are also responsible for hypoglycemia. There are also alimentary and idiopathic hypoglycemias. Alimentary hypoglycemia appears to be caused by an increase in the release of insulin in response to rapid absorption of nutrients after a meal or the rapid secretion of insulin-releasing gastric factors. Idiopathic postprandial hypoglycemia is a controversial diagnosis that may be overused.[7]

ROLE OF LABORATORY IN DIFFERENTIAL DIAGNOSIS AND MANAGEMENT OF PATIENTS WITH GLUCOSE METABOLIC ALTERATIONS

The demonstration of hyperglycemia or hypoglycemia under specific conditions is used to diagnose diabetes mellitus and hypoglycemic conditions. Other laboratory tests have been developed to identify insulinomas and to monitor glycemic control and the development of renal complications.

CASE STUDY 14-6

Laboratory tests were performed on a 50-year-old lean white woman during an annual physical examination. She had no family history of diabetes or any history of elevated glucose levels during pregnancy.

LABORATORY RESULTS

Fasting blood glucose	90 mg/dL
Cholesterol	140 mg/dL
HDL	40 mg/dL
Triglycerides	90 mg/dL

Questions

1. What is the probable diagnosis of this patient?

2. Describe the proper follow-up for this patient?

3. What are the appropriate screening tests for diabetes in nonpregnant adults?

4. What are the risk factors that would indicate a potential of this patient's developing diabetes?

Methods of Glucose Measurement

Glucose can be measured from serum, plasma, or whole blood. Today, most glucose measurements are performed on serum or plasma. The glucose concentration in whole blood is approximately 11% lower than the glucose concentration in plasma. Serum or plasma must be refrigerated and separated from the cells within 1 hour to prevent substantial loss of glucose by the cellular fraction, particularly if the white blood cell count is elevated. Sodium fluoride ions (gray-top tubes) are often used as an anticoagulant and preservative of whole blood, particularly if analysis is delayed. The fluoride inhibits glycolytic enzymes. However, although fluoride maintains long-term glucose stability, the rates of decline of glucose in the first hour after sample collection in tubes with and without fluoride are virtually identical. Therefore, the plasma should be separated from the cells as soon as possible. Fasting blood glucose (FBG) should be obtained in the morning after an approximately 8- to 10-hour fast (not longer than 16 h). Fasting plasma glucose values have a diurnal variation with the mean FBG higher in the morning than in the afternoon.[8] Diabetes in patients tested in the afternoon may be missed because of this variation. Cerebrospinal fluid and urine can also be analyzed. Urine glucose measurement is not used in diabetes diagnosis; however, some patients use this measurement for monitoring purposes.

CASE STUDY 14-7

For three consecutive quarters, a fasting glucose and glycosylated hemoglobin were performed on a patient. The results are as follows:

	QUARTER 1	QUARTER 2	QUARTER 3
Plasma glucose, fasting	280 mg/dL	85 mg/dL	91 mg/dL
Glycosylated hemoglobin	7.8%	15.3%	8.5%

Questions

1. In which quarter was the patient's glucose best controlled? The least controlled?

2. Do the fasting plasma glucose and glycosylated hemoglobin match? Why or why not?

3. What methods are used to measure glycosylated hemoglobin?

4. What potential conditions might cause erroneous results?

The ability of glucose to function as a reducing agent has been useful in the detection and quantitation of carbohydrates in body fluids. Glucose and other carbohydrates are capable of converting cupric ions in alkaline solution to cuprous ions. The solution loses its deep-blue color and a red precipitate of cuprous oxide forms. Benedict's and Fehling's reagents, which contain an alkaline solution of cupric ions stabilized by citrate or tartrate, respectively, have been used to detect reducing agents in urine and other body fluids. Another chemical characteristic that used to be exploited to quantitate carbohydrates is the ability of these molecules to form Schiff bases with aromatic amines. O-Toluidine in a hot acidic solution will yield a colored compound with an absorbance maximum at 630 nm. Galactose, an aldohexose, and mannose, an aldopentose, will also react with O-toluidine and produce a colored compound that can interfere with the reaction. The Schiff base reaction with O-toluidine is of historical interest only and has been replaced by more specific enzymatic methods, which are discussed in the following section.

The most common methods of glucose analysis use the enzyme glucose oxidase or hexokinase (Table 14-10). Glucose oxidase is the most specific enzyme reacting with only β-D-glucose. Glucose oxidase converts β-D-glucose to gluconic acid. Mutarotase may be added to the reaction to facilitate the conversion of α-D-glucose to β-D-glucose. Oxygen is consumed and hydrogen peroxide (H_2O_2) is produced. The reaction can be monitored polarographically either by measuring the rate of disappearance of oxygen using an oxygen electrode or by consuming H_2O_2 in a side reaction. Horseradish peroxidase is used to catalyze the second reaction, and the H_2O_2 is used to oxidize a dye compound. Two commonly used chromogens are 3-methyl-2-benzothiazolinone hydrazone and N,N-dimethylaniline. The shift in absorbance can be monitored spectrophotometrically and is proportional to the amount of glucose present in the specimen. This coupled reaction is known as the Trinder reaction. However, the peroxidase coupling reaction used in the glucose oxidase method is subject to positive and negative interference. Increased levels of uric acid, bilirubin, and ascorbic acid can cause falsely decreased values as a result of these substances being oxidized by peroxidase, which then prevents the oxidation and detection of the chromogen. Strong oxidizing substances, such as bleach, can cause falsely increased values. An oxygen consumption electrode can be used to perform the direct measurement of oxygen by the polarographic technique, which avoids this interference. Oxygen depletion is measured and is proportional to the amount of glucose present. Polarographic glucose analyzers measure the rate of oxygen consumption because glucose is oxidized under first-order conditions using glucose oxidase reagent. The H_2O_2 formed must be eliminated in a side reaction

TABLE 14-10	METHODS OF GLUCOSE MEASUREMENT

Glucose oxidase	$Glucose + O_2 + H_2O \xrightarrow{\text{glucose oxidase}} gluconic\ acid + H_2O_2$
	$H_2O_2 + reduced\ chromogen \xrightarrow{\text{peroxidase}} oxidized\ chromogen + H_2O$
Hexokinase	$Glucose + ATP \xrightarrow{\text{hexokinase}} glucose\text{-}6\text{-}PO_4 + ADP$
	$Glucose\text{-}6\text{-}PO_4 + NADP^+ \xrightarrow{\text{G-6-PD}} NADPH + 6\text{-}phosphogluconate$
Clinitest	$Cu^{2+} \xrightarrow{\text{Reducing substance}} Cu^{1+}O$

to prevent the reaction from reversing. Molybdate can be used to catalyze the oxidation of iodide to iodine by H_2O_2 or catalase can be used to catalyze oxidation of ethanol by H_2O_2, forming acetaldehyde and H_2O.

The hexokinase method is considered more accurate than the glucose oxidase methods because the coupling reaction using glucose-6-phosphate dehydrogenase is highly specific; therefore, it has less interference than the coupled glucose oxidase procedure. Hexokinase in the presence of ATP converts glucose to glucose-6-phosphate. Glucose-6-phosphate and the cofactor $NADP^+$ are converted to 6-phosphogluconate and NADPH by glucose-6-phosphate dehydrogenase. NADPH has a strong absorbance maximum at 340 nm, and the rate of appearance of NADPH can be monitored spectrophotometrically and is proportional to the amount of glucose present in the sample. Generally accepted as the reference method, this method is not affected by ascorbic acid or uric acid. Gross hemolysis and extremely elevated bilirubin may cause a false decrease in results. The hexokinase method may be performed on serum or plasma collected using heparin, ethylenediaminetetraacetic acid (EDTA), fluoride, oxalate, or citrate. The method can also be used for urine, cerebrospinal fluid, and serous fluids.

Nonspecific methods of measuring glucose are still used in the urinalysis section of the laboratory primarily to detect reducing substances other than glucose. The method given next is the Benedict's modification, also called the Clinitest reaction.

Self-Monitoring of Blood Glucose

The ADA has recommended that individuals with diabetes monitor their blood glucose levels in an effort to maintain levels as close to normal as possible. For persons with type 1 diabetes, the recommendation is three to four times per day; for persons with type 2 diabetes, the optimal frequency is unknown. It is important that patients be taught how to use control solutions and calibrators to ensure the accuracy of their results.[9] Urine glucose testing should be replaced by self-monitoring of

blood glucose; however, urine ketone testing will remain for type 1 and gestational diabetes.

Glucose Tolerance and 2-Hour Postprandial Tests

Guidelines for the performance and interpretation of the 2-hour postprandial test were set by the Expert Committee. A variation of this test is to use a standardized load of glucose. A solution containing 75 g of glucose is administered, and a specimen for plasma glucose measurement is drawn 2 hours later. Under this criterion, the patient drinks a standardized (75 g) glucose load and a glucose measurement is taken 2 hours later. If that level is ≥200 mg/dL and is confirmed on a subsequent day by either an increased random or fasting glucose level, the patient is diagnosed with diabetes (see earlier discussion).

The OGTT is not recommended for routine use under the ADA guidelines. This procedure is inconvenient to patients and is not being used by physicians for diagnosing diabetes. However, if OGTT is used, the WHO recommends the criteria listed in Table 14-7. It is important that proper patient preparation be given before this test is performed. The patient should be ambulatory and on a normal-to-high carbohydrate intake for 3 days before the test. The patient should be fasting for at least 10 hours and not longer than 16 hours, and the test should be performed in the morning because of the hormonal diurnal effect on glucose. Just before tolerance and while the test is in progress, patients should refrain from exercise, eating, drinking (except that the patient may drink water), and smoking. Factors that affect the tolerance results include medications such as large doses of salicylates, diuretics, anticonvulsants, oral contraceptives, and corticosteroids. Also, gastrointestinal problems, including malabsorption problems, gastrointestinal surgery, and vomiting and endocrine dysfunctions, can affect the OGTT results. The guidelines recommend that only the fasting and the 2-hour sample be measured, except when the patient is pregnant. The adult dose of glucose solution (glucola) is 75 g; children receive 1.75 g/kg of glucose to a maximum dose of 75 g.

CASE STUDY 14-8

A 25-year-old healthy female patient complained of dizziness and shaking 1 hour after eating a large, heavy-carbohydrate meal. The result of a random glucose test performed via fingerstick was 60 mg/dL.

Questions

1. Identify the characteristics of hypoglycemia in this case study.

2. What test(s) should be performed next to determine this young woman's problem?

3. To which category of hypoglycemia would this individual belong?

4. What criteria would be used to diagnose a potential insulinoma?

Glycosylated Hemoglobin/HbA₁c

The aim of diabetic management is to maintain the blood glucose concentration within or near the nondiabetic range with a minimal number of fluctuations. Serum or plasma glucose concentrations can be measured by laboratories in addition to patient self-monitoring of whole blood glucose concentrations. Long-term blood glucose regulation can be followed by measurement of glycosylated hemoglobin.

Glycosylated hemoglobin is the term used to describe the formation of a hemoglobin compound produced when glucose (a reducing sugar) reacts with the amino group of hemoglobin (a protein). The glucose molecule attaches nonenzymatically to the hemoglobin molecule to form a ketoamine. The rate of formation is directly proportional to the plasma glucose concentrations. Because the average red blood cell lives approximately 120 days, the glycosylated hemoglobin level at any one time reflects the average blood glucose level over the previous 2 to 3 months. Therefore, measuring the glycosylated hemoglobin provides the clinician with a time-averaged picture of the patient's blood glucose concentration over the past 3 months.

HbA₁c, the most commonly detected glycosylated hemoglobin, is a glucose molecule attached to one or both N-terminal valines of the β-polypeptide chains of normal adult hemoglobin.[10] HbA₁c is a more reliable method of monitoring long-term diabetes control than random plasma glucose. Normal values range from 4.0% to 6.0%. Studies have shown that there is a strong linear relationship between average blood glucose and HbA₁c. Using a linear regression model, Nathan et al.[11] determined that an estimated average glucose (eAG) can be calculated from the HbA₁c reported value

using the equation eAG (mg/dL) = 28.7 × HbA₁c − 46.7 (Table 14-11). However, this information needs to be used carefully, as another study has shown that the relationship between average plasma glucose and HbA₁c can differ substantially depending on the glycemic control of the population studied.[12] It is also important to remember that two factors determine the glycosylated hemoglobin levels: the average glucose concentration and the red blood cell life span. If the red blood cell life span is decreased because of another disease state such as hemoglobinopathies, the hemoglobin will have less time to become glycosylated and the glycosylated hemoglobin level will be lower.

Current ADA guidelines recommend that an HbA₁c test be performed at least two times a year with patients who are meeting treatment goals and who have stable glycemic control. For patients whose therapy has changed or who are not meeting glycemic goals, a quarterly HbA₁c test is recommended. The use of point-of-care testing for HbA₁c allows for more timely decisions on therapy changes and has been shown to result in tighter glycemic control.[13] Lowering HbA₁c to an average of <7% has clearly been shown to reduce the microvascular, retinopathic, and neuropathic complications of diabetes. Therefore, the HbA₁c goal for nonpregnant adults in general is <7%. Further studies have shown a small benefit to lowering HbA₁c to <6%, making this a goal for selected individual patients if possible without significant hypoglycemia.

The specimen requirement for HbA₁c measurement is an EDTA whole blood sample. Before analysis, a hemolysate must be prepared. The methods of measurement are grouped into two major categories: (1) based on charge differences between glycosylated and nonglycosylated

TABLE 14-11	TRANSLATING THE A₁C ASSAY INTO ESTIMATED AVERAGE GLUCOSE VALUES GLUCOSE LEVELS AND A₁C LEVELS[12]	
AVERAGE PLASMA GLUCOSE	**A₁C (%)**
97 mg/dL (5.4 mmol/L)	5
126 mg/dL (7.0 mmol/L)	6
154 mg/dL (8.6 mmol/L)	7
183 mg/dL (10.2 mmol/L)	8
212 mg/dL (11.8 mmol/L)	9
240 mg/dL (13.4 mmol/L)	10
269 mg/dL (14.9 mmol/L)	11
298 mg/dL (16.5 mmol/L)	12

Source: Nathan DM, Kuenen J, Borg R, Zheng H, Schoenfeld D, Heine RJ. Translating the A1C assay into estimated average glucose values. *Diabetes Care.* August 2008;31(8):1473-1478.

TABLE 14-12	METHODS OF GLYCATED HEMOGLOBIN MEASUREMENT	
METHODS BASED ON STRUCTURAL DIFFERENCES		
Immunoassays	Polyclonal or monoclonal antibodies toward the glycated N-terminal group of the β-chain of hemoglobin	
Affinity chromatography	Separates based on chemical structure using borate to bind glycosylated proteins	Not temperature dependent Not affected by other hemoglobins
METHODS BASED ON CHARGE DIFFERENCES		
Ion-exchange chromatography	Positive-charge resin bed	Highly temperature dependent Affected by hemoglobinopathies
Electrophoresis	Separation is based on differences in charge	Hemoglobin F values > 7% interfere
Isoelectric focusing	Type of electrophoresis using isoelectric point to separate	Pre-HbA$_1$c interferes
High-pressure liquid chromatography	A form of ion-exchange chromatography	Separates of all forms of glyco-Hb: A$_1$a, A$_1$b, A$_1$c

hemoglobin (cation exchange chromatography, electrophoresis, and isoelectric focusing) and (2) structural characteristics of glycogroups on hemoglobin (affinity chromatography and immunoassay).

In the clinical laboratory, affinity chromatography is the preferred method of measurement. In this method, the glycosylated hemoglobin attaches to the boronate group of the resin and is selectively eluted from the resin bed using a buffer. This method is not temperature dependent and not affected by hemoglobin F, S, or C. Another method of measurement uses cation exchange chromatography in which the negatively charged hemoglobins attach to the positively charged resin bed. The glycosylated hemoglobin is selectively eluted from the resin bed using a buffer of specific pH in which the glycohemoglobins are the most negatively charged and elute first from the column. However, this method is highly temperature dependent and affected by hemoglobinopathies. The presence of hemoglobin F yields false increased levels, and the presence of hemoglobins S and C yields false decreased levels. A common point-of-care instrument HbA$_1$c assay is based on a latex immunoagglutination inhibition methodology. In this method, both the concentration of HbA$_1$c specifically and the concentration of total hemoglobin are measured, and the ratio reported as percent HbA$_1$c. In this method, glycated hemoglobin F is not measured, so at a very high level of hemoglobin F (>10%), the amount of HbA$_1$c will be lower than expected because a greater proportion of the glycated hemoglobin will be in the form of glycated hemoglobin F. High-performance liquid chromatography (HPLC) and electrophoresis methods are also used to separate the various forms of hemoglobin. With HPLC, all forms of glycosylated hemoglobin—A$_1$a, A$_1$b, and A$_1$c—can be separated.

Standardization of glycosylated hemoglobin has been a continuing problem; there was no consensus on the reference method and no single standard is available to be used in the assays. Because of this, HbA$_1$c values vary with the method and laboratory performing them (Table 14-12). The International Federation of Clinical Chemistry and Laboratory Medicine (IFCC) developed a common definition for HbA$_1$c and a reference method that specifically measures the concentration of only one molecular species of glycated A$_1$c, the glycated N-terminal residue of the β-chain of hemoglobin. This method, using either HPLC/electrospray mass spectrometry or HPLC/capillary electrophoresis, is only used to standardize A$_1$c assays and cannot be used for the clinical measurement of HbA$_1$c.[14] International consensus groups have determined that HbA$_1$c results will be represented worldwide in IFCC units (mmol/mol) and derived NGSP units (%) using the IFCC–NGSP master equation.[15] (Note: The relationship between the NGSP network and IFCC networks was originally expressed as NGSP = [0.9148 × IFCC] + 2.152. In 2007, the IFCC recommended that IFCC HbA1c be expressed as mmol HbA1c/mol Hb. With these new units, the master equation changed to NGSP = [0.09148 × IFCC] + 2.152). This change in units avoids any confusion between NGSP and IFCC results. HbA$_1$c reagent and instrument manufacturers are required to document their traceability to the IFCC reference system with both the IFCC units (mmol/mol) and derived NGSP units (%). In the United States, the NGSP, with the Diabetes Control and Complications Trial (DCCT) HPLC method, is used as a primary reference method. With these developments, HbA$_1$c measurement has become a more reliable indicator of the long-term patient blood glucose regulation

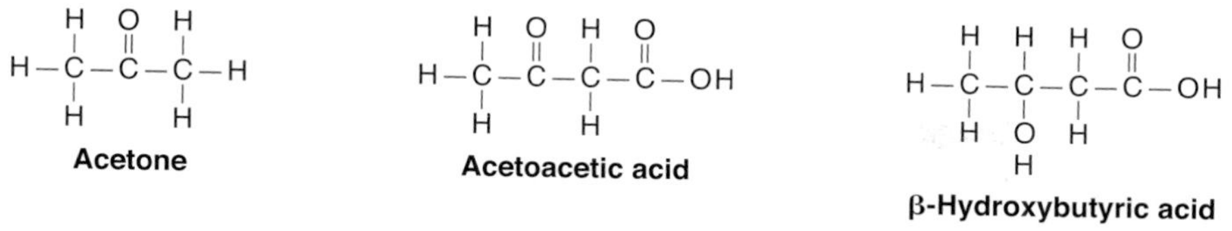

FIGURE 14-9 The three ketone bodies.

with more consistency in the results from laboratory to laboratory.

Ketones

Ketone bodies are produced by the liver through metabolism of fatty acids to provide a ready energy source from stored lipids at times of low carbohydrate availability. The three ketone bodies are acetone (2%), acetoacetic acid (20%), and 3-β-hydroxybutyric acid (78%). A low level of ketone bodies is present in the body at all times. However, in cases of carbohydrate deprivation or decreased carbohydrate use such as diabetes mellitus, starvation/fasting, high-fat diets, prolonged vomiting, and glycogen storage disease, blood levels increase to meet the energy needs. The term *ketonemia* refers to the accumulation of ketones in blood, and the term *ketonuria* refers to the accumulation of ketones in urine (Fig. 14-9). The measurement of ketones is recommended for patients with type 1 diabetes during acute illness, stress, pregnancy, or elevated blood glucose levels above 300 mg/dL or when the patient has signs of ketoacidosis.

The specimen requirement is *fresh* serum or urine; the sample should be tightly stoppered and analyzed immediately. No method used for the determination of ketones reacts with all three ketone bodies. The historical test (Gerhardt's) that used ferric chloride reacted with acetoacetic acid to produce a red color. The procedure had many interfering substances, including salicylates. A more common method using sodium nitroprusside ($NaFe[CN]_5NO$) reacts with acetoacetic acid in an alkaline pH to form a purple color. If the reagent contains glycerin, then acetone is also detected. This method is used with the urine reagent strip test and Acetest tablets. A newer enzymatic method adapted to some automated instruments uses the enzyme 3-hydroxybutyrate dehydrogenase to detect either 3-β-hydroxybutyric acid or acetoacetic acid, depending on the pH of the solution. A pH of 7.0 causes the reaction to proceed to the right

(decreasing absorbance) and a pH of 8.5 to 9.5 causes the reaction to proceed to left (increasing absorbance; Table 14-13).

Microalbuminuria

Diabetes mellitus causes progressive changes to the kidneys and ultimately results in diabetic renal nephropathy. This complication progresses over years and may be delayed by aggressive glycemic control. An early sign that nephropathy is occurring is an increase in urinary albumin. Microalbumin measurements are useful to assist in diagnosis at an early stage and before the development of proteinuria. An annual assessment of kidney function by the determination of urinary albumin excretion is recommended for diabetic patients. Microalbuminuria is defined as persistent albuminuria in two out of three urine collections of 30 to 300 mg/24 h, 20 to 200 µg/min, or an albumin–creatinine ratio of 30 to 300 µg/mg creatinine. Clinical proteinuria or macroalbuminuria is established with an albumin–creatinine ratio ≥ 300 mg/24 h, >200 µg/min, or ≥300 µg/mg.

Although three methods for microalbuminuria screening are available, the use of a random spot collection for the measurement of the albumin–creatinine ratio is the preferred method.[16] Using the spot method, without the simultaneous creatinine measurement, may result in false-positive and false-negative results because of variation in urine concentration. The two other alternatives, a 24-hour collection and a timed 4-hour overnight collection, which are more burdensome to the patient and add little to prediction or accuracy, are seldom required. A patient is determined to have microalbuminuria when two of three specimens collected within a 3- to 6-month period are abnormal. Factors that may elevate the urinary excretion of albumin include exercise within 24 hours, infection, fever, congestive heart failure, marked hyperglycemia, and marked hypertension.[17]

TABLE 14-13	METHODS OF KETONE MEASUREMENT
Nitroprusside	Acetoacetic acid + nitroprusside —alkaline pH→ purple color
Enzymatic	3-β-Hydroxybutyrate + NAD+ —3-HBD→ acetoacetate + H+ + NADH

Islet Autoantibody and Insulin Testing

The presence of autoantibodies to the β-islet cells of the pancreas is characteristic of type 1 diabetes. However, islet autoantibody testing is not currently recommended for routine screening for diabetes diagnosis. In the future, this testing might identify at-risk, prediabetic patients. Insulin measurements are not required for the diagnosis of diabetes mellitus, but in certain hypoglycemic states, it is important to know the concentration of insulin in relation to the plasma glucose concentration.

CASE STUDY 14-9

A nurse caring for patients with diabetes performed a fingerstick glucose test on the Accu-Chek glucose monitor and obtained a value of 200 mg/dL. A plasma sample, collected at the same time by a phlebotomist and performed by the laboratory, resulted in a glucose value of 225 mg/dL.

Questions

1. Are these two results significantly different?

2. Explain.

For additional student resources please visit thePoint at http://thepoint.lww.com. **thePoint**※

QUESTIONS

1. Which of the following hormones promotes gluconeogenesis?
   a. Growth hormone
   b. Hydrocortisone
   c. Insulin
   d. Thyroxine

2. Glucose oxidase oxidizes glucose to gluconic acid and
   a. H_2O_2
   b. CO_2
   c. HCO_3
   d. H_2O

3. From glucose and ATP, hexokinase catalyzes the formation of
   a. Acetyl-CoA
   b. Fructose-6-phosphate
   c. Glucose-6-phosphate
   d. Lactose

4. What is the preferred specimen for glucose analysis?
   a. EDTA plasma
   b. Fluoride oxalate plasma
   c. Heparinized plasma
   d. Serum

5. Hyperglycemic factor produced by the pancreas is
   a. Epinephrine
   b. Glucagon
   c. Insulin
   d. Growth hormone

6. Polarographic methods of glucose assay are based on which principle?
   a. Nonenzymatic oxidation of glucose
   b. Rate of oxygen depletion measured
   c. Chemiluminescence caused by the formation of ATP
   d. Change in electrical potential as glucose is oxidized

7. Select the enzyme that is most specific for β-D-glucose:
   a. Glucose oxidase
   b. Glucose-6-phosphate dehydrogenase
   c. Hexokinase
   d. Phosphohexose isomerase

8. Select the coupling enzyme used in the hexokinase method for glucose:
   a. Glucose dehydrogenase
   b. Glucose-6-phosphatase
   c. Glucose-6-phosphate dehydrogenase
   d. Peroxidase

9. All of the following are characteristic of von Gierke disease EXCEPT
   a. Hypoglycemia
   b. Hypolipidemia
   c. Increased plasma lactate
   d. Subnormal response to epinephrine

10. The preferred screening test for diabetes in nonpregnant adults is measurement of
    a. Fasting plasma glucose
    b. Random plasma glucose

c. Glycohemoglobin

d. Depends on the patient factors

11. Following the 2012 ADA guidelines, the times of measurement for plasma glucose levels during an OGTT in nonpregnant patients are

a. Fasting, 1 hour, and 2 hours

b. Fasting and 60 minutes

c. 30, 60, 90, and 120 minutes

d. Fasting, 30, 60, 90, and 120 minutes.

12. Monitoring the levels of ketone bodies in the urine via nitroprusside reagents provides a semi-quantitative measure of

a. Acetoacetate

b. 3-β-Hydroxybutyrate

c. Acetone

d. All three ketone bodies

13. A factor, other than average plasma glucose values, that can affect the HbA$_1$c level is

a. Serum ketone bodies level

b. Red blood cell life span

c. Ascorbic acid intake

d. Increased triglyceride levels

14. Monitoring the levels of ketone bodies in the urine is

a. Considered essential on a daily basis for all diabetic patients

b. A reliable method of assessing long-term glycemic control

c. Recommended for patients with type 1 diabetes on sick days

d. Not recommended by the ADA

15. A urinalysis identifies a positive result for reducing sugars, yet the test for glucose (glucose oxidase reaction) was negative on the dipstick. What do these results suggest?

a. This is commonly observed with ascorbic acid interference.

b. This may suggest the patient has a deficiency in galactose-1-phosphate uridyl transferase.

c. This may suggest a pancreatic beta cell tumor.

d. This may suggest a deficiency in glycogen debrancher enzyme.

e. It is not possible to obtain these results and there is an analytic error in testing.

16. Urinalysis of a diabetic patient identified the following:

Year 1: Urine albumin was 15 mg/24 h

Year 2: Urine albumin was 56 mg/24 h

Year 3: Urine albumin was 156 mg/24 h

What do these clinical data suggest?

a. These levels of albumin in the urine are normal and no follow-up is necessary.

b. These levels of albumin in the urine suggest that kidney function is compromised and follow-up is necessary.

c. As these values of urinary albumin are not greater than 300 mg/24 h, the patient is not likely to have compromised kidney function.

d. An additional urinary albumin test is required in Year 4 to verify diminishing kidney function.

REFERENCES

1. National Diabetes Data Group. Classification and diagnosis of diabetes mellitus and other categories of glucose tolerance. *Diabetes.* 1979;28:1039-1057.

2. Expert Committee on the Diagnosis and Classification of Diabetes Mellitus. Report of the Expert Committee on the Diagnosis and Classification of Diabetes Mellitus. *Diabetes Care.* 2003;26(suppl 1):S7.

3. Malchoff CD. Diagnosis and classification of diabetes mellitus. *Conn Med.* 1991;55(11):625.

4. American Diabetes Association. *Diabetes Care.* 2012;35:S64-S71.

5. Service FJ. Classification of hypoglycemic disorders. *Endocrinol Metab Clin.* 1999;28(3):501-517.

6. Service FJ. Medical progress: hypoglycemic disorders. *N Engl J Med.* 1995;332(17):1144-1152.

7. Cryer PE. Glucose homeostasis and hypoglycemia. In: Wilson JD, Foster DW, eds. *Williams Textbook of Endocrinology.* Philadelphia, PA: WB Saunders; 1992.

8. Troisi RJ, Cowie CC, Harris MI. Diurnal variation in fasting plasma glucose: implications for diagnosis of diabetes in patients examined in the afternoon. *JAMA.* 2000;284:3157-3159.

9. American Diabetes Association. Tests of glycemia in diabetes. *Diabetes Care.* 2004;27(suppl 1):S91-S93.

10. Eckfeldt JH, Bruns DE. Another step towards standardization of methods for measuring hemoglobin A$_{1c}$. *Clin Chem.* 1997;43(10):1811-1813.

11. Nathan DM, Kuenen J, Borg R, Zheng H, Schoenfeld D, Heine RJ. Translating the A1C assay into estimated average glucose values. *Diabetes Care.* 2008;31:1473-1478.

12. Kilpatrick ES, Rigby AS, Atkin SL. Variability in the relationship between mean plasma glucose and HbA$_1$c: implications for the assessment of glycemic control. *Clin Chem.* 2007;53:897-901.

13. American Diabetes Association. Standards of medical care in diabetes—2012. *Diabetes Care.* January 2012;35(suppl 1):S11-S63.

14. Jeppsson JO, Kobold U, Barr J, et al.; International Federation of Clinical Chemistry and Laboratory Medicine (IFCC): Approved IFCC reference method for the measurement of HbA1c in human blood. *Clin Chem Lab Med.* 2002;40:78-89.

15. Geistanger A, Arends S, Berding C, et al. Statistical methods for monitoring the relationship between the IFCC reference measurement procedure for hemoglobin A1c and the designated comparison methods in the United States, Japan, and Sweden. *Clin Chem.* 2008;54:1379-1385.

16. KDOQI Clinical Practice Guidelines and Clinical Practice Recommendations for Diabetes and Chronic Kidney Disease. *Am J Kidney Dis.* 2007;49(2 suppl 2):S12-S154.

17. Sacks DB, Arnold M, Bakris GL, et al. Guidelines and recommendations for laboratory analysis in the diagnosis and management of diabetes mellitus. *Clin Chem.* 2011;57:p.e1-p.e47. Published May 26, 2011.

Lipids and Lipoproteins

RAFFICK A. R. BOWEN, AMAR A. SETHI,
G. RUSSELL WARNICK, ALAN T. REMALEY

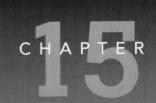

CHAPTER
15

CHAPTER OUTLINE

Chapter Objectives

Upon completion of this chapter, the clinical laboratorian should be able to do the following:

• Explain lipoprotein physiology and metabolism.
• Describe the structure of fatty acids, phospholipids, triglycerides, cholesterol, and the various types of lipoprotein particles.
• Describe the laboratory tests used to assess lipids and lipoproteins, including principles and procedures.

• Identify common lipid disorders from clinical and laboratory data.
• Discuss the incidence and types of lipid and lipoprotein abnormalities.
• Identify the reference ranges for the major serum lipids.
• Relate the clinical significance of lipid and lipoprotein values in the assessment of coronary heart disease.
• Describe the role of standardization in the measurement of lipids and lipoproteins.

KEY TERMS

Arteriosclerosis
Cholesterol
Chylomicrons
Dyslipidemias
Endogenous pathway

Exogenous pathway
Fatty acids
Friedewald equation
HDL
LDL

Lipoprotein
Lp(a)
Phospholipids
Triglycerides
VLDL

Lipoproteins constitute the body's "petroleum industry." Like the great oil tankers that travel the oceans of the world transporting petroleum for fuel needs, chylomicrons are large, lipid-rich transport vessels that ferry their cargo dietary triglycerides, the main oil in the body, throughout the circulatory system to cells, finally docking at the liver as chylomicron remnants. The very low density lipoproteins (VLDLs) are like tanker trucks, redistributing dietary and hepatic synthesized triglycerides to peripheral cells for energy needs or storage as fat. The low-density lipoproteins (LDLs), rich in cholesterol, are like nearly empty tankers that just deliver cholesterol to peripheral cells and liver after their main cargo triglycerides have been off-loaded. The high-density lipoproteins (HDLs) are the cleanup crew, gathering up excess cholesterol for transport back to the liver. Cholesterol is used by the body for such useful functions as facilitating triglyceride transport by lipoproteins and maintaining the normal structure and integrity of cell membranes and as a precursor for steroid hormone synthesis, but when in excess, it can lead to cardiovascular disease.

Lipids and lipoproteins, which are central to the energy metabolism of the body, have become increasingly important in clinical practice, primarily because of their association with coronary heart disease (CHD). Numerous epidemiologic studies have demonstrated that, especially in affluent countries with high fat consumption, there is a clear association between the blood lipid levels and the development of atherosclerosis. Decades of basic research have also contributed to knowledge about the nature of the lipoproteins and their lipid and protein constituents, as well as their role in the pathogenesis of the atherosclerotic process.

The accurate measurement of the various lipid and lipoprotein parameters is critical in the diagnosis and treatment of patients with dyslipidemia. International efforts to reduce the impact of CHD on public health have focused attention on improving the reliability and convenience of the lipid and lipoprotein assays. Expert panels have developed guidelines for the detection and treatment of high cholesterol, as well as laboratory performance goals of accuracy and precision for the measurement of the lipid and lipoprotein analytes. This chapter begins with a review of lipid chemistry and lipoprotein metabolism, followed by the diagnosis and treatment of dyslipidemia. Finally, the clinical laboratory measurement of lipids and lipoproteins will be discussed in the context of the guidelines from the National Cholesterol Education Program (NCEP).

LIPID CHEMISTRY

Lipids, commonly referred to as fats, are ubiquitous constituents of all living cells and have a dual role. First, because they are composed of mostly carbon–hydrogen (C–H) bonds, they are a rich source of energy and an efficient way for the body to store excess calories. Because of their unique physical properties, lipids are also an integral part of cell membranes and, therefore, also play an important structural role in cells. Lipids are also precursors for the steroid hormones, prostaglandins, leukotrienes, and lipoxins. The lipids transported by lipoproteins, namely triglycerides, phospholipids, cholesterol, and cholesteryl esters, are also the principal lipids found in cells and the main focus of this section.

Fatty Acids

Fatty acids, as seen in the structure shown in Figure 15-1, are simply linear chains of C–H bonds that terminate with a carboxyl group (–COOH).[1] In plasma, only a relatively small amount of fatty acids exists in the free or unesterified form, most of which are non-covalently bound to albumin. The majority of plasma fatty acids are instead found as a constituent of triglycerides or phospholipids (Fig. 15-1). Fatty acids are covalently attached to the glycerol backbone of triglycerides and phospholipids by an ester bond that forms between the carboxyl group on the fatty acid and the hydroxyl group (–OH) on glycerol (Fig. 15-1). Fatty acids are variable in length and can be classified as short-chain (4 to 6 carbon atoms), medium-chain (8 to 12 carbon atoms), or long-chain (more than 12 carbon atoms) fatty acids. Most fatty acids in our diet are of the long-chain variety and contain an even number of carbon atoms, such as palmitic acid (16 carbons), stearic, oleic, linoleic, and linolenic acids (18 carbons). Not all of the carbon atoms in fatty acids are fully saturated or bonded with hydrogen atoms; some of them may instead form carbon–carbon (C=C) double bonds. Depending on the number of C=C double bonds, fatty acids can be classified as being saturated (no double bonds) like palmitic acid, monounsaturated (one double bond) like oleic acid, or polyunsaturated (two or more double bonds) like linoleic and linolenic acids. The C=C double bonds of unsaturated fatty acids are typically arranged in the cis form, with both hydrogen atoms on the same side of the C=C double bond, which causes a bend in their molecular structure (Fig. 15-1). These bends increase the space that unsaturated fatty acids require when packed in a lipid layer, and as a result, these fatty acids are more fluid because they do not as readily self-associate and pack together tightly. Fatty acid C=C double bonds can also occur in the trans configuration, with both hydrogen atoms on opposite sides of the C=C double bond. Because of the spatial orientation of their double bonds, trans fatty acids do not bend and have physical properties more similar to saturated fatty acids. The trans fatty acids are not commonly found in nature; however, they are present in our diet because of the chemical hydrogenation treatment used in food processing to increase the viscosity of oils (harden fat)

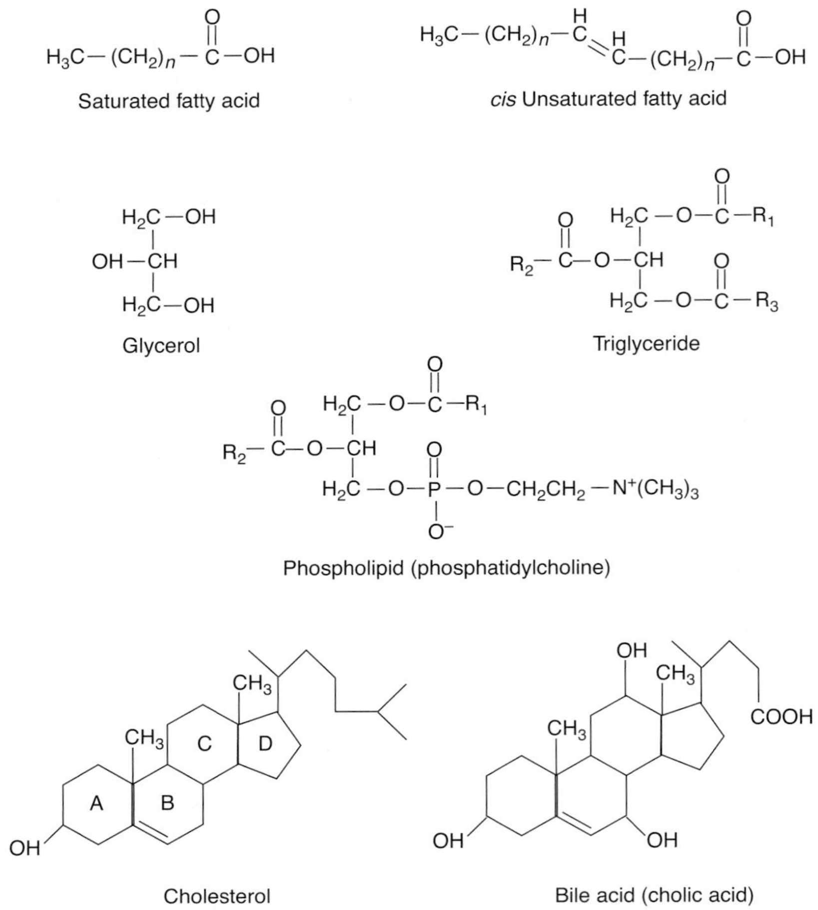

FIGURE 15-1 Chemical structures of lipids. Fatty acids are abbreviated as (R) for triglycerides and phospholipids.

by converting polyunsaturated plant oils into solid margarine, which introduces trans double bonds. The major dietary trans fatty acid is elaidic acid, an 18-carbon fatty acid with one double bond. Both metabolic and epidemiological studies have shown that the consumption of trans fatty acids increases the risk of CHD and hence the recent public health measures to reduce the content of trans fatty acids in our foods.[2] The adverse effects of trans fatty acids are attributed to an elevation of LDL and a decrease in HDL.[2] Most fatty acids are synthesized in the body from carbohydrate precursors, except linoleic and linolenic acids, which are referred to as essential fatty acids.[3] These two fatty acids are found in plants and must be ingested in the diet. Both of these essential fatty acids are important for growth, maintenance, and proper functioning of many physiological processes.

The polyunsaturated fatty acids are classified into omega-3, omega-6, and omega-9 families, depending on the position of the first double bond from the terminal (omega) methyl group of the fatty acid chain. Polyunsaturated fatty acids are precursors for the synthesis of eicosanoids that include prostaglandins, thromboxanes, prostacyclins, and leukotrienes. These fatty acids play a vital role in the structure and function of most biological membranes; and some fatty acids like omega-3 polyunsaturated fatty acids are beneficial in lowering the risk of cardiovascular disease.

Triglycerides

As can be inferred from the name, triglycerides contain three fatty acid molecules attached to one molecule of glycerol by ester bonds[4] in one of three stereochemically distinct bonding positions, referred to as sn-1, sn-2, and sn-3 (Fig. 15-1). Each fatty acid in the triglyceride molecule can potentially be different in structure, thus producing many possible types of triglycerides. Triglycerides containing saturated fatty acids, which do not have bends in their structure (Fig. 15-1), pack together more closely and tend to be solid at room temperature. In contrast, triglycerides, containing cis unsaturated fatty acids (Fig. 15-1), typically form oils at room temperature. Most triglycerides from plant sources, such as corn, sunflower seeds, and safflower seeds, are rich in polyunsaturated fatty acids and are oils, whereas triglycerides from animal sources contain mostly saturated fatty acids and are usually solid at room temperature. As can be seen by inspecting the structure of triglycerides (Fig. 15-1), there are no charged groups or polar hydrophilic groups, making it very hydrophobic and virtually water insoluble. Because it has no charge, triglyceride is classified as a neutral lipid.

Phospholipids

Phospholipids are similar in structure to triglycerides except that they only have two esterified fatty acids (Fig. 15-1).[5] The third position on the glycerol backbone instead contains a phospholipid head group. There are several types of phospholipid head groups, such as choline, inositol, inositol phosphates, glycerol, serine, and ethanolamine, which are all hydrophilic in nature. The various types of phospholipids are named based on the type of phospholipid head group present. Phosphatidylcholine (often referred as lecithin) (Fig. 15-1) has a choline head group and is the most common phospholipid found on lipoproteins and in cell membranes. The two asymmetrically positioned fatty acids in phospholipids are typically 14 to 24 carbon atoms long, with one fatty acid commonly saturated and the other unsaturated.

Because phospholipids contain both hydrophobic fatty acid C–H chains and a hydrophilic head group, they are by definition amphipathic lipid molecules and, as such, are found on the surface of lipid layers. The polar hydrophilic head group faces outward toward the aqueous environment, whereas the fatty acid chains face inward away from the water in a perpendicular orientation with respect to the lipid surface. Phospholipids are synthesized in the cytosolic compartment of all organs of the body, especially the liver with phosphatidylcholine and phosphatidylethanolamine being the most abundant phospholipids in the body.[6]

Cholesterol

Cholesterol is an unsaturated steroid alcohol containing four rings (A, B, C, and D), and it has a single C–H side chain tail similar to a fatty acid in its physical properties (Fig. 15-1).[7] The only hydrophilic part of cholesterol is the hydroxyl group in the A-ring. Cholesterol is, therefore, also an amphipathic lipid and is found on the surface of lipid layers along with phospholipids. Cholesterol is oriented in lipid layers so that the four rings and the side chain tail are buried in the membrane in a parallel orientation to the fatty acid acyl chains on adjacent phospholipid molecules. The polar hydroxyl group on the cholesterol A-ring faces outward, away from the lipid layer, allowing it to interact with water by noncovalent hydrogen bonding.

Cholesterol can also exist in an esterified form called cholesteryl ester, with the hydroxyl group conjugated by an ester bond to a fatty acid, in the same way as in triglycerides. In contrast to free cholesterol, there are no polar groups on cholesteryl esters, making them very hydrophobic. Because it is not charged, cholesteryl esters are classified as a neutral lipid and are not found on the surface of lipid layers but instead are located in the center of lipid drops and lipoproteins, along with triglycerides.

Cholesterol is almost exclusively synthesized by animals, but plants do contain other sterols (called phytosterols) similar in structure to cholesterol. Dietary phytosterols are known to   lower plasma total cholesterol and LDL cholesterol (LDL-C) and raise HDL cholesterol (HDL-C) levels most likely by interfering with the intestinal absorption of cholesterol.[8]

Cholesterol is synthesized in most tissues of the body from acetyl-CoA in the microsomal and cytosolic compartments of the cell. More than 25 enzymes are involved in the formation of cholesterol from acetyl-CoA. The principal steps include the conversion of acetyl-CoA derived from either the β-oxidation of fatty acids or the oxidative decarboxylation of pyruvate to β-hydroxy β-methyl glutaryl CoA (HMG-CoA).[9] HMG-CoA is then converted to mevalonic acid by the enzyme HMG-CoA reductase, the rate-limiting enzyme in cholesterol biosynthesis.[9] Mevalonic acid is phosphorylated, isomerized, and converted to geranyl- and farnesyl pyrophosphate, which, in turn, forms squalene.[9] Cyclization of squalene occurs with oxidation, methyl group transfer reactions, saturation of the side chain, and double bond shifting to produce cholesterol.[9]

Cholesterol is also unique in that, unlike other lipids, it is not readily catabolized by most cells and, therefore, does not serve as a source of fuel. Cholesterol can, however, be converted in the liver to primary bile acids, such as cholic acid (Fig. 15-1) and chenodeoxycholic acid, which promote fat absorption in the intestine by acting as detergents. A small amount of cholesterol can also be converted by some tissue, such as the adrenal gland, testis, and ovary, to steroid hormones, such as glucocorticoids, mineralocorticoids, and estrogens. Finally, a small amount of cholesterol, after first being converted to 7-dehydrocholesterol, can also be transformed to vitamin D_3 in the skin by irradiation from sunlight.

GENERAL LIPOPROTEIN STRUCTURE

The prototypical structure of a lipoprotein particle is shown in Figure 15-2. Lipoproteins are typically spherical in shape and range in size from 10 to 1,200 nm (Table 15-1) As the name implies, lipoproteins are composed of both lipids and proteins, called apolipoproteins.[10-12] The amphipathic cholesterol and phospholipid molecules are primarily found on the surface of lipoproteins as a single monolayer, whereas the

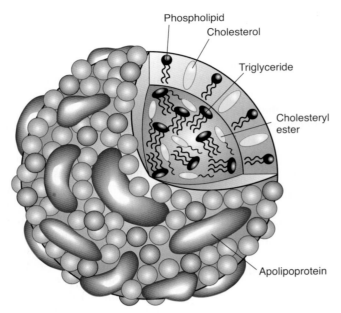

FIGURE 15-2 Model of lipoprotein structure.

hydrophobic and neutral triglyceride and cholesteryl ester molecules are found in the central or core region (Fig. 15-2). Because the main role of lipoproteins is the delivery of fuel to peripheral cells, the core of the lipoprotein particle essentially represents the cargo that is being transported by lipoproteins. The size of the lipoprotein particle correlates with its lipid content. The larger lipoprotein particles have correspondingly larger core regions and, therefore, contain relatively more triglyceride and cholesteryl ester. The larger lipoprotein particles also contain more lipid relative to protein and thus are lighter in density. The various lipoprotein particles were originally separated by ultracentrifugation into different density fractions (chylomicrons [chylos], VLDL, LDL, and HDL), which still form the basis for the most commonly used lipoprotein classification system (Table 15-1).

Apolipoproteins are primarily located on the surface of lipoprotein particles (Table 15-2). They help maintain the structural integrity of lipoproteins and also serve as ligands for cell receptors and as activators and inhibitors of the various enzymes that modify lipoprotein particles (Table 15-2). Apolipoproteins contain a structural motif called an amphipathic helix,[13] which accounts for the ability of these proteins to bind to lipids. Amphipathic helices are protein segments arranged in coils so that the hydrophobic amino acid residues interact with lipids, whereas the part of the helix containing hydrophilic amino acids faces away from the lipids and toward the aqueous environment.

Apolipoprotein (apo) A-I, the major protein of HDL, is frequently used as a measure of the amount of the antiatherogenic HDL present in plasma.[14] Apo B is a large protein with a molecular weight of

TABLE 15-1	CHARACTERISTICS OF THE MAJOR HUMAN LIPOPROTEINS			
CHARACTERISTICS	**CHYLOS**	**VLDL**	**LDL**	**HDL**
Density (g/mL)	<0.93	0.93–1.006	1.019–1.063	1.063–1.21
Molecular weight (kD)	$(0.4–30) \times 10^9$	$(10–80) \times 10^6$	2.75×10^6	$(1.75–3.6) \times 10^5$
Diameter (nm)	80–1,200	30–80	18–30	5–12
Total lipid (% by weight)	98	89–96	77	50
Triglycerides (% by weight)	84	44–60	11	3
Total cholesterol (% by weight)	7	16–22	62	19

CHYLOS, chylomicrons; VLDL, very low density lipoprotein; LDL, low-density lipoprotein; HDL, high-density lipoprotein.

TABLE 15-2	CHARACTERISTICS OF THE MAJOR HUMAN APOLIPOPROTEINS			
APOLIPOPROTEIN	**MOLECULAR WEIGHT (kD)**	**PLASMA CONCENTRATION (mg/dL)**	**MAJOR LIPOPROTEIN LOCATION**	**FUNCTION**
Apo A-I	28,000	100–200	HDL	Structural, LCAT activator, ABCA1 lipid acceptor
Apo A-II	17,400	20–50	HDL	Structural
Apo A-IV	44,000	10–20	Chylos, VLDL, HDL	Structural
Apo B-100	5.4×10^5	70–125	LDL, VLDL	Structural, LDL receptor ligand
Apo B-48	2.6×10^5	<5	Chylos	Structural, remnant receptor ligand
Apo C-I	6,630	5–8	Chylos, VLDL,HDL	Structural
Apo C-II	8,900	3–7	Chylos, VLDL, HDL	Structural, LPL cofactor
Apo C-III	9,400	10–12	Chylos, VLDL, HDL	Structural, LPL inhibitor
Apo E	34,400	3–15	VLDL, HDL	Structural, LDL receptor ligand
Apo(a)	$(3–7) \times 10^5$	<30	Lp(a)	Structural, plasminogen inhibitor

HDL, high-density lipoprotein; Chylos, chylomicrons; LCAT, lecithin:cholesterol acyltransferase; VLDL, very low density lipoprotein; LDL, low-density lipoprotein; LPL, lipoprotein lipase.

approximately 500 kD and the principal protein of LDL, VLDL, and chylomicrons.[15] Apo B exists in two forms: apo B-100 and apo B-48. Apo B-100 is found in LDL and VLDL and is a ligand for the LDL receptor,[16] and it is, therefore, critical in the uptake of LDL by cells. Apo B-48, exclusively found in chylomicrons, is essentially the first 48% or half of the apo B molecule and is produced by posttranscriptional editing of the apo B-100 mRNA found in chromosome 2.[17] Apo B-100 can also be found covalently linked to apo (a),[18] a plasminogen-like protein that is found in a proatherogenic lipoprotein particle called lipoprotein (a) (Lp(a)). Apo E, another important apolipoprotein found in many types of lipoproteins (LDL, VLDL, and HDL), also serves as a ligand for the LDL receptor and the chylomicron remnant receptor.[19] There are three major isoforms of apo E: apo E2, E3, and E4. The apo E isoforms affect lipoprotein metabolism because they differ in their ability to interact with the LDL receptor.[20,21] For example, patients who are homozygous for the apo E2 isoform are at an increased risk for developing type III hyperlipoproteinemia. The connection with lipid metabolism is not completely understood, but individuals with the apo E4 isoform have been shown to have an increased risk of developing Alzheimer's disease.[22,23]

Chylomicrons

Chylomicrons, which contain apo B-48, are the largest and the least dense of the lipoprotein particles, having diameters as large as 1,200 nm[19] (Table 15-1). Because of their large size, they scatter light, which accounts for the turbidity or milky appearance of postprandial plasma. Because they are so light, they also readily float to the top of plasma when stored for hours or overnight at 4°C and form a creamy layer. Chylomicrons are produced by the intestine, where they are packaged with absorbed dietary lipids and apolipoproteins. Once they enter the circulation, triglycerides and cholesteryl esters in chylomicrons are rapidly hydrolyzed by lipases and, within a few hours, are transformed into chylomicron remnant particles, which are recognized by proteoglycans and remnant receptors in the liver, facilitating their uptake.[19] The principal role of chylomicrons is the delivery of dietary lipids to hepatic and peripheral cells.

Very Low Density Lipoproteins

VLDL is produced primarily by the liver and contains apo B-100, the main apolipoprotein, apo E, and apo Cs; like chylomicrons, they are also rich in triglycerides.[24,25] They are the major carriers of endogenous (hepatic-derived) triglycerides and transfer triglycerides from the liver to peripheral tissue for energy utilization and storage. Like chylomicrons, they also reflect light and account for most of the turbidity observed in fasting hyperlipidemic plasma specimens, although they do not form a creamy top layer like chylomicrons, because they are smaller and less buoyant (Table 15-1). Excess dietary intake of carbohydrate, saturated fatty acids, and trans fatty acids enhances the hepatic synthesis of triglycerides, which in turn increases VLDL production.

Intermediate-Density Lipoproteins

Intermediate-density lipoproteins (IDLs), also referred to as VLDL remnants, normally only exist transiently during the conversion of VLDL to LDL.[26] The triglyceride and cholesterol contents of IDL are intermediate between those of VLDL and LDL.[26] Normally, the conversion of VLDL to IDL proceeds so efficiently that appreciable quantities of IDL usually do not accumulate in the plasma after an overnight fast; thus, IDLs are not typically present in normal plasma.[26] In patients with type III hyperlipoproteinemia (dysbetalipoproteinemia or broad beta disease), a rare inborn error of metabolism, elevated levels of IDLs can be found in plasma. This defect is due to an abnormal form of apo E that delays the clearance of IDL.[26] Individuals with this disorder are at a significant risk for peripheral vascular disease (PVD) and coronary artery disease (CAD).[26]

Low-Density Lipoproteins

LDL primarily contains apo B-100 and is more cholesterol rich than other apo B–containing lipoproteins (Table 15-1). They form as a consequence of the lipolysis of VLDL. LDL is readily taken up by cells via the LDL receptor in the liver and peripheral cells.[27] In addition, because LDL particles are significantly smaller than VLDL particles and chylomicrons, they can infiltrate into the extracellular space of the vessel wall, where they can be oxidized and taken up by macrophages through various scavenger receptors.[28] Macrophages that take up too much lipid become filled with intracellular lipid drops and turn into foam cells,[29] which is the predominant cell type of fatty streaks, an early precursor of atherosclerotic plaques.

LDL particles can exist in various sizes and compositions and have been separated into as many as eight subclasses through density ultracentrifugation or gradient gel electrophoresis.[30-32] The LDL subclasses differ largely in their content of core lipids; the smaller particles are denser and have relatively more triglyceride than cholesteryl esters. Recently, there has been great interest in measuring LDL subfractions, because small, dense, LDL particles have been shown to be more proatherogenic and may be a better marker for CHD risk.[33]

Lipoprotein (a)

Lp(a) particles are LDL-like particles that contain one molecule of apo (a) linked to apo B-100 by a single disulfide bond.[18,34] Lp(a) particles are heterogeneous in both size and density, as a result of a differing number of repeating peptide sequences, called kringles, in the apo (a) portion of the molecule. Lp(a) is larger than LDL and has a higher lipid content and a slightly lower density. The concentration of Lp(a) is inversely related to the size of the isoform; the larger size isoforms are not as efficiently secreted from the liver. Plasma levels of Lp(a) vary widely among individuals in the general population but remain relatively constant within an individual. Lp(a) appears to be poorly cleared by the LDL receptor, but the kidney has been postulated as the site of removal.[35]

Elevated levels of Lp(a) (>30 mg/dL) are thought to confer increased risk of premature CHD and stroke. Because the kringle domains of Lp(a) have a high level of homology with plasminogen, a precursor of plasmin that promotes clot lysis via fibrin cleavage, it has been proposed that Lp(a) may compete with plasminogen for binding sites on endothelium and on fibrin, thereby promoting clotting. Clinical studies have demonstrated increasing risk of both myocardial infarction and stroke with increasing Lp(a) concentration; however, the measurement of Lp(a) is not typically part of the routine evaluation of lipid disorders. Its utility is limited by the fact that its contribution to the overall risk is not clear, the accurate measurement of Lp(a) is difficult, there are wide interindividual and intraindividual variations, and specific therapies for reducing its concentration in blood are limited.[27,29] Measuring Lp(a) is thought to be useful in patients with a strong family history of CHD, particularly in the absence of other known risk factors, such as increased LDL-C.

High-Density Lipoproteins

HDL, the smallest and most dense lipoprotein particle, is synthesized by both the liver and the intestine (Table 15-1).[14,36] HDL can exist as either disk-shaped particles or, more commonly, spherical particles.[14] Discoidal HDL typically contains two molecules of apo A-I, which form a ring around a central lipid bilayer of phospholipid and cholesterol. Discoidal HDL is believed to represent nascent or newly secreted HDL and is the most active form in removing excess cholesterol from peripheral cells. The ability of HDL to remove cholesterol from cells, called reverse cholesterol transport, is one of the main mechanisms proposed to explain the antiatherogenic property of HDL. When discoidal HDL has acquired an additional lipid, cholesteryl esters and triglycerides form a core region between its phospholipid bilayer, which transforms discoidal HDL into spherical HDL. HDL is highly heterogeneous and is separable into as many as 13 or 14 different subfractions. There are two major types of spherical HDL based on density differences: HDL$_2$ (1.063 to 1.125 g/mL) and HDL$_3$ (1.125 to 1.21 g/mL). HDL$_2$ particles are larger in size, less dense, and richer in lipid than HDL$_3$ and may be more efficient in the delivery of lipids to the liver.[37,38]

Lipoprotein X

Lipoprotein X is an abnormal lipoprotein present in patients with biliary cirrhosis or cholestasis and in patients with mutations in lecithin:cholesterol acyltransferase (LCAT), the enzyme that esterifies cholesterol.[39] Lipoprotein X is different from other lipoproteins in the endogenous pathway due to the lack of apo B-100.[39] Phospholipids and non-esterified cholesterol are the lipid components (~90% by weight) and albumin and apo C are the main protein components (<10% by weight).[40] Lipoprotein X is mainly removed by the reticuloendothelial system of the liver and the spleen.[40] Other organs, such as the kidney, also actively clear lipoprotein X from the plasma.[40] Lipoprotein X is typically included in the LDL-C value as calculated by the Friedewald equation, as well as in some direct methods for LDL-C but can be separated by LDL-C by ultracentrifugation.[41]

LIPOPROTEIN PHYSIOLOGY AND METABOLISM

The four major pathways involved in lipoprotein metabolism are shown in Figure 15-3. The lipid absorption pathway, the exogenous pathway, and the endogenous pathway all depend on apo B–containing lipoprotein particles and can be viewed as the process to transport dietary lipid and hepatic-derived lipid to peripheral cells. In terms of energy metabolism, these three pathways are critical in the transport to peripheral cells of fatty acids, which are generated during the lipolysis of triglycerides and, to a lesser degree, cholesteryl esters on lipoproteins. In regard to the pathogenesis of

atherosclerosis, the net result of these three pathways is also the net delivery or forward transport of cholesterol to peripheral cells, which can lead to atherosclerosis when the cells in the vessel wall accumulate too much cholesterol.[27,29] Peripheral cells are prone to accumulating cholesterol because they also synthesize their own cholesterol, and, unlike liver cells, they do not have the enzymatic pathways to catabolize cholesterol. Furthermore, cholesterol is relatively water insoluble and cannot readily diffuse away from its site of deposition or synthesis.

The principal way that peripheral cells maintain their cholesterol equilibrium is the reverse cholesterol transport pathway (Fig. 15-3), which is mediated by HDL. In this pathway, excess cholesterol from peripheral cells is transported back to the liver, where it can be excreted into the bile as free cholesterol or after being converted to bile acids. The liver is, therefore, involved in both forward and reverse cholesterol transport pathways and, in many ways, acts as a buffer in helping the body maintain its overall cholesterol homeostasis. There are several genetic defects in the genes that encode for proteins in the forward and reverse cholesterol transport pathways, which result in a predisposition for atherosclerosis.[42,43] The majority of individuals with CAD, however, do not have a clear, single, genetic defect but instead have multiple genetic variations or gene polymorphisms that most likely interact with various lifestyle habits,[44] such as exercise, diet, and smoking, leading to a predisposition for disease.

Lipid Absorption

Because fats are water insoluble, special mechanisms are required to facilitate the intestinal absorption of the 60 to 130 g of fat consumed per day in a typical Western diet. During the process of digestion, pancreatic lipase, by cleaving off fatty acids, first converts dietary lipids into more polar compounds with amphipathic properties.[45] Thus, triglycerides are transformed into monoglycerides and diglycerides; cholesterol esters are transformed into free cholesterol; and phospholipids are transformed into lysophospholipids. These amphipathic lipids in the intestinal lumen form large aggregates with bile acids called micelles. Lipid absorption occurs when the micelles come in contact with the microvillus membranes of the intestinal mucosal cells. Absorption of some of these lipids may occur via a passive transfer process; however, recent evidence suggests that, in some cases, it might also be facilitated by specific transporters, such as the NPC1L-1 transporter for cholesterol.[46,47] Short-chain free fatty acids, with 10 or fewer carbon atoms, can readily pass directly into the portal circulation and are carried by albumin to the liver. The absorbed long-chain fatty acids, monoglycerides, and diglycerides are

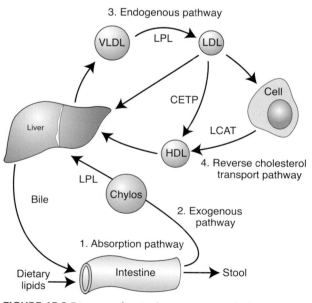

FIGURE 15-3 Diagram of major lipoprotein metabolism pathways.

reesterified in intestinal cells to form triglycerides and cholesteryl esters. The newly formed triglycerides and cholesteryl esters are then packaged into chylomicrons, along with apo B-48.

Triglyceride absorption is efficient; greater than 90% of dietary triglycerides are taken up by the intestine. In contrast, only about half of the 500 mg of cholesterol in the typical diet is absorbed each day. Even a smaller fraction of plant sterols are absorbed by the intestine. Recently, a specific transport system, involving the ABCG5 and ABCG8 transporters, has been described that prevents excess absorption of dietary cholesterol and plant sterols.[48] Individuals with defective ABCG5 or ABCG8 transporters have a disease called sitosterolemia and have a predisposition for atherosclerosis and xanthomatosis because of increased cholesterol and plant sterol absorption.[48] ABCG5 and ABCG8 are also present in the liver and defects in these proteins also impair the elimination of plant sterols into bile for removal from the body.[49]

Exogenous Pathway

The newly synthesized chylomicrons in the intestine (Fig. 15-3) are initially secreted into the lacteals and then pass into the lymphatic ducts and eventually enter the circulation by way of the thoracic duct.[19,50,51] After entering the circulation, chylomicrons interact with proteoglycans, such as heparan sulfate, on the luminal surface of capillaries in various tissues, such as skeletal muscle, heart, and adipose tissue. The proteoglycans on capillaries also promote the binding of lipoprotein lipase (LPL),[52] which hydrolyzes triglycerides on chylomicrons. The free fatty acids and glycerol generated by the hydrolysis of triglycerides by LPL can then be taken up by cells and used as a source of energy. Excess fatty acids, particularly in fat cells (adipocytes), are reesterified into triglycerides for long-term energy storage in intracellular lipid drops. A key protein in triglyceride metabolism is apo C-II, which is found on VLDL and is critical in the activation of LPL. Hormone-sensitive lipase, another lipase that is found inside adipose cells, releases free fatty acids from triglycerides in stored fat when energy sources from carbohydrates are insufficient for the body's energy needs. The hormones epinephrine and cortisol play a key role in the mobilization and hydrolysis of triglycerides from adipocytes, whereas insulin prevents lipolysis by adipocytes and promotes fat storage and glucose utilization.

During lipolysis of chylomicrons, there is a transfer of lipid (mainly triglyceride) and apolipoproteins (apo A-I and C-II) onto HDL, and chlyomicrons are converted within a few hours after a meal into chylomicron remnant particles. Chylomicron remnants are rapidly taken up by the liver through interaction of apo E with the LDL receptor and another receptor on the surface of liver cells called LDL-related receptor protein.[53] Once in the liver, lysosomal enzymes break down the remnant particles to release free fatty acids, free cholesterol, and amino acids. Some cholesterol is converted to bile acids. Both bile acids and free cholesterol are directly excreted into the bile but not all of the excreted cholesterol and bile salt exit the body. As previously described, approximately half of the excreted biliary cholesterol is reabsorbed by the intestine, with the remainder appearing in the stool, as fecal neutral steroids. In the case of bile acids, almost all of the bile acids are reabsorbed and reused by the liver for bile production.

Endogenous Pathway

Most triglycerides in the liver that are packaged into VLDL are derived from the diet after recirculation from adipose tissue.[24,54] Normally, only a small fraction is synthesized de novo in the liver from dietary carbohydrate. VLDL particles, once secreted into the circulation, undergo a lipolytic process similar to that of chylomicrons (Fig. 15-3). VLDL loses core lipids, causing dissociation and transfer of apolipoproteins and phospholipids to other lipoprotein particles like HDL, primarily by the action of LPL, resulting in the conversion of VLDL to denser particles, called IDLs. IDL persists for short periods of time and receives cholesterol esters from HDL in exchange for triglycerides via cholesteryl ester transport protein. As with chylomicron remnants, IDL is transported and taken up by the liver via apo E and the LDL receptor and the triglyceride in IDL are removed by hepatic triglyceride lipase, located on hepatic endothelial cells, producing LDL. During this process, VLDL is converted to VLDL remnants, which can be further transformed by lipolysis into LDL. About half of VLDL is eventually completely converted to LDL, and the remainder is taken up as VLDL remnants by the liver remnant receptors.

LDL particles are the major lipoproteins responsible for the delivery of exogenous cholesterol to peripheral cells due to the efficient uptake of LDL by the LDL receptors.[16] LDL can pass between capillary endothelial cells and bind to LDL receptors on cell membranes that recognize apo B-100. Once bound to LDL receptors, they are endocytosed by cells and transported to the lysosome, where they are degraded. The triglycerides in LDL are converted by acid lipase into free fatty acids and glycerol and further metabolized by the cell for energy or are reesterified and stored in lipid drops for later use. Free cholesterol derived from degraded LDL can be used for membrane biosynthesis, and excess cholesterol is converted by acyl-CoA:cholesterol acyltransferase (ACAT) into cholesteryl esters and stored in intracellular lipid drops.[55] The regulation of cellular cholesterol biosynthesis is, in part, coordinated by the availability of cholesterol delivered by the LDL receptor.[16] Many enzymes in the cholesterol biosynthetic pathway (e.g., HMG-CoA reductase, the main target for the cholesterol-lowering statin-type drugs) are downregulated, along with the LDL receptor, when there is excess cellular cholesterol by a complex mechanism involving both gene regulation and posttranscriptional gene regulation.[56]

Abnormalities in LDL receptor function result in elevation of LDL in the circulation and lead to hypercholesterolemia and premature atherosclerosis.[16,57] Patients who are heterozygous for a disease called familial hypercholesterolemia (FH), with an incidence of approximately 1:500, have only approximately half the normal LDL receptors, which results in decreased hepatic uptake of LDL by the liver and increased hepatic cholesterol biosynthesis. The LDL that accumulates in the plasma of these individuals often leads to the development of CHD by mid-adulthood in heterozygotes and even earlier for homozygotes.[16,57]

Individuals can be classified into two distinct phenotypes based on LDL, namely type A and B. Type A individuals have large buoyant LDL particles, whereas in type B LDL particles are smaller.[58,59] Elevated VLDL is associated with an exchange of VLDL triglycerides for cholesterol esters in HDL, resulting in HDL with decreased cholesterol content.[58,59] Cholesterol esters in LDL are also exchanged for VLDL triglycerides.[58,59] The triglycerides in LDL are subsequently removed by the action of lipases, producing smaller, more dense cholesterol-containing particles.[58,59] These small, dense LDL particles have been found to be an independent predictor of CHD and is also associated with increased risk of metabolic syndrome, which is a group of interrelated metabolic risk factors that appear to promote the development of atherosclerotic cardiovascular disease.[58,59] Small, dense LDL particles have a longer half-life in circulation than normal LDL and are more likely to be modified and taken up by scavenger receptors on macrophage, which will develop into foam cells, one of the critical steps in the development of atheroma.[58,59] It is difficult to define the degree of increased risk with small, dense LDL particles quantitatively because of the common association between small LDLs with other risk factors of atherogenic dyslipidemia.

Reverse Cholesterol Transport Pathway

As previously described, one of the major roles of HDL is to maintain the equilibrium of cholesterol in peripheral cells by the reverse cholesterol transport pathway (Fig. 15-3).[60,61] HDL is believed to remove excess cholesterol from cells by multiple pathways. In the aqueous diffusion pathway,[62] HDL acts as a sink for the small amount of cholesterol that can diffuse away from the cells. Although cholesterol is relatively water insoluble, because it is an amphipathic lipid, it is soluble in plasma

in micromolar amounts and can spontaneously dissociate from the surface of cell membranes and enter the extracellular fluid. Some free cholesterol will then bind to nascent HDL in the extracellular space, and once bound, it becomes trapped in lipoproteins after it is converted to cholesteryl ester by the enzyme LCAT,[63] which resides on nascent HDL and is activated by its cofactor, apo A-I. The nascent HDL is first converted to HDL_3. The formation of cholesteryl ester via LCAT increases the capacity of the surface of HDL_3 particle to absorb more free cholesterol from cell membranes along with apo C-I, C-II, C-III, and E and phospholipids from VLDL and chylomicrons and is converted to HDL_2.[64] HDL_2 can then directly deliver cholesterol to the liver by the scavenger receptor type B1 (SR-B1)[63] and, possibly, other receptors.[10] HDL particles can also transfer cholesteryl esters to chylomicrons and VLDL remnants to be transported to liver. Approximately half of the cholesterol on HDL is returned to the liver by the LDL receptor, after first being transferred from HDL to LDL by the cholesteryl ester transfer protein (CETP),[65] which connects the forward and reverse cholesterol transport pathways (Fig. 15-3). Cholesterol that reaches the liver is then directly excreted into the bile or first converted to a bile acid before excretion.

Another pathway in which HDL mediates the removal of cholesterol from cells involves the ABCA1 transporter.[66] The ABCA1 transporter is a member of the ATP-binding cassette transporter family,[67] which pumps various ligands across the plasma membrane. Defects in the gene for the ABCA1 transporter lead to Tangier disease, a disorder associated with low HDL and a predisposition to premature CHD.[68] The exact substrate for the ABCA1 transporter is not known, but it is believed that the transporter modifies the plasma membrane by transferring a lipid, which then enables apo A-I that has dissociated from HDL to bind to the cell membrane. In a detergent-like extraction mechanism, apo A-I then removes excess cholesterol and phospholipid from the plasma membrane of cells to form a discoidal-shaped HDL particle.[69] The newly formed HDL is then competent to accept additional cholesterol by the aqueous diffusion pathway and is eventually converted into spherical HDL by the action of LCAT (Fig. 15-3). Recently, ABCG1 and ABCG5, which are other ABC transporters, have been described to facilitate the efflux of cholesterol to lipid-rich spherical HDL via a mechanism that appears to be different than the ABCA1 transporter.[70]

LIPID AND LIPOPROTEIN POPULATION DISTRIBUTIONS

Serum lipoprotein concentrations differ between adult men and women, primarily as a result of differences in sex hormone levels, with women having, on average, higher HDL-C levels and lower total cholesterol and triglyceride levels than men.[71] The difference in total cholesterol, however, disappears after menopause as estrogen decreases.[72] Men and women both show a tendency toward increased total cholesterol, LDL-C, and triglyceride concentrations with age. HDL-C concentrations generally remain stable after the onset of puberty and do not drop in women with the onset of menopause. General adult reference ranges are shown in Table 15-3.

Circulating levels of total cholesterol, LDL-C, and triglycerides in young children are generally much lower than those seen in adults.[73] In addition, concentrations do not significantly differ between boys and girls. HDL-C levels for both boys and girls are comparable to those of adult women. At the onset of puberty, however, HDL-C concentrations in boys fall to adult male levels, a drop of approximately 20%, whereas those of girls do not change. It is the lower concentration of HDL-C in men, combined with their higher LDL-C and triglyceride levels, that accounts for much of the increased risk of premature heart disease in men.

The incidence of heart disease is strongly associated with serum cholesterol concentration, particularly LDL-C.[74] Comparisons across different societies show that eating less animal fat and more grains, fruits, and vegetables, as is common in many Asian populations, is associated with lower LDL-C and lower rates of heart disease compared with societies that ingest more fat, particularly animal fat, and are more sedentary.[75,76] These differences can be attributed to both genetic and lifestyle factors in the various countries and ethnic groups. The importance of diet was clearly shown in a study that compared the dietary patterns and heart disease rates in Japanese men living in Japan, Hawaii, and California.[77] In this study, as dietary intake became more westernized, with increased consumption of fat and cholesterol, the LDL-C concentrations increased, as did the rates of heart disease. Japanese men living in California were found to have much higher rates of heart disease than Japanese men living in Japan; those in Hawaii were intermediate. Within societies in which diet tends to be more homogeneous, LDL-C levels become somewhat less discriminatory as a

TABLE 15-3	ADULT REFERENCE RANGES FOR LIPIDS
ANALYTE	**REFERENCE RANGE**
Total cholesterol	140–200 mg/dL (3.6–5.2 mmol/L)
HDL-C	40–75 mg/dL (1.0–2.0 mmol/L)
LDL-C	50–130 mg/dL (1.3–3.4 mmol/L)
Triglycerides	60–150 mg/dL (0.7–1.7 mmol/L)

HDL-C, high-density lipoprotein cholesterol; LDL-C, low-density lipoprotein cholesterol.

CASE STUDY 15-1

A 52-year-old man went to his physician for a physical examination. The patient had been a district manager for an automobile insurance company for the past 10 years and was 24 pounds overweight. He had missed his last two appointments with the physician because of business. The urinalysis dipstick finding was not remarkable. His blood pressure was elevated. The blood chemistry results are listed in Case Study Table 15-1.1.

CASE STUDY TABLE 15-1.1
LABORATORY RESULTS

ANALYTE	PATIENT VALUE	REFERENCE RANGE
Na^+	151	135–143 mmol/L
K^+	4.5	3.0–5.0 mmol/L
Cl^-	106	98–103 mmol/L
CO_2 content	13	22–27 mmol/L
Total protein	5.7	6.5–8.0 g/dL
Albumin	1.6	3.5–5.0 g/dL
Ca^{2+}	7.9	9.0–10.5 mg/dL
Cholesterol	210	140–200 mg/dL
Uric acid	6.2	3.5–7.9 mg/dL
Creatinine	2.5	0.5–1.2 mg/dL
BUN	95	7–25 mg/dL
Glucose	88	75–105 mg/dL
Total bilirubin	1.2	0.2–1.0 mg/dL
Alkaline phosphatase	27	7–59 IU/L
Lactate dehydrogenase	202	90–190 IU/L
Aspartate transaminase	39	8–40 IU/L
Amylase	152	76–375 IU/L

Questions

1. Given the abnormal tests, what additional information would you like to have?

2. If this patient had triglycerides of 100 mg/dL (1.1 mmol/L) and an HDL-C of 23 mg/dL (0.6 mmol/L), what would be his calculated LDL-C value?

3. If, however, his triglycerides were 476 mg/dL (5.4 mmol/L), with an HDL-C of 23 mg/dL (0.6 mmol/L), what would be his calculated LDL-C value?

TABLE 15-4	CORONARY HEART DISEASE RISK FACTORS DETERMINED BY THE NCEP ADULT TREATMENT PANELS

POSITIVE RISK FACTORS

- Age: ≥ 45 y for men; ≥ 55 y or premature menopause for women
- Family history of premature CHD
- Current cigarette smoking
- Hypertension (blood pressure ≥ 140/90 mm Hg or taking antihypertensive medication)
- LDL-C concentration ≥ 160 mg/dL (≥ 4.1 mmol/L), with ≤ 1 risk factor
- LDL-C concentration ≥ 130 mg/dL (3.4 mmol/L), with ≥ 2 risk factors
- LDL-C concentration ≥ 100 mg/dL (2.6 mmol/L), with CHD or risk equivalent
- HDL-C concentration < 40 mg/dL (< 1.0 mmol/L)
- Diabetes mellitus = CHD risk equivalent
- Metabolic syndrome (multiple metabolic risk factors)

NEGATIVE RISK FACTORS

- HDL-C concentration ≥ 60 mg/dL (≥ 1.6 mmol/L)
- LDL-C concentration < 100 mg/dL (< 2.6 mmol/L)

CHD, coronary heart disease; LDL-C, low-density lipoprotein cholesterol; HDL-C, high-density lipoprotein cholesterol.

risk factor, and HDL-C levels become more important as a negative risk factor.

The NCEP was formed to alert the American population to the risk factors associated with heart disease. The NCEP has used panels of experts, including Adult Treatment Panels (ATPs), the Children and Adolescents Treatment Panel, and the Laboratory Standardization Panel, to produce various recommendations.[73,78-81] In 1988, the first NCEP ATP developed a list of heart disease risk factors. These guidelines were most recently updated by ATP III in 2002.[81] The current list of risk factors is shown in Table 15-4. ATP III also has recommended that all adults (20 years and older) have a fasting lipoprotein profile performed (total cholesterol, LDL-C, and HDL-C and triglycerides) once every 5 years and has developed guidelines for the diagnosis and follow-up treatment of individuals with abnormal levels (Table 15-5). The Children and Adolescents Treatment Panel has developed similar guidelines for the pediatric population.[73]

The NCEP Laboratory Standardization Panel and its successor, the Lipoprotein Measurement Working Group,[78-80] set laboratory guidelines for acceptable precision and accuracy when measuring total cholesterol, triglycerides, and lipoprotein cholesterol (HDL-C and LDL-C) (Table 15-6).

Obviously, the best way to reduce the prevalence of heart disease is through prevention. Learning and practicing good dietary and exercise patterns early in life, maintaining these patterns throughout life,[71] refraining from

smoking, and controlling blood pressure are important means for reducing the incidence of CHD and stroke.[82] Lipoprotein profile measurements provide a method of identifying individuals who may have levels that put them at risk so that they can receive appropriate treatment. Treatment of other diseases that may affect lipoproteins, such as diabetes mellitus, hypothyroidism, and renal disease, is also important. A prudent diet, low in fat and cholesterol, with a caloric intake adjusted to meet and maintain ideal body weight, along with regular exercise, can significantly reduce the risk of heart disease, stroke, diabetes, and cancer.[83] Dietary intake of fat and cholesterol has been shown to have a synergistic effect, such that dietary cholesterol is more efficiently absorbed when in the presence of dietary fat. Additionally, saturated fat is more atherogenic than unsaturated fat.[71] The American Heart Association has recommended dietary guidelines for the intake of fat and cholesterol for most adult Americans (Table 15-7).

DIAGNOSIS AND TREATMENT OF LIPID DISORDERS

Diseases associated with abnormal lipid concentrations are referred to as dyslipidemias. They can be caused directly by genetic abnormalities or through environmental/lifestyle imbalances, or they can develop secondarily, as a consequence of other diseases.[84,85] Dyslipidemias are generally defined by the clinical

TABLE 15-5	TREATMENT GUIDELINES ESTABLISHED BY THE NCEP ADULT TREATMENT PANELS (INITIAL TESTING SHOULD CONSIST OF FASTING FOR ≥12 H)

RISK CATEGORY AND ACTION

Total cholesterol (TC), <200 mg/dL (<5.2 mmol/L); triglycerides (TG), <150 mg/dL (<1.7 mmol/L); low-density lipoprotein cholesterol (LDL-C), <130 mg/dL (<3.4 mmol/L); high-density lipoprotein cholesterol (HDL-C), ≥40 mg/dL (≥1.0 mmol/L)

Repeat within 5 years

Provide risk reduction information

TC, 200–239 mg/dL (5.2–6.2 mmol/L); TG, 150–199 mg/dL (1.7–2.2 mmol/L); LDL-C, 130–159 mg/dL (3.4–4.1 mmol/L); HDL-C, ≥40 mg/dL (≥1.0 mmol/L); and 0–1 risk factors

Provide therapeutic lifestyle changes diet and physical activity information and reevaluate in 1 y

Provide risk reduction information

TC, ≥200 mg/dL (≥5.2 mmol/L); TG, ≥200 mg/dL (≥2.2 mmol/L); LDL-C, 130–159 mg/dL (3.4–4.1 mmol/L); HDL-C, <40 mg/dL (<1.0 mmol/L); and ≥2 risk factors

Do clinical evaluation, including family history

Start dietary therapy (see below)

TC, ≥240 mg/dL (6.2 mmol/L)

Perform lipoprotein (LDL-C) analysis (see below)

TREATMENT DECISIONS

RISK CATEGORY	ACTION LEVEL	GOAL
DIETARY THERAPY		
No coronary heart disease (CHD); 0–1 risk factors	≥160 mg/dL (4.1 mmol/L)	<160 mg/dL (4.1 mmol/L)
No CHD; ≥2 risk factors (10-y risk, ≥20%)	≥130 mg/dL (3.4 mmol/L)	<130 mg/dL (3.4 mmol/L)
CHD; CHD risk equivalent (10-y risk, >20%)	>100 mg/dL (2.6 mmol/L)	<100 mg/dL (2.6 mmol/L)
DRUG THERAPY		
No CHD; 0–1 risk factors	≥190 mg/dL (4.9 mmol/L)	<160 mg/dL (4.1 mmol/L)
No CHD; 2 risk factors (10-y risk, ≤10%)	≥160 mg/dL (4.1 mmol/L)	<130 mg/dL (3.4 mmol/L)
No CHD; ≥2 risk factors (10-y risk, 10–20%)	≥130 mg/dL (4.1 mmol/L)	<100 mg/dL (3.4 mmol/L)
CHD; CHD risk equivalent	≥130 mg/dL (3.4 mmol/L)	<100 mg/dL (2.6 mmol/L)

characteristics of patients and the results of laboratory tests and are not necessarily defined by the specific genetic defect associated with the abnormality. Many, but not all, dyslipidemias, regardless of etiology, are associated with CHD, or arteriosclerosis.

Arteriosclerosis

In the United States and many other developed countries, arteriosclerosis is the single leading cause of death and disability. The mortality rate has leveled off and started to decrease in the United States in the past three decades, partly as a result of advances in diagnosis and treatment but also because of changes in lifestyle in the American population. This increased awareness of the importance of diet and exercise in preventing CHD has resulted in an overall decrease in the average serum cholesterol concentration and in a lower prevalence of heart disease; however, it still exceeds all other causes of death combined. Although as many women as men develop arteriosclerosis, they typically develop it 10 years later than men, and unfortunately, it sometimes

TABLE 15-6	NCEP ANALYTIC PERFORMANCE GOALS		
	PRECISION	**BIAS**	**TOTAL ERROR**
Total cholesterol	3% CV	±3%	±8.9%
HDL-C			
≥42 mg/dL	4% CV	±5%	±12.8%
<42 mg/dL	SD	<1.7 mg/dL	
LDL-C	4% CV	±4%	±11.8%
Triglycerides	5% CV	±5%	±14.8%

CV, coefficient of variation; HDL-C, high-density lipoprotein cholesterol; SD, standard deviation; LDL-C, low-density lipoprotein cholesterol.

goes unrecognized because of lack of awareness and because symptoms of myocardial infarction are sometimes more subtle in women.

The relationship between heart disease and dyslipidemias stems from the deposition of lipids, mainly in the form of esterified cholesterol, in artery walls. This lipid deposition first results in fatty streaks, which are thin streaks of excess fat in macrophages in the subendothelial space. Autopsy studies have shown that fatty streaks occur in almost everyone older than age 15.[86] Fatty streaks can develop over time into plaques that contain increased number of smooth muscle cells, extracellular lipid, calcification, and fibrous tissue, which can partially block or occlude blood flow. Also, established plaque for unknown reasons can become vulnerable to rupture or erosion, triggering a thrombosis that can block circulation. When plaque develops in arteries of the arms or legs, it is called PVD; when it develops in the heart, it is referred to as CAD; and, when it develops in the vessels of the brain, it is called cerebrovascular disease (CVD). CAD is associated with angina and myocardial infarction, and CVD is associated with stroke. Many genetic and acquired dyslipidemias may also lead to lipid deposits in the liver and kidney, resulting in impaired function of these vital organs. Lipid deposits in skin form nodules called xanthomas, which are often a clue to the presence of an underlying genetic abnormality.

Plaque formation involves repeated cycles of cell injury, followed by infiltration and cell proliferation to repair the site. LDL is believed to play a central role in initiating and promoting plaque formation. It is deposited into the subendothelial space where it is taken up by various cells, including macrophages. This alters the gene and protein expression pattern of these cells and can promote an inflammatory response, particularly when LDL becomes oxidized.[87] Injury signals from the evolving plaque trigger the expression of adhesion

TABLE 15-7	COMPOSITION OF THE THERAPEUTIC LIFESTYLE CHANGES DIET RECOMMENDED BY THE NCEP ADULT TREATMENT PANEL III (COMPARED WITH THE AVERAGE AMERICAN DIET)	
DIETARY NUTRIENT	**TLC DIET**	**AVERAGE AMERICAN DIET**
Total fat	25–35%	36% (% total calories)
Saturated	<7%	15%
Monounsaturated	≤20%	15%
Polyunsaturated	≤10%	6%
Cholesterol		>400 mg/d
Carbohydrate	50–60%	
Fiber	20–30 g/d	
Protein	<15%	

TLC, therapeutic lifestyle changes.

CASE STUDY 15-2

A 30-year-old man with chest pain was brought to the emergency department after a softball game. He was placed in the coronary care unit when his ECG showed erratic waves in the ST region. A family history revealed that his father died of a heart attack at the age of 45 years. The patient had always been athletic in high school and college, so he had not concerned himself with a routine physical. The laboratory tests listed in Case Study Table 15-2.1 were run.

CASE STUDY TABLE 15-2.1
LABORATORY RESULTS

PATIENT ANALYTE	VALUES	RANGE
Na$^+$	139	135–143 mmol/L
K$^+$	4.1	3.0–5.0 mmol/L
Cl$^-$	101	98–103 mmol/L
CO$_2$ content	29	22–27 mmol/L
Total protein	6.9	6.5–8.0 g/dL
Albumin	3.2	3.5–5.0 g/dL
Ca^{2+}	9.3	9.0–10.5 mg/dL
Cholesterol	278	140–200 mg/dL
Uric acid	5.9	3.5–7.9 mg/dL
Creatinine	1.1	0.5–1.2 mg/dL
BUN	20	7–25 mg/dL
Glucose	97	75–105 mg/dL
Total bilirubin	0.8	0.2–1.0 mg/dL
Alkaline phosphatase	20	7–59 IU/L
Lactate dehydrogenase	175	90–190 IU/L
Aspartate transaminase	35	8–40 IU/L
Amylase	98	76–375 IU/L

Questions

1. Given the symptoms and the family history, what additional tests should be recommended?

2. If his follow-up total cholesterol remains in the same range after he is released from the hospital, and his triglycerides and HDL-C are within the normal range, what course of treatment should be recommended?

proteins on endothelial cells and the production of soluble chemotactic proteins from resident macrophages, which promotes the attachment and infiltration of additional macrophages, lymphocytes, and platelets to the plaque. Continual injury and repair lead to additional narrowing of the vessel opening, or lumen, causing the blood to circulate in a nonlaminar manner under greater and greater pressure, which further aggravates plaque formation. The final event leading to complete occlusion of blood flow occurs when there is a hemorrhage into the plaque, which results in the formation of a thrombus that blocks blood flow and precipitates a myocardial infarction.

Because lipid deposits in the vessel walls are frequently associated with increased serum concentrations of LDL-C or decreased HDL-C, lowering LDL is an important step in preventing and treating CHD.[88-90] It is estimated that for every 1% decrease in LDL-C concentration, there is a 2% decrease in the risk of developing arteriosclerosis.[91] For patients with established heart disease, studies have shown that aggressive treatment to reduce LDL-C levels below 100 mg/dL (2.6 mmol/L) or even lower is effective in the stabilization and sometimes regression of plaques.[92] Stabilization of plaque is thought to be at least as important as plaque regression in terms of rupture potential.[93]

In some individuals, high levels of blood cholesterol or triglycerides are caused by genetic abnormalities in which either too much is synthesized or too little is removed.[94-97] High levels of cholesterol and/or triglycerides in most people, however, are a result of increased consumption of foods rich in fat and cholesterol, smoking, and lack of exercise or a result of other disorders or disease states that affect lipid metabolism, such as diabetes, hypertension, hypothyroidism, obesity, liver and kidney diseases, and alcoholism. Low levels of HDL-C are also associated with increased risk of heart disease, but there are currently limited ways to pharmacologically raise HDL-C levels. Existing drugs for increasing HDL-C are primarily fibric acid derivatives (fibrates) and niacin-containing compounds.[98,99] Newer drugs that raise HDL-C by inhibiting CETP may play a role in the future; however, a recent clinical trial with the first CETP inhibitor drug unexpectedly showed increased CHD events.[100] Other drugs using reconstituted HDL particles or administration of apo A-I mimetic peptides is also being actively investigated.[101]

Laboratory analyses are an important adjunct to managing patients with dyslipidemia, because accurate measurement of total cholesterol, HDL-C, and LDL-C and triglyceride levels is needed to determine the most appropriate diet or diet and drug therapy. As shown in Table 15-5, individuals on a low-fat diet, who continue to have LDL-C levels of 190 mg/dL (4.9 mmol/L) or higher on repeated measurement will likely benefit from drug intervention. If they have two or more CAD risk factors and continue to have LDL-C levels of 160 mg/dL (4.1 mmol/L) or higher, they also would benefit from drug therapy. And, if they have already been previously diagnosed with heart disease, drug therapy should be considered when the LDL-C level is 130 mg/dL (3.4 mmol/L) or higher. The average of at least two measurements, taken 1 to 8 weeks apart, should be used to determine the best treatment approach.[81]

Classic bile acid sequestrant drug treatments, such as cholestyramine, colesevelam, and colestipol, work by sequestering cholesterol in the gut so that it is not absorbed; this action enhances conversion of cholesterol into bile acids in the liver, reduces hepatic cholesterol content, and enhances the activity of LDL receptors, and until recently, these were considered to be the only safe drugs for use in children.[91] These bile acid sequestrants lower LDL-C concentrations by 15% to 30%, but may increase triglycerides.[102,103] It is important to note that these agents interfere with the absorption of fat-soluble vitamins and some drugs like digoxin, warfarin, and thyroid supplements, resulting in altered blood concentrations of these drugs and prothrombin times.[102,103] Bile acid sequestrants are contraindicated in individuals with triglyceride levels greater than 400 mg/dL (4.5 mmol/L).[102,103] Bile acid sequestrants have uncomfortable adverse effects such as bloating and constipation and are poorly tolerated.

The most effective class of drugs for managing patients with dyslipidemia are the HMG-CoA reductase drug inhibitors, such as lovastatin, simvastatin, pravastatin, fluvastatin, atorvastatin, and rosuvastatin. These drugs, commonly known as statins, block intracellular cholesterol synthesis by inhibiting HMG-CoA reductase, a rate-limiting enzyme in cholesterol biosynthesis. The reduced level of cholesterol in hepatocytes increases the expression of the LDL receptor, which removes LDL from the circulation, thus reducing the deposition of LDL into vessels and the formation of plaques. All statins are identical in mechanism but differ in dose–response curves. The major safety issues with statins are myositis and hepatotoxic effects; however, patient monitoring in clinical trials has shown that fewer than 2% of patients have sustained increases in liver enzymes. Routine monitoring of serum transaminases for potential hepatotoxicity and creatine kinase for myopathy is still required. These drugs typically reduce LDL-C by as much as 20% to 40%, raise HDL-C by 5% to 10%, and can lower triglyceride by 7% to 43%, depending on the initial triglyceride level.[88,104] Statins are generally well tolerated, with maximum effects observed after 4 to 6 weeks.[88,104] Clinical trials have shown that statin is beneficial for both the primary and secondary prevention of CHD.[81]

Niacin or nicotinic acid at high doses (~2 to 6 g/d) is also a potent drug for reducing LDL-C levels (by 5%

to 25%) and is the only effective drug at this time for significantly raising HDL-C levels (by 15% to 35%).[105] Niacin can also lower triglyceride levels by 20% to 50%[106]; however, it causes flushing, pruritus, hyperuricemia, and diarrhea in many patients and can be hepatotoxic.[107] The precise mechanism of action for niacin is not known, although it appears to act in the liver to reduce the formation of LDL and VLDL by inhibiting lipolysis of triglyceride in adipose tissue and triglyceride synthesis in the liver.[108-110] This action is sufficient to control severe hypertriglyceridemia. Newer slow-release formulations of niacin and combination drugs reduce incidence of flushing.[98]

Fibric acid derivatives, such as clofibrate, gemfibrozil, fenofibrate, and etiofibrate, are most often used to reduce triglyceride by 20% to 50% and increase HDL-C levels by 10% to 20%.[99,107] The effects of fibric acid derivatives on LDL-C concentrations are less predictable and depend on the individual's level of triglyceride.[111] Individuals receiving fibric acid agents should have liver function tests monitored, because these drugs are associated with elevations in transaminases, as well as creatine kinase for patients complaining of muscle ache.[112] Patients on fibrates and warfarin should also have their prothrombin time monitored, because fibrates can displace warfarin from their protein-binding sites.[103]

Ezetimibe is a new drug that inhibits the absorption of cholesterol by inhibiting the Niemann-Pick C1-Like 1 (NPC1-L1) transporter in the intestine without impacting the absorption of fat-soluble nutrients. Ezetimibe therapy has been shown to decrease LDL-C concentrations by approximately 20%.[113] Ezetimibe in conjunction with statins results in greater reductions in LDL-C concentration than with statin alone.[45] As with the use of statin drugs, liver function tests should be performed on individuals taking ezetimibe.[113]

Fish oil products that contain omega-3 fatty acids, eicosapentaenoic and docosahexaenoic acids, can be used to lower triglyceride levels (up to 45%) and raise HDL-C (up to 13%) in patients, although the mechanism of action is not fully understood; it has been shown that fish oils decrease hepatic triglyceride synthesis[114] via inhibition of diacylglycerol acyltransferase, fatty acid synthase, and acetyl-CoA carboxylase enzyme activities. Fish oils also enhance fatty acid β-oxidation by stimulating peroxisome proliferator–activated receptors. In addition, fish oils decrease the hepatic pool of triglycerides by suppressing transcription of the SREBP-1c gene, thereby inhibiting de novo synthesis of fatty acids and triglycerides.[115] However, elevations in LDL-C concentrations (up to 40%) have been observed in some patients receiving omega-3 fatty acids,[116] but LDL-C changes from small, dense atherogenic particles to larger, more buoyant and less atherogenic particles. Clinically, this cholesterol change could offset the increase in LDL-C that may occur. Also, the rise in LDL-C is usually less than the decrease in VLDL cholesterol (VLDL-C).[117] In addition, elevations in serum transaminases have been reported and these enzymes should be monitored periodically for those patients taking omega-3 fatty acids.

Hyperlipoproteinemia

Disease states associated with abnormal serum lipids are generally caused by malfunctions in the synthesis, transport, or catabolism of lipoproteins.[107,118] Dyslipidemias can be subdivided into two major categories: hyperlipoproteinemias, which are diseases associated with elevated lipoprotein levels, and hypolipoproteinemias, which are associated with decreased lipoprotein levels. The hyperlipoproteinemias can be subdivided into hypercholesterolemia, hypertriglyceridemia, and combined hyperlipidemia, with elevations of both cholesterol and triglycerides.

Hypercholesterolemia

Hypercholesterolemia is the lipid abnormality most closely linked to heart disease.[74] One form of the disease, which is associated with genetic abnormalities that predispose affected individuals to elevated cholesterol levels, is called FH. Homozygotes for FH are fortunately rare (1:1 million in the population) and can have total cholesterol concentrations as high as 800 to 1,000 mg/dL (20 to 26 mmol/L). These patients can have their first heart attack when still in their teenage years.[119] Heterozygotes for the disease are seen much more frequently (1:500 in the population) because it is an autosomal codominant disorder; a defect in just one of the two copies of the LDL receptor can adversely affect lipid levels. Heterozygotes tend to have total cholesterol concentrations in the range of 300 to 600 mg/dL (8 to 15 mmol/L) and, if not treated, become symptomatic for heart disease in their twenties to fifties. Approximately 5% of patients younger than age 50 with CAD are FH heterozygotes. Other symptoms associated with FH include tendinous and tuberous xanthomas, which are cholesterol deposits under the skin, and arcus, which are cholesterol deposits in the cornea.[118]

In both homozygotes and heterozygotes, the cholesterol elevation is primarily associated with an increase in LDL-C. These individuals synthesize intracellular cholesterol normally but lack, or are deficient in, active LDL receptors. There are several classes of defects in the LDL receptor gene that are associated with FH. Class 1 mutations result in null allele where no LDL receptor protein is identified. Class 2 mutation, which accounts for the majority of clinical mutations in FH, creates a membrane protein that is synthesized but not transported to the Golgi in a timely manner and, thus, is degraded. Class 3 mutations result in an LDL receptor that cannot bind LDL. Class 4 mutations create an LDL receptor that cannot internalize the

CASE STUDY 15-3

A 43-year-old white man was diagnosed with hyperlipidemia at age 13 years, when his father died of a myocardial infarction at age 34 years. The man's grandfather had died at age 43 years, also of a myocardial infarction. Currently, the man is active and asymptomatic with regard to CHD. He is taking 40 mg of lovastatin (Mevacor), 2 times/d (maximum dose). He had previously taken niacin but could not tolerate it because of flushing and gastrointestinal distress, nor could he tolerate cholestyramine resin (Questran). His physical examination is remarkable for bilateral Achilles tendon thickening/xanthomas and a right carotid bruit (Case Study Table 15-3.1).

CASE STUDY TABLE 15-3.1
LABORATORY RESULTS

Triglycerides	91 mg/dL
Total cholesterol	269 mg/dL
HDL-C	47 mg/dL
LDL-C	204 mg/dL
Aspartate aminotransferase	34 U/L
Alanine aminotransferase	36 U/L
Alkaline phosphatase	53 U/L
Electrolytes and fasting glucose	Normal

Questions

1. What is his diagnosis?

2. Does he need further workup?

3. What other laboratory tests should be done?

4. Does he need further drug treatment? If so, what?

LDL and transport it to the Golgi, and class 5 mutations create LDL receptors that do not recyle.[120] Mutations in the LDL receptor gene promoter region have also been described.[121] Consequently, LDL builds up in the circulation because there are insufficient receptors to bind the LDL and transfer the cholesterol into the cells. Cells, however, which require cholesterol for use in cell membrane and hormone production, synthesize cholesterol intracellularly at an increased rate to compensate for the lack of cholesterol from the receptor-mediated mechanism.

In FH heterozygotes and other forms of hypercholesterolemia, reduction in the rate of internal cholesterol synthesis, by inhibition of HMG-CoA reductase with statin drugs, stimulates the production of additional LDL receptors, particularly in the liver, which removes LDL from the circulation. Homozygotes, however, do not usually benefit as much from this type of therapy, because they do not have enough functional receptors to stimulate. Homozygotes can be treated by a technique called LDL pheresis, a method similar to the dialysis treatment, in which blood is periodically drawn from the patient, processed to remove LDL, and returned to the patient.[119,122]

Most individuals with elevated LDL-C levels do not have FH but are still at increased risk for premature CHD[74,81,91] and should be maintained on a low-fat, low-cholesterol diet and receive statin treatment when necessary (Table 15-5). Regular physical activity should also be incorporated, with drug therapy (Table 15-5).

Hypertriglyceridemia

The NCEP ATP has identified borderline high triglycerides as levels of 150 to 200 mg/dL (1.7 to 2.3 mmol/L), high as 200 to 500 mg/dL (2.3 to 5.6 mmol/L), and very high as greater than 500 mg/dL (>5.6 mmol/L).[81] Hypertriglyceridemia can be a consequence of genetic abnormalities, called familial hypertriglyceridemia, or the result of secondary causes, such as hormonal abnormalities associated with the pancreas, adrenal glands, and pituitary, or of diabetes mellitus or nephrosis. Diabetes mellitus leads to increased shunting of glucose into the pentose pathway, causing increased fatty acid synthesis. Renal failure depresses the removal of large-molecular-weight constituents like triglycerides, causing increased serum levels. Hypertriglyceridemia is generally a result of an imbalance between synthesis and clearance of VLDL in the circulation.[122-124] In some studies, hypertriglyceridemia has not been shown as an independent risk factor for CHD, but many CHD patients have moderately elevated triglycerides in conjunction with decreased HDL-C levels.[125] It is often difficult to separate the risk associated with increased triglycerides from that of decreased HDL-C, but hypertriglyceridemia is now generally considered an important and potentially treatable risk factor for CHD.

Triglycerides are influenced by a number of hormones, such as insulin, glucagon, pituitary growth hormone, adrenocorticotropic hormone (ACTH), thyrotropin, and adrenal medulla epinephrine and norepinephrine from the nervous system. Epinephrine and norepinephrine influence serum triglyceride levels by triggering production of hormone-sensitive lipase, which is located in adipose tissue.[126] Other body processes that trigger hormone-sensitive lipase activity are cell growth (growth hormone), adrenal stimulation (ACTH), thyroid stimulation (thyrotropin), and fasting (glucagon). Each process, through its action on hormone-sensitive lipase, results in an increase in serum triglyceride values.

Although severe hypertriglyceridemia (>500 mg/dL [>5.6 mmol/L]) is usually not associated with high risk of CHD, it is a potentially life-threatening abnormality because it can cause acute and recurrent pancreatitis.[107,127] It is, therefore, imperative that these patients be diagnosed and treated with low-fat diets and triglyceride-lowering medication. Severe hypertriglyceridemia is generally caused by a deficiency of LPL located on chromosome 8 or by a deficiency in apo C-II located on chromosome 19, which is a necessary cofactor for LPL activity.[128] Normally, LPL hydrolyzes triglycerides carried in chylomicrons and VLDL to provide cells with free fatty acids for energy from exogenous and endogenous triglyceride sources. A deficiency in LPL or apo C-II activity keeps chylomicrons from being cleared and serum triglycerides remain extremely elevated, even when the patient has fasted for longer than 12 to 14 hours.

Treatment of hypertriglyceridemia consists of dietary modifications, fish oil, and/or triglyceride-lowering drugs (primarily, fibric acid derivatives) in cases of severe hypertriglyceridemia or when accompanied with low HDL-C.[129,130] It is possible that a certain subspecies of chylomicrons and VLDL are atherogenic. Remnants of chylomicrons and VLDL represent subspecies that have been partially hydrolyzed by lipases and are thought to be potentially atherogenic.[131]

Combined Hyperlipoproteinemia

Combined hyperlipoproteinemia is generally defined as the presence of elevated levels of serum total cholesterol and triglycerides. Individuals presenting with this syndrome are considered at increased risk for CHD. In one genetic form of this condition, called familial combined hyperlipoproteinemia (FCH), individuals from an affected kindred may only have elevated cholesterol, whereas others only have elevated triglycerides, and yet others, elevations of both. FCH is due in part to excessive hepatic synthesis of apoprotein B, leading to increased VLDL secretion and increased production of LDL from VLDL. These patients may have eruptive xanthomata and are at high risk for developing CHD. Another rare genetic form of combined hyperlipoproteinemia is called familial dysbetalipoproteinemia, or type III hyperlipoproteinemia. The name type III hyperlipoproteinemia is a holdover from a lipoprotein typing system developed by Fredrickson et al.,[132] which otherwise is generally no longer used. The disease results from an accumulation of cholesterol-rich VLDL and chylomicron remnants as a result of defective catabolism of those particles. The disease is associated with the presence of a relatively rare form of apo E, called apo E2/2. The apo E2/2 cannot bind with hepatic E receptor and therefore VLDL and chylomicron remnant uptake is impaired.[132-134] Individuals with type III will frequently have total cholesterol values

CASE STUDY 15-4

A 60-year-old woman came to her physician because she was having problems with urination. Her previous history included hypertension and episodes of edema. The physician ordered various laboratory tests on blood drawn in his office. The results are shown in Case Study Table 15-4.1.

CASE STUDY TABLE 15-4.1
LABORATORY RESULTS

PATIENT ANALYTE	VALUES	REFERENCE RANGE
Na^+	149	135–143 mmol/L
K^+	4.5	3.0–5.0 mmol/L
Cl^-	120	98–103 mmol/L
CO_2 content	12	22–27 mmol/L
Total protein	5.7	6.5–8.0 g/dL
Albumin	2.3	3.5–5.0 g/dL
Ca^{2+}	7.6	9.0–10.5 mg/dL
Cholesterol	201	140–200 mg/dL
Uric acid	15.4	3.5–7.9 mg/dL
Creatinine	4.5	0.5–1.2 mg/dL
BUN	87	7–25 mg/dL
Glucose	88	75–105 mg/dL
Total bilirubin	1.3	0.2–1.0 mg/dL
Triglycerides	327	65–157 mg/dL
Lactate dehydrogenase	200	90–190 IU/L
Aspartate transaminase	45	8–40 IU/L
Amylase	380	76–375 IU/L

Questions

1. What are the abnormal results in this case?

2. Why do you think the triglycerides are abnormal?

3. What is the primary disease exhibited by this patient's laboratory data?

of 200 to 300 mg/dL (5 to 8 mmol/L) and triglycerides of 300 to 600 mg/dL (3 to 7 mmol/L). This disorder is associated with an increased risk of PVD and coronary disease.[133] Patients often have palmar xanthomas and tuberoeruptive xanthomas.[134] To distinguish them from other forms of combined hyperlipoproteinemias, it is first necessary to isolate the VLDL fraction with ultracentrifugation. A ratio derived from the cholesterol concentration in VLDL to total serum triglycerides will be greater than >0.30 in the presence of type III hyperlipoproteinemia. If the VLDL fraction is analyzed by agarose electrophoresis, the particles will migrate in a broad β region, rather than in the normal pre-β region. Definitive diagnosis requires a determination of apo E isoforms by isoelectric focusing or DNA typing, resulting in either apo E2/2 homozygosity or, rarely, apo E mutation or deficiency. As with other dyslipidemias, these patients can be treated with a combination of drugs, such as niacin, gemfibrozil, HMG-CoA reductase inhibitors, and low-fat diets. Because of the cholesterol-enriched composition of these particles, use of the Friedewald equation[135] to calculate LDL-C levels will result in an underestimation of VLDL-C and, therefore, an overestimation of LDL-C, compared with beta-quantification ultracentrifugation procedure.[136]

Lp(a) Elevation

Elevations in the serum concentration of Lp(a), especially in conjunction with elevations of LDL, increase the risk of CHD and CVD.[137,138] Higher Lp(a) levels have been observed more frequently in patients with CHD than in normal control subjects,[139] although prospective studies have not conclusively determined this positive association.[140] Lp(a) are variants of LDL with an extra apolipoprotein, called apo (a); the size and serum concentrations of Lp(a) are largely genetically determined.[141] Because apo (a) has a high degree of homology with the coagulation factor plasminogen,[142] it has been proposed that it competes with plasminogen for fibrin binding sites, thus increasing plaque formation.[143,144] Most LDL-lowering drugs have no effect on Lp(a) concentration, even when LDL-C is significantly lowered. The two drugs shown to have some effect are niacin and estrogen replacement in postmenopausal women, but the value of specifically treating patients for high Lp(a) is unclear, and instead lowering LDL-C should probably be the first goal.

Non–HDL Cholesterol

Although LDL-C is widely recognized as an established risk marker for CVD, many studies have demonstrated that LDL-C alone does not provide sufficient measure of atherogenesis, especially in hypertriglyceridemic patients. To address this issue, the calculation of non–HDL-C has been employed. Non–HDL-C reflects total cholesterol minus HDL-C and encompasses all cholesterol present in potentially atherogenic, apo B–containing lipoproteins [LDL, VLDL, IDL, and Lp(a)].[145] Unlike LDL-C, which can be incorrectly calculated using the Friedewald equation in the presence of postprandial hypertriglyceridemia, non–HDL-C is reliable when measured in the non-fasting state.[145] On average, non–HDL-C levels are approximately 30 mg/dL higher than LDL-C levels.[81,146] Recent studies have shown that elevated levels of non–HDL-C are associated with increased CVD risk, even if the LDL-C levels are normal.[147] In clinical studies, non–HDL-C has been found to be an independent predictor of CVD and for diabetes patients; it may be a stronger predictor than LDL-C and triglycerides.[147] The NCEP ATP III has recommended the use of non–HDL-C as a secondary target of lipid lowering, after achieving adequate control of LDL-C and if triglycerides are elevated (≥200 mg/dL [2.3 mmol/L]).[81]

Hypobetalipoproteinemia

Hypobetalipoproteinemia is associated with isolated low levels of LDL-C as a result of a defect in the Apo B gene, but because it is not generally associated with CHD, unless in the homozygous state, it is not discussed further here. Abetalipoproteinemia, which is due to a defect in the microsomal transfer protein used in the synthesis and secretion of VLDL, can also present with low LDL and apo B like hypobetalipoproteinemia. It is an autosomal recessive disorder and like hypobetalipoproteinemia patients, they are not at an increased risk of cardiovascular disease but can develop several neurologic and ophthalmologic problems from fat-soluble vitamin deficiencies.

Hypoalphalipoproteinemia

Hypoalphalipoproteinemia indicates an isolated decrease in circulating HDL, currently defined by the NCEP as an HDL-C concentration less than 40 mg/dL (1.0 mmol/L),[81] without the presence of hypertriglyceridemia. The term alpha denotes the region in which HDL migrates on agarose electrophoresis. There are several defects, often genetically determined, that are associated with hypoalphalipoproteinemia, such as LCAT, apo A-I, and ABCA1 transporter gene mutations.[148,149] Virtually all of these defects are associated with increased risk of premature CHD. An extreme form of hypoalphalipoproteinemia, Tangier disease, is associated with HDL-C concentrations as low as 1 to 2 mg/dL (0.03 to 0.05 mmol/L) in homozygotes, accompanied by total cholesterol concentrations of 50 to 80 mg/dL (1.3 to 2.1 mmol/L).

Treatment options of individuals with isolated decreases of HDL-C are limited. Niacin is somewhat effective but can have adverse effects, such as flushing or even hepatotoxicity, although newer, timed-release preparations may ameliorate those effects.[107,118,150] Lifestyle modifications and treatment of any coexisting disorders that increase CHD risk are also important in these patients.

Acute, transitory hypoalphalipoproteinemia can also be seen in cases of severe physiologic stress, such as acute infections (primarily viral), other acute illnesses, and surgical procedures. HDL-C, as well as total cholesterol, concentrations can be significantly reduced under these conditions but will return to normal levels as recovery proceeds. For this reason, lipoprotein concentrations drawn during hospitalization or with a known disease state should be reassessed in the healthy, nonhospitalized state before intervention is considered.

LIPID AND LIPOPROTEIN ANALYSES

Lipid Measurement

Lipids and lipoproteins are important indicators of CHD risk, which is a major reason for their measurement in research, as well as in clinical practice. It is impractical for individual laboratories or diagnostic manufacturers to establish their own cutpoints, as is commonly done for other analytes. Rather, decision cutpoints used to characterize CHD risk have been developed by the NCEP based on consideration of population distributions from large epidemiologic studies, intervention studies that demonstrated the efficacy of treatment regimens and cost-effectiveness.[81] To improve the reliability of the analytic measurements, standardization programs have been implemented for the research laboratories performing the population and intervention studies, which helped to make results comparable among laboratories and over time.[151] More recently, standardization programs have been extended to diagnostic manufacturers and routine clinical laboratories to facilitate reliable classification of patients using the national decision cutpoints. Thus, accuracy and standardization of results are especially important with the lipid and lipoprotein analytes.

Cholesterol Measurement

Serum or plasma specimens collected from patients in blood collection tubes who have fasted for at least 12 hours are preferred for total cholesterol testing and required for triglyceride testing. If analysis is delayed, the serum/plasma specimen can be refrigerated at 4°C for several days. The lipid workup traditionally has begun with measurement of total serum cholesterol. Early analytic methods used strong acids (e.g., sulfuric and acetic) sometimes together with other chemicals (e.g., acetic anhydride or ferric chloride) to produce a measurable color with cholesterol.[152] Because the strong acid reactions are relatively nonspecific, partial or full extraction by organic solvents was sometimes used to improve specificity. In the past, the reference method for cholesterol involved hexane extraction after hydrolysis with alcoholic KOH followed by reaction with

Liebermann-Burchard color reagent, which comprises sulfuric and acetic acids and acetic anhydride.[153,154] Recently, the reference method has changed to a gas chromatography–mass spectrometry (GC–MS) method that now specifically measures cholesterol and does not detect related sterols. This method shows good agreement with the gold standard method developed and applied at the U.S. National Institute of Standards and Technology, the so-called Definitive Method, using isotope dilution mass spectrometry.[155]

Enzymatic reagents have generally replaced strong acid chemistries in the routine laboratory. Enzymes, selected for specificity to the analyte of interest, provide reasonably accurate quantitation without the necessity for extraction or other pretreatment. Enzymatic reagents are mild compared with the earlier acid reagents and better suited for automated chemistry analyzers. The lipoproteins, HDL and LDL, are generally quantified based on their cholesterol content. Thus, the common lipid panel, including measurements of total cholesterol, LDL-C, and HDL-C, together with triglycerides, can be completed routinely using chemistry analyzers.

Although several enzymatic reaction sequences have been described, one sequence (Fig. 15-4) is most common for measuring cholesterol.[156] The enzyme cholesteryl ester hydrolase cleaves the fatty acid residue from cholesteryl esters, which comprise about two-thirds of circulating cholesterol, converting them to unesterified or free cholesterol. The free cholesterol is reacted by the second enzyme, cholesterol oxidase, producing hydrogen peroxide (H_2O_2), a substrate for a common enzymatic color reaction using horseradish peroxidase to couple two colorless chemicals into a colored compound. The intensity of the resulting color, proportional to the amount of cholesterol, can be measured by a spectrophotometer, usually at a wavelength around 500 nm. Enzymes and reagents have improved so that most appropriately calibrated commercial reagents can be expected to give reliable results. This reaction sequence is generally used on serum without an extraction step but can be subject to interference. For example, vitamin C and bilirubin are reducing agents that could interfere with the peroxidase-catalyzed color reaction, unless appropriate additional enzyme systems are added to eliminate the interference.[157]

Triglyceride Measurement

Measurement of serum triglycerides in conjunction with cholesterol is useful in detecting certain genetic and other types of metabolic disorders, as well as in characterizing the risk of CVDs. The triglyceride value is also commonly used in the estimation of LDL-C by the Friedewald equation. Several enzymatic reaction sequences are available for triglyceride measurement, all including lipases to cleave fatty acids from the glycerol backbone.[158] The freed glycerol participates in any one of several enzymatic sequences. One of the more common earlier reactions, ending in a product measured in the ultraviolet (UV) region, used glycerol kinase and pyruvate kinase, culminating in the conversion of NADH to NAD^+, with an associated decrease in absorbance.[159] This reaction is susceptible to interference and side reactions. The UV endpoint is also less convenient for modern analyzers, so this and other UV reaction sequences have been replaced by a second sequence (Fig. 15-5), involving glycerol kinase and glycerophosphate oxidase, coupled to the same peroxidase color reaction described for cholesterol.[160]

The enzymatic triglyceride reaction sequences also react with any endogenous free glycerol, which is universally present in serum and can be a significant source of interference.[161] In most specimens, the endogenous free glycerol contributes a 10 to 20 mg/dL (0.11 to 0.023 mmol/L) overestimation of triglycerides. About 20% of specimens will have higher glycerol, with levels increased in certain conditions, such as diabetes and liver disease, or from glycerol-containing medications. Reagents are available that correct for endogenous free glycerol and are used by many research laboratories, but such methods are less efficient and hence uncommon in clinical laboratories. The most common correction, designated "double-cuvette blank," is accomplished with a second parallel measurement using the triglyceride reagent without the lipase enzyme to quantify only the free glycerol blank. The glycerol blank measurement is subtracted from the total glycerol measurement obtained with the complete reagent to determine a net or blank-corrected triglyceride result.[162] Another approach, designated "single-cuvette

1. Cholesteryl ester + H_2O $\xrightarrow{\text{Cholesteryl esterase}}$ Cholesterol + Fatty acid

2. Cholesterol + O_2 $\xrightarrow{\text{Cholesterol oxidase}}$ Cholestenone + H_2O_2

3. H_2O_2 + Dye $\xrightarrow{\text{Peroxidase}}$ Color

FIGURE 15-4 Enzymatic assay sequence—cholesterol.

1. Triglyceride + H_2O $\xrightarrow{\text{Bacterial lipase}}$ Fatty acid + Glycerol

2. Glycerol + ATP $\xrightarrow{\text{Glycerokinase}}$ Glycerophosphate + ADP

3. Glycerophosphate + O_2 $\xrightarrow{\text{Glycerophosphate oxidase}}$ Dihydroxyacetone + H_2O_2

4. H_2O_2 + Dye $\xrightarrow{\text{Peroxidase}}$ Color

FIGURE 15-5 Enzymatic assay sequence—triglycerides.

blank," begins with the lipase-free reagent. After a brief incubation, a blank reading is taken to measure only endogenous free glycerol. The lipase enzyme is then added as a second separate reagent and, after additional incubation, a final reading is taken that, after correcting for the blank by the instrument, gives a net or glycerol-blanked triglyceride value.[163] A convenient and easily implemented alternative that does not increase cost—designated calibration blanking—can be done by simply adjusting the calibrator set points to net or blank-corrected values, compensating for the average free glycerol content of specimens. This approach, which is used by some diagnostic reagent companies, is usually reasonably accurate because free glycerol levels are generally relatively low and fairly consistent in most specimens. Most specimens will be blank-corrected reasonably well and only a few specimens will be undercorrected but will still be better than without the calibration adjustment.

Until recently, the triglyceride reference method involved alkaline hydrolysis, solvent extraction, and a color reaction with chromotropic acid,[164] an assay that is tedious, poorly characterized, and was largely only done by the lipid standardization laboratory at the Centers for Disease Control and Prevention (CDC). Like the reference method for cholesterol, the CDC has recently switched to a GC–MS method that involves the hydrolysis of fatty acids on triglycerides and the measurement of glycerol. However, it must be noted that accuracy in triglyceride measurements for clinical purposes might be considered less relevant than that for cholesterol because the physiologic variation is so large, with the coefficient of variation (CV) in the range of 25% to 30%, making the contribution of analytic variation relatively insignificant.

Lipoprotein Methods

Various methods have been used for the separation and quantitation of serum lipoproteins, taking advantage of physical properties, such as density, size, charge, and apolipoprotein content. The range in density observed among the lipoprotein classes is a function of the relative lipid and protein content and enables fractionation by density, using ultracentrifugation. Electrophoretic separations take advantage of differences in charge and size. Chemical precipitation methods, once common in clinical laboratories and now primarily used in research laboratories, depend on particle size, charge, and differences in the apolipoprotein content. Antibodies specific to apolipoproteins can be used to bind and separate lipoprotein classes. Chromatographic methods take advantage of size differences in molecular sieving methods or composition in affinity methods, using, for example, heparin sepharose. Most common in clinical laboratories are direct homogeneous reagents designed for fully automated use with chemistry analyzers, using combinations of detergents and, in some cases, antibodies to selectively assay cholesterol in lipoprotein classes.

Many ultracentrifugation methods have been used in the research laboratory, but ultracentrifugation is uncommon in the clinical laboratory. The most common approach, called preparative ultracentrifugation, uses sequential density adjustments of serum to fractionate major and minor lipoprotein classes.[165] Density gradient methods, either nonequilibrium techniques in which separations are based on the rate of flotation or equilibrium techniques in which the lipoproteins separate based on their density, permit fractionation of several or all classes in a single run.[31,166,167] The available methods use different types of ultracentrifuge rotors: swinging bucket, fixed angle, vertical, and zonal. Newer methods have trended toward smaller scale separations in small rotors, using tabletop ultracentrifuges.[168,169] Ultracentrifugation, although tedious, expensive, and technically demanding, remains a workhorse for separation of lipoproteins for quantitative purposes and preparative isolations. Ultracentrifugation is also used in the reference methods for lipoprotein quantitation, because lipoproteins are classically defined in terms of hydrated density.

Electrophoretic methods allow separation and quantitation of major lipoprotein classes, as well as subclasses, and provide a visual display useful in detecting unusual or variant patterns.[170,171] Agarose gel has been the most common medium for separation of intact lipoproteins, providing a clear background and convenience in use.[172,173] Electrophoretic methods, in general, were considered useful for qualitative analysis but less than desirable for lipoprotein quantitation because of poor precision and large systematic biases, compared with other methods.[174] Using newer commercial automated electrophoretic systems, lipoprotein determinations can be precise and accurate.[175]

Electrophoresis in polyacrylamide gels is used for separation of lipoprotein classes,[176] subclasses, and the apolipoproteins.[177] Of particular interest are methods that fractionate LDL subclasses to characterize the more atherogenic smaller, denser, lipid-depleted fractions versus the larger, lighter subclasses.[178]

Chemical precipitation, usually with polyanions, such as heparin and dextran sulfate, together with divalent cations, such as manganese or magnesium, can be used to separate any of the lipoproteins but are most common for HDL.[179,180] Apo B in VLDL and LDL is rich in positively charged amino acids, which preferentially form complexes with polyanions. The addition of divalent cations neutralizes the charged groups on the lipoproteins, making them aggregate and become insoluble, resulting in their precipitation leaving HDL in solution. At appropriate concentrations of polyanion and divalent cation, the separation is reasonably specific.

Immunochemical methods, using antibodies specific to epitopes on the apolipoproteins, have been useful in both research and routine methods.[181,182] Antibodies have been immobilized on solid supports, such as a column matrix or latex beads. For example, the apo B–containing lipoproteins as a group can be bound by antibodies to apo B. Selectivity within the apo B–containing lipoproteins, such as removing VLDL while retaining LDL, can be obtained by including antibodies to minor apolipoproteins. HDL can be selectively bound using antibodies to apo A-I, the major protein of HDL. As another example, immobilized monoclonal antibodies have been used to separate a fraction of remnant lipoproteins designated RLP (remnant-like particles), shown to be particularly atherogenic.[183]

HDL Methods

The measurement of HDL-C has assumed progressively greater importance in the NCEP treatment guidelines. In the earliest guidelines, HDL-C was measured as a risk factor but otherwise was not considered in treatment decisions. Following recommendations of a National Institutes of Health–sponsored consensus panel,[89] the 1993 NCEP ATP II guidelines included HDL-C measurement with total cholesterol in the first medical workup, which was reinforced by the 2002 ATP III guidelines.[81] Because the risk associated with HDL-C is expressed over a relatively small concentration range, accuracy in the measurement is especially important.

For routine diagnostic purposes, HDL for many years was separated almost exclusively by chemical precipitation, involving a two-step procedure with manual pretreatment. A precipitation reagent added to serum or

CASE STUDY 15-5

A 49-year-old woman was referred for a lipid evaluation by her dermatologist after she developed a papular rash over her trunk and arms. The rash consisted of multiple, red, raised lesions with yellow centers. She had no previous history of such a rash and no family history of lipid disorders or CHD. She is postmenopausal, on standard estrogen replacement therapy, and otherwise healthy (Case Study Table 15-5.1).

CASE STUDY TABLE 15-5.1
LABORATORY RESULTS

SERUM	GROSSLY LIPEMIC
Triglycerides	6,200 mg/dL
Total cholesterol	458 mg/dL
Fasting glucose	160 mg/dL
Liver function tests and electrolytes	Normal

Questions

1. What is the rash? What is the cause of her rash?

2. Is her oral estrogen contributing?

3. Is her glucose contributing?

4. What treatments are warranted, and what is her most acute risk?

plasma aggregated non-HDLs, which were sedimented by centrifugation, at forces of approximately 1,500g (gravity) with lengthy centrifugation times of 10 to 30 minutes or higher forces of 10,000 to 15,000g, decreasing centrifugation times to 3 minutes. HDL is then quantified as cholesterol in the supernate, usually by one of the enzymatic assays modified for the lower HDL-C range.

The earliest common precipitation method used heparin in combination with manganese to precipitate the apo B–containing lipoproteins.[184,185] Because manganese interfered with enzymatic assays, alternative reagents were developed.[186] Sodium phosphotungstate[187] with magnesium became commonly used, but because of its sensitivity to reaction conditions and greater variability, it was largely replaced by dextran sulfate (a synthetic heparin) with magnesium.[188] The earliest dextran sulfate methods used material of 500 kD, which was replaced by a 50 kD material, considered to be more specific.[179] Polyethylene glycol also precipitates lipoproteins, but it requires 100-fold higher reagent concentrations with highly viscous reagents, which are difficult to pipet precisely.[189] Numerous commercial versions of these precipitation reagents became available, which in earlier years often gave quite different results but gradually became more comparable as standardization programs were implemented.

A significant problem with HDL precipitation methods is interference from elevated triglyceride levels.[190] When triglyceride-rich VLDL and chylomicrons are present, the low density of the aggregated lipoproteins may prevent them from sedimenting or may even cause floating during centrifugation. This incomplete sedimentation, indicated by cloudiness, turbidity, or particulate matter floating in the supernate, results in overestimation of HDL-C. High-speed centrifugation reduces the proportion of turbid supernate. Predilution of the specimen promotes clearing but may lead to errors in the cholesterol analysis. Turbid supernates may also be cleared by ultrafiltration, a method that is reliable but tedious and inefficient. Because of these drawbacks and the fact that the laborious pretreatment step is not amenable to full automation, the precipitation methods became increasingly out of step with the modern automated clinical laboratory.

The result has been development of a new class of direct, sometimes termed homogeneous, methods, which automate the HDL quantification, making them better suited for the modern chemistry laboratory. Specific polymers, detergents, and even modified enzymes are used to suppress the enzymatic cholesterol reaction in lipoproteins other than HDL.[191] In general, a first reagent is added to "block" non-HDLs, followed by a second reagent with the enzymes to quantify the accessible (HDL) cholesterol. Homogeneous assays, which appear to be highly precise and reasonably accurate, have generally replaced pretreatment methods in the routine laboratory.[192] However, the methods have been shown to lack specificity for HDL in unusual specimens, for example, from patients with liver or kidney conditions.[193] Also, the reagents have been subject to frequent modifications by the manufacturers in an effort to improve performance, which can affect results in long-term studies. For these reasons, the methods have not been recommended for use in research laboratories.

The accepted reference method for HDL-C is a three-step procedure developed at the CDC. This method involves ultracentrifugation to remove VLDL, heparin manganese precipitation from the 1.006 g/mL infranate to remove LDL, and analysis of supernatant cholesterol by the Abell-Kendall assay.[154] Because this method is tedious and expensive, a simpler, direct precipitation method has been validated by the CDC Network Laboratory Group as a designated comparison method, using direct dextran sulfate (50 kD) precipitation of serum with Abell-Kendall cholesterol analysis.[151]

LDL Methods

LDL-C, well validated as a treatable risk factor for CHD, is the primary basis for treatment decisions in the NCEP clinical guidelines.[81] The most common research method for LDL-C quantitation and the basis for the reference method has been designated beta-quantification, in which beta designation refers to the electrophoretic term for LDL. Beta-quantification combines ultracentrifugation and chemical precipitation.[185,194] Ultracentrifugation of serum at the native density of 1.006 g/mL is used to float VLDL and any chylomicrons for separation. The fractions are recovered by pipeting after separating the fractions by slicing the tube. Ultracentrifugation has been preferred for VLDL separation because other methods, such as precipitation, are not as specific for VLDL and may be subject to interference from chylomicrons. In general, ultracentrifugation is a robust but tedious technique that can give reliable results, provided the technique is meticulous.

In a separate step, chemical precipitation is used to separate HDL from either the whole serum or the infranate obtained from ultracentrifugation. Cholesterol is quantified in serum, in the 1.006 g/mL infranate, and in the HDL supernate by enzymatic or other assay methods. LDL-C is calculated as the difference between cholesterol measured in the infranate and in the HDL fraction. VLDL-C is usually calculated as the difference between that in whole serum and the amount in the infranate fraction. The requirement for the need of an ultracentrifuge has generally limited beta-quantification to lipid specialty laboratories. Beta-quantification is also the basis for the accepted reference method for LDL. The method is the same as that described for HDL above, with the measured HDL-C subtracted from that in the bottom fraction to obtain LDL-C.

A more common approach, bypassing ultracentrifugation and commonly used in routine and sometimes research laboratories, is calculating LDL-C by the Friedewald calculation.[135] HDL-C is quantified either after precipitation or using one of the direct methods, and total cholesterol and triglycerides are measured in the serum. VLDL-C is estimated as the triglyceride level divided by 5 (when using mg/dL units), an approximation that works reasonably well in most normolipemic specimens. The presence of elevated triglycerides (400 mg/dL [4.52 mmol/L] is the accepted limit), chylomicrons, and β-VLDL characteristic of the rare type III hyperlipoproteinemia precludes this estimation. The estimated VLDL-C and measured HDL-C are subtracted from total serum cholesterol to estimate or derive LDL-C. Thus, LDL-C = total cholesterol − HDL − Trig/5. This method, commonly performed as the lipid panel, is widely used in estimating LDL-C in routine clinical practice, having been recommended in the NCEP guidelines. Investigations in lipid specialty laboratories have suggested that the method is reasonably reliable for patient classification, provided the underlying measurements are made with appropriate accuracy and precision.[195] There has been concern about the reliability in routine laboratories, however, because the error in calculating LDL-C combines the error in the underlying measurements: total cholesterol, triglycerides, and HDL-C. The NCEP Laboratory Expert Panel, considering performance as represented by proficiency surveys, concluded that the level of analytic performance required to derive LDL-C accurately enough to meet clinical needs was beyond the capability of most routine laboratories. To meet the NCEP precision goal of 4% CV for LDL-C (Table 15-6), a laboratory would be required to achieve half the NCEP goals for each of the underlying measurements. The NCEP panel concluded that better methods are needed for routine diagnostic use, preferably methods that directly separate LDL for cholesterol quantitation.[79]

In response to the NCEP request, direct LDL-C methods have been developed or refined for general use, similar to the homogeneous assays for HDL-C.[194,196] Besides achieving full automation of the challenging LDL-C separation, these assays have the potential to streamline the measurement while improving precision. However, separating LDL with adequate specificity from other lipoproteins in this manner is more challenging even than that for HDL, and the few evaluations of the direct methods have not been encouraging.[197] More experience will be required, especially with specimens of unusual composition, to judge the adequacy of the homogeneous separations.[198]

Compact Analyzers

The common lipids and lipoproteins can be measured with compact analysis systems designed for use in point-of-care testing at the patient's bedside, in the physician's office, in wellness centers, and even in the home.[194] These compact devices that are used outside the clinical laboratory are considered waived from the Clinical Laboratory Improvement Amendments. The earliest systems, introduced in the 1980s, were relatively large and measured cholesterol and triglycerides as well as other common analytes, usually separately and sequentially. Newer systems have become smaller and more sophisticated, offering integrated separation of HDL and analysis of cholesterol and triglycerides simultaneously from fingerstick blood. Systems can measure cholesterol, triglycerides, HDL-C, and glucose simultaneously from a fingerstick sample. Noninstrumented systems are also available. These new technologies offer the capability of measuring lipids and lipoproteins with reasonable reliability outside the conventional laboratory.

Apolipoprotein Methods

Lipids by nature tend to be insoluble in the aqueous environment of the circulation; hence, the lipoproteins include various protein constituents, designated apolipoproteins, that enhance solubility, as well as playing other functional roles (Table 15-2). Apolipoproteins are commonly measured in research and some specialty laboratories supporting cardiovascular practices or clinical studies measure them routinely in addition to the lipoproteins. For clinical diagnostic purposes, three apolipoproteins in particular have been of interest. Apo B, the major protein of LDL and VLDL, is an indicator of combined LDL and VLDL concentration that can be measured directly in serum by immunoassay.[199] Studies suggest that apo B may be a better indicator of atherogenic particles than LDL-C.[200] Apo A-I, as the major protein of HDL, could be measured directly in serum in place of separation and analysis of HDL-C; however, because quantification in terms of cholesterol content is more common, the latter practice has prevailed. Lp(a), the variant of LDL, shown to be an independent indicator of CHD risk, is sometimes determined in managing patients. Measurement of these three apolipoproteins, considered to be emerging markers, can be useful in patient management by experienced practitioners.

Lp(a) has pre-β mobility on agarose electrophoresis and can be quantified by this technique. However, the apolipoproteins are commonly measured by immunoassays of various types, with several commercial kit methods available.[201] Most common in routine laboratories are turbidimetric assays for chemistry analyzers or nephelometric assays for dedicated nephelometers. Especially for apo B and Lp(a), these light-scattering assays may be subject to interference from the larger triglyceride-rich lipoproteins (chylomicrons) and VLDL. Enzyme-linked immunosorbent assay (ELISA), radial immunodiffusion (RID), and radioimmunoassay (RIA) methods have also been available, but the latter two methods are becoming less common. Antibodies used in the immunoassays may be polyclonal or monoclonal. International efforts to develop reference materials and standardization programs for the assays are in progress. Because Lp(a) is genetically heterogeneous and the levels and CHD risk correlate with the isoform size, qualitative assessment of isoform distribution may also be useful.[141]

Phospholipid Measurement

Quantitative measurements of phospholipids are primarily done for research but not as part of routine laboratory assessments of lipids and lipoproteins, because they have not been shown to add any value for cardiovascular risk prediction. The choline-containing phospholipids lecithin, lysolecithin, and sphingomyelin, which account for at least 95% of total phospholipids in serum, can be measured by an enzymatic reaction sequence using phospholipase D, choline oxidase, and horseradish peroxidase.[202]

Fatty Acid Measurement

Although studies suggest that fatty acids have potential in assessing CHD risk (e.g., the n-3 fatty acids), analysis is also primarily used in research laboratories for studies of diet. Less common is their measurement in the diagnosis of rare genetic conditions. Fatty acids are commonly analyzed by gas–liquid chromatography—after extraction, alkaline hydrolysis, and conversion to methyl esters of diazomethane. A reference standard typically contains laurate, myristate, palmitate, palmitoleate, phytanate, stearate, oleate, linoleate, arachidate, and arachidonate.[203]

STANDARDIZATION OF LIPID AND LIPOPROTEIN ASSAYS

Precision

Precision is a prerequisite for accuracy; a method may have no overall systematic error or bias, but if it is imprecise, it will still be inaccurate on some individual measurements. With the shift to modern automated analyzers, analytic variation has generally become less of a concern than biologic and other sources of preanalytic variation. Cholesterol levels are affected by many factors that can be categorized into biologic, clinical, and sampling sources.[204] Changes in lifestyle that affect diet, exercise, weight, and smoking patterns can result in fluctuations in the observed cvholesterol and triglyceride values and the distribution of the lipoproteins. Similarly, the presence of clinical conditions, various diseases, or the medications used in their treatment can affect the circulating lipoproteins. Conditions present during blood collection, such as fasting status, posture, the choice of anticoagulant in the collection tube, and storage conditions, can alter the measurements. Typical observed biologic variation for more than 1 year for total cholesterol averages approximately 6.1% CV. In the average patient, measurements made over the course of a year would fall 66% of the time within ±6.1% of the mean cholesterol concentration and 95% of the time within twice this range. Some patients may exhibit substantially more biologic variation. Thus, preanalytic variation is generally relatively large in relation to the usual analytic variation, which is typically less than 3% CV, and must be considered in interpreting cholesterol results. Some factors, such as posture and blood collection, can be standardized to minimize the variation. The NCEP guidelines recommend averaging at least two successive measurements to reduce the effects of both preanalytic and analytic sources.[81] The use of stepped cutpoints also reduces the practical effect of variation.

CASE STUDY 15-6

Three patients are seen in clinic:
- Patient 1 is a 40-year-old man with hypertension, who also smokes, but has not been previously diagnosed with CHD. His father developed CHD at age 53 years. He is fasting, and the results of his lipids include a total cholesterol concentration of 210 mg/dL, triglycerides of 150 mg/dL, and an HDL-C value of 45 mg/dL. He has a fasting glucose level of 98 mg/dL.
- Patient 2 is a 60-year-old woman with no family history of CHD and who is normotensive and does not smoke, with a total cholesterol concentration of 220 mg/dL, triglycerides of 85 mg/dL, and an HDL-C value of 80 mg/dL. Her fasting glucose level is 85 mg/dL.
- Patient 3 is a 49-year-old man with no personal or family history of CHD and who is not hypertensive and does not smoke. His fasting total cholesterol level is 260 mg/dL, his triglycerides are 505 mg/dL, his HDL-C is 25 mg/dL, and his glucose level is 134 mg/dL

Questions

For each patient seen in clinic:
1. What is the LDL-C level, as calculated using the Friedewald calculation?
2. Which patient, if any, should have his or her LDL-C measured, rather than calculated? Why?
3. How many known CHD risk factors does each patient have?
4. Based on what is known, are these patients recommended for lipid therapy (diet or drug) and, if so, on what basis?

Accuracy

Accuracy or trueness is ensured by demonstrating traceability or agreement through calibration to the respective "gold standard" reference system. With cholesterol, the reference system is advanced and complete, having served as a model for standardization of other laboratory analytes.[151,156] The definitive method at the National Institute of Standards and Technology provides the ultimate accuracy target but is too expensive and complicated for frequent use.[155] The reference method developed and applied at the CDC, and calibrated by an approved primary reference standard to the definitive method, provides a transferable, practical reference link.[154] The reference method has been made conveniently accessible through a network of standardized laboratories, the Cholesterol Reference Method Laboratory Network. This network was established in the United States and other countries to extend standardization to manufacturers and clinical laboratories.[151] The network provides accuracy comparisons leading to certification of performance using fresh native serum specimens, necessary for reliable accuracy transfer because of analyte–matrix interaction problems on processed reference materials.[205,206]

Matrix Interactions

In the early stages of cholesterol standardization, which were directed toward diagnostic manufacturers and routine laboratories, commercial lyophilized or freeze-dried materials were used. These materials, made in large quantities, often with spiking or artificial addition of analytes, were assayed by the definitive and/or reference methods and distributed widely for accuracy transfer. Subsequently, biases were observed with some systems on fresh patient specimens even though they appeared to be accurate on the reference materials. Although such manufactured reference materials are convenient, stable, and amenable to shipment at ambient temperatures, the manufacturing process, especially spiking and lyophilization, altered the measurement properties in enzymatic assays such that results were not representative of those on patient specimens. To achieve reliable feedback on accuracy and facilitate transfer of the accuracy base, direct comparisons with the reference methods on actual patient specimens were determined to be necessary.[151] In response to these problems, the College of American Pathologists, a major provider of proficiency testing, now offers Accuracy-Based Lipid survey, which is made of fresh frozen serum and is commutable and without any matrix problems. Lipid and lipoprotein values are assigned to the material using reference methods.

CDC Cholesterol Reference Method Laboratory Network

The CDC cholesterol reference method laboratory network program was organized to improve the accuracy of lipid and lipoprotein testing. (Information is available at http://www.cdc.gov/labstandards/crmln.html.) The network offers formal certification programs for total cholesterol, HDL-C, and LDL-C and triglycerides whereby laboratories and manufacturers can document traceability to the national reference systems.[151] Through this program, clinical laboratories are able to identify certified commercial methods. Certification does not ensure all aspects of quality in a reagent system but primarily ensures that the accuracy is traceable to reference methods within accepted limits and that precision can meet the NCEP targets. The certification process is somewhat tedious and, thus, most efficient through manufacturers, but individual laboratories desiring to confirm the performance of their systems can complete a scaled-down certification protocol for cholesterol.

Analytic Performance Goals

The NCEP laboratory panels have established analytic performance goals based on clinical needs for routine measurements (Table 15-6).[78-80,156] For analysis of total cholesterol, the performance goal for total error is 8.9%. That is, the overall error should be such that each individual cholesterol measurement falls within ±8.9% of the reference method value. Actually, because the goals are based on 95% certainty, 95 of 100 measurements should fall within the total error limit. One can assay a specimen many times and calculate the mean to determine the usual value or the central tendency. The scatter or random variation around the mean is described by the standard deviation, an interval around the mean that includes, by definition, two-thirds of the observations. In the laboratory, because the scatter or imprecision is often proportional to the concentration, random variation is usually specified in relative terms as CV—the coefficient of variation or relative standard deviation, calculated as the standard deviation divided by the mean. Overall accuracy or systematic error is described as bias or trueness, the difference between the mean and the true value. Bias is primarily a function of the method's calibration and may vary by concentration. Of greatest concern in this context is bias at the NCEP decision cutpoints. The bias and CV targets presented in Table 15-6 are representative of performance that will meet the NCEP goals for total error.

Quality Control

Achieving acceptable analytic performance requires the use of reliable quality control materials, which should preferably closely emulate actual patient specimens. Commercial control materials have improved in recent years but may not approximate results with patients' specimens. Control materials can also be prepared in-house from freshly collected patient serum, aliquoted into securely sealed vials, quick frozen, and stored at −70°C. Such pools of fresh frozen serum are less subject to matrix interactions than the usual commercial materials, which is most important in monitoring accuracy in lipoprotein separation and analysis and preferable for monitoring cholesterol and other lipid measurements. At least two pools should be analyzed, preferably with levels at or near decision points for each analyte.

Specimen Collection

Serum, usually collected in serum separator vacuum tubes with clotting enhancers, has been the fluid of choice for lipoprotein measurement in the routine clinical laboratory. Ethylenediaminetetraacetic acid (EDTA) plasma was the traditional choice in lipid research laboratories, especially for lipoprotein separations, because the anticoagulant was thought to enhance stability by chelating metal ions. EDTA, however, has potential disadvantages that discourage routine use. Microclots, which can form in plasma during storage, could plug the sampling probes on the modern chemistry analyzers. EDTA also osmotically draws water from red cells, diluting the plasma constituents, and the dilution effect can vary depending on such factors as fill volume, the analyte being measured, and the extent of mixing. Because the NCEP cutpoints are based on serum values, cholesterol measurements made on EDTA plasma require correction by the factor of 1.03.

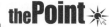

For additional student resources please visit thePoint at **http://thepoint.lww.com**.

QUESTIONS

1. Which of the following methods for lipoprotein electrophoresis depends on charge *and* molecular size?
   a. Polyacrylamide gel
   b. Paper
   c. Cellulose acetate
   d. Agarose

2. Which of the following statements concerning chylomicrons is FALSE?
   a. The major lipid transported by this lipoprotein is cholesterol.
   b. This lipoprotein is produced in the intestinal mucosa.
   c. The primary function is to carry dietary (exogenous) lipids to the liver.
   d. It remains at the origin (point of application) during lipoprotein electrophoresis.

3. The lipoprotein that contains the greatest amount of protein is called
   a. HDL
   b. Chylomicrons
   c. VLDL
   d. LDL

4. True or False? Pre-beta (VLDL) lipoproteins migrate further toward the anode on polyacrylamide gel than they do on cellulose acetate or agarose.

5. Several enzymatic triglyceride methods measure the production or consumption of
   a. NADH
   b. Fatty acids
   c. Glycerol
   d. Diacetyl lutidine

6. The most likely cause for serum/plasma to appear "milky" is the presence of
   a. Chylomicrons
   b. VLDL
   c. LDL
   d. HDL

7. In the colorimetric determination of cholesterol using the enzyme cholesterol oxidase, the agent that oxidizes the colorless organic compound 4-aminoantipyrine to a pink complex is
   a. Hydrogen peroxide
   b. Cholest-4-ene-3-one
   c. NAD
   d. Phenol

8. Which lipoprotein is the major carrier of cholesterol *to* peripheral tissue?
   a. LDL
   b. Chylomicrons
   c. VLDL
   d. HDL

9. True or false? Increased levels of apo A-I are associated with increased risk of CAD.

10. A patient is admitted to the hospital with intense chest pains. The patient's primary care physician requests the emergency department doctor to order several tests, including a lipid profile with cholesterol fractionation. Given the patient's results provided below, what would be the LDL-C for this patient?

Total cholesterol = 400 mg/dL; triglycerides = 300 mg/dL; HDL-C = 100 mg/dL; LP electrophoresis, pending

    a. 240 mg/dL
    b. 160 mg/dL
    c. 200 mg/dL
    d. 300 mg/dL

11. A patient is admitted to the hospital with intense chest pains. The patient's primary care physician requests the emergency department doctor to order several tests, including a lipid profile with cholesterol fractionation. Given the patient's results provided below, what would be this patient's LDL-C status?

Total cholesterol = 400 mg/dL; triglycerides = 300 mg/dL; HDL-C = 100 mg/dL; LP electrophoresis, pending

    a. High
    b. Optimal
    c. Desirable
    d. Borderline

12. As part of a lipoprotein phenotyping, it is necessary to perform total cholesterol and triglyceride determinations, as well as lipoprotein electrophoresis. The test results obtained from such studies were

- Triglyceride, 340 mg/dL (reference range, <150 mg/dL)
- Total cholesterol, 180 mg/dL (reference range, <200 mg/dL)
- Pre-beta-lipoprotein fraction increased
- Beta-lipoprotein fraction normal
- No chylomicrons present
- Serum appearance turbid

The best explanation for these results would be that the patient exhibits a phenotype indicative of

    a. Type IV hyperlipoproteinemia
    b. Type I hyperlipoproteinemia
    c. Type II hyperlipoproteinemia
    d. Type III hyperlipoproteinemia
    e. Type V hyperlipoproteinemia

13. Which of the following results is the most consistent with high risk of CHD?

    a. 20 mg/dL HDL-C and 250 mg/dL total cholesterol
    b. 35 mg/dL HDL-C and 200 mg/dL total cholesterol
    c. 50 mg/dL HDL-C and 190 mg/dL total cholesterol
    d. 55 mg/dL HDL-C and 180 mg/dL total cholesterol
    e. 60 mg/dL HDL-C and 170 mg/dL total cholesterol

14. What is the presumed defect in most cases of familial type IIa hyperlipoproteinemia?

    a. Defective receptors for LDL
    b. Deficiency of hydroxymethylglutaryl (HMG)-CoA reductase
    c. Deficiency of cholesterol esterase
    d. Deficiency of LPL
    e. Defective esterifying enzymes LCAT and ACAT

15. Hyperchylomicronemia (type I) in childhood has been associated with which of the following?

    a. A deficiency of apo C-II
    b. A deficiency of LCAT
    c. A deficiency of LPL
    d. A deficiency of apo A-I

REFERENCES

1. Laposata M. Fatty acids. Biochemistry to clinical significance. *Am J Clin Pathol.* 1995;104(2):172-179.
2. Muller H, Kirkhus B, Pedersen JI. Serum cholesterol predictive equations with special emphasis on trans and saturated fatty acids. An analysis from designed controlled studies. *Lipids.* 2001;36(8):783-791.
3. Cunnane SC. Problems with essential fatty acids: time for a new paradigm? *Prog Lipid Res.* 2003;42(6):544-568.
4. Kritchevsky D. Effects of triglyceride structure on lipid metabolism. *Nutr Rev.* 1988;46:177-181.
5. Ridgway ND, Byers DM, Cook HW, Storey MK. Integration of phospholipid and sterol metabolism in mammalian cells. *Prog Lipid Res.* 1999;38(4):337-360.
6. van Hellemond JJ, Slot JW, Geelen MJ, van Golde LM, Vermeulen PS. Ultrastructural localization of CTP: phosphoethanolamine cytidylyltransferase in rat liver. *J Biol Chem.* 1994;269(22):15415-15418.
7. Barenholz Y. Cholesterol and other membrane active sterols: from membrane evolution to "rafts". *Prog Lipid Res.* 2002;41(1):1-5.
8. Ostlund RE Jr. Phytosterols, cholesterol absorption and healthy diets. *Lipids.* 2007;42(1):41-45.
9. Jones PJ. Regulation of cholesterol biosynthesis by diet in humans. *Am J Clin Nutr.* 1997;66(2):438-446.
10. Pauciullo P. Lipoprotein transport and metabolism: a brief update. *Nutr Metab Cardiovasc Dis.* 2002;12(2):90-97.
11. Gursky O. Apolipoprotein structure and dynamics. *Curr Opin Lipidol.* 2005;16(3):287-294.
12. Hevonoja T, Pentikainen MO, Hyvonen KT, Kovanen PT, Ala-Korpela M. Structure of low density lipoprotein (LDL) particles: basis for understanding molecular changes in modified LDL. *Biochim Biophys Acta.* 2000;1488(3):189-210.
13. Anantharamaiah GM, Brouillette CG, Engler JA, et al. Role of amphipathic helixes in HDL structure/function. *Adv Exp Med Biol.* 1991;285:131-140.

14. Segrest JP, Li L, Anantharamaiah GM, Harvey SC, Liadaki KN, Zannis V. Structure and function of apolipoprotein A-I and high-density lipoprotein. *Curr Opin Lipidol.* 2000;11(2): 105-115.

15. Burnett JR, Barrett PH. Apolipoprotein B metabolism: tracer kinetics, models, metabolic studies. *Crit Rev Clin Lab Sci.* 2002;39(2): 89-137.

16. Javitt NB. Cholesterol homeostasis: role of the LDL receptor. *FASEB J.* 1995;9(13):1378-1381.

17. Law SW, Lackner KJ, Hospattankar AV, et al. Human apo-lipoprotein B-100: cloning, analysis of liver mRNA, assignment of the gene to chromosome 2. *Proc Natl Acad Sci U S A.* 1985;82(24):8340-8344.

18. Kostner KM, Kostner GM. Lipoprotein(a): still an enigma? *Curr Opin Lipidol.* 2002;13(4):391-396.

19. Cooper AD. Hepatic uptake of chylomicron remnants. *J Lipid Res.* 1997;38(11):2173-2192.

20. Mahley RW, Rall SC Jr. Apolipoprotein E: far more than a lipid transport protein. *Annu Rev Genomics Hum Genet.* 2000;1:507-537.

21. Walden CC, Hegele RA. Apolipoprotein E in hyperlipidemia. *Ann Intern Med.* 1994;120(12):1026-1036.

22. Lane RM, Farlow MR. Lipid homeostasis and apolipoprotein E in the development and progression of Alzheimer's disease. *J Lipid Res.* 2005;46(5):949-968.

23. Corder EH, Lannfelt L, Bogdanovic N, Fratiglioni L, Mori H. The role of APOE polymorphisms in late-onset dementias. *Cell Mol Life Sci.* 1998;54(9):928-934.

24. Gruffat D, Durand D, Graulet B, Bauchart D. Regulation of VLDL synthesis and secretion in the liver. *Reprod Nutr Dev.* 1996;36(4):375-389.

25. Griffin BA, Packard CJ. Metabolism of VLDL and LDL subclasses. *Curr Opin Lipidol.* 1994;5(3):200-206.

26. Packard CJ, Shepherd J. Lipoprotein heterogeneity and apolipoprotein B metabolism. *Arterioscler Thromb Vasc Biol.* 1997;17(12):3542-3556.

27. Ginsberg HN. Lipoprotein metabolism and its relationship to atherosclerosis. *Med Clin North Am.* 1994;78(1):1-20.

28. Kruth HS. Sequestration of aggregated low-density lipoproteins by macrophages. *Curr Opin Lipidol.* 2002;13(5):483-488.

29. Plenz G, Robenek H. Monocytes/macrophages in atherosclerosis. *Eur Cytokine Netw.* 1998;9(4):701-703.

30. Warnick GR, McNamara JR, Boggess CN, Clendenen F, Williams PT, Landolt CC. Polyacrylamide gradient gel electrophoresis of lipoprotein subclasses. *Clin Lab Med.* 2006;26(4):803-846.

31. Kulkarni KR. Cholesterol profile measurement by vertical auto profile method. *Clin Lab Med.* 2006;26(4):787-802.

32. McNamara JR, Small DM, Li Z, Schaefer EJ. Differences in LDL subspecies involve alterations in lipid composition and conformational changes in apolipoprotein B. *J Lipid Res.* 1996;37(9):1924-1935.

33. Carmena R, Duriez P, Fruchart JC. Atherogenic lipoprotein particles in atherosclerosis. *Circulation.* 2004;109(23 suppl 1):III2-III7.

34. Erbagci AB, Tarakcioglu M, Aksoy M, et al. Diagnostic value of CRP and Lp(a) in coronary heart disease. *Acta Cardiol.* 2002;57(3):197-204.

35. Albers JJ, Koschinsky ML, Marcovina SM. Evidence mounts for a role of the kidney in lipoprotein(a) catabolism. *Kidney Int.* 2007;71(10):961-962.

36. Lund-Katz S, Liu L, Thuahnai ST, Phillips MC. High density lipoprotein structure. *Front Biosci.* 2003;8:d1044-d1054.

37. Morgan J, Carey C, Lincoff A, Capuzzi D. High-density lipoprotein subfractions and risk of coronary artery disease. *Curr Atheroscler Rep.* 2004;6(5):359-365.

38. Patsch JR, Prasad S, Gotto AM, Jr., Bengtsson-Olivecrona G. Postprandial lipemia. A key for the conversion of high density lipoprotein2 into high density lipoprotein3 by hepatic lipase. *J Clin Invest.* 1984;74(6):2017-2023.

39. Soros P, Bottcher J, Maschek H, Selberg O, Muller MJ. Lipoprotein-X in patients with cirrhosis: its relationship to cholestasis and hypercholesterolemia. *Hepatology.* 1998;28(5): 1199-1205.

40. Nishiwaki M, Ikewaki K, Bader G, et al. Human lecithin:cholesterol acyltransferase deficiency: in vivo kinetics of low-density lipoprotein and lipoprotein-X. *Arterioscler Thromb Vasc Biol.* 2006;26(6):1370-1375.

41. Matas C, Cabre M, La Ville A, et al. Limitations of the Friedewald formula for estimating low-density lipoprotein cholesterol in alcoholics with liver disease. *Clin Chem.* 1994;40(3):404-406.

42. Lusis AJ, Mar R, Pajukanta P. Genetics of atherosclerosis. *Annu Rev Genomics Hum Genet.* 2004;5:189-218.

43. Seo DM, Goldschmidt-Clermont PJ. Unraveling the genetics of atherosclerosis: implications for diagnosis and treatment. *Expert Rev Mol Diagn.* 2007;7(1):45-51.

44. Fruchart JC, Nierman MC, Stroes ES, Kastelein JJ, Duriez P. New risk factors for atherosclerosis and patient risk assessment. *Circulation.* 2004;109(23 suppl 1):III15-III19.

45. Levy E, Spahis S, Sinnett D, et al. Intestinal cholesterol transport proteins: an update and beyond. *Curr Opin Lipidol.* 2007;18(3): 310-318.

46. Davis HR, Veltri EP. Zetia: inhibition of Niemann-Pick C1 Like 1 (NPC1L1) to reduce intestinal cholesterol absorption and treat hyperlipidemia. *J Atheroscler Thromb.* 2007;14(3):99-108.

47. Huff MW, Pollex RL, Hegele RA. NPC1L1: evolution from pharmacological target to physiological sterol transporter. *Arterioscler Thromb Vasc Biol.* 2006;26(11):2433-2438.

48. Lee MH, Lu K, Patel SB. Genetic basis of sitosterolemia. *Curr Opin Lipidol.* 2001;12(2):141-149.

49. Graf GA, Yu L, Li WP, et al. ABCG5 and ABCG8 are obligate heterodimers for protein trafficking and biliary cholesterol excretion. *J Biol Chem.* 2003;278(48):48275-48282.

50. van Greevenbroek MM, de Bruin TW. Chylomicron synthesis by intestinal cells in vitro and in vivo. *Atherosclerosis.* 1998;141 (suppl 1):S9-S16.

51. Zannis VI, Chroni A, Kypreos KE, et al. Probing the pathways of chylomicron and HDL metabolism using adenovirus-mediated gene transfer. *Curr Opin Lipidol.* 2004;15(2):151-166.

52. Mead JR, Irvine SA, Ramji DP. Lipoprotein lipase: structure, function, regulation, role in disease. *J Mol Med (Berl).* 2002;80 (12):753-769.

53. Vaziri ND. Causes of dysregulation of lipid metabolism in chronic renal failure. *Semin Dial.* 2009;22(6):644-651.

54. Parhofer KG, Barrett PH. Thematic review series: patient-oriented research. What we have learned about VLDL and LDL metabolism from human kinetics studies. *J Lipid Res.* 2006;47(8): 1620-1630.

55. Akopian D, Medh JD. Genetics and molecular biology: macrophage ACAT depletion—mechanisms of atherogenesis. *Curr Opin Lipidol.* 2006;17(1):85-88.

56. Osborne TF. Cholesterol homeostasis: clipping out a slippery regulator. *Curr Biol.* 1997;7(3):R172-R174.

57. Hobbs HH, Brown MS, Goldstein JL. Molecular genetics of the LDL receptor gene in familial hypercholesterolemia. *Hum Mutat.* 1992;1(6):445-466.

58. Le NA. Small, dense low-density lipoprotein: risk or myth? *Curr Atheroscler Rep.* 2003;5(1):22-28.

59. Rizzo M, Berneis K. Small, dense low-density-lipoproteins and the metabolic syndrome. *Diabetes Metab Res Rev.* 2007;23(1):14-20.

60. Lewis GF, Rader DJ. New insights into the regulation of HDL metabolism and reverse cholesterol transport. *Circ Res.* 2005;96(12):1221-1232.

61. Toth PP. Reverse cholesterol transport: high-density lipoprotein's magnificent mile. *Curr Atheroscler Rep.* 2003;5(5):386-393.

62. Rothblat GH, de la Llera-Moya M, Atger V, Kellner-Weibel G, Williams DL, Phillips MC. Cell cholesterol efflux: integration of old and new observations provides new insights. *J Lipid Res.* 1999;40(5):781-796.

63. Zannis VI, Chroni A, Krieger M. Role of apoA-I, ABCA1, LCAT, SR-BI in the biogenesis of HDL. *J Mol Med (Berl).* 2006;84(4): 276-294.

64. Nestel PJ. High-density lipoprotein turnover. *Am Heart J.* 1987;113 (2 pt 2):518-521.

65. Yamashita S, Hirano K, Sakai N, Matsuzawa Y. Molecular biology and pathophysiological aspects of plasma cholesteryl ester transfer protein. *Biochim Biophys Acta.* 2000;1529(1-3):257-275.

66. Cavelier C, Lorenzi I, Rohrer L, von Eckardstein A. Lipid efflux by the ATP-binding cassettetransporters ABCA1 and ABCG1. *Biochim Biophys Acta.* 2006; 1761(7):655-666.

67. Dean M, Hamon Y, Chimini G. The human ATP-binding cassette (ABC) transporter superfamily. *J Lipid Res.* 2001;42(7): 1007-1017.

68. Nofer JR, Remaley AT. Tangier disease: still more questions than answers. *Cell Mol Life Sci.* 2005;62(19-20):2150-2160.

69. Vedhachalam C, et al. Mechanism of ATP-binding cassette transporter A1-mediated cellular lipid efflux to apolipoprotein A-I and formation of high density lipoprotein particles. *J Biol Chem.* 2007;282(34):25123-25130.

70. Wang N, Lan D, Chen W, Matsuura F, Tall AR. ATP-binding cassette transporters G1 and G4 mediate cellular cholesterol efflux to high-density lipoproteins. *Proc Natl Acad Sci U S A.* 2004;101(26):9774-9779.

71. Schaefer EJ, Lichtenstein AH, Lamon-Fava S, McNamara JR, Ordovas JM. Lipoproteins, nutrition, aging, atherosclerosis. *Am J Clin Nutr.* 1995;61(3 suppl):726S-740S.

72. Hall G, Collins A, Csemiczky G, Landgren BM. Lipoproteins and BMI: a comparison between women during transition to menopause and regularly menstruating healthy women. *Maturitas.* 2002;41(3):177-185.

73. Expert panel on integrated guidelines for cardiovascular health and risk reduction in children and adolescents: summary report. *Pediatrics.* 2011;128 suppl 5:S213-S256.

74. Castelli WP, Garrison RJ, Wilson PW, Abbott RD, Kalousdian S, Kannel WB. Incidence of coronary heart disease and lipoprotein cholesterol levels. The Framingham Study. *JAMA.* 1986; 256(20):2835-2838.

75. Stamler J, Stamler R, Shekelle RB. Regional differences in prevalence, incidence, mortality from atherosclerotic coronary heart disease. In: deHaas JH, Hemker HC, Snellen HA, eds. *Ischemic Heart Disease.* Leiden, the Netherlands: Leiden University Press; 1970:84-92.

76. Thom TJ, Epstein FH, Feldman JJ. *Total Mortality and Mortality from Heart Disease, Cancer, Stroke from 1950–1987 in 27 Countries.* Washington, DC: National Institutes of Health; 1992.

77. Kato H, Tillotson J, Nichaman MZ, Rhoads GG, Hamilton HB. Epidemiologic studies of coronary heart disease and stroke in Japanese men living in Japan, Hawaii and California. *Am J Epidemiol.* 1973;97(6):372-385.

78. Warnick GR, Wood PD. National Cholesterol Education Program recommendations for measurement of high-density lipoprotein cholesterol: executive summary. The National Cholesterol Education Program Working Group on Lipoprotein Measurement. *Clin Chem.* 1995;41(10):1427-1433.

79. Bachorik PS, Ross JW. National Cholesterol Education Program recommendations for measurement of low-density lipoprotein cholesterol: executive summary. The National Cholesterol Education Program Working Group on Lipoprotein Measurement. *Clin Chem.* 1995;41(10):1414-1420.

80. Stein EA, Myers GL. National Cholesterol Education Program recommendations for triglyceride measurement: executive summary. The National Cholesterol Education Program Working Group on Lipoprotein Measurement. *Clin Chem.* 1995;41(10): 1421-1426.

81. Third Report of the National Cholesterol Education Program (NCEP). Expert Panel on Detection, Evaluation, Treatment of High Blood Cholesterol in Adults (Adult Treatment Panel III) final report. *Circulation.* 2002;106(25):3143-3421.

82. Rea TD, Heckbert SR, Kaplan RC, Smith NL, Lemaitre RN, Psaty BM. Smoking status and risk for recurrent coronary events after myocardial infarction. *Ann Intern Med.* 2002;137(6):494-500.

83. Niebauer J, Hambrecht R, Velich T, et al. Attenuated progression of coronary artery disease after 6 years of multifactorial risk intervention: role of physical exercise. *Circulation.* 1997;96(8):2534-2541.

84. Coleman MP, Key TJ, Wang DY, et al. A prospective study of obesity, lipids, apolipoproteins and ischaemic heart disease in women. *Atherosclerosis.* 1992;92(2-3):177-185.

85. Genest JJ Jr., Martin-Munley SS, McNamara JR, et al. Familial lipoprotein disorders in patients with premature coronary artery disease. *Circulation.* 1992;85(6):2025-2033.

86. Stary HC. Macrophages, macrophage foam cells, eccentric intimal thickening in the coronary arteries of young children. *Atherosclerosis.* 1987;64(2-3):91-108.

87. Keaney JF Jr. Atherosclerosis: from lesion formation to plaque activation and endothelial dysfunction. *Mol Aspects Med.* 2000;21(4-5):99-166.

88. Randomised trial of cholesterol lowering in 4444 patients with coronary heart disease: the Scandinavian Simvastatin Survival Study (4S). *Lancet.* 1994;344(8934):1383-1389.

89. National Institutes of Health Consensus Conference. Triglyceride, HDL cholesterol and coronary heart disease. *JAMA.* 1993;269:505.

90. Shepherd J, Cobbe SM, Ford I, et al. Prevention of coronary heart disease with pravastatin in men with hypercholesterolemia. *Atheroscler Suppl.* 2004;5(3):91-97.

91. The Lipid Research Clinics Coronary Primary Prevention Trial Results. I. Reduction in incidence of coronary heart disease. *JAMA.* 1984;251(3):351-364.

92. Matthan NR, Giovanni A, Schaefer EJ, Brown BG, Lichtenstein AH. Impact of simvastatin, niacin, and/or antioxidants on cholesterol metabolism in CAD patients with low HDL. *J Lipid Res.* 2003;44(4):800-806.

93. Yamagishi M, Terashima M, Awano K, et al. Morphology of vulnerable coronary plaque: insights from follow-up of patients examined by intravascular ultrasound before an acute coronary syndrome. *J Am Coll Cardiol.* 2000;35(1):106-111.

94. Genest JJ Jr, Ordovas JM, McNamara JR, et al. DNA polymorphisms of the apolipoprotein B gene in patients with premature coronary artery disease. *Atherosclerosis.* 1990;82(1-2):7-17.

95. Schaefer EJ, McNamara JR. Overview of the diagnosis and treatment of lipid disorders. In: Rifai N, Warnick GR, eds. *Handbook of Lipoprotein Testing.* Washington, DC: AACC Press; 1997:25-48.

96. Clee SM, Zwinderman AH, Engert JC, et al. Common genetic variation in ABCA1 is associated with altered lipoprotein levels and a modified risk for coronary artery disease. *Circulation.* 2001;103(9):1198-1205.

97. Russo GT, Meigs JB, Cupples LA, et al. Association of the Sst-I polymorphism at the APOC3 gene locus with variations in lipid levels, lipoprotein subclass profiles and coronary heart disease risk: the Framingham offspring study. *Atherosclerosis.* 2001;158(1):173-181.

98. Guyton JR. Niacin in cardiovascular prevention: mechanisms, efficacy, safety. *Curr Opin Lipidol.* 2007;18(4):415-420.

99. Rubins HB, Robins SJ, Collins D, et al. Gemfibrozil for the secondary prevention of coronary heart disease in men with low levels of high-density lipoprotein cholesterol. Veterans Affairs High-Density Lipoprotein Cholesterol Intervention Trial Study Group. *N Engl J Med.* 1999;341:410-418.

100. Nissen SE, Tardif JC, Nicholls SJ, et al. Effect of torcetrapib on the progression of coronary atherosclerosis. *N Engl J Med.* 2007;356(13):1304-1316.

101. Sethi AA, Amar M, Shamburek RD, Remaley AT. Apolipoprotein AI mimetic peptides: possible new agents for the treatment of atherosclerosis. *Curr Opin Investig Drugs.* 2007;8(3):201-212.

102. Grundy SM. Bile acid resins: mechanisms of action. In: *Pharmacological Control of Hyperlipidemia.* R. Fears, editor. Barcelona: JR Prous Science Publishers; 1986:3-19.

103. Gotto AM. Management of dyslipidemia. *Am J Med.* 2002;112(suppl):10S-18S.

104. Shepherd J, Cobbe SM, Ford I, et al. Prevention of coronary heart disease with pravastatin in men with hypercholesterolemia. West of Scotland Coronary Prevention Study Group. *N Engl J Med.* 1995;333(20):1301-1307.

105. Ganji SH. Kamanna VS, Kashyap ML. Niacin and cholesterol: role in cardiovascular disease. *J Nutr Biochem.* 2003;14:298-305.

106. Knopp RH, Drug treatment of lipid disorders. *N Engl J Med.* 1999;341(7):498-511.

107. Batiste MC, Schaefer EJ. Diagnosis and management of lipoprotein abnormalities. *Nutr Clin Care.* 2002;5(3):115-123.

108. Tavintharan S, Kashyap ML. The benefits of niacin in atherosclerosis. *Curr Atheroscler Rep.* 2001;3:74-82.

109. Tunaru S, Kero J, Schaub A. PUMA-G and HM74 are receptors for nicotinic acid and mediate its anti-lipolytic effect. *Nat Med.* 2003;9:352-355.

110. Grundy SM, Mok HY, Zech L, Berman M. Influence of nicotinic acid on metabolism of cholesterol and triglycerides in man. *J Lipid Res.* 1981;22:24-36.

111. Hunninghake DB, Peters JR. Effect of fibric acid derivatives on blood lipid and lipoprotein levels. *Am J Med.* 1987;83(5B):44-49.

112. Rader DJ, Haffner SM. Role of fibrates in the management of hypertriglyceridemia. *Am J Cardiol.* 1999;83(9B):30F-35F.

113. Kosoglou T, Statkevich P, Johnson-Levonas AO, Paolini JF, Bergman AJ, Alton KB. Ezetimibe: a review of its metabolism, pharmacokinetics and drug interactions. *Clin Pharmacokinet.* 2005;44(5):467-494.

114. Nestel PJ, Connor WE, Reardon MF, Connor S, Wong S, Boston R. Suppression by diets rich in fish oil of very low density lipoprotein production in man. *J Clin Invest.* 1984;74:82-89.

115. Price PT, Nelson CM, Clarke SD. Omega 3 polyunsaturated fatty acid regulation of gene expression.. *Curr Opin Lipidol.* 2000;11:3-7.

116. McKenney JM, Sica D. Role of prescription omega-3 fatty acids in the treatment of hypertriglyceridemia. *Pharmacotherapy.* 2007;27(5):715-728.

117. Bays H. Clinical overview of Omacor: a concentrated formulation of omega-3 polyunsaturated fatty acids. *Am J Cardiol.* 2006;98(suppl):71i-76i.

118. Schaefer EJ, Warnick GR, eds. *Handbook of Lipoprotein Testing.* Washington, DC: AACC Press; 1997.

119. Marais AD, Firth JC, Blom DJ. Homozygous familial hypercholesterolemia and its management. *Semin Vasc Med.* 2004;4(1):43-50.

120. Chang JH, Pan JP, Tai DY, et al. Identification and characterization of LDL receptor gene mutations in hyperlipidemic Chinese. *J Lipid Res.* 2003;44(10):1850-1858.

121. Mozas P, Galetto R, Albajar M, Ros E, Pocovi M, Rodriguez-Rey JC. A mutation (-49C>T) in the promoter of the low density lipoprotein receptor gene associated with familial hypercholesterolemia. *J Lipid Res.* 2002;43(1):13-18.

122. Palcoux JB, Meyer M, Jouanel P, Vanlieferinghen P, Malpuech G. Comparison of different treatment regimens in a case of homozygous familial hypercholesterolemia. *Ther Apher.* 2002;6(2):136-139.

123. Kovar, J, Havel RJ. Sources and properties of triglyceride-rich lipoproteins containing apoB-48 and apoB-100 in postprandial blood plasma of patients with primary combined hyperlipidemia. *J Lipid Res.* 2002;43(7):1026-1034.

124. Couillard C, Bergeron N, Pascot A, et al. Evidence for impaired lipolysis in abdominally obese men: postprandial study of apolipoprotein B-48- and B-100-containing lipoproteins. *Am J Clin Nutr.* 2002;76(2):311-318.

125. Genest J Jr, Cohn J. Plasma triglyceride-rich lipoprotein and high density lipoproteins disorders associated with atherosclerosis. *J Investig Med.* 1998;46(8):351-358.

126. Reynisdottir S, Eriksson M, Angelin B, Arner P. Impaired activation of adipocyte lipolysis in familial combined hyperlipidemia. *J Clin Invest.* 1995;95(5):2161-2169.

127. Yadav, D, Pitchumoni CS. Issues in hyperlipidemic pancreatitis. *J Clin Gastroenterol.* 2003;36(1):54-62.

128. Jackson RL, McLean LR, Demel RA. Mechanism of action of lipoprotein lipase and hepatic triglyceride lipase. *Am Heart J.* 1987;113(2 pt 2):551-554.

129. Pschierer V, Richter WO, Schwandt P. Primary chylomicronemia in patients with severe familial hypertriglyceridemia responds to long-term treatment with (n-3) fatty acids. *J Nutr.* 1995;125(6):1490-1494.

130. Santamarina-Fojo S. The familial chylomicronemia syndrome. *Endocrinol Metab Clin North Am.* 1998;27(3):551-567, viii.

131. McNamara JR, Shah PK, Nakajima K, et al. Remnant-like particle (RLP) cholesterol is an independent cardiovascular disease risk factor in women: results from the Framingham Heart Study. *Atherosclerosis.* 2001;154(1):229-236.

132. Fredrickson DS, Levy RI, Lees RS. Fat transport in lipoproteins—an integrated approach to mechanisms and disorders. *N Engl J Med.* 1967;276(5):273-281.

133. Civeira F, Pocovi M, Cenarro A, et al. Apo E variants in patients with type III hyperlipoproteinemia. *Atherosclerosis.* 1996;127(2):273-282.

134. Sijbrands EJ, Hoffer MJ, Meinders AE, et al. Severe hyperlipidemia in apolipoprotein E2 homozygotes due to a combined effect of hyperinsulinemia and an SstI polymorphism. *Arterioscler Thromb Vasc Biol.* 1999;19(11):2722-2729.

135. Friedewald WT, Levy RI, Fredrickson DS. Estimation of the concentration of low-density lipoprotein cholesterol in plasma, without use of the preparative ultracentrifuge. *Clin Chem.* 1972;18(6):499-502.

136. Jialal I, Hirany SV, Devaraj S, Sherwood TA. Comparison of an immunoprecipitation method for direct measurement of LDL-cholesterol with beta-quantification (ultracentrifugation). *Am J Clin Pathol.* 1995;104(1):76-81.

137. Schaefer EJ, Lamon-Fava S, Jenner JL, et al. Lipoprotein(a) levels and risk of coronary heart disease in men. The Lipid Research Clinics Coronary Primary Prevention Trial. *JAMA.* 1994;271(13):999-1003.

138. Hopkins PN, Hunt SC, Schreiner PJ, et al. Lipoprotein(a) interactions with lipid and non-lipid risk factors in patients with early onset coronary artery disease: results from the NHLBI Family Heart Study. *Atherosclerosis.* 1998;141(2):333-345.

139. Kamstrup PR, Benn M, Tybjaerg-Hansen A, Nordestgaard BG. Extreme lipoprotein(a) levels and risk of myocardial infarction in the general population: the Copenhagen City Heart Study. *Circulation.* 2008;117(2):176-184.

140. Ridker PM, Hennekens CH, Stampfer MJ. A prospective study of lipoprotein(a) and the risk of myocardial infarction. *JAMA.* 1993;270(18):2195-2199.

141. Marcovina SM, Koschinsky ML. Lipoprotein(a): structure, measurement, and clinical significance. In: Rifai N, Warnick GR, Dominczak MH, eds. *Handbook of Lipoprotein Testing,* 2nd ed. Washington, D.C.: AACC Press, 2000:345.

142. McLean JW, Tomlinson JE, Kuang WJ, et al. cDNA sequence of human apolipoprotein(a) is homologous to plasminogen. *Nature.* 1987;330(6144):132-137.

344 PART 2 ▪ CLINICAL CORRELATIONS AND ANALYTIC PROCEDURES

143. Miles LA, Fless GM, Levin EG, Scanu AM, Plow EF. A potential basis for the thrombotic risks associated with lipoprotein(a). *Nature.* 1989;339(6222):301-303.

144. Hajjar KA, et al. Lipoprotein(a) modulation of endothelial cell surface fibrinolysis and its potential role in atherosclerosis. *Nature.* 1989;339(6222):303-305.

145. Bittner V. Non-high-density lipoprotein cholesterol and cardiovascular disease. *Curr Opin Lipidol.* 2003;14(4):367-371.

146. Mora S, Rifai N, Buring JE, Ridker PM. Fasting compared with nonfasting lipids and apolipoproteins for predicting incident cardiovascular events. *Circulation.* 2008;118(10):993-1001.

147. Charlton-Menys V, Betteridge DJ, Colhoun H, et al. Targets of statin therapy: LDL cholesterol, non-HDL cholesterol, apolipoprotein B in type 2 diabetes in the Collaborative Atorvastatin Diabetes Study (CARDS). *Clin Chem.* 2009;55(3):473-480.

148. Mott S, Yu L, Marcil M, Boucher B, Rondeau C, Genest J, Jr. Decreased cellular cholesterol efflux is a common cause of familial hypoalphalipoproteinemia: role of the ABCA1 gene mutations. *Atherosclerosis.* 2000;152(2):457-468.

149. Baldassarre D, Amato M, Pustina L, et al. Increased carotid artery intima-media thickness in subjects with primary hypoalphalipoproteinemia. *Arterioscler Thromb Vasc Biol.* 2002;22:317-322.

150. McCormack PL, Keating GM. Prolonged-release nicotinic acid: a review of its use in the treatment of dyslipidaemia. *Drugs.* 2005;65(18):2719-2740.

151. Myers GL, Cooper GR, Greenberg N, et al. Standardization of lipid and lipoprotein measurements. In: Rifai N, Warnick GR, Dominczak MH, eds. *Handbook of Lipoprotein Testing.* 2nd ed. Washington, DC: AACC Press; 2000:717.

152. Zak B. Cholesterol methodologies: a review. *Clin Chem.* 1977;23(7):1201-1214.

153. Abel LL, et al. A simplified method for the estimation of total cholesterol in serum and demonstration of its specificity. *J Biol Chem.* 1952;195(1):357-366.

154. Duncan IW, Mather A, Cooper GR. The procedure for the proposed cholesterol reference method. Atlanta, GA: Division of Environmental Health Laboratory Sciences, Center for Environmental Health, Centers for Disease Control and Prevention; 1985.

155. Cohen A, Hertz HS, Mandel J, et al. Total serum cholesterol by isotope dilution/mass spectrometry: a candidate definitive method. *Clin Chem.* 1980;26(7):854-860.

156. National Institutes of Health. *Recommendations for Improving Cholesterol Measurement. A Report from the Laboratory Standardization Panel of the National Cholesterol Education Program.* Bethesda, MD: National Institutes of Health; 1990: NIH publication no. 90-2964.

157. McGowan MW, Artiss J, Zak B. Spectrophotometric study on minimizing bilirubin interference in an enzyme reagent mediated cholesterol reaction. *Microchem J.* 1983;27:564.

158. Klotzsch SG, McNamara JR. Triglyceride measurements: a review of methods and interferences. *Clin Chem.* 1990;36(9):1605-1613.

159. Bucolo G, Yabut J, Chang TY. Mechanized enzymatic determination of triglycerides in serum. *Clin Chem.* 1975;21(3):420-424.

160. McGowan MW, Artiss JD, Strandbergh DR, Zak B. A peroxidase-coupled method for the colorimetric determination of serum triglycerides. *Clin Chem.* 1983;29(3):538-542.

161. Stinshoff K, Weisshaar D, Staehler F, Hesse D, Gruber W, Steier E. Relation between concentrations of free glycerol and triglycerides in human sera. *Clin Chem.* 1977; 23(6):1029-1032.

162. Warnick GR. Enzymatic methods for quantification of lipoprotein lipids. *Methods Enzymol.* 1986;129:101-123.

163. Sullivan DR, Kruijswijk Z, West CE, Kohlmeier M, Katan MB. Determination of serum triglycerides by an accurate enzymatic method not affected by free glycerol. *Clin Chem.* 1985;31(7):1227-1228.

164. Lofland HB Jr. A semiautomated procedure for the determination of triglycerides in serum. *Anal Biochem.* 1964;9:393-400.

165. Havel RJ, Eder HA, Bragdon JH. The distribution and chemical composition of ultracentrifugally separated lipoproteins in human serum. *J Clin Invest.* 1955;34(9):1345-1353.

166. Chapman MJ, Goldstein S, Lagrange D, Laplaud PM. A density gradient ultracentrifugal procedure for the isolation of the major lipoprotein classes from human serum. *J Lipid Res.* 1981;22(2):339-358.

167. Patsch JR, Patsch W. Zonal ultracentrifugation. *Methods Enzymol.* 1986;129:3-26.

168. Brousseau T, Clavey V, Bard JM, Fruchart JC. Sequential ultracentrifugation micromethod for separation of serum lipoproteins and assays of lipids, apolipoproteins, lipoprotein particles. *Clin Chem.* 1993;39(6):960-964.

169. Wu LL, Warnick GR, Wu JT, Williams RR, Lalouel JM. A rapid micro-scale procedure for determination of the total lipid profile. *Clin Chem.* 1989;35(7):1486-1491.

170. Lewis LA, Opplt JJ. *CRC Handbook of Electrophoresis.* Boca Raton, FL: CRC Press; 1980.

171. Schmitz G, Boettcher A, Barlage S. New approaches to the use of lipoprotein electrophoresis in the clinical laboratory. In: Rifai N, Warnick GR, Dominczak MH, eds. *Handbook of Lipoprotein Testing.* 2nd ed. Washington, DC: AACC Press; 2000:593.

172. Warnick GR, Benderson J, Albers JJ. Lipoprotein quantification: an electrophoretic method compared with the Lipid Research Clinics method. *Clin Chem.* 1982;28(10):2116-2120.

173. Greenspan P, Mao FW, Ryu BH, Gutman RL, et al. Advances in agarose gel electrophoresis of serum lipoproteins. *J Chromatogr A.* 1995;698(1-2):333-339.

174. Rifai N, et al. Measurement of low-density-lipoprotein cholesterol in serum: a status report. *Clin Chem.* 1992;38(1):150-160.

175. Warnick GR, Leary E, Goetsch J. Electrophoretic quantification of LDL-cholesterol using the Helena REP. *Clin Chem.* 1993;39:1122.

176. Muniz N. Measurement of plasma lipoproteins by electrophoresis on polyacrylamide gel. *Clin Chem.* 1977;23(10):1826-1833.

177. Li Z, et al. Analysis of high density lipoproteins by a modified gradient gel electrophoresis method. *J Lipid Res.* 1994;35(9):1698-1711.

178. Krauss RM, Lindgren FT, Ray RM. Interrelationships among subgroups of serum lipoproteins in normal human subjects. *Clin Chim Acta.* 1980;104(3):275-290.

179. Warnick GR, Benderson J, Albers JJ. Dextran sulfate-Mg2+ precipitation procedure for quantitation of high-density-lipoprotein cholesterol. *Clin Chem.* 1982;28(6):1379-1388.

180. Burstein, M, Legmann P. Lipoprotein precipitation. *Monogr Atheroscler.* 1982;11:1-131.

181. Kerscher L, et al. Precipitation methods for the determination of LDL-cholesterol. *Clin Biochem.* 1985;18(2):118-125.

182. Schumaker VN, et al. Anti-apoprotein B monoclonal antibodies detect human low density lipoprotein polymorphism. *J Biol Chem.* 1984;259(10):6423-6430.

183. Nakajima K, et al. Cholesterol in remnant-like lipoproteins in human serum using monoclonal anti apo B-100 and anti apo A-I immunoaffinity mixed gels. *Clin Chim Acta.* 1993;223(1-2):53-71.

184. Fredrickson DS, Levy RI, Lindgren FT. A comparison of heritable abnormal lipoprotein patterns as defined by two different techniques. *J Clin Invest.* 1969;47(11):2446-2457.

185. National Institutes of Health. Manual of laboratory operations, L.R.C.P., lipid and lipoprotein analysis. Washington, DC: U.S. Department of Health and Human Services; 1983.

186. Steele BW, et al. Enzymatic determinations of cholesterol in high-density-lipoprotein fractions prepared by a precipitation technique. *Clin Chem.* 1976;22(1):98-101.

187. Lopes-Virella MF, et al. Cholesterol determination in high-density lipoproteins separated by three different methods. *Clin Chem.* 1977;23(5):882-884.

188. Warnick GR, Cheung MC, Albers JJ. Comparison of current methods for high-density lipoprotein cholesterol quantitation. *Clin Chem.* 1979;25(4):596-604.

189. Demacker PN, et al. Measurement of high-density lipoprotein cholesterol in serum: comparison of six isolation methods combined with enzymic cholesterol analysis. *Clin Chem.* 1980;26(13):1780-1786.

190. Warnick GR, et al. Multilaboratory evaluation of an ultrafiltration procedure for high density lipoprotein cholesterol quantification in turbid heparin-manganese supernates. *J Lipid Res.* 1981;22(6):1015-1020.

191. Sugiuchi H, et al. Direct measurement of high-density lipoprotein cholesterol in serum with polyethylene glycol-modified enzymes and sulfated alpha-cyclodextrin. *Clin Chem.* 1995;41(5):717-723.

192. Harris N, Galpchian V, Rifai N. Three routine methods for measuring high-density lipoprotein cholesterol compared with the reference method. *Clin Chem.* 1996;42(5):738-743.

193. Warnick GR, Nauck M, Rifai N. Evolution of methods for measurement of HDL-cholesterol: from ultracentrifugation to homogeneous assays. *Clin Chem.* 2001;47(9):1579-1596.

194. Bachorik PS. Lipid and lipoprotein analysis with desktop analyzers. In: Rifai N, Warnick G, Dominczak MH, eds. *Handbook of Lipoprotein Testing.* 2nd ed. Washington, DC: AACC Press; 2000:265.

195. Warnick GR, Wood PD. Estimating low-density lipoprotein cholesterol by the Friedewald equation is adequate for classifying patients on the basis of nationally recommended cutpoints. *Clin Chem.* 1990;36(1):15-19.

196. Sugiuchi H, Irie T, Uji Y, et al. Homogeneous assay for measuring low-density lipoprotein cholesterol in serum with triblock copolymer and alpha-cyclodextrin sulfate. *Clin Chem.* 1998;44(3):522-531.

197. Rifai N, Iannotti E, DeAngelis K, Law T. Analytical and clinical performance of a homogeneous enzymatic LDL-cholesterol assay compared with the ultracentrifugation-dextran sulfate-Mg2+ method. *Clin Chem.* 1998;44(6 pt 1):1242-1250.

198. Nauck M, Warnick GR, Rifai N. Methods for measurement of LDL-cholesterol: a critical assessment of direct measurement by homogeneous assays versus calculation. *Clin Chem.* 2002;48(2):236-254.

199. Bhatnager D, Durrington PN. Measurement and clinical significance of apolipoproteins A-1 and B. In: Rifai N, Warnick GR, Dominczak MH, eds. *Handbook of Lipoprotein Testing.* 2nd ed. Washington, DC: AACC Press; 2000:287.

200. Barter PJ, Ballantyne CM, Carmena R, et al. Apo B versus cholesterol in estimating cardiovascular risk and in guiding therapy: report of the thirty-person/ten-country panel. *J Intern Med.* 2006;259(3):247-258.

201. Bhatnager D, Warnick GR, Dominczak MH, eds. *Handbook of Lipoprotein Testing.* 2nd ed. Washington, DC: AACC Press; 2000.

202. McGowan MW, Artiss JD, Zak B. A procedure for the determination of high-density lipoprotein choline-containing phospholipids. *J Clin Chem Clin Biochem.* 1982;20(11):807-812.

203. Hellerstein MK. Methods for measurement of fatty acid and cholesterol metabolism. *Curr Opin Lipidol.* 1995;6(3):172-181.

204. Cooper GR, Myers GL, Smith SJ, Schlant RC. Blood lipid measurements. Variations and practical utility. *JAMA.* 1992;267(12):1652-1660.

205. Bernert JT Jr, et al. Factors influencing the accuracy of the national reference system total cholesterol reference method. *Clin Chem.* 1991;37(12):2053-2061.

206. Eckfeldt JH, Copeland KR. Accuracy verification and identification of matrix effects. The College of American Pathologists' Protocol. *Arch Pathol Lab Med.* 1993;117(4):381-386.

Electrolytes

GEORGE A. HARWELL

CHAPTER 16

CHAPTER OUTLINE

- ◆ WATER
  Osmolality
- ◆ THE ELECTROLYTES
  Sodium
  Potassium
  Chloride
  Bicarbonate
  Magnesium

Calcium
Phosphate
Lactate
- ◆ ANION GAP
- ◆ ELECTROLYTES AND RENAL FUNCTION
- ◆ QUESTIONS
- ◆ REFERENCES

Chapter Objectives

Upon completion of this chapter, the clinical laboratorian should be able to do the following:

- Define electrolyte, osmolality, anion gap, anion, and cation.
- Discuss the physiology of each electrolyte described in the chapter.
- State the clinical significance of each of the electrolytes mentioned in the chapter.
- Calculate osmolality, osmolal gap, and anion gap and discuss the clinical usefulness of each.

- Discuss the analytic techniques used to assess electrolyte concentrations.
- Correlate the information with disease state, given patient data.
- Identify the reference ranges for sodium, potassium, chloride, bicarbonate, magnesium, and calcium.
- State the specimen of choice for the major electrolytes.
- Discuss the role of the kidney in electrolyte excretion and conservation in a healthy individual.
- Discuss the usefulness of urine electrolyte results: sodium, potassium, calcium, and osmolality.

KEY TERMS

Active transport
Anion
Anion gap (AG)
Cation
Diffusion
Electrolyte
Extracellular fluid (ECF)
Hypercalcemia
Hyperchloremia
Hyperkalemia
Hypermagnesemia
Hypernatremia
Hyperphosphatemia

Hypocalcemia
Hypochloremia
Hypokalemia
Hypomagnesemia
Hyponatremia
Hypophosphatemia
Hypovolemia
Intracellular fluid (ICF)
Osmolal gap
Osmolality
Osmolarity
Osmometer
Polydipsia
Tetany

Electrolytes, by definition, are ions capable of carrying an electric charge. They are classified as anions or cations based on the type of charge they carry. These names were determined years ago based on how the ion migrates in an electric field. Those electrolytes with a positive charge are cations that move toward the cathode, and those with a negative charge are anions that move toward the anode.

Electrolytes are an essential component in numerous processes, including volume and osmotic regulation (sodium [Na^+], chloride [Cl^-], potassium [K^+]); myocardial rhythm and contractility (K^+, magnesium

[Mg^{2+}], calcium [Ca^{2+}]); cofactors in enzyme activation (e.g., Mg^{2+}, Ca^{2+}, zinc [Zn^{2+}]); regulation of adenosine triphosphatase (ATPase) ion pumps (Mg^{2+}); acid–base balance (bicarbonate HCO$_3^-$, K$^+$, Cl$^-$); blood coagulation (Ca^{2+}, Mg^{2+}); neuromuscular excitability (K$^+$, Ca^{2+}, Mg^{2+}); and the production and use of ATP from glucose (e.g., Mg^{2+}, phosphate PO$_4^-$). Because many of these functions require electrolyte concentrations to be held within narrow ranges, the body has complex systems for monitoring and maintaining electrolyte concentrations.

This chapter explores both the metabolic physiology and regulation of each electrolyte and relates these factors to the clinical significance of electrolyte measurements. In addition, methodologies used in determining concentrations of the individual analytes are discussed.

WATER

The average water content of the human body varies from 40% to 75% of total body weight, with values declining with age and especially with obesity. Women have lower average water content than men as a result of a higher fat content. Water is the solvent for all processes in the human body. It transports nutrients to cells, determines cell volume by its transport into and out of cells, removes waste products by way of urine, and acts as the body's coolant by way of sweating. Water is located in intracellular and extracellular compartments. Intracellular fluid (ICF) is the fluid inside the cells and accounts for about two-thirds of total body water. Extracellular fluid (ECF) accounts for the other one-third of total body water and can be subdivided into the *intravascular ECF (plasma)* and the *interstitial cell fluid* that surrounds the cells in the tissue. Normal plasma is about 93% water, with the remaining volume occupied by lipids and proteins. The concentrations of ions within cells and in plasma are maintained both by energy-consuming active transport processes and by diffusion or passive transport processes.

Active transport is a mechanism that requires energy to move ions across cellular membranes. For example, maintaining a high intracellular concentration of K$^+$ and a high extracellular (plasma) concentration of Na$^+$ requires use of energy from ATP in ATPase-dependent ion pumps. Diffusion is the passive movement of ions across a membrane. It depends on the size and charge of the ion being transported and on the nature of the membrane through which it is passing. The rate of diffusion of various ions also may be altered by physiologic and hormonal processes.

Distribution of water in the various body fluid compartments is controlled by maintaining the concentration of electrolytes and proteins in the individual compartments. Because most biologic membranes are freely permeable to water but not to ions or proteins, the concentration of ions and proteins on either side of the membrane will influence the flow of water across a membrane (an osmoregulator). In addition to the osmotic effects of Na$^+$, other ions, proteins, and blood pressure influence the flow of water across a membrane.

Osmolality

Osmolality is a physical property of a solution that is based on the concentration of solutes (expressed as millimoles) per kilogram of solvent (w/w). Osmolality is related to several changes in the properties of a solution relative to pure water, such as freezing point depression and vapor pressure decrease. These colligative properties (see Chapter 5) are the basis for routine measurements of osmolality in the laboratory. The term osmolarity is still occasionally used, with results reported in milliosmoles per liter (w/v), but it is inaccurate in cases of hyperlipidemia or hyperproteinemia; for urine specimens; or in the presence of certain osmotically active substances, such as alcohol or mannitol. Both the sensation of thirst and arginine vasopressin hormone (AVP), formerly called antidiuretic hormone (ADH), secretion are stimulated by the hypothalamus in response to an increased osmolality of blood. The natural response to the thirst sensation is to consume more fluids, increasing the water content of the ECF, diluting the elevated solute (Na$^+$) levels, and decreasing the osmolality of the plasma. Thirst, therefore, is important in mediating fluid intake. The other means of controlling osmolality is by secretion of AVP. This hormone is secreted by the posterior pituitary gland and acts on the cells of the collecting ducts in the kidneys to increase water reabsorption. As water is conserved, osmolality decreases, turning off AVP secretion.[1]

Clinical Significance of Osmolality

Osmolality in plasma is important because it is the parameter to which the hypothalamus responds. The regulation of osmolality also affects the Na$^+$ concentration in plasma, largely because Na$^+$ and its associated anions account for approximately 90% of the osmotic activity in plasma. Another important process affecting the Na$^+$ concentration in blood is the regulation of blood volume. As discussed later, although osmolality and volume are regulated by separate mechanisms (except for AVP and thirst), they are related because osmolality (Na$^+$) is regulated by changes in water balance, whereas volume is regulated by changes in Na$^+$ balance.[1]

To maintain a normal plasma osmolality ($\approx$275 to 295 mOsm/kg of plasma H$_2$O), osmoreceptors in the hypothalamus respond quickly to small changes in osmolality. A 1% to 2% increase in osmolality causes a fourfold increase in the circulating concentration of AVP, and a 1% to 2% decrease in osmolality shuts off AVP production. AVP acts by increasing the reabsorption of water in the cortical and medullary collecting tubules. AVP has a half-life in the circulation of only 15 to 20 minutes.

Renal water regulation by AVP and thirst play important roles in regulating plasma osmolality. Renal water excretion is more important in controlling water excess, whereas thirst is more important in preventing water deficit or dehydration. Consider what happens in several conditions.

Water Load
As excess intake of water (e.g., in polydipsia) begins to lower plasma osmolality, both AVP and thirst are suppressed. In the absence of AVP, water is not reabsorbed, causing a large volume of dilute urine to be excreted, as much as 10 to 20 L daily, well above any normal intake of water. Therefore, hypoosmolality and hyponatremia usually occur only in patients with impaired renal excretion of water.[1]

Water Deficit
As the deficit of water begins to increase plasma osmolality, both AVP secretion and thirst are activated. Although AVP contributes by minimizing renal water loss, thirst is the major defense against hyperosmolality and hypernatremia. Although hypernatremia rarely occurs in a person with a normal thirst mechanism and access to water, it becomes a concern in infants, unconscious patients, or anyone who is unable to either drink or ask for water. Osmotic stimulation of thirst progressively diminishes in people who are older than age 60. In the older patient with illness and diminished mental status, dehydration becomes increasingly likely. As an example of the effectiveness of thirst in preventing dehydration, a patient with diabetes insipidus (no AVP) may excrete 10 L of urine per day; however, because thirst persists, water intake matches output and plasma Na^+ remains normal.[1]

Regulation of Blood Volume
Adequate blood volume is essential to maintain blood pressure and ensure good perfusion to all tissue and organs. Regulation of both Na^+ and water is interrelated in controlling blood volume. The renin–angiotensin–aldosterone system responds primarily to a decreased blood volume. Renin is secreted near the renal glomeruli in response to decreased renal blood flow (decreased blood volume or blood pressure). Renin converts angiotensinogen to angiotensin I, which then becomes angiotensin II. Angiotensin II causes vasoconstriction, which quickly increases blood pressure, and secretion of aldosterone, which increases retention of Na^+ and the water that accompanies the Na^+. The effects of blood volume and osmolality on Na^+ and water metabolism are shown in Figure 16-1. Changes in blood volume (actually pressure) are initially detected by a series of stretch receptors located in areas such as the cardiopulmonary circulation, carotid sinus, aortic arch, and glomerular arterioles. These receptors then activate a series of responses (effectors) that restore volume by appropriately varying vascular resistance, cardiac output, and renal Na^+ and water retention.[1]

Four other factors affect blood volume: (1) atrial natriuretic peptide (ANP), released from the myocardial atria in response to volume expansion, promotes Na^+ excretion in the kidney (B-type natriuretic peptide and ANP act together in regulating blood pressure and fluid balance); (2) volume receptors independent of osmolality stimulate the release of AVP, which conserves water by renal reabsorption; (3) glomerular filtration rate (GFR) increases with volume expansion and decreases with volume depletion; and (4) all other things equal, an increased plasma Na^+ will increase urinary Na^+ excretion and vice versa. The normal reabsorption of 98% to 99% of filtered Na^+ by the tubules conserves nearly all of the 150 L of glomerular filtrate produced daily. A 1% to 2% reduction in tubular reabsorption of Na^+ can increase water loss by several liters per day.

Urine osmolality values may vary widely depending on water intake and the circumstances of collection. However, it is generally decreased in diabetes insipidus (inadequate AVP) and polydipsia (excessive H_2O intake) and increased in conditions such as the syndrome of inappropriate ADH (AVP) secretion (SIADH) and hypovolemia (although urinary Na^+ is usually decreased).

Determination of Osmolality

Specimen
Osmolality may be measured in serum or urine. Major electrolyte concentrations, mainly sodium, chloride, and bicarbonate, provide the largest contribution to the osmolality value of serum. Plasma use is not recommended because osmotically active substances may be introduced into the specimen from the anticoagulant.

Discussion
The methods for determining osmolality are based on properties of a solution that are related to the number of molecules of solute per kilogram of solvent (colligative properties), such as changes in freezing point and vapor pressure. An increase in osmolality decreases the freezing point temperature and the vapor pressure. Measurements of freezing point depression and vapor pressure decrease (actually, the dew point) are the two most frequently used methods of analysis. For detailed information on theory and methodology, consult Chapter 5 or the operator's manual of the instrument being used.

Samples must be free of particulate matter to obtain accurate results. Turbid serum and urine samples should be centrifuged before analysis to remove any extraneous particles. If reusable sample cups are used, they should be thoroughly cleaned and dried between each use to prevent contamination.

Osmometers that operate by freezing point depression are standardized using sodium chloride reference solutions. After calibration, the appropriate amount of sample is pipetted into the required cuvette or sample cup and placed in the analyzer. The sample is then supercooled to −7°C and seeded to initiate the freezing process. When temperature equilibrium has been reached, the freezing point is measured, with results for serum and urine osmolality reported as milliosmoles per kilogram.

Calculation of osmolality has some usefulness either as an estimate of the true osmolality or to determine the osmolal gap, which is the difference between the measured osmolality and the calculated osmolality. The osmolal gap indirectly indicates the presence of osmotically active substances other than Na^+, urea, or glucose, such as ethanol, methanol, ethylene glycol, lactate, or β-hydroxybutyrate.

Two formulas are presented, each having theoretic advantages and disadvantages. Both are adequate for the purpose previously described. For more discussion, the reader may consult other references.[2]

$$2\,Na + \frac{glucose\ (mg/dL)}{20} + \frac{BUN\ (mg/dL)}{3}$$
$$1.86\,Na + \frac{glucose}{18} + \frac{BUN}{2.8} + 9 \qquad \text{(Eq. 16-1)}$$

Reference Ranges

See Table 16-1.[3]

THE ELECTROLYTES

Sodium

Na^+ is the most abundant cation in the ECF, representing 90% of all extracellular cations, and largely determines the osmolality of the plasma. A normal plasma osmolality is approximately 295 mmol/L, with 270 mmol/L being the result of Na^+ and associated anions.

Na^+ concentration in the ECF is much larger than inside the cells. Because a small amount of Na^+ can diffuse through the cell membrane, the two sides would eventually reach equilibrium. To prevent equilibrium from occurring, active transport systems, such as ATPase ion pumps, are present in all cells. K^+ (see section "Potassium") is the major intracellular cation. Like Na^+, K^+ would eventually diffuse across the cell membrane until equilibrium is reached. The Na^+, K^+-ATPase ion pump moves three Na^+ ions out of the cell in exchange for two K^+ ions moving into the cell as ATP is converted

to ADP. Because water follows electrolytes across cell membranes, the continual removal of Na^+ from the cell prevents osmotic rupture of the cell by also drawing water from the cell.

Regulation

The plasma Na^+ concentration depends greatly on the intake and excretion of water and, to a somewhat lesser degree, on the renal regulation of Na^+. Three processes are of primary importance: (1) the intake of water in response to thirst, as stimulated or suppressed by plasma osmolality; (2) the excretion of water, largely affected by AVP release in response to changes in either blood volume or osmolality; and (3) the blood volume status, which affects Na^+ excretion through aldosterone, angiotensin II, and ANP. The kidneys have the ability to conserve or excrete large amounts of Na^+, depending on the Na^+ content of the ECF and the blood volume. Normally, 60% to 75% of filtered Na^+ is reabsorbed in the proximal tubule; electroneutrality is maintained by either Cl^- reabsorption or hydrogen ion (H^+) secretion. Some Na^+ is also reabsorbed in the loop and distal tubule and (controlled by aldosterone) exchanged for K^+ in the connecting segment and cortical collecting tubule. The regulation of osmolality and volume has been summarized in Figure 16-1.

CASE STUDY 16-1

A 32-year-old woman was admitted to the hospital following 2½ days of severe vomiting. Before this episode, she was reportedly well. Physical findings revealed decreased skin turgor and dry mucous membranes. Admission study results were as follows:

SERUM

- Na^+: 129 mmol/L
- K^+: 5.0 mmol/L
- Cl^-: 77 mmol/L
- HCO_3^-: 9 mmol/L
- Osmolality: 265 mOsm/kg

URINE

- Na^+: 8 mmol/d
- Ketones: trace

Questions

1. What is the cause for each abnormal plasma electrolyte result?

2. What is the significance of the urine sodium and serum osmolality results?

TABLE 16-1	REFERENCE RANGES FOR OSMOLALITY
Serum	275–295 mOsm/kg
Urine (24 h)	300–900 mOsm/kg
Urine/serum ratio	1.0–3.0
Random urine	50–1200 mOsm/kg
Osmolal gap	5–10 mOsm/kg

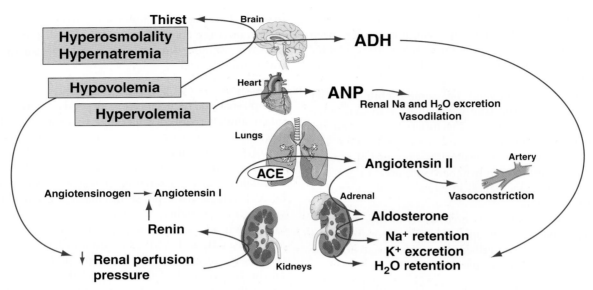

FIGURE 16-1 Responses to changes in blood osmolality and blood volume. ANP, atrial natriuretic peptide; ADH, antidiuretic hormone; ACE, angiotensin-converting enzyme. The primary stimuli are shown in *boxes* (e.g., hypovolemia).

Clinical Applications

Hyponatremia

Hyponatremia is defined as a serum/plasma level less than 135 mmol/L.[4] Hyponatremia is one of the most common electrolyte disorders in hospitalized and non-hospitalized patients.[5,6] Levels below 130 mmol/L are clinically significant. Hyponatremia can be assessed by the cause for the decrease or with the osmolality level.

Decreased levels may be caused by increased Na^+ loss, increased water retention, or water imbalance (Table 16-2). *Increased Na^+ loss* in the urine can occur with decreased aldosterone production, certain diuretics (thiazides), ketonuria (Na^+ lost with ketones), or a salt-losing nephropathy (with some renal tubular disorders). K^+ deficiency also causes Na^+ loss because of the inverse relationship of the two ions in the renal tubules. When serum K^+ levels are low, the tubules will conserve K^+ and excrete Na^+ in exchange for the loss of the monovalent cation. Each disorder results in an increased urine Na^+ level ($\geq$20 mmol/d), which exceeds the amount of water loss.[7]

Prolonged vomiting or diarrhea or severe burns can result in Na^+ loss. Urine Na^+ levels are usually less than 20 mmol/d in these disorders, which can be used to differentiate among causes for urinary loss.

Increased water retention causes dilution of serum/plasma Na^+ as with acute or chronic renal failure. In nephrotic syndrome and hepatic cirrhosis, plasma proteins are decreased, resulting in a decreased colloid osmotic pressure in which intravascular fluid migrates to the tissue (edema results). The low plasma volume causes AVP to be produced, causing fluid retention and resulting in dilution of Na^+. This compensatory mechanism is also seen with congestive heart failure (CHF) as a result of increased venous pressure. Urine Na^+ levels can be used to differentiate the cause for increased water retention. When urine Na^+ is $\geq$20 mmol/d, acute or chronic renal failure is the likely cause. When urine levels are less than

TABLE 16-2	CAUSES OF HYPONATREMIA
INCREASED SODIUM LOSS	
Hypoadrenalism	
Potassium deficiency	
Diuretic use	
Ketonuria	
Salt-losing nephropathy	
Prolonged vomiting or diarrhea	
Severe burns	
INCREASED WATER RETENTION	
Renal failure	
Nephrotic syndrome	
Hepatic cirrhosis	
Congestive heart failure	
WATER IMBALANCE	
Excess water intake	
SIADH	
Pseudohyponatremia	

SIADH, syndrome of inappropriate arginine vasopressin hormone secretion.

20 mmol/d, water retention may be a result of nephrotic syndrome, hepatic cirrhosis, or CHF.[7]

Water imbalance can occur as a result of excess water intake, as with polydipsia (increased thirst). The increased intake must be chronic before water imbalance occurs, which may cause mild or severe hyponatremia. In a normal individual, excess intake will not affect Na^+ levels. SIADH causes an increase in water retention because of increased AVP (ADH) production. A defect in AVP regulation has been associated with pulmonary disease, malignancies, central nervous system (CNS) disorders, infections (e.g., *Pneumocystis carinii* pneumonia), or trauma.[7] Pseudohyponatremia can occur when Na^+ is measured using indirect ion-selective electrodes (ISEs) in a patient who is hyperproteinemic or hyperlipidemic. An indirect ISE dilutes the sample prior to analysis and as a result of plasma/serum water displacement; the ion levels are falsely decreased. (For detailed information on the theory of water displacement with indirect ISEs, consult Chapter 5.)

Hyponatremia can also be *classified according to plasma/serum osmolality* (Table 16-3). Because Na^+ is a major contributor to osmolality, both levels can assist in identifying the cause of hyponatremia. There are three categories of hyponatremia—low osmolality, normal osmolality, or high osmolality.[4] Most instances of hyponatremia occur *with decreased osmolality*. This may be a result of Na^+ loss or water retention, as previously mentioned.

TABLE 16-3	CLASSIFICATION OF HYPO-NATREMIA BY OSMOLALITY

WITH LOW OSMOLALITY
Increased sodium loss
Increased water retention

WITH NORMAL OSMOLALITY
Increased nonsodium cations
Lithium excess
Increased γ-globulins—cationic (multiple myeloma)
Severe hyperkalemia
Severe hypermagnesemia
Severe hypercalcemia
Pseudohyponatremia
Hyperlipidemia
Hyperproteinemia
Pseudohyperkalemia as a result of in vitro hemolysis

WITH HIGH OSMOLALITY
Hyperglycemia
Mannitol infusion

TABLE 16-4	CAUSES OF HYPERNATREMIA

EXCESS WATER LOSS
Diabetes insipidus
Renal tubular disorder
Prolonged diarrhea
Profuse sweating
Severe burns

DECREASED WATER INTAKE
Older persons
Infants
Mental impairment

INCREASED INTAKE OR RETENTION
Hyperaldosteronism
Sodium bicarbonate excess
Dialysis fluid excess

Hyponatremia with a normal osmolality may be a result of a high increase in nonsodium cations as listed in Table 16-4. In multiple myeloma, the cationic γ-globulins replace some Na^+ to maintain the electroneutrality; however, because it is a multivalent cation, it has little affect on osmolality.

Pseudohyponatremia, as mentioned earlier, may also be seen with in vitro hemolysis, considered the most common cause for a false decrease.[4] When red blood cells (RBCs) lyse, Na^+, K^+, and water are released. Na^+ concentration is lower in RBCs, resulting in a false decrease. *Hyponatremia with a high osmolality* is associated with hyperglycemia. The elevated levels of glucose increase the serum osmolality and cause a shift of water from the cells to the blood, resulting in a dilution of Na^+.

Symptoms of hyponatremia. Symptoms depend on the serum level. Between 125 and 130 mmol/L, symptoms are primarily gastrointestinal (GI). More severe neuropsychiatric symptoms are seen below 125 mmol/L, including nausea and vomiting, muscular weakness, headache, lethargy, and ataxia. More severe symptoms also include seizures, coma, and respiratory depression.[7] A level below 120 mmol/L for 48 hours or less (acute hyponatremia) is considered a medical emergency.[8] Serum and urine electrolytes are monitored as treatment to return Na^+ levels to normal occurs.[9]

Treatment of hyponatremia. Treatment is directed at correction of the condition that caused either water loss or Na^+ loss in excess of water loss. In addition, the onset of hyponatremia—acute or chronic (less than or more than 48 hours)—and the severity of hyponatremia are considered in treatment. Conventional treatment of hyponatremia involves fluid restriction and providing hypertonic saline and/or other pharmacologic agents that may take several days to reach the desired effect and may have deleterious side effects.[5] Correcting severe hyponatremia too rapidly can cause cerebral myelinolysis and too slowly can cause cerebral edema.[9] Appropriate management of fluid administration is critical. Fluid administration and monitoring are required during treatment of the underlying cause of the hyponatremia.

A newer type of pharmacologic agent, an AVP receptor antagonist, has been found to be an effective treatment for euvolemic or hypervolemic hyponatremia. Conivaptan has been approved by the U.S. Food and Drug Administration for use in the United States and blocks the action of AVP in the collecting ducts of the nephron, thus decreasing water reabsorption.[10] This AVP receptor antagonist tends to restore Na⁺ levels within 24 hours.[5] Euvolemic hypernatremia is associated with SIADH, hypothyroidism, and adrenal insufficiency.[6] Hypervolemic hyponatremia is associated with liver cirrhosis with ascites, CHF, and overhydrated postoperative patients.[8] Conivaptan is not an effective treatment with hypovolemic hyponatremia because the increased water loss would accentuate the volume depletion problem.[10]

Hypernatremia
Hypernatremia (increased serum Na⁺ concentration) results from excess loss of water relative to Na⁺ loss, decreased water intake, or increased Na⁺ intake or retention. Hypernatremia is less commonly seen in hospitalized patients than hyponatremia.[7]

Loss of hypotonic fluid may occur either by the kidney or through profuse sweating, diarrhea, or severe burns.

Hypernatremia may result from loss of water in diabetes insipidus, either because the kidney cannot respond to AVP (nephrogenic diabetes insipidus) or because AVP secretion is impaired (central diabetes insipidus). Diabetes insipidus is characterized by copious production of dilute urine (3 to 20 L/d). Because people with diabetes insipidus drink large volumes of water, hypernatremia usually does not occur unless the thirst mechanism is also impaired. Partial defects of either AVP release or the response to AVP may also occur. In such cases, urine is concentrated to a lesser extent than appropriate to correct the hypernatremia. Excess water loss may also occur in renal tubular disease, such as acute tubular necrosis, in which the tubules become unable to fully concentrate the urine.

The measurement of urine osmolality is necessary to evaluate the cause of hypernatremia. With renal loss of water, the urine osmolality is low or normal. With extrarenal fluid losses, the urine osmolality is increased. Interpretation of the urine osmolality in hypernatremia is shown in Table 16-5.

TABLE 16-5	HYPERNATREMIA (150 mmol/L) RELATED TO URINE OSMOLALITY
URINE OSMOLALITY <300 mOsm/kg	
Diabetes insipidus (impaired secretion of AVP or kidneys cannot respond to AVP)	
URINE OSMOLALITY 300–700 mOsm/kg	
Partial defect in AVP release or response to AVP	
Osmotic diuresis	
URINE OSMOLALITY >700 mOsm/kg	
Loss of thirst	
Insensible loss of water (breathing, skin)	
Gastrointestinal loss of hypotonic fluid	
Excess intake of sodium	

AVP, arginine vasopressin hormone.

Water loss through the skin and by breathing (insensible loss) accounts for about 1 L of water loss per day in adults. Any condition that increases water loss, such as fever, burns, diarrhea, or exposure to heat, will increase the likelihood of developing hypernatremia. Commonly, hypernatremia occurs in those persons who may be thirsty but who are unable to ask for or obtain water, such as adults with altered mental status and infants. When urine cannot be fully concentrated (e.g., in neonates, young children, older persons, and certain patients with renal insufficiency), a relatively lower urine osmolality may occur.

Chronic hypernatremia in an alert patient is indicative of hypothalamic disease, usually with a defect in the osmoreceptors rather than from a true resetting of the osmostat. A reset osmostat may occur in primary hyperaldosteronism, in which excess aldosterone induces mild hypervolemia that retards AVP release, shifting plasma Na⁺ upward by approximately 3 to 5 mmol/L.[1]

Hypernatremia may be from excess ingestion of salt or administration of hypertonic solutions of Na⁺, such as sodium bicarbonate or hypertonic dialysis solutions. Neonates are especially susceptible to hypernatremia from this cause. In these cases, AVP response is appropriate, resulting in urine osmolality of greater than 800 mOsm/kg (Table 16-5).

Symptoms of hypernatremia. Symptoms most commonly involve the CNS as a result of the hyperosmolar state. These symptoms include altered mental status, lethargy, irritability, restlessness, seizures, muscle twitching, hyperreflexes, fever, nausea or vomiting, difficult respiration, and increased thirst. Serum Na⁺ of more than 160 mmol/L is associated with a mortality rate of 60% to 75%.[7]

Treatment of hypernatremia. Treatment is directed at correction of the underlying condition that caused the water depletion or Na^+ retention. The speed of correction depends on the rate with which the condition developed. Hypernatremia must be corrected gradually because too rapid a correction of serious hypernatremia ($\geq$160 mmol/L) can induce cerebral edema and death; the maximal rate should be 0.5 mmol/L/h.[1]

Determination of Sodium

Specimen
Serum, plasma, and urine are all acceptable for Na^+ measurements. When plasma is used, lithium heparin, ammonium heparin, and lithium oxalate are suitable anticoagulants. Hemolysis does not cause a significant change in serum or plasma values as a result of decreased levels of intracellular Na^+. However, with marked hemolysis, levels may be decreased as a result of a dilutional effect.

Whole blood samples may be used with some analyzers. Consult the instrument operation manual for acceptability. The specimen of choice in urine Na^+ analyses is a 24-hour collection. Sweat is also suitable for analysis. Sweat collection and analysis are discussed in Chapter 29.

Methods
Through the years, Na^+ has been measured in various ways, including chemical methods, flame emission spectrophotometry, atomic absorption spectrophotometry (AAS), and ISEs. Chemical methods are outdated because of large sample volume requirements and lack of precision. ISEs are the most routinely used method in clinical laboratories.

The ISE method uses a semipermeable membrane to develop a potential produced by having different ion concentrations on either side of the membrane. In this type of system, two electrodes are used. One electrode has a constant potential, making it the reference electrode. The difference in potential between the reference and measuring electrodes can be used to calculate the "concentration" of the ion in solution. However, it is the activity of the ion, not the concentration that is being measured (see Chapter 5). Most analyzers use a glass ion-exchange membrane in its ISE system for Na^+ measurement (Fig. 16-2). There are two types of ISE measurement, based on sample preparation: direct and indirect. Direct measurement provides an undiluted sample to interact with the ISE membrane. With the indirect method, a diluted sample is used for measurement. There is no significant difference in results, except when samples are hyperlipidemic or hyperproteinemic. Excess lipids or proteins displace plasma water, which leads to a falsely decreased measurement of ionic activity in millimoles per liter of plasma, whereas the direct method measures in plasma water only. In these cases, direct ISE is more accurate.

One source of error with ISEs is protein buildup on the membrane through continuous use. The protein-coated

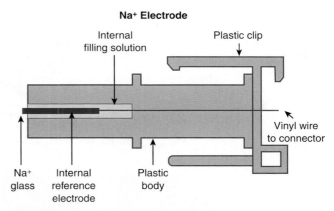

Na⁺ Electrode

FIGURE 16-2 Diagram of sodium ion-selective electrode with glass capillary membrane. (Courtesy of Nova Biomedical, Waltham, MA.)

membranes cause poor selectivity, which results in poor reproducibility of results. A routine maintenance of these ISEs requires removal of this protein buildup to ensure quality results.

Vitros analyzers (Ortho-Clinical Diagnostics) use a single-use direct ISE potentiometric system. Each disposable slide contains a reference and measuring electrode (Fig. 16-3). A drop of sample fluid and a drop of reference fluid are simultaneously applied to the slide, and the potential difference between the two is measured, which is proportional to the Na^+ concentration.[11]

Reference Ranges
See Table 16-6.[3]

Potassium

Potassium (K^+) is the major intracellular cation in the body, with a concentration 20 times greater inside the cells than outside. Many cellular functions require that the body maintain a low ECF concentration of K^+ ions. As a result, only 2% of the body's total K^+ circulates in the plasma. Functions of K^+ in the body include regulation of neuromuscular excitability, contraction of the heart, ICF volume, and H^+ concentration.[1]

The K^+ concentration has a major effect on the contraction of skeletal and cardiac muscles. An elevated plasma K^+ decreases the resting membrane potential (RMP) of the cell (the RMP is closer to zero), which decreases the net difference between the cell's resting potential and threshold (action) potential. A lower than normal difference increases cell excitability, leading to muscle weakness. Severe hyperkalemia can ultimately cause a lack of muscle excitability (as a result of a higher RMP than action potential), which may lead to paralysis or a fatal cardiac arrhythmia.[1] Hypokalemia decreases cell excitability by increasing the RMP, often resulting in an arrhythmia or paralysis.[1] The heart may cease to contract in extreme cases of either hyperkalemia or hypokalemia.

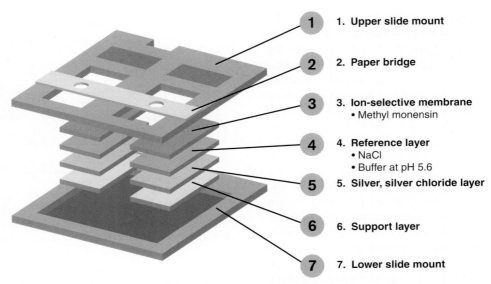

1. **Upper slide mount**
2. **Paper bridge**
3. **Ion-selective membrane**
   • Methyl monensin
4. **Reference layer**
   • NaCl
   • Buffer at pH 5.6
5. **Silver, silver chloride layer**
6. **Support layer**
7. **Lower slide mount**

FIGURE 16-3 Schematic diagram of the ion-selective electrode system for the potentiometric slide on the Vitros. (Courtesy of OCD, a Johnson & Johnson company, Rochester, NY.)

K^+ concentration also affects the H^+ concentration in the blood. For example, in hypokalemia (low serum K^+), as K^+ is lost from the body, Na^+ and H^+ move into the cell. The H^+ concentration is, therefore, decreased in the ECF, resulting in alkalosis.

Regulation
Renal function related to tubular reabsorption and secretion is important in the regulation of potassium balance. Initially, the proximal tubules reabsorb nearly all the K^+. Then, under the influence of aldosterone, additional K^+ is secreted into the urine in exchange for Na^+ in both the distal tubules and the collecting ducts. Thus, the distal nephron is the principal determinant of urinary K^+ excretion. Most individuals consume far more K^+ than needed; the excess is excreted in the urine but may accumulate to toxic levels if renal failure occurs.

K^+ uptake from the ECF into the cells is important in normalizing an acute rise in plasma K^+ concentration due to an increased K^+ intake. Excess plasma K^+ rapidly enters the cells to normalize plasma K^+. As the cellular K^+ gradually returns to the plasma, it is removed by urinary excretion. Note that chronic loss of cellular K^+ may result in cellular depletion before there is an appreciable change in the plasma K^+ concentration because excess K^+ is normally excreted in the urine.

Three factors that influence the distribution of K^+ between cells and ECF are as follows: (1) K^+ loss frequently occurs whenever the Na^+, K^+-ATPase pump is inhibited by conditions such as hypoxia, hypomagnesemia, or digoxin overdose; (2) insulin promotes acute entry of K^+ into skeletal muscle and liver by increasing Na^+, K^+-ATPase activity; and (3) catecholamines, such as epinephrine (β_2-stimulator), promote cellular entry of K^+, whereas propanolol (β-blocker) impairs cellular entry of K^+. Dietary deficiency or excess is rarely a primary cause of hypokalemia or hyperkalemia. However, with a pre-existing condition, dietary deficiency (or excess) can enhance the degree of hypokalemia (or hyperkalemia).

Exercise
K^+ is released from muscle cells during exercise, which may increase plasma K^+ by 0.3 to 1.2 mmol/L with mild to moderate exercise and by as much as 2 to 3 mmol/L with exhaustive exercise. These changes are usually reversed after several minutes of rest. Forearm exercise during venipuncture can cause erroneously high plasma K^+ concentrations.[12]

Hyperosmolality
Hyperosmolality, as with uncontrolled diabetes mellitus, causes water to diffuse from the cells, carrying K^+ with the water, which leads to gradual depletion of K^+ if kidney function is normal.

Cellular Breakdown
Cellular breakdown releases K^+ into the ECF. Examples are severe trauma, tumor lysis syndrome, and massive blood transfusions.

TABLE 16-6	REFERENCE RANGES FOR SODIUM	
Serum, plasma	136–145 mmol/L	
Urine (24 h)	40–220 mmol/d, varies with diet	
Cerebrospinal fluid	136–150 mmol/L	

TABLE 16-7	CAUSES OF HYPOKALEMIA

GASTROINTESTINAL LOSS

Vomiting

Diarrhea

Gastric suction

Intestinal tumor

Malabsorption

Cancer therapy—chemotherapy, radiation therapy

Large doses of laxatives

RENAL LOSS

Diuretics—thiazides, mineralocorticoids

Nephritis

Renal tubular acidosis

Hyperaldosteronism

Cushing's syndrome

Hypomagnesemia

Acute leukemia

CELLULAR SHIFT

Alkalosis

Insulin overdose

DECREASED INTAKE

Clinical Applications

Hypokalemia

Hypokalemia is a plasma K^+ concentration below the lower limit of the reference range. Hypokalemia can occur with GI or urinary loss of K^+ or with increased cellular uptake of K^+. Common causes of hypokalemia are shown in Table 16-7. Of these, therapy with thiazide-type diuretics is the most common.[13] GI loss occurs when GI fluid is lost through vomiting, diarrhea, gastric suction, or discharge from an intestinal fistula. Increased K^+ loss in the stool also occurs with certain tumors, malabsorption, cancer therapy (chemotherapy or radiation therapy), and large doses of laxatives.

Renal loss of K^+ can result from kidney disorders such as K^+-losing nephritis and renal tubular acidosis (RTA). In RTA, as tubular excretion of H^+ decreases, K^+ excretion increases. Because aldosterone promotes Na^+ retention and K^+ loss, hyperaldosteronism can lead to hypokalemia and metabolic alkalosis.[1] Hypomagnesemia can lead to hypokalemia by promoting urinary loss of K^+. Mg^{2+} deficiency also diminishes the activity of Na^+, K^+-ATPase and enhances the secretion of aldosterone. Effective treatment requires supplementation with both Mg^{2+} and K^+.[1] Renal K^+ loss also occurs with acute myelogenous leukemia, acute myelomonocytic leukemia, and acute lymphocytic leukemia.[13] Although reduced dietary intake of K^+ rarely causes hypokalemia

in healthy persons, decreased intake may intensify hypokalemia caused by use of diuretics, for example.

Increased cellular uptake of potassium is encountered in alkalemia and with elevated levels of insulin via therapeutic treatment of diabetes. Both alkalemia and insulin increase the cellular uptake of K^+. Because alkalemia promotes intracellular loss of H^+ to minimize elevation of intracellular pH, both K^+ and Na^+ enter cells to preserve electroneutrality. Plasma K^+ decreases by about 0.4 mmol/L per 0.1 unit rise in pH.[1] Insulin promotes the entry of K^+ into skeletal muscle and liver cells. Because insulin therapy can sometimes uncover an underlying hypokalemic state, plasma K^+ should be monitored carefully whenever insulin is administered to susceptible patients.[1] A rare cause of hypokalemia is associated with a blood sample from a leukemic patient with a significantly elevated white blood cell count. The K^+ present in the sample is taken up by the white cells if the sample is left at room temperature for several hours.[13]

Symptoms of hypokalemia. Symptoms (e.g., weakness, fatigue, and constipation) often become apparent as plasma K^+ decreases below 3 mmol/L. Hypokalemia can lead to muscle weakness or paralysis, which can interfere with breathing. The dangers of hypokalemia concern all patients, but especially those with cardiovascular disorders because of an increased risk of arrhythmia, which may cause sudden death in certain patients. Mild hypokalemia (3.0 to 3.4 mmol/L) is usually asymptomatic.

Treatment of hypokalemia. Treatment typically includes oral KCl replacement of K^+ over several days. In some instances, intravenous (IV) replacement may be indicated. In some cases, chronic mild hypokalemia may be corrected simply by including food in the diet with high K^+ content, such as dried fruits, nuts, bran cereals, bananas, and orange juice. Plasma electrolytes are monitored as treatment to return K^+ levels to normal occurs.

Hyperkalemia

The most common causes of hyperkalemia are shown in Table 16-8. Patients with hyperkalemia often have an underlying disorder, such as renal insufficiency, diabetes mellitus, or metabolic acidosis, that contributes to hyperkalemia.[12] For example, during administration of KCl, a person with renal insufficiency is far more likely to develop hyperkalemia than is a person with normal renal function. The most common cause of hyperkalemia in hospitalized patients is due to therapeutic K^+ administration. The risk is greatest with IV K^+ replacement.[12]

In healthy persons, an acute oral load of K^+ will briefly increase plasma K^+ because most of the absorbed K^+ rapidly moves intracellularly. Normal cellular processes gradually release this excess K^+ back into the plasma, where it is normally removed by renal excretion. Impairment of urinary K^+ excretion is usually associated with chronic hyperkalemia.[1]

TABLE 16-8	CAUSES OF HYPERKALEMIA

DECREASED RENAL EXCRETION

Acute or chronic renal failure (GFR < 20 mL/min)

Hypoaldosteronism

Addison's disease

Diuretics

CELLULAR SHIFT

Acidosis

Muscle/cellular injury

Chemotherapy

Leukemia

Hemolysis

INCREASED INTAKE

Oral or intravenous potassium replacement therapy

ARTIFACTUAL

Sample hemolysis

Thrombocytosis

Prolonged tourniquet use or excessive fist clenching

GFR, glomerular filtration rate.

If a shift of K^+ from cells into plasma occurs too rapidly to be removed by renal excretion, acute hyperkalemia develops. In diabetes mellitus, insulin deficiency promotes cellular loss of K^+. Hyperglycemia also contributes by producing a hyperosmolar plasma that pulls water and K^+ from cells, promoting further loss of K^+ into the plasma.[1]

In metabolic acidosis, as excess H^+ moves intracellularly to be buffered, K^+ leaves the cell to maintain electroneutrality. Plasma K^+ increases by 0.2 to 1.7 mmol/L for each 0.1 unit reduction of pH.[1] Because cellular K^+ often becomes depleted in cases of acidosis with hyperkalemia (including diabetic ketoacidosis), treatment with agents such as insulin and bicarbonate can cause a rapid intracellular movement of K^+, producing severe hypokalemia.

Various drugs may cause hyperkalemia, especially in patients with either renal insufficiency or diabetes mellitus. These drugs include captopril (inhibits angiotensin-converting enzyme), nonsteroidal anti-inflammatory agents (inhibit aldosterone), spironolactone (K^+-sparing diuretic), digoxin (inhibits Na^+–K^+ pump), cyclosporine (inhibits renal response to aldosterone), and heparin therapy (inhibits aldosterone secretion).

Hyperkalemia may result when K^+ is released into the ECF during enhanced tissue breakdown or catabolism, especially if renal insufficiency is present. Increased cellular breakdown may be caused by trauma, administration of cytotoxic agents, massive hemolysis, tumor lysis syndrome, and blood transfusions. In banked blood, K^+ is gradually released from erythrocytes during storage, often causing elevated K^+ concentration in plasma supernatant.

Patients on cardiac bypass may develop mild elevations in plasma K^+ during warming after surgery because warming causes cellular release of K^+. Hypothermia causes movement of K^+ into cells.

Symptoms of hyperkalemia. Hyperkalemia can cause muscle weakness, tingling, numbness, or mental confusion by altering neuromuscular conduction. Muscle weakness does not usually develop until plasma K^+ reaches 8 mmol/L.[1]

Hyperkalemia disturbs cardiac conduction, which can lead to cardiac arrhythmias and possible cardiac arrest. Plasma K^+ concentrations of 6 to 7 mmol/L may alter the electrocardiogram (ECG), and concentrations more than 10 mmol/L may cause fatal cardiac arrest.[1]

Treatment of hyperkalemia. Treatment should be immediately initiated when serum K^+ is 6.0 to 6.5 mmol/L or greater or if there are ECG changes.[12] To offset the effect of K^+, which lowers the resting potential of myocardial cells, Ca^{2+} may be given to reduce the threshold potential of myocardial cells. Therefore, Ca^{2+} provides immediate but short-lived protection to the myocardium against the effects of hyperkalemia. Substances that acutely shift K^+ back into cells, such as sodium bicarbonate, glucose, or insulin, may also be administered. K^+ may be quickly removed from the body by use of diuretics (loop), if renal function is adequate, or sodium polystyrene sulfonate (Kayexalate) enemas, which bind to K^+ secreted in the colon. Hemodialysis can be used if other measures fail.[12] Patients treated with these agents must be monitored carefully to prevent hypokalemia as K^+ moves back into cells or is removed from the body.

Collection of Samples

Proper collection and handling of samples for K^+ analysis is extremely important because there are many causes of artifactual hyperkalemia. First, the coagulation process releases K^+ from platelets, so that serum K^+ may be 0.1 to 0.7 mmol/L higher than plasma K^+ concentrations.[2] If the patient's platelet count is elevated (thrombocytosis), serum K^+ may be further elevated. Second, if a tourniquet is left on the arm too long during blood collection or if patients excessively clench their fists or otherwise exercise their forearms before venipuncture, cells may release K^+ into the plasma. The first situation may be avoided by using a heparinized tube to prevent clotting of the specimen and the second by using proper care in the drawing of blood. Third, because storing blood on ice promotes the release of K^+ from cells,[14] whole blood samples for K^+ determinations should be stored at room temperature (never iced) and analyzed promptly or centrifuged to remove the cells. Fourth, if hemolysis occurs after the blood is drawn, K^+ may be falsely elevated—the most common cause of artifactual hyperkalemia. Slight hemolysis (≈50 mg/dL of hemoglobin) can cause an increase of approximately 3% while gross hemolysis (>500 mg/dL of hemoglobin) can cause an increase of up to 30%.[2]

Determination of Potassium

Specimen

Serum, plasma, and urine may be acceptable for analysis. Hemolysis must be avoided because of the high K^+ content of erythrocytes. Heparin is the anticoagulant of choice. Whereas serum and plasma generally give similar K^+ levels, serum reference intervals tend to be slightly higher. Significantly elevated platelet counts may result in the release of K^+ during clotting from rupture of these cells, causing a spurious hyperkalemia. In this case, plasma is preferred. Whole blood samples may be used with some analyzers. Consult the instrument's operations manual for acceptability. Urine specimens should be collected over a 24-hour period to eliminate the influence of diurnal variation.

Methods

As with Na^+, the current method of choice is ISE. For ISE measurements, a valinomycin membrane is used to selectively bind K^+, causing an impedance change that can be correlated to K^+ concentration. KCl is the inner electrolyte solution.

Reference Ranges
See Table 16-9.[3]

Chloride

Chloride (Cl^-) is the major extracellular anion. Its precise function in the body is not well understood;

TABLE 16-9	REFERENCE RANGES FOR POTASSIUM
Serum	3.5–5.1 mmol/L
Plasma	Males: 3.5–4.5 mmol/L
	Females: 3.4–4.4 mmol/L
Urine (24 h)	25–125 mmol/d

however, it is involved in maintaining osmolality, blood volume, and electric neutrality. In most processes, Cl^- shifts secondarily to a movement of Na^+ or HCO_3^-.

Cl^- ingested in the diet is almost completely absorbed by the intestinal tract. Cl^- is then filtered out by the glomerulus and passively reabsorbed, in conjunction with Na^+, by the proximal tubules. Excess Cl^- is excreted in the urine and sweat. Excessive sweating stimulates aldosterone secretion, which acts on the sweat glands to conserve Na^+ and Cl^-.

Cl^- maintains electrical neutrality in two ways. First, Na^+ is reabsorbed along with Cl^- in the proximal tubules. In effect, Cl^- acts as the rate-limiting component, in that Na^+ reabsorption is limited by the amount of Cl^- available. Electroneutrality is also maintained by Cl^- through the *chloride shift*. In this process, CO_2 generated by cellular metabolism within the tissue diffuses out into both the plasma and the red cell. In the red cell, CO_2 forms carbonic acid (H_2CO_3), which splits into H^+ and HCO_3^- (bicarbonate). Deoxyhemoglobin buffers H^+, whereas the HCO_3^- diffuses out into the plasma and Cl^- diffuses into the red cell to maintain the electric balance of the cell (Fig. 16-4).

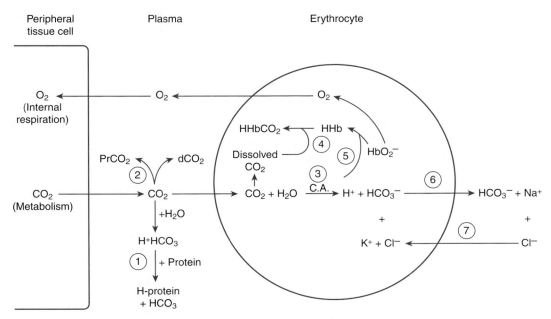

FIGURE 16-4 Chloride shift mechanism. See text for details. (Reprinted with permission from Burtis CA, Ashwood ER, eds. *Tietz Textbook of Clinical Chemistry.* 2nd ed. Philadelphia, PA: WB Saunders; 1994.)

Clinical Applications

Cl^- disorders are often a result of the same causes that disturb Na^+ levels because Cl^- passively follows Na^+. There are a few exceptions. Hyperchloremia may also occur when there is an excess loss of HCO_3^- as a result of GI losses, RTA, or metabolic acidosis. Hypochloremia may also occur with excessive loss of Cl^- from prolonged vomiting, diabetic ketoacidosis, aldosterone deficiency, or salt-losing renal diseases such as pyelonephritis. A low serum level of Cl^- may also be encountered in conditions associated with high serum HCO_3^- concentrations, such as compensated respiratory acidosis or metabolic alkalosis.

Determination of Chloride

Specimen

Serum or plasma may be used, with lithium heparin being the anticoagulant of choice. Hemolysis does not cause a significant change in serum or plasma values as a result of decreased levels of intracellular Cl^-. However, with marked hemolysis, levels may be decreased as a result of a dilutional effect.

Whole blood samples may be used with some analyzers. Consult the instrument's operation manual for acceptability. The specimen of choice in urine Cl^- analyses is 24-hour collection because of the large diurnal variation. Sweat is also suitable for analysis. Sweat collection and analysis are discussed in Chapter 29.

Methods

There are several methodologies available for measuring Cl^-, including ISEs, amperometric-coulometric titration, mercurimetric titration, and colorimetry. The most commonly used is ISE. For ISE measurement, an ion-exchange membrane is used to selectively bind Cl^- ions.

Amperometric-coulometric titration is a method using coulometric generation of silver ions (Ag^+), which combine with Cl^- to quantitate the Cl^- concentration.

$$Ag^{2+} + 2Cl^- \rightarrow AgCl_2 \qquad \text{(Eq. 16-2)}$$

When all Cl^- in a patient is bound to Ag^+, excess or free Ag^+ is used to indicate the endpoint. As Ag^+ accumulates, the coulometric generator and timer are turned off. The elapsed time is used to calculate the concentration of Cl^- in the sample. The digital (Cotlove) chloridometer (Labconco Corporation) uses this principle in Cl^- analysis.

Reference Ranges

See Table 16-10.[3]

TABLE 16-10	REFERENCE RANGES FOR CHLORIDE
Plasma, serum	98–107 mmol/L
Urine (24 h)	110–250 mmol/d, varies with diet

Bicarbonate

Bicarbonate is the second most abundant anion in the ECF. Total CO_2 comprises the bicarbonate ion (HCO_3^-), H_2CO_3, and dissolved CO_2, with HCO_3^- accounting for more than 90% of the total CO_2 at physiologic pH. Because HCO_3^- composes the largest fraction of total CO_2, total CO_2 measurement is indicative of HCO_3^- measurement.

HCO_3^- is the major component of the buffering system in the blood. Carbonic anhydrase in RBCs converts CO_2 and H_2O to H_2CO_3, which dissociates into H^+ and HCO_3^-.

$$CO_2 + H_2O \underset{}{\overset{CA}{\longleftrightarrow}} H_2CO_3 \underset{}{\overset{CA}{\longleftrightarrow}} H^+ + HCO_3^-$$

(Eq. 16-3)

where CA is carbonic anhydrase. HCO_3^- diffuses out of the cell in exchange for Cl^- to maintain ionic charge neutrality within the cell (chloride shift; see Fig. 16-4). This process converts potentially toxic CO_2 in the plasma to an effective buffer: HCO_3^-. HCO_3^- buffers excess H^+ by combining with acid, then eventually dissociating into H_2O and CO_2 in the lungs where the acidic gas CO_2 is eliminated.

Regulation

Most of the HCO_3^- in the kidneys (85%) is reabsorbed by the proximal tubules, with 15% being reabsorbed by the distal tubules. Because tubules are only slightly permeable to HCO_3^-, it is usually reabsorbed as CO_2. This happens as HCO_3^-, after filtering into the tubules, combines with H^+ to form H_2CO_3, which then dissociates into H_2O and CO_2. The CO_2 readily diffuses back into the ECF. Normally, nearly all the HCO_3^- is reabsorbed from the tubules, with little lost in the urine. When HCO_3^- is filtered in excess of H^+ available, almost all excess HCO_3^- flows into the urine.

In alkalosis, with a relative increase in HCO_3^- compared with CO_2, the kidneys increase excretion of HCO_3^- into the urine, carrying along a cation such as Na^+. This loss of HCO_3^- from the body helps correct pH.

Among the responses of the body to acidosis is an increased excretion of H^+ into the urine. In addition, HCO_3^- reabsorption is virtually complete, with 90% of the filtered HCO_3^- reabsorbed in the proximal tubule and the remainder in the distal tubule.[1]

Clinical Applications

Acid–base imbalances cause changes in HCO_3^- and CO_2 levels. A decreased HCO_3^- may occur from metabolic acidosis as HCO_3^- combines with H^+ to produce CO_2, which is exhaled by the lungs. The typical response to metabolic acidosis is compensation by hyperventilation, which lowers pco_2. Elevated total CO_2 concentrations occur in metabolic alkalosis as HCO_3^- is retained, often with increased

pco_2 as a result of compensation by hypoventilation. Typical causes of metabolic alkalosis include severe vomiting, hypokalemia, and excessive alkali intake.

Determination of CO₂

Specimen

This chapter deals specifically with venous serum or plasma determinations. For discussion of arterial and whole blood pco_2 measurements, refer Chapter 17.

Serum or lithium heparin plasma is suitable for analysis. Although specimens should be anaerobic for the highest accuracy, many current analyzers (excluding blood gas analyzers) do not permit anaerobic sample handling. In most instances, the sample is capped until the serum or plasma is separated and the sample is analyzed immediately. If the sample is left uncapped before analysis, CO_2 escapes. Levels can decrease by 6 mmol/L/h.[2]

CO_2 measurements may be obtained in several ways; however, the actual portion of the total CO_2 being measured may vary with the method used. Two common methods are ISE and an enzymatic method.

One type of ISE for measuring total CO_2 uses an acid reagent to convert all the forms of CO_2 to CO_2 gas and is measured by a pco_2 electrode (see Chapter 5).

The enzyme method alkalinizes the sample to convert all forms of CO_2 to HCO_3^-. HCO_3^- is used to carboxylate phosphoenolpyruvate (PEP) in the presence of PEP carboxylase, which catalyzes the formation of oxaloacetate:

$$\text{Phosphoenolpyruvate} + HCO_3^- \xrightarrow{\text{PEF carboxylate}}$$
$$\text{Oxalocetate} + H_2PO_4^- \qquad \text{(Eq. 16-4)}$$

This is coupled to the following reaction, in which NADH is consumed as a result of the action of malate dehydrogenase (MDH):

$$\text{Oxaloacetate} + NADH + H^+ \xrightarrow{\text{MDH}} \text{Malate} + NAD^+$$
$$\text{(Eq. 16-5)}$$

The rate of change in absorbance of NADH is proportional to the concentration of HCO_3^-.

Reference Ranges

CO_2, venous 23 to 29 mmol/L (plasma, serum).[3]

Magnesium

Magnesium Physiology

Magnesium (Mg^{2+}) is the fourth most abundant cation in the body and second most abundant intracellular ion. The average human body (70 kg) contains 1 mol (24 g) of Mg^{2+}. Approximately 53% of Mg^{2+} in the body is found in bone, 46% in muscle and other organs and soft tissue, and less than 1% is present in serum and RBCs.[15] Of the Mg^{2+} present in serum, about one-third is bound to protein, primarily albumin. Of the remaining two-thirds, 61% exists in the free or ionized state and about 5% is complexed with other ions, such as PO_4^- and citrate. Similar to Ca^{2+}, it is the free ion that is physiologically active in the body.[16]

The role of Mg^{2+} in the body is widespread. It is an essential cofactor of more than 300 enzymes, including those important in glycolysis; transcellular ion transport; neuromuscular transmission; synthesis of carbohydrates, proteins, lipids, and nucleic acids; and the release of and response to certain hormones.

The clinical usefulness of serum Mg^{2+} levels has greatly increased in the past 10 years as more information about the analyte has been discovered. The most significant findings are the relationship between abnormal serum Mg^{2+} levels and cardiovascular, metabolic, and neuromuscular disorders. Although serum levels may not reflect total body stores of Mg^{2+}, they are useful in determining acute changes in the ion.

Regulation

Rich sources of Mg^{2+} in the diet include raw nuts, dry cereal, and "hard" drinking water; other sources include vegetables, meats, fish, and fruit.[15] Processed foods, an ever-increasing part of the average U.S. diet, have low levels of Mg^{2+} that may cause an inadequate intake. This in turn may increase the likelihood of Mg^{2+} deficiency. The small intestine may absorb 20% to 65% of the dietary Mg^{2+}, depending on the need and intake.

The overall regulation of body Mg^{2+} is controlled largely by the kidney, which can reabsorb Mg^{2+} in deficiency states or readily excrete excess Mg^{2+} in overload states. Of the nonprotein-bound Mg^{2+} that gets filtered by the glomerulus, 25% to 30% is reabsorbed by the proximal convoluted tubule (PCT), unlike Na^+, in which 60% to 75% is absorbed in the PCT. Henle's loop is the major renal regulatory site, where 50% to 60% of filtered Mg^{2+} is reabsorbed in the ascending limb. In addition, 2% to 5% is reabsorbed in the distal convoluted tubule.[17] The renal threshold for Mg^{2+} is approximately 0.60 to 0.85 mmol/L ($\approx$1.46 to 2.07 mg/dL). Because this is close to normal serum concentration, slight excesses of Mg^{2+} in serum are rapidly excreted by the kidneys. Normally, only about 6% of filtered Mg^{2+} is excreted in the urine per day.[15]

Mg^{2+} regulation appears to be related to that of Ca^{2+} and Na^+. Parathyroid hormone (PTH) increases the renal reabsorption of Mg^{2+} and enhances the absorption of Mg^{2+} in the intestine. However, changes in ionized Ca^{2+} have a far greater effect on PTH secretion. Aldosterone and thyroxine apparently have the opposite effect of PTH in the kidney, increasing the renal excretion of Mg^{2+}.[16]

Clinical Applications

Hypomagnesemia

Hypomagnesemia is most frequently observed in hospitalized individuals in intensive care units (ICUs) or those receiving diuretic therapy or digitalis therapy. These

TABLE 16-11	CAUSES OF HYPOMAGNESEMIA

REDUCED INTAKE

Poor diet/starvation

Prolonged magnesium-deficient intravenous therapy

Chronic alcoholism

DECREASED ABSORPTION

Malabsorption syndrome

Surgical resection of small intestine

Nasogastric suction

Pancreatitis

Vomiting

Diarrhea

Laxative abuse

Neonatal

Primary

Congenital

INCREASED EXCRETION—RENAL

Tubular disorder

Glomerulonephritis

Pyelonephritis

INCREASED EXCRETION—ENDOCRINE

Hyperparathyroidism

Hyperaldosteronism

Hyperthyroidism

Hypercalcemia

Diabetic ketoacidosis

INCREASED EXCRETION—DRUG INDUCED

Diuretics

Antibiotics

Cyclosporin

Digitalis

MISCELLANEOUS

Excess lactation

Pregnancy

Adapted from Polancic JE. Magnesium: metabolism, clinical importance, and analysis. *Clin Lab Sci.* 1991;4(2):105-109.

patients most likely have an overall tissue depletion of Mg^{2+} as a result of severe illness or loss, which leads to low serum levels. Hypomagnesemia is rare in nonhospitalized individuals.[16]

There are many causes of hypomagnesemia; however, it can be grouped into general categories (Table 16-11). Reduced intake is least likely to cause severe deficiencies in the United States. A Mg^{2+}-deficient diet as a result of starvation, chronic alcoholism, or Mg^{2+}-deficient IV therapy can cause a loss of the ion.

Various GI disorders may cause decreased absorption by the intestine, which can result in an excess loss of Mg^{2+} via the feces. Malabsorption syndromes; intestinal resection or bypass surgery; nasogastric suction; pancreatitis; and prolonged vomiting, diarrhea, or laxative use may lead to an Mg^{2+} deficiency. Neonatal hypomagnesemia has been reported as a result of various surgical procedures. A primary deficiency has also been reported in infants as a result of a selective malabsorption of the ion.[16] A chronic congenital hypomagnesemia with secondary hypocalcemia (autosomal recessive disorder) has also been reported; molecular studies have revealed a specific transport protein defect in the intestine.[18]

Mg^{2+} loss due to increased excretion by way of urine can occur as a result of various renal and endocrine disorders or the effects of certain drugs on the kidneys. Renal tubular disorders and other select renal disorders may result in excess amounts of Mg^{2+} being lost through the urine because of decreased tubular reabsorption.

Several endocrine disorders can cause a loss of Mg^{2+}. Hyperparathyroidism and hypercalcemia may cause increased renal excretion of Mg^{2+} as a result of excess Ca^{2+} ions. Excess serum Na^+ levels caused by hyperaldosteronism may also cause increased renal excretion of Mg^{2+}. A pseudohypomagnesemia may also be the result of hyperaldosteronism caused by increased water reabsorption. Hyperthyroidism may result in an increased renal excretion of Mg^{2+} and may also cause an intracellular shift of the ion. In persons with diabetes, excess urinary loss of Mg^{2+} is associated with glycosuria. Hypomagnesemia can aggravate the neuromuscular and vascular complications commonly found in this disease. Some studies have shown a relationship between Mg^{2+} deficiency and insulin resistance; however, Mg^{2+} is not thought to play a role in the pathophysiology of diabetes mellitus. The American Diabetes Association has issued a statement regarding dietary intake of Mg^{2+} and measurement of serum Mg^{2+} in patients with diabetes.[19]

Several drugs, including diuretics, gentamicin, cisplatin, and cyclosporine, increase renal loss of Mg^{2+} and frequently result in hypomagnesemia. The loop diuretics, such as furosemide, are especially effective in increasing renal loss of Mg^{2+}. Thiazide diuretics require a longer period of use to cause hypomagnesemia. Cisplatin has a nephrotoxic effect that inhibits the ability of the renal tubule to conserve Mg^{2+}. Cyclosporine, an immunosuppressant, severely inhibits the renal tubular reabsorption of Mg^{2+} and has many adverse effects, including nephrotoxicity, hypertension, hepatotoxicity, and neurologic symptoms such as seizures and tremors. Cardiac glycosides, such as digoxin and digitalis, can interfere with Mg^{2+} reabsorption. The resulting hypomagnesemia is a significant finding because the decreased level of Mg^{2+} can amplify the symptoms of digitalis toxicity.[16]

Excess lactation has been associated with hypomagnesemia as a result of increased use and loss through milk production. Mild deficiencies have been reported in pregnancy, which may cause a hyperexcitable uterus, anxiety, and insomnia.

Symptoms of hypomagnesemia. A patient who is hypomagnesemic may be asymptomatic until serum levels fall below 0.5 mmol/L.[16] A variety of symptoms can occur. The most frequent involve cardiovascular, neuromuscular, psychiatric, and metabolic abnormalities (Table 16-12). The cardiovascular and neuromuscular symptoms result primarily from the ATPase enzyme's requirement for Mg^{2+}. Mg^{2+} loss leads to decreased intracellular K^+ levels because of a faulty $Na^+–K^+$ pump (ATPase). This change in cellular RMP causes increased excitability that may lead to cardiac arrhythmias. This condition may also lead to digitalis toxicity.

Muscle contraction also requires Mg^{2+} and ATPase for normal Ca^{2+} uptake following contraction. Normal nerve and muscle cell stimulation requires Mg^{2+} to assist with the regulation of acetylcholine, a potent neurotransmitter. Hypomagnesemia can cause a variety of symptoms from weakness to tremors, tetany, paralysis, or coma. The CNS can also be affected, resulting in psychiatric disorders that range from subtle changes to depression or psychosis.

Metabolic disorders are associated with hypomagnesemia. Studies have indicated that approximately 40% of hospitalized patients with hypokalemia are also hypomagnesemic.[17] In addition, 20% to 30% of patients with hyponatremia, hypocalcemia, or hypophosphatemia are also hypomagnesemic.[17] Mg^{2+} deficiency can impair PTH release and target tissue response, resulting in hypocalcemia. Replenishing any of these deficient ions alone often does not remedy the disorder unless Mg^{2+} therapy is provided. Mg^{2+} therapy alone may restore both ion levels to normal; serum levels of the ions must be monitored during treatment.

Treatment of hypomagnesemia. The preferred form of treatment is by oral intake using magnesium lactate, magnesium oxide, or magnesium chloride or an antacid that contains Mg^{2+}. In severely ill patients, an $MgSO_4$ solution is given parenterally. Before initiation of therapy, renal function must be evaluated to avoid inducing hypermagnesemia during treatment.[17]

TABLE 16-12	SYMPTOMS OF HYPOMAGNESEMIA
CARDIOVASCULAR	**PSYCHIATRIC**
Arrhythmia	Depression
Hypertension	Agitation
Digitalis toxicity	Psychosis
NEUROMUSCULAR	**METABOLIC**
Weakness	Hypokalemia
Cramps	Hypocalcemia
Ataxia	Hypophosphatemia
Tremor	Hyponatremia
Seizure	
Tetany	
Paralysis	
Coma	

Adapted from Polancic JE. Magnesium: metabolism, clinical importance, and analysis. *Clin Lab Sci.* 1991;4(2):105-109.

CASE STUDY 16-2

A 60-year-old man entered the emergency department after 2 days of "not feeling so well." History revealed a myocardial infarction 5 years ago, when he was prescribed digoxin. Two years ago, he was prescribed a diuretic after periodic bouts of edema. An ECG at time of admission indicated a cardiac arrhythmia. Admitting lab results are shown in Case Study Table 16-2.1.

CASE STUDY TABLE 16-2.1 LABORATORY RESULTS

VENOUS BLOOD

Digoxin: 1.4 ng/mL, therapeutic 0.5–2.2 (1.8 nmol/L, therapeutic 0.6–2.8)

Na^+: 137 mmol/L

K^+: 2.5 mmol/L

Cl^-: 100 mmol/L

HCO_3^-: 25 mmol/L

Mg^{2+}: 0.4 mmol/L

Ion/free Ca^{2+}: 1.0 mmol/L

Questions

1. Because the digoxin level is within the therapeutic range, what may be the cause for the arrhythmia?

2. What is the most likely cause for the hypomagnesemia?

3. What is the most likely cause for the decreased potassium and ionized calcium levels?

4. What type of treatment would be helpful?

TABLE 16-13	CAUSES OF HYPERMAGNESEMIA

DECREASED EXCRETION

Acute or chronic renal failure

Hypothyroidism

Hypoaldosteronism

Hypopituitarism (↓growth hormone)

INCREASED INTAKE

Antacids

Enemas

Cathartics

Therapeutic—eclampsia, cardiac arrhythmia

MISCELLANEOUS

Dehydration

Bone carcinoma

Bone metastases

Adapted from Polancic JE. Magnesium: metabolism, clinical importance, and analysis. *Clin Lab Sci.* 1991;4(2):105-109.

TABLE 16-14	SYMPTOMS OF HYPERMAGNESEMIA

CARDIOVASCULAR	NEUROMUSCULAR
Hypotension	Decreased reflexes
Bradycardia	Dysarthria
Heart block	Respiratory depression
	Paralysis
DERMATOLOGIC	**METABOLIC**
Flushing	Hypocalcemia
Warm skin	
GASTROINTESTINAL	**HEMOSTATIC**
Nausea	Decreased thrombin generation
Vomiting	Decreased platelet adhesion
NEUROLOGIC	
Lethargy	
Coma	

Adapted from Polancic JE. Magnesium: metabolism, clinical importance, and analysis. *Clin Lab Sci.* 1991;4(2):105-109.

Hypermagnesemia

Hypermagnesemia is observed less frequently than hypomagnesemia.[16] Causes for elevated serum Mg^{2+} levels are summarized in Table 16-13; the most common is renal failure (GFR < 30 mL/min). The most severe elevations are usually a result of the combined effects of decreased renal function and increased intake of commonly prescribed Mg^{2+}-containing medications, such as antacids, enemas, or cathartics. Nursing home patients are at greatest risk for this occurrence.[16]

Hypermagnesemia has been associated with several endocrine disorders. Thyroxine and growth hormone cause a decrease in tubular reabsorption of Mg^{2+}, and a deficiency of either hormone may cause a moderate elevation in serum Mg^{2+}. Adrenal insufficiency may cause a mild elevation as a result of decreased renal excretion of Mg^{2+}.[16]

$MgSO_4$ may be used therapeutically with preeclampsia, cardiac arrhythmia, or myocardial infarction. Mg^{2+} is a vasodilator and can decrease uterine hyperactivity in eclamptic states and increase uterine blood flow. This therapy can lead to maternal hypermagnesemia, as well as neonatal hypermagnesemia due to the immature kidney of the newborn. Premature infants are at greater risk to develop actual symptoms.[16] Studies have shown that IV Mg^{2+} therapy in myocardial infarction patients may reduce early mortality.[15]

Dehydration can cause a pseudohypermagnesemia, which can be corrected with rehydration. Because of increased bone loss, mild serum Mg^{2+} elevations can occur in individuals with multiple myeloma or bone metastases.

Symptoms of hypermagnesemia. Symptoms of hypermagnesemia typically do not occur until the serum level exceeds 1.5 mmol/L.[16] The most frequent symptoms involve cardiovascular, dermatologic, GI, neurologic, neuromuscular, metabolic, and hemostatic abnormalities (Table 16-14). Mild to moderate symptoms, such as hypotension, bradycardia, skin flushing, increased skin temperature, nausea, vomiting, and lethargy may occur when serum levels are 1.5 to 2.5 mmol/L.[16] Life-threatening symptoms, such as ECG changes, heart block, asystole, sedation, coma, respiratory depression or arrest, and paralysis, can occur when serum levels reach 5.0 mmol/L.[16]

Elevated Mg^{2+} levels may inhibit PTH release and target tissue response. This may lead to hypocalcemia and hypercalcuria.[16] Normal hemostasis is a Ca^{2+}-dependent process that may be inhibited as a result of competition between increased levels of Mg^{2+} and Ca^{2+} ions. Thrombin generation and platelet adhesion are two processes in which interference may occur.[16]

Treatment of hypermagnesemia. Treatment of Mg^{2+} excess associated with increased intake is to discontinue the source of Mg^{2+}. Severe symptomatic hypermagnesemia requires immediate supportive therapy for cardiac, neuromuscular, respiratory, or neurologic abnormalities. Patients with renal failure require hemodialysis. Patients with normal renal function may be treated with a diuretic and IV fluid.

Determination of Magnesium

Specimen

Nonhemolyzed serum or lithium heparin plasma may be analyzed. Because the Mg^{2+} concentration inside erythrocytes is 10 times greater than that in the ECF, hemolysis should be avoided and the serum should be separated from the cells as soon as possible. Oxalate, citrate, and ethylenediaminetetraacetic acid (EDTA) anticoagulants are unacceptable because they will bind with Mg^{2+}. A 24-hour urine sample is preferred for analysis because of a diurnal variation in excretion. The urine must be acidified with HCl to avoid precipitation.

Methods
The three most common methods for measuring total serum Mg^{2+} are colorimetric: calmagite, formazan dye, and methylthymol blue. In the calmagite method, Mg^{2+} binds with calmagite to form a reddish-violet complex that may be read at 532 nm. In the formazan dye method, Mg^{2+} binds with the dye to form a colored complex that may be read at 660 nm. In the methylthymol blue method, Mg^{2+} binds with the chromogen to form a colored complex. Most methods use a Ca^{2+} shelter to prohibit interference from this divalent cation. The reference method for measuring Mg^{2+} is AAS.

Although the measurement of total Mg^{2+} concentrations in serum remains the usual diagnostic test for detection of Mg^{2+} abnormalities, it has limitations. First, because approximately 25% of Mg^{2+} is protein bound, total Mg^{2+} may not reflect the physiologically active free ionized Mg^{2+}. Second, because Mg^{2+} is primarily an intracellular ion, serum concentrations will not necessarily reflect the status of intracellular Mg^{2+}. Even when tissue and cellular Mg^{2+} is depleted by as much as 20%, serum Mg^{2+} concentrations may remain normal.

Reference Ranges
See Table 16-15.[3]

TABLE 16-15	REFERENCE RANGE FOR MAGNESIUM
Serum, colorimetric	0.63–1.0 mmol/L (1.26–2.10 mmol/L)

Calcium

Calcium Physiology
In 1883, Ringer[20] showed that Ca^{2+} was essential for myocardial contraction. While attempting to study how bound and free forms of Ca^{2+} affected frog heart contraction, McLean and Hastings[21] showed that the ionized/free Ca^{2+} concentration was proportional to the amplitude of frog heart contraction, whereas protein-bound and citrate-bound Ca^{2+} had no effect. From this observation, they developed the first assay for ionized/free Ca^{2+} using isolated frog hearts. Although the method had poor precision by today's standards, the investigators were able to show that blood-ionized Ca^{2+} was closely regulated and had a mean concentration in humans of about 1.18 mmol/L. Because decreased ionized Ca^{2+} impairs myocardial function, it is important to maintain ionized Ca^{2+} at a near-normal concentration during surgery and in critically ill patients. Decreased ionized Ca^{2+} concentrations in blood can cause neuromuscular irritability, which may become clinically apparent as irregular muscle spasms, called tetany.

Regulation
Three hormones, PTH, vitamin D, and calcitonin, are known to regulate serum Ca^{2+} by altering their secretion rate in response to changes in ionized Ca^{2+}. The actions of these hormones are shown in Figure 16-5.

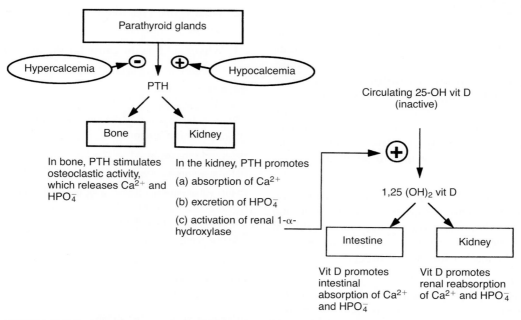

FIGURE 16-5 Hormonal response to hypercalcemia and hypocalcemia. PTH, parathyroid hormone; 25-OH vit D, 25-hydroxy vitamin D; 1,25(OH)₂ vit D, dihydroxy vitamin D.

PTH secretion in blood is stimulated by a decrease in ionized Ca^{2+}, and conversely, PTH secretion is stopped by an increase in ionized Ca^{2+}. PTH exerts three major effects on both bone and kidney. In the bone, PTH activates a process known as *bone resorption*, in which activated osteoclasts break down bone and subsequently release Ca^{2+} into the ECF. In the kidneys, PTH conserves Ca^{2+} by increasing tubular reabsorption of Ca^{2+} ions. PTH also stimulates renal production of active vitamin D.

Vitamin D_3, a cholecalciferol, is obtained from the diet or exposure of skin to sunlight. Vitamin D_3 is then converted in the liver to 25-hydroxycholecalciferol (25-OH-D_3), still an inactive form of vitamin D. In the kidney, 25-OH-D_3 is specifically hydroxylated to form 1,25-dihydroxycholecalciferol (1,25-$[OH]_2$-D_3), the biologically active form. This active form of vitamin D increases Ca^{2+} absorption in the intestine and enhances the effect of PTH on bone resorption.

Calcitonin, which originates in the medullary cells of the thyroid gland, is secreted when the concentration of Ca^{2+} in blood increases. Calcitonin exerts its Ca^{2+}-lowering effect by inhibiting the actions of both PTH and vitamin D. Although calcitonin is apparently not secreted during normal regulation of the ionized Ca^{2+} concentration in blood, it is secreted in response to a hypercalcemic stimulus.

Distribution

About 99% of Ca^{2+} in the body is part of bone. The remaining 1% is mostly in the blood and other ECF. Little is in the cytosol of most cells. In fact, the concentration of ionized Ca^{2+} in blood is 5,000 to 10,000 times higher than in the cytosol of cardiac or smooth muscle cells. Maintenance of this large gradient is vital to maintain the essential rapid inward flux of Ca^{2+}.

Ca^{2+} in blood is distributed among several forms. About 45% circulates as free Ca^{2+} ions (referred to as ionized Ca^{2+}), 40% is bound to protein, mostly albumin, and 15% is bound to anions, such as HCO_3^-, citrate, HCO_3^-, and lactate. Clearly, this distribution can change in disease. It is noteworthy that concentrations of citrate, HCO_3^-, lactate, HCO_3^-, and albumin can change dramatically during surgery or critical care. This is why ionized Ca^{2+} cannot be reliably calculated from total Ca^{2+} measurements, especially in acutely ill individuals.

Clinical Applications

Tables 16-16 and 16-17 summarize causes of hypocalcemic and hypercalcemic disorders. Although both total Ca^{2+} and ionized Ca^{2+} measurements are available in many laboratories, ionized Ca^{2+} is usually a more sensitive and specific marker for Ca^{2+} disorders.

Hypocalcemia

When PTH is not present, as with *primary hypoparathyroidism*, serum Ca^{2+} levels are not properly regulated. Bone tends to "hang on" to its storage pool and the

CASE STUDY 16-3

An 84-year-old nursing home resident was seen in the emergency department with the following symptoms: nausea, vomiting, decreased respiration, hypotension, and low pulse rate (46 bpm). Physical examination showed the skin was warm to the touch and flushed. Admission laboratory data are found in Case Study Table 16-3.1.

CASE STUDY TABLE 16-3.1
LABORATORY RESULTS

		RESULT	REFERENCE RANGE
Serum	Total protein	5.6 g/dL	6.0–8.0 g/dL
	Albumin	3.0 g/dL	3.5–5.0 g/dL
	Total Ca^{2+}	8.2 mg/dL	8.6–10.0 mg/dL
	BUN	45 mg/dL	5–20 mg/dL
	Creatinine	2.3 mg/dL	0.7–1.5 mg/dL
	Mg^{2+}	4.0 mmol/L	0.63–1.0 mmol/L
Plasma	Na^+	129 mmol/L	136–145 mmol/L
	K^+	5.3 mmol/L	3.4–5.0 mmol/L
	Cl^-	96 mmol/L	98–107 mmol/L
	HCO_3^-	16 mmol/L	22–29 mmol/L

Questions

1. What is the most likely cause for the patient's symptoms?

2. What is the most likely cause for the hypermagnesemia?

3. What could be the cause for the hypocalcemia?

TABLE 16-16 CAUSES OF HYPOCALCEMIA

Primary hypoparathyroidism—glandular aplasia, destruction, or removal

Hypomagnesemia

Hypermagnesemia

Hypoalbuminemia (total only, ionized calcium not affected by)—chronic liver disease, nephrotic syndrome, malnutrition

Acute pancreatitis

Vitamin D deficiency

Renal disease

Rhabdomyolysis

Pseudohypoparathyroidism

TABLE 16-17   CAUSES OF HYPERCALCEMIA

Primary hyperparathyroidism—adenoma or glandular hyperplasia

Hyperthyroidism

Benign familial hypocalciuria

Malignancy

Multiple myeloma

Increased vitamin D

Thiazide diuretics

Prolonged immobilization

kidney increases excretion of Ca^{2+}. Because PTH is also required for normal vitamin D metabolism, the lack of vitamin D's effects also leads to a decreased level of Ca^{2+}. Parathyroid gland aplasia, destruction, and removal are obvious reasons for primary hypoparathyroidism.

Because hypomagnesemia has become more frequent in hospitalized patients, chronic hypomagnesemia has also become recognized as a frequent cause of hypocalcemia. Hypomagnesemia may cause hypocalcemia by three mechanisms: (1) it inhibits the glandular secretion of PTH across the parathyroid gland membrane, (2) it impairs PTH action at its receptor site on bone, and (3) it causes vitamin D resistance.[15] Elevated Mg^{2+} levels may inhibit PTH release and target tissue response, perhaps leading to hypocalcemia and hypercalciuria.[16]

When total Ca^{2+} is the only result reported, hypocalcemia can appear with hypoalbuminemia. Common causes are associated with chronic liver disease, nephrotic syndrome, and malnutrition. In general, for each 1 g/dL decrease in serum albumin, there is a 0.2 mmol/L (0.8 mg/dL) decrease in total Ca^{2+} levels.[22]

About one-half of the patients with acute pancreatitis develop hypocalcemia. The most consistent cause appears to be a result of increased intestinal binding of Ca^{2+} as increased intestinal lipase activity occurs.[22] Vitamin D deficiency and malabsorption can cause decreased absorption, which leads to increased PTH production or secondary hyperparathyroidism.

Patients with renal disease caused by glomerular failure often have altered concentrations of Ca^{2+}, PO_4^-, albumin, Mg^{2+}, and H^+ (pH). In chronic renal disease, secondary hyperparathyroidism frequently develops as the body tries to compensate for hypocalcemia caused either by hyperphosphatemia (PO_4^- binds and lowers ionized Ca^{2+}) or altered vitamin D metabolism. Monitoring and controlling ionized Ca^{2+} concentrations may avoid problems due to hypocalcemia, such as osteodystrophy, unstable cardiac output or blood pressure, or problems arising from hypercalcemia, such as renal stones and other calcifications. Rhabdomyolysis, as with major crush injury and muscle damage, may cause hypocalcemia as a result of increased PO_4^- release from cells, which bind to Ca^{2+} ions.[22]

Pseudohypoparathyroidism is a rare hereditary disorder in which PTH target tissue response is decreased (end organ resistance). PTH production responds normally to loss of Ca^{2+}; however, without normal response (decreased cAMP [cyclic adenosine 3′,5′-phosphate] production), Ca^{2+} is lost in the urine or remains in the bone storage pool. Patients often have common physical features, including short stature, obesity, shortened metacarpals and metatarsals, and abnormal calcification.

Surgery and intensive care. Because appropriate Ca^{2+} concentrations promote good cardiac output and maintain adequate blood pressure, the maintenance of a normal ionized Ca^{2+} concentration in blood is beneficial to patients in either surgery or intensive care. Controlling Ca^{2+} concentrations may be critical in open heart surgery when the heart is restarted and during liver transplantation because large volumes of citrated blood are given.

Because these patients may receive large amounts of citrate, HCO_3^-, Ca^{2+} salts, or fluids, the greatest discrepancies between total Ca^{2+} and ionized Ca^{2+} concentrations may be seen during major surgical operations. Consequently, ionized Ca^{2+} measurements are the Ca^{2+} measurement of greatest clinical value.

Hypocalcemia occurs commonly in critically ill patients, that is, those with sepsis, thermal burns, renal failure, or cardiopulmonary insufficiency. These patients frequently have abnormalities of acid–base regulation and losses of protein and albumin, which are best suited to monitoring Ca^{2+} status by ionized Ca^{2+} measurements. Normalization of ionized Ca^{2+} may have beneficial effects on cardiac output and blood pressure.

Neonatal monitoring. Typically, blood-ionized Ca^{2+} concentrations in neonates are high at birth and then rapidly decline by 10% to 20% after 1 to 3 days. After about 1 week, ionized Ca^{2+} concentrations in the neonate stabilize at levels slightly higher than in adults.[23]

The concentration of ionized Ca^{2+} may decrease rapidly in the early neonatal period because the infant may lose Ca^{2+} rapidly and not readily reabsorb it. Several possible etiologies have been suggested: abnormal PTH and vitamin D metabolism, hypercholesterolemia, hyperphosphatemia, and hypomagnesemia.

Symptoms of hypocalcemia. Neuromuscular irritability and cardiac irregularities are the primary groups of symptoms that occur with hypocalcemia. Neuromuscular symptoms include paresthesia, muscle cramps, tetany, and seizures. Cardiac symptoms may include arrhythmia or heart block. Symptoms usually occur with severe hypocalcemia, in which total Ca^{2+} levels are below 1.88 mmol/L (7.5 mg/dL).[22]

Treatment of hypocalcemia. Oral or parenteral Ca^{2+} therapy may occur, depending on the severity of the decreased level and the cause. Vitamin D may sometimes be administered in addition to oral Ca^{2+} to increase absorption. If hypomagnesemia is a concurrent disorder, Mg^{2+} therapy should also be provided.

Hypercalcemia

Primary hyperparathyroidism is the main cause of hypercalcemia.[22] Hyperparathyroidism, or excess secretion of PTH, may show obvious clinical signs or may be asymptomatic. The patient population seen most frequently with primary hyperparathyroidism is older women.[22] Although either total or ionized Ca^{2+} measurements are elevated in serious cases, ionized Ca^{2+} is more frequently elevated in subtle or asymptomatic hyperparathyroidism. In general, ionized Ca^{2+} measurements are elevated in 90% to 95% of cases of hyperparathyroidism, whereas total Ca^{2+} is elevated in 80% to 85% of cases.

The second leading cause of hypercalcemia is associated with various types of malignancy, with hypercalcemia sometimes being the sole biochemical marker for disease.[22] Many tumors produce PTH-related peptide (PTH-rP), which binds to normal PTH receptors and causes increased Ca^{2+} levels. Assays to measure PTH-rP are available because this abnormal protein is not detected by most PTH assays.

Because of the proximity of the parathyroid gland to the thyroid gland, hyperthyroidism can sometimes cause hyperparathyroidism. A rare, benign, familial hypocalciuria has also been reported. Thiazide diuretics increase Ca^{2+} reabsorption, leading to hypercalcemia. Prolonged immobilization may cause increased bone resorption. Hypercalcemia associated with immobilization is further compounded by renal insufficiency.

Symptoms of hypercalcemia. A mild hypercalcemia (2.62 to 3.00 mmol/L [10.5 to 12 mg/dL]) is often asymptomatic.[22] Moderate or severe Ca^{2+} elevations include neurologic, GI, and renal symptoms. Neurologic symptoms may include mild drowsiness or weakness, depression, lethargy, and coma. GI symptoms may include constipation, nausea, vomiting, anorexia, and peptic ulcer disease. Hypercalcemia may cause renal symptoms of nephrolithiasis and nephrocalcinosis. Hypercalciuria can result in nephrogenic diabetes insipidus, which causes polyuria that results in hypovolemia, which further aggravates the hypercalcemia.[22] Hypercalcemia can also cause symptoms of digitalis toxicity.

Treatment of hypercalcemia. Treatment of hypercalcemia depends on the level of hypercalcemia and the cause. Often people with primary hyperparathyroidism are asymptomatic. Estrogen deficiency in postmenopausal women has been implicated in primary hyperparathyroidism in older women.[22] Often, estrogen replacement therapy reduces Ca^{2+} levels. Parathyroidectomy may be necessary in some hyperparathyroid patients. Patients with moderate to severe hypercalcemia are treated to reduce Ca^{2+} levels. Salt and water intake is encouraged to increase Ca^{2+} excretion and avoid dehydration, which can compound the hypercalcemia. Thiazide diuretics should be discontinued. Bisphosphonates (a derivative of pyrophosphate) are the main drug class used to lower Ca^{2+} levels, achieved by its binding action to bone, which prevents bone resorption.[22]

Determination of Calcium

Specimen

The preferred specimen for total Ca^{2+} determinations is either serum or lithium heparin plasma collected without venous stasis. Because anticoagulants such as EDTA or oxalate bind Ca^{2+} tightly and interfere with measurement, they are unacceptable for use.

The proper collection of samples for ionized Ca^{2+} measurements requires greater care. Because loss of CO_2 will increase pH, samples must be collected anaerobically. Although heparinized whole blood is the preferred sample, serum from sealed evacuated blood collection tubes may be used if clotting and centrifugation are done quickly (<30 minutes) and at room temperature. No liquid heparin products should be used. Most heparin anticoagulants (Na^+ and lithium) partially bind to Ca^{2+} and lower ionized Ca^{2+} concentrations. A heparin concentration of 25 IU/mL, for example, decreases ionized Ca^{2+} by about 3%. Dry heparin products are available titrated with small amounts of Ca^{2+} or Zn^{2+} or with small amounts of heparin dispersed in an inert "puff" that essentially eliminates the interference by heparin.

For analysis of Ca^{2+} in urine, an accurately timed urine collection is preferred. The urine should be acidified with 6 mol/L HCl, with approximately 1 mL of the acid added for each 100 mL of urine.

Methods

The two commonly used methods for total Ca^{2+} analysis use either ortho-cresolphthalein complexone (CPC) or arsenazo III dye to form a complex with Ca^{2+}. Prior to the dye-binding reaction, Ca^{2+} is released from its protein carrier and complexes by acidification of the sample. The CPC method uses 8-hydroxyquinoline to prevent Mg^{2+} interference. AAS remains the reference method for total Ca^{2+}, although it is rarely used in the clinical setting.

Current commercial analyzers that measure ionized/free Ca^{2+} use ISEs for this measurement. These systems may use membranes impregnated with special molecules that selectively, but reversibly, bind Ca^{2+} ions. As Ca^{2+} binds to these membranes, an electric potential develops across the membrane that is proportional to the ionized Ca^{2+} concentration. A diagram of one such electrode is shown in Figure 16-6.

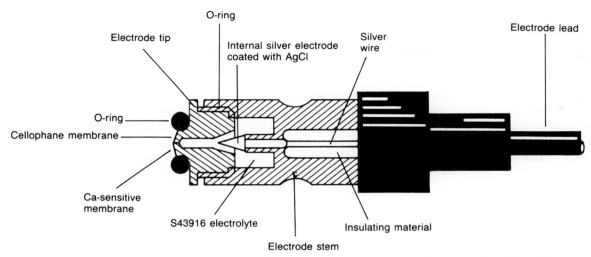

FIGURE 16-6 Diagram of ionized calcium electrode for the ionized calcium analyzer. (Courtesy of Radiometer America, Westlake, OH.)

Reference Ranges

For total Ca^{2+}, the reference range varies slightly with age.[3] In general, Ca^{2+} concentrations are higher through adolescence when bone growth is most active. Ionized/free Ca^{2+} concentrations can change rapidly from day 1 to day 3 of life. Following this, they stabilize at relatively high levels, with a gradual decline through adolescence; see Table 16-18.

Phosphate

Phosphate Physiology

Found everywhere in living cells, phosphate compounds participate in many of the most important biochemical processes. The genetic materials deoxyribonucleic acid and ribonucleic acid are complex phosphodiesters. Most

TABLE 16-18	REFERENCE RANGES FOR CALCIUM
TOTAL CALCIUM—SERUM, PLASMA	
Child, <12 y	2.20–2.70 mmol/L (8.8–10.8 mg/dL)
Adult	2.15–2.50 mmol/L (8.6–10.0 mg/dL)
IONIZED CALCIUM—SERUM	
Child	1.20–1.38 mmol/L (4.8–5.5 mg/dL)
Adult	1.16–1.32 mmol/L (4.6–5.3 mg/dL)
IONIZED CALCIUM—PLASMA	
Adult	1.03–1.23 mmol/L (4.1–4.9 mg/dL)
IONIZED CALCIUM—WHOLE BLOOD	
Adult	1.15–1.27 mmol/L (4.6–5.1 mg/dL)
TOTAL CALCIUM— URINE (24 H)	2.50–7.50 mmol/d (100–300 mg/d), varies with diet

coenzymes are esters of phosphoric or pyrophosphoric acid. The most important reservoirs of biochemical energy are ATP, creatine phosphate, and PEP. Phosphate deficiency can lead to ATP depletion, which is ultimately responsible for many of the clinical symptoms observed in hypophosphatemia.

Alterations in the concentration of 2,3-bisphosphoglycerate (2,3-BPG) in RBCs affect the affinity of hemoglobin for oxygen, with an increase facilitating the release of oxygen in tissue and a decrease making oxygen bound to hemoglobin less available. By affecting the formation of 2,3-BPG, the concentration of inorganic phosphate indirectly affects the release of oxygen from hemoglobin.

Understanding the cause of an altered phosphate concentration in the blood is often difficult because transcellular shifts of phosphate are a major cause of hypophosphatemia in blood. That is, an increased shift of phosphate into cells can deplete phosphate in the blood. Once phosphate is taken up by the cell, it remains there to be used in the synthesis of phosphorylated compounds. As these phosphate compounds are metabolized, inorganic phosphate slowly leaks out of the cell into the blood, where it is regulated principally by the kidney.

Regulation

Phosphate in blood may be absorbed in the intestine from dietary sources, released from cells into blood, and lost from bone. In healthy individuals, all these processes are relatively constant and easily regulated by renal excretion or reabsorption of phosphate.

Disturbances to any of these processes can alter phosphate concentrations in the blood; however, the loss of regulation by the kidneys will have the most profound effect. Although other factors, such as vitamin D, calcitonin, growth hormone, and acid–base status, can affect renal regulation of phosphate, the most important factor is PTH, which overall lowers blood concentrations by increasing renal excretion.

Vitamin D acts to increase phosphate in the blood. Vitamin D increases both phosphate absorption in the intestine and phosphate reabsorption in the kidney.

Growth hormone, which helps regulate skeletal growth, can affect circulating concentrations of phosphate. In cases of excessive secretion or administration of growth hormone, phosphate concentrations in the blood may increase because of decreased renal excretion of phosphate.

Distribution

Although the concentration of all phosphate compounds in blood is about 12 mg/dL (3.9 mmol/L), most of that is organic phosphate and only about 3 to 4 mg/dL is inorganic phosphate. Phosphate is the predominant intracellular anion, with intracellular concentrations varying, depending on the type of cell. About 80% of the total body pool of phosphate is contained in bone, 20% in soft tissues, and less than 1% is active in the serum/plasma.

Clinical Applications

Hypophosphatemia

Hypophosphatemia occurs in about 1% to 5% of hospitalized patients.[24] The incidence of hypophosphatemia increases to 20% to 40% in patients with the following disorders: diabetic ketoacidosis, chronic obstructive pulmonary disease, asthma, malignancy, long-term treatment with total parenteral nutrition, inflammatory bowel disease, anorexia nervosa, and alcoholism. The incidence increases to 60% to 80% in ICU patients with sepsis. In addition, hypophosphatemia can also be caused by increased renal excretion, as with hyperparathyroidism, and decreased intestinal absorption, as with vitamin D deficiency or antacid use.[24]

Although most cases are moderate and seldom cause problems, severe hypophosphatemia (<1.0 g/dL or 0.3 mmol/L) requires monitoring and possible replacement therapy. There is a 30% mortality rate in those who are severely hypophosphatemic versus a 15% rate in those with normal or mild hypophosphatemia.[24]

Hyperphosphatemia

Patients at greatest risk for hyperphosphatemia are those with acute or chronic renal failure.[24] An increased intake of phosphate or increased release of cellular phosphate may also cause hyperphosphatemia. Because they may not yet have developed mature PTH and vitamin D metabolism, neonates are especially susceptible to hyperphosphatemia caused by increased intake, such as from cow's milk or laxatives. Increased breakdown of cells can sometimes lead to hyperphosphatemia, as with severe infections, intensive exercise, neoplastic disorders, or intravascular hemolysis. Because immature lymphoblasts have about four times the phosphate content of mature lymphocytes,

patients with lymphoblastic leukemia are especially susceptible to hyperphosphatemia. Hypoparathyroidism may also cause hyperphosphatemia.

Determination of Inorganic Phosphorus

Specimen

Serum or lithium heparin plasma is acceptable for analysis. Oxalate, citrate, or EDTA anticoagulants should not be used because they interfere with the analytic method. Hemolysis should be avoided because of the higher concentrations inside the red cells. Circulating phosphate levels are subject to circadian rhythm, with highest levels in late morning and lowest in the evening. Urine analysis for phosphate requires a 24-hour sample collection because of significant diurnal variations.

Methods

Most of the current methods for phosphorus determination involve the formation of an ammonium phosphomolybdate complex. This colorless complex can be measured by ultraviolet absorption at 340 nm or can be reduced to form molybdenum blue, a stable blue chromophore, which is read between 600 and 700 nm.

Reference Ranges

Phosphate values vary with age. Divided into age groups, the ranges are shown in Table 16-19.

Lactate

Lactate Biochemistry and Physiology

Lactate is a by-product of an emergency mechanism that produces a small amount of ATP when oxygen delivery is severely diminished. Pyruvate is the normal end product of glucose metabolism (glycolysis). The conversion of pyruvate to lactate is activated when a deficiency of oxygen leads to an accumulation of excess NADH (Fig. 16-7). Normally, sufficient oxygen maintains a favorably high ratio of NAD to NADH. Under these conditions, pyruvate is converted to acetyl-coenzyme A (CoA), which enters the citric acid cycle and produces 38 mol of ATP for each mole of glucose oxidized. However, under hypoxic conditions, acetyl-CoA formation does not occur and NADH accumulates, favoring the conversion of pyruvate to lactate through anaerobic metabolism. As a result, only

TABLE 16-19	REFERENCE RANGES FOR INORGANIC PHOSPHORUS
SERUM	
Neonate	1.45–2.91 mmol/L (4.5–9.0 mg/dL)
Child ≤15 y	1.07–1.74 mmol/L (3.3–5.4 mg/dL)
Adult	0.78–1.42 mmol/L (2.4–4.4 mg/dL)
Urine (24 h)	13–42 mmol/d (0.4–1.3 g/d)

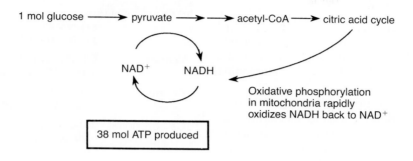

Aerobic Metabolism

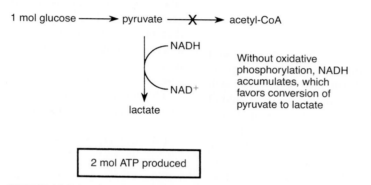

Anaerobic Metabolism

FIGURE 16-7 Aerobic vs. anaerobic metabolism of glucose.

2 mol of ATP are produced for each mole of glucose metabolized to lactate, with the excess lactate released into the blood. This release of lactate into blood has clinical importance because the accumulation of excess lactate in blood is an early, sensitive, and quantitative indicator of the severity of oxygen deprivation (Fig. 16-8).

Regulation

Because lactate is a by-product of anaerobic metabolism, it is not specifically regulated, as with K^+ or Ca^{2+}, for example. As oxygen delivery decreases below a critical level, blood lactate concentrations rise rapidly and indicate tissue hypoxia earlier than pH. The liver is the major

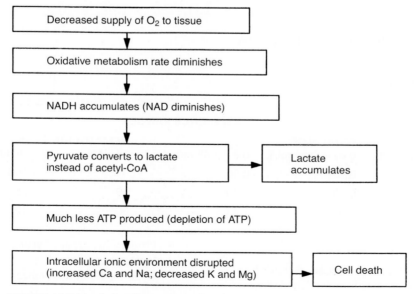

FIGURE 16-8 Metabolic effects of hypoxia, leading to cell death.

organ for removing lactate by converting lactate back to glucose by a process called *gluconeogenesis*.

Clinical Applications

Measurements of blood lactate are useful for metabolic monitoring in critically ill patients, for indicating the severity of the illness, and for objectively determining patient prognosis.

There are two types of lactic acidosis. Type A is associated with hypoxic conditions, such as shock, myocardial infarction, severe CHF, pulmonary edema, or severe blood loss. Type B is of metabolic origin, such as with diabetes mellitus, severe infection, leukemia, liver or renal disease, and toxins (ethanol, methanol, or salicylate poisoning).

Determination of Lactate

Specimen Handling

Special care should be practiced when collecting and handling specimens for lactate analysis. Ideally, a tourniquet should not be used because venous stasis will increase lactate levels. If a tourniquet is used, blood should be collected immediately and the patient should not exercise the hand before or during collection.[14] After sample collection, glucose is converted to lactose by way of anaerobic glycolysis and should be prevented. Heparinized blood may be used but must be delivered on ice and the plasma must be quickly separated. Iodoacetate and fluoride, which inhibit glycolysis without affecting coagulation, are usually satisfactory additives, but the specific method directions must be consulted.

Methods

Although lactate is a sensitive indicator of inadequate tissue oxygenation, the use of blood lactate measurements

TABLE 16-20	REFERENCE RANGES FOR LACTATE	
	ENZYMATIC METHOD, PLASMA	COLORIMETRIC, WHOLE BLOOD
Venous	0.5–2.2 mmol/L (4.5–19.8 mg/dL)	0.9–1.7 mmol/L (8.1–15.3 mg/dL)
Arterial	0.5–1.6 mmol/L (4.5–14.4 mg/dL)	<1.3 mmol/L (<11.7 mg/dL)
Cerebrospinal fluid	1.0–2.9 mmol/L (9–26 mg/dL)	

has been hindered because older methods were slow and laborious. Other means of following perfusion or oxygenation have been used, such as indwelling catheters that measure blood flow, pulse oximeters, base-excess determinations, and measurements of oxygen consumption (Vo_2). Current enzymatic methods make lactate determination readily available.

The most commonly used enzymatic method uses lactate oxidase to produce pyruvate and H_2O_2:

$$Lactate + O_2 \xrightarrow{\text{Lactate oxidase}} pyruvate + H_2O_2 \quad \text{(Eq. 16-6)}$$

One of two couple reactions may then be used. Peroxidase may be used to produce a colored chromogen from H_2O_2:

$$H_2O_2 + H \text{ donar} + chromogen \xrightarrow{\text{Peroxidase}}$$
$$colored\ dye + 2H_2O \quad \text{(Eq. 16-7)}$$

Reference Ranges

See Table 16-20.[3]

CASE STUDY 16-4

Consider the following laboratory results from three adult patients (Case Study Table 16-4.1):

CASE STUDY TABLE 16-4.1 LABORATORY RESULTS

			REFERENCE RANGES		
CASE	ION CA²⁺ 1.16–1.32 mmol/L	TOTAL MG²⁺ 0.63–1.0 mmol/L	PO₄⁻ 0.87–1.45 mmol/L	HEMATOCRIT 35–45%	INTACT PARATHYROID HORMONE 13–64 ng/L
A	1.44	0.90	0.85	42	100
B	1.08	0.50	0.90	40	25
C	1.70	0.98	1.43	30	12

Questions

1. Which set of laboratory results (Case A, B, or C) is most likely associated with each of the following diagnoses?

- Primary hyperparathyroidism
- Malignancy
- Hypomagnesemic hypocalcemia

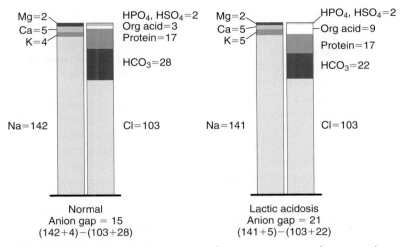

FIGURE 16-9 Demonstration of anion gap from concentrations of anions and cations in normal state and in lactic acidosis.

ANION GAP

Routine measurement of electrolytes usually involves only Na^+, K^+, Cl^-, and HCO_3^- (as total CO_2). These values may be used to approximate the anion gap (AG), which is the difference between unmeasured anions and unmeasured cations. There is never a "gap" between total cationic charges and anionic charges. The AG is calculated by the concentration difference between commonly measured cations (Na+K) and commonly measured anions (Cl+HCO3), as shown in Figure 16-9. AG is useful in indicating an increase in one or more of the unmeasured anions in the serum and also as a form of quality control for the analyzer used to measure these electrolytes. Consistently abnormal AGs in serum from healthy persons may indicate an instrument problem.

There are two commonly used methods for calculating the AG. The first equation is

$$Ag^{2+} = Na^+ - (Cl^- + HCO_3^-) \qquad \text{(Eq. 16-8)}$$

It is equivalent to unmeasured anions minus the unmeasured cations in this way:

$$(PO_4^- + 2SO_4^{2-}) - (K^+ + 2Ca^{2+} + Mg^{2+}) \qquad \text{(Eq. 16-9)}$$

The reference range for the Ag^{2+} using this calculation is 7 to 16 mmol/L.[3] The second calculation method is

$$Ag^{2+} = (Na^+ + K^+) - (Cl^- + HCO_3^-) \qquad \text{(Eq. 16-10)}$$

It has a reference range of 10 to 20 mmol/L.[3]

An *elevated AG* may be caused by uremia/renal failure, which leads to PO_4^- and SO_4^2 retention; ketoacidosis, as seen in cases of starvation or diabetes; methanol, ethanol, ethylene glycol, or salicylate poisoning; lactic acidosis; hypernatremia; and instrument error. *Low AG* values are rare but may be seen with hypoalbuminemia (decrease in unmeasured anions) or severe hypercalcemia (increase in unmeasured cations).

ELECTROLYTES AND RENAL FUNCTION

The kidney is central to the regulation and conservation of electrolytes in the body. For a review of kidney structure, refer Figure 16-10 and Chapter 27. The following is

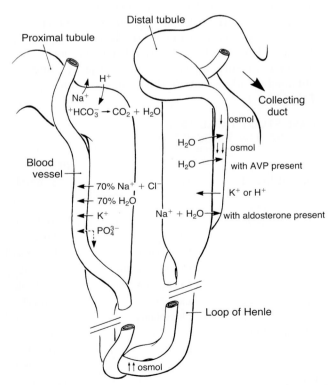

FIGURE 16-10 Summary of electrolyte movements in the renal tubules. AVP, arginine vasopressin hormone.

a summary of electrolyte excretion and conservation in a healthy individual:

1. Glomerulus: This portion of the nephron acts as a filter, retaining large proteins and protein-bound constituents while most other plasma constituents pass into the filtrate. The concentrations in the filtered plasma should be approximately equal to ECF without protein.
2. Renal tubules:
   a. Phosphate reabsorption is inhibited by PTH and increased by 1,25-$[OH]_2$-D_3. Excretion of Po_4 is stimulated by calcitonin.
   b. Ca^{2+} is reabsorbed under the influence of PTH and 1,25-$[OH]_2$-D_3. Calcitonin stimulates excretion of Ca^{2+}.
   c. Mg^{2+} reabsorption occurs largely in the thick ascending limb of Henle's loop.
   d. Sodium reabsorption can occur through three mechanisms:

   Approximately 70% of the Na^+ in the filtrate is reabsorbed in the proximal tubules by iso-osmotic reabsorption. It is limited, however, by the availability of Cl^- to maintain electrical neutrality.

Na^+ is reabsorbed in exchange for H^+. This reaction is linked with HCO_3^- and depends on carbonic anhydrase.

Stimulated by aldosterone, Na^+ is reabsorbed in exchange for K^+ in the distal tubules. (H^+ competes with K^+ for this exchange.)

   e. Cl^- is reabsorbed, in part, by passive transport in the proximal tubule along the concentration gradient created by Na^+.
   f. K^+ is reabsorbed by two mechanisms:
   Active reabsorption in the proximal tubule almost completely conserves K^+.
   Exchange with Na^+ is stimulated by aldosterone. H^+ competes with K^+ for this exchange.
   g. Bicarbonate is recovered from the glomerular filtrate and converted to CO_2 when H^+ is excreted in the urine.

   Henle's loop: With normal AVP function, it creates an osmotic gradient that enables water reabsorption to be increased or decreased in response to body fluid changes in osmolality.

   Collecting ducts: Also under AVP influence, this is where final adjustment of water excretion is made.

CASE STUDY 16-5

A 15-year-old girl in a coma was brought to the emergency department by her parents. She has diabetes and has been insulin dependent for 7 years. Her parents stated that there have been several episodes of hypoglycemia and ketoacidosis in the past and that their daughter has often been "too busy" to take her insulin injections. The laboratory results obtained on admission are shown in Case Study Table 16-5.1.

Questions

1. What is the diagnosis?

2. Calculate the anion gap. What is the cause of the anion gap result in this patient?

3. Why are chloride and bicarbonate decreased? What is the significance of the elevated potassium value?

4. What is the significance of the plasma osmolality?

CASE STUDY TABLE 16-5.1
LABORATORY RESULTS

		RESULT	REFERENCE RANGE
Venous blood	Na^+	145 mmol/L	136–145 mmol/L
	K^+	5.8 mmol/L	3.4–5.0 mmol/L
	Cl^-	87 mmol/L	98–107 mmol/L
	HCO_3^-	8 mmol/L	22–29 mmol/L
	Glucose	1,050 mg/dL	70–110 mg/dL
	Urea nitrogen	35 mg/dL	7–18 mg/dL
	Creatinine	1.3 mg/dL	0.5–1.3 mg/dL
	Lactate	5 mmol/L	0.5–2.2 mmol/L
	Osmolality	385 mOsm/kg	275–295 mOsm/kg
Arterial blood	pH	7.11	7.35–7.45
	po_2	98 mm Hg	83–100 mm Hg
	pco_2	20 mm Hg	35–45 mm Hg
Urine		Normal	
	Glucose	4+	Negative
	Ketones	4+	Negative

For additional student resources please visit thePoint at http://thepoint.lww.com. **the Point** ☀

QUESTIONS

1. What is the major intracellular cation?
   a. Potassium
   b. Calcium
   c. Magnesium
   d. Sodium

2. What is the major extracellular cation?
   a. Sodium
   b. Chloride
   c. Magnesium
   d. Calcium

3. Osmolality can be defined as a measure of the concentration of a solution based on the
   a. Number of dissolved particles
   b. Number of ionic particles present
   c. Number and size of the dissolved particles
   d. Density of the dissolved particles

4. Hyponatremia may be caused by each of the following EXCEPT
   a. Hypomagnesemia
   b. Aldosterone deficiency
   c. Prolonged vomiting or diarrhea
   d. Acute or chronic renal failure

5. Hypokalemia may be caused by each of the following EXCEPT
   a. Acidosis
   b. Prolonged vomiting or diarrhea
   c. Hypomagnesemia
   d. Hyperaldosteronism

6. Hyperkalemia may be caused by each of the following EXCEPT
   a. Alkalosis
   b. Acute or chronic renal failure
   c. Hypoaldosteronism
   d. Sample hemolysis

7. The main difference between a direct and indirect ISE is
   a. Sample is diluted in the indirect method, not in the direct method
   b. The type of membrane that is used
   c. Direct ISEs use a reference electrode, whereas indirect ISEs do not
   d. Whole blood samples can be measured with the direct method and not with the indirect method

8. Which method of analysis will provide the most accurate electrolyte results if a grossly lipemic sample is used?
   a. Direct ISE
   b. Indirect ISE
   c. Flame emission photometry
   d. Atomic absorption

9. The most frequent cause of hypermagnesemia is due to
   a. Renal failure
   b. Increased intake of magnesium
   c. Hypoaldosteronism
   d. Acidosis

10. A hemolyzed sample will cause falsely increased levels of each of the following EXCEPT
    a. Sodium
    b. Potassium
    c. Phosphate
    d. Magnesium

11. The largest portion of total body water is found in which tissue?
    a. Intracellular fluid
    b. Extracellular fluid
    c. Intravascular extracellular fluid
    d. Interstitial cell fluid
    e. Plasma

12. Osmoreceptors in the hypothalamus are key to regulating blood osmolality. Typically, a 1% to 2% shift in osmolality causes a _____ change in circulating concentration of ADH.
    a. Twofold
    b. Fourfold
    c. Eightfold
    d. Tenfold

13. The quantitative relationship between changes in blood osmolality and the normal expected response by ADH is best described as a(n):
    a. Indirect relationship
    b. Direct relationship
    c. Logarithmic relationship
    d. There is no quantitative relationship

14. The sample of choice for measuring blood osmolality is:
    a. Serum
    b. Plasma

c. Whole blood

d. Serum or plasma may both be used

15. With increased water loss, burn patients are most likely to also experience:
    a. Hypernatremia
    b. Hyponatremia
    c. Hypomagnesemia
    d. Hypoosmolality

16. Which plasma electrolyte has the most narrow reference range and is MOST strictly regulated by the body?

a. Sodium
b. Magnesium
c. Calcium
d. Chloride
e. Potassium

17. True or False? Red blood cells are key for oxygen transport, carbon dioxide transport, and maintaining electroneutrality in the blood.

REFERENCES

1. Rose BD, ed. *Clinical Physiology of Acid-Base and Electrolyte Disorders.* 5th ed. New York, NY: McGraw-Hill; 2001:163-228, 241-257, 372-402, 696-793, 836-930.

2. Burtis CA, Ashwood ER, Bruns DE, eds. *Tietz Textbook of Clinical Chemistry and Molecular Diagnostics.* 4th ed. St. Louis, MO: Elsevier Saunders; 2006:49, 985, 991-992.

3. Wu HB, ed. *Tietz Clinical Guide to Laboratory Tests.* 4th ed. St. Louis, MO: Elsevier Saunders; 2006:118, 214, 198-200, 234-237, 650-653, 706-707, 786-789, 852-855, 880-883, 992-996.

4. Oh MS. Pathogenesis and diagnosis of hyponatremia. *Nephron.* 2002;92(suppl 1):2-8.

5. Munger MA. New agents for managing hyponatremia in hospitalized patients. *Am J Health Syst Pharm.* 2007;64:253-265.

6. Oh MS. Management of hyponatremia and clinical use of vasopressin antagonists. *Am J Med Sci.* 2007;333:101-105.

7. Kumar S, Tomas B. Sodium. *Lancet.* 1998;352:220-228.

8. Patel GP, Balk RA. Recognition and treatment of hyponatremia in acutely ill hospitalized patients. *Clin Ther.* 2007;29:211-229.

9. Crook M. The investigation and management of severe hyponatremia. *J Clin Pathol.* 2002;55:883.

10. Verbalis JG, Goldsmith SR, Greenberg A, Schrier RW, Sterns RH. Hyponatremia treatment guidelines 2007: expert panel recommendations. *Am J Med.* 2007;120:S1-S21.

11. *Vitros Na+ Package Insert, Version 4.0.* Rochester, NY: Ortho-Clinical Diagnostics; 2004.

12. Gennari FJ. Disorders of potassium homeostasis: hypokalemia and hyperkalemia. *Crit Care Clin.* 2002;18:273-288.

13. Gennari FJ. Hypokalemia. *N Engl J Med.* 1998;339:451-458.

14. Burtis CA, Ashwood ER, Bruns DE, eds. *Tietz Fundamentals of Clinical Chemistry.* 6th ed. St. Louis, MO: Elsevier Saunders; 2008:394, 433.

15. Elin RJ. Magnesium: The fifth but forgotten electrolyte. *Am J Clin Pathol.* 1994;102:616-622.

16. Polancic JE. Magnesium: metabolism, clinical importance, and analysis. *Clin Lab Sci.* 1991;4:105-109.

17. Whang R. Clinical disorders of magnesium metabolism. *Comp Ther.* 1997;23:168-173.

18. Schlingmann KP, Weber S, Peters M, et al. Hypomagnesemia with secondary hypocalcemia is caused by mutations in TRPM6, a new member of the TRPM gene family. *Nat Genet.* 2002;31:166-170.

19. Whang R, Sims G. Magnesium and potassium supplementation in the prevention of diabetic vascular disease. *Med Hypotheses.* 2000;55:263-265.

20. Ringer S. A further contribution regarding the influence of different constituents of blood on contractions of the heart. *J Physiol.* 1883;4:29.

21. McLean FC, Hastings AB. A biological method for estimation of calcium ion concentration. *J Biol Chem.* 1934;107:337.

22. Bushinsky DA, Monk RD. Calcium. *Lancet.* 1998;352:23.

23. Wandrup J. Critical analytical and clinical aspects of ionized calcium in neonates. *Clin Chem.* 1989;35:2027.

24. Shiber JR, Mattu A. Serum phosphate abnormalities in the emergency department. *J Emerg Med.* 2002;23:395-400.

Blood Gases, pH, and Buffer Systems

SHARON S. EHRMEYER, JOHN J. ANCY

CHAPTER

17

CHAPTER OUTLINE

Chapter Objectives

Upon completion of this chapter, the clinical laboratorian should be able to do the following:

• Describe the principles involved in the measurement of pH, pCO_2, pO_2, and the various hemoglobin species.
• Outline the interrelationship of the buffering mechanisms of bicarbonate, carbonic acid, and hemoglobin.
• Explain the clinical significance of the following pH and blood gas parameters: pH, pCO_2, pO_2, actual bicarbonate, carbonic acid, base excess, oxygen saturation, fractional oxyhemoglobin, hemoglobin oxygen (binding) capacity, oxygen content, and total CO_2.
• Determine whether data are normal or represent metabolic or respiratory acidosis or metabolic or respiratory alkalosis using the Henderson-Hasselbalch equation and blood gas data. Identify whether the data represent uncompensated or compensated conditions.
• Identify some common causes of nonrespiratory acidosis and alkalosis, respiratory acidosis and alkalosis, and mixed abnormalities. State how the body attempts to compensate (kidney and lungs) for the various conditions.

• Describe the significance of the hemoglobin–oxygen dissociation curve and the impact of pH, 2,3-diphospho-glycerate (2,3-DPG), temperature, pH, and pCO_2 on its shape and release of O_2 to the tissues.
• Discuss problems and precautions in collecting and handling samples for pH and blood gas analysis. Include syringes, anticoagulants, mixing, icing, and capillary and venous samples as well as arterial samples in the discussion.
• Describe instrumental approaches to measuring various hemoglobin species and pH and blood gas parameters.
• Describe approaches to quality assurance, including quality control, proficiency testing, and delta checks to assess analytic quality.
• Discuss the reasons for possible discrepancies, given oxygen saturation data calculated by the blood gas analyzer and measured by the CO-oximeter.
• Calculate partial pressures of pCO_2 and pO_2 for various percentages of carbon dioxide and oxygen. In doing these calculations, account for the barometric pressure and vapor pressure of water.

An important aspect of clinical biochemistry is information on a patient's acid–base balance and blood gas homeostasis. These data often are used to assess patients in life-threatening situations. Because the test parameters are interrelated, test sites are expected to provide panels of tests frequently supplemented with calculated parameters. Focusing on only one test result can be misleading.

This chapter discusses exchange of gases, carbon dioxide and oxygen, together with the body's mechanisms to maintain acid–base balance. The interpretation of data, from measurement of pH and other blood gas parameters, and the techniques and instrumentation used in these measurements are also described. Preanalytic considerations—sample collection and handling—that greatly affect the quality of test results are addressed. Quality assurance approaches to blood gas analysis are also presented.

DEFINITIONS: ACID, BASE, AND BUFFER

A discussion of acid–base balance requires a review of several basic concepts—acid, base, buffer, pH, and pK_a—and the principles of equilibrium and the law of mass action.

An *acid* is a substance that can yield a hydrogen ion (H^+) or hydronium ion when dissolved in water. A *base* is a substance that can yield hydroxyl ions (OH^-). The relative strengths of acids and bases, their ability to dissociate in water, are described by their dissociation constant (also ionization constant K value). Tables can be found in most biochemistry texts. The pK_a defined as the negative log of the ionization constant, is also the pH in which the protonated and unprotonated forms are present in equal concentrations. Strong acids have pK_a values of less than 3.0, whereas strong bases have pK_a values greater than 9.0. For acids, raising the pH above the pK_a will cause the acid to dissociate and yield an H^+. For bases, lowering the pH below the pK_a will cause the base to release OH^-. Many species have more than one pK_a meaning they can accept or donate more than one H^+.

A *buffer*, the combination of a weak acid or weak base and its salt, is a system that resists changes in pH. The effectiveness of a buffer depends on the pK_a of the buffering system and the pH of the environment in which it is placed. In plasma, the bicarbonate–carbonic acid system, having a pK_a of 6.1, is one of the principal buffers:

$$H_2CO_3 \leftrightarrow HCO_3^- + H^+ \qquad \text{(Eq. 17-1)}$$
Carbonic acid   Bicarbonate

The reference value for blood plasma pH is 7.40. Weisberg cited an example to demonstrate the effectiveness of the blood buffers.[1] If the pH of 100 mL of distilled water is 7.35 and one drop of 0.05 mol/L HCl is added, the pH will change to 7.00. To change 100 mL of normal blood from a pH of 7.35 to 7.00, approximately 25 mL of 0.05 mol/L HCl is needed. With 5.5 L of blood in the average body, more than 1,300 mL of HCl would be required to make this same change in pH.

ACID–BASE BALANCE

Maintenance of H^+

The normal concentration of H^+ in the extracellular body fluid ranges from 36 to 44 nmol/L (pH 7.34 to 7.44); however, through metabolism, the body produces much greater quantities of H^+. Through exquisite mechanisms that involve the lungs and kidneys, the body controls and excretes H^+ in order to maintain pH homeostasis. Any H^+ value outside this range will cause alterations in the rates of chemical reactions within the cell and affect the many metabolic processes of the body and can lead to alterations in consciousness, neuromuscular irritability, tetany, coma, and death.

The logarithmic pH scale expresses H^+ concentration (c is concentration):

$$pH = \log \frac{1}{cH^+} = -\log cH^+ \qquad \text{(Eq. 17-2)}$$

The reference value for arterial blood pH is 7.40 and is equivalent to an H^+ concentration of 40 nmol/L. Because pH is the negative log of the cH^+, an increase in H^+ concentration decreases the pH, whereas a decrease in H^+ concentration increases the pH. A pH below the reference range <7.34 is referred to as acidosis, whereas a pH above the reference range >7.44 is referred to as alkalosis. Technically, the suffix *-osis* refers to a process in the body; the suffix *-emia* refers to the corresponding state in blood (*-osis* is the cause of the *-emia*).

The arterial pH is controlled by systems that regulate the production and retention of acids and bases. These include buffers, the respiratory center and lungs, and the kidneys.

Buffer Systems: Regulation of H+

The body's first line of defense against extreme changes in H+ concentration is the buffer systems present in all body fluids. All buffers consist of a weak acid, such as carbonic acid (H_2CO_3), and its salt or conjugate base, bicarbonate (HCO_3^-), for the bicarbonate–carbonic acid buffer system. H_2CO_3 is a weak acid because it does not completely dissociate into H+ and HCO_3^-. (In contrast, a strong acid, such as HCl, completely dissociates into H+ and Cl− in solution.) When an acid is added to the bicarbonate–carbonic acid system, the HCO_3^- will combine with the H+ from the acid to form H_2CO_3. When a base is added, H_2CO_3 will combine with the OH− group to form H_2O and HCO_3^-. In both cases, there is a smaller change in pH that would result from adding the acid or base to an unbuffered solution.

Although the bicarbonate–carbonic acid system has low buffering capacity, it is still an important buffer for three reasons: (1) H_2CO_3 dissociates into CO_2 and H_2O, allowing CO_2 to be eliminated by the lungs and H+ as water; (2) changes in CO_2 modify the ventilation (respiratory) rate; and (3) HCO_3^- concentration can be altered by the kidneys. In addition, this buffering system immediately counters the effects of fixed nonvolatile acids (H+A−) by binding the dissociated hydrogen ion (H+A− + HCO_3^- = H_2CO_3 + A−). The resultant H_2CO_3 then dissociates, and the H+ is neutralized by the buffering capacity of hemoglobin. Figure 17-1 shows the interrelationship of hemoglobin in the red blood cells and the H+ from the bicarbonate buffering system.

Other buffers are also important. The phosphate buffer system (HPO_4^{2-} – $H_2PO_4^-$) plays a role in plasma and red blood cells and is involved in the exchange of sodium ion in the urine H+ filtrate. Plasma protein, especially the imidazole groups of histidine, also forms an important buffer system in plasma. Most circulating proteins have a net negative charge and are capable of binding H+.

The lungs and kidneys play important roles in regulating blood pH. The interrelationship of the lungs and kidneys in maintaining pH is depicted by the Henderson-Hasselbalch equation (Eq. 17-4). The numerator (HCO_3^-) denotes the kidney function, whereas the denominator (pCO_2, which represents H_2CO_3) denotes the lung function. The lungs regulate pH through retention or elimination of CO_2 by changing the rate and volume of ventilation. The kidneys regulate pH by excreting acid, primarily in the ammonium ion, and by reclaiming HCO_3^- from the glomerular filtrate.

Regulation of Acid–Base Balance: Lungs and Kidneys

Carbon dioxide, the end product of most aerobic metabolic processes, easily diffuses out of the tissue where it is produced and into the plasma and red cells in the surrounding capillaries. In plasma, a small amount of CO_2 is physically dissolved or combined with proteins to form carbamino compounds. Most of the CO_2 combines with H_2O to form H_2CO_3, which quickly dissociates into H+ and HCO_3^- (Fig. 17-1). The reaction is accelerated by the enzyme carbonic anhydrase found in the red cell membrane. The dissociation of H_2CO_3 causes the HCO_3^- concentration to increase in the red cells and diffuse into the plasma. To maintain electroneutrality (the same number of positively and negatively charged ions on each side of the red cell membrane), chloride diffuses into the cell. This is known as the *chloride shift*. Plasma proteins and plasma buffers combine with the freed H+ to maintain a stable pH.

In the lungs, the process is reversed. Inspired O_2 diffuses from the alveoli into the blood and is bound to hemoglobin, forming oxyhemoglobin (O_2Hb). The H+ that was carried on the (reduced) hemoglobin in the venous blood is released to recombine with HCO_3^- to form H_2CO_3, which dissociates into H_2O and CO_2. The CO_2 diffuses into the alveoli and is eliminated through ventilation. The net effect of the interaction of these two buffering systems is a minimal change in H+ concentration between the venous and arterial circulation. When the lungs do not remove CO_2 at the rate of its production (as a result of decreased ventilation or disease), it accumulates in the blood, causing an increase in H+ concentration. If, however, CO_2 removal is faster than production (hyperventilation), the H+ concentration will be decreased. Consequently, ventilation affects the pH of the blood. A change in the H+ concentration of blood

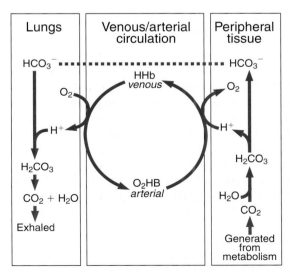

FIGURE 17-1 Interrelationship of the bicarbonate and hemoglobin buffering systems.

that results from nonrespiratory disturbances causes the respiratory center to respond by altering the rate of ventilation in an effort to restore the blood pH to normal. The lungs, by responding within seconds, together with the buffer systems, provide the first line of defense to changes in acid–base status.

The kidneys are also able to excrete variable amounts of acid or base, making them an important player in the regulation of acid–base balance. The kidney's main role in maintaining acid–base homeostasis is to reclaim HCO_3^- from the glomerular filtrate. Without this reclamation, the loss of HCO_3^- in the urine would result in an excessive acid gain in the blood. The main site for HCO_3^- reclamation is the proximal tubules (Fig. 17-2). The glomerular filtrate contains essentially the same HCO_3^- levels as plasma. The process is not a direct transport of HCO_3^- across the tubule membrane into the blood. Instead, sodium (Na^+) in the glomerular filtrate is exchanged for H^+ in the tubular cell. The H^+ combines with HCO_3^- in the filtrate to form H_2CO_3, which is converted into H_2O and CO_2 by carbonic anhydrase. The CO_2 easily diffuses into the tubule and reacts with H_2O to reform H_2CO_3 and then HCO_3^-, which is reabsorbed into the blood along with sodium. With alkalotic conditions, the kidney excretes HCO_3^- to compensate for the elevated blood pH. The exchange between H^+ and Na^+ suggests, in part, why clinicians order pH and blood gases together, along with electrolytes (Na^+, K^+, and Cl^-), to assess the patient. (*Reabsorption* or *reclamation* refers to the process of re-entering the blood. *Secretion* or *excretion* by the tubule cells concentrate or remove substances from the filtrate. These reactions determine the pH of the urine, as well as the pH of the blood.)

Under normal conditions, the body produces a net excess (50 to 100 mmol/L) of acid (H^+) each day that must be excreted by the kidney. Because the minimum urine pH is approximately 4.5, the kidney excretes little nonbuffered H^+. The remainder of the urinary H^+ combines with monohydrogen phosphate (HPO_4^{2-}) and ammonia (NH_3) and is excreted as dihydrogen phosphate ($H_2PO_4^-$) and ammonium (NH_4^+). The amount of HPO_4^{2-} available for combining with H^+ is fairly constant; therefore, the daily excretion of H^+ in urine largely depends on the amount of NH_4^+ formed. Because the renal tubular cells are able to generate NH_3 from glutamine and other amino acids, the concentration of NH_3 will increase in response to a decreased blood pH.

Various factors affect the reabsorption of HCO_3^-. When the blood or plasma HCO_3^- level is higher than 26 to 30 mmol/L, HCO_3^- will be excreted. It is unlikely that the plasma will exceed an HCO_3^- value of 30 mmol/L unless these excretory capabilities fail (e.g., kidney failure occurs). However, a frequent exception to this is compensatory retention of HCO_3^- in chronic **hypercarbia** as seen with chronic lung disease.

The HCO_3^- level may increase if an excessive amount of lactate, acetate, or HCO_3^- is intravenously infused. It may also increase if there is an excessive loss of chloride without replacement (as occurs with sweating, vomiting, or prolonged nasogastric suction) because the HCO_3^- will be retained by the tubule to preserve electroneutrality.

Several factors may result in decreased HCO_3^- levels. Most diuretics, regardless of the mechanism of action, favor the excretion of HCO_3^-. Reduced HCO_3^- reabsorption also occurs in conditions in which there is an excessive loss of cations. In kidney dysfunction (such as chronic nephritis or infections), HCO_3^- reabsorption may be impaired.

ASSESSMENT OF ACID–BASE HOMEOSTASIS

The Bicarbonate Buffering System and the Henderson-Hasselbalch Equation

In assessing acid–base homeostasis, components of the bicarbonate buffering system are measured and calculated. From the data, inferences can be made pertaining to the other buffers and the systems that regulate the production, retention, and excretion of acids and bases. For the bicarbonate buffering system, the dissolved CO_2 (dCO_2) is in equilibrium with CO_2 gas, which can be expelled by the lungs. Therefore, the bicarbonate buffering system is referred to as an *open* system, and the dCO_2, which is controlled by the lungs, is the *respiratory component*. The lungs participate rapidly in the regulation of blood pH through hypoventilation or hyperventilation. Mainly, the kidneys, the nonrespiratory or formerly known as the metabolic component, control the bicarbonate concentration.

The *Henderson-Hasselbalch equation* expresses acid–base relationships in a mathematical formula:

$$pH = pK_a' + \log \frac{cA^-}{cHA} \qquad \text{(Eq. 17-3)}$$

where A^- is the proton acceptor or base (e.g., HCO_3^-); HA is the proton donor or weak acid (e.g., H_2CO_3); and pK_a' is the pH at which there is an equal concentration of protonated and unprotonated species. Knowing any of the three variables allows for the calculation of the fourth.

In plasma and at body temperature (37°C), the pK_a' of the bicarbonate buffering system is 6.1. The equilibrium between H_2CO_3 and CO_2 in plasma is approximately 1:800. The concentration of H_2CO_3 is proportional to the partial pressure exerted by the dCO_2. In plasma at 37°C, the value for the combination of the solubility constant for pCO_2 and the factor to convert mm Hg to mmol/L is 0.0307 mmol/L/mm Hg. Temperature and the solvent affect the constant. If either of these changes, the solubility constant also will change. Both pH and pCO_2

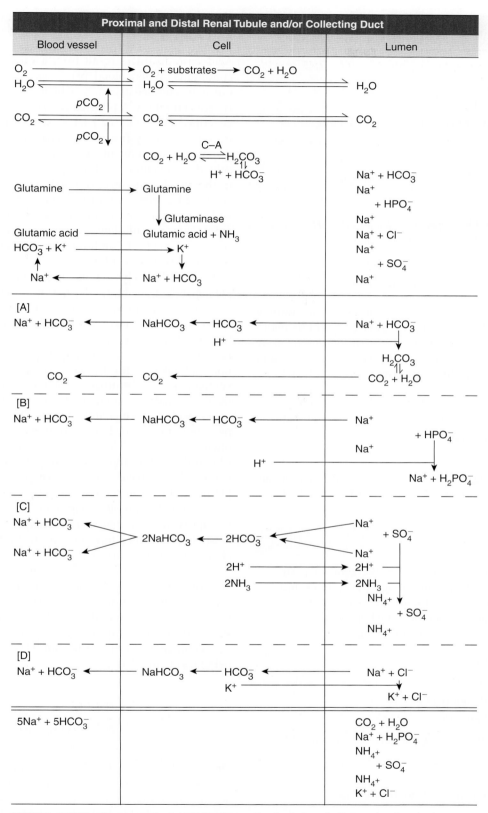

FIGURE 17-2 Bicarbonate reabsorption by the proximal tubule cell. C–A, carbonic anhydrase.

TABLE 17-1	ARTERIAL BLOOD GAS REFERENCE RANGE AT 37°C
pH	7.35–7.45
pCO_2 (mm Hg)	35–45
HCO_3^- (mmol/L)	22–26
Total CO_2 content (mmol/L)	23–27
pO_2 (mmol/L)	80–110
SO_2 (%)	>95
O_2Hb (%)	>95

are measured in blood gas analysis, and the pK_a' is a constant; therefore, HCO_3^- can be calculated:

$$pH = pK_a' + \log \frac{cHCO_3^-}{0.0307 \times pCO_2} \quad \text{(Eq. 17-4)}$$

In health, when the kidneys and lungs are functioning properly, a 20:1 ratio of HCO_3^- to H_2CO_3 will be maintained (resulting in a pH of 7.40). This is illustrated by substituting normal values (Table 17-1) for HCO_3^- and pCO_2 into the preceding equation:

$$\frac{24 \text{ mmol/L}}{(0.0307 \text{ mmol/L} - \text{mm Hg}) \times 40 \text{ mm Hg}}$$

$$= \frac{24}{1.2} = \frac{20}{1} \quad \text{(Eq. 17-5)}$$

Adding the log of 20 (1.3) to the pK_a' of the bicarbonate system yields a normal pH of 7.40 (7.40 = 6.1 + 1.3).

CASE STUDY 17-1

A 50-year-old man came to the emergency department after returning from foreign travel. His symptoms included persistent diarrhea (over the past 3 days) and rapid respiration (tachypnea). Blood gases were drawn with the following results:

pH	7.21
pCO_2	19 mm Hg
pO_2	96 mm Hg
HCO_3^-	7 mmol/L
SO_2	96% (calculated) (reference range, >95%)

Question

1. What is the patient's acid–base status?

2. Why is the HCO_3^- level so low?

3. Why does the patient have rapid respiration?

Acid–Base Disorders: Acidosis and Alkalosis

Acid–base disorders result from a variety of pathologic conditions. When blood pH is less than the reference range, it is termed acidemia, which reflects excess acid or H^+ concentration. A pH greater than the reference range is termed alkalemia or excess base. A disorder caused by ventilatory dysfunction (a change in the pCO_2, the respiratory component) is termed *primary respiratory acidosis* or *alkalosis*. A disorder resulting from a change in the bicarbonate level (a renal or metabolic function) is termed a *nonrespiratory disorder*. Mixed respiratory and nonrespiratory disorders occasionally arise from more than one pathologic process and represent the most serious of medical conditions as compensation for the primary disorder is failing.

Because the body's cellular and metabolic activities are pH dependent, the body tries to restore acid–base homeostasis whenever an imbalance occurs. This action by the body is termed compensation—the body accomplishes this by altering the factor *not primarily* affected by the pathologic process. For example, if the imbalance is of nonrespiratory origin, the body compensates by altering ventilation. For disturbances of the respiratory component, the kidneys compensate by selectively excreting or reabsorbing anions and cations. The lungs can compensate immediately, but the response is short term and often incomplete. The kidneys are slower to respond (2 to 4 days), however, but the response is long term and potentially complete. *Fully compensated* implies that the pH has returned to the normal range (the 20:1 ratio has been restored); *partially compensated* implies that the pH is approaching normal. While compensation may successfully return the ratio to the normal 20:1, the primary abnormality is not corrected.

Acidosis may be caused by a primary nonrespiratory abnormality or by a primary respiratory problem. In primary nonrespiratory acidosis, there is a decrease in bicarbonate (<24 mmol/L), resulting in a decreased pH as a result of the ratio for the nonrespiratory to respiratory component in the Henderson-Hasselbalch equation being less than 20:1:

$$pH \propto \frac{\downarrow cHCO_3^-}{N(0.0307 \times pCO_2)} < \frac{20}{1} \quad \text{(Eq. 17-6)}$$

where N is normal value and $\propto$ indicates proportional.

Nonrespiratory acidosis may be caused by the direct administration of an acid-producing substance, such as ammonium chloride and calcium chloride, or by excessive formation of organic acids as seen with diabetic ketoacidosis and starvation. Nonrespiratory acidosis is also seen with reduced excretion of acids, as in renal

CASE STUDY 17-2

An 80-year-old woman fell on the ice and fractured her femur. After several hours, when she arrived at the emergency department, she was anxious, panting, and complaining of severe chest pain and not being able to breathe. Her pulse was rapid (tachycardia) as was her respiration rate (tachypnea). Blood gases were drawn and yielded the following results:

pH	7.31
pCO_2	27 mm Hg
pO_2	62 mm Hg
HCO_3^-	12 mmol/L
SO_2	78% (calculated) (reference range, >95%)

Question

1. What is the patient's acid–base status?

2. Why is the HCO_3^- level so low?

3. What caused the acid–base imbalance?

tubular acidosis, and with excessive loss of bicarbonate from diarrhea or drainage from a biliary, pancreatic, or intestinal fistula.

The body compensates for nonrespiratory acidosis through *hyperventilation*, which is an increase in the rate or depth of breathing. By "blowing off" CO_2, the base-to-acid ratio will return toward normal. Secondary compensation occurs when the "original" organ (the kidneys, in this case) begins to correct the ratio by retaining bicarbonate.

Primary *respiratory acidosis* results from a decrease in alveolar ventilation (*hypoventilation*), causing a decreased elimination of CO_2 by the lungs:

$$pH \propto \frac{NcHCO_3^-}{\uparrow(0.0307 \times pCO_2)} < \frac{20}{1} \quad \text{(Eq. 17-7)}$$

Respiration is regulated in the medulla of the brain. Chemoreceptors present in the aortic arch and the carotid sinus respond to the levels of H^+ (pH), O_2, and CO_2 in the blood and cerebrospinal fluid. There are several situations, including many lung diseases, in which CO_2 is not effectively removed from the blood. In certain patients with chronic obstructive pulmonary disease (COPD), for example, destructive changes in the airways and alveolar walls increase the size of the alveolar air spaces, with the resultant reduction of

the lung surface area available for gas exchange. As a result, CO_2 is retained in the blood, causing chronic hypercarbia (elevated pCO_2). In bronchopneumonia, gas exchange is impeded because of the secretions, white blood cells, bacteria, and fibrin in the alveoli. Hypoventilation caused by drugs such as barbiturates, morphine, and alcohol will increase blood pCO_2 levels, as will mechanical obstruction or asphyxiation (strangulation or aspiration). Decreased cardiac output, such as that seen with congestive heart failure, also will result in less blood being presented to the lungs for gas exchange and, therefore, an elevated pCO_2.

In primary respiratory acidosis, the compensation occurs through nonrespiratory processes. The kidneys increase the excretion of H^+ and increase the reclamation of HCO_3^-. Although the renal compensation begins immediately, it takes days to weeks for maximal compensation to occur. When the HCO_3^- in the blood increases as a result of the action of the kidneys, the base-to-acid ratio will be altered and the pH will return toward normal.

As with acidosis, alkalosis can result from nonrespiratory and respiratory causes. Primary *nonrespiratory alkalosis* results from a gain in HCO_3^-, causing an increase in the nonrespiratory component and pH:

$$pH \propto \frac{\uparrow cHCO_3^-}{N(0.0307 \times pCO_2)} > \frac{20}{1} \quad \text{(Eq. 17-8)}$$

This condition may result from the excess administration of sodium bicarbonate or through ingestion of bicarbonate-producing salts, such as sodium lactate, citrate, and acetate. Excessive loss of acid through vomiting, nasogastric suctioning, or prolonged use of diuretics that augment renal excretion of H^+ can produce an apparent increase in HCO_3^-. The body responds by depressing the respiratory center. The resulting hypoventilation increases the retention of CO_2.

Primary *respiratory alkalosis* from an increased rate of alveolar ventilation causes excessive elimination of CO_2 by the lungs:

$$pH \propto \frac{NcHCO_3^-}{\downarrow(0.0307 \times pCO_2)} > \frac{20}{1} \quad \text{(Eq. 17-9)}$$

The causes of respiratory alkalosis include hypoxemia; chemical stimulation of the respiratory center by drugs, such as salicylates; an increase in the environmental temperature; fever; hysteria (hyperventilation); pulmonary emboli; and pulmonary fibrosis. The kidneys compensate by excreting HCO_3^- in the urine and reclaiming H^+ to the blood. The popular treatment for hysterical hyperventilation, breathing into a paper bag, is self-explanatory.

CASE STUDY 17-3

A 24-year-old graduate student was brought to the emergency department in a comatose state after being found unconscious in his room. A bottle of secobarbital was there on his bed stand. He did not respond to painful stimuli, his respiration was barely perceptible, and his pulse was weak. Blood gases were drawn and yielded the following results:

pH	7.10
pCO_2	70 mm Hg
pO_2	58 mm Hg
HCO_3^-	20 mmol/L
O_2Hb	80% (reference range, >95%)

Question

1. What is the patient's acid–base status?

2. What caused the profound hypoventilation?

3. Once the respiratory component returns to normal, what will be the patient's expected acid–base status?

CASE STUDY 17-4

A 24-year-old Himalayan man was accepted to graduate school in the United States. Before leaving home, he had an extensive physical exam that included various blood tests. When the medical staff at the US university reviewed his medical records, it was noted that all test results were normal except the HCO_3^-, which was 15 mmol/L (reference range, 22 to 26 mmol/L). The HCO_3^- was done separately on a serum sample. It was not part of a blood gas panel. To rule out nonrespiratory acidosis, the university physician wanted the HCO_3^- repeated. The repeated value was 24 mmol/L.

Question

1. Was the initial assumption of a nonrespiratory acidosis valid?

2. What would be a better description of the acid–base disturbance?

3. Why, on repeat testing, did the HCO_3^- return to normal?

OXYGEN AND GAS EXCHANGE

Oxygen and Carbon Dioxide

The role of oxygen in metabolism is crucial to all life. In cell mitochondria, electron pairs from the oxidation of NADH and $FADH_2$ are transferred to molecular oxygen, causing release of the energy used to synthesize ATP from the phosphorylation of ADP. Although measurement of intracellular O_2 is not feasible with current technology, evaluation of a patient's oxygen status is possible using pO_2 measured along with pH and pCO_2 in the blood gas analysis.

For adequate tissue oxygenation, the following seven conditions are necessary: (1) available atmospheric oxygen, (2) adequate ventilation, (3) gas exchange between the lungs and arterial blood, (4) loading of O_2 onto hemoglobin, (5) adequate hemoglobin, (6) adequate transport (cardiac output), and (7) release of O_2 to the tissue. Any disturbances in these conditions can result in poor tissue oxygenation.

The amount of O_2 available in atmospheric air depends on the barometric pressure (BP). At sea level, the BP is 760 mm Hg. (In the International System of Units, 1 mm Hg = 0.133 kPa, where 1 Pa = 1 N/m^2.) Dalton's law states that total atmospheric pressure is the sum of the individual gas pressures. One atmosphere exerts 760 mm Hg pressure and is made up of O_2 (20.93%), CO_2 (0.03%), nitrogen (78.1%), and inert gases (approximately 1%). The percentage for each gas is the same at all altitudes; the *partial pressure* for each gas in the atmosphere is equal to the BP at a particular altitude times the appropriate percentage for each gas. The vapor pressure of water (47 mm Hg at 37°C) must be accounted for in calculating the partial pressure for the individual gases (Fig. 17-3). In the body, these gases are always fully saturated with water. For example:

Partial pressure of O_2 at sea level (in the body)
= (760 mm Hg − 47 mm Hg) × 20.93%
= 149 mm Hg (at 37°C)

Partial pressure of CO_2 at sea level (in the body)
= (760 mm Hg − 47 mm Hg) × 0.03%
= 2 mm Hg (at 37°C)

Air is moved into the lungs through expansion of the thoracic cavity, which creates a temporary negative pressure gradient, causing air to move into the numerous tracheal branches and the alveoli. At the beginning of inspiration, these airways are still filled with air (gas) retained from the previously expired breath. This air, termed *dead space air*, dilutes the air being inspired. The inspired air, in addition to being somewhat diluted, is warmed to 37°C and fully saturated with water vapor causing the pO_2 in the alveoli to average at sea level about 110 mm Hg instead of the anticipated 149 mm Hg. Three other factors—the percentage of O_2 in inspired air, the

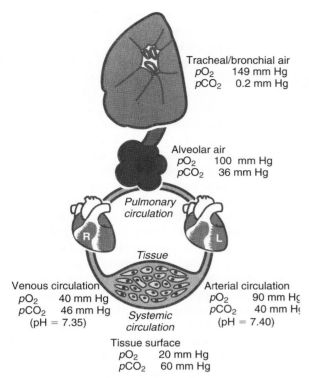

Tracheal/bronchial air
pO_2 149 mm Hg
pCO_2 0.2 mm Hg

Alveolar air
pO_2 100 mm Hg
pCO_2 36 mm Hg

Pulmonary circulation

R   L

Tissue

Venous circulation
pO_2 40 mm Hg
pCO_2 46 mm Hg
(pH = 7.35)

Arterial circulation
pO_2 90 mm Hg
pCO_2 40 mm Hg
(pH = 7.40)

Systemic circulation

Tissue surface
pO_2 20 mm Hg
pCO_2 60 mm Hg

FIGURE 17-3 Gas content in lungs and pulmonary and systemic circulation.

amount of pCO_2 in the expired air, and the ratio of the volume of inspired air to the volume of the dead space air—influence pO_2 in the alveoli. The percentage of O_2 in inspired air, or fraction of inspired oxygen (FiO_2), can be increased by breathing gas mixtures up to 100% O_2. Clinical conditions influence the amount of pCO_2 in the expired air that dilutes inspired air. For example, a patient with increased metabolism, as seen in hyperthermia, may produce more CO_2 than can be eliminated, causing pCO_2 in both the blood and expired gas to increase and a greater dilution of the inspired air. While the ratio of the volume of inspired air to the volume of dead space air is usually constant, people with shallow breaths have less "fresh" air entering the lungs than those breathing deeply.

There are many factors that can influence the amount of O_2 that moves through the alveoli into the blood and then to the tissue. Among the more common are as follows:

- *Destruction of the alveoli.* The normal surface area of the alveoli is as big as a tennis court. When the surface area is destroyed to a critically low value by diseases such as emphysema, an inadequate amount of O_2 will move into the blood.
- *Pulmonary edema.* Gas diffuses from the alveoli to the capillary through a small space. With pulmonary edema, fluid "leaks" into this space, increasing the

distance between the alveoli and capillary walls and causing a barrier to diffusion.
- *Airway blockage.* Airways can be blocked, preventing the air from the atmosphere from reaching the alveoli. Asthma and bronchitis are more common causes of this type of problem.
- *Inadequate blood supply.* When the blood supply to the lung is inadequate, O_2 enters the blood in the lungs, but not enough blood is being carried away to the tissue where it is needed. This may be the consequence of a blockage in a pulmonary blood vessel (pulmonary embolism), pulmonary hypertension, or a failing heart.
- *Diffusion of CO_2 and O_2.* Because O_2 diffuses 20 times slower than CO_2, it is more sensitive to problems with diffusion. Structural or physiologic alterations to the alveolar-capillary bed impair O_2 uptake with minimal alteration of CO_2 excretion. This type of hypoxemia is generally treated with supplemental O_2. The percentage of O_2 can be increased temporarily when needed; however, 60% or higher O_2 concentrations must be used with caution because it can be toxic to the lungs.

Oxygen Transport

Most O_2 in arterial blood is transported to the tissue by hemoglobin. Each adult hemoglobin (A_1) molecule can combine reversibly with up to four molecules of O_2. The actual amount of O_2 loaded onto hemoglobin depends on the availability of O_2; concentration and type(s) of hemoglobin present; presence of interfering substances, such as carbon monoxide (CO); pH; temperature of the blood; and levels of pCO_2 and 2,3-diphosphoglycerate (2,3-DPG). With adequate atmospheric and alveolar O_2 available and normal diffusion of O_2 to the arterial blood, more than 95% of "functional" hemoglobin (hemoglobin capable of *reversibly* binding O_2) will bind O_2. Increasing FiO_2 further saturates the hemoglobin. However, once the hemoglobin is 100% saturated, an increase in O_2 to the alveoli serves only to increase the concentration of dO_2 in the arterial blood. Prolonged administration of high concentrations of O_2 may cause oxygen toxicity and, in some cases, decreased ventilation that leads to hypercarbia. The ability of hemoglobin to carry O_2 can be affected significantly by other molecules. Normally, blood hemoglobin exists in one of four conditions:

1. O_2Hb describes O_2 reversibly bound to hemoglobin.
2. Deoxyhemoglobin (HHb; reduced hemoglobin) is hemoglobin not bound to O_2 but capable of forming a bond when O_2 is available.
3. Carboxyhemoglobin (COHb) is hemoglobin bound to CO. The bond between CO and Hb is reversible

but is 200 times as strong as the bond between O_2 and Hb.

4. Methemoglobin (MetHb) is hemoglobin unable to bind O_2 because iron (Fe) is in an oxidized rather than reduced state. The Fe^{3+} can be reduced by the enzyme methemoglobin reductase, which is found in red blood cells.

Dedicated spectrophotometers (CO-oximeters), which are discussed later in this chapter, are used to determine the relative concentrations (relative to total hemoglobin) of each of these species of hemoglobin.

Quantities Associated with Assessing a Patient's Oxygen Status

Four parameters commonly used to assess a patient's oxygen status are oxygen saturation (SO_2); measured fractional (percent) oxyhemoglobin (FO_2Hb); trends in oxygen saturation assessed by transcutaneous (TC), pulse oximetry (SpO_2) assessments; and the amount of O_2 dissolved in plasma (pO_2).

Oxygen saturation SO_2 represents the ratio of O_2 that is bound to the carrier protein, hemoglobin, compared with the total amount of hemoglobin capable of binding O_2:[2]

$$SO_2 = \frac{cO_2Hb}{(cO_2Hb + cHHb)} \times 100 \qquad \text{(Eq. 17-10)}$$

Software included with blood gas instruments applies algorithms to calculate SO_2 from pO_2, pH, and temperature of the sample. These calculated results, however, can differ significantly from those determined by direct CO-oximeter measurement due to the assumption that only adult hemoglobin is present and the oxyhemoglobin dissociation curve has a specific shape and location. These algorithms do not account for the presence of other hemoglobin species, such as COHb and MetHb, that are incapable of reversibly binding O_2. Because of the potential for generating erroneous information, calculated SO_2 should not be used to assess oxygenation status.[2,3]

Fractional (or percent) oxyhemoglobin (FO_2Hb) is the ratio of the concentration of oxyhemoglobin to the concentration of total hemoglobin ($ctHb$):

$$FO_2Hb = \frac{cO_2Hb}{ctHb} = \frac{cO_2Hb}{cO_2Hb + cHHb + cdysHb} \qquad \text{(Eq. 17-11)}$$

where the $cdysHb$ represents hemoglobin derivatives, such as COHb, that cannot reversibly bind with O_2 but are still part of the "total" hemoglobin measurement.

These two terms, SO_2 and FO_2Hb, can be confused because, in most healthy individuals (and even those individuals with some disease states), the numeric values for SO_2 are close to those for FO_2Hb. However, the values for FO_2Hb and SO_2 will deviate when dyshemoglobins are present and even when the patient is a smoker, owing to the preferential binding of CO to hemoglobin and the resultant loss of hemoglobin to bind O_2.

Partial pressure of oxygen dissolved in plasma (pO_2) accounts for little of the body's O_2 stores. A healthy adult breathing room air will have a pO_2 of 90 to 95 mm Hg. For an adult blood volume of 5 L, only 13.5 mL of O_2 will be available from pO_2 in plasma, compared with more than 1,000 mL of O_2 carried as O_2Hb.

Noninvasive measurements for following "trends" in oxygenation are attained with *pulse oximetry (SpO_2)*. These devices pass light of two or more wavelengths through the tissue in the capillary bed of the toe, finger, or ear. Until recently, pulse oximetry technology could *not* measure COHb and MetHb. For those pulse oximeters that calculate oxyhemoglobin saturation based only on oxyhemoglobin and deoxyhemoglobin, oxyhemoglobin saturation will be overestimated when one or more dyshemoglobins are present. In addition, the accuracy of pulse oximetry can be compromised by many factors, including poor perfusion and severe anemia.

The maximum amount of O_2 that can be carried by hemoglobin in a given quantity of blood is the *hemoglobin oxygen (binding) capacity*. The molecular weight of tetramer hemoglobin is 64,458 g/mol. One mole of a perfect gas occupies 22,414 mL. Therefore, each gram of hemoglobin carries 1.39 mL of O_2:

$$\frac{22,414 \text{ mL/mol}_4}{64,458 \text{ g/mol}} = 1.39 \text{ mL/g} \qquad \text{(Eq. 17-12)}$$

When the total hemoglobin (tHb) is 15 g/dL and the hemoglobin is 100% saturated with O_2, the O_2 capacity is

$$15 \text{ g/100 mL} \times 1.39 \text{ mL/g}$$
$$= 20.8 \text{ mL O}_2/100 \text{ mL of blood} \qquad \text{(Eq. 17-13)}$$

Oxygen content is the total O_2 in blood and determined from the sum of the O_2 bound to hemoglobin (O_2Hb) and the amount dissolved in the plasma (pO_2). (Because pO_2 and pCO_2 are only indices of gas exchange efficiency in the lungs, they do not reveal the *content* of either gas in the blood.) For every mm Hg pO_2, 0.00314 mL of O_2 will be dissolved in 100 mL of plasma at 37°C. For example, if the pO_2 is 100 mm Hg, 0.3 mL of O_2 will be dissolved in every 100 mL of blood plasma. The amount of dissolved O_2 is usually not clinically significant. However, with low tHb or at hyperbaric conditions, it may become a significant source of O_2 to the tissue. Normally, 97% to 99% of the available hemoglobin is saturated with O_2. Assuming a tHb of 15 g/dL, the O_2 content for every 100 mL of blood plasma becomes

$$0.3 \text{ mL} + (20.8 \text{ mL} \times 0.97) = 20.5 \text{ mL} \qquad \text{(Eq. 17-14)}$$

Hemoglobin–Oxygen Dissociation

In addition to adequate ventilation and gas exchange with the pulmonary circulation, hemoglobin, which transports O_2 to the tissues, must release it. The increased H^+ concentration and pCO_2 levels at the tissue from cellular metabolism change the molecular configuration of O_2Hb, facilitating O_2 release.

Oxygen dissociates from adult hemoglobin (A_1) in a characteristic fashion. If this dissociation is graphed (Fig. 17-4) with pO_2 on the x-axis and percent SO_2 on the y-axis, the resulting curve is sigmoid, or slightly S-shaped. Hemoglobin "holds on" to O_2 until the O_2 tension in the tissue is reduced to about 60 mm Hg. Below this tension, the O_2 is released rapidly. The position of the oxygen dissociation curve reflects the *affinity* that hemoglobin has for O_2 and affects the rate of this dissociation.

Hydrogen ion activity, pCO_2 and CO levels, body temperature, and 2,3-DPG can affect the position and shape of the oxygen dissociation curve as well as the affinity of hemoglobin for O_2. In actively metabolizing tissue, the conditions in the microenvironment promote release of oxygen. Oxidative metabolism increases the temperature, H^+, CO_2, and 2,3-DPG concentrations, which results in a right shift of the dissociation curve. This decreased affinity of hemoglobin for O_2 promotes release of oxygen to the tissue and allows patients, even those with low pO_2 and hemoglobin levels, to benefit. In the lungs, temperature, H^+, pCO_2, and 2,3-DPG decrease relative to tissue levels, shifting the oxygen dissociation curve slightly to the left. This enhances O_2 binding to hemoglobin and improves O_2 uptake. The metabolic by-product, 2,3-DPG, is also involved in two seemingly unrelated adaptations to potentially hypoxic conditions. When the β-chains of the hemoglobin molecule bind 2,3-DPG, oxyhemoglobin dissociation shifts to the right, with subsequent enhancement of oxygen release. Many patients with slow onset of anemia demonstrate elevated levels of 2,3-DPG, which may partially explain why patients with extremely low hemoglobin values are able to function. In addition, 2,3-DPG levels increase as an adaptation to high altitude.

Hemoglobin is a remarkable molecule. Its unique structure allows it to act as both an acid–base buffer and O_2 buffer. As hemoglobin moves through the body, exposure to the various microenvironments promotes appropriate association and dissociation of O_2, CO_2, and H^+. In tissue, exposure to elevated CO_2 and H^+ results in enhanced O_2 release (oxygen buffering). This release of oxygen from hemoglobin accelerates the uptake of CO_2 and H^+ by hemoglobin (acid–base buffering). In the lungs, the microenvironment promotes uptake of O_2 and release of CO_2.

Dyshemoglobins, such as COHb or MetHb, can also affect oxyhemoglobin dissociation. An elevation in CO from cigarette smoking or CO exposure causes the curve to shift to the left. As the percentage of COHb increases, the shape of the curve loses some of its sigmoid characteristics and shifts to the left, making the release of O_2 bound to hemoglobin much more difficult.

The preceding discussion refers to normal adult (A_1) hemoglobin. In patients with hemoglobinopathies and in newborns, the pattern of dissociation may differ. For example, fetal hemoglobin causes a shift to the left, but with little change in the sigmoid shape.

MEASUREMENT

Spectrophotometric (CO-Oximeter) Determination of Oxygen Saturation

The *actual percent oxyhemoglobin* (O_2Hb) can be determined spectrophotometrically using a CO-oximeter designed to directly measure the various hemoglobin species. Each species of hemoglobin has a characteristic absorbance curve (Fig. 17-5). The number of hemoglobin species measured will depend on the number and specific wavelengths incorporated into the instrumentation. For example, two-wavelength instrument systems can measure only two hemoglobin species (i.e., O_2Hb and HHb), which are expressed as a fraction or percentage of the total hemoglobin.

Instruments, at a minimum, should have four wavelengths for measurements of HHb, O_2Hb, and the two most common dyshemoglobins, COHb and MetHb. Instruments with more than four wavelengths can recognize dyes and pigments, turbidity, other hemoglobin species, and abnormal proteins. Some newer CO-oximeters employ hundreds of wavelengths, which has greatly reduced measurement interferences. Microprocessors control the sequencing of multiple wavelengths of light

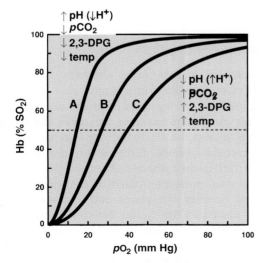

FIGURE 17-4 Oxygen dissociation curves. Curve *B* is the normal human curve. Curves *A* and *C* are from blood with increased affinity and decreased affinity, respectively. 2,3-DPG, 2,3-diphosphoglycerate.

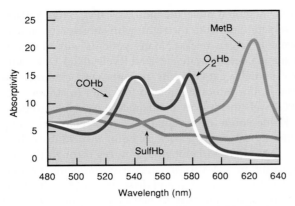

FIGURE 17-5 Optical absorption of hemoglobin fractions. (Reproduced with permission from Clin Chem News 1990 [January].).

through the sample and apply the necessary matrix equations after absorbance readings are made to calculate the percentage of the individual hemoglobin species:

$$O_2HB = a_1A_1 + a_2A_2 + \cdots + a_nA_n$$

$$HHb = b_1A_1 + \cdots + b_nA_n$$

$$COHB = c_1A_1 + c_2A_2 + \cdots + c_nA_n$$

$$MetHb = d_1A_1 + d_2A_2 + d_nA_n \qquad \text{(Eq. 17-15)}$$

where a_1, a_n, b_n, etc., are coefficients that are analogues of the absorption constant (a) that are derived from established methods, and A_1, A_2, and so on are the absorbances of the sample. The matrix equations will change depending on the number of wavelengths of light (which is manufacturer specific) passed through the sample. (The "calculation" made by these instruments should not be confused with a calculated SO_2 from a blood gas analyzer, which, in reality, *estimates* the value from a measured pO_2 and an empirical equation for the location and shape of the oxygen–hemoglobin dissociation curve. Only measured O_2Hb values reflect the patient's true status because calculated SO_2 and O_2Hb values will be vastly different in the presence of dyshemoglobins. In CO poisoning, for example, SO_2 will likely be normal with a significantly decreased O_2Hb value.)

As with any spectrophotometric measurement, potential sources of error exist, including faulty calibration of the instrument and spectral-interfering substances. The presence of any substances absorbing light at the wavelengths used in the measurement of any hemoglobin pigment has the potential of being a source of error. Product claims for specific instruments must be consulted for specific interferences.

Because the primary purpose of determining O_2Hb is to assess oxygen transport from the lungs, it is best to stabilize the patient's ventilation status before blood sample collection. An appropriate waiting period before the sample is drawn should follow changes in supplemental O_2 or mechanical ventilation. All blood samples should be collected under anaerobic conditions and mixed immediately with heparin or other appropriate anticoagulant. All samples should be analyzed promptly to avoid changes in saturation resulting from the consumption of oxygen by metabolizing cells.[2,4]

Blood Gas Analyzers: pH, pCO_2, and pO_2

Blood gas analyzers use *electrodes* (macroelectrochemical or microelectrochemical sensors) as sensing devices to measure pO_2, pCO_2, and pH. The pO_2 measurement is amperometric, meaning that the amount of current flow is an indication of the oxygen present. The pCO_2 and pH measurements are potentiometric, in which a change in voltage indicates the activity of each analyte. Advances in microsensor technology have greatly expanded the analytic menus of whole blood analyzers. In addition to pH and blood gas measurements, many manufacturers include hemoglobin and/or hematocrit, electrolytes, metabolites (glucose, lactate, creatinine, and blood urea nitrogen), and CO-oximetry with their instrumentation.

The *cathode* can be defined in at least three ways: (1) the negative electrode, (2) a site to which cations tend to travel, or (3) a site at which reduction occurs. *Reduction* is the gain of electrons by a particle (atom, molecule, or ion). The *anode* is the positive electrode, the site to which anions migrate or the site at which oxidation occurs. *Oxidation* is the loss of electrons by a particle. An *electrochemical cell* is formed when two opposite electrodes are immersed in a liquid that will conduct the current. The blood gas analyzer can calculate several additional parameters: bicarbonate, total CO_2, base excess, and SO_2.

Measurement of pO_2

pO_2 electrodes, called *Clarke electrodes*, measure the amount of current flow in a circuit that is related to the amount of O_2 being reduced at the cathode. A gas-permeable membrane covering the tip of the electrode selectively allows the O_2 to diffuse into an electrolyte and contact the cathode. Electrons are drawn from the anode surface to the cathode surface to reduce the O_2. A small, constant polarizing potential (typically, −0.65 V) is applied between the anode and cathode. A *micro-ammeter* placed in the circuit between the anode and cathode measures the movement of electrons (current). Four electrons are drawn for every mole of O_2 reduced, making it possible to determine pO_2. The semipermeable membrane will also allow other gases to pass, such as CO_2 and N_2, but these gases will not be reduced at the cathode if the polarizing voltage is tightly controlled.

CASE STUDY 17-5

A 37-year-old man was admitted to the emergency department. He was short of breath, dizzy, flushed (hyperemic), sweating (diaphoretic), and nauseous. Shortly after being admitted, blood gases were drawn:

pH	7.48
pCO_2	32 mm Hg
pO_2	96 mm Hg
HCO_3^-	24 mmol/L
SO_2	98% (calculated)
SpO_2	99% (pulse oximetry oxygen saturation)

After a few hours, the patient's symptoms diminished and he was released. Two weeks later, the same patient was again admitted to the emergency department with the same symptoms. This time, arterial blood was drawn for both blood gases and CO-oximetry measurements. The results were as follows:

pH	7.49
pCO_2	33 mm Hg
pO_2	95 mm Hg
HCO_3^-	23 mmol/L
SO_2	98% (calculated) (reference range, >95%)
SpO_2	99% (pulse oximetry oxygen saturation) (reference range, >95%)

Spectrophotometric (CO-oximeter) measurement of hemoglobin species:

Hb	13.5 g/L
O_2Hb	73% (reference range, >95%)
COHb	22% (reference range, <2%; higher with smokers)
MetHb	1% (reference range, <1.5%)

Question

1. Is the patient hypoxic on the first admission to the ED?

2. Considering the new laboratory data, is this patient hypoxic on the second admission to the ED?

3. Why is there discrepancy between calculated SO_2, SpO_2, and O_2Hb?

4. What is a possible cause of this patient's shortness of breath and low O_2Hb?

The primary source of error for pO_2 measurement is associated with the buildup of protein material on the surface of the membrane. This buildup retards diffusion and slows the electrode response. Bacterial contamination within the measuring chamber, although uncommon, will consume O_2 and cause low and drifting values. Other errors are mostly associated with a system malfunction, such as incorrect calibration.

Nonanalytic concerns, including sample collection and handling, are addressed later in this chapter. However, it is particularly important not to expose the sample to room air when collecting, transporting, and making O_2 measurements. Contamination of the sample with room air ($pO_2 > 150$ mm Hg) can result in significant error. Even after the sample is drawn, leukocytes continue to metabolize O_2. Unless the sample is analyzed immediately after being drawn, low pO_2 values may be seen with high white blood cell counts.

Continuous measurements for pO_2 are also possible using TC *electrodes* placed directly on the skin. Measurement depends on oxygen diffusing from the capillary bed through the tissue to the electrode. Although most commonly used with neonates and infants, this noninvasive approach is not without problems. Skin thickness and tissue perfusion with arterial blood can significantly affect the results. Heating the electrode placed on the skin can enhance diffusion of O_2 to the electrode; however, burns can result unless the electrodes are moved regularly. Although pO_2 measured by these electrodes may *reflect* the arterial pO_2, the two values are not equivalent. Oxygen consumption by tissue at the electrode site, the effects of heating the tissue, and possible hypoperfusion from cardiovascular instability can all contribute to the unpredictability of the arterial tissue O_2 gradient.

Measurement of pH and pCO_2

To understand potentiometric measurements, it is helpful to think of atoms and ions as having a chemical energy. An increased concentration or *activity* of the ions leads to an increase in the force exerted by those ions.

To measure how much force—energy or potential—a given ion possesses, certain elements in the measuring device are required; namely, two electrodes (the measuring electrode responsive to the ion of interest and the reference electrode) and a voltmeter, which measures the potential difference (ΔE) between the two electrodes. The potential difference is related to the concentration of the ion of interest by the Nernst equation:

$$\Delta E = \Delta E^\circ + \frac{0.05916}{n} \log a_1 \text{ at } 25^\circ C \qquad \text{(Eq. 17-16)}$$

CASE STUDY 17-6

A 48-year-old man with diabetes with a history of alcohol abuse was admitted to the emergency department. He had an elevated heart rate (tachycardia) and was experiencing extreme shortness of breath. Blood was drawn for glucose and blood gases and urine collected for ketones:

Glucose	570 mg/dL
Urinary ketones	Large (reference range, negative)
pH	7.00
pCO_2	48 mm Hg
pO_2	68 mm Hg
HCO_3^-	12 mmol/L
SO_2	81% (calculated)
tHb	10 g/dL

Question

1. Is the patient's acidemia a result of respiratory or nonrespiratory disturbances or a combination of both?

2. If the patient was not having respiratory problems, how would you classify the acid–base disturbance?

3. What is the significance of shortness of breath, tachycardia, and elevated pCO_2?

4. What is the significance of the urinary ketones that result in terms of identifying the type of diabetes?

where $\Delta E°$ is standard potential of the electrochemical cell, n is charge of the analyte ion i, and a_i is activity of the analyte ion i.

To measure pH, a glass membrane sensitive to H^+ is placed around an internal Ag–AgCl electrode to form a measuring electrode. The potential that develops at the glass membrane as a result of H^+ from the unknown solution diffusing into the membrane's surface is proportional to the difference in cH^+ between the unknown sample and the buffer solution inside the electrode. For the potential developed at the glass membrane to be measured, a reference electrode must be introduced into the solution and both electrodes must be connected to a pH (volt) meter. The reference electrode (commonly either a calomel [Hg–HgCl] or an Ag–AgCl half-cell) provides a steady reference voltage against which voltage changes from the measuring electrode are compared. The pH meter reflects the potential difference between the two electrodes.

For the cell described, the Nernst equation predicts that a change of +59.16 mV, at 25°C, is the result of a 10-fold increase in H^+ activity or a decrease of an entire pH unit (e.g., pH 7.0 to 6.0). Changing the temperature affects the response. At 37°C, a change of 1 pH unit elicits a 61.5 mV change. The glass membrane of the measuring electrode must be kept free from protein buildup because coating of the membrane causes sluggish or erratic responses.

pCO_2 is determined with a modified pH electrode, called a *Severinghaus electrode*. An outer semipermeable membrane that allows CO_2 to diffuse into a layer of electrolyte, usually a bicarbonate buffer, covers the glass pH electrode. The CO_2 that diffuses across the membrane reacts with the buffer, forming *carbonic acid*, which then dissociates into bicarbonate plus H^+. The change in activity of the H^+ is measured by the pH electrode and related to pCO_2.

As with the other electrodes, the buildup of protein material on the membrane will affect diffusion and cause errors. pCO_2 electrodes are the slowest to respond because of the chemical reaction that must be completed. Other error sources include erroneous calibration caused by incorrect or contaminated calibration materials.

Types of Electrochemical Sensors

Macroelectrode sensors have been used in blood gas instruments since the beginning of the clinical measurement of blood gases. These have been modified over time in an effort to simplify their use and minimize the required sample volume and maintenance. *Microelectrodes* basically are miniaturized macroelectrodes. Miniaturization became possible with better manufacturing capabilities and with the development of the sophisticated electronics required to handle minute changes in signal.

Thick and thin film technology is a further modification of electrochemical sensors. Although the measurement principle is identical, the sensors are reduced to tiny wires embedded in a printed circuit card. The special card has etched grooves to separate components. A special paste material containing the required components (similar in function to the electrolytes of macroelectrodes) is spread over the sensors. To reduce the required sample volume, several sensors can be placed on a single small card. These sensors are disposable and less expensive to manufacture, which reduces maintenance.

Optical Sensors

Another technology for blood gas measurements is based on the fact that certain fluorescent dyes will react predictably with specific chemicals, such as O_2, CO_2, and H^+. The dye is separated from the sample by a membrane, as with electrodes, and the analyte diffuses into the dye, causing either an increase in or a quenching of fluorescence proportional to the amount of analyte. Calibration is used to establish the relationship between concentration and fluorescence. Normally, a single calibration will suffice for long periods because this technology is not subject to the drifts seen in electrochemical technology.

Optical technology has been applied to indwelling blood gas systems. Fiberoptic bundles carry light to sensors positioned at the tip of catheters and other bundles carry light back, allowing changes in fluorescence to be measured in a catheter within the patient's arterial system. The commercial development of indwelling systems has been limited by the increased probability of thrombogenesis and protein buildup on the membrane, separating the sample from the fluorescing dyes. This buildup impedes free sample diffusion into the measuring chamber.

Calibration

Temperature is an important factor in the measurement of pH and blood gases. The Nernst equation specifies the expected voltage output of an electrochemical cell at a given temperature. If the temperature of the measurement system changes, the output (voltage) will change. The solubility of gases in a liquid medium also depends on the temperature: as the temperature goes down, the solubility of the gas increases. Because pH and blood gas measurements are extremely sensitive to temperature, it is critical that the electrode sample chamber be maintained at constant temperature for all measurements. All blood gas analyzers have electrode chambers thermostatically controlled to $37°C \pm 0.1°C$.

The pH electrode is usually calibrated with two buffer solutions traceable to standards prepared by the National Institute of Standards and Technology (NIST). *Traceable* usually means that the actual value of the calibrator has been determined using an NIST standard as a reference. Usually, one calibrator is near 6.8 and the other is near 7.38 because most pH electrodes produce "0" voltage at this point. The calibrators must be stored at the stated temperature and not exposed to room air because pH changes with the absorption of CO_2.

Calibration of any blood gas analyzer will vary depending on the manufacturer. Normally, two gas mixtures are used for pCO_2 and pO_2. One gas has no O_2 to set the zero point of the O_2 electrode (which is usually a stable point). The same gas has approximately 5% CO_2 because this is the null (zero potential and stable) point for the CO_2 electrode. The other gas sets the gain, that is, the amount of change in the electrode signal relative to the change for the analyte. The gas can have any value.

Most instruments are self-calibrating (calibrate automatically at specified time intervals) and are programmed to indicate a calibration error if the electronic signal from the electrode is inconsistent with the programmed expected value. For example, if the value(s) obtained during calibration exceed(s) a programmed tolerance

CASE STUDY 17-7

A 64-year-old woman with COPD was admitted to the emergency department with extreme shortness of breath. She had a bluish color that was particularly pronounced on her lips and nail beds and she displayed a weak and persistent cough with diminished, but rattling breath sounds. Home medications included bronchodilators, steroids, Lasix (a loop diuretic that does not conserve plasma potassium), and digitalis. Vital signs: heart rate, 148 bpm; blood pressure, 100/88 mm Hg; temperature, 37°C; and respiratory rate, 38/min. Initial blood gas results on room air were the following:

pH	7.289
pCO_2	91 mm Hg
pO_2	53 mm Hg
HCO_3^-	43 mmol/L

Questions

1. What is the patient's acid–base status?

2. Would the pH be normal if the patient was able to decrease her pCO_2 to 50 mm Hg?

3. In addition to COPD, what condition likely contributed to her poor gas exchange (hypercarbia and hypoxemia)?

She was treated with a bolus of Lasix intravenously and two albuterol (bronchodilator) respiratory treatments. Her vital signs improved: heart rate, 124 bpm; blood pressure, 120/80 mm Hg; and respiratory rate, 22/min. Blood gases were repeated with the patient breathing 28% O_2 ($FiO_2 = 0.28$)

pH	7.306
pCO_2	75 mm Hg
pO_2	78 mm Hg
HCO_3^-	36 mmol/L

Questions

1. Should more oxygen be administered to this patient?

2. How did Lasix administration and respiratory treatment benefit the patient?

3. Which critical electrolyte should be closely monitored in the management of this case?

limit, flagging of a *drift* error will occur at the time of calibration, and corrective action will need to be taken before patient samples can be analyzed.

Calculated Parameters

Several acid–base parameters can be calculated from measured pH and pCO_2 values. Manufacturers of blood gas instruments include algorithms to perform the calculations. No calculated parameter is universally used; many physicians have "favorite" parameters for identifying various pathologies.

The calculation of HCO_3^- is based on the Henderson-Hasselbalch equation. This can be calculated when pH and pCO_2 are known. One basic assumption is that the pK_a of the bicarbonate buffer system in plasma at 37°C is 6.1.

Carbonic acid concentration can be calculated using the solubility coefficient of CO_2 in plasma at 37°C. The solubility constant to convert pCO_2 to mmol/L of H_2CO_3 is 0.0307. If the temperature or the composition of plasma changes (e.g., an increase in lipids, in which gases are more soluble), the constant will change.

Total carbon dioxide content ($ctCO_2$) is the bicarbonate plus the dCO_2 (carbonic acid) plus the associated CO_2 with proteins (carbamates). A blood gas analyzer approximates $ctCO_2$ by adding the bicarbonate and carbonic acid values ($ctCO_2 = cHCO_3^- + [0.0307\ pCO_2]$).

Some clinicians use *base excess* to assess the nonrespiratory component of a patient's acid–base disorder. Base excess is calculated from an algorithm that uses the patient's pH, pCO_2, and hemoglobin. A positive value (base excess) indicates an excess of bicarbonate or relative deficit of noncarbonic acid and suggests *nonrespiratory alkalosis*. A negative value (base deficit) indicates a deficit of bicarbonate or relative excess of noncarbonic acids and suggests *nonrespiratory acidosis*. Because the indicated nonrespiratory alkalosis or acidosis may be a result of primary disturbances or compensatory mechanisms, base excess values should not be used alone in assessing a patient's acid–base status.

Correction for Temperature

Values for pH, pCO_2, and pO_2 are temperature dependent. By convention, all of these measurements are made at 37°C. The question becomes, "When the patient's body temperature differs from 37°C, should the blood gas values be 'corrected' to the actual temperature of the patient?." Although the blood gas instrument software can easily perform the correction, the data may be confusing because appropriate reference ranges *for the patient's temperature* must be used for proper result interpretation and these may be difficult to find or may be controversial. When results are reported at actual patient temperature, results should also be reported at 37°C for the purpose evaluating relative to euthermic reference range.

QUALITY ASSURANCE

Preanalytic Considerations

Blood gas measurements, like all laboratory measurements, are subject to preanalytic, analytic, and postanalytic errors. Few other measurements, however, are as affected by preanalytic errors—those introduced during the collection and transport of samples before analysis.[2,4]

Figure 17-6 depicts the quality assurance cycle. The steps included in the analytic area are under the direct control of the laboratory. Because much of the quality assurance cycle lies outside the laboratory, the laboratorian must take an active role in educating *all* people involved in developing policies and procedures for controlling all the processes in the cycle to ensure quality. The preanalytic considerations start with proper patient identification, which is absolutely essential before any blood specimen is collected. Once collected the specimen must be correctly labeled and accompanied by accurate information, e.g., FiO_2, needed for result interpretation.

Only personnel who have experience with the drawing equipment and technique and have knowledge of the possible sources of error should draw samples for pH and blood gas analyses. Because arterial blood collection may

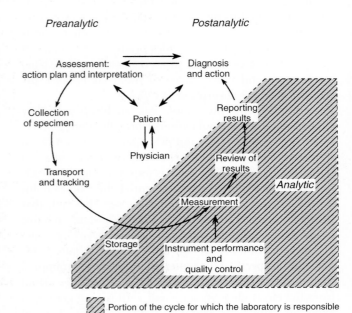

FIGURE 17-6 Blood gas analysis quality assurance cycle. (Courtesy of Robert F. Moran.)

be painful and result in patient hyperventilation, which lowers the pCO_2 and increases the pH, the ability to reassure the patient is essential. The choice of site—radial, brachial, femoral, or temporal artery—is usually customary within an institution, depending on the predominant patient population (e.g., pediatric patients, burn patients, and outpatients). The Clinical and Laboratory Standards Institute (CLSI) publication *Procedures for the Collection of Arterial Blood Specimens* is an excellent reference.[4]

While arterial samples for pH and blood gas studies are recommended, peripheral venous samples can be used if pulmonary function or O_2 transport is not being assessed. For venous samples, the source of the specimen must be clearly identified and the appropriate (venous) reference ranges included with the results for data interpretation. Depending on the patient, capillary blood may need to be collected to assess pH and pCO_2. Although the correlation with arterial blood is good for pH and pCO_2, capillary pO_2 values, even with warming of the skin before drawing the sample, do not correlate well with arterial pO_2 values as a result of sample exposure to room air. Central venous (pulmonary artery) blood samples are obtained to assess O_2 consumption, which is calculated from the O_2 content of arterial and pulmonary artery blood and the cardiac output. For sample collection from an indwelling arterial line, an appropriate blood volume must initially be withdrawn and discarded from the line to assure that the actual sample collected contains only arterial blood. The proper flushing procedure minimizes the chance of specimen contamination with solutions (i.e., liquid heparin, medication, or electrolyte fluids) that may be in the line.[2]

Sources of error in the collection and handling of blood gas specimens include the collection device, form and concentration of heparin used for anticoagulation, speed of syringe filling, maintenance of the anaerobic environment, mixing of the sample to ensure dissolution and distribution of the heparin, and transport and storage time before analysis. For proper interpretation of blood gas results, the patient's status—ventilation (on room air or supplemental O_2) and body temperature—at the time of sample collection must be documented.

In most instances, the ideal collection device for arterial blood sampling is a 1- to 3-mL self-filling, plastic, disposable syringe, containing the appropriate type and amount of anticoagulant. Evacuated collection tubes are not appropriate for blood gases. While both dry (lyophilized) and liquid heparin are acceptable anticoagulants, the liquid form is not recommended because excessive amounts can dilute the sample and possibly alter the sample due to equilibration with room air.[2,4] Once drawn, the blood in the syringe must be mixed thoroughly with the heparin to prevent microclots from forming. Adequate mixing is also important immediately

CASE STUDY 17-8

A 23-year-old woman with a history of asthma was brought to the emergency department by ambulance. She was extremely short of breath. Her level of consciousness was diminished greatly, and she was only able to respond to questions with nods or one-word responses. She had a weak cough, with nearly inaudible breath sounds. After drawing blood gases, she was placed on supplemental oxygen. Vital signs: heart rate, 160 bpm; blood pressure, 120/84 mm Hg; temperature, 37°C; and respiratory rate, 36/min. Her initial blood gas and total hemoglobin results were as follows:

pH	7.330
pCO_2	25 mm Hg
pO_2	58 mm Hg
HCO_3^-	13 mmol/L
tHb	12.4 g/L

Questions

1. What is the patient's acid–base and oxygenation status?
2. What is the cause of the acid–base disturbance?
3. Would the pH be normal if the patient's pCO_2 increased to 40 mm Hg?
4. Does asthma typically present in this manner?
5. What clinical findings are most indicative of this patient's impending failure?

before analysis to resuspend the settled cells. Although sodium and lithium salts of heparin are recommended for pH and blood gas analysis, other forms are available: ammonium, zinc, electrolyte balanced, and calcium titrated. Selection of the proper type of heparin is particularly important with instruments combining blood gas, electrolyte, and metabolite measurements. It is important to consult the manufacturer's product insert.

Slow filling of the syringe may be caused by a mismatch of syringe and needle sizes. Although too small a needle reduces patient's pain and, therefore, the likelihood of arteriospasm and hematoma, it may produce bubbles that affect pCO_2 and pO_2 values as well as hemolysis, which is important when potassium is measured along with pH and blood gases. Maintenance of an anaerobic environment is critical to correct results. Any air trapped in the syringe during the draw should be immediately expelled at the completion of the draw.

Transport time prior to analysis should be minimal to reduce cell metabolism, which results in oxygen and glucose consumption and carbon dioxide and lactate production. While placing the filled syringe in an ice water slurry immediately after the draw minimizes metabolism, there is a potential for pO_2 to increase due to oxygen diffusing from the water through the pores of the plastic syringe. In addition, lower temperatures cause increased oxygen solubility in blood and a left-shift in the oxyhemoglobin curve resulting in more oxygen combining with hemoglobin. As a consequence when the sample is heated by the blood gas analyzer, the measured pO_2 is falsely elevated.[5] The best practice in avoiding many of the preanalytic errors is to analyze the sample as quickly as possible. Oxygen and carbon dioxide levels in blood kept at cool room temperatures for 20 to 30 minutes or less are minimally affected except in the presence of an elevated leukocyte or platelet count. The CLSI guidelines advocate samples be kept at room temperature and analyzed in less than 30 minutes.[2] Consideration should be given to the additional sources of preanalytic errors for samples that are to be analyzed on multi-analyte instruments. For example, prolonged ice water slurry storage can result in falsely elevated potassium in whole blood samples. Consult manufacturer manuals for preanalytic considerations.

Because sample procurement and handling are the source of many possible errors in blood gas analysis, it is necessary that procedures and policies are carefully constructed and adherence monitored to ensure quality. At this time, no quality assessment approach can detect all preanalytic problems associated with blood gas analysis.

Analytic Assessments: Quality Control and Proficiency Testing

Quality control (QC) assesses the analytic phase of the three-part—preanalytic, analytic, and postanalytic—testing process. Ideally, to evaluate the performance of a test method, a control should closely mimic actual patient samples; this is impossible for blood gases. There are several approaches for blood gas QC.[2] All have limitations.

Surrogate liquid control materials are the basis of most of the traditional QC practices.[6] Usually, these are sold in sealed glass ampules or bags that contain solutions equilibrated with gases of known concentration. The ampules can be snapped and the contents analyzed by the analyst like a patient's sample or the instrument can automatically assess the liquid at programmed intervals for analysis. Surrogate liquid controls are typically available in at least three levels, corresponding to values observed with low, expected or "normal," and elevated values for each of the measured analytes, which may include additional analytes, such as sodium, potassium,

chloride, lactate, ionized calcium and magnesium, and glucose. The materials vary in stability and are susceptible to temperature variation in storage and handling. Each must be handled as described by the manufacturer to eliminate precision errors caused by improper handling of the material. Because liquid control materials have significantly different matrices than fresh whole blood, the laboratorian must be aware that they may not detect problems that affect patient samples or they may detect errors induced by improper handling of the commercial controls. Aqueous-based controls, the most commonly used QC material, have low O_2 solubility, making them sensitive to factors, particularly when manually analyzed, that affect pO_2. Aqueous controls must be at room temperature for analysis and manufacturer recommendations must be followed closely or pO_2 values may be unreliable. Hemoglobin-containing and emulsion-based controls have increased O_2 solubility to better resist O_2 changes. Several manufacturers have devised onboard QC systems that greatly reduce operator handling errors. Advances in computer technology and software monitoring algorithms now can automatically analyze QC products, continuously monitor instrument performance, and detect some preanalytical problems (i.e., microclots and hemolysis) for improved reliability and error detection in blood gas and multi-analyte instruments.

Tonometry is the equilibration of a fluid with gases of known concentration and under controlled conditions, such as constant temperature, BP, and humidification.[2] When whole blood is used, it is considered the reference procedure to establish the accuracy for pCO_2 and pO_2. However, tonometry is rarely used today because the technique is considered to be too cumbersome and time consuming and it can be potentially hazardous when whole blood is used.

Duplicate assays using two or more instruments for simultaneous analysis of a patient sample is another technique. The delta checks, or the difference in values obtained on the two instruments, often pick up problems that might be missed by routine QC. The allowable difference in duplicates should be tighter than those observed with surrogate liquid controls, and discrepancies between results provide no clue regarding which data point is wrong or which instrument is malfunctioning. Consequently, the duplicate assay approach cannot be used as the sole method of QC, but it can be a useful technique for detecting errors and also for troubleshooting instruments.

Nonsurrogate QC is becoming particularly popular for testing devices used at the point of care. This category includes a variety of quality assurance mechanisms that are integrated into the design of the device, such as electronic QC (which simulates sensor signals to test electronic components), automated procedural controls (which ensure that certain steps of the method occur appropriately), and automated internal checks (which may, for example, ensure the quality of a raw electronic signal). Such controls may check all, but usually just a portion, of the test system's analytic components each time the test is performed.

Whatever the QC approach, the QC needs of the blood gas laboratory contrast sharply with those of the general laboratory, which analyzes many patient samples as a group and includes multiple control specimens with each run. In the blood gas laboratory, the critical nature of the measurements and the limited patient sample volume do not always allow for repeat analyses, if problems exist. Consequently, the blood gas laboratory must perform *prospective* QC because instruments must be *prequalified* to ensure proper performance before the patient sample arrives for analysis.

Participating in external, interlaboratory surveys or proficiency testing programs is another essential component of ensuring the quality of blood gas measurements.[7] Ongoing comparisons of results through proficiency testing help ensure that systematic (accuracy) errors do not slowly increase and go undetected by internal QC procedures. A rigorous internal QC program ensures internal consistency. Good performance in a proficiency testing program ensures the absence of significant bias relative to other laboratories and further confirms the validity of a laboratory's patient results. If an individual analyzer does not produce proficiency testing results consistent with its peer laboratories (those using the same method/instrument) or if the differences between values change over time, suspicion of the instrument's performance is warranted.

Interpretation of Results

Laboratory professionals need certain knowledge, attitudes, and skills for obtaining and analyzing specimens for pH and blood gases. Although the patient's physician assimilates all results—laboratory, radiology, nuclear medicine, surgical pathology findings, and so on, along with the patient's clinical history—laboratory personnel must immediately assess patient results and make preliminary judgments about the "fit," that is, do the results make sense? Simple evaluation of the data may reveal an instrument problem (possible bubble in the sample chamber or fibrin plug) or a possible sample handling problem (pO_2 out of line with previous results and current inspired FiO_2 levels). The application of knowledge saves time. The ability to correlate data quickly reduces turnaround time and prevents mistakes.

For additional student resources please visit thePoint at http://thepoint.lww.com. **thePoint**✳

QUESTIONS

1. The presence of dyshemoglobins will cause a calculated % SO_2 result to be falsely (elevated, decreased) and a pulse oximeter % SpO_2 value to be falsely (elevated, decreased).
   a. Elevated, elevated
   b. Decreased, decreased
   c. Elevated, decreased
   d. Decreased, elevated

2. The anticoagulant of choice for arterial blood gas measurements is _____ in the _____ state.
   a. Lithium heparin; dry
   b. EDTA; dry
   c. Potassium oxalate; liquid
   d. Sodium citrate; dry

3. At a pH of 7.10, the H^+ concentration is equal to
   a. 80 nmol/L
   b. 20 nmol/L
   c. 40 nmol/L
   d. 60 nmol/L

4. The kidneys compensate for respiratory alkalosis by (excretion, retention) of bicarbonate and (increased, decreased) excretion of NaH_2PO_4.
   a. Excretion, decreased
   b. Excretion, increased
   c. Retention, increased
   d. Retention, decreased

5. The normal ratio of carbonic acid to bicarbonate in arterial blood is
   a. 1:20
   b. 7.4:6.1
   c. 0.003:1.39
   d. 20:1

6. When arterial blood from a normal patient is exposed to room air:
   a. pCO_2 increases; pO_2 decreases
   b. pCO_2 decreases; pO_2 increases
   c. pCO_2 decreases; pO_2 decreases
   d. pCO_2 increases; pO_2 increases

7. A patient's arterial blood gas results are as follows: pH 7.37; pCO_2, 75 mm Hg; HCO_3^-, 37 mmol/L. These values are consistent with
   a. Compensated respiratory acidosis
   b. Compensated nonrespiratory acidosis
   c. Uncompensated respiratory alkalosis
   d. Uncompensated nonrespiratory alkalosis

8. A patient's arterial blood gas results are as follows: pH 7.48; pCO_2, 54 mm Hg; HCO_3^-, 38 mmol/L. These values are consistent with
   a. Compensated nonrespiratory alkalosis
   b. Compensated respiratory alkalosis
   c. Uncompensated respiratory alkalosis
   d. Uncompensated nonrespiratory alkalosis

9. In the circulatory system, bicarbonate leaves the red blood cells and enters the plasma through an exchange mechanism with _____ to maintain electroneutrality.
   a. Chloride
   b. Carbonic acid
   c. Lactate
   d. Sodium

10. Hypoventilation can compensate for
    a. Nonrespiratory acidosis
    b. Mixed alkalosis
    c. Mixed acidosis
    d. Nonrespiratory alkalosis

11. The hemoglobin oxygen binding capacity for a blood sample that is 100% saturated with O_2 and has a total hemoglobin value of 12 g/dL is approximately
    a. 17 mL O_2/dL
    b. 4 mL O_2/dL
    c. 8 mL O_2/dL
    d. 34 mL O_2/dL

12. Carbonic acid concentration in blood plasma equals
    a. 0.0307 mmol/L/mm Hg times the pCO_2 value in mm Hg
    b. Apparent pK_a of carbonic acid, 6.1, plus the pCO_2 value in mm Hg
    c. pCO_2 value in mm Hg plus HCO_3^- value in mm Hg
    d. Bicarbonate concentration divided by the pCO_2 value in mm Hg

13. Oxygen content in blood reflects
    a. pO_2 value
    b. O_2Hb only
    c. O_2 dissolved in blood plasma only
    d. The patient's total hemoglobin value
    e. All of these

REFERENCES

1. Weisberg HF. *Water, Electrolyte, and Acid-Base Balance.* 2nd ed. Baltimore, MD: Williams & Wilkins; 1962.
2. D'Orazio P, Ehrmeyer SS, Jacobs E, Toffaletti JG, Wandrup JH. *Blood Gas and pH Analysis and Related Measurements.* Wayne, PA: Clinical and Laboratory Standards Institute; 2009:Publication no. C46-A2.
3. Ehrmeyer S, Ancy J, Laessig R. Oxygenation: measure the right thing. *Respir Ther.* 1998;11(3):25-28.
4. Blonshine S, Alberti R, Olesinski RL, National Committee for Clinical Laboratory Standards. *Procedures for the Collection of Arterial Blood Specimens.* Wayne, PA: Clinical and Laboratory Standards Institute; 2004:Publication no. H11-A4.
5. Ancy J. Preventing preanalytical error in blood gas analysis. The Blood Gas Laboratory. http://www.foocus.com/pdfs/Articles/MarApr06/John%20Ancy.pdf
6. Westgard JO, Gregory Miller W, Allen K, et al. *Statistical Quality Control for Quantitative Measurements: Principles and Definitions.* Wayne, PA: Clinical and Laboratory Standards Institute; 2006:Publication no. C24-A3.
7. Ehrmeyer SS, Laessig RH: Benefits of voluntary proficiency testing. *Adv Lab Admin.* 2006;15(8):10-12.

Trace and Toxic Elements

FREDERICK G. STRATHMANN, ELZBIETA (ELA) BAKOWSKA, ALAN L. ROCKWOOD

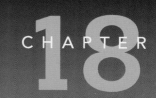

CHAPTER 18

CHAPTER OUTLINE

Chapter Objectives

Upon completion of this chapter, the clinical laboratorian should be able to do the following:

- Define metalloprotein, metalloenzyme, cofactor, trace element, ultratrace element, essential trace element, and nonessential trace element.
- State the biologic functions of selected essential trace elements.
- Distinguish between essential and nonessential trace elements.
- Discuss the clinical significance of selected trace elements and the consequences of deficiency and toxic states.
- Discuss specimen collection considerations and laboratory determination.
- Describe instrumentation used for trace element analysis

KEY TERMS

Atomic absorption
Atomic emission
Cold vapor atomic absorption spectroscopy
Emission spectrum
Essential element

Inductively coupled plasma
Mass-to-charge ratio
Mass spectrometry
Metalloenzyme
Metalloprotein
Nonessential element

Almost half of the elements listed in the periodic table have been found in the human body.[1] An element is considered essential if a deficiency impairs a biochemical or functional process, and replacement of the element corrects this impairment. Decreased intake, impaired absorption, increased excretion, and genetic abnormalities are all examples of conditions that could result in deficiency of one or several trace elements. The World Health Organization has established the dietary requirement for nutrients as the smallest amount of the nutrient needed to maintain optimal function and health. Any element that is not considered essential is classified as nonessential. Nonessential trace elements are of medical interest primarily because many of them are toxic.

The trace and toxic elements included in this chapter all have biochemical importance, whether minor or major. The essential trace elements are often associated with an enzyme (metalloenzyme) or another protein (metalloprotein) as a cofactor. Deficiencies typically impair one or more biochemical functions and excess concentrations are associated with at least some degree of toxicity. Although trace elements, such as iron, copper, and zinc, are found in milligram per liter or parts per million concentrations, ultratrace elements, such as selenium, chromium, and manganese, are found in microgram per liter or parts per billion concentrations.

This chapter provides an overview of the trace and toxic elements frequently encountered in the clinical laboratory. The absorption, transport, distribution, metabolism (if relevant), and elimination will be described and related to the clinical significance of disease states or toxicity. In addition, an introduction to the most common testing methodologies is provided. No reference intervals have been included in the chapter text; however, several excellent sources for toxic element thresholds and trace element reference intervals are included in the bibliography. As always, the use of published thresholds and reference intervals as more than general guidelines must be done with caution, as variations in geographical location, testing methodologies, and population differences can often compromise their validity.

METHODS AND INSTRUMENTATION

For many years, the most commonly used instrumentation for trace and toxic metal analysis has been the atomic absorption (AA) spectrometer, either with flame atomic absorption spectroscopy (FAAS) or flameless (i.e., graphite furnace atomic absorption spectroscopy [GFAAS]) atomization. Atomic emission spectrometry is also useful for some elements, particularly if used in the form of inductively coupled plasma atomic emission spectroscopy (ICP-AES) for atomization and excitation. Recently, inductively coupled plasma mass spectrometry (ICP-MS) is becoming more widely used because of its sensitivity, wide range of elements covered, and relative freedom from interferences. No single technique is best for all purposes. A summary of the relative advantages and disadvantages of the main techniques is given in Table 18-1.

Sample Collection and Processing

Specimens for the analysis of trace elements must be collected with scrupulous attention to details such as anticoagulant, collection apparatus, and specimen type (urine, serum, plasma, or blood). Because of the low concentration in biologic specimens and the ubiquitous presence

TABLE 18-1	RELATIVE ADVANTAGES AND DISADVANTAGES OF MAIN TECHNIQUES FOR ELEMENTAL ANALYSIS			
	FLAME AA	**GFAA**	**ICP-AES**	**ICP-MS**
Sensitivity	Moderate	Excellent	Moderate	Excellent
Selectivity	Excellent	Good	Poor	Good
Elemental coverage	Moderate	Good	Good	Excellent
Speed for one analyte	Fast	Slow	Fast	Fast
Multi-element capabilities	No	No	Yes	Yes
Initial cost of instrument	Low	Moderate	Moderate	High
Cost of consumables	Very low	Very high	Low	Moderate
Ease of operation	Excellent	Poor	Moderate	Moderate

in the environment, extraordinary measures are required to prevent contamination of the specimen. This includes using special sampling and collection devices, specially cleaned glassware, and water and reagents of high purity. The selection of needles, evacuated blood collection tubes, anticoagulants and other additives, water and other reagents, pipettes, and sample cups must be carefully evaluated for use in trace and ultratrace analyses. In addition, the laboratory environment must be carefully controlled. Recommended measures include placing the trace elements laboratory in a separate room incorporating rigorous contamination control features, such as sticky mats at doors, non-shedding ceiling tiles, carefully controlled air flow to minimize particulate contamination, disposable booties worn over shoes, and particle monitoring equipment. Many useful measures are borrowed from those employed in semiconductor clean rooms.

Atomic Emission Spectroscopy

The simplified principle of the atomic emission spectroscopy (AES) instruments is presented in Figure 18-1.

The three most important components of atomic emission spectrophotometer are as follows:

1. A source, in which the sample is atomized at a sufficient temperature to produce an excited-state species. Those species will emit radiation upon relaxation back to the ground state.
2. A wavelength selecting device (monochromator), for the spectral dispersion of the radiation and separation of the analytical line from other radiation.
3. A detector permitting measurement of radiation intensity.

A liquid sample, containing element(s) of interest, is converted into an aerosol and delivered into the source, where it receives energy sufficient to emit radiation.

The intensity of the emitted radiation is correlated to the concentration of an analyte and is the basis for quantitation. The most commonly used sources in AES are flame and inductively coupled plasma (ICP). Flames are capable of producing temperatures up to 3,000 K. Typical fuel gases include hydrogen and acetylene, while oxidant gases include air, oxygen, and nitrous oxide.

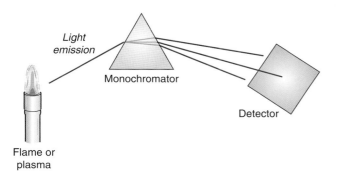

FIGURE 18-1 Simplified schematic of AES.

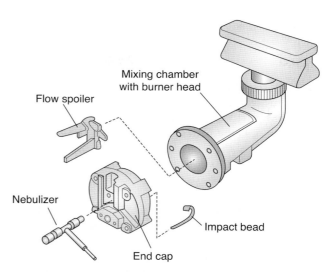

FIGURE 18-2 Mixing chamber burner for flame AA. (Courtesy of Perkin-Elmer, Waltham, MA.)

The gases are combined in a specially designed mixing chamber. A sample is also introduced into the mixing chamber using a nebulizer that converts liquid into a fine spray. The mixing chamber and burner assembly are shown in Figure 18-2. The same assembly can be used for AA instrumentation.

In AES, both atomic and ionic excited states can be produced (depending on the element and the source), which leads to the production of complicated emission spectra. The "emission spectrum" of an element is composed of a series of very narrow peaks (sometimes known as "lines"), with each line at a different wavelength and each line matched to a specific transition. Each element has its own characteristic emission spectrum. For example, sodium can be detected by tuning the monochromator to a wavelength of 589 nm. Ideally, each emission line of a given element would be distinct from all other emission lines of other elements. However, there are many cases where emission lines from distinct elements overlap resulting in interferences. The choice of interference-free wavelength (atomic or ionic line) may be challenging. While there are several possible wavelengths for a given element, wavelengths producing suitable analytical performance, such as limit of quantitation, freedom from interferences, and robustness, are selected.

The first detectors in AES used photographic film. Contemporary AES instruments feature photomultiplier tubes or array-based detector systems.

Atomic Absorption Spectroscopy

Atomic absorption spectroscopy (AAS) is an analytical procedure for the quantitative determination of elements through the absorption of optical radiation by free atoms in the gas phase. The spectra of the atoms are line spectra that are specific for the absorbing elements.

Absorption is governed by the Beer-Lambert law:

$$A = -\log_{10}\left(\frac{I_1}{I_0}\right) \varepsilon L C_g \qquad \text{(Eq. 18-1)}$$

where A is the absorbance of the sample, I_0 is the incident light intensity, I_1 is the transmitted light intensity, ε is the molar absorptivity of the target analyte for the wavelength being used, L is the path length, and C_g is the gas-phase concentration of the target analyte. Under some simplifying assumptions, this equation takes the form

$$A = KC \qquad \text{(Eq. 18-2)}$$

where K is a constant determined by calibration and C is the solution-phase concentration of the analyte.

The simplified principle of the AAS instruments is presented in Figure 18-3.

The four most important components of AA spectrophotometer are as follows:

1. Radiation (light) source, which emits the spectrum of the analyte element.
2. Atomizer, in which the atoms of the element of interest in the sample are formed.
3. Monochromator for the spectral dispersion of the radiation and separation of the analytical line from other radiation.
4. Detector permitting measurement of radiation intensity.

Typical radiation sources for AAS are hollow cathode lamps (HCLs) and electrodeless discharge lamps (EDLs). The HCL contains a quantity of the target element in the form of a hollow cylinder. During operation, a small quantity of the target element is vaporized, and some of the gas-phase atoms of the target element become electronically excited and emit photons with the right wavelength to be absorbed by atoms of the target element in the atomizer. While HCLs are an ideal source for determining most elements by AA, for volatile elements the use of EDLs is recommended.

The most common sources in AAS are FAAS and GFAAS (also called flameless or electrothermal AAS).

The mixing chamber burner, which produces laminar flames of high optical transparency, was already described in the section on AES in this chapter. Copper, iron, and zinc are often measured by FAAS.

The graphite tubes are the most commonly used atomizers in flameless AAS. Tubes are made of high-purity polycrystalline electrographite and coated with pyrolytic graphite and can be heated to a high temperature by an electrical current. A small aliquot (usually 20 µL) of liquid sample is placed in the tube at the ambient temperature. The heating program (specifying the temperatures and times) is designed to first dry the sample, then pyrolyze, vaporize, and atomize the sample, followed by a cleaning step.

Selenium, cadmium, and lead are often measured by GFAAS. GFAAS allows for measurements of both liquid and solid samples. A common problem in GFAAS is that analyte volatility depends on the molecular form of the analyte and the sample matrix. To overcome this limitation, chemical modifiers (palladium nitrate, magnesium nitrate, or a mixture of both) are frequently added to samples, calibrators, and controls.

Inductively Coupled Plasma Mass Spectrometry

ICP-MS is a state-of-the-art analytical technique for elemental analysis. The term *plasma* in ICP refers to an ionized gas (typically argon), in which a certain proportion of electrons are free.

Like other mass spectrometers, the ICP-MS measures the mass-to-charge ratio (molecular mass divided by ionic charge [m/z]) of selected analyte ions) and includes the following components: (1) an ion source, (2) a mass analyzer, and (3) an ion detector. A simplified schematic of an ICP-MS is given in Figure 18-4.

The argon plasma induced by commercial ICP instruments (both ICP-AES and ICP-MS) generates temperatures ranging from 6,000 to 10,000 K and serves several purposes. First, it dries and then vaporizes the droplets produced by the nebulizer. This step is followed by

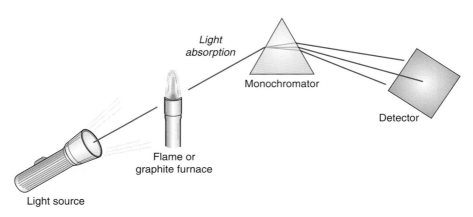

FIGURE 18-3 Simplified schematic of AAS instrumentation.

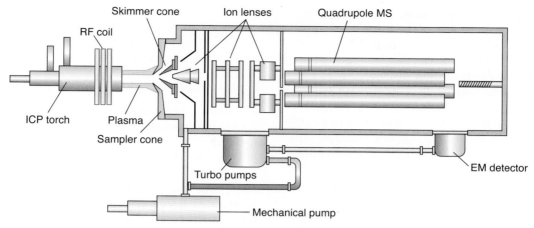

FIGURE 18-4 Simplified schematic of ICP-MS instrumentation. ICP, inductively coupled plasma; RF, radiofrequency; MS, mass spectrometer.

atomization of any molecular species. Finally, atoms are thermally ionized, at which point they are ready for introduction into the mass spectrometer.

Nearly, all ICP torches consist of three concentric quartz tubes surrounded by a coil carrying radiofrequency (RF) power. The middle tube of the torch carries the argon (Ar) that forms the plasma.

Quantitative analysis for clinical samples is best performed with the use of an internal standard. All patient samples, calibrators, and controls are diluted with an internal standard, usually a solution of an uncommon element such as yttrium. Rather than using the raw signal level of the target elements as the basis for quantitation, the signal for each of the target elements is divided by the signal of the internal standard to give signal ratios (i.e., normalized intensities).

Quadrupole Mass Spectrometers

The typical mass spectrometer used for ICP-MS is a quadrupole mass spectrometer. The analyzer consists of four parallel conducting rods arranged in a square array. Applying RF and constant (DC) voltages to the rods, the instrument can be tuned so that only ions of a specific m/z ratio can pass through the device to reach the detector. This type of instrument tends to be relatively simple to use and maintain, but the resolution (the ability to discriminate between closely spaced m/z values) is limited, being able to well resolve peaks separated by one m/z unit but not able to resolve peaks separated by a small fraction of an m/z unit.

High-Resolution Mass Spectrometers

Other ICP-MS instruments incorporate high-resolution mass spectrometers. These are usually "double focusing sector field" instruments. Such instruments separate ions of different m/z values via deflection in a magnetic field, with ions of greater m/z being deflected to a lesser degree than those of lower m/z. The magnetic field is adjusted to allow only ions of a selected m/z to reach the detection system at any given point in time. A second device known as an electrostatic analyzer corrects for certain nonideal effects, allowing the instrument to achieve high resolution. Commercially available high-resolution ICP-MS instruments are capable of a resolution of 10,000 (10% valley). This is enough to resolve, for example $^{75}As^+$ from $^{75}ArCl^+$, both nominally 75 m/z units, but which differ by 1×10^3 units when viewed at high resolution. However, magnetic sector instruments are not able to resolve elemental isobaric interferences such as $^{115}Sn/^{115}In$ and $^{40}Ca/^{40}Ar$, which would require resolution much higher than 10,000.

Interferences

In general, the interferences in elemental analysis are classified as spectroscopic or nonspectroscopic.

Spectroscopic

Spectral interferences generally result from a spectral overlap with the spectrum of the target analyte. For example, in AA certain molecular species may have broad absorption spectra that may overlap the line spectra of the elements of interest, leading to false elevations of the target element concentrations. A much less common occurrence would be for the absorption spectrum of one element to overlap with that of another.

Various strategies are used to deal with spectral interferences in AAS. A continuum source background corrector may be included in the instrument design at the cost of some instrument complication. Another alternative is Zeeman background correction, which relies on shifting the atomic spectral lines by the application of a magnetic field.

In ICP-MS, spectral interferences include polyatomic species whose m/z may overlap m/z of the target analyte. For example, $^{56}(ArO^+)$ has the same nominal m/z as $^{56}Fe^+$.

The argon oxide ion, which can be a significant component of plasma generated by an ICP torch, can potentially interfere with iron analysis by ICP-MS. Another well-known polyatomic interference is argon chloride ion $^{75}(ArCl)^+$ on determination of $^{75}As^+$. An extensive table of polyatomic interferences in ICP-MS has been published.[2]

Several approaches are used to deal with polyatomic interferences in ICP-MS. One applies algebraic equations, together with relative isotopic abundance information, to mathematically correct for interferences.[3] Another approach interposes a reaction cell or collision cell between the main ion lenses and the mass analyzer.[4] A small amount of a gas such as helium or ammonia introduced into the cell removes interferences, either by chemical reaction or by an energy filtering process, using the fact that polyatomic species, with their larger collisional cross sections, lose energy faster than atomic ions. High-resolution mass spectrometers provide a third way to remove interferences as discussed in an earlier section.

A second source of spectral interferences in ICP-MS arises from nearby elements in the periodic table. For example, tin (Sn) and cadmium (Cd) both have isotopes at 114 Da (atomic mass unit), so they could potentially interfere with each other if the instrument is set to measure 114 m/z. This can usually be handled by using a different isotope for the analysis. For example, cadmium also has an isotope at 111 Da that is free from isobaric elemental interferences.

A third source of spectral interferences in ICP-MS comes from doubly charged ions. For example, $^{136}Ba^{2+}$ appears at the same m/z as $^{68}Zn^+$ (136/2 equals 68/1). These are relatively uncommon and can usually be avoided, such as by choosing a different isotope for analysis or tuning the torch to reduce multiply charged ions.

Nonspectroscopic
Matrix interferences involve the bulk physical properties of the sample to be analyzed. The aqueous samples may behave differently than organic and biological specimens, depending upon the technology used and the analyte of interest. The properties of significance are viscosity, presence of easily ionized elements, and presence of carbon. Matrix matching of the calibrators, controls, and specimens helps to overcome matrix interferences. Dilution of the specimens helps minimize matrix effect, but it is only applicable to certain analytical techniques and to the determination of analytes with higher concentrations.

Anything that could interfere with atomization of the sample could be classified as a nonspectral interference. For example, in AA, a flame may not be hot enough for efficient atomization. Difference in sample viscosity between standards and unknown samples, resulting in differing rates of sample introduction, is another example of a nonspectral interference. In AES, anything that would prevent the efficient excitation or emission of spectral lines used for the analysis would constitute a nonspectral interference.

Elemental Speciation

The toxicity of elements may depend on their chemical forms. For example, arsenobetaine is a relatively nontoxic form of arsenic. Methylated forms of arsenic are intermediate in toxicity, and inorganic arsenic, such as As(V) and As(III), are highly toxic. In the medical evaluation of patients, it can be important to know whether an elevated arsenic level is due to relatively innocuous forms, such as arsenobetaine, perhaps from a seafood meal ingested up to 3 days before the specimen collection, or by dangerous forms such as inorganic arsenic. In addition, the concentrations of methylated forms may be useful information for monitoring recovery from toxic exposure. The methodologies for elemental analysis discussed in previous sections are generally not capable of specifying the chemical form of the target elements.

The so-called hyphenated techniques allow for speciation determinations. In a hyphenated analysis, the combination of two or more complementary analytical techniques is used to measure the specific form of an analyte. A classic example of this approach is liquid chromatography-ICP-MS (LC-ICP-MS). The sample is injected into a liquid chromatograph which separates the different chemical forms of the analyte producing a characteristic retention time. Concurrently, the eluting sample is continuously analyzed by a mass spectrometer. The retention time partially identifies the analytes, and the mass spectrometer further identifies the element. In some cases, AA may substitute for MS in elemental speciation schemes. Methods for elemental speciation are becoming more common, especially in Europe. Despite clinical matrices being among the most difficult for speciation, several applications are reported; some among them are as follows:

Arsenic speciation in urine by LC-ICP-MS and HG-GFAAS

Copper in urine by size exclusion chromatography (SEC)-ICP-MS

Copper in red blood cells (RBCs) by SEC-ICP-MS

Lead in blood by gas chromatography (GC)-GFAAS

Selenium in serum by SEC-GFAAS

Zinc in urine by anion exchange chromatography ICP-MS

Alternative Analytical Techniques

Voltammetric methods, such as anodic stripping voltammetry (ASV) and adsorptive stripping voltammetry, can be used in determination of selected metals and are the basis for some point-of-care devices.[5] Ion chromatography can be used for the determination of copper, iron, and zinc in blood, serum, and plasma and for the determination of zinc in urine.

Gas chromatography–mass spectrometry (GC-MS) is capable of determination of cadmium, chromium, cobalt, copper, lead, and selenium in urine, copper in serum, and lead in blood.

The methods accommodating direct analysis of solid samples, for instance, laser ablation ICP-MS (LA-ICP-MS), are gaining recognition for selected clinical applications.

ALUMINUM

Introduction

Aluminum (Al) is a crystalline silver-white ductile metal. Aluminum is the most abundant metal in the earth's crust (~8%). It is always found combined with other elements such as oxygen, silicon, and fluorine. Aluminum as the metal is obtained from aluminum-containing minerals.

Due to its good conductivity of heat and electricity, ease of welding, tensile strength, light weight, and corrosion-resistant oxide coat, aluminum is applicable to a wide variety of industrial and household uses. Aluminum is used for beverage cans, pots and pans, airplanes, siding and roofing, and foil. Aluminum is often mixed with small amounts of other metals to form aluminum alloys, which are stronger and harder than aluminum alone.

Aluminum compounds have many different uses, for example, as alums in water treatment and alumina in abrasives and furnace linings. They are also found in consumer products such as antacids, astringents, buffered aspirin, food additives, cosmetics, and antiperspirants.

Absorption, Transport, and Excretion

The average adult in the United States ingests about 7 to 9 mg aluminum per day in their food.[6] The human organism can absorb aluminum and its compounds orally, by inhaling, and parenterally. There is no indication of dermal absorption. Approximately 1.5% to 2% of inhaled and 0.01% to 5% of ingested aluminum is absorbed. The absorption efficiency is dependent on chemical form, particle size (inhalation), and concurrent dietary exposure to chelators such as citric acid or lactic acid.[6,7]

After a relatively quick uptake of aluminum into the intestinal walls, its passage into the blood is much slower. In plasma, aluminum is bound to carrier proteins such as transferrin.[8] Aluminum binds to various ligands in the blood and distributes to every organ, with highest concentrations ultimately found in bone (~50% of the body burden) and lung tissues (~25% of the body burden). Aluminum levels in lungs increase with age.[6]

Urine accounts for 95% of aluminum excretion with 2% eliminated in the bile.

Health Effects and Toxicity

The mechanism by which aluminum applies its toxicity is not well understood, though aluminum has been shown to interfere with a variety of enzymatic processes,[9] and administration of aluminum to experimental animals is known to produce encephalopathy similar to that seen in Alzheimer disease in man.[10] Although aluminum-containing over-the-counter oral products are considered safe in healthy individuals at recommended doses, some adverse effects have been observed following long-term use in some individuals. Workers who breathe large amounts of aluminum dusts can have lung problems, such as coughing or changes that show up in chest X-rays.

Signs and symptoms of aluminum toxicity include encephalopathy (stuttering, gait disturbance, myoclonic jerks, seizures, coma, and abnormal EEG); osteomalacia or aplastic bone disease (painful spontaneous fractures, hypercalcemia, and tumorous calcinosis); proximal myopathy; increased risk of infection; microcytic anemia; and increased left ventricular mass and decreased myocardial function.[7]

Aluminum toxicity occurs in people with renal insufficiencies who are treated by dialysis with aluminum-contaminated solutions or oral agents that contain aluminum. The clinical manifestations of aluminum toxicity include anemia, bone disease, and progressive dementia with increased concentrations of aluminum in the brain. Prolonged intravenous feeding of preterm infants with solutions containing aluminum is associated with impaired neurologic development.

Laboratory Evaluation

Aluminum is primarily measured using ICP-MS or GFAAS. Accurate measurements are often complicated by the increased risk of environmental contamination of specimens. Urine and serum levels are useful in determining toxic exposures, monitoring exposure over time, and monitoring chelation therapy.[11]

ARSENIC

Introduction

Arsenic (As) is a ubiquitous element displaying both metallic and non-metallic properties. Its content in the earth's crust is estimated at 1.5 to 2.0 mg/kg. For most people, food is the largest source of arsenic exposure (about 25 to 50 µg/d), with lower amounts coming from drinking water and air.[12] Anthropogenic sources of arsenic (production of metals, burning of coil, fossil fuels, timber and its use in agriculture) release three times more of arsenic than natural sources. The main current use of arsenic is as a wood preservative. Other current and past uses of arsenic include pesticides, pigments, poison gases, ammunition manufacturing, semiconductor processing, and medicines.[13]

Health Effects and Toxicity

The relation of clinical signs and symptoms to arsenic exposure depends on the duration and extent of the exposure to inorganic and methylated species of arsenic, as well as the underlying clinical status of the patient. For acute arsenic exposure, the symptoms may include gastrointestinal (nausea, emesis, abdominal pain, and rice water diarrhea), bone marrow (pancytopenia, anemia, and basophilic stippling), cardiovascular (ECG changes), central nervous system (encephalopathy and polyneuropathy), renal (renal insufficiency and renal failure), and hepatic (hepatitis) systems. For chronic arsenic exposure, systems and symptoms may include dermatologic (Mees' lines, hyperkeratosis, hyperpigmentation, and alopecia), hepatic (cirrhosis and hepatomegaly), cardiovascular (hypertension and peripheral vascular disease [PVD]), central nervous system ("socks and glove" neuropathy and tremor), and malignancies (squamous cell, hepatocellular, skin, bladder, lung, and renal carcinomas). Chronic arsenic exposure has been shown to cause blackfoot disease, a severe form of PVD which leads to gangrenous changes.

The white powder of arsenic trioxide is odorless, tasteless, and one of the most common poisons in human history. Doses of 0.01 to 0.05 g produce toxic symptoms. The lethal dose is reported to be between 0.12 and 0.3 g; however, recoveries from higher doses have been reported.[13] Immediate treatment of expected exposure consists of lavage and use of activated charcoal to reduce arsenic absorption. The most effective antidotes for arsenic poisoning are the following chelating agents: dimercaprol (a.k.a British anti-Lewisite), penicillamine, and succimer.[14]

In 2000, the US FDA approved the use of arsenic trioxide for the treatment of acute promyelocytic leukemia,[15] which is diagnosed in approximately 1,500 people in the United States every year.

Absorption, Transport, and Excretion of Arsenic

The main routes of exposure are ingestion of arsenic-containing foods, water, and beverages or inhalation of contaminated air; however, arsenic toxicity is a complex topic. Organic forms of arsenic such as arsenocholine and arsenobetaine are commonly found in fish and seafood, are considered relatively non-toxic, and are cleared rapidly (1 to 2 d).[16] Inorganic species of arsenic are highly toxic and occur naturally in rocks, soil, and

CASE STUDY 18-1

An 11-year-old child visiting family in Seattle was suspected of ingesting an unknown quantity of ant killer thought to contain arsenic trioxide. The initial total arsenic urine level was found to be 340 µg/L shortly after presentation to the emergency department. Reflexive arsenic speciation indicated <10 µg/L As, total inorganic, <10 µg/L As, total methylated, and 320 µg/L of As, organic.

Questions

1. Discuss the metabolism of arsenic after inorganic arsenic ingestion.

2. What is a likely cause of the elevated total arsenic result?

3. Would blood arsenic levels have helped in the diagnosis?

groundwater. They are also found in many synthetic products, poisons, and industrial processes. Methylated species are intermediate in toxicity and arise primarily from metabolism of inorganic species, but small amounts may arise directly from food. Organic methylated arsenic compounds such as monomethylarsonic acid (MMA) and dimethylarsenic acid (DMA) are formed by hepatic metabolism of $As(3^+)$ and $As(5^+)$. The methylated inorganic forms are considered less toxic than $As(3^+)$ and $As(5^+)$; however, they are eliminated slowly (1 to 3 wk). The Biological Exposure Index established by the American Conference of Governmental Industrial Hygienists for the sum of inorganic and methylated metabolites of arsenic in urine is 35 µg/L. However, clinical symptoms may not be evident at 35 µg/L.[14]

Laboratory Evaluation

Arsenic is primarily measured using ICP-MS, GFAAS, or HG-AAS. In most cases, arsenic is best detected by urine due to the short half-life of arsenic in blood. When arsenic speciation is desired (typically following a high total urine arsenic value reported by ICP-MS or AA), a separation method is employed either online or off-line prior to elemental analysis.

CADMIUM

Introduction

Cadmium (Cd) is a soft, bluish-white metal, which is easily cut with a knife. Principal industrial uses of cadmium include manufacture of pigments and batteries, as well as in the metal-plating and plastics industries. In the United States, the burning of fossil fuels such as coal and oil and the incineration of municipal waste materials constitute the largest sources of airborne cadmium exposure, along with zinc, lead, and copper smelters in some locations. Cadmium-containing waste products and soil contamination, primarily as a result of human activity, are becoming of concern, and the US Environmental Protection Agency (EPA) has established loading rates of 20 kg/ha for high cation exchange capacity soils with a pH of 6.5 and a lower rate of 5 kg/ha for acid soils.[17]

Absorption, Transport, and Excretion

Based on renal function (development of proteinuria), the reference dose for cadmium in drinking water is 0.0005 mg/kg/d and the dose for dietary exposure to cadmium is 0.001 mg/kg/d.[18] Absorption of cadmium is higher in females than in males due to differences in iron stores. The absorption of inhaled cadmium in air is 10% to 50% with gastrointestinal absorption of cadmium estimated to be 5%. The absorption of cadmium in cigarette smoke is 10% to 50% and smokers of tobacco products have about twice the cadmium abundance in their bodies as nonsmokers. For nonsmokers, the primary exposure to cadmium is through ingested food.[19] About 90% of ingested cadmium is excreted in the feces due to the low absorbance of cadmium from the gut.[20]

Health Effects and Toxicity

Cadmium has no known role in normal human physiology. Toxicity is believed to be a result of protein-Cd adducts causing denaturation of the associated proteins, resulting in a loss of function.[20] Ingestion of high amounts of cadmium may lead to a rapid onset with severe nausea, vomiting, and abdominal pain.[20] Renal dysfunction is a common presentation for chronic cadmium exposure, often resulting in slow-onset proteinuria. Acute effects of inhalation of fumes containing cadmium include respiratory distress due to chemical pneumonitis and edema and can cause death. Breathing of cadmium vapors can also result in nasal epithelial damage and lung damage similar to emphysema.[20] Cadmium exposure can affect the liver, bone, immune, blood, and nervous systems.[19,21]

EDTA (ethylenediaminetetraacetic acid) can be used as a chelating agent in cadmium poisoning.

Laboratory Evaluation

Cadmium is usually quantified by GFAAS and ICP-MS; ICP-AES is also used. In blood, cadmium is found mostly (70%) in the RBCs. Cadmium in blood reflects the average uptake during the past few months and can be used for monitoring purposes but does not accurately reflect a recent exposure. Urinary excretion is about 0.001% and 0.01% of the body burden per 24 hours. At low exposure, urine cadmium reflects the total accumulation.[22]

CHROMIUM

Introduction

Chromium (Cr), from the Greek word *chroma* ("color"), makes rubies red and emeralds green. Chromium is the 21st most abundant element in the earth's crust and is used in the manufacturing of stainless steel. Occupational exposure to chromium occurs in wood treatment, stainless steel welding, chrome plating, the leather tanning industry, and the use of lead chromate or strontium chromate paints. Chromium exists in two main valency states: trivalent and hexavalent.

Absorption, Transport, and Excretion

$Cr(6^+)$ is better absorbed and much more toxic than $Cr(3^+)$.[22] Both transferrin and albumin are involved in chromium absorption and transport.[23] Transferrin binds the newly absorbed chromium at site B, while albumin acts as an acceptor and transporter of chromium if the transferrin sites are saturated.[24] Other plasma proteins, including β- and γ-globulins and lipoproteins, bind chromium.

Health Effects, Deficiency, and Toxicity

$Cr(3^+)$ is an essential dietary element and plays a role in maintaining normal metabolism of glucose, fat, and cholesterol. The estimated safe and adequate daily intake of chromium for adults is in the range of 50 to 200 μg/d, although data are insufficient to establish a recommended daily allowance.[25]

Dietary chromium deficiency is relatively uncommon and most cases occur in persons with specific clinical situations such as total parenteral nutrition, diabetes, and malnutrition. Chromium deficiency is characterized by glucose intolerance, glycosuria, hypercholesterolemia, decreased longevity, decreased sperm counts, and impaired fertility.[25]

$Cr(6^+)$ compounds are powerful oxidizing agents and are more toxic systemically than $Cr(3^+)$ compounds, given similar amounts and solubilities. At physiological pH, $Cr(6^+)$ forms $CrO4^{2-}$ and readily passes through cell membranes due to its similarity to essential phosphate and sulfate oxyanions. Intracellularly, $Cr(6^+)$ is reduced to reactive intermediates, producing free radicals and oxidizing deoxyribonucleic acid (DNA), both potentially inducing cell death.[26] Severe dermatitis and skin ulcers can result from contact with $Cr(6^+)$ salts. Up to 20% of chromium workers develop contact dermatitis. Allergic dermatitis with eczema has been reported in printers, cement workers, metal workers, painters, and leather tanners. Data suggest that a $Cr(3^+)$–protein complex is responsible for the allergic reaction.[25]

When inhaled, $Cr(6^+)$ is a respiratory tract irritant, resulting in airway irritation, airway obstruction, and possibly lung cancer. The target organ of inhaled chromium is the lung; the kidneys, liver, skin, and immune system may also be affected.

Low-dose, chronic chromium exposure typically results only in transient renal effects. Elevated urinary β2-microglobulin levels (an indicator of renal tubular damage) have been found in chrome platers, and higher levels have generally been observed in younger persons exposed to higher $Cr(6^+)$ concentrations.[25]

In May 2011, the FDA issued orders for postmarket surveillance studies to manufacturers of metal-on-metal (MoM) hip replacement systems in response to an increasing concern over failed implant devices reported in Europe.[27] In the United States, no guidelines have been established for the assessment of metal ions in asymptomatic patients due to a lack of knowledge regarding the prevalence of adverse events in the US population and no clear threshold levels associated with an adverse event.

Laboratory Evaluation

Chromium may be determined by GFAAS, NAA, or ICP-MS. Plasma, serum, and urine do not indicate the total body status of the individual, whereas urine levels may be useful for metabolic studies.[23] In the setting of suspected failure of MoM hip implants that use a cobalt–chrome alloy femoral head, serum is the preferred specimen type for both chromium and cobalt analysis.[28]

COPPER

Introduction

Copper (Cu) is a relatively soft yet tough metal with excellent electrical and heat conducting properties. Copper is widely distributed in nature both in its elemental form and in compounds. Copper forms alloys with zinc (brass), tin (bronze), and nickel (cupronickel, widely used in coins). Copper is an essential trace element found in four oxidation states, $Cu(0)$, $Cu(1^+)$, $Cu(2^+)$, and $Cu(3^+)$, with $Cu(2^+)$ the most stable of all oxidation states.[29] Copper is an important cofactor for several metalloenzymes and is critical for the reduction of iron in heme synthesis.

Absorption, Transport, and Excretion

The copper content in the normal human adult is 50 to 120 mg. Copper is distributed through the body with the highest concentrations found in liver, brain, heart, and kidneys. Hepatic copper accounts for about 10% of the total copper in the body.[30] Copper is also found in the cornea, spleen,

intestine, and lung. The amount of copper absorbed from the intestine is 50% to 80% of ingested copper.[25] The average daily intake is approximately 10 mg or more of copper.[30] The exact mechanisms by which copper is absorbed and transported by the intestine are unknown, but an active transport mechanism at low concentrations and passive diffusion at high concentrations have been proposed. Copper is transported to the liver and bounds to albumin, transcuprein, and low-molecular-weight components in the portal system. In the liver, copper is incorporated into ceruloplasmin for distribution throughout the body.[29] Ceruloplasmin is an α2-globulin, and each 132,000 Da molecular weight molecule contains six atoms of copper.[30]

In a normal physiological state, 98% of copper excretion is through the bile, with copper losses in the urine and sweat comprising approximately 2% of dietary intake.[25] Menstrual losses of copper are minor.

Health Effects, Deficiency, and Toxicity

Copper is a component of several metalloenzymes, including ceruloplasmin, cytochrome C oxidase, superoxide dismutase, tyrosinase, metallothionein, dopamine hydroxylase, lysyl oxidase, clotting factor V, and an unknown enzyme that cross-links keratin in hair.

Copper deficiency is observed in premature infants and copper absorption is impaired in severe diffuse diseases of small bowel, lymphosarcoma, and scleroderma.[30] Copper deficiency is related to malnutrition, malabsorption, chronic diarrhea, hyperalimentation, and prolonged feeding with low copper, total-milk diets. Signs of copper deficiency include (1) neutropenia and hypochromic anemia in the early stages, (2) osteoporosis and various bone and joint abnormalities that reflect deficient copper-dependent cross-linking of bone collagen and connective tissue, (3) decreased pigmentation of the skin and general pallor, and (4), in the later stages, possible neurologic abnormalities (hypotonia, apnea, and psychomotor retardation).[25]

Subclinical copper depletion contributes to an increased risk of coronary heart disease. An extreme form of copper deficiency is seen in Menkes disease, with symptoms usually appear at the age of 3 months and death usually occurring by the age of 5. This invariably fatal, progressive brain disease is characterized by peculiar hair, called kinky or steely, and retardation of growth. Clinical signs include progressive mental deterioration, coarse feces, disturbance of muscle tone, seizures, and episodes of severe hypothermia.

Copper toxicity has been associated with living near copper-producing facilities, using water from copper pipes or cooking with copper-lined vessels or exposure to algaecides, herbicides, pyrotechnics, ceramic glazes, electrical wiring, or welding supplies. Because of its redox potential, copper is an irritant to epithelia and mucous membranes and can cause hepatic and renal damage with hemolysis.[31] Copper-induced emesis has a characteristic blue-green color.

Wilson's disease is a genetically determined copper accumulation disease that usually presents between the ages of 6 and 40 years. Clinical findings include neurologic disorders, liver dysfunction, and Kayser-Fleischer rings (green-brown discoloration) in the cornea caused by copper deposition. Early diagnosis of Wilson's disease is important because complications can be effectively prevented and in some cases the disease can be halted with the use of zinc acetate or chelation therapy.[25] Serum ceruloplasmin levels and the direct measurement of free copper are key diagnostic steps in the diagnosis of Wilson's disease.[32]

Laboratory Evaluation

Copper is measured by flame AAS, ICP-MS, ICP-AES, and ASV. Serum copper and urine copper are used to monitor for nutritional adequacy and subacute management of copper toxicity. Direct measurement of free copper and ceruloplasmin in serum is used to screen for Wilson's disease. Common trends in laboratory testing seen in various diseases states are summarized in Table 18-2.

IRON

Introduction

Iron (Fe) is the fourth most abundant element in the earth's crust and the most abundant transition metal. Methods of extracting iron from ore have been known for centuries. The physical properties of iron alloys can be varied over an enormous range by appropriate alloying and heat treating methods, giving a range of strength, hardness, toughness, corrosion resistance (in the form of stainless steels), and magnetic properties and ability to take and hold a sharp edge.

Although highly abundant in the earth's crust, iron is classified as a trace element in the body. Iron ions are able to participate in redox chemistry in both the ferrous [Fe^{2+}] and ferric [Fe^{3+}] states, allowing iron to fill numerous biochemical roles as a carrier of other biochemically active substances (e.g., oxygen) and as an agent in redox and electron transfer reactions (e.g., via various cytochromes). Iron's high activity is a double-edged sword, and free iron ions in the body also participate in destructive chemistry, primarily in catalyzing the formation of toxic free radicals. As a result, very little free iron is normally found in the body.

Absorption, Transport, and Excretion

Absorption of iron from the intestine is the primary means of regulating the amount of iron within the body. Typically, only about 10% of the 1 g/d of dietary iron is absorbed. To be absorbed by intestinal cells, iron must be in the ferrous oxidation state and bound to protein. Because Fe^{3+} is the predominant form of iron in foods, it must first be reduced to Fe^{2+} by agents such as vitamin C or ferric reductases present in the intestinal epithelium before it can be absorbed. In the intestinal mucosal cell, Fe^{2+} can be bound by ferritin for storage and eliminated after sloughing off or be exported to the basolateral side. From there, iron is oxidized to Fe^{3+} and bound by apotransferrin for transport throughout the body. The peptide hormone hepcidin regulates iron absorption in the upper gastrointestinal tract by modulating the export of iron from cells by ferroportin.[33] After about 120 days in circulation, red cells are degraded by the spleen, liver, and macrophages, which return Fe to the circulation for reuse. Absorption and transport capacity can be increased in conditions such as iron deficiency, anemia, or hypoxia. Iron is lost primarily by desquamation and red cell loss to urine and feces. With each menstrual cycle, women lose approximately 20 to 40 mg of iron.

Health Effects, Deficiency, and Toxicity

Of the 3 to 5 g of iron in the body, approximately 2 to 2.5 g of iron is in hemoglobin, mostly in RBCs and red cell precursors. A moderate amount of iron (~130 mg) is

TABLE 18-2	INTERPRETATION OF COPPER TESTING RESULTS[7]	
	SERUM COPPER	**URINE COPPER**
Nutritional deficiency	↓	↓
Menkes syndrome	↓	↑
Acute copper toxicity	↑ or ↑↑	↑
Chronic copper toxicity	↑	↑
Wilson's disease	N or ↓	↑ or ↑↑
Smoking, inflammatory conditions	↑ or ↑↑	N
Estrogen, pregnancy	↑ or ↑↑	N

N, normal; ↓, decreased; ↑, increased; ↑↑, Significantly increased.

in myoglobin, the oxygen-carrying protein of muscle. A small (8 mg) but extremely important pool is bound in tissue to enzymes that require iron for full activity. These include peroxidases, cytochromes, and many of the Krebs cycle enzymes. Iron is also stored as ferritin and hemosiderin, primarily in the bone marrow, spleen, and liver. Only 3 to 5 mg of iron is found in plasma, almost all of it associated with transferrin, albumin, and free hemoglobin.[34]

Iron deficiency affects about 15% of the worldwide population. Those with a higher than average risk of iron deficiency anemia include pregnant women, young children, adolescents, and women of reproductive age.[35] Increased blood loss, decreased dietary iron intake, or decreased release from ferritin may result in iron deficiency. Reduction in iron stores usually precedes both a reduction in circulating iron and anemia, as demonstrated by a decreased RBC count, mean corpuscular hemoglobin concentration, and microcytic RBCs.

Iron overload states are collectively referred to as hemochromatosis, whether or not tissue damage is present. Primary Fe overload is most frequently associated with hereditary hemochromatosis (HH). HH is a single-gene homozygous recessive disorder leading to abnormally high Fe absorption, culminating in Fe overload. HH causes tissue accumulation of iron, affects liver function, and often leads to hyperpigmentation of the skin. Some conditions associated with severe hemochromatosis include diabetes mellitus, arthritis, cardiac arrhythmia or failure, cirrhosis, hypothyroidism, impotence, and liver cancer. Treatment may include therapeutic phlebotomy or administration of *chelators*, such as deferoxamine. Transferrin can be administered in the case of atransferrinemia.[33]

Secondary Fe overload may result from excessive dietary, medicinal, or transfusional Fe intake or due to metabolic dysfunction. Hemosiderosis has been used to specifically designate a condition of iron overload as demonstrated by an increased serum iron and total iron-binding capacity (TIBC) or transferrin, in the absence of demonstrable tissue damage.

Iron may play a role as a *prooxidant*, contributing to lipid peroxidation,[36,37] atherosclerosis,[37,38] DNA damage,[36–38] carcinogenesis,[39,40] and neurodegenerative diseases.[41,42] Fe(3+), released from binding proteins, can enhance the production of free radicals to cause oxidative damage. In iron-loaded individuals with thalassemia who are treated with chelators to bind and mobilize iron, intake of ascorbic acid may actually promote the generation of free radicals.[43]

Laboratory Evaluation

Disorders of iron metabolism are evaluated primarily by packed cell volume, hemoglobin, red cell count and indices, total iron and TIBC, percent saturation, transferrin, and ferritin.[44] Common trends in laboratory testing seen in various disease states are summarized in Table 18-3.

Total Iron Content (Serum Iron)
Measurement of serum iron concentration refers specifically to the $Fe(3^+)$ bound to transferrin and not to the iron circulating as free hemoglobin in serum. The specimen may be collected as serum without anticoagulant or as plasma with heparin. Oxalate, citrate, and EDTA bind Fe ions and all are unacceptable anticoagulants. Early morning sampling is preferred because of the diurnal variation in iron concentration. Specimens with visible hemolysis should be rejected.

Total Iron-Binding Capacity
TIBC refers to the theoretical amount of iron that could be bound if transferrin and other minor iron-binding proteins present in the serum or plasma sample were saturated. Typically, only one-third of the iron-binding sites on transferrin are saturated.

Percent Saturation
The percent saturation, also called the transferrin saturation, is the ratio of serum iron to TIBC. The normal range for this is approximately 20% to 50%, but it varies with age and sex.

TABLE 18-3	LABORATORY MARKERS OF IRON STATUS IN SEVERAL DISEASE STATES[7]				
CONDITION	**SERUM IRON**	**TRANSFERRIN**	**FERRITIN**	**PERCENT SATURATION**	**TIBC**
Iron deficiency	↓	↑	↓	↓	↑
Iron overdose	↑	↓	↑	↑	↓
Hemochromatosis	↑	Slightly ↓	↑	↑	↓
Malnutrition	↓	↓	↓	Variable	↓
Chronic infection	↓	↓	↑	↓	↓
Acute liver disease	↑	Variable	↑	↑	Variable
Chronic anemia	↓	N or ↓	N or ↑	↓	N or ↓

N, normal; ↑, decreased; ↓, increased.

Transferrin and Ferritin

Transferrin is measured by immunochemical methods such as nephelometry. Transferrin is increased in iron deficiency and decreased in iron overload and hemochromatosis. Transferrin may also be decreased in chronic infections and malignancies.

Ferritin is measured in serum by various immunochemical methods. Ferritin is decreased in iron deficiency anemia and increased in iron overload and hemochromatosis. Ferritin is often increased in several other conditions, including chronic infections, malignancy, and viral hepatitis.

A liver biopsy sample can be digested and analyzed for iron by AAS or ICP-MS as a follow-up to abnormal blood tests consistent with an HH diagnosis.[45] Iron quantification in liver is not used for the evaluation of acute iron toxicity. Hepcidin testing has not yet been shown to be clinically useful.

CASE STUDY 18-2

A 42-year-old woman with a history of diabetes was seen by her physician for weight loss, anorexia, and general fatigue. As part of the physical examination, both "bronze" skin pigmentation and an enlarged liver were noted. Her initial chemistry panel showed the following relevant results (reference intervals provided in parentheses):

Albumin	3.7 g/dL (3.8–5.0)
AST	180 U/L (14–50)
ALT	200 U/L (10–60)
Total bilirubin	2.5 mg/dL (0.2–1.2)
Serum iron	180 µg/dL (45–150)

Further testing for the elevated iron showed the following:

Serum iron	170 µg/dL (45–150)
Transferrin	210 mg/dL (200–380)
Ferritin	300 µg/L (10–250)
% Transferrin saturation	80 (20–50)

Genetic testing confirmed the patient had an *HFE 3* mutation and was diagnosed with HH.

Questions

1. Are the test results consistent with iron deficiency or toxicity?

2. Are this patient's conditions and symptoms typical of hemochromatosis?

3. What is a treatment plan for iron overload and what is the main goal?

LEAD

Introduction

Metallic lead (Pb) is soft, bluish white, highly malleable, and ductile. It is a poor conductor of electricity and heat and is resistant to corrosion. Lead is widely distributed in the earth's crust and the main lead ores are galena, cerrusite, and anglesite.[46] Lead is used in the production of storage batteries, ammunition, solder, and foils. Tetraethyl lead was once used extensively as an additive in gasoline (petrol) for its ability to increase the fuel's octane rating and is present in many paints manufactured before 1970. The manufacture of lead-based household paints was banned in the United States in 1972 but is still used in paints intended for nondomestic use. Toxic concentrations of lead can be found in areas adjacent to homes painted with lead-based paints and around highways where it has accumulated from the past use of leaded gasoline. In recent years, there have been massive recalls of toys and costume jewelry produced in China, due to concerns over elevated lead content. Lead plays no known role in normal human physiology.

Absorption, Transport, and Excretion

Exposure to lead is primarily respiratory or gastrointestinal. Inhalation results in 30% to 40% of absorption efficiency. Gut absorption depends on a variety of factors, including age and nutritional status, with enhanced gastrointestinal absorption occurring in children younger than 6 years of age. Certain substances, such as iron, calcium, magnesium, alcohol, and fat, may weaken lead absorption while low dietary zinc, ascorbic acid, and citric acid can enhance the absorption of lead.[46] About 99% of absorbed lead is taken up by erythrocytes where it interferes with heme synthesis. Lead distributes to soft tissues, such as liver, kidneys, and brain, with the skeletal lead concentrations containing greater than 90% of the body burden of lead.[47] Absorbed lead is excreted primarily in urine (76%) and feces (16%), and the remaining 8% is excreted in hair, sweat, nails, and others.[46]

Health Effects and Toxicity

The clinical presentation of lead toxicity is variable. In children, obvious symptoms are usually seen at blood levels of 60 µg/dL or higher with 45 µg/dL as the typical threshold for acute, clinical intervention. IQ declines are seen in children with blood lead levels (BLLs) of 10 µg/dL or higher. Other central nervous system symptoms of lead toxicity in children may include clumsiness, gait abnormalities, headache, behavioral changes, seizures, and severe cognitive and behavioral problems. Gastrointestinal symptoms include abdominal pain, constipation, and colic. Other conditions may include acute nephropathy and anemia. The US Centers for Disease

Control and Prevention (CDC) estimates an incidence of more than 450,000 for children with BLLs higher than 10 µg/dL. In adults, the following symptoms may be observed: peripheral neuropathies, motor weakness, chronic renal insufficiency and systolic hypertension, and anemia.

Lead exposure primarily arises in two settings: childhood exposure, usually through paint chips, and adult occupational exposure in the smelting, mining, ammunitions, soldering, plumbing, ceramic glazing, and construction industries. Other sources include lead-glazed ceramics and certain Asian herbal remedies. The US government web sites contain extensive information on the health and environmental impacts of lead.[48]

Laboratory Evaluation

The most common specimen type is whole venous blood, the result of which is commonly referred to as the BLL. This is preferred over plasma and serum as circulating lead is predominantly associated with RBCs. Elevated lead levels in capillary blood specimens should be confirmed with a venous specimen to avoid the potential contribution of external contamination.

Urine lead may be useful for detecting recent exposures to lead or to monitor chelation therapy. Other testing, such as plasma aminolevulinic acid, whole blood zinc protoporphyrin, and free erythrocyte protoporphyrins, may be useful for screening in occupational exposures. Noninvasive measurements of lead in bone may be available radiographically. Removal of further lead exposure and parental education are essential parts to the management for patients with elevated BLLs.[31]

ICP-MS is a preferred method of analysis, although ICP-AES and GFAAS are also used.

CASE STUDY 18-3

An asymptomatic 1-year-old African-American male had a BLL of 39 µg/dL during a follow-up visit scheduled after a 44 µg/dL routine capillary blood test 5 days prior. The child shows no signs of developmental delay and has been staying with relatives since the initial BLL result.

Questions

1. What is a common source of lead exposure for children?

2. Discuss the various methods for chelation after toxic lead exposure.

3. Is chelation therapy indicated in this case?

MERCURY

Introduction

Mercury (Hg), also called quicksilver, is a heavy, silvery metal. Along with bromine, mercury is one of only two elements that are liquid at room temperature and pressure. There are three naturally occurring oxidation states of mercury: Hg(0), Hg(1$^+$), and Hg(2$^+$). Organic mercury refers to various forms of mercury bound to a carbon atom, with mercury usually in the +2 oxidation state.

Mercury is released to the atmosphere as a product of the natural degassing of rock (30,000 tons/yr) and through various human activities (20,000 tons/yr). Mercury is used in dental amalgams, electronic switches, germicides, fungicides, and fluorescent light bulbs.[49] The use of mercury in medicine has greatly declined in all respects; however, mercury compounds are found in some over-the-counter drugs, including topical antiseptics, stimulant laxatives, diaper-rash ointment, eye drops, and nasal sprays. Mercury is widely used in the production of eye cosmetics, especially mascara.

Absorption, Transport, and Excretion

Routes of exposure include (1) inhalation, primarily as elemental mercury vapor but occasionally as dimethyl mercury; (2) ingestion of $HgCl_2$ and mercury-containing foods such as predatory fish species; (3) cutaneous absorption of methyl mercury (MeHg) through the skin and even through latex gloves; (4) injection of relatively inert liquid mercury and mercury-containing tattoo pigments; and (5) dental amalgams. Inhaled mercury vapor is retained in the lungs to about 80%, whereas liquid metallic mercury passes through the gastrointestinal tract largely unabsorbed.[50]

Mercury enters the food chain primarily by volcanic activity and manmade sources such as coal combustion and smelting. Most of the dietary intake comes from consumption of meat and fish products, with estimates of dietary intake varying based upon geographical location and dietary sources.[49] The kidney is the major storage organ after elemental or inorganic mercury exposure. MeHg is efficiently absorbed from the gastrointestinal tract, and distribution to tissues, including the brain, appears complete in 48 hours. Movement of MeHg across the blood–brain barrier appears to be dependent on coupling with the amino acid cysteine.[51]

There is relatively little bioaccumulation of inorganic and elemental mercury. Half-lives vary according to the route of exposure and form of mercury, from 5 days in blood for phenylmercury to 90 days in urine for chronic exposure to inorganic mercury. Normally, the highest accumulation of mercury is in the kidney, liver, spleen, and brain. Mercury can accumulate in pituitary and thyroid glands, the pancreas, and the reproductive organs.

The bulk of mercury accumulated in the body is eliminated in approximately 60 days; however, organic forms of mercury can accumulate in brain and may take up to several years to be eliminated.

Fecal and urinary excretions are the main elimination routes for inorganic and organic mercury. A special form of elimination is the transfer of mercury from the fetus through the placenta.

Health Effects and Toxicity

Mercury has no known function in normal human physiology. Toxicities have been observed following inhalation, ingestion, and dermal absorption of mercury compounds. Mercurial salts were historically used as diuretics, topical disinfectants, and laxatives before mercury toxicity was well understood. Since the 1930s, some vaccines contained the preservative thimerosal, a mercury-containing compound metabolized into ethylmercury. Although it was widely speculated that this mercury-based preservative can cause or trigger autism in children, scientific studies showed no evidence supporting any such link. Nevertheless, thimerosal has been removed from or reduced to trace amounts in all US vaccines recommended for children of 6 years and younger, with the exception of the inactivated influenza vaccine.

Organic mercury and elemental mercury vapor are toxic to both the central and peripheral nervous systems. Mercury attacks the central nervous system well before a victim shows symptoms. Professor Karen Wetterhahn, the founding director of Dartmouth College's Toxic Metals Research Program and an expert in the mechanisms of metal toxicity, died in 1997, at the age of 48, because of a tragic laboratory accident involving the use of dimethylmercury.

Elemental mercury readily vaporizes, and its inhalation can produce harmful effects on the nervous, digestive, and immune systems and the lungs and kidneys. The inorganic salts of mercury can affect the skin, eyes, gastrointestinal tract, and kidneys.

The toxicity of mercury is primarily through reaction with protein sulfhydryl groups (MSH), resulting in dysfunction and inactivation. Liquid elemental mercury is poorly absorbed and relatively nontoxic but elemental mercury vapor is highly absorbed and is highly toxic. Inorganic, ionized forms of mercury are toxic. Further bioconversion to an alkyl mercury, such as MeHg, yields a very toxic species of mercury that is highly selective for lipid-rich mediums such as the brain.[52]

Mercury intoxication can manifest in many signs and symptoms that affect several organ systems, including headache, tremor, impaired coordination, abdominal cramps, diarrhea, dermatitis, polyneuropathy, proteinuria, and hepatic dysfunction.[53] Because many of these are relatively nonspecific signs and symptoms, laboratory testing provides a key role in assessing mercury intoxication.

Laboratory Evaluation

Mercury is usually determined as total mercury levels in blood and urine without regard to chemical form. Analytical methods include ICP-MS and cold vapor AAS.

MANGANESE

Introduction

As the 12th most abundant element in the earth's crust, manganese (Mn) is found in over 250 minerals, of which 15 have commercial importance. Nearly all the elemental manganese is used in the production of the alloy ferromanganese widely used in steel production. Other uses of elemental manganese include a scavenger role in copper and aluminum alloys and in a production of dry cell batteries. Various manganese compounds are widely used in fertilizers, animal feeds, pharmaceutical products, dyes, paint dryers, catalysts, and wood preservatives and in production of glass and ceramics. The manganese-based compound methylcyclopentadienyl manganese tricarbonyl is a fuel supplement used to increase the octane level of gasoline and though banned in 1977 is currently approved for use in the United States.[54]

Absorption, Transport, and Excretion

Roughly, 2% to 15% of dietary manganese is absorbed in the small intestine. Dietary factors that affect manganese absorption include iron, calcium, phosphates, and fiber.[25] Manganese absorption is age dependent, with infants retaining higher levels of manganese than adults do. Manganese is a normal component in tissue with the highest levels found in fat and bone. Though accumulation of manganese in the healthy population has not been observed, chronic liver disease or other types of liver dysfunction can reduce manganese elimination and promote accumulation in various regions of the brain.[54] Manganese elimination occurs predominately through the bile.

Health Effects, Deficiency, and Toxicity

Manganese is biochemically essential as a constituent of metalloenzymes and as an enzyme activator. Manganese-containing enzymes include arginase, pyruvate carboxylase, and manganese superoxide dismutase in the mitochondria. Manganese-activated enzymes include hydrolases, kinases, decarboxylases, and transferases. Many of these activations are not specific to manganese and other metal ions (magnesium, iron, or copper) can replace manganese as an activator and mask the effects of manganese deficiency.[25]

Blood clotting defects, hypocholesterolemia, dermatitis, and elevated serum calcium, phosphorus, and alkaline phosphatase activity have been observed in some subjects who underwent experimental manganese depletion.[25] Low levels of manganese have been associated with epilepsy,[7] hip abnormalities, joint disease, congenital malformation,[25] heart and bone problems, and stunted growth in children.[55]

Manganese toxicity causes nausea, vomiting, headache, disorientation, memory loss, anxiety, and compulsive laughing or crying. Chronic manganese toxicity resembles Parkinson's disease with akinesia, rigidity, tremors, and mask-like faces.[7] A clinical condition named *locura manganica* (manganese madness) was described in Chilean manganese miners with acute manganese aerosol intoxication.[56]

Laboratory Evaluation

Manganese is measured by ICP-MS and GFAAS. Urine manganese is used in conjunction with serum manganese to evaluate possible toxicity or deficiency.

MOLYBDENUM

Introduction

Molybdenum (Mo) is a hard, silvery white metal occurring naturally as molybdenite, wulfenite, and powelite. Most molybdenum is used for the production of alloys, as well as catalysts, corrosion inhibitors, flame retardants, smoke depressants, lubricants, and molybdenum blue pigments. Molybdenum is an essential trace element with the importance of molybdenum-containing organic compounds in biological systems identified over 80 years ago.[57]

Absorption, Transport, and Excretion

Between 25% and 80% of ingested molybdenum is absorbed predominately in the stomach and small intestine,[25] with the majority of absorbed molybdenum retained in the liver, skeleton, and kidney. In blood, molybdenum is extensively bound to α2-macroglobulin and RBC membranes.[57] Molybdenum can cross the placental barrier, and increased intake of molybdenum in the diet of the mother can increase its level in the liver of the neonate.[58]

Health Effects, Deficiency, and Toxicity

Molybdenum is vital to human health through its inclusion in at least three enzymes: xanthine oxidase, aldehyde oxidase, and sulfite oxidase. The active site of these enzymes binds molybdenum in the form of a cofactor "molybdopterin."[7]

Dietary molybdenum deficiency is rare with a single case reported because of total parenteral nutrition in a man with Crohn's disease.[57] Molybdenum cofactor deficiency is a recessively inherited error of metabolism due to a lack of functional molybdopterin. The symptoms include seizures, anterior lens dislocation, decreased brain weight, and usually death prior to 1 year of age.[7]

Molybdenum toxicity is rarely reported, as there are few known cases of human exposure to excess molybdenum. High dietary and occupational exposures to molybdenum have been linked to elevated uric acid in blood and an increased incidence of gout.[25]

Molybdenum is rapidly eliminated in both urine and bile, with urine excretion predominating when intake is high.[57]

Laboratory Evaluation

Molybdenum levels are measured by ICP-MS and GFAAS. Blood levels are less than 60 μg/L.[57]

SELENIUM

Introduction

Selenium (Se) is a naturally occurring metalloid with many chemical and physical properties similar to those of sulfur. Selenium is an essential trace element and a major constituent of 40 minerals and a minor constituent of 37 others.[59] Most processed selenium is used in the electronics industry; however, other uses include nutritional supplements, pigments, pesticides, rubber production, anti-dandruff shampoos, and fungicides.

Absorption, Transport, and Excretion

Selenium is well absorbed from the gastrointestinal tract (~50%). Selenium exposure occurs primarily from food but can be found in drinking water, usually in the form of inorganic sodium selenate or sodium selenite. Selenium homeostasis is largely achieved by excretion via urine and feces. Other routes of elimination include sweat and, at very high intakes, exhalation of volatile forms of selenium.[60]

Health Effects, Deficiency, and Toxicity

In the 1930s, selenium was considered a toxic element; in the 1940s, a carcinogen; in the 1950s, it was declared as an essential element; and since the 1960s and especially the 1970s, it has been viewed as an anticarcinogen. Glutathione peroxidase (in the form of selenocysteine) is part of the cellular antioxidant defense system against free radicals.[25] and selenium is also involved in the metabolism of thyroid hormones[61] (e.g., deiodinase enzymes and thioredoxin reductase).[60]

Selenium deficiency has been associated with cardiomyopathy, skeletal muscle weakness, and osteoarthritis. A significant negative correlation was observed between selenium intakes and the rate of cancer of the large intestine, rectum, prostate, breast, ovary, and lungs and leukemia.[59]

Keshan disease, an endemic cardiomyopathy that affects mostly children and women in childbearing age in certain areas in China, has been associated with selenium deficiency. Symptoms include dizziness, malaise, loss of appetite, nausea, chills, abnormal electrocardiograms, cardiogenic shock, cardiac enlargements, and congestive heart failure. Selenium supplementation has been shown to effectively control Keshan disease.[25] Kashin-Beck disease, an endemic osteoarthritis that occurs during adolescent and preadolescent years, is another disease linked to low selenium status in northern China, North Korea, and eastern Siberia.[62]

Acute oral exposure to extremely high levels of selenium may produce gastrointestinal symptoms (nausea, vomiting, and diarrhea) and cardiovascular symptoms such as tachycardia. Chronic exposure to very high levels can cause dermal effects, including diseased nails and skin and hair loss, as well as neurologic problems such as unsteady gait or paralysis.[60] In 1984, 12 cases of selenium toxicity were reported to the FDA and CDC, because of the ingestion of selenium supplements, containing levels almost 200 times higher than stated on the label. The most common symptoms reported in these cases were nausea and vomiting, nail changes, hair loss, fatigue, abdominal cramps, watery diarrhea, and garlicky breath. No abnormalities of blood chemistry were seen in 67% of the victims, and renal and liver functions were normal.[63]

The EPA has determined that one specific form of selenium, selenium sulfide, is a probable human carcinogen. Selenium sulfide is a very different chemical from the organic and inorganic selenium compounds found in foods and in the environment.[62] In Hubei Province (China) during 1961 through 1964, almost half of the population of many villages died from chronic selenosis. The most common signs of selenium poisoning were loss of hair and nails, skin lesions, tooth decay, and abnormalities of the nervous system.[59]

Laboratory Evaluation

Selenium is most often determined by ICP-MS or GFAAS. The determination of urinary and blood selenium is an useful measure of selenium status.

ZINC

Introduction

Zinc (Zn) is a bluish white, lustrous metal that is stable in dry air and becomes covered with a white coating when exposed to moisture. Zinc is used in a production of alloys, especially brass (with copper), in galvanizing steel, in die casting, in paints, in skin lotions, as treatment for Wilson's disease, and in many over-the-counter medications. Zinc is an essential trace element and deficiency is common throughout life, especially in individuals that do not ingest meat.

Absorption, Transport, and Excretion

The body content in a normal individual varies substantially with age and is predominantly distributed in the muscle (60%) and skeleton (30%). The remaining 10% is distributed in various other tissues with highest concentrations found in the eyes, prostate, and hair. Zinc absorption mainly occurs in the small intestine and especially in the jejunum.[64] Factors increasing zinc absorption include the presence of animal proteins[65] and amino acids in a meal,[66] intake of calcium,[67] and unsaturated fatty acids.[68] Conversely, factors decreasing zinc absorption include the intake of iron,[69,70] taking zinc on empty stomach,[68] presence of copper at high levels,[71] and age.[72] In blood, the absorbed zinc is distributed between RBCs (80%), plasma (17%), and white blood cells (3%).[73] In normal dietary circumstances, about 90% of zinc is excreted in feces.[74]

Health Effects, Deficiency, and Toxicity

Zinc is second only to iron in importance as an essential trace element. The main biochemical role of zinc is seen in its influence on the activity of more than 300 enzymes in classes such as oxidoreductases, transferases, hydrolases, leases, isomerases, and lipases. As a result of the importance of zinc for the structure, regulation, and catalytic action of various enzymes, zinc is indirectly involved in the synthesis and metabolism of DNA and RNA, the synthesis and metabolism of proteins, the metabolism of glucose and cholesterol, membrane structure maintenance, insulin function, and growth factor affects.[64] Chronic oral zinc supplementation interferes with copper absorption and may cause copper deficiency forming the basis for using zinc to treat Wilson's disease.

Zinc deficiency causes growth retardation, slows skeletal maturation, causes testicular atrophy, and reduces taste perception. Old age, pregnancy, lactation, and alcoholism are also associated with poor zinc nutrition.[25] Infants with acrodermatitis enteropathica (zinc malabsorption) first develop a characteristic facial and diaper rash. If untreated, symptoms progress and include growth retardation, diarrhea, impaired T-cell immunity, insufficient wound healing, infections, delayed testicular development in adolescence, and early death.[7] Zn deficiency in adolescents is manifested by slow growth or weight loss, altered taste, delayed puberty, dwarfism, impaired dark adaptation, alopecia, emotional instability, and tremors. In severe cases, lymphopenia and death can result from an overwhelming infection.[7]

Zinc is relatively nontoxic. Nevertheless, high doses (1 g) or repetitive doses of 100 mg/d for several months may lead to gastrointestinal tract symptoms, decrease in heme synthesis due to an induced copper deficiency, and hyperglycemia.[64] Exposure to ZnO fumes and dust may cause "zinc fume fever," with symptoms including chemically induced pneumonia, severe pulmonary inflammation, fever, hyperpnea, coughing, pains in legs and chest, and vomiting.[64]

Laboratory Evaluation

Zinc is measured by FAAS, ICP-AES, and ICP-MS. Low urine zinc levels in the presence of low serum zinc levels usually confirm zinc deficiency.[7] Low serum zinc in an apparently healthy (nonstressed and nonseptic) patient who has normal serum albumin levels can be used as evidence of zinc deficiency, especially if urine zinc levels are also low. Normal

serum zinc cannot be interpreted as evidence of normal zinc stores. Zinc concentration in RBCs is approximately 10 times that in serum.[25] Copper status should be monitored in patients undergoing long-term zinc therapy.[7,72]

For additional student resources please visit thePoint at http://thepoint.lww.com. **thePoint**

QUESTIONS

1. Extreme copper deficiency is seen in what fatal condition?
   a. Menkes disease
   b. Klinefelter's syndrome
   c. Meese disease
   d. Kayser-Fleischer rings

2. Suppose the controller on a GFAAS is defective and the furnace is running cold. What effect will this likely have on the number of photons absorbed in the measurements?
   a. It will decrease the number of photons absorbed
   b. It will increase the number of photons absorbed
   c. It will have little effect
   d. It is not a relevant question because AAS relies on emission of light from electronically excited atoms

3. Why would a clinical chemist develop an arsenic method that combines liquid chromatography with ICP-MS?
   a. To separate and quantitate several different arsenic-containing species in the same sample
   b. To eliminate interference by sodium from the analysis
   c. To shorten the run time of the measurement
   d. To lower the coefficient of variation for total arsenic measurements

4. Select the answer that designates three techniques widely used for elemental analysis, identified according to the initials for the techniques.
   a. AAS, ICP-MS, AES
   b. NMR, ICP-MS, AES
   c. GC-MS, ICP-MS, AES
   d. HPLC-ICP-MS, AAS, FTIR

5. One of the calcium isotopes (^{40}Ca) has an atomic weight of 40. At what positions in a mass spectrum would singly and doubly charged ions of this isotope of calcium appear? Assume that singly charged Ca is listed first.

a. 40 and 20
b. 40 and 60
c. 40 and 80
d. 40 and 40

6. What primary purposes does the torch serve in ICP-MS?
   a. Vaporization, atomization, and ionization
   b. Vaporization, atomization, and electronic excitation
   c. Nebulization, atomization, and photon absorption
   d. Droplet transport, vaporization, and ion detection

7. Manganese toxicity resembles the following disease:
   a. Parkinson's disease
   b. Wilson's disease
   c. Alzheimer's disease
   d. Menkes disease

8. Iron is physiologically active only in the ferrous form in
   a. Hemoglobin
   b. Cytochromes
   c. Ferritin
   d. Transferrin

9. A metal ion required for optimal enzyme activity is best termed a(an)
   a. Cofactor
   b. Accelerator
   c. Coenzyme
   d. Catalyst

10. Which trace metal is contained in glucose tolerance factor?
    a. Chromium
    b. Copper
    c. Selenium
    d. Zinc

11. What metal may be used as a treatment for Wilson's disease?

    a. Zinc

    b. Copper

    c. Molybdenum

    d. Fluorine

12. The metal ion essential for the activity of xanthine oxidase and xanthine dehydrogenase is

    a. Molybdenum

    b. Iron

    c. Zinc

    d. Manganese

BIBLIOGRAPHY

Holstege CP, Heavy metals. In: Holstege CP, Borloz MP, Benner JP, eds. *Toxicology Recall*. Baltimore, MD: Lippincott William & Wilkins; 2009:256-310.

Jacobs DS, DeMott WR, Oxley DK. *Jacobs & DeMott Laboratory Test Handbook*. 5th ed. Lexi-Comp's Clinical Reference Library. Hudson, OH: Lexi-Comp; 2001:1031.

Nordberg G, Fowler B, Nordberg M, Friberg L, eds. *Handbook on the Toxicology of Metals*. Amsterdam; Boston, MA: Academic Press; 2007:xlvii, 975 p.

Pais I, Jones JB. *The Handbook of Trace Elements*. Boca Raton, FL: St. Lucie Press; 1997:xv, 223.

Seiler HG, Sigel A, Sigel H. *Handbook on Metals in Clinical and Analytical Chemistry*. New York, NY: Marcel Dekker; 1994: xx, 753.

Thomas R. *Practical Guide to ICP-MS: A Tutorial for Beginners*. 2nd ed. Practical Spectroscopy. Boca Raton, FL: CRC Press; 2008:xxv, 347.

REFERENCES

1. Rodushkin I, Odman F, Branth S, et al. Multielemental analysis of whole blood by high resolution inductively coupled plasma mass spectrometry. *Fresenius Chem*. 1999;364 SRC:338-346.

2. May T, Wiedmeyer R. A table of polyatomic interferences in ICP-MS. *Atom Spectrosc*. 1998;19(5):150-155.

3. Vaughan M, Horlick G. Correction procedures for rare earth analysis in inductively coupled plasma-mass spectrometry. *Appl Spectrosc*. 1990;44:587-593.

4. Thomas R. *Practical Guide to ICP-MS: A Tutorial for Beginners*. 2nd ed. Practical Spectroscopy. Boca Raton, FL: CRC Press; 2008:xxv, 347.

5. Sobin C, Parisi N, Schaub T, et al. A Bland–Altman comparison of the Lead Care® System and inductively coupled plasma mass spectrometry for detecting low-level lead in child whole blood samples. *J Med Toxicol*. 2011;7(1):24-32.

6. Agency for Toxic Substances & Disease Registry. Aluminum. Toxic Substances Portal 2012 [cited 2012 January]. http://www.atsdr.cdc.gov/toxfaqs/tf.asp?id=190&tid=34. Accessed March 3, 2011.

7. Jacobs DS, DeMott WR, Oxley DK. *Jacobs & DeMott Laboratory Test Handbook*. 5th ed. Lexi-Comp's Clinical Reference Library. Hudson, OH: Lexi-Comp; 2001:1031.

8. Schaller K, Letzel S, Angerer J. Aluminum. In: Seiler H, Sigel A, Sigel H, eds. *Handbook on Metals in Clinical and Analytical Chemistry*. New York, NY: Marcel Dekker; 1994: 217-226.

9. Alfrey A. Aluminum. In: Mertz W, Underwood EJ, eds. *Trace Elements in Human and Animal Nutrition*. St. Louis, MO: Academic Press; 1986:399-413.

10. Baselt R. In: Baselt R, ed. *Disposition of Toxic Drugs and Chemicals in Man*. Seal Beach, CA: Biomedical Publications; 2004:39-41.

11. Sjögren B, Iregren A, Elinder C, et al. Aluminum. In: Nordberg G, et al. eds. *Handbook on the Toxicology of Metals*. Amsterdam; Boston, MA: Academic Press; 2007:339-352.

12. U.S. Environmental Protection Agency. *Arsenic Compounds*. 2012 11/6/2007 [cited 2012 January]. www.epa.gov/ttn/atw/hlthef/arsenic.html.

13. Iffland R. Arsenic. In: Seiler H, Sigel A, Sigel H, eds. *Handbook on Metals in Clinical and Analytical Chemistry*. New York, NY: Marcel Dekker; 1994:237-253.

14. Fowler B, Chou C-HS, Jones R, et al. Arsenic. In: Nordberg G, et al. eds. *Handbook on the Toxicology of Metals*. Amsterdam; Boston, MA: Academic Press; 2007:367-406.

15. Kamimura T, Miyamoto T, Harada M, et al. Advances in therapies for acute promyelocytic leukemia. *Cancer Sci*. 2011;102(11): 1929-1937.

16. Anke M. Arsenic. In: Mertz W, Underwood EJ, eds. *Trace Elements in Human and Animal Nutrition*. St. Louis, MO: Academic Press; 1986:347-372.

17. Pais I, Jones JB. *The Handbook of Trace Elements*. Boca Raton, FL: St. Lucie Press; 1997:xv, 223.

18. U.S. Environmental Protection Agency. *Cadmium*. Integrated Risk Information System 2012 [cited 2012 January]. http://www.epa.gov/iris/subst/0141.htm.

19. Agency for Toxic Substances & Disease Registry. *Cadmium*. Toxic Substances Portal 2012 [cited 2012 January]. http://www.atsdr.cdc.gov/substances/toxsubstance.asp?toxid=15. March 3, 2011.

20. Moyer T, Burritt M, Butz J. Toxic metals. In: Burtis CA, Ashwood ER, Bruns DE, eds. *Tietz Textbook of Clinical Chemistry and Molecular Diagnostics*. Philadelphia, PA: Elsevier Saunders; 2006:1377-1378.

21. Herber RFM. Cadmium. In: Seiler HG, et al. eds. *Handbook on Metals in Clinical and Analytical Chemistry*. New York, NY: Marcel Dekker; 1994:283-297.

22. Nordberg G, Nogawa K, Nordberg M, et al. Cadmium. In: Nordberg G, et al. eds. *Handbook on the Toxicology of Metals*. Amsterdam; Boston, MA: Academic Press; 2007:445-486.

23. Herold DA, Fitzgerald RL. Chromium. In: Seiler H, Sigel A, Sigel H, eds. *Handbook on Metals in Clinical and Analytical Chemistry*. New York, NY: Marcel Dekker; 1994: 321-332.

24. Offenbacher EG, Pi-Sunyer FX. Chromium in human nutrition. *Ann Rev Nutr*. 1988;8:543-563.

25. Shenkin A, Baines M, Lyon T. Vitamins and trace elements. In: Burtis CA, Ashwood ER, Bruns DE, eds. *Tietz Textbook of Clinical Chemistry and Molecular Diagnostics*. Philadelphia, PA: Elsevier Saunders; 2006:1075-1164.

26. Langård S, Costa M. Chromium. In: Nordberg G, et al. eds. *Handbook on the Toxicology of Metals*. Amsterdam; Boston, MA: Academic Press; 2007:487-510.

27. U.S. Food and Drug Administration. *Information for All Health Care Professionals who Provide Treatment to Patients with a Metalon-Metal Hip Implant System*. 2011 [cited 2012 January]. http://www.fda.gov/MedicalDevices/ProductsandMedicalProcedures/ImplantsandProsthetics/MetalonMetalHipImplants/ucm241744.htm. Accessed January 11, 2012.

28. Walter LR, Marel E, Harbury R, et al. Distribution of chromium and cobalt ions in various blood fractions after resurfacing hip arthroplasty. *J Arthroplasty*. 2008;23(6):814-821.

29. Ellingsen D, Horn N, Aaseth J. Copper. In: Nordberg G, et al. eds. *Handbook on the Toxicology of Metals*. Amsterdam; Boston, MA: Academic Press; 2007:529-546.

30. Sarkar B. Copper. In: Seiler HG, Sigel A, Sigel H, eds. *Handbook on Metals in Clinical and Analytical Chemistry.* New York, NY: Marcel Dekker; 1994:339-347.

31. Holstege CP, Heavy metals. In: Holstege CP, Borloz MP, Benner JP, eds. *Toxicology Recall.* Baltimore, MD: Lippincott William & Wilkins; 2009:256-310.

32. McMillin GA, Travis JJ, Hunt JW. Direct measurement of free copper in serum or plasma ultrafiltrate. *Am J Clin Pathol.* 2009;131(2):160-165.

33. Higgins T, Beutler E, Doumas B. Hemoglobin, iron, and bilirubin. In: Burtis CA, Ashwood ER, Bruns DE, eds. *Tietz Textbook of Clinical Chemistry and Molecular Diagnostics.* Philadelphia, PA: WB Saunders; 2006:1165-1208.

34. Rossi E. Hepcidin—the iron regulatory hormone. *Clin Biochem Rev.* 2005;26(3):47-49.

35. Beard JL, Dawson H, Piñero DJ. Iron metabolism: a comprehensive review. *Nutr Rev.* 1996;54(10):295-317.

36. Meneghini R. Iron homeostasis, oxidative stress, and DNA damage. *Free Rad Biol Med.* 1997;23(5):783-792.

37. Smith C, Mitchinson MJ, Aruoma OI, et al. Stimulation of lipid peroxidation and hydroxyl-radical generation by the contents of human atherosclerotic lesions. *Biochem J.* 1992;286(pt 3):901-905.

38. Schwartz CJ, Valente AJ, Sprague EA, et al. The pathogenesis of atherosclerosis: an overview. *Clin Cardiol.* 1991;14(2 suppl 1):I1-I16.

39. Anghileri LJ. Iron, intracellular calcium ion, lipid peroxidation and carcino-genesis. *Anticancer Res.* 1995;15(4):1395-1400.

40. Weinberg ED. Cellular iron metabolism in health and disease. *Drug Metab Rev.* 1990;22(5):531-579.

41. McCord JM. Iron, free radicals, and oxidative injury. *Semin Hematol.* 1998;35(1):5-12.

42. Smith MA, Perry G. Free radical damage, iron, and Alzheimer's disease. *J Neurol Sci.* 1995;134(suppl):92-94.

43. Herbert V, Shaw S, Jayatilleke E. Vitamin C-driven free radical generation from iron. *J Nutr.* 1996;126(4 suppl):1213S-1220S.

44. Tofaletti JG. Trace elements. In: Bishop ML, Fody EP, Schoeff LE, eds. *Clinical Chemistry: Principles, Procedures, Correlations.* Philadelphia, PA: Lippincott Williams & Wilkins; 2004:403-423.

45. ARUP Laboratories I. Hemochromatosis. ARUP's Laboratory Test Directory 2012 [cited 2012 January]. http://www.arupconsult.com/Topics/Hemochromatosis.html. Accessed January 7, 2012.

46. Christensen J, Kristiansen J. Lead. In: Seiler H, Sigel A, Sigel H, eds. *Handbook on Metals in Clinical and Analytical Chemistry.* New York, NY: Marcel Dekker; 1994:425-440.

47. Skerfving S, Bergdahl I. Lead. In: Nordberg G, et al. eds. *Handbook on the Toxicology of Metals.* Amsterdam; Boston, MA: Academic Press; 2007:599-643.

48. Boffetta P, Nyberg F. Contribution of environmental factors to cancer risk. *Br Med Bull.* 2003;68:71-94.

49. Berlin M, Zalups R, Fowler B. Mercury. In: Nordberg G, et al. eds. *Handbook on the Toxicology of Metals.* Amsterdam; Boston, MA: Academic Press; 2007:675-729.

50. Drash G. Mercury. In: Seiler H, Sigel A, Sigel H, eds. *Handbook on Metals in Clinical and Analytical Chemistry.* New York, NY: Marcel Dekker; 1994:479-493.

51. Goyer R, Klaassen CD, Waalkes MP. Nervous system. In: Goyer R, Klaassen CD, Waalkes MP, eds. *Metal Toxicology.* San Diego, CA: Academic Press; 1995:199-235.

52. Porter W, Moyer T. Clinical toxicology. In: Burtis CA, Ashwood ER, eds. *Tietz Fundamentals of Clinical Chemistry.* Philadelphia, PA: WB Saunders; 2006:427-456.

53. Ashwood E. *Clinical Testing.* New York, NY: ARUP Laboratories; 2004:101-102.

54. Šarić M, Lucchini R. Manganese. In: Nordberg G, et al. eds. *Handbook on the Toxicology of Metals.* Amsterdam; Boston, MA: Academic Press; 2007:645-674.

55. Kaiser J. State Court to rule on manganese fume claims. *Science (New York, NY).* 2003;300(5621):927.

56. Donaldson J. The physiopathologic significance of manganese in brain: its relation to schizophrenia and neurodegenerative disorders. *Neurotoxicology.* 1987;8(3):451-462.

57. Turnlund J, Friberg L. Molybdenum. In: Nordberg G, et al. eds. *Handbook on the Toxicology of Metals.* Amsterdam; Boston, MA: Academic Press; 2007:731-741.

58. Anke M, Giel M. Molybdenum. In: Seiler H, Sigel A, Sigel H, eds. *Handbook on Metals in Clinical and Analytical Chemistry.* New York, NY: Marcel Dekker; 1994:495-501.

59. Magee R, James B. Selenium. In: Seiler H, Sigel A, Sigel H, eds. *Handbook on Metals in Clinical and Analytical Chemistry.* New York, NY: Marcel Dekker; 1994:551-562.

60. Högberg J, Alexander J. Selenium. In: Nordberg G, et al. eds. *Handbook on the Toxicology of Metals.* Amsterdam; Boston, MA: Academic Press; 2007:783-807.

61. Gladyshev VN, Jeang KT, Stadtman TC. Selenocysteine, identified as the penultimate C-terminal residue in human T-cell thioredoxin reductase, corresponds to TGA in the human placental gene. *Proc Natl Acad Sci U S A.* 1996;93(12):6146-6151.

62. Agency for Toxic Substances & Disease Registry. *Selenium.* Toxic Substances Portal 2012 [cited 2012 January]. http://www.atsdr.cdc.gov/substances/toxsubstance.asp?toxid=28. Accessed March 3, 2011.

63. Levander O. Selenium. In: Mertz W, Underwood EJ, eds. *Trace Elements in Human and Animal Nutrition.* St. Louis, MO: Academic Press; 1986:209-279.

64. Thunus L, Lejeune R. Zinc. In: Seiler H, Sigel A, Sigel H, eds. *Handbook on Metals in Clinical and Analytical Chemistry.* New York, NY: Marcel Dekker; 1994:667-674.

65. Solomons NW. Biological availability of zinc in humans. *Am J Clin Nutr.* 1982;35(5):1048-1075.

66. Sandstrom B, Cederblad A. Zinc absorption from composite meals. II. Influence of the main protein source. *Am J Clin Nutr.* 1980;33(8):1778-1783.

67. Sandstrom B, Arvidsson B, Cederblad A, et al. Zinc absorption from composite meals. I. The significance of wheat extraction rate, zinc, calcium, and protein content in meals based on bread. *Am J Clin Nutr.* 1980;33(4):739-745.

68. Cunnane SC. Maternal essential fatty acid supplementation increases zinc absorption in neonatal rats: relevance to the defect in zinc absorption in acrodermatitis enteropathica. *Pediatr Res.* 1982;16(8):599-603.

69. Solomons NW. Competitive interaction of iron and zinc in the diet: consequences for human nutrition. *J Nutr.* 1986;116(6):927-935.

70. Sandström B, Davidsson L, Cederblad A, et al. Oral iron, dietary ligands and zinc absorption. *J Nutr.* 1985;115(3):411-414.

71. Lönnderdal B. Iron-zinc-copper interactions. In: *Micronutrient Interactions. Impact on Child Health and Nutrition.* Washington, DC: International Life Sciences Institute; 1996:3-10.

72. Bales CW, Steinman LC, Freeland-Graves JH, et al. The effect of age on plasma zinc uptake and taste acuity. *Am J Clin Nutr.* 1986;44(5):664-669.

73. Fisher GL. Function and homeostasis of copper and zinc in mammals. *Sci Tot Environ.* 1975;4(4):373-412.

74. Hambridge K, Casey C, Krebs N. Zinc. In: Mertz W, Underwood EJ, eds. *Trace Elements in Human and Animal Nutrition.* St. Louis, MO: Academic Press; 1986:1-137.

Porphyrins and Hemoglobin

LOUANN W. LAWRENCE, LARRY A. BROUSSARD

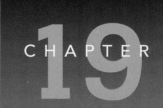

CHAPTER OUTLINE

- ◆ **PORPHYRINS**
  Role in the Body
  Chemistry of Porphyrins
  Porphyrin Synthesis
  Clinical Significance and Disease Correlation
  Methods of Analyzing Porphyrins
- ◆ **HEMOGLOBIN**
  Role in the Body
  Structure of Hemoglobin
  Synthesis and Degradation of Hemoglobin

Clinical Significance and Disease Correlation
Methodology
DNA Technology
- ◆ **MYOGLOBIN**
  Structure and Role in the Body
  Clinical Significance
  Methodology
- ◆ **QUESTIONS**
- ◆ **REFERENCES**

Chapter Objectives

Upon completion of this chapter, the clinical laboratorian should be able to do the following:

- Describe the chemical nature and structure of porphyrins and hemoglobin.
- Relate the role of porphyrins in the body.
- Outline the biochemical pathway of porphyrin and heme synthesis.
- Discuss the clinical significance of the porphyrias.
- Compare and contrast the porphyrias with regard to enzyme deficiency, clinical symptoms, and clinical laboratory data.

- Explain the principles of the basic qualitative and quantitative porphyrin tests, to include PBG, ALA, uroporphyrin, coproporphyrin, and protoporphyrin.
- Describe the degradation of hemoglobin.
- Discuss the clinical significance and laboratory data associated with the hemoglobinopathies and thalassemias.
- Identify the tests used in the diagnosis of hemoglobinopathies and thalassemias.
- Discuss the structure and clinical significance of myoglobin in the body.

KEY TERMS

Cytochrome
Hemoglobinopathy
Myoglobin
Porphyrias

Porphyrin
Porphyrinogen
Porphyrinuria
Pyrrole
Thalassemia

Because of chemical similarities, porphyrins, hemoglobin, and myoglobin are discussed together in this chapter. These compounds all contain the porphyrin ring, which comprises four pyrrole groups bonded by methene bridges (Fig. 19-1). Porphyrins are able to chelate metals to form the functional groups that participate in oxidative metabolism. The analysis of porphyrins in the laboratory aids in the diagnosis of a group of disorders resulting from disturbances in heme synthesis called the porphyrias.

Each defective enzyme that causes porphyria may be assayed by various methods. Hemoglobin molecules are specially designed to bind, deliver, and release oxygen. Qualitative defects in the hemoglobin molecule result in a group of disorders called hemoglobinopathies, such as sickle cell anemia. Quantitative defects in the production of normal hemoglobin molecules lead to another group of disorders, called thalassemias. Analytic methods to diagnose these disorders are discussed. Myoglobin is a

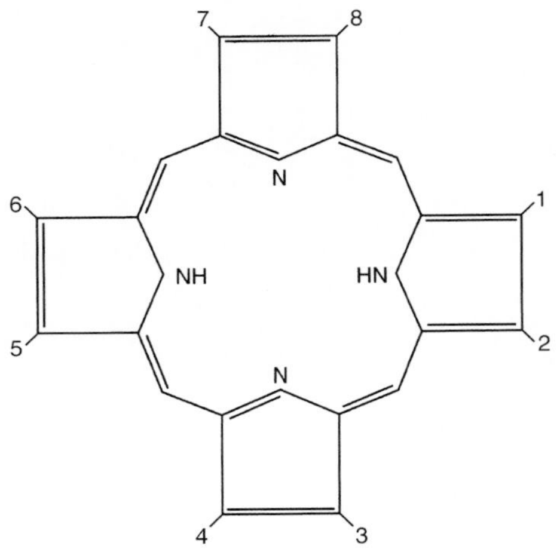

FIGURE 19-1 Basic structure of porphyrins.

simple heme protein found only in skeletal and cardiac muscle, which may be analyzed to aid in the diagnosis of acute myocardial infarction (AMI).

PORPHYRINS

Role in the Body

Porphyrins are chemical intermediates in the synthesis of hemoglobin, myoglobin, and other respiratory pigments called cytochromes. They also form part of the peroxidase and catalase enzymes, which contribute to the efficiency of internal respiration. Iron is chelated within porphyrins to form heme. Heme is then incorporated into proteins to become biologically functional hemoproteins. Porphyrins are analyzed in clinical chemistry to aid in the diagnosis of *porphyrias*, which result from disturbances in heme synthesis. Excess amounts of these intermediate compounds in urine, feces, or blood indicate a metabolic block in heme synthesis.

Chemistry of Porphyrins

The porphyrins found in nature are all compounds in which the side chains are substituted for the eight hydrogen atoms found in the four pyrrole rings that make up porphyrin (Fig. 19-1). Because of the wide variety of substitutions, many porphyrins have been described in nature. The pigment chlorophyll is a magnesium porphyrin and is essential for plants to use light energy to synthesize carbohydrates. Four basic isomers may exist for every porphyrin compound; however, only type I and type III occur in nature. The difference between type I and type III isomers is in the arrangement of side chains. Only type III isomers form heme; however, in some disorders, the functionless type I isomers may be present in excess in the tissue. Porphyrins are stable compounds, red-violet to red-brown in color, that

fluoresce red when excited by light near 400 nm. Only three porphyrin compounds are clinically significant in humans: protoporphyrin (PROTO), uroporphyrin (URO), and coproporphyrin (COPRO). Their presence in excess in biologic fluids is a clinical sign of abnormal heme synthesis. The three compounds have different solubility properties and different degrees of ionization determined by the addition of various carboxyl groups to the basic porphyrin structure. This allows for separate assays of each. URO is excreted primarily in the urine, PROTO in the feces, and COPRO in either, depending on the rate of formation of the urine and its pH.

The reduced forms of porphyrins are termed porphyrinogens, the functional form of the compound that must be used in heme synthesis. Porphyrinogens are highly unstable and colorless and do not fluoresce, which makes them more difficult to analyze. With light, oxygen, or oxidizing agents, porphyrinogens are readily oxidized to the corresponding porphyrin form. Therefore, the porphyrin form is routinely analyzed in clinical laboratories as a result of the increased stability and ease of detection by various common clinical laboratory systems.

Porphyrin Synthesis

All cells contain hemoproteins and can synthesize heme; however, the bone marrow and liver are the main sites. The series of irreversible reactions is outlined in Figure 19-2. Some steps occur in the mitochondria of the cell and some steps occur in the cytoplasm. The transport of substrates across the mitochondrial membrane is a complex process and a potential point for interruptions in heme synthesis.

Control of the rate of heme synthesis in the cells in the liver is achieved largely through regulation of the enzyme δ-aminolevulinic acid synthase (ALAS). The main mechanism is repression of synthesis of new enzyme. A negative feedback mechanism exists in which increases in the pool of hepatic heme diminish the production of ALAS. Conversely, ALAS production is increased with a depletion of heme. The size of the regulatory heme pool may be affected by the requirement for hemoproteins in the liver. Drugs and other compounds appear to induce ALAS production via several different mechanisms, but all result in a depletion of the regulatory heme pool. Therefore, the rate of heme synthesis is flexible and can change rapidly in response to a wide variety of external stimuli. In bone marrow erythrocytes, other enzymes in the pathway and the rate of cellular iron uptake seem to control the rate of heme synthesis.

Clinical Significance and Disease Correlation

The porphyrias are inherited or acquired enzyme deficiencies that result in overproduction of heme precursors

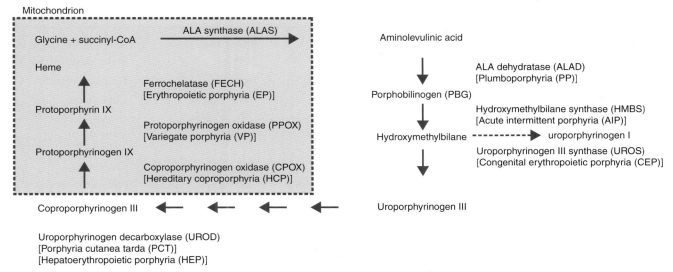

FIGURE 19-2 Synthesis of heme. *Brackets* indicate diseases associated with enzyme deficiencies.

in the bone marrow (erythropoietic porphyrias [EPs]) or the liver (hepatic porphyrias). Disease states corresponding to enzyme deficiencies have been identified in every step of heme synthesis except for ALAS. Some patients demonstrate an enzyme deficiency but do not show clinical or biochemical manifestations of porphyria, indicating that other factors, such as demand for increased heme biosynthesis, are also important in causing disease expression. An excess of the early precursors in the pathway of heme synthesis (ALA, porphobilinogen [PBG], or both) causes neuropsychiatric symptoms, including abdominal pain, vomiting, constipation, tachycardia, hypertension, psychiatric symptoms, fever, leukocytosis, and paresthesia. Porphyrias in this category include ALA dehydratase (ALAD) deficiency porphyria (ADP) or plumboporphyria and acute intermittent porphyria (AIP). Excesses of the later intermediates (UROs, COPROs, and PROTOs) may cause cutaneous symptoms, including photosensitivity, blisters, excess facial hair, and hyperpigmentation. Porphyria cutanea tarda (PCT), hepatoerythropoietic porphyria (HEP), EP, and congenital erythropoietic porphyria (CEP) are associated with cutaneous symptoms. Porphyrin-induced photosensitivity manifests by increased fragility of light-exposed skin, as in PCT, or by burning of light-exposed skin, as in EP. The photosensitizing effects of the porphyrins are attributable to absorption of light. There may also be excesses of both early and late intermediates, causing neurocutaneous symptoms. Hereditary coproporphyria (HCP) and variegate porphyria (VP) fall into this category. All porphyrias are inherited as autosomal dominant (one altered gene) traits producing about a 50% reduction in enzyme levels, except for ADP and CEP, which are autosomal recessive (altered gene from each parent).[1] Reduction in enzyme

levels results in excess production of one or more precursors causing development of symptoms. Residual enzyme activity is sufficient to produce enough heme to prevent anemia.

The diagnosis of porphyrias is made by a combination of history and physical and laboratory findings. The cutaneous porphyrias are easier to diagnose because photosensitivity is usually the presenting symptom. Laboratory diagnosis, if necessary, is made by analysis of the appropriate sample for intermediates in heme synthesis (Table 19-1). The differentiation of neurologic porphyrias from other disorders is more difficult based on history and physical examination and must be verified by laboratory findings.

Inherited ADP, an autosomal recessive disorder, is extremely rare, with only seven cases reported worldwide.[2] The affected ALAD gene is located on chromosome 9q33.1 and at least 10 mutations have been identified.[3] Urinary ALA is significantly elevated with normal PBG excretion. Increased urinary coproporphyrin III may provide supporting evidence for the diagnosis, but this also occurs in lead poisoning, which is the most common cause of low ALAD activity and must be ruled out before making a diagnosis of ADP. ADP may be distinguished from lead poisoning by the in vitro addition of dithiothreitol or other sulfhydryl reagents. This results in restoration of erythrocyte ALAD activity to normal in patients with lead poisoning but no change in the reduced ALAD activity in ADP patients.[4]

AIP results from a deficiency of the enzyme hydroxymethylbilane synthase (HMBS), also known as PBG deaminase. The estimated frequency of acute attacks of AIP in most developed countries is 1 to 2 per 100,000, with a higher prevalence in Scandinavian countries.[4]

TABLE 19-1	METABOLITES FOUND IN EXCESS IN THE PORPHYRIAS			
PORPHYRIA	**URINE**	**FECES**	**ERYTHROCYTES**	**SYMPTOMS**
ADP (PP)	ALA, COPRO III	Normal	ZPP	Neuropsychiatric
AIP	ALA, PBG, URO I	Normal	Normal	Neuropsychiatric
CEP	URO I, COPRO I	URO I	URO, COPRO I, ZPP, PROTO	Cutaneous
PCT	URO I, ISOCOPRO, HEPTA	ISOCOPRO	Normal	Cutaneous
HEP	URO, COPRO	ISOCOPRO	ZPP	Cutaneous
HCP	[a]ALA, [a]PBG, [a]COPRO III	COPRO, HARDERO	Normal	Neurocutaneous
VP	[a]ALA, [a]PBG, [a]COPRO III	PROTO > COPRO	Normal	Neurocutaneous
EP	Normal	PROTO	PROTO	Cutaneous

[a]Indicates during acute attacks; ADP, ALA dehydratase (ALAD) deficiency porphyria; ALA, aminolevulinic acid; COPRO, coproporphyrin; ZPP, zinc protoporphyrin; AIP, acute intermittent porphyria; PBG, porphobilinogen; URO, uroporphyrin; CEP, congenital erythropoietic porphyria; PROTO, protoporphyrin; PCT, porphyria cutanea tarda; ISOCOPRO, isocoproporphyrin; HARDERO, harderoporphyrin; HEPTA, heptacarboxylate porphyrin; HEP, hepatoerythropoietic porphyria; HCP, hereditary coproporphyria; VP, variegate porphyria; EP, erythropoietic porphyria.

HMBS is located on chromosome 11q23, with more than 300 mutations of this gene described.[3] Although the inheritance is autosomal dominant, only about 10% of patients with the deficiency suffer attacks of the disease, so other etiologic factors are involved. Drugs are the most common precipitating cause of the disease, especially barbiturates and sulfonamides; however, a wide variety of drugs are potentially hazardous. This disease is characterized by multiple neurologic symptoms with colicky stomach pain and, occasionally, fever and vomiting. The characteristic laboratory findings are a marked elevation of ALA and PBG in the urine, although these test results may be normal between attacks. A patient's urine with clinically manifest AIP may turn red or dark brown due to nonenzymatic conversion to uroporphyrin I, a process that may be delayed with refrigeration, protection from light, and alkaline adjustment to pH 8.0 to 9.0. Electrolyte abnormalities, including hyponatremia during acute attacks, may help suggest the diagnosis.[4] Measurement of levels of erythrocyte or lymphoblast HMBS may be performed to confirm the diagnosis.[5]

CEP, a deficiency of uroporphyrinogen III cosynthase (UROS), is one of the rarest porphyrias with fewer than 200 cases reported. UROS is located on chromosome 10q25.2-q26.3 and more than 35 mutations have been found.[3] CEP usually appears shortly after birth, with the first signs often being red-brown urine staining of diapers and cutaneous photosensitivity.[5] It is also known as *Günther's disease*. The teeth will fluoresce red under ultraviolet light and exhibit a red or brownish discoloration under normal light as a result of porphyrin deposits in the dentin. Urine and fecal porphyrins, URO I and COPRO I, are significantly elevated. The urine is often red because of the presence of URO and COPRO.

Photosensitivity is a major clinical problem, resulting in lesions that may become infected and leave the patient scarred or with multiple occurrences that may lead to mutilation of the ears, nose, or digits. Abnormal hair growth is often seen in exposed areas. It is thought that the disfigurements of this disorder and the tendency to avoid daylight (hence, only coming outside at night) led to the legend of the werewolf.[6] Patients may also develop a hemolytic anemia and splenomegaly with hemolysis serving as a stimulus for increased porphyrin production in the bone marrow. Allogeneic bone marrow transplantation has proved curative in patients with CEP.[3]

Deficiency of uroporphyrinogen decarboxylase (UROD) occurs in PCT, the most common porphyria, and in the rarer HEP. PCT is subdivided into two types: sporadic type I, in which decreased UROD activity is restricted to the liver and there is no family history of the disease; and familial type II, characterized by UROD deficiency in all tissue and an autosomal dominant inheritance pattern. Genetic studies have shown that PCT is not a single monogenic disorder but rather a group of diseases characterized by more than 50 mutations to the gene (mapped on chromosome *1p34*) coding for UROD and possibly to other genes outside the UROD locus.[3,7] PCT usually presents in adulthood with cutaneous blistering and fragility in light-exposed areas, typically the hands, along with some abnormal hair growth. Liver biopsy specimens from these patients show fluorescence, hemosiderosis, fatty infiltration, and variable degrees of necrosis and fibrosis. PCT is differentiated from all other porphyrias by three features: (1) association of skin lesions with severe deficiency of UROD, resulting in increased excretion of uroporphyrin, heptacarboxylic porphyrin, isocoproporphyrin, and other porphyrins; (2)

remission following low-dose chloroquine or iron depletion; and (3) some degree of liver cell damage in almost all patients.[8] In genetically predisposed patients, PCT may be induced by multiple factors, including alcohol, estrogen, halogenated aromatic hydrocarbons (hexachlorobenzene and 2,3,7,8-tetrachlorodibenzo-p-dioxin), infection by hepatitis C and human immunodeficiency virus, thalassemia, hepatic tumors, hemodialysis, and bone marrow transplantation.[7,9] In laboratory tests, PCT is characterized by increased levels of urinary URO, COPRO, and 7-carboxyl porphyrin III, plasma URO, and fecal isocoproporphyrins (ISOCOPROs).[5] Other laboratory findings that may also be seen in this disease are elevated serum iron, ferritin, and liver enzymes.

At least 10 mutations in the UROD gene have been associated with HEP, a condition in which the enzyme activity is reduced by 90% or more.[3] Clinical features are similar to those of CEP, including photosensitivity beginning in childhood. Patients are severely affected and develop excess facial hair and scarring of the hands and face. The severity of photosensitivity improves somewhat with age, but hepatic disease follows. Urine and fecal porphyrin levels are similar to those found in PCT. Erythrocyte zinc protoporphyrin (ZPP) levels are increased in HEP and normal in PCT.[5]

HCP, a deficiency of coproporphyrinogen oxidase (CPOX), is a fairly mild condition with primarily neurologic manifestations and cutaneous photosensitivity in about 30% of patients.[5] The CPOX gene is located on chromosome 3q12 and at least 45 mutations have been identified.[3] Attacks have been precipitated by exposure to certain drugs, hormones, and nutritional changes.[4] The hallmark of HCP is significantly increased excretion of COPRO III in urine and feces. In harderoporphyria, a rare erythropoietic variant form of HCP, harderoporphyrin, a three-carboxyl porphyrin, is also present in feces. Increased plasma COPRO also occurs. During acute attacks, urinary excretion of COPRO III, ALA, and PBG is increased.

VP is prevalent in South Africa and can be traced to a single couple that emigrated from the Netherlands in 1688. The cause is a deficiency of protoporphyrinogen oxidase activity (PPOX). The PPOX gene is located on chromosome 1q22 and more than 130 mutations have been identified.[3] Clinical manifestations include acute attacks of neurologic dysfunction (such as those in AIP), photodermatitis (as in HCP and PCT), or both. Hallmark laboratory findings are increased levels of COPRO and PROTO in feces, with levels of PROTO exceeding those of COPRO and COPRO III levels higher than COPRO I levels. Porphyrin–protein complexes specific for VP (X-porphyrins) are present in plasma.[5] During acute attacks, urinary ALA and PBG excretion is increased; however, in asymptomatic subjects, the excretion is often normal.

EPP, the second most common porphyria, results from a deficiency of ferrochelatase (FECH), the last enzyme in the heme pathway. The FECH gene is located on the long (q) arm of chromosome 18 and more than 110 mutations have been identified in individuals with EPP.[3] The major clinical symptom is photosensitivity, which is usually present from infancy. Patients complain of burning, itching, or pain in the skin on exposure to sunlight. Some patients also have severe liver disease. The diagnosis of EPP is made by demonstrating increased levels of PROTO in erythrocytes, plasma, and stool, along with normal urinary porphyrins or increased COPRO I. High levels of free protoporphyrin (not bound to zinc) in erythrocytes and plasma occur in EPP. Clinical expression of the disease is highly variable. Some individuals have no clinical manifestations of the disease but have increased levels of erythrocyte PROTO. Coinheritance of a second weak mutation of the FECH gene (in addition to the primary mutations detected) may explain the significant individual differences in clinical expression.[3,4]

Treatment of the inherited porphyrias is aimed at modifying the biochemical abnormalities causing clinical symptoms. The cutaneous symptoms are treated by avoiding sunlight, using sun-blocking agents, and using oral beta-carotene, which acts as a singlet oxygen trap, preventing skin damage. Reduction of the heme load can be accomplished by phlebotomy or by giving desferrioxamine to chelate iron. Intravenous hematin may be used to counteract acute attacks of neurologic dysfunction. Hematin, an enzyme inhibitor, limits the synthesis of porphyrins in cells in the bone marrow. Cessation of precipitating factors, such as ingestion of alcohol or estrogens, should be the first line of PCT treatment.[10] Gene therapy (adding the normal gene to a patient's bone marrow stem cells, such as addition of the normal FECH gene to an EPP patient's cells) appears to be a feasible future treatment of porphyrias.[10]

The term *secondary porphyrias*, or porphyrinurias, is given to acquired conditions in which a mild to moderate increase in the excretion of urinary porphyrins is seen. In this case, the disorders are not the result of an inherited biochemical defect in heme synthesis but a result of another disorder, toxin, or drug interfering with heme synthesis. Symptoms may be similar to the inherited porphyrias in some cases. Various anemias, liver diseases, and toxins, such as lead and alcohol, fit into this category. Lead is known to inhibit both the activity of ALAD and the incorporation of iron into heme. Secondary porphyrias can be distinguished from true porphyrias by measuring levels of urinary ALA and PBG. In secondary porphyria, ALA levels are increased in the urine, whereas PBG excretion usually remains normal. Lead poisoning also classically exhibits increased COPRO in the urine and erythrocyte ZPP, as well as increased ALA. However, determination of blood lead is the most accurate method to detect lead poisoning.

CASE STUDY 19-1

A 58-year-old man with a history of alcoholism complained of increased skin fragility and skin lesion formation on his hands, forehead, neck, and ears on exposure to the sun. Also noted on physical examination were hyperpigmentation and hypertrichosis. Laboratory findings showed an increase in urinary uroporphyrin and a slight increase in coproporphyrin, with normal levels of ALA and porphobilinogen. Isocoproporphyrin was elevated in the feces. Serum ferritin and serum transaminase were increased. Erythrocyte ZPP and FEP levels were normal.

Questions

1. What is the most probable disorder?

2. What confirmatory test should be done?

3. What is the most probable precipitating factor?

4. What are other causes of acquired cases of this type of porphyria?

5. How is this case differentiated from the homozygous deficiency of this enzyme?

6. How is this type of porphyria differentiated from other porphyrias causing cutaneous symptoms?

Methods of Analyzing Porphyrins

There are individual enzyme assays available for each defective enzyme that causes porphyria. These procedures typically include addition of substrate under conditions close to physiologic pH and temperature, cessation of the reaction by addition of protein-precipitating agents, and separation (usually by high-performance liquid chromatography [HPLC] or ion-exchange chromatography), followed by fluorometric identification and quantitation of porphyrin products.[5] However, most are still limited to use in specialized laboratories and are not discussed here. Screening tests can be performed easily and may be beneficial in emergency situations, but care should be taken in interpretation because false negatives and false positives occur.[11,12] Quantitative assays should follow all screening tests. Quantitative assays of the three porphyrins (URO, PROTO, and COPRO) and two porphyrin precursors (ALA and PBG) will serve to classify most porphyrias. The complexity of testing and interpretation of test results is illustrated by the fact that the American Porphyria Foundation web site (www.porphyriafoundation.com) contains a short list of laboratories with the following comment: "There are only a few laboratories in the United States that can perform the complex analysis to diagnose Porphyria."

CASE STUDY 19-2

A few days after a laparotomy for "intestinal obstruction," a young nurse from South Africa became emotionally disturbed and appeared to be hysterical. For longer than 1 week before the operation, she had taken barbiturate capsules to help her sleep. When first seen, she complained of severe abdominal and muscle pain and general weakness. Her tendon reflexes were absent, and she was vomiting and constipated. Her urine was dark in color on standing and gave a brilliant pink fluorescence when viewed in ultraviolet light. Within 24 hours, she was completely paralyzed, and within 2 days she died.

Questions

1. What possible condition did this young woman have, and why did it manifest at this time?

2. Would any members of her family have a similar disease?

3. What enzyme defect did she have?

4. What other confirmatory tests, if any, could be done?

Tests for Urinary PBG and ALA

The two most common screening tests for urinary PBG are the Watson-Schwartz and the Hoesch tests.[4,13] Ideally, these screening tests should be quantitative and not qualitative. Both tests are based on the principle of PBG forming a red-orange color when mixed with Ehrlich's reagent (acidic *p*-dimethylaminobenzaldehyde). In the Watson-Schwartz test, an extraction with chloroform or butanol is performed to differentiate PBG from interfering substances such as urobilinogen or indole. If a cherry-red color remains in the aqueous phase after addition of chloroform or butanol, this indicates a positive test for PBG. The reagent in the Hoesch test does not react with urobilinogen; therefore, it is sometimes used to confirm the results of the Watson-Schwartz test. PBG and ALA are determined quantitatively by successive separation on two ion-exchange columns.[4] An aliquot of urine is loaded on an anion-exchange or alumina column that retains PBG while ALA passes through. Following washes to remove interfering substances, PBG is eluted with acetic acid and measured spectrophotometrically using Ehrlich's reagent. The eluate from the first column is loaded on a cation-exchange column to retain ALA and then eluted with sodium acetate. The eluted ALA is reacted with Ehrlich's reagent after first being condensed with acetylacetone to form a pyrrole and then measured spectrophotometrically.[5]

Tests for Porphyrins

Screening and quantitative tests for porphyrins in urine, blood (erythrocytes and plasma), and feces are based on the enhanced fluorescence of these compounds in acidic solution. Typically, an aliquot of specimen is extracted into an organic solvent and then back-extracted into an acidified aqueous layer. For screening procedures, samples containing porphyrins will exhibit a pink or red fluorescence in the aqueous layer when viewed under a Wood's (ultraviolet) lamp. Quantitative procedures include fluorometric measurements usually at an excitation wavelength of 400 to 405 nm and an emission wavelength of 594 to 598 nm. Standard solutions of coproporphyrin, uroporphyrin, and, possibly, protoporphyrin are used to calculate the porphyrin concentrations in the samples. Each porphyrin exhibits different excitation and emission wavelengths (solvent dependent) and some procedures use average wavelengths, whereas other procedures include multiple measurements and calculation of levels of each porphyrin. To verify positive results and eliminate possible interferences, fluorescence scan with comparison to scans of standards is recommended. Fluorometric procedures are more sensitive than those measuring the absorbance of porphyrins.

Other tests for porphyrins use chromatographic separation and quantitation of the individual porphyrins with spectrophotometry or fluorometry. Reversed-phase HPLC and ion-exchange chromatography are common methods for separating porphyrins. Capillary zone electrophoresis (CZE), which separates compounds based on charge/mass ratio (modified by pH adjustment), is another chromatographic technique used for quantitation of porphyrins. This technique is as sensitive as HPLC with fluorescence detection and has the advantages of simpler instrumentation, minimum use of organic solvent, and lower reagent consumption.[5]

Zinc protoporphyrin, a normal metabolite formed by the chelation of zinc instead of iron with protoporphyrin during heme biosynthesis, is another porphyrin that may be measured. Increased zinc protoporphyrin formation occurs during periods of iron insufficiency or impaired iron use. Clinically, ZPP has been advocated as a valuable test for evaluating iron nutrition and metabolism in various settings, including pediatrics, obstetrics, and blood banking, as well as a screening test for iron deficiency anemia and lead exposure in adults.[14] A rapid screening method for determination of ZPP includes measurement of the fluorescence of whole blood and washed erythrocytes using a hematofluorometer. It is recommended that ZPP concentrations be reported as a ratio to the heme concentration (per mole of heme).[14]

Molecular diagnostic techniques are becoming useful in the diagnosis of porphyrias.[4,15] Most of the genes that encode the enzymes of heme synthesis have been identified and mutations, which cause various porphyrias,

have been discovered. The use of these techniques to aid in the diagnosis of porphyrias has certain advantages over traditional biochemical assays. The interpretation of the traditional tests is complicated by the fact that analytes being measured may be normal except during an acute attack, and the amount of porphyrin excreted in the various disorders is highly variable, causing significant overlap between affected and normal patients. By testing for the disease-causing mutation, these problems of biologic variability and disease activity can be overcome. However, perhaps the most important application of molecular testing is its use in detecting asymptomatic gene carriers, which are not easily identified by standard laboratory testing.[15]

HEMOGLOBIN

Role in the Body

Hemoglobin has many important functions in the body. Its major role is oxygen transport to the tissue and CO_2 transport back to the lungs. The hemoglobin molecule is designed to take up oxygen in areas of high oxygen tension and release oxygen in areas of low oxygen tension. Hemoglobin is carried to all tissues of the body by erythrocytes. Hemoglobin is also one of the major buffering systems of the body.

Structure of Hemoglobin

Hemoglobin is a large, complex protein molecule with a molecular weight of approximately 68,000 daltons. It is roughly spherical in shape and comprises two major parts: heme, which makes up 3% of the molecule, and globin proteins, which make up the remaining 97%. The heme portion comprises a porphyrin ring with iron chelated in the center. The iron atom is the site of reversible oxygen attachment. The protein portion comprises two pairs of globin chains that are twisted together so that the heme groups are exposed on the exterior of the molecule (Fig. 19-3). The complete hemoglobin molecule contains four heme groups attached to each of four globin chains and may carry up to four molecules of oxygen. Each globin chain contains 141 or more amino acids.

The structure of each chain is fourfold. The primary structure consists of the individual amino acids and their sequences. Their sequences vary and are the basis of chain nomenclature: α, β, δ, and γ. The secondary structure is the three-dimensional arrangement of the amino acids making up the polypeptide chain. Regions of amino acids may form helixes or a pleated structure. The tertiary structure is a larger fold superimposed on the helical or pleated forms. It represents the position taken by each chain or subunit in three-dimensional space. The quaternary structure represents the relationship of the four subunits to one another, particularly at the points of

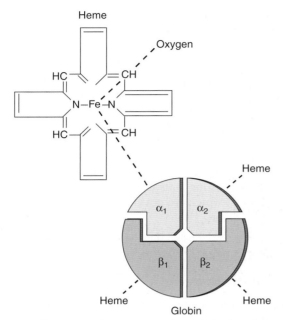

FIGURE 19-3 Hemoglobin A: structure of the hemoglobin molecule.

contact. Mutations at particular points of contact result in altered specific functional properties of the molecule, such as its oxygen affinity.

The majority of hemoglobin in normal adults is designated as hemoglobin A, or A_1, which contains two α and two β chains (Fig. 19-3). Hemoglobin A_2, which comprises two α and two δ chains, makes up less than 3% of normal adult hemoglobin. The remainder is composed of hemoglobin F, which contains two α and two γ chains. Two types of γ chains may be present in hemoglobin F, $γ^G$ and $γ^A$. These two types of chains are functionally identical but differ in the amino acid present at the 136th position, glycine or alanine, respectively. Hemoglobin F is the main hemoglobin during fetal life and is about 60% of normal hemoglobin at birth. There is a gradual switch from production of γ chains to β chains, and by about age 9 months, hemoglobin F usually constitutes less than 1% of total hemoglobin. Hemoglobin F has a greater affinity for oxygen than hemoglobin A; therefore, it is a more efficient oxygen carrier for the fetus. Hemoglobin F is more resistant to alkali than hemoglobin A, and this is the basis of one laboratory test to differentiate these two types of hemoglobin.

Two other hemoglobin chains, designated ζ and ε, are present only in embryonic life. Production of these chains stops by week 8 of gestation, and γ chain production takes over. The three embryonic hemoglobins are identified as Gower I, two ζ chains and two ε chains; Gower II, two α chains and two ε chains; and Portland I, two ζ chains and two γ chains.

Genetic control of hemoglobin synthesis occurs in two areas: control of structure and control of rate and quantity of production. Defects in structure produce a group of diseases called the *hemoglobinopathies*. Defects in rate and quantity of production lead to disorders called the *thalassemias*. Structurally, each globin chain has its own genetic locus; therefore, it is the individual chains, not the whole hemoglobin molecule, that are under genetic control. The genes for the globin chains can be divided into two major groups: the α genes, located on chromosome 16, and the non–α genes, located on chromosome 11. In most persons, the α gene locus is duplicated—there are two α chain genes per haploid set of chromosomes, designated $α_1$ and $α_2$. The α gene and, hence, its polypeptide chains are identical in hemoglobins A, A_2, and F. The non–α genes for the β, δ, and γ chains are sufficiently close in genetic terms to be subjected to nonhomologous crossover, with the resulting production of fused or hybrid globin chains, such as hemoglobin Lepore (δβ-globin chain) and Kenya (γβ-globin chain).

Based on the genetics of the globin chain production, the structural abnormalities, or *hemoglobinopathies*, can be divided into four groups:

1. Amino acid substitutions (e.g., hemoglobins S, C, D, E, O, and G)
2. Amino acid deletion—deletions of three or multiples of three nucleotides in deoxyribonucleic acid (DNA; e.g., hemoglobin Gun Hill)
3. Elongated globin chains resulting from chain termination, frame shift, or other mutations (e.g., hemoglobin Constant Spring)
4. Fused or hybrid chains resulting from nonhomologous crossover (e.g., hemoglobins Lepore and Kenya)

The amino acid substitutions are the most common abnormalities, with several hundred described so far. Approximately two-thirds of the hemoglobinopathies have an affected β chain. They may be clinically silent or they may cause severe damage, as with hemoglobin S. Amino acid substitutions, for the majority of defects, result from a single-base nucleotide substitution in DNA.

Absent or diminished synthesis of one of the polypeptide chains of human hemoglobin characterizes the *thalassemias*, a heterogeneous group of inherited disorders. In α-thalassemia, α-globin chain synthesis is absent or reduced; in β-thalassemia, β-globin chain synthesis is absent ($β^0$-thal) or partially reduced ($β^+$-thal).

Synthesis and Degradation of Hemoglobin

Hemoglobin synthesis occurs in the immature red blood cells (RBCs) in the bone marrow: 65% in the nucleated cells and 35% in reticulocytes. Normal synthesis depends on adequate iron supply as well as normal synthesis of

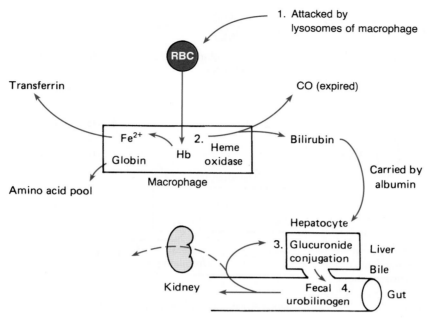

FIGURE 19-4 Extravascular degradation of hemoglobin.

heme and protein synthesis to form the globin portion. Heme is synthesized in the mitochondria of the cells. Iron is transported to the developing RBCs by transferrin, a plasma protein. Iron traverses the cell membrane and the mitochondria, where it is inserted into the PROTO ring to form heme. Protein synthesis of the globin chains occurs in the cytoplasmic polyribosomes. Heme leaves the mitochondria and is joined to the globin chains in the cytoplasm in the final step.

Two possible pathways degrade hemoglobin. The normal pathway is called extravascular because it occurs outside of the circulatory system within the phagocytic cells of the spleen, liver, and bone marrow. Within the splenic phagocytic cells, or macrophages, hemoglobin loses its iron to transferrin, its α carbon is expired as CO, the globin chains return to the amino acid pool, and the rest of the molecule is converted to bilirubin, which undergoes further metabolism. Normally, 80% to 90% of all hemoglobin is degraded in this manner (Fig. 19-4).

Normally, 10% to 20% of erythrocyte destruction occurs intravascularly. Hemoglobin is released directly into the bloodstream and dissociated into α and β dimers. Greater amounts are released during hemolytic episodes. The dimers are bound to haptoglobin, which prevents renal excretion of plasma hemoglobin and stabilizes the heme–globin bond. This complex is then removed from the circulation by the liver and processed in a fashion similar to extravascular degradation. If the amount of circulating haptoglobin is decreased, as during a hemolytic episode, the unbound dimers go through the kidneys and are reabsorbed, and the iron is stored as

hemosiderin. Some hemoglobin dimers may be excreted in the urine, resulting in hemoglobinuria. If the storage limit of the kidneys is exceeded, cells lining the renal tubules may be shed and free hemoglobin, methemoglobin, and/or hemosiderin will appear in the urine.[16]

Hemoglobin that is not entirely bound by haptoglobin or processed by the kidneys is oxidized to methemoglobin. Heme groups are released and taken up by the protein hemopexin. The heme–hemopexin complex is cleared by the liver and catabolized. Then, heme groups present in excess of the binding capacity of the hemopexin complex combine with albumin to form methemalbumin and are held by this protein until additional hemopexin becomes available for shuttle to the liver (Fig. 19-5). Laboratory measurement of any of these hemoglobin degradation products can help to determine increased RBC destruction, such as in a hemolytic anemia.

Clinical Significance and Disease Correlation

Hemoglobin Qualitative Defects: The Hemoglobinopathies

Hemoglobin S

The amino acid defect in hemoglobin S is at the sixth position on the β chain, where glutamic acid is substituted by valine, giving the hemoglobin a less negative charge than hemoglobin A. This is the most common hemoglobinopathy in the United States.

Individuals have either sickle cell trait (HbAS, the heterozygous state) or sickle cell disease (HbSS, the homozygous state). Black Africans and African Americans have

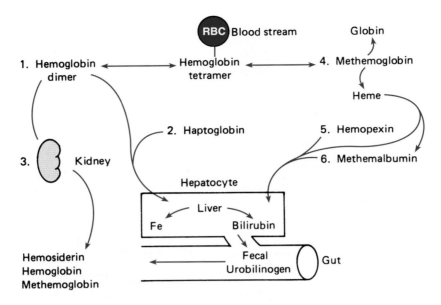

Intravascular Breakdown of Hemoglobin <10%

FIGURE 19-5 Intravascular breakdown of hemoglobin.

CASE STUDY 19-3

A 32-year-old African American woman came to the obstetrics and gynecology clinic of her local hospital because she was feeling a little weak. A CBC showed hemoglobin of 9.9 g/dL (reference range 11.7 to 15.7 g/dL), with an MCV of 87 fL (reference range 80 to 100 fL). The physician ordered a hemoglobin electrophoresis as a follow-up. The cellulose acetate pattern showed a peak of 58% at the hemoglobin A position, a peak of 35% at the hemoglobin S position, and a peak of 5% at the A_2 position. Further studies indicated a positive dithionite solubility test result and a hemoglobin F value of 1%.

Questions

1. What is the best possible diagnosis for this woman?

2. Does this condition require further follow-up and treatment?

3. What implications does this disease have for her unborn child?

4. Are the values for hemoglobins A_2 and F normal for this condition?

Because of the high mortality and morbidity associated with homozygous expression of the gene, the frequency of the mutant gene would be expected to decline in the gene pool. However, a phenomenon known as balanced polymorphism exists, which indicates that the heterozygous state (HbAS) has a selective advantage over either of the homozygous states (HbAA or HbSS). It appears that the heterozygous condition offers protection from parasites, particularly *Plasmodium falciparum*, especially in children. When infected with *P. falciparum*, children with sickle cell trait have a lower parasite count, the infection is shorter in duration, and the incidence of death is low. It is thought that the infected RBCs are preferentially sickled and, therefore, efficiently destroyed by phagocytic cells.[17]

When hemoglobin S is deoxygenated in vitro under near-physiologic conditions, it becomes relatively insoluble as compared with hemoglobin A and aggregates into long, rigid polymers called *tactoids*. These cells appear as sickle- or crescent-shaped forms on stained blood films. Sickled cells may return to their original shape when oxygenated; however, after several sickling episodes, irreversible membrane damage occurs and cells are phagocytized by macrophages in the spleen, liver, or bone marrow, causing anemia. The severity of the hemolytic process is directly related to the number of damaged cells in circulation. The rigid sickled cells are unable to deform and circulate through small capillaries, resulting in blockage. Tissue hypoxia results, causing extreme pain and leading to tissue death. Infarctions in the spleen are common, causing excessive necrosis and scarring, leading to a nonfunctional spleen in most adults with

the highest incidence: 1 of 500 infants have sickle cell anemia and 8% to 10% carry the HbAS trait. It is also found in Mediterranean countries, such as Greece, Italy, and Israel, as well as in Saudi Arabia and India.

sickle cell anemia. This is referred to as *autosplenectomy*. The amount of sickling is related to the amount of hemoglobin S in the cells. The reported inhibitory effect of hemoglobins A and F is due to a dilutional effect. There is also a lower tendency for hemoglobin F to copolymerize with hemoglobin S than with hemoglobin A. This is considered responsible for the observed protective effect of elevated hemoglobin F levels in individuals with sickle cell anemia.

Laboratory findings in the homozygous disease include a normocytic, normochromic anemia, increased reticulocyte count, and variation in size and shape of RBCs with target cells and sickle cells present. Polychromatophilia and nucleated RBCs are common. The heterozygous disease is clinically asymptomatic and usually has a normal blood film. The solubility test for hemoglobin S will be positive in both homozygous and heterozygous forms but should always be confirmed with hemoglobin electrophoresis. On cellulose acetate electrophoresis at an alkaline pH, hemoglobin S moves in a position between hemoglobin A and A_2. Of total hemoglobin, 85% to 100% will be hemoglobin S in the homozygous state and usually less than 50% in the heterozygous state. Hemoglobins D and G migrate in the same position as hemoglobin S, but both would be negative with the solubility test. Electrophoresis on citrate agar at an acid pH is necessary to separate these hemoglobins from hemoglobin S (see Fig. 19-7).

Hemoglobin C

The glutamic acid in the sixth position of the β chain is replaced by lysine, resulting in a net positive charge. Hemoglobin C is found in West Africa in the vicinity of North Ghana in 17% to 28% of the population and in 2% to 3% of African Americans.

The heterozygous form, hemoglobin AC, is asymptomatic. The homozygous form usually causes a mild, well-compensated anemia characterized by abdominal pain and splenomegaly. The most prominent laboratory feature is the presence of target cells. There is a tendency to form large, oblong, hexagonal crystalloid structures within the red cell. These structures are most prominent in patients who have undergone splenectomy.

A differential diagnosis is obtained by cellulose acetate electrophoresis. Hemoglobin C moves with hemoglobin A_2 and is negative with the solubility test. In the heterozygous form, hemoglobin C falls in the range of 35% to 48%. Hemoglobins E, O, and C_{Harlem} migrate with hemoglobin C. These hemoglobin variants can be readily distinguished from hemoglobin C by citrate agar electrophoresis at an acid pH.

Hemoglobin SC

Hemoglobin SC disease is the most common *mixed hemoglobinopathy*. One β gene codes for β-S chains and the other β gene codes for β-C chains, leaving no normal β chains to produce hemoglobin A. Clinically, this disease is less severe than homozygous sickle cell anemia but has similar clinical symptoms. The blood film characteristically shows many target cells and occasional abnormal shapes resembling the sickle cell, the hexagonal hemoglobin C crystal, and a combination of the two. The solubility test is positive, and electrophoresis on cellulose acetate shows about equal amounts of hemoglobin S and hemoglobin C.

Hemoglobin E

Hemoglobin E is an amino acid substitution of lysine for glutamic acid in the 26th position of the β chain, resulting in a net positive charge. Hemoglobin E is somewhat unstable when subjected to oxidizing agents.

Found in Asia, it is estimated to occur in about 20 million individuals, 80% of whom live in Southeast Asia. In the homozygous form, there is a mild anemia with microcytosis and target cells. In the heterozygous form, the patient is asymptomatic. The differential diagnosis is obtained by electrophoresis. On cellulose acetate, hemoglobin E moves with A_2, C, and O. It is present in the heterozygous form in amounts varying from 30% to 45%, which is somewhat lower than the percentage for hemoglobin C. This is probably a result of the somewhat unstable nature of hemoglobin E. On citrate agar, hemoglobin E migrates with A. It is more common to find this defect in association with both α- and β-thalassemia. E-β-thalassemia is a more severe disorder, with moderate anemia and splenomegaly.

Hemoglobin D

The letter D is given to any hemoglobin variant with an electrophoretic mobility on cellulose acetate similar to that of hemoglobin S but that has a negative solubility test. Hemoglobin $D_{Los Angeles}$ and its identical variant, hemoglobin D_{Punjab}, are the most common, with glycine substituted for glutamic acid at the 121st position of the β chain. Hemoglobin D_{Punjab} is found in Northwest India but occasionally can be seen in English, Portuguese, and French individuals because of the close historical connection of these countries with East India. Hemoglobin $D_{Los Angeles}$ is found in 0.02% of African Americans.

The homozygous state is rare. There is a mild anemia and/or splenomegaly and only a slight anisocytosis. The oxygen affinity is higher than in normal blood. Heterozygous individuals are asymptomatic. Differential diagnosis is accomplished with electrophoresis. On cellulose acetate, hemoglobin D migrates with hemoglobin S in proportions of 35% to 50%. On citrate agar, hemoglobin D migrates with A.

Hemoglobin Quantitative Defects: The Thalassemias

The thalassemias are a group of diseases in which a defect causes reduced synthesis of one or more of the hemoglobin chains, but the chains are structurally

CASE STUDY 19-4

A 54-year-old African American woman was admitted to the hospital with the chief complaint of left hip pain and lethargy. She had a long history of multiple emergency department visits for hip pain requiring medication. She previously had been found to have a positive solubility test for hemoglobin S, but denied a history of sickle cell disease. There was family history of sickle cell trait. She had a mastectomy for breast cancer 10 years before. Admission laboratory values were as follows:

		REFERENCE RANGE
Hemoglobin	5.3 g/dL	11.7–15.7 g/dL
Hematocrit	17%	35–47%
MCV	82 fL	80–100 fL
MCHC	31%	32–36%
WBC	12.0×10^9/L	$3.5–11.0 \times 10^9$/L
Platelet count	53.0×10^9/L	$150–440 \times 10^9$/L
Differential	Normal	
Reticulocyte count	6.4% (corrected, 2.4%)	0.5–1.5%
RBC morphology	Target cells; spherocytes; schistocytes; basophilic stippling; and bizarre forms, including elongated, block-shaped, and more densely stained cells	

A hemoglobin electrophoresis was ordered. Patterns from the cellulose acetate and citrate agar electrophoresis are shown in Case Study Figure 19-4.1. Chest x-ray showed a right lower lobe infiltrate with pulmonary vascular congestion and an enlarged spleen. Fluid aspirated from the nasogastric tube was positive for blood.

The patient was given medication for an aspiration pneumonia, gastrointestinal bleeding, and congestive heart failure. She was given packed RBCs; fresh, frozen plasma; and platelets, but her condition continued to worsen. Six hours later, laboratory tests confirmed disseminated intravascular coagulation. A bone marrow biopsy was performed and revealed extensive necrosis of marrow elements. Three hours later, the patient died of cardiac arrest.

Questions

1. What hemoglobinopathy is indicated by the hemoglobin electrophoresis patterns?

2. What clinical feature of this disease differs from the typical picture in sickle cell anemia?

3. What other hemoglobins interact with hemoglobin S, and how can these be differentiated from hemoglobin C?

4. Was this patient's death due to the hemoglobinopathy? Is it unusual for hemoglobin SC to be life shortening?

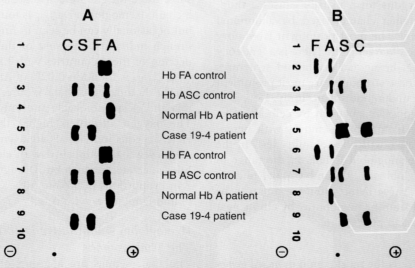

FIGURE 19-4.1 Hemoglobin electrophoretic patterns. (A) Cellulose acetate at pH 8.4. (B) Citrate agar at pH 6.2. • = origin (Case study data courtesy of Margaret Uthman, MD, University of Texas Medical School at Houston.)

normal. Interaction among a large number of different molecular defects is the cause for decreased or absent globin chain synthesis.[18] The two most common types are α-thalassemia, resulting from defective production of α chains, and β-thalassemia, resulting from a defect in the production of β chains. Defects in the production of the δ and γ chains have been described, but these are not involved in the production of hemoglobin A and are, therefore, not clinically significant. Rarely, combinations of gene deletions, such as δ and β, may lead to clinical disease. Any form of unbalanced production of globin chains causes the erythrocytes to be small, hypochromic, and sometimes deformed. Intracellular accumulation of unmatched chains in the developing erythrocytes causes precipitation of the proteins, which leads to cell destruction in the bone marrow. Although erythropoiesis is occurring, it is ineffective because mature cells do not reach the peripheral blood to carry oxygen.

Thalassemia is inherited as an autosomal dominant disorder with heterogeneous expression of the disease. One of the most common hereditary disorders, it is distributed worldwide. The prevalence of the thalassemia gene has been attributed to the protection it offers against falciparum malaria. The heterozygous state produces a disorder called *thalassemia minor*, which is clinically asymptomatic and resembles iron deficiency. The homozygous state, *thalassemia major*, is usually lethal before birth or in childhood. Early and continuous treatment of some forms of the disease allows survival to young adulthood, but complications are many.

α-Thalassemias

Two α genes are located on each chromosome 16, one inherited from the mother and one from the father, yielding a total of four α genes. There are four principal clinical types of different severity known to occur in the population, and these four types can be explained, respectively, by deletions of four, three, two, or one of the α-globin gene loci (Fig. 19-6). α-Thalassemia occurs with high frequency in Asian populations, but is also seen in the Black African, African American, Indian, and Middle Eastern populations. The type of α-thalassemia found in Black Africans and African Americans is also associated with deletion of the α-globin genes but in a different pattern than is found in the Asian population (Fig. 19-6). The four clinical types of α-thalassemia in order of most deletions to least deletions are the following:

1. Hydrops fetalis is the most clinically severe form of α-thalassemia because of the total absence of α chain synthesis. Hemoglobin Bart's, which is a tetramer of γ chains, is the main hemoglobin found in the red cells of affected infants. Hemoglobin Bart's has an extremely high O_2 affinity and allows almost no oxygen transport to the tissue. These infants are either stillborn or die of hypoxia shortly after birth.

Thalassemias

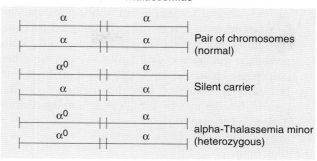

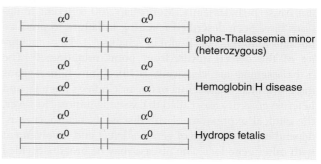

α = Normal a gene locus α^0 = Deleted a gene locus

FIGURE 19-6 Deletions of α-globin gene loci on chromosome 16 in α-thalassemia.

2. Hemoglobin H disease has α chain synthesis at about one-third the amount of β chain synthesis. As a result, β chains accumulate and form tetramers, which are called *hemoglobin H*. β chain precipitates (hemoglobin H inclusions) alter the shape and ability of the cell to deform, significantly shortening the life span of the cells. These individuals have a moderate hemolytic anemia, with 5% to 30% hemoglobin H, 1% hemoglobin A_2, and the remainder hemoglobin A. Hemoglobin H inclusions can be seen in the red cells with a supravital stain. Cord blood contains 10% to 20% hemoglobin Bart's.

3. α-Thalassemia trait results from two gene deletions, either on the same (—/αα) or on different chromosomes (–α/–α). The deletion on two separate chromosomes is more common in Black Africans and African Americans (Fig. 19-6). These individuals have a mild, microcytic, hypochromic anemia. Occasionally, excess β chains may form hemoglobin H inclusions. Cord blood contains 2% to 10% hemoglobin Bart's; however, after age 3 months, electrophoresis is normal.

4. Silent carriers are missing only one α gene, and the remaining genes direct production of sufficient α chains for normal hemoglobin production. This state is often characterized by expression of 1% to 2% of hemoglobin Bart's in a neonate. If hemoglobin Bart's

is not detected in a neonate or prior to 3 months of age by standard testing, it can only be detected by by standard testing, it can only be detected by more specialized testing, such as gene mapping, α:β-globin messenger ribonucleic acid (mRNA) ratio, or other polymerase chain reaction (PCR)–based methods.[18,19] It has been estimated that the frequency of this genetic disorder may be as high as 27% in the African American population.[18]

β-Thalassemias

In contrast to α-thalassemia, gene deletions usually do not cause β-thalassemia. More than 200 different mutations have been described resulting in failure to produce normal amounts of β-globin chains. A large majority of the defects result from point mutations.[18] The β-thalassemias are classically divided into homozygous disease, called thalassemia major or Cooley's anemia, and heterozygous disease, called thalassemia minor. However, the clinical expression of the disease is heterogeneous, depending on the type of genetic defect and involvement with other gene loci. The disease may be broadly divided into two major subtypes according to genetic expression: β^+, in which β chains are produced in reduced amounts, and β^0, which is complete absence of β chains.

β^+-Thalassemia is the most common type. There is some synthesis of β-globin chains but in significantly reduced amounts (5% to 30%) of normal. The biochemical defect shows a quantitative deficiency of β-globin mRNA. The hemoglobin electrophoresis pattern and hemoglobin F and A_2 quantitation show about 2% to 8% hemoglobin A_2, an elevated but varying amount of hemoglobin F, and the remainder hemoglobin A. The mean cell volume (MCV) is low, with severe anemia, reticulocytes, nucleated RBCs, basophilic stippling, target cells, extreme poikilocytosis, and anisocytosis.

β^0-Thalassemia accounts for 10% of homozygous β-thalassemia, with a total absence of β chain synthesis but intact synthesis of γ chains. In the homozygous form, there is 1% to 6% hemoglobin A_2 and 95% hemoglobin F. The hemoglobin concentration is low, with a severe anemia. The heterozygous form appears clinically the same as homozygous β^+-thalassemia.

Homozygous β-thalassemia—β-thalassemia major— either β^+ or β^0, is a crippling disease of childhood. This is unlike α-thalassemia, in which the child either dies shortly after birth or leads a normal life. The hypochromic, microcytic anemia is a result of both the defect of functional hemoglobin tetramer synthesis and the premature destruction of RBCs, both intramedullary and extramedullary, due to increased α chains. The bone marrow compensates by enormously expanding in size, sometimes causing structural bone abnormalities. Treatment of severe forms of the disease include regular transfusion therapy, iron chelation drugs to remove excess iron, and folic acid supplements.[20] Bone marrow transplantation has been successful if an HLA-identical donor is available.[18] Gene therapy is being studied as an alternative treatment of the future.[21-23]

Heterozygous β-thalassemia—thalassemia minor— may be caused by inheritance of one thalassemia gene, either β^+ or β^0. The other gene directing β chain production is normal and RBC survival is not shortened. About 1% of African Americans are affected and it also commonly occurs in individuals of Mediterranean and Arabic descent. Clinically, the condition is usually asymptomatic but may sometimes cause a mild microcytic anemia. The hematologic laboratory values resemble those of iron deficiency anemia, and it is important to distinguish the two because quite different treatments are required. The RBC count in thalassemia minor is usually higher than would be expected with the accompanying hemoglobin concentration, and a few target cells or occasional basophilic stippling may be seen on a stained smear. The red cell distribution width (RDW) parameter on automated instruments, which is a quantitative measure of RBC variation in size, may be helpful to distinguish the two disorders. It is typically normal in thalassemia and increased in iron deficiency as a result of the heterogeneity of the RBCs. Hemoglobin electrophoresis of thalassemia minor characteristically shows an increase in hemoglobin A_2. Quantitation of hemoglobin A_2 by column chromatography usually reveals values between 3.5% and 7%.

δ-β-thalassemia is a rare type characterized by total absence of both β chain synthesis of hemoglobin A and δ chain synthesis of hemoglobin A_2. Homozygous patients have 100% hemoglobin F. Heterozygous individuals usually have less than 90% hemoglobin A, 2–3% hemoglobin A_2 and 5–20% hemoglobin F.

Patients are anemic and show a thalassemic phenotype because the γ chain synthesis of hemoglobin F is not equal to α chain synthesis. There is approximately one-third as much γ chain produced as α chain. Hemoglobin F is heterogeneously distributed among the erythrocytes, as revealed by the acid elution stain procedure.

Hereditary persistence of fetal hemoglobin (HPFH) is genetically and hematologically heterogeneous. In African Blacks and African Americans, there is a total absence of β as well as δ chain synthesis because of deletions in chromosome 11. γ chain synthesis is present in the adult at a high level and, in contrast to synthesis of hemoglobin F in β-thalassemia or δ-β-thalassemia, is uniformly distributed. In heterozygotes, there is no imbalance of globin chain synthesis. There is 17% to 33% hemoglobin F. The patients are clinically normal. In homozygotes, there is 100% hemoglobin F, with no synthesis of hemoglobin A or A_2.

There are no significant hematologic abnormalities, other than erythrocytosis, and these patients are also asymptomatic.

Methodology

Most hemoglobinopathies and thalassemias can be diagnosed by use of the complete blood count (CBC), blood film evaluation, solubility test, and cellulose acetate electrophoresis. Citrate agar electrophoresis may be necessary for confirmation of some abnormal hemoglobins. Thalassemias may require quantitation of hemoglobin A_2 or F by more definitive methods. A serum ferritin may be helpful to distinguish thalassemia minor from iron deficiency anemia. Hemoglobinopathies may also be

diagnosed rapidly and accurately using newer automated techniques such as HPLC and isoelectric focusing.[24] The more complicated cases may require more specialized procedures, such as α/β-globin chain analysis,[25] cation-exchange HPLC,[25,26] or DNA technology testing.[25-27]

Solubility Test (Screening Test for Sickling Hemoglobins)

The solubility test is based on the principle that sickling hemoglobin, in the deoxygenated state, is relatively insoluble and forms a precipitate when placed in a high-molarity phosphate buffer solution.[27,28] The precipitate appears because the deoxygenated hemoglobin molecules form tactoids that refract and deflect light rays, producing a turbid solution. A small amount of packed RBCs is

CASE STUDY 19-5

A 5-year-old white boy was seen by a physician for an upper respiratory tract infection and splenomegaly was noted. A CBC was ordered and, subsequently, a hemoglobin electrophoresis. The following were the results:

		REFERENCE RANGE
Hemoglobin	8.5 g/dL	11.7–15.7 g/dL
Hematocrit	27%	35–47%
RBC	4.3×10^{12}/L	$3.8–5.2 \times 10^{12}$/L
MCV	62.3 fL	80–100 fL
MCHC	32.0%	32–36%
RDW	18.5%	11.5–14.5%
Platelet	538×10^9/L	$150–440 \times 10^9$/L
WBC	10.7×10^9/L	$3.5–11.0 \times 10^9$/L
Reticulocyte count	5.6%	0.5–1.5%
WBC differential	Normal except for 1 nucleated RBC/100 WBCs	
RBC morphology	Moderate anisocytosis, moderate microcytosis, slight polychromasia, slight target cells, slight schistocytes	

Hemoglobin electrophoresis (cellulose acetate)

Hemoglobin C   89%

Hemoglobin F   11%

A hemoglobin electrophoresis by citrate agar method confirmed hemoglobins C and F. Hemoglobin F was determined by the alkali denaturation method to be 7.5%. Hemoglobin A_2 could not be quantitated due to the presence of hemoglobin C. The patient's father had been previously told that he was slightly anemic due to a blood disorder called thalassemia. The patient's mother and four older siblings were healthy and unaware of any abnormal hemoglobin.

Questions

1. What combination of disorders did the patient most probably inherit?

2. Why were the mother and the other siblings unaware of an abnormality?

3. Why was the patient unable to produce hemoglobin A?

4. What caused the discrepancy in values for hemoglobin F from electrophoresis and the alkali denaturation test?

5. Why was it unusual to find hemoglobin C in a white family?

placed in a buffered solution of sodium dithionite with saponin to lyse the RBCs in a 12×75 mm glass tube. After mixing well and incubating at room temperature for 5 minutes, the tube containing the solution is placed approximately 1 in. in front of a heavy, black-lined index card. If there is no sickling hemoglobin present, the lines on the card will be easily seen. If sickling hemoglobin is present, the lines will be indistinct or impossible to read. The test is reported as positive or negative for sickling hemoglobin. A positive and a negative control should be run with each test batch.

Outdated reagents and reagents not at room temperature interfere with the test. False-negative tests may be due to anemia or recent transfusions or may occur in infants younger than age 6 months because of high concentrations of hemoglobin F. If whole blood is used instead of packed RBCs, false-positive results may occur due to erythrocytosis, hyperglobulinemia, extreme leukocytosis, or hyperlipidemia and false-negative results may occur in anemia. This test does not differentiate between the homozygous and heterozygous presence of hemoglobin S, and other rare sickling variants, such as hemoglobin C_{Harlem}, may give a positive test. Commonly used as a screening test for sickling hemoglobin in adults, this test may also be used as a confirmatory test for sickling hemoglobin after initial evaluation with cellulose acetate electrophoresis.

Cellulose Acetate Hemoglobin Electrophoresis

A fresh hemolysate made from a packed RBC sample is applied to a cellulose acetate plate using a buffer of alkaline pH (8.4 to 8.6) and electrophoresis is performed.[28-30] After electrophoresis, the membrane is stained and cleared. The patient's hemoglobin migration is compared with that of a control for test interpretation. A rough estimate of proportions of different hemoglobins may be made using a densitometer.

The order of electrophoretic mobility, from slowest to fastest, is hemoglobins C, S, F, and A (Fig. 19-7). (There are several mnemonic devices for remembering the migration pattern, such as **A**ccelerated, **F**ast, **S**low, and **C**rawl.) Hemoglobin that migrates beyond hemoglobin A is termed *fast hemoglobin*. Hemoglobin Bart's and hemoglobin H both migrate here. Any abnormal hemoglobin or any normal hemoglobin present in increased amounts, such as hemoglobin A_2 and F, should be confirmed. If there is abnormal hemoglobin, confirm with citrate agar electrophoresis and solubility test if hemoglobin S is suspected. If an increased amount of A_2 or F occurs, then quantify the amount. Hemoglobin D and G comigrate with hemoglobin S in this method.

Universal newborn screening for hemoglobinopathies has become the norm since it was shown that early diagnosis and comprehensive care can reduce morbidity and mortality in infants with sickle cell disease. For

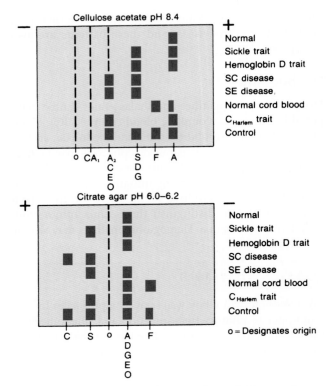

FIGURE 19-7 Comparison of various hemoglobin samples on cellulose acetate and citrate agar.

mass screening, isoelectric focusing and HPLC have replaced cellulose acetate electrophoresis in most cases due to their automation and high throughput.[17]

Citrate Agar Electrophoresis

Citrate agar electrophoresis is performed at an acid pH (6.0 to 6.2) after abnormal hemoglobin is detected on cellulose acetate electrophoresis.[28,31] In this method, an important factor in determining the mobility of hemoglobin is solubility. Hemoglobin F, with the fastest cathodal mobility, is also the most soluble, probably because it is most resistant to denaturation at pH 6.0. Adult hemoglobins with solubility similar to that of hemoglobin A, such as D, E, G, O, and I, move with hemoglobin A. The relatively insoluble hemoglobin S moves behind hemoglobin A, and the even more insoluble hemoglobin C moves behind hemoglobin S (Fig. 19-7).

Hemoglobin A_2 Quantitation

The quantity of hemoglobin A_2 may be estimated by hemoglobin electrophoresis; however, this yields only a rough estimate. Quantitation is best accomplished by microcolumn chromatography[28,32] or HPLC.[25,26,28]

Acid Elution Stain for Hemoglobin F

Erythrocytes containing an increased amount of hemoglobin F can be distinguished from normal adult cells by the acid elution technique.[28,33] This method may be helpful in the diagnosis of HPFH or to detect fetal cells in maternal circulation during problem pregnancies. In the microscopic method, adult hemoglobin, hemoglobin A, is eluted from the erythrocytes by incubation in an acid buffer. Hemoglobin F remains behind and is stained with eosin. Adult cells are negative and have no staining because they contain no hemoglobin F. Fetal RBCs may also be detected by flow cytometric assay methods.[34]

Hemoglobin F Quantitation

Fetal hemoglobin may be quantitated based on the principle that it is resistant to alkali denaturation in 1.25 mol/L NaOH for 2 minutes. Denatured hemoglobin A is precipitated out with ammonium sulfate and removed by filtration. The optical density of the clear supernatant solution is read at 540 nm, and the percentage of fetal hemoglobin is calculated against the optical density of the total hemoglobin solutions.[28] HPLC has been recommended as the method of choice for quantitation of fetal hemoglobin.[26]

The average adult has less than 1.5% fetal hemoglobin. However, elevated levels may be found in several inherited and acquired diseases. The HPFH should be suspected in individuals who possess 10% or more fetal hemoglobin with no other apparent clinical abnormalities.

The importance of accurate quantitation of hemoglobin F may increase in the future due to its use in experimental methods as a cure for hemoglobinopathies and thalassemia syndromes.[24,35] The protective effect of hemoglobin F in sickle cell disease is a main focus of current research for effective therapy. Investigation of the cellular and molecular mechanisms of the fetal to adult (γ to β) switch during the perinatal period and search for antiswitching drugs to maintain high levels of hemoglobin F is promising.[24]

DNA Technology

The definitive diagnosis of some hemoglobinopathies and thalassemias that involve combinations of genetic defects may require DNA analysis. With increased use and efficiency of the PCR technique, the DNA sequence of interest may be easily analyzed from whole blood or spots of dried blood on filter paper. With currently available automated sequencing methods, the time required to perform this type of analysis is not significantly greater than that for standard methodology. Disadvantages of these methods are higher cost and lack of availability in most routine laboratories. The advantages are that it provides definitive information on the genotype of individuals tested, and in some cases, direct detection of the molecular lesions is possible. Specific techniques are discussed elsewhere.[25,27]

A special strength of the DNA technology is in the prenatal diagnosis of thalassemia major. Because the globin genes are represented in all tissue, including those in which they are not active, prenatal diagnosis of thalassemic states may be made by sampling tissue that is relatively easy to obtain, such as chorionic villi or amniotic fluid cells, rather than fetal blood, which is obtained with much greater difficulty and at a much greater risk to the fetus.[27] Two new techniques for analysis of fetal DNA with even lower risk are the isolation of fetal cells from maternal blood by flow cytometry and the use of cell-free fetal DNA from the maternal serum. Maternal DNA molecules are longer than fetal-derived ones, allowing for accurate sepatation.[18,36] DNA technology also has been used in the prenatal diagnosis of sickle cell anemia. Fetal cells obtained by amniocentesis or chorionic villus sampling may be analyzed using similar techniques as in the thalassemias. PCR is the method of choice for prenatal diagnosis, if available.[24] Hemoglobin electrophoresis on a hemolysate of fetal blood cells can also be used in

CASE STUDY 19-6

A 22-year-old white woman of Italian heritage had been told that she was slightly anemic and had been treated with iron periodically throughout her life. She was a student in a clinical laboratory science program and had a CBC performed as a part of a hematology class.

Laboratory values were as follows:

		REFERENCE RANGE
Hemoglobin	11.0 g/dL	11.7–15.7 g/dL
Hematocrit	34%	35–47%
RBC	5.8×10^{12}/L	$3.8–5.2 \times 10^{12}$/L
MCV	59.4 fL	80–100 fL
MCHC	31.9%	32–36%
RDW	14.2%	11.5–14.5%

From these values, the hematology instructor suspected an inherited disorder instead of iron deficiency and suggested that the student contact her physician for further testing. A hemoglobin electrophoresis revealed slightly increased amounts of hemoglobins F and A_2, which were subsequently quantitated to reveal hemoglobin F of 3.2% and hemoglobin A_2 of 4.2%. Iron studies were normal.

Questions

1. What is the most probable disorder?

2. What CBC values caused the instructor to suggest further testing?

3. Why is it important for this disorder to be correctly diagnosed?

cases in which DNA technology is unavailable or when rapid results are needed, owing to a patient's advanced gestational age. Prenatal diagnosis is a major factor in controlling these severe genetic diseases because there is no effective cure at this time, other than HLA-matched allogeneic bone marrow transplant.[36]

MYOGLOBIN

Structure and Role in the Body

Myoglobin is a heme protein found in the skeletal and cardiac muscle. It can reversibly bind oxygen in a manner similar to the hemoglobin molecule; however, myoglobin is unable to release oxygen, except under low oxygen tension. Myoglobin is a simple heme protein containing one polypeptide chain and one heme group per molecule. The polypeptide chain contains 153 amino acids, making it slightly larger than one chain in the hemoglobin molecule. Therefore, its size is slightly larger than one-fourth that of a hemoglobin molecule, with a molecular weight of approximately 17,000. The iron atom in the center of the heme group is the site of reversible oxygen binding, identical to the hemoglobin molecule. In the body, myoglobin acts as an oxygen carrier in the cytoplasm of the muscle cell. Transport of oxygen from the muscle cell membrane to the mitochondria is its main role. Myoglobin serves as an extra reserve of oxygen to help exercising muscle maintain activity longer.

Clinical Significance

Damage to muscles often results in elevated levels of serum and urine myoglobin (Table 19-2). Renal clearance is rapid, and myoglobinemia following a single injury tends to be transient. High concentrations of myoglobin may cause acute renal failure (ARF). Measurement of myoglobin in serum and urine can be used to calculate a myoglobin clearance rate. The combination of a high serum myoglobin (≥400 ng/mL) and a low clearance rate (≤4 mL/min) indicates a high risk of ARF.[37] Myoglobin in urine will cross-react with the hemoglobin test on the dipstick and cause a positive reaction. Confirmation of myoglobinuria by a more specific assay, such as an immunoassay, allows differentiation from hemoglobinuria. Myoglobin measurement in urine or serum may be performed when rhabdomyolysis or any disease/injury resulting in muscle damage is suspected.

Currently the primary use of serum myoglobin testing is in the investigation of chest pain to diagnose or rule out AMI. The combined use of myoglobin and troponin or the MB isoenzyme of creatine kinase (CK-MB) is useful for the early exclusion of AMI.[38] Damaged heart muscle cells release myoglobin within the first few hours of onset of myocardial infarction, and peak values are reached within 2 to 3 hours and as early as 30 minutes. Myoglobin, therefore, is the first cardiac marker to rise, sooner than CK-MB or troponin (T or I). Although an increase of myoglobin in the circulation provides an early indicator of myocardial infarction, false-positive results may occur from any injury to skeletal muscle that also contains myoglobin. The use of myoglobin as an early marker should be followed by use of a definitive marker, such as troponin (T or I), that is more cardiac specific but does not appear in the blood as early. In cases in which thrombolytic therapy is used in the treatment of myocardial infarction, myoglobin levels combined with CK-MB and clinical indications may be used as monitors of reperfusion of the occluded artery.[39] Myoglobin also has been investigated to aid in the diagnosis and differentiation of the different types of hereditary progressive muscular dystrophy.[40] Myoglobin levels in urine are normally not detected or very low. Elevated levels of urine myoglobin indicate an increased risk of renal damage and failure. Myoglobin is discussed in greater detail in Chapter 11.

Methodology

There are several immunoassay methods for measurement and identification of myoglobin. These procedures incorporate the binding of specific antibodies to myoglobin, with a resulting chemical or physical change (e.g., fluorescence, chemiluminescence, and immunochromatic) that can be measured and correlated to myoglobin concentration. These methods have been adapted to point-of-care devices for rapid assessment of chest pain, as well as conventional methods for multianalyte analyzer platforms.[41,42] Although plasma is the specimen of choice for cardiac marker analysis, there is evidence that different anticoagulants have different effects on particular commercial assays for myoglobin.[41] It has also been shown that there are precision and reference range differences between the different myoglobin assays.[41]

TABLE 19-2	CAUSES OF MYOGLOBIN ELEVATIONS	
Acute myocardial	Angina without infarction
Rhabdomyolysis	Multiple fractures; muscle trauma
Renal failure	Myopathies
Vigorous exercise	Intramuscular injections
Open heart surgery	Tonic–clonic seizures
Electric shock	Arterial thrombosis
Certain toxins	Malignant hyperthermia
Muscular dystrophy	Systemic lupus erythematosus

For additional student resources please visit thePoint at **http://thepoint.lww.com.**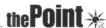

QUESTIONS

1. The main purpose of porphyrins in the body is to
   a. Contribute to the synthesis of heme
   b. Carry oxygen to the tissue
   c. Transport iron
   d. Combine with free hemoglobin

2. The two main sites in the body for accumulation of excess porphyrins are
   a. Liver and bone marrow
   b. Heart and lung
   c. Muscle and blood
   d. Liver and spleen

3. The two main classes of porphyrias, according to symptoms, are
   a. Neurologic and cutaneous
   b. Erythropoietic and hepatic
   c. Congenital and acquired
   d. Hematologic and muscular

4. Porphobilinogen is most commonly quantitated in the urine by
   a. Ion-exchange column
   b. The Watson-Schwartz method
   c. Thin-layer chromatography
   d. Electrophoresis

5. Extremely high levels of ALA and PBG in the urine with normal porphyrin levels in the feces and blood most likely indicate
   a. Acute intermittent porphyria (AIP)
   b. Erythropoietic porphyria (EP)
   c. Hereditary coproporphyria (HCP)
   d. Porphyria cutanea tarda (PCT)

6. Inherited disorders in which a genetic defect causes abnormalities in rate and quantity of synthesis of structurally normal polypeptide chains of the hemoglobin molecule are called
   a. Thalassemias
   b. Hemoglobinopathies
   c. Porphyrias
   d. Molecular dyscrasias

7. Increased intravascular hemolysis is indicated by a decrease in
   a. Haptoglobin
   b. Methemoglobin
   c. Methemalbumin
   d. Hemopexin

8. Which of the following abnormal hemoglobins, found frequently in individuals from Southeast Asia, migrates with hemoglobin A_2 on cellulose acetate electrophoresis?
   a. Hemoglobin E
   b. Hemoglobin D
   c. Hemoglobin C
   d. Hemoglobin Lepore

9. Which type of alpha-thalassemia results from deletion of three genes and produces a moderate hemolytic anemia?
   a. Hemoglobin H disease
   b. Hemoglobin Bart's
   c. Hydrops fetalis
   d. Thalassemia trait

10. The most effective way to quantitate hemoglobin A_2 is by
    a. Column chromatography
    b. Densitometry
    c. Citrate agar electrophoresis
    d. Alkali denaturation test

11. Serum or plasma myoglobin levels are used as
    a. An early marker of acute myocardial infarction
    b. Liver function tests
    c. Lead poisoning indicator
    d. Indicator of congestive heart failure

12. Which of the following is the best test to differentiate beta-thalassemia minor from iron deficiency anemia?
    a. Hemoglobin A_2 quantitation
    b. Hemoglobin electrophoresis (cellulose acetate, alkaline pH)
    c. Solubility test
    d. Complete blood count

13. Which is the correct sequence of electrophoretic migration of hemoglobins from slowest to fastest on cellulose acetate at an alkaline pH?
    a. C, S, F, A
    b. C, A, S, F
    c. C, S, A, F
    d. A, F, S, C

14. The primary route(s) of excretion for protoporphyrin (PROTO), uroporphyrin (URO), and coproporphyrin (COPRO) are
    a. URO is excreted primarily in the urine, PROTO in the feces, and COPRO in either.

b. URO is excreted primarily in the feces, PROTO in the urine, and COPRO in either.

c. URO is excreted primarily in the urine, PROTO and COPRO in the feces.

d. URO is excreted primarily in the feces, PROTO and COPRO in urine.

15. Control of the rate of heme synthesis in the liver cells is achieved largely through regulation of the enzyme
    a. ALA synthase
    b. ALA dehydratase
    c. PBG deaminase
    d. Ferrochelatase

16. The two main sites of production of heme are
    a. Liver and bone marrow
    b. Heart and lung
    c. Muscle and blood
    d. Liver and spleen

17. The relationship between precursors in the heme synthesis pathway and the type of porphyria resulting from excess buildup of these precursors is
    a. Excess of early precursors causes neurologic porphyrias and excess of late precursors causes cutaneous porphyrias.
    b. Excess of early precursors causes cutaneous porphyrias and excess of late precursors causes neurologic porphyrias.
    c. Excess of early precursors causes both neurologic and cutaneous porphyrias, whereas excess of late precursors causes only cutaneous porphyrias.
    d. Excess of early precursors causes both neurologic and cutaneous porphyrias whereas excess of late precursors causes only neurologic porphyrias.

18. Secondary porphyrias not due to an inherited biochemical defect in heme synthesis can be distinguished from true porphyrias by measuring levels of
    a. Urinary ALA and PBG
    b. Urinary COPRO and blood lead

c. Urinary URO and COPRO
d. Fecal URO and urinary COPRO

19. Which hemoglobin is resistant to alkali denaturation in NaOH?
    a. Hb F
    b. Hb A
    c. Hb C
    d. Hb S

20. A patient has an abnormal hemoglobin band that migrates with Hb S on cellulose acetate (pH 8.4) hemoglobin electrophoresis. The solubility test is negative. What test should be performed next?
    a. Citrate agar (pH 6.2) electrophoresis
    b. HbA$_2$ quantitation
    c. Acid elution stain
    d. Blood film evaluation

21. Silent carriers of alpha-thalassemia are missing how many alpha genes?
    a. 1
    b. 2
    c. 3
    d. 4

22. Which hemoglobin contains four gamma chains and has an extremely high affinity for oxygen?
    a. Hb Barts
    b. Hb Gower I
    c. Hb Portland I
    d. Hb F

23. A patient with Southeast Asian heritage is found to have a mild microcytic anemia and a few target cells. Hemoglobin electrophoresis on cellulose acetate at pH 8.4 reveals a major band that migrates with Hb A$_2$ and no Hb A. On citrate agar electrophoresis, the band travels in the position of Hb A. What is the most probable abnormal hemoglobin present?
    a. Hb E
    b. Hb A
    c. Hb C
    d. Hb D

REFERENCES

1. Deacon AC, Elder GH. Front line tests for the investigation of suspected porphyria. *J Clin Pathol.* 2000;54:500.
2. Maruno M, Furuyama K, Akagi R, et al. Highly heterogenous nature of δ-aminolevulinate dehydratase (ALAD) deficiencies in ALAD porphyria. *Blood.* 2001;97:2972.
3. Genetics Home Reference Web Site. http://ghr.nlm.nih.gov/condition/porphyria. Accessed February 1, 2012.
4. Sassa S, Kappas A. Molecular aspects of the inherited porphyrias. *J Intern Med.* 2000;247:169.
5. Zaider E, Bickers DR. Clinical laboratory methods for diagnosis of the porphyrias. *Clin Dermatol.* 1998;16:277.
6. Nuttall KL. Porphyrins and disorders of porphyrin metabolism. In: Burtis CA, Ashwood ER, eds. *Tietz Fundamentals of Clinical Chemistry.* 4th ed. Philadelphia, PA: WB Saunders; 1996:731.
7. Elder GH. Porphyria cutanea tarda. *Semin Liver Dis.* 1998;18:67.

8. Elder GH. Alcohol intake and porphyria cutanea tarda. *Clin Dermatol.* 1999;17:431.

9. Rich M. Porphyria cutanea tarda. *Postgrad Med.* 1999;105:208.

10. Mathews-Roth MM. Treatment of the cutaneous porphyrias. *Clin Dermatol.* 1998;16:295.

11. Nuttall KL. Porphyrins and disorders of porphyrin metabolism. In: Burtis CA, Ashwood ER, eds. *Tietz Textbook of Clinical Chemistry.* 2nd ed. Philadelphia, PA: WB Saunders; 1994:2073.

12. Buttery JE, Chamberlain BR, Beng CG. A sensitive method of screening for urinary porphobilinogen. *Clin Chem.* 1989;35:2311.

13. Watson CJ, Schwartz S. A simple test for urinary porphobilinogen. *Proc Soc Exp Biol Med.* 1941;47:393.

14. Labbe RF, Vreman HJ, Stevenson DK. Zinc protoporphyrin: a metabolite with a mission. *Clin Chem.* 1999;45:2060.

15. Sassa S. Modern diagnosis and management of the porphyrias. *Br J Haematol.* 2006;135:281.

16. Glader B. Destruction of erythrocytes. In: Greer JP, Foerster J, Rodgers GM, et al., eds. *Wintrobe's Clinical Hematology.* 12th ed. Philadelphia, PA: Wolters Kluwer Health/Lippincott Williams & Wilkins; 2009:161.

17. Wang WC. Sickle cell anemia and other sickling syndromes. In: Greer JP, Foerster J, Rodgers GM, et al., eds. *Wintrobe's Clinical Hematology.* 12th ed. Philadelphia, PA: Wolters Kluwer Health/Lippincott Williams & Wilkins; 2009:1038, 1062-1063.

18. Borgna-Pignatti C, Galanello R. The thalassemias and related disorders: quantitative disorders of hemoglobin synthesis. In: Greer JP, Foerster J, Rodgers GM, et al., eds. *Wintrobe's Clinical Hematology.* 12th ed. Philadelphia, PA: Wolters Kluwer Health/Lippincott Williams & Wilkins; 2009:1083, 1093.

19. Galanello R, Sollaine C, Paglietti E, et al. α-Thalassemia carrier identification by DNA analysis in the screening for thalassemia. *Am J Hematol.* 1998;59:273.

20. Harrison CR. Hemolytic anemias: intracorpuscular defects, IV. Thalassemia. In: Harmening DM, ed. *Clinical Hematology and Fundamentals of Hemostasis.* 4th ed. Philadelphia, PA: FA Davis; 2002:194.

21. Herzog RW, Hagstrom JN. Gene therapy for hereditary hematological disorders. *Am J Pharmacogenomics.* 2001;1:137.

22. Tisdale J, Sadelain M. Toward gene therapy for disorders of globin synthesis. *Semin Hematol.* 2001;38:382.

23. Quek L, Thein SL. Molecular therapies in beta-thalassemia. *Br J Haematol.* 2007;136:353-365.

24. Natarajan K, Townes TM, Kutlar A. Chapter 48. Disorders of hemoglobin structure: sickle cell anemia and related abnormalities. In: Prchal JT, Kaushansky K, Lichtman MA, Kipps TJ, Seligsohn U, eds. *Williams Hematology.* 8th ed. New York, NY: McGraw-Hill; 2010. http://0-www.accessmedicine.com.innopac.lsuhsc.edu/content.aspx?aID=6130552. Accessed January 30, 2012.

25. Tuzmen S, Schecter AN. Genetic diseases of hemoglobin: diagnostic methods for elucidating β-thalassemia mutations. *Blood Rev.* 2001;15:19.

26. Clarke GM, Higgins TN. Laboratory investigation of hemoglobinopathies and thalassemias: review and update. *Clin Chem.* 2000;46:1284.

27. Arcasoy MO, Gallagher PG. Molecular diagnosis of hemoglobinopathies and other red blood cell disorders. *Semin Hematol.* 1999;36:328.

28. Elghetany MT, Davey FR. Erythrocytic disorders. In: Henry JB, ed. *Clinical Diagnosis and Management by Laboratory Methods.* 20th ed. Philadelphia, PA: WB Saunders; 2001:562-563.

29. Briere RO, Golias T, Gatsakis JG. Rapid qualitative and quantitative hemoglobin fractionation. *Am J Clin Pathol.* 1965;44:695.

30. Graham JL, Grunbaum BW. A rapid method for microelectrophoresis and quantitation of hemoglobins on cellulose acetate. *Am J Clin Pathol.* 1963;39:567.

31. Milner PF, Gooden H. Rapid citrate-agar electrophoresis in routine screening for hemoglobinopathies using a simple hemolysate. *Am J Clin Pathol.* 1975;64:58.

32. Huisman THJ, Schroeder WA, Brodie AN, et al. Microchromatography of hemoglobins: II. A simplified procedure for the determination of hemoglobin A$_2$. *J Lab Clin Med.* 1975;86:700.

33. Clayton E, Foster BE, Clayton EP. New stain for fetal erythrocytes in peripheral blood smears. *Obstet Gynecol.* 1970;35:642.

34. Clinical and Laboratory Standards Institute (CLSI). *Fetal Red Cell Detection: Approved Guideline.* Wayne, PA: CLSI; 2001 (Document H52-A).

35. Mosca A, Paleari R, Ivaldi G. The relevance of hemoglobin F measurement in the diagnosis of thalassemias and related hemoglobinopathies. *Clin Biochem.* 2009;42:1798.

36. Harteveld CL, Kleanthous M, Traeger-Synodinos J. Prenatal diagnosis of hemoglobin disorders: present and future strategies. *Clin Biochem.* 2009;42:1768.

37. Wu AH, Laios I, Green S, et al. Immunoassays for serum and urine myoglobin: myoglobin clearance assessed as a risk factor for acute renal failure. *Clin Chem.* May 1994;40(5):796-802.

38. Morrow DA, Cannon CP, Jesse RL, et al. National Academy of Clinical Biochemistry laboratory medicine practice guidelines: clinical characteristics and utilization of biochemical markers in acute coronary syndromes. *Clin Chem.* 2007;53:552.

39. Christenson RH, Azzazy HME. Biochemical markers of the acute coronary syndromes. *Clin Chem.* 1998;44:1855.

40. Poche H, Kattner E, Beckmann R, et al. Hereditary progressive muscular dystrophies: serum myoglobin pattern in patients with different types of muscular dystrophies. *Clin Physiol Biochem.* 1989;7:40.

41. Zaninotto M, Pagani F, Altinier S, et al. Multicenter evaluation of five assays for myoglobin determination. *Clin Chem.* October 2000;46(10):1631-1637.

42. Apple FS, Christenson RH, Valdes R Jr, et al. Simultaneous rapid measurement of whole blood myoglobin, creatine kinase MB, and cardiac troponin I by the triage cardiac panel for detection of myocardial infarction. *Clin Chem.* February 1999;45(2):199-205.

Assessment of Organ System Functions

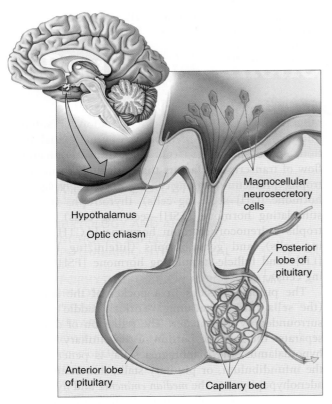

FIGURE 20-1 Relational anatomy of the pituitary and hypothalamus. (Reproduced with permission from Bear MF, Connors BW, Paradiso MA. *Neuroscience: Exploring the Brain.* 2nd ed. Baltimore, MD: Lippincott Williams & Wilkins; 2001:501.)

similar for each specific pituitary hormone and characterized by open-loop negative feedback mechanisms, pulsatility, and cyclicity. Negative feedback resembles a typical servomechanism and forms the basis of our understanding of hypothalamic–pituitary function. An example of negative feedback is the relationship between a thermostat and a home heating unit. The thermostat is set to a given temperature. As the temperature in the home falls below this set point, the thermostat sends an electrical impulse to the furnace and turns the furnace on. Heat is restored to the room and, when the temperature in the room exceeds the predetermined set point, the thermostat turns off the furnace. Because the thermostat set point can be adjusted for the comfort of the occupants, the furnace–thermostat functional relationship is termed an *open-loop negative feedback system*. Most endocrine feedback loops are of the open-loop variety, meaning that they are subject to external modulation and generally influenced or modified by higher neural input or other hormones.

A simple example of an endocrine feedback loop is the hypothalamic–pituitary–thyroidal axis. The hypothalamus produces the hypophysiotropic hormone,

thyrotropin-releasing hormone (TRH), and releases it into the portal system where it directs the thyrotrophs (or TSH-producing cells) in the anterior pituitary to secrete TSH. TSH circulates to the thyroid and stimulates several steps in the thyroid that are critical in the production and release of thyroid hormone (thyroxine). Thyroxine is released in the blood and circulates to the hypothalamus and pituitary to suppress further TRH and TSH production. This axis can be partially inhibited by adrenal steroids (glucocorticoids) and by cytokines; as a result, thyroid hormone production may decline during periods of severe physiologic stress.[4] The feedback of thyroxine at the level of the pituitary is called a *short feedback loop*, and feedback at the level of the hypothalamus is called a *long feedback loop*. Feedback between the pituitary and hypothalamus (when present) is called an *ultrashort feedback loop*. Figure 20-2 illustrates this simple feedback loop.

All anterior pituitary hormones are secreted in a pulsatile fashion. The pulse frequency of secretion is generally regulated by neural modulation and is specific for each hypothalamic–pituitary–end-organ unit. Perhaps the best example of pituitary pulsatility is the secretion of the hormones that regulate gonadal function (LH and FSH). In normal male subjects, the median interpulse interval for LH is 55 minutes, and the average LH peak duration is 40 minutes.[5,6] The pulse frequency of the regulatory hypothalamic hormone, gonadotropin-releasing hormone (GnRH), has profound effects on LH secretion profiles—increasing the frequency of GnRH pulses reduces the gonadotrope secretory response and decreasing the GnRH pulse frequency increases the amplitude of the subsequent LH pulse.[7,8]

Another feature of the hypothalamic–pituitary unit is the cyclic nature of hormone secretion. The nervous system usually regulates this function through external signals, such as light–dark changes or the ratio of daylight

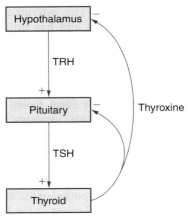

FIGURE 20-2 Simple feedback loop. TRH, thyrotropin-releasing hormone; TSH, thyroid-stimulating hormone.

to darkness. The term *zeitgeber* ("time giver") refers to the process of entraining or synchronizing these external cues into the function of internal biologic clocks. As a result, many pituitary hormones are secreted in different amounts, depending on the time of day. These circadian, or diurnal, rhythms are typified by ACTH, or TSH secretion. With ACTH, the nadir of secretion is between 11:00 P.M. and 3:00 A.M., and the peak occurs on awakening or around 6:00 to 9:00 A.M.[9,10] The circadian rhythm of ACTH is a result of variations in pulse amplitude and not alterations in pulse frequency.[11] The nocturnal levels of TSH are approximately twice the daytime levels, the nocturnal rise in TSH is a result of increased pulse amplitude.[12]

HYPOPHYSIOTROPIC OR HYPOTHALAMIC HORMONES

The hypothalamus produces many different products; however, only those that have a direct effect on classic pituitary function will be discussed in this chapter. Most products are peptides; however, bioactive amines are also synthesized and transported from the hypothalamus. Hypothalamic hormones may have multiple actions. For example, TRH stimulates the secretion of both TSH and prolactin; GnRH stimulates both LH and FSH production; and somatostatin (SS) inhibits GH and TSH release from the pituitary. In addition to its effects on water metabolism, vasopressin (ADH) can also stimulate *ACTH* secretion. The main stimulus for ACTH secretion is corticotropin-releasing hormone. These hypophysiotropic hormones are found throughout the central nervous system and various other tissues, including the gut, pancreas, and other endocrine glands. Their function outside the hypothalamus and pituitary is poorly understood. The action of hypophysiotropic hormones on anterior pituitary function is summarized in Table 20-1.

ANTERIOR PITUITARY HORMONES

The hormones secreted from the anterior pituitary are larger and more complex than those synthesized in the hypothalamus. These pituitary hormones are either *tropic*, meaning their actions are specific for another endocrine gland, or they are direct effectors, because they act directly on peripheral tissue. TSH and its unique role in regulating thyroid function provide an example of tropic; an example of a direct effector is GH. GH has direct effects on substrate metabolism in numerous tissues and also stimulates the liver to produce growth factors that are critical in enhancing linear growth. The tropic hormones are LH, which directs testosterone production from Leydig cells in men and ovulation in women; FSH, which is responsible for ovarian recruitment and early folliculogenesis in women and spermatogenesis in men; TSH, which directs thyroid hormone production from the thyroid; and ACTH, which regulates adrenal steroidogenesis. Both GH and prolactin are direct effectors. A general summary of relationships among anterior pituitary hormones and their target organs and feedback effectors is provided in Table 20-2.

The actions of the tropic hormones are discussed in other chapters devoted to the specific target gland.

PITUITARY TUMORS

According to autopsy studies, up to 20% of people harbor clinically silent pituitary adenomas, and findings consistent with pituitary tumors are observed in 10% to 30% of normal individuals undergoing MRI examinations. In addition, pituitary tumors account for 91% of the lesions removed from carefully selected patients who have undergone transsphenoidal surgery.[13,14] Close medical follow-up is recommended if the incidentally discovered lesion is hormonally silent and is less than 1 cm in diameter. Prolactin-secreting pituitary tumors

TABLE 20-1	HYPOPHYSIOTROPIC HORMONES	
HORMONE	**STRUCTURE**	**ACTION**
TRH	3 amino acids	Releases TSH and prolactin
GnRH	10 amino acids	Releases LH and FSH
CRH	41 amino acids	Releases ACTH
GHRH	44 amino acids	Releases GH
Somatostatin	14 and 28 amino acids	Inhibits GH and TSH release (additional effects on gut and pancreatic function)
Dopamine (prolactin inhibitory factor)	1 amino acid	Inhibits prolactin release

TRH, thyrotropin-releasing hormone; TSH, thyroid-stimulating hormone; GnRH, gonadotropin-releasing hormone; LH, luteinizing hormone; FSH, follicle-stimulating hormone; CRH, corticotropin-releasing hormone; ACTH, adrenocorticotropin hormone; GHRH, growth hormone–releasing hormone.

TABLE 20-2	ANTERIOR PITUITARY HORMONES		
PITUITARY HORMONE	**TARGET GLAND**	**STRUCTURE**	**FEEDBACK HORMONE**
LH	Gonad (tropic)	Dimeric glycoprotein	Sex steroids (E_2/T)
FSH	Gonad (tropic)	Dimeric glycoprotein	Inhibin
TSH	Thyroid (tropic)	Dimeric glycoprotein	Thyroid hormones (T_4/T_3)
ACTH	Adrenal (tropic)	Single peptide derived from POMC	Cortisol
Growth hormone	Multiple (direct effector)	Single peptide	IGF-I
Prolactin	Breast (direct effector)	Single peptide	Unknown

LH, luteinizing hormone; FSH, follicle-stimulating hormone; TSH, thyroid-stimulating hormone; ACTH, adrenocorticotropin hormone; T_4, thyroxine; T_3, triiodothyronine; E_2, estradiol; T, testosterone; POMC, pro-opiomelanocortin; IGF-I, insulin-like growth factor.

are the most common, followed by nonfunctioning or null cell tumors, and tumors that secrete GH, gonadotropins, ACTH, or TSH account for the remainder. The WHO defined "atypical pituitary tumors" as tumors that have an MIB-1 proliferative index greater than 3%, excessive p53 immunoreactivity, and increased mitotic activity.[15,16] Most of these "atypical" tumors are macroadenomas (i.e., >1 cm in diameter) and show invasion into surrounding structures like the cavernous sinuses. They may or may not be hormonally active and, interestingly, tend to stain commonly for GH or ACTH even though they may not produce clinically evident syndromes.[15] MIB-1 is a monoclonal antibody that is used to detect the Ki-67 antigen, a marker of cell proliferation, and a high "proliferation index" suggests higher degree of atypia.[17]

Physiologic enlargement of the pituitary can be seen during puberty and pregnancy. The enlargement seen during pregnancy is due to lactotroph hyperplasia. Thyrotroph and lactotroph or gonadotroph hyperplasia can also be seen in longstanding primary thyroidal or gonadal failure, respectively.

GROWTH HORMONE

The pituitary is vital for normal growth. Growth ceases if the pituitary is removed, and if the hormonal products from other endocrine glands that are acted on by the pituitary are replaced (thyroxine, adrenal steroids, and gonadal steroids), growth is not restored until GH is administered. However, if GH is given in isolation without the other hormones, growth is not promoted. Therefore, it takes complete functioning of the pituitary to establish conditions ripe for growth of the individual. It also takes adequate nutrition, normal levels of insulin, and overall good health to achieve a person's genetic growth potential.

GH, also called *somatotropin*, is structurally related to prolactin and human placental lactogen. A single peptide with two intramolecular disulfide bridges, it belongs to the direct effector class of anterior pituitary hormones. The somatotrophs, pituitary cells that produce GH, comprise over one-third of normal pituitary weight. Release of somatotropin from the pituitary is stimulated by the hypothalamic peptide growth hormone–releasing hormone (GHRH); somatotropin's secretion is inhibited by SS.[18,19] GH is secreted in pulses, with an average interpulse interval of 2 to 3 hours, with the most reproducible peak occurring at the onset of sleep.[20,21] Between these pulses, the level of GH may fall below the detectable limit, resulting in the clinical evaluation of GH deficiency being based on a single, challenging measurement.

No other hypothalamic–hypophyseal system more vividly illustrates the concept of an open-loop paradigm than that seen with GH. The on-and-off functions of GHRH/SS and the basic pattern of secretory pulses of GH are heavily modulated by other factors (Table 20-3).[22]

Actions of GH

GH has many diverse effects on metabolism; it is considered an amphibolic hormone because it directly influences both anabolic and catabolic processes. One major effect of GH is that it allows an individual to effectively transition from a fed state to a fasting state without experiencing a shortage of substrates required for normal intracellular oxidation. GH directly antagonizes the effect of insulin on glucose metabolism, promotes hepatic gluconeogenesis, and stimulates lipolysis.[19,23] From a teleologic viewpoint, this makes perfect sense—enhanced lipolysis provides oxidative substrate for peripheral tissue, such as skeletal muscle, and yet conserves glucose for the central nervous system by stimulating the hepatic delivery of glucose and opposing insulin-mediated glucose disposal. Indeed, GH deficiency in children may be accompanied by hypoglycemia[24,25]; in adults, hypoglycemia may occur if both GH and ACTH are deficient.

The anabolic effects of GH are reflected by enhanced protein synthesis in skeletal muscle and other tissues.

TABLE 20-3	OTHER MODIFIERS OF GROWTH HORMONE SECRETION

STIMULATE GROWTH HORMONE SECRETION	INHIBIT GROWTH HORMONE SECRETION
Sleep	Glucose loading
Exercise	β-Agonists (e.g., epinephrine)
Physiologic stress	α-Blockers (e.g., phentolamine)
Amino acids (e.g., arginine)	Emotional/psychogenic stress
Hypoglycemia	Nutritional deficiencies
Sex steroids (e.g., estradiol)	Insulin deficiency
α-Agonists (e.g., norepinephrine)	Thyroxine deficiency
β-Blockers (e.g., propranolol)	

This is translated into a positive nitrogen balance and phosphate retention.

Although GH has direct effects on many tissues, it also has indirect effects that are mediated by factors that were initially called *somatomedins*. In early experiments, it became apparent that GH supplementation in hypophysectomized animals induced the production of an additional factor that stimulated the incorporation of sulfate into cartilage.[26-31] As this "protein" was purified, it was evident that there was more than one somatomedin, and because of their structural homology to proinsulin, the nomenclature shifted to insulin-like growth factor (IGF).[32,33] For example, somatomedin C, the major growth factor induced by GH, is now IGF-I.[32] IGFs also have cell surface receptors that are distinct from insulin; however, supraphysiologic levels of IGF-II can "bleed" over on the insulin receptor and cause hypoglycemia,[34-36] and hyperinsulinemia can partially activate IGF-I receptors.[37,38] GH stimulates the production of IGF-I from the liver, and as a result, IGF-I becomes a biologic amplifier of GH levels. IGFs are complexed to specific serum *binding proteins* that have been shown to affect the actions of IGFs in multifaceted ways.[39] IGF binding protein 3 (IGFBP-3) is perhaps the best studied member of the IGFBP family. Recently, IGFBPs and specifically IGFBP-3 have been shown to directly play a role in the pathophysiology of several human cancers (this may be independent of IGF-1 and IGF-1 receptor–mediated pathways).[40,41] P53 tumor suppressor gene was recently shown to upregulate active IGFBP-3 secretion, which inhibits IGF-1 signaled mutagenesis, and, thus, inhibits neoplastic cell proliferation.[42] Low levels of IGFBP-3 were positively correlated with higher rates of colorectal cancer risk (in men) in a nested case–control study from the Physicians Health Study cohort.[43]

Testing

As noted above, a single, random measurement of GH is rarely diagnostic. The current testing paradigms for GH are soundly based on the dynamic physiology of the GH axis. For example, circulating levels of IGF-I and, perhaps, IGFBP-3 reasonably integrate the peaks of GH secretion, and elevated levels of both are consistent with a sustained excess of GH.[44] Other conditions, however, notably hepatomas, can be associated with high levels of IGF-I, and levels of IGFBP-3 may be inappropriately normal in some people with active acromegaly.[45] Conversely, low IGF-I levels may reflect inadequate production of GH; however, low IGF levels are also seen in patients with poorly controlled diabetes, malnutrition, or other chronic illnesses.[46,47]

Definitive testing for determining the autonomous production of GH relies upon the normal suppressibility of GH by oral glucose loading.[48-50] This test is performed after an overnight fast, and the patient is given a 100 g oral glucose load. GH is measured at time zero and at 60 and 120 minutes after glucose ingestion. Following oral glucose loading, GH levels are undetectable in normal individuals; however, in patients with acromegaly, GH levels fail to suppress and may even paradoxically rise.

Testing patients for suspected GH deficiency is more complicated. There are several strategies to stimulate GH, and new protocols are currently evolving. Once considered the gold standard, insulin-induced hypoglycemia is being replaced by less uncomfortable testing schemes.[51] Combination infusions of GHRH and the amino acid l-arginine or an infusion of l-arginine coupled with oral l-DOPA are the most widely used.[52] If GH levels rise above 3 to 5 ng/mL, it is unlikely that the patient is GH deficient[51]; however, a lower threshold may be adopted because of improved sensitivity of the newer two-site GH assays.[53] On the other hand, several studies have shown that provocative GH testing may not be necessary in patients with low IGF-1 levels and otherwise documented panhypopituitarism.[46,54]

Acromegaly

Acromegaly results from pathologic or autonomous GH excess and, in the vast majority of patients, is a result of a pituitary tumor. There have been isolated case reports of

CASE STUDY 20-1

A 48-year-old man seeks care for evaluation of muscle weakness, headaches, and excessive sweating. He has poorly controlled hypertension and, on questioning, admits to noticing a gradual increase in both glove and shoe size, as well as a reduction in libido. A review of older photographs of the man documents coarsening of facial features, progressive prognathism, and broadening of the nose. Acromegaly is suspected.

Questions

1. What screening tests are available?

2. What is the definitive test for autonomous growth hormone production?

3. Because the patient complains of reduced libido, hypogonadism is suspected. What evaluation is appropriate?

tumors causing acromegaly as a result of the ectopic production of GHRH,[55-58] and although exceedingly interesting or instructive, the ectopic production of GHRH or GH (one case) remains rare.[56] Recent reports have documented mutations in the aryl hydrocarbon–interacting protein gene (AIP)[59] in cases of familial acromegaly and polymorphisms in the SS receptor type 5 gene in sporadic cases.[60] If a GH-producing tumor occurs before epiphyseal closure, the patient develops gigantism[61] and may grow to an impressive height; otherwise, the patient develops classical, but insidious, features of bony and soft tissue overgrowth.[62] These features include progressive enlargement of the hands and feet as well as growth of facial bones, including the mandible and bones of the skull. In advanced cases, the patient may develop significant gaps between their teeth. Diffuse (not longitudinal if the condition occurred following puberty) overgrowth of the ends of long bones or the spine can produce a debilitating form of arthritis.[63] Because GH is an insulin antagonist, glucose intolerance or overt diabetes can occur. Hypertension; accelerated atherosclerosis; and proximal muscle weakness, resulting from acquired myopathy,[64] may be seen late in the illness. Sleep apnea is common. Organomegaly, especially thyromegaly, is common, but hyperthyroidism is exceedingly rare unless the tumor cosecretes TSH. GH excess is also a hypermetabolic condition, and as a result, acromegalic patients may complain of excessive sweating or heat intolerance. The features of acromegaly develop slowly over time, and the patient (or even their family) may be oblivious that changes in physiognomy have occurred. In these cases, the patient's complaints may center on the local effects of

the tumor (headache or visual complaints) or symptoms related to the loss of other anterior pituitary hormones (hypopituitarism). A careful, retrospective review of older photographs may be crucial in differentiating coarse features due to inheritance from the classical consequences of acromegaly. If left untreated, acromegaly shortens life expectancy because of increased risk of heart disease, resulting from the combination of hypertension, coronary artery disease, and diabetes/insulin resistance. Because patients with acromegaly also have a greater lifetime risk of developing cancer, cancer surveillance programs (especially regular colonoscopy) are recommended.[48]

Cosecretion of prolactin can be seen in up to 40% of patients with acromegaly.[65] Only a few TSH/GH-secreting tumors have also been reported.[66]

Confirming the diagnosis of acromegaly is relatively easy; however, some patients with acromegaly have normal random levels of GH. An elevated level of GH that does not suppress normally with glucose loading equates to an easy diagnosis. In those patients with normal, but inappropriately sustained, random levels of GH, elevated levels of IGF-I are helpful; however, nonsuppressibility of GH to glucose loading is the definitive test.[49,50]

Treatment of acromegaly can be challenging. The goal of treatment is tumor ablation, with continued function of the remainder of the pituitary. Transsphenoidal adenomectomy is the procedure of choice.[48] If normal GH levels and kinetics (normal suppressibility to glucose) are restored following surgery, the patient is likely cured. Unfortunately, GH-producing tumors may be too large or may invade into local structures that preclude complete surgical extirpation, and the patient is left with a smaller, but hormonally active, tumor. External beam or focused irradiation is frequently used at this point, but it may take several years before GH levels decline.[67,68] In the interim, efforts are made to suppress GH. Three different classes of agents, SS analogs (octreotide and lanreotide), dopaminergic agonists (cabergoline and bromocriptine), and GH receptor antagonists (pegvisomant) may be employed for GH suppression.[69,70]

GH Deficiency

GH deficiency occurs in both children and adults. In children, it may be familial or it may be due to tumors, such as craniopharyngiomas. In adults, it is a result of structural or functional abnormalities of the pituitary (see the section on *hypopituitarism* in this chapter); however, a decline in GH production is an inevitable consequence of aging and the significance of this phenomenon is poorly understood.[71,72]

Although GH deficiency in children is manifest by growth failure, not all patients with short stature have GH deficiency (see above). There have been several genetic defects identified in the GH axis. The more common type is a recessive mutation in the GHRH gene that causes a failure of GH secretion. A rarer mutation, loss of the GH gene itself, has also been observed. Mutations that cause GH insensitivity have also been reported. These mutations may involve the GH receptor, IGF-I biosynthesis, IGF-I receptors, or defects in GH signal transduction. Patients with GH insensitivity do not respond normally to exogenously administered GH. Finally, structural lesions of the pituitary or hypothalamus may also cause GH deficiency and may be associated with other anterior pituitary hormone deficiencies.[73]

An adult GH deficiency syndrome has been described in patients who have complete or even partial failure of the anterior pituitary. The symptoms of this syndrome are extremely vague and include social withdrawal, fatigue, loss of motivation, and a diminished feeling of well-being,[74] but several studies have documented increased mortality in adults who are GH deficient although this relationship is less clear in adults.[75] Osteoporosis and alterations in body composition (i.e., reduced lean body mass) are frequent concomitants of adult GH deficiency.[76]

GH replacement therapy has become relatively simple with the advent of recombinant human GH.[77] Currently, the cost of GH is the major limiting factor for replacement.

PROLACTIN

Prolactin is structurally related to GH and human placental lactogen. Considered a stress hormone, it has vital functions in relationship to reproduction. Prolactin is classified as a direct effector hormone (as opposed to a tropic hormone) because it has diffuse target tissue and lacks a single endocrine end organ.

Prolactin is unique among the anterior pituitary hormones because its major mode of hypothalamic regulation is tonic inhibition rather than intermittent stimulation. Prolactin inhibitory factor (PIF) was once considered a polypeptide hormone capable of inhibiting prolactin secretion; dopamine, however, is the only neuroendocrine signal that inhibits prolactin and is now considered to be the elusive PIF. Any compound that affects dopaminergic activity in the median eminence of the hypothalamus will also alter prolactin secretion.[78] Examples of medications that cause hyperprolactinemia include phenothiazines, butyrophenones, metoclopramide, reserpine, tricyclic antidepressants, α-methyldopa, and antipsychotics that antagonize the dopamine D2 receptor. Any disruption of the pituitary stalk (e.g., tumors, trauma, or inflammation) causes an elevation in prolactin as a result of interruption of the flow of dopamine from the hypothalamus to the lactotrophs, the pituitary prolactin-secreting cells. TRH directly stimulates prolactin secretion, and increases in TRH (as seen in primary hypothyroidism) elevate prolactin levels.[79,80] Estrogens also directly stimulate lactotrophs to synthesize prolactin. Pathologic stimulation of the neural suckling reflex is the likely explanation of hyperprolactinemia associated with chest wall injuries. Hyperprolactinemia may also be seen in renal failure and polycystic ovary syndrome. Physiologic stressors, such as exercise and seizures, also elevate prolactin. The feedback effector for prolactin is unknown. Although the primary regulation of prolactin secretions is tonic inhibition (e.g., dopamine), it is also regulated by several hormones, including GnRH, TRH, and vasoactive intestinal polypeptide. Stimulation of breasts, as in nursing, causes the release of prolactin-secreting hormones from the hypothalamus through a spinal reflex act.

As mentioned, the physiologic effect of prolactin is lactation. The usual consequence of prolactin excess is hypogonadism, either by suppression of gonadotropin secretion from the pituitary or by inhibition of gonadotropin action at the gonad.[81] The suppression of ovulation seen in lactating postpartum mothers is related to this phenomenon.

Prolactinoma

A prolactinoma is a pituitary tumor that directly secretes prolactin, and it represents the most common type of functional pituitary tumor. The clinical presentation of a patient with a prolactinoma depends on the age and gender of the patient and the size of the tumor. Premenopausal women most frequently complain of menstrual irregularity/amenorrhea, infertility, or galactorrhea; men or postmenopausal women generally present with symptoms of a pituitary mass, such as headaches or visual complaints. Occasionally, a man may present with reduced libido or complaints of erectile dysfunction. The reason(s) for the varied presentations of a prolactinoma are somewhat obscure but likely relate to the dramatic, noticeable alteration in menses or the

CASE STUDY 20-2

A 23-year-old woman has experienced recent onset of a spontaneous, bilateral breast discharge and gradual cessation of menses. She reports normal growth and development and has never been pregnant.

Questions

1. What conditions could be causing her symptoms?

2. What medical conditions (other than a prolactinoma) are associated with hyperprolactinemia?

3. Which medications raise prolactin?

4. How would your thinking change if she had galactorrhea but normal levels of prolactin?

abrupt onset of a breast discharge in younger women. By contrast, the decline in reproductive function in older patients may be overlooked as an inexorable consequence of "aging." One recently recognized complication of prolactin-induced hypogonadism is osteoporosis.[82]

Other Causes of Hyperprolactinemia

There are many physiologic, pharmacologic, and pathologic causes of hyperprolactinemia, and a common error by clinicians is to ascribe any elevation in prolactin to a "prolactinoma." Generally, substantial elevations in prolactin (>150 ng/mL) indicate prolactinoma, and the degree of elevation in prolactin is correlated with tumor size.[83,84] Modest elevations in prolactin (25 to 100 ng/mL) may be seen with pituitary stalk interruption, use of dopaminergic antagonist medications, or other medical conditions such as primary thyroidal failure, renal failure, or polycystic ovary syndrome. Breast or genital stimulation may also modestly elevate prolactin. Significant hyperprolactinemia is also encountered during pregnancy. Under most circumstances, the principal form of prolactin is a 23-kD peptide; however, a 150-kD form may also be secreted. This larger prolactin molecule has a markedly reduced biologic potency and does not share the reproductive consequences of the 23-kD variety. If the 150-kD form of prolactin predominates, this is called macroprolactinemia, and the clinical consequences are unclear, but most patients are relatively asymptomatic.[84] The prevalence of macroprolactinemia has been estimated at 10% to 22% of hyperprolactinemic samples[85] and can be excluded by precipitating serum samples with polyethylene glycol prior to measuring prolactin.

Clinical Evaluation of Hyperprolactinemia

A careful history and physical examination are usually sufficient to exclude most common, nonendocrine causes of hyperprolactinemia. It is essential to obtain TSH and free T_4 (or total thyroxine and T_3 resin uptake) to eliminate primary hypothyroidism as a cause for the elevated prolactin. If a pituitary tumor is suspected, a careful assessment of other anterior pituitary function (basal cortisol, LH, FSH, and gender-specific gonadal steroid [either estradiol or testosterone]) and an evaluation of sellar anatomy with a high-resolution MRI should be obtained.

Management of Prolactinoma

The therapeutic goals are correction of symptoms that result from local invasion or extension of the tumor by reducing tumor mass, restoration of normal gonadal function and fertility, prevention of osteoporosis, and preservation of normal anterior and posterior pituitary function. The different therapeutic options include simple observation, surgery, radiotherapy, or medical management with dopamine agonists.[86] However, the management of prolactinoma also depends on the size of the tumor (macroadenomas [tumor size >10 mm] are less likely to be "cured" than are microadenomas [tumor size < 10 mm])[87] and the preferences of the patient.

Dopamine agonists are the most commonly used therapy for microprolactinomas. Tumor shrinkage is noted in more than 90% of patients treated with either bromocriptine mesylate (Parlodel) or cabergoline (Dostinex), dopamine receptor agonists. Both drugs also shrink prolactin-secreting macroadenomas.[88] A resumption of menses and restoration of fertility is also frequently seen during medical therapy. The adverse effects of bromocriptine include orthostatic hypotension, dizziness, and nausea. The gastrointestinal adverse effects of bromocriptine can be ameliorated through intravaginal administration, and its efficacy is otherwise uncompromised.[89] Cabergoline has fewer adverse effects and may be administered biweekly because of its longer duration of action. By virtue of its ability to interact with the 5-hydroxytryptamine $(5-HT)_{2B}$ serotonergic receptor, cabergoline has been linked to the development of valvular heart disease,[90] although the doses of cabergoline required to elicit the risk of valvular damage are in vast excess to the doses used in the management of prolactinomas. Either agent should be discontinued during pregnancy unless tumor regrowth has been documented.

Neurosurgery is not a primary mode of prolactinoma management. The indications for neurosurgical intervention include pituitary tumor apoplexy (hemorrhage), acute visual loss due to macroadenoma, cystic prolactinoma, or intolerance to medical therapy. Surgical cure rates are inversely proportional to tumor size and the degree of prolactin elevation. External beam radiotherapy is generally reserved for high surgical risk patients with locally aggressive macroadenomas who are unable to tolerate dopamine agonists.

Idiopathic Galactorrhea

Lactation occurring in women with normal prolactin levels is defined as *idiopathic galactorrhea*. This condition is usually seen in women who have been pregnant several times and has no pathologic implication. It is to be remembered that this is a diagnosis of exclusion.

HYPOPITUITARISM

The failure of either the pituitary or the hypothalamus results in the loss of anterior pituitary function. Complete loss of function is termed *panhypopituitarism*; however, there may be a loss of only a single pituitary hormone, which is referred to as a *monotropic hormone deficiency*. The loss of a tropic hormone (ACTH, TSH, LH, and FSH) is reflected in function cessation of the affected endocrine gland. Loss of the direct effectors (GH and prolactin) may not be readily apparent. This section

CASE STUDY 20-3

A 60-year-old man presented with intractable headaches. MRI was requested to evaluate this complaint, and a 2.5 cm pituitary tumor was discovered. In retrospect, he noted an unexplained 20 kg weight loss, cold intolerance, fatigue, and loss of sexual desire.

Questions

1. How would you approach the evaluation of his anterior pituitary function?

2. What additional testing may be required to confirm a loss in anterior pituitary function?

TABLE 20-4	CAUSES OF HYPOPITUITARISM
1. Pituitary tumors	
2. Parapituitary/hypothalamic tumors	
3. Trauma	
4. Radiation therapy/surgery	
5. Infarction	
6. Infection	
7. Infiltrative disease	
8. Immunologic	
9. Familial	
10. Idiopathic	

concentrates on the causes of hypopituitarism and certain subtleties involved in the therapy of panhypopituitarism; more detailed descriptions of various hormone deficiency states are covered in other chapters.

The laboratory diagnosis of hypopituitarism is relatively straightforward. In contrast to the primary failure of an endocrine gland that is accompanied by dramatic increases in circulating levels of the corresponding pituitary tropic hormone, secondary failure (hypopituitarism) is associated with low or normal levels of tropic hormone. In primary hypothyroidism, for example, the circulating levels of thyroxine are low and TSH levels may exceed 200 μU/mL (normal, 0.4 to 5.0 μU/mL). As a result of pituitary failure in hypothyroidism, TSH levels are inappropriately low and typically less than 1.0 μU/mL in association with low free thyroxine levels.

There are several important issues in distinguishing between primary and secondary hormone deficiency states. To differentiate between primary and secondary deficiencies, both tropic and target hormone levels should be measured when there is any suspicion of pituitary failure or as part of the routine evaluation of gonadal or adrenal function. If one secondary deficiency is documented, it is essential to search for other deficiency states and the cause for pituitary failure. For example, failure to recognize secondary hypoadrenalism may have catastrophic consequences if the patient is treated with thyroxine. Similarly, initially overlooking a pituitary or hypothalamic lesion could preclude early diagnosis and treatment of a potentially aggressive tumor.

Etiology of Hypopituitarism

The many causes of hypopituitarism are listed in Table 20-4. Direct effects of pituitary tumors, or the sequelae of treatment of tumors, are the most common causes of pituitary failure. Pituitary tumors may cause panhypopituitarism by compressing or replacing normal

tissue or interrupting the flow of hypothalamic hormones by destroying the pituitary stalk. Large, nonsecretory pituitary tumors (chromophobe adenomas or null cell tumors) or macroprolactinomas are most commonly associated with this phenomenon. Parasellar tumors (meningiomas and gliomas), metastatic tumors (breast and lung), and hypothalamic tumors (craniopharyngiomas or dysgerminomas) can also cause hypopituitarism through similar mechanisms. Hemorrhage into a pituitary tumor (pituitary tumor apoplexy) is rare; however, when it occurs, it frequently causes complete pituitary failure.[91] Postpartum ischemic necrosis of the pituitary following a complicated delivery (Sheehan's syndrome) typically presents as profound, unresponsive shock or as failure to lactate in the puerperium. Infiltrative diseases, such as hemochromatosis, sarcoidosis, or histiocytosis, can also affect pituitary function. Fungal infections, tuberculosis, and syphilis can involve the pituitary or hypothalamus and may cause impairment of function. Lymphocytic hypophysitis,[92] an autoimmune disease of the pituitary, may only affect a single cell type in the pituitary, resulting in a monotropic hormone deficiency, or can involve all cell types, yielding total loss of function. Ipilimumab, a monoclonal antibody that blocks cytotoxic T-lymphocyte–associated antigen 4 (CTLA-4) and proven to increase survival in melanoma patients, has been associated with lymphocytic hypophysitis in up to 5% of treated patients.[93] Severe head trauma may shear the pituitary stalk or may interrupt the portal circulation. Similarly, surgery involving the pituitary may compromise the stalk and/or blood supply to the pituitary or may iatrogenically diminish the mass of functioning pituitary tissue. Panhypopituitarism can result from radiotherapy used to treat a primary pituitary tumor or a pituitary that was inadvertently included in the radiation port; loss of function, however, may be gradual and may occur over several years. There have been rare instances of familial panhypopituitarism or monotropic hormone

CASE STUDY 20-4

An 18-year-old woman was admitted to the neurologic intensive care unit following a severe closed head injury. Her course stabilized after 24 hours, but the nursing staff noticed a dramatic increase in the patient's urine output, which exceeded 1,000 mL/h.

Questions

1. What caused her increased urine production?

2. How could you prove your suspicions?

3. Could she have other possible endocrinologic problems?

deficiencies. In Kallmann syndrome, for example, GnRH is deficient and the patient presents with secondary hypogonadism. Last, there may not be an apparent identified cause for the loss of pituitary function, and the patient is classified as having idiopathic hypopituitarism, although one recent case report emphasized the need to continue the search for a cause.[94]

Treatment of Panhypopituitarism

In the average patient, replacement therapy for panhypopituitarism is the same as for primary target organ failure. Patients are treated with thyroxine, glucocorticoids, and gender-specific sex steroids. It is less clear about GH replacement in adults, and additional studies are needed to clarify this issue.[95,96] Replacement becomes more complicated in panhypopituitary patients who desire fertility. Pulsatile GnRH infusions have induced puberty and restored fertility in patients with Kallmann syndrome,[97] and gonadotropin preparations have restored ovulation/spermatogenesis in people with gonadotropin deficiency.[98]

POSTERIOR PITUITARY HORMONES

The posterior pituitary is an extension of the forebrain and represents the storage region for vasopressin (also called ADH) and oxytocin. Both of these small peptide hormones are synthesized in the supraoptic and paraventricular nuclei of the hypothalamus and transported to the neurohypophysis via their axons in the hypothalamoneurohypophyseal tract. This tract transits the median eminence of the hypothalamus and continues into the posterior pituitary through the pituitary stalk. The synthesis of each of these hormones is tightly linked to the production of neurophysin,[99] a larger protein whose function is poorly understood. Both hormones are synthesized outside of the hypothalamus in various tissues, and it is plausible they have an autocrine or a paracrine function.

Oxytocin

Oxytocin is a cyclic nonapeptide, with a disulfide bridge connecting amino acid residues 1 and 6. As a posttranslational modification, the C-terminus is amidated. Oxytocin has a critical role in lactation[100] and likely plays a major role in labor and parturition.[101] Synthetic oxytocin, Pitocin, is used in obstetrics to induce labor. Recent studies have linked oxytocin to maternal nurturing behavior and mother–infant bonding.[102] In addition to its reproductive and prosocial effects, oxytocin has been shown to have effects on pituitary, renal, cardiac, and immune function.

Vasopressin

Structurally similar to oxytocin, vasopressin is a cyclic nonapeptide with an identical disulfide bridge; it differs from oxytocin by only two amino acids. Vasopressin's major action is to regulate renal free water excretion and, therefore, has a central role in water balance. The vasopressin receptors in the kidney (V_2) are concentrated in the renal collecting tubules and the ascending limb of the loop of Henle. They are coupled to adenylate cyclase, and once activated, they induce insertion of aquaporin-2, a water channel protein, into the tubular luminal membrane.[103] Vasopressin is also a potent pressor agent and effects blood clotting[104] by promoting factor VII release from hepatocytes and von Willebrand factor release from the endothelium. These vasopressin receptors (V_{1a} and V_{1b}) are coupled to phospholipase C.

Hypothalamic osmoreceptors and vascular baroreceptors regulate the release of vasopressin from the posterior pituitary. The osmoreceptors are extremely sensitive to even small changes in plasma osmolality, with an average osmotic threshold for vasopressin release in humans of 284 mOsm/kg. As plasma osmolality increases, vasopressin secretion increases. The consequence is a reduction in renal free water clearance, a lowering of plasma osmolality, and a return to homeostasis. The vascular baroreceptors (located in the left atrium, aortic arch, and carotid arteries) initiate vasopressin release in response to a fall in blood volume or blood pressure. A 5% to 10% fall in arterial blood pressure in normal humans will trigger vasopressin release; however, in contrast to an osmotic stimulus, the vasopressin response to a baroreceptor-induced stimulus is exponential. In fact, baroreceptor-induced vasopressin secretion will override the normal osmotic suppression of vasopressin secretion.

Diabetes insipidus (DI), characterized by copious production of urine (polyuria) and intense thirst (polydipsia), is a consequence of vasopressin deficiency. However, total vasopressin deficiency is unusual, and the typical patient presents with a partial deficiency. The causes of hypothalamic DI include apparent autoimmunity to vasopressin-secreting neurons, trauma, diseases affecting pituitary stalk function, and various central nervous system or pituitary tumors. A sizable percentage of patients (up to 30%) will have idiopathic DI.[105]

Depending on the degree of vasopressin deficiency, diagnosis of DI can be readily apparent or may require extensive investigation. Documenting an inappropriately low vasopressin level with an elevated plasma osmolality would yield a reasonably secure diagnosis of DI. In less obvious cases, the patient may require a water deprivation test in which fluids are withheld from the patient and serial determinations of serum and urine osmolality are performed in an attempt to document the patient's ability to conserve water. Under selected

circumstances, a health-care provider may simply offer a therapeutic trial of vasopressin or a synthetic analog such as desmopressin (dDAVP), and assess the patient's response. In this circumstance, amelioration of both polyuria and polydipsia would be considered a positive response, and a presumptive diagnosis of DI is made. However, if the patient has primary polydipsia (also known as compulsive water drinking), a profound hypo-osmolar state (water intoxication) can ensue due to the continued ingestion of copious amounts of fluids and a reduced renal excretion of free water. This scenario illustrates the importance of carefully evaluating each patient prior to therapy.

Recently, conivaptan and tolvaptan,[106] vasopressin V_2 receptor antagonists, have been approved for the management of euvolemic hyponatremia due to vasopressin excess.

For additional student resources please visit thePoint at http://thepoint.lww.com. **thePoint**

QUESTIONS

1. Open-loop negative feedback refers to the phenomenon of
   a. Negative feedback with a modifiable set point
   b. Blood flow in the hypothalamic–hypophyseal portal system
   c. Blood flow to the pituitary via dural-penetrating vessels
   d. Negative feedback involving an unvarying, fixed set point

2. The specific feedback effector for FSH is
   a. Inhibin
   b. Activin
   c. Progesterone
   d. Estradiol

3. Which anterior pituitary hormone lacks a stimulatory hypophysiotropic hormone?
   a. Prolactin
   b. Growth hormone
   c. Vasopressin
   d. ACTH

4. The definitive suppression test to prove autonomous production of growth hormone is
   a. Oral glucose loading
   b. Somatostatin infusion
   c. Estrogen priming
   d. Dexamethasone suppression

5. Which of the following is influenced by growth hormone?
   a. All of these
   b. IGF-I

   c. IGFBP-III
   d. Lipolysis

6. What statement concerning vasopressin secretion is NOT true?
   a. All of these
   b. Vasopressin secretion is closely tied to plasma osmolality.
   c. Changes in blood volume also alter vasopressin secretion.
   d. A reduction in effective blood volume overrides the effects of plasma osmolality in regulating vasopressin secretion.

7. What are the long-term sequelae of untreated or partially treated acromegaly?
   a. An increased risk of colon and lung cancer
   b. A reduced risk of heart disease
   c. Enhanced longevity
   d. Increased muscle strength

8. TRH stimulates the secretion of
   a. Prolactin and TSH
   b. Prolactin
   c. Growth hormone
   d. TSH

9. Estrogen influences the secretion of which of the following hormones?
   a. All of these
   b. Growth hormone
   c. Prolactin
   d. Luteinizing hormone

10. What is the difference between a tropic hormone and a direct effector hormone?
  a. Tropic and direct effector hormones are both similar in that both act directly on peripheral tissue.
  b. Tropic and direct effector hormones are both similar in that both act directly on another endocrine gland.
  c. Tropic hormones act on peripheral tissue while direct effector hormones act on endocrine glands.
  d. Tropic hormones act on endocrine glands while direct effector hormones act on peripheral tissues.

11. A deficiency in vasopressin can lead to which of the following?
  a. Euvolemic hypokalemia
  b. Euvolemic hyponatremia
  c. Diabetes insipidus
  d. Primary hypothyroidism

REFERENCES

1. Kelberman D, Rizzoti K, Lovell-Badge R, Robinson IC, Dattani MT. Genetic regulation of pituitary gland development in human and mouse. *Endocr Rev.* 2009;30(7):790-829.
2. Frohman LA. Diseases of the anterior pituitary. In: Felig P, Baxter JD, Broadus AE, Frohman LA, eds. *Endocrinology and Metabolism.* 2nd ed. New York, NY: McGraw-Hill; 1981:247-337.
3. Asa SL, Horvath E, Kovacs KT. Functional pituitary anatomy and histology. In: Melmed S, ed. *Endocrinology.* 4th ed. Philadelphia, PA: WB Saunders; 2001:167-182.
4. Adler SM, Wartofsky L. The nonthyroidal illness syndrome. *Endocrinol Metab Clin North Am.* 2007;36(3):657-672.
5. Veldhuis JD, Keenan DM, Pincus SM. Regulation of complex pulsatile and rhythmic neuroendocrine systems: the male gonadal axis as a prototype. *Prog Brain Res.* 2010;181:79-110.
6. Urban RJ, Evans WS, Rogol AD, et al. Contemporary aspects of discrete pulse detection algorithms. I. The paradigm of the LH pulse signal in men. *Endocr Rev.* 1988;9:3-37.
7. Crowley WF Jr, Whitcomb RN, Jameson JL, et al. The neuroendocrine control of reproduction in the male. *Recent Prog Horm Res.* 1991;47:27-62.
8. Stojilkovic SS, Reinhart J, Catt KJ. Gonadotropin-releasing hormone receptors: structure and signal transduction pathways. *Endocr Rev.* 1994;15(4):462-499.
9. Dijk DJ, Duffy JF, Silva EJ, et al. Amplitude reduction and phase shifts of melatonin, cortisol and other circadian rhythms after a gradual advance of sleep and light exposure in humans. *PLoS One.* 2012;7(2):e30037.
10. Follenius M, Brandenberger G. Plasma free cortisol during secretory episodes. *J Clin Endocrinol Metab.* 1986;62:609-612.
11. Veldhuis JD, Iranmanesh A, Johnson ML, Lizarralde G. Amplitude, but not frequency, modulation of adrenocorticotropin secretory bursts gives rise to the nyctohemeral rhythm of the corticotropic axis in man. *J Clin Endocrinol Metab.* 1990;71:452-463.
12. Samuels MH, Veldhuis JD, Henry P, Ridgeway EC. Pathophysiology of pulsatile and copulsatile release of thyroid stimulating hormone, luteinizing hormone, follicle stimulating hormone and alpha-subunit. *J Clin Endocrinol Metab.* 1990;71:425-432.
13. Freda PU, Post KD. Differential diagnosis of sellar masses. *Endocrinol Metab Clin North Am.* 1999;28:81-117.
14. Couldwell WT, Altay T, Krisht K, Couldwell WT. Sellar and parasellar metastatic tumors. *Int J Surg Oncol.* 2012:Article ID 647256.
15. Zada G, Woodmansee WW, Ramkissoon S, et al. Atypical pituitary adenomas: incidence, clinical characteristics, and implications. *J Neurosurg.* 2011;114:336-344.
16. DeLellis R, Lloyd RV, Heitz P, Eng C, eds. *World Health Organization Classification of Tumours: Tumours of Endocrine Organs.* Lyon: IARC Press; 2004.
17. Marrelli D, Pinto E, Nari A, et al. Mib-1 proliferation index is an independent predictor of lymph node metastasis in invasive breast cancer: a prospective study on 675 patients. *Oncol Rep.* 2006;15(2):425-429.
18. Tannenbaum GS, Bowers CY. Interactions of growth hormone secretagogues and growth hormone-releasing hormone/somatostatin. *Endocrine.* 2001;14(1):21-27.
19. Casanueva FF. Physiology of growth hormone secretion and action. *Endocrinol Metab Clin North Am.* 1992;21:483-517.
20. Ribeiro-Oliveira A, Barkan AL. Growth hormone pulsatility and its impact on growth and metabolism in humans. *Growth Hormone Relat Dis Ther. Contemp Endocrinol.* 2011;pt 1:33-56.
21. Van Cauter E, Plat L, Copinschi G. Interrelations between sleep and the somatotropic axis. *Sleep.* 1998;21:553-566.
22. Herman-Bonert VS, Prager D, Melmed S. Growth hormone. In: Melmed S, ed. *The Pituitary.* Cambridge, MA: Blackwell Science; 1995:98-135.
23. Møller N, Jørgensen JO. Effects of growth hormone on glucose, lipid, and protein metabolism in human subjects. *Endocr Rev.* 2009;30(2):152-177.
24. Pinto G, Adan L, Souberbielle JC, et al. Idiopathic growth hormone deficiency: presentation, diagnosis and treatment during childhood. *Ann Endocrinol (Paris).* 1999;60:224-231.
25. Freemark M, Oden J, Kelly PA, et al. Roles of the lactogens and somatogens in perinatal and postnatal metabolism and growth: studies of a novel mouse model combining lactogen resistance and growth hormone deficiency. *Endocrinology.* 2005;146(1):103-112.
26. Salmon WD, Daughaday WH. A hormonally controlled serum factor which stimulates sulfate incorporation by cartilage in vitro. *J Lab Clin Med.* 1957;49:825-826.
27. Murphy WR, Daughaday WH, Hartnett C. The effect of hypophysectomy and growth hormone on the incorporation of labeled sulfate into tibial epiphyseal and nasal cartilage of the rat. *J Lab Clin Med.* 1956;47:715-722.
28. Denko CW, Bergenstal DM. The effect of hypophysectomy and growth hormone on cartilage sulfate metabolism. *Proc Soc Exp Biol Med.* 1955;84:603-605.
29. Daughaday WH, Reeder C. Synchronous activation of DNA synthesis in hypophysectomized rat cartilage by growth hormone. *J Lab Clin Med.* 1966;68:357-368.
30. LeRoith D, Bondy C, Yakar S, Liu JL, Butler A. The somatomedin hypothesis: 2001. *Endocr Rev.* 2001;22(1):53-74.
31. Daughaday WH, Hall K, Raben MS, et al. Somatomedin: proposed designation for sulphation factor. *Nature.* 1972;235:107.
32. Klapper DG, Svoboda ME, Van Wyk JJ. Sequence analysis of somatomedin-C: confirmation of identity with insulin-like growth factor I. *Endocrinology.* 1983;112:2215-2217.
33. Rinderknecht E, Humbel RE. The amino acid sequence of human insulin-like growth factor I and its structural homology with proinsulin. *J Biol Chem.* 1978;253:2769-2776.
34. Teale JD, Marks V. Inappropriately elevated plasma insulin-like growth factor II in relation to suppressed insulin-like growth

factor I in the diagnosis of non-islet cell hypoglycemia. *Clin Endocrinol (Oxf)*. 1990;33:87-98.

35. Daughaday WH, Kapadia M. Significance of abnormal serum binding of insulin-like growth factor II in the development of hypoglycemia in patients with non-islet-cell tumors. *Proc Natl Acad Sci U S A*. September 1989;86(17):6778-6782.

36. Ron D, Powers AC, Pandian MR, et al. Increased insulin-like growth factor II production and consequent suppression of growth hormone secretion: a dual mechanism for tumor-induced hypoglycemia. *J Clin Endocrinol Metab*. 1989;68(4):701-706.

37. Blakesley VA, Scrimgeour A, Esposito D, LeRoith D. Signaling via the insulin-like growth factor I receptor. Does it differ from insulin receptor signaling. *Cytokine Growth Factor Rev*. 1996;7:153-159.

38. Schäffer L, Kjeldson T, Anderson AS, et al. Interactions of a hybrid insulin/insulin-like growth factor-I analog with chimeric insulin/type I insulin-like growth factor receptors. *J Biol Chem*. 1993;268(5):3044-3047.

39. Clemmons DR. Insulin-like growth factor-I and its binding proteins. In: Melmed S, ed. *Endocrinology*. 4th ed. Philadelphia, PA: WB Saunders; 2001:439-460.

40. Jogie-Brahim S, Feldman D, Oh Y. Unraveling insulin-like growth factor binding protein-3 actions in human disease. *Endocr Rev*. 2009;30(5):417-437.

41. Firth SM, Baxter RC. Cellular actions of the insulin-like growth factor binding proteins. *Endocr Rev*. 2002;23(6):824-854.

42. Buckbinder L, Talbott R, Velasco-Miguel S, et al. Induction of the growth inhibitor IGF-binding protein 3 by p53. *Nature*. 1995;377:646-649.

43. Jing M, Pollack MN, Giovannucci E, et al. Prospective study of colorectal cancer risk in men and plasma levels of insulin-like growth factor (IGF)-I and IGF-binding protein-3. *J Natl Cancer Inst*. 1999;91(7):620-625.

44. Marzullo M, Somma C, Pratt KL, et al. Usefulness of different biochemical markers of the insulin-like growth factor (IGF) family in diagnosing growth hormone excess and deficiency in adults. *J Clin Endocrinol Metab*. 2001;86(7):3001-3008.

45. de Herder WW, van der Lely AJ, Janssen JA, et al. IGFBP-3 is a poor parameter for assessment of clinical activity in acromegaly. *Clin Endocrinol (Oxf)*. 1995;43:501-505.

46. Kwan AYM, Hartman ML. IGF-I measurements in the diagnosis of adult growth hormone deficiency. *Pituitary*. 2007;10(2):151-157.

47. Clemmons DR. Value of insulin-like growth factor system markers in the assessment of growth hormone status. *Endocrinol Metab Clin North Am*. 2007;36(1):109-129.

48. Melmed S, Colao A, Barkan A, et al. Guidelines for acromegaly management: an update. *J Clin Endocrinol Metab*. 2009;94(5):1509-1517.

49. Ben-Shlomo A, Melmed S. Acromegaly. *Endocrinol Metab Clin North Am*. 2008;37(1):101-122.

50. Melmed S. Medical progress: acromegaly. *N Engl J Med*. 2006;355(24):2558-2573.

51. Molitch ME, Clemmons DR, Malozowski S, et al. Evaluation and treatment of adult growth hormone deficiency: an Endocrine Society clinical practice guideline. *J Clin Endocrinol Metab*. 2011;96(6):1587-1609.

52. Murad MH, Elamin MB, Malaga G, et al. The accuracy of diagnostic tests for GH deficiency in adults: a systematic review and meta-analysis. *Eur J Endocrinol*. 2011;165:841-849.

53. Bidlingmaier M, Freda PU. Measurement of human growth hormone by immunoassays: current status, unsolved problems and clinical consequences. *Growth Horm IGF Res*. 2010;20(1):19-25.

54. Hartman ML, Crowe BJ, Biller BM, et al. Which patients do not require a GH stimulation test for the diagnosis of adult growth hormone deficiency? *J Clin Endocrinol Metab*. 2002;87:477-485.

55. Faglia G, Arosio M, Bazzoni N. Ectopic acromegaly. *Endocrinol Metab Clin North Am*. 1992;21:575-596.

56. Ezzat S, Ezrin C, Yamashita S, Melmed S. Recurrent acromegaly resulting from ectopic growth hormone gene expression by a metastatic pancreatic tumor. *Cancer*. 1993;71:66-70.

57. Gola M, Doga M, Bonadonna S, et al. Neuroendocrine tumors secreting growth hormone-releasing hormone: pathophysiological and clinical aspects. *Pituitary*. 2006;9(3):221-229.

58. Sano T, Asa SL, Kovacs K. Growth hormone-releasing hormone-producing tumors: clinical, biochemical, and morphological manifestations. *Endocr Rev*. 1988;9(3):357-373.

59. Chahal HS, Stals K, Unterländer M, et al. AIP mutation in pituitary adenomas in the 18th century and today. *N Engl J Med*. 2011;364:43-50.

60. Ciganoka D, Balcere I, Kapa I, et al. Identification of somatostatin receptor type 5 gene polymorphisms associated with acromegaly. *Eur J Endocrinol*. 2011;165:517-525.

61. de Herder WW. Acromegaly and gigantism in the medical literature. Case descriptions in the era before and the early years after the initial publication of Pierre Marie (1886). *Pituitary*. 2009;12(3):236-244.

62. Reddy R, Hope S, Wass J. Acromegaly. *BMJ*. 2010;341:c4189.

63. Killinger Z, Rovenský J. Arthropathy in acromegaly. *Rheum Dis Clin North Am*. 2010;36(4):713-720.

64. McNab TL, Khandwala HM. Acromegaly as an endocrine form of myopathy: case report and review of literature. *Endocr Pract*. 2005;11(1):18-22.

65. Lopes MB. Growth hormone-secreting adenomas: pathology and cell biology. *Neurosurg Focus*. 2010;29(4):E2.

66. Beck-Peccoz P, Brucker-Davis F, Persani L, et al. Thyrotropin-secreting pituitary tumors. *Endocr Rev*. 1996;17:610-638.

67. Del Porto LA, Liubinas SV, Kaye AH. Treatment of persistent and recurrent acromegaly. *J Clin Neurosci*. 2011;18(2):181-190.

68. Rowland NC, Aghi MK. Radiation treatment strategies for acromegaly. *Neurosurg Focus*. 2010;29(4):E12.

69. Sherlock M, Woods C, Sheppard MC. Medical therapy in acromegaly. *Nat Rev Endocrinol*. 2011;7(5):291-300.

70. Brue T, Castinetti F, Lundgren F, et al. Which patients with acromegaly are treated with pegvisomant? An overview of methodology and baseline data in ACROSTUDY. *Eur J Endocrinol*. 2009;161(suppl 1):S11-S17.

71. Giordano R, Arvat E. Somatopause reflects age-related changes in the neural control of GH/IGF-I axis. *J Endocrinol Invest*. 2005;28(3 suppl):94-98.

72. Bartke A. Growth hormone and aging: a challenging controversy. *Clin Interv Aging*. 2008;3(4):659-665.

73. Rosenfeld RG. Growth hormone deficiency in children. In: Melmed S, ed. *Endocrinology*. 4th ed. Philadelphia, PA: WB Saunders; 2001:503-519.

74. de Boer H, Blok GJ, Van der Veen EA. Clinical aspects of growth hormone deficiency in adults. *Endocr Rev*. 1995;16(1):63-86.

75. Friedrich N, Schneider H, Dörr M, et al. All-cause mortality and serum insulin-like growth factor I in primary care patients. *Growth Horm IGF Res*. 2011;21(2):102-106.

76. Woodhouse LJ, Mukerjee A, Shalet SM, Ezzat S. The influence of growth hormone status on physical impairments, functional limitations, and health-related quality of life in adults. *Endocr Rev*. 2006;27(3):287-317.

77. Svensson J, Bengtsson BA. Safety aspects of GH replacement. *Eur J Endocrinol*. November 2009;161(suppl 1):S65-S74.

78. Ben-Jonathan N, Hnasko R. Dopamine as a prolactin (PRL) inhibitor. *Endocr Rev*. 2001;22(6):724-763.

79. Hekimsoy Z, Kafesçiler S, Güçlü F, Ozmen B. The prevalence of hyperprolactinaemia in overt and subclinical hypothyroidism. *Endocr J*. 2010;57(12):1011-1015.

80. Meier C, Christ-Crain M, Guglielmetti M, et al. Prolactin dysregulation in women with subclinical hypothyroidism: effect of levothyroxine replacement therapy. *Thyroid*. 2003;13(10):979-985.

81. Shibli-Rahhal A, Schlechte J. Hyperprolactinemia and infertility. *Endocrinol Metab Clin North Am.* 2011;40(4):837-846.

82. Shibli-Rahhal A, Schlechte J. The effects of hyperprolactinemia on bone and fat. *Pituitary.* 2009;12(2):96-104.

83. Faglia G. Prolactinomas and hyperprolactinemic syndrome. In: Melmed S, ed. *Endocrinology.* 4th ed. Philadelphia, PA: WB Saunders; 2001:329-342.

84. Chahal J, Schlechte J. Hyperprolactinemia. *Pituitary.* 2008;11(2): 141-146.

85. Gibney J, Smith TP, McKenna TJ. The impact on clinical practice of routine screening for macroprolactin. *J Clin Endocrinol Metab.* 2005;90:3927-3932.

86. Melmed S, Montori VM, Schlechte JA, et al; Endocrine Society. Diagnosis and treatment of hyperprolactinemia: an Endocrine Society clinical practice guideline. *J Clin Endocrinol Metab.* 2011;96(2):273-288.

87. Dekkers OM, Lagro J, Burman P, et al. Recurrence of hyperprolactinemia after withdrawal of dopamine agonists: systematic review and meta-analysis. *J Clin Endocrinol Metab.* 2010;95(1):43-51.

88. Bevan JS, Webster J, Burke CW, Scanlon MF. Dopamine agonists and pituitary tumor shrinkage. *Endocr Rev.* 1992;13(2):220-240.

89. Ricci G, Nucera G, Pozzobon C, Guaschino S. Pregnancy in hyperprolactinemic infertile women treated with vaginal bromocriptine: report of two cases and review of the literature. *Gynecol Obstet Invest.* 2001;51(4):266-270.

90. Delgado V, Biermasz NR, van Thiel SW, et al. Changes in heart valve structure and function in patients treated with dopamine agonists for prolactinomas, a 2-year follow-up study. *Clin Endocrinol (Oxf).* 2011;doi:10.1111/j.1365-2265.

91. Nawar RN, Abdelmannan D, Selman WR, Arafah BM. Pituitary tumor apoplexy: a review. *J Intensive Care Med.* 2008;23:75-90.

92. Caturegli P, Newschaffer C, Olivi A, et al. Autoimmune hypophysitis. *Endocr Rev.* 2005;26(5):599-614.

93. Hodi FS, O'Day SJ, McDermott DF, et al. Improved survival with ipilimumab in patients with metastatic melanoma. *N Engl J Med.* 2010;363:711-723.

94. Katz BJ, Jones RE, Digre KB, et al. Panhypopituitarism as an initial manifestation of primary central nervous system non-Hodgkin's lymphoma. *Endocr Pract.* 2003;9:296-300.

95. Isley WL. Growth hormone therapy for adults: not ready for prime time? *Ann Intern Med.* 2002;137:190-196.

96. Cook DM. Shouldn't adults with growth hormone deficiency be offered growth hormone replacement therapy? *Ann Intern Med.* 2002;137:197-201.

97. Fechner A, Fong S, McGovern P. A review of Kallmann syndrome: genetics, pathophysiology, and clinical management. *Obstet Gynecol Surv.* 2008;63(3):189-194.

98. Delemarre-van de Waal HA. Application of gonadotropin releasing hormone in hypogonadotropic hypogonadism—diagnostic and therapeutic aspects. *Eur J Endocrinol.* 2004;151(suppl 3):U89-U94.

99. Elphick MR. NG peptides: a novel family of neurophysin-associated neuropeptides. *Gene.* 2010;458(1-2):20-26.

100. Nishimori K, Young LJ, Guo Q, et al. Oxytocin is required for nursing but is not essential for parturition or reproductive behavior. *Proc Natl Acad Sci U S A.* 1996;93:11699-11704.

101. Vrachnis N, Iliodromiti Z. The oxytocin-oxytocin receptor system and its antagonists as tocolytic agents. *Int J Endocrinol.* 2011;2011:350546.

102. Ross HE, Young LJ. Oxytocin and neural mechanisms regulating social cognition and affiliative behavior. *Front Neuroendocrinol.* 2009;30:534-547.

103. Nielsen MA, Frøkiaer J, Marples D, et al. Aquaporins in the kidney: from molecules to medicine. *Physiol Rev.* 2002; 82(1):205-244.

104. Ozier Y, Bellamy L. Pharmacological agents: antifibrinolytics and desmopressin. *Best Pract Res Clin Anaesthesiol.* 2010;24(1): 107-119.

105. Jane JA Jr, Vance ML, Laws ER. Neurogenic diabetes insipidus. *Pituitary.* 2006;9(4):327-329.

106. Cassagnol M, Shogbon AO, Saad M. The therapeutic use of vaptans for the treatment of dilutional hyponatremia. *J Pharm Pract.* 2011;24(4):391-399.

Adrenal Function

T. CREIGHTON MITCHELL, A. WAYNE MEIKLE

CHAPTER OUTLINE

Chapter Objectives

Upon completion of this chapter, the clinical laboratorian should be able to do the following:

- Explain how the adrenal gland functions to maintain blood pressure, potassium, and glucose homeostasis.
- Describe steroid biosynthesis, regulation, and actions according to anatomic location within the adrenal gland.
- Discuss the pathophysiology of adrenal cortex disorders, namely Cushing's syndrome and Addison's disease.
- Differentiate the adrenal enzyme deficiencies and their blocking pathways in establishing a diagnosis.

- Describe the synthesis, storage, and metabolism of catecholamines.
- State the most useful measurements in supporting the diagnosis of pheochromocytoma.
- List the clinical findings associated with hypertension that suggest an underlying adrenal etiology is causing high blood pressure.
- List the appropriate laboratory tests to differentially diagnose primary and secondary Cushing's syndrome and Addison's disease.

KEY TERMS

Adrenocorticotropic hormone (ACTH)
Aldosterone
Angiotensin-converting enzyme (ACE)
Antidiuretic hormone (ADH)
Atrial natriuretic peptide (ANP)
Cardiovascular disease
Catechol methyltransferase
Congenital adrenal hyperplasia

Corticotropin-releasing hormone (CRH)
Dehydroepiandrosterone (DHEA)
5-Dihydrotestosterone
11-Deoxycortisol
Epinephrine (EPI)
Homovanillic acid
17-Hydroxycorticosteroid
Monoamine oxidase (MAO)
Norepinephrine (NE)

Phenylethanolamine *N*-methyltransferase
Pheochromocytoma
Renin–angiotensin system (RAS)
Vasoactive inhibitory peptide

Vesicular monoamine transporters (VMATs)
Zona fasciculata (F-zone)
Zona glomerulosa (G-zone)
Zona reticularis (R-zone)

THE ADRENAL GLAND: AN OVERVIEW

The adrenal gland is a multifunctional organ that produces the steroid hormones and neuropeptides essential for life. Despite the complex effects of adrenal hormones, most pathologic conditions of the adrenal gland are linked by their impact on blood pressure and electrolyte balance.[1] As such, an adrenal etiology should be considered in the differential diagnosis of all patients with high blood pressure accompanied by electrolyte abnormalities, unexplained change in weight, inappropriate virilization, anxiety, weakness, orthostasis, palpitations, headache, chest pain, or abdominal pain.

In clinical practice, patients often present with states of diminished production or overproduction of one or more adrenal hormones. Hypofunction is generally treated with exogenous hormone replacement, and hyperfunction is generally treated with pharmacologic suppression or surgery.

EMBRYOLOGY AND ANATOMY

The adrenal gland is composed of two embryologically distinct, but conjoined, glands—the outer adrenal cortex and inner adrenal medulla. The cortex is derived from mesenchymal cells located near the urogenital ridge that differentiate into three structurally and functionally distinct zones (Fig. 21-1). The medulla arises from neural crest cells that invade the cortex during the second month of fetal development. By adulthood, the medulla contributes 10% of total adrenal weight. To date, mechanisms involved in maintaining adrenal size and function are poorly understood.[2]

Adult adrenal glands are shaped like pyramids, located superiorly and medially to the kidneys in the retroperitoneal space (suprarenal glands). On gross sectioning, both regions remain distinct; the cortex appears yellow, the medulla is dark mahogany.

Adrenal arterial supply is symmetric. Small arterioles branch to form a dense subcapsular plexus that drains into the sinusoidal plexus of the cortex. There is no direct arterial blood supply to middle and inner zones. In contrast, venous drainage from the central vein displays laterality. After crossing the medulla, the right adrenal vein empties into the inferior vena cava, and the left adrenal vein drains into the left renal vein. There is a separate capillary sinusoidal network from the medullary arterioles that also drains into the central vein and limits the exposure of cortical cells to medullary venous blood. Glucocorticoids from the cortex are carried directly to the adrenal medulla via the portal system, where they stimulate enzyme production of epinephrine (EPI) (see Fig. 21-17).

Sympathetic and parasympathetic axons reach the medulla through the cortex. En route, these axons release neurotransmitters (e.g., catecholamines and neuropeptide Y) that modulate cortex blood flow, cell growth, and function. Medullary projections into the cortex have been found to contain cells that also synthesize and release neuropeptides, such as vasoactive inhibitory peptide, adrenomedullin, and atrial natriuretic peptide (ANP), and potentially influence cortex function.

THE ADRENAL CORTEX BY ZONE

The major cortex hormones, aldosterone, cortisol, and *dehydroepiandrosterone sulfate (DHEAS)*, are uniquely synthesized from a common precursor cholesterol by cells located in one of three functionally distinct zonal layers of the adrenal cortex. These zonal layers are zona glomerulosa, zona fasciculata, and zona reticularis (Fig. 21-1).

Zona glomerulosa (G-zone) cells (outer 10%) synthesize mineralocorticoids (aldosterone) critical for sodium retention (volume), potassium, and acid–base homeostasis. They have low cytoplasmic-to-nuclear ratios and small nuclei with dense chromatin with intermediate lipid inclusions.

Zona fasciculata (F-zone) cells (middle 75%) synthesize glucocorticoids, such as cortisol and cortisone critical to blood glucose homeostasis and blood pressure. Fasciculata cells are cords of clear cells, with a high cytoplasmic-to-nuclear ratio and lipids laden with "foamy" cytoplasm. The fasciculata cells also generate androgen precursors such as dehydroepiandrosterone (DHEA), which is sulfated in the innermost *zona reticularis (R-zone)*. Subcapsular adrenal cortex remnants can regenerate into fasciculate adrenals, metastasize, and survive in ectopic locations such as the liver, gallbladder wall, broad ligaments, celiac plexus, ovaries, scrotum, and cranium.

Zona reticularis cells (inner 15%) sulfate DHEA to DHEAS, which is the main adrenal androgen. The zone is sharply demarcated with lipid-deficient cords of irregular, dense cells with lipofuscin deposits.

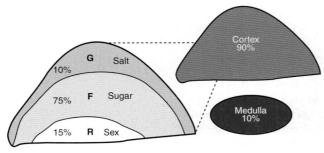

FIGURE 21-1 Adrenal gland by layer.

Adrenal cell types are presumed to arise from stem cells. A proposed tissue layer between the zona glomerulosa and fasciculata may serve as a site for progenitor cells to regenerate zonal cells.[3]

Cortex Steroidogenesis

Control of steroid hormone biosynthesis is complex, including adrenocorticotropic hormone (ACTH) and angiotensin (Ang) II. It occurs via substrate availability, enzyme activities, and inhibitory feedback loops that are layer specific. Defining adrenal cortex biosynthesis and actions in terms of three layers simplifies its complexity.

All adrenal steroids are derived by sequential enzymatic conversion of a common substrate, cholesterol. Adrenal parenchymal cells accumulate and store circulating low-density lipoproteins (LDLs). The adrenal gland can also synthesize additional cholesterol using acetyl-CoA, ensuring that adrenal steroidogenesis remains normal in patients with variable lipid disorders and in patients on lipid-lowering agents.

Only free cholesterol can enter steroidogenic pathways in response to ACTH. The availability of free intracellular cholesterol is metabolically regulated by LDL negatively and ACTH positively through multiple mechanisms. Corticotropin-releasing hormone (CRH)

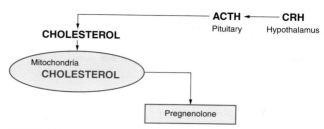

FIGURE 21-2 Conversion of cholesterol to pregnenolone. ACTH, adrenocorticotropic hormone; CRH, corticotropin-releasing hormone.

is secreted from the hypothalamus in response to circadian signals, serum cortisol, and stress, causing release of stored ACTH, which stimulates transport of free cholesterol into adrenal mitochondria, initiating steroid production.

Conversion of cholesterol to pregnenolone is a rate-limiting step in steroid biosynthesis: six carbons are removed from cholesterol by mitochondrial membrane cytochrome P450 (CYP450) enzyme (Fig. 21-2). Newly synthesized pregnenolone is then returned to the cytosol for subsequent zonal conversion by microsomal enzymes in each layer by F-zone enzymes and/or androgens by enzymes in the R-zone (Fig. 21-3).

Because F-zone glucocorticoids powerfully suppress ACTH release, cortisol is the primary feedback regulator

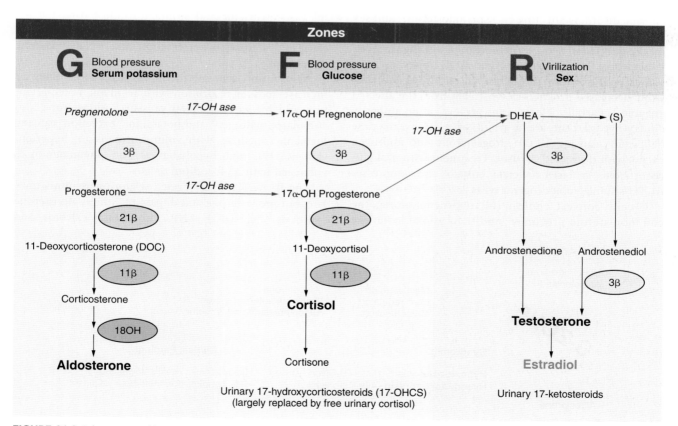

FIGURE 21-3 Adrenocorticol hormone synthesis by zone.

Enzyme Defect	New Classification	HTN	Virilization	High Lab Value
3β-Hydroxysteroid dehydrogenase	3β-HSD II	N	Slight	DHEA
17α-Hydroxylase	CYP17	Y	No	Aldosterone
11β-Hydroxylase	CYP11B1GF	Y	Marked	11-DOC
21β-Hydroxylase	CYP21A2	N	Marked	17-OH-progesterone

FIGURE 21-4 Congenital adrenal hyperplasia syndromes.

of ACTH-stimulated hormone production in the adrenal cortex. ACTH generally does not significantly impact G-zone aldosterone synthesis, although certain glucocorticoids have mineralocorticoid actions.

Decreased activity of any enzyme required for biosynthesis can occur as an acquired or inherited (autosomal recessive) trait. Defects that decrease the production of cortisol cause increases in ACTH and CRH secretion in an attempt to stimulate cortisol levels and lead to adrenal hyperplasia or overproduction of androgens, depending on the affected enzyme.

Evaluation of adrenal function requires measuring relevant adrenal hormones, metabolites, and regulatory secretagogues. Diagnosis is based on the correlation of clinical and laboratory findings.[4]

Congenital Adrenal Hyperplasia

Congenital adrenal hyperplasia is an inherited family of enzyme disorders affecting cortisol, aldosterone, and sex steroid production. The clinical presentation depends on the affected enzyme as demonstrated in Figure 21-4. Laboratory findings reveal increased upstream substrates with overflow through open pathways and relatively decreased products downstream from the affected enzyme.[5] Partial defects can present after puberty. Ninety-five percent are a result of a 21-hydroxylase deficiency, causing 17-OH progesterone and androgen excess with decreased cortisol. Treatment with oral glucocorticoids replaces deficient cortisol and suppresses ACTH-stimulated androgen excess.[6]

G-cells convert cholesterol to pregnenolone, the common steroid precursor, and then into aldosterone (50 to 250 µg/d) (Fig. 21-3). G-zone-specific aldosterone synthesis occurs for several reasons. Low G-cell 17α-hydroxylase activity prevents substrate diversion into other pathways and low aldosterone synthase activity in other zones ensures the final oxidation of corticosterone to aldosterone is G-cell specific (Fig. 21-3).

Aldosterone secretion is mainly regulated by the renin–angiotensin system (RAS), which functions to regulate blood pressure and sodium balance. Volume depletion, reduced sodium load, and sympathetic nerve stimulation are sensed by juxtaglomerular cells in the kidney and stimulate renin production. Renin is a proteolytic enzyme made by cells in the juxtaglomerular apparatus and is secreted directly into the circulation, resulting in conversion of angiotensinogen to angiotensin I (Ang I). Angiotensin-converting enzyme (ACE) converts Ang I to Ang II, which acts as a powerful vasoconstrictor and stimulates aldosterone release. Chronic Ang II stimulation or dietary salt restriction can cause aldosterone hypersecretion and isolated G-zone hypertrophy.[7]

Aldosterone acts on the tubules of the kidney to increase sodium resorption with resultant water retention and increase in blood pressure. Aldosterone also stimulates hydrogen$^+$ and potassium$^+$ excretion, causing metabolic alkalosis with volume expansion, hypertension (HTN), and hypokalemia. The phenomenon is enhanced with high-sodium diets.

Ang II, ACTH, and elevated serum potassium stimulate, but progesterone and dopamine inhibit aldosterone synthesis (Fig. 21-5). ANP, intracellular calcium, and

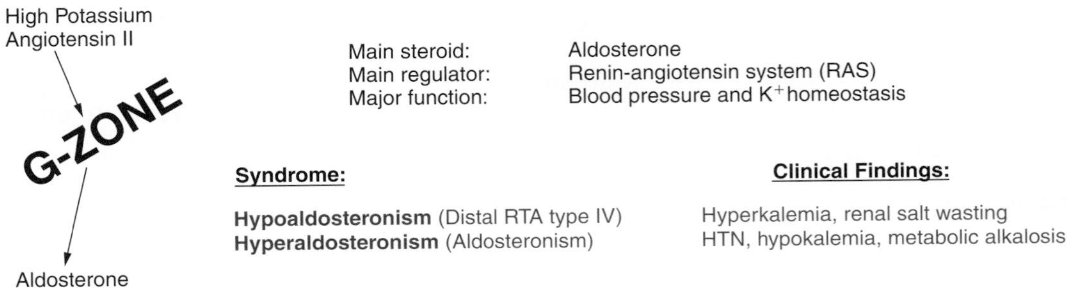

High Potassium
Angiotensin II

G-ZONE

Aldosterone

Main steroid: Aldosterone
Main regulator: Renin-angiotensin system (RAS)
Major function: Blood pressure and K$^+$ homeostasis

Syndrome:

Hypoaldosteronism (Distal RTA type IV)
Hyperaldosteronism (Aldosteronism)

Clinical Findings:

Hyperkalemia, renal salt wasting
HTN, hypokalemia, metabolic alkalosis

FIGURE 21-5 G-zone function and pathology. HTN, hypertension.

- Easy fatigability
- Muscle weakness (paralysis)
- Polyuria (loss of renal concentration ability and renal cysts)
- Palpitations (increased ventricular ectopy)
- Autonomic dysregulation (hypotension without reflex tachycardia)
- Impaired insulin secretion (decreased glucose tolerance)
- Aldosterone suppression

FIGURE 21-6 Signs and symptoms of hypokalemia.

certain drugs are aldosterone suppressors, including ketoconazole, ACE inhibitors, nonsteroidal anti-inflammatory drugs, and heparin.

Isolated Hypoaldosteronism

Insufficient aldosterone secretion is seen with adrenal gland destruction, chronic heparin therapy, following unilateral adrenalectomy (transient), and with G-zone enzyme deficiencies. Most hypoaldosteronism occurs in patients with mild renal insufficiency such as persons with diabetes who present with mild metabolic acidosis, high serum potassium$^+$, low urinary potassium$^+$ excretion (urine K$^+$ < urine Na$^+$), and low renin. Treatment is with dietary changes and Florinef (a synthetic mineralocorticoid), which enhances salt retention and the secretion of potassium$^+$ and hydrogen$^+$.

Hyperaldosteronism

Patients with excess aldosterone production may develop metabolic alkalosis, HTN, and hypokalemia. They may present with HTN and symptoms caused by low serum potassium$^+$, as outlined in Figure 21-6.

Causes of HTN and unprovoked hypokalemia include

- Primary aldosteronism (low renin)—autonomous oversecretion of aldosterone
- Secondary aldosteronism (elevated renin)—RAS-activated aldosterone secretion
- Pseudoaldosteronism (variable renin and aldosterone levels)—renal tubular diseases causing urinary potassium loss by aldosterone-independent mechanisms. In most cases, aldosterone is low; however, two syndromes are associated with high aldosterone levels: Bartter's syndrome (bumetanide-sensitive chloride channel mutation) and Gitelman's syndrome (thiazide-sensitive transporter mutation).

Documenting excess aldosterone excretion establishes the diagnosis of aldosteronism (urine measurements are superior to plasma measurements) but cannot always distinguish between underlying etiologies. Plasma renin activity (PRA) measurements reflect the state of RAS activation and are helpful diagnostically. Because PRA varies with volume status, upright or supine position, and dietary sodium intake, an isolated PRA measurement has limited clinical value. Plasma aldosterone (PA) relative to PRA helps distinguish primary from other forms of aldosteronism.

Types of aldosteronism are diagrammed in Figure 21-7 according to their PA (y-axis) and PRA (x-axis) values.

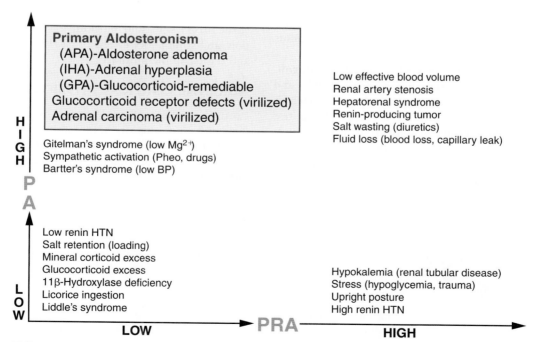

FIGURE 21-7 Types of aldosteronism according to plasma aldosterone (PA):plasma renin activity (PRA) ratio. HTN, hypertension.

DIAGNOSIS OF PRIMARY ALDOSTERONISM

Because 25% of hypertensive patients have low renin, the diagnosis of primary aldosteronism relies on the following criteria[8]:

- PA/PRA greater than 25
- Low plasma renin that fails to increase with volume depletion
- High aldosterone that fails to decrease with saline or angiotensin inhibition

Diagnosis Algorithm

Urinary potassium excretion measured in patients with HTN and unprovoked hypokalemia is a cost-effective screening test for aldosteronism. Urine potassium$^+$ greater than 30 mmol/d is inappropriate in hypokalemic patients and strongly suggests hyperaldosteronism (spot urine $K^+ > Na^+$ is also suggestive). Urine potassium less than 30 mmol/d reflects renal potassium$^+$ retention, as seen with prior diuretic use or gastrointestinal loss.

Upright PA/PRA ratio measured in a fluid-deprived patient (overnight dehydration increases PRA) is definitive in distinguishing primary from other causes of aldosteronism, particularly when repeated following volume expansion (2 L of normal saline over 4 h), which normally suppresses aldosterone. A PA/PRA ratio greater than 25 suggests primary aldosteronism. Most clinicians then recommend abdominal imaging with computed tomography (CT) or magnetic resonance imaging (MRI) to evaluate for the presence of an adrenal mass.

Captopril suppression is often confirmatory. Within 3 hours of taking 50 mg of captopril (1 mg/kg), PA remains high in primary aldosteronism (PA:PRA ratio >25 before and after test) but is suppressed in patients with other forms of HTN.

18-Hydroxycorticosterone levels greater than 100 ng/dL suggest an *aldosterone-producing adenoma (APA)* and levels less than this suggest idiopathic hyperaldosteronism (IHA). However, because the accuracy of this test is poor, its clinical utility is limited. Surgery is curative for an autonomous functioning adenoma or unilateral hyperplasia; otherwise, drug therapy is used to antagonize aldosterone actions (e.g., spironolactone or amiloride with thiazide for IHA) or suppress aldosterone secretion (e.g., cortisone for glucocorticoid-responsive hyperaldosteronism).

Adrenal imaging (CT or MRI) is used to visualize adrenal gland anatomy. Structural abnormalities should complement functional findings to establish a diagnosis. Pathology based on imaging studies alone can be misleading. Adrenal adenomas (nonsecreting) are routinely found in 10% of healthy patients; adrenal nodules can be normal structural variants or result from abnormal gland stimulation. Occasionally, aldosterone-secreting adenomas are missed because they are too small to visualize or are obscured within hyperplastic glands. If imaging is negative, the scan can be repeated in 6 to 12 months.

Adrenal vein sampling is used to differentiate between unilateral adenoma and bilateral hyperplasia. It is superior to adrenal CT. In one study, 50% of patients diagnosed with APA by venous sampling had hyperplasia by CT.[8]

ACTH is secreted in a pulsatile fashion by the pituitary gland and regulates cortisol production. Diurnal variation results in ACTH and cortisol levels that are highest in the early morning (8:00 AM) and lowest at night (10:00 PM to 12:00 AM). ACTH pulse amplitude (not frequency) rises between 2:00 and 4:00 AM. ACTH peaks can also be observed following protein-rich meals and stimulation with antidiuretic hormone (ADH) or CRH. Hypoglycemia indirectly stimulates ACTH by increasing CRH and ADH release. In addition, acute stress (physical and psychological) directly stimulates ACTH secretion, causing cortisol levels to rise. Elevated glucocorticoids (endogenous and exogenous), in turn, suppress ACTH through feedback inhibition, decreasing pro-opiomelanocortin gene transcription in pituitary corticotroph cells and blocking the production, secretion, and stimulatory effects of CRH on ACTH synthesis and release in the pituitary.

ADRENAL CORTICAL PHYSIOLOGY

Cortisol synthesis (8 to 15 mg/d) is critical to hemodynamics and glucose homeostasis. F-zone disorders manifest with blood pressure and glucose abnormalities (Fig. 21-8). Glucocorticoids maintain blood glucose by inducing lipolysis and causing amino acid release from

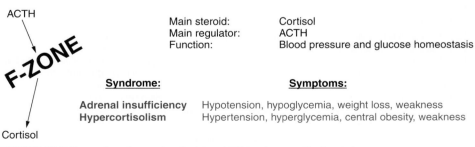

FIGURE 21-8 F-zone function and pathology. ACTH, adrenocorticotropic hormone.

muscle for conversion into glucose (gluconeogenesis) and storage as liver glycogen.

ADRENAL INSUFFICIENCY (ADDISON'S DISEASE)

Adrenal insufficiency (low cortisol) results from a primary adrenal disorder (destruction of 90% of the adrenal cortex) or is secondary to ACTH deficiency (abnormality at the hypothalamic–pituitary level).[9]

Symptoms of deficiency can be vague and misleading (Fig. 21-9). As cortisol is critical to normal glucose homeostasis and maintenance of vascular tone, deficiency produces symptoms resembling failure to thrive, such as weakness, fatigue, anorexia, nausea, diarrhea, and abdominal pain accompanied by physical findings such as weight loss. Abnormal laboratory values depend on the underlying cause of low cortisol production and include hyponatremia, hyperkalemia, hypercalcemia, prerenal azotemia, and mild metabolic acidosis. Mineralocorticoid deficiency is usually not observed in secondary adrenal insufficiency.

Autoimmune adrenalitis accounts for 70% of the cases of primary adrenal insufficiency; however, other conditions, including infectious diseases such as fungal infection, human immunodeficiency virus infection, and tuberculosis; bilateral adrenal hemorrhage; adrenoleukodystrophy; infiltrative processes; and metastasis, can also destroy the adrenal gland. Glucocorticoid therapy is the most common cause of secondary adrenal insufficiency; however, tumors, hemorrhage, infiltrative processes, developmental abnormalities, and malignancies also interfere with ACTH production by the pituitary gland.

Diagnosis of Adrenal Insufficiency

Low baseline cortisol levels (8:00 AM, supine) and an elevated ACTH greater than 200 pg/mL are suggestive of adrenal primary insufficiency. Random cortisol levels are only useful in excluding the diagnosis when elevated (>20 μg/dL). Cosyntropin is a synthetic stimulator of cortisol and aldosterone secretion, which tests the capacity of the adrenal gland to increase hormone production in response to stimulation. It is safe and offers reliable

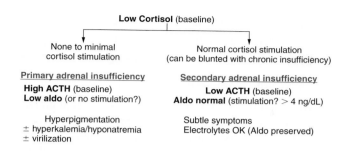

FIGURE 21-10 Differential diagnosis of low cortisol states. ACTH, adrenocorticotropic hormone.

results regardless of food intake or time of day. Lower serum concentrations of ACTH and cortisol are consistent with secondary adrenal failure. Hypoglycemia is also a potent stimulator of cortisol secretion but is potentially dangerous. A stimulated plasma cortisol level less than 20 μg/dL indicates impaired adrenal function.

Following a blood draw for baseline cortisol, ACTH, and aldosterone levels, cosyntropin (IV/IM) is given. Repeat samples are drawn at 30 and 60 minutes poststimulation. ACTH and aldosterone responses to cosyntropin aid in the differential diagnosis of low cortisol states as illustrated in Figure 21-10. Although good at identifying primary adrenal insufficiency, most causes of chronic secondary insufficiency (central) are associated with abnormal cortisol response to cosyntropin stimulation, but the test is not diagnostic of secondary adrenal insufficiency.

Metyrapone is used as an alternate diagnostic or confirmatory test for secondary causes of adrenal insufficiency. Metyrapone administered orally at midnight will, in normal individuals, block 11β-hydroxylase (Fig. 21-3), increasing 11-deoxycortisol (>7 μg/dL) while cortisol decreases (<5 μg/dL). Secondary adrenal insufficiency is suggested in patients with a near-normal response to a 250-μg cosyntropin test but with an abnormal response to metyrapone. Patients suspected of having secondary adrenal insufficiency should be screened with MRI of the brain to assess for pituitary disease unless they have a history of chronic exogenous glucocorticoid use.

The cause of primary adrenal gland destruction can often be distinguished by 21-hydroxylase antibody titers and/or a distinctive appearance on imaging. Autoimmune disease is suggested by small adrenal glands, infection by large adrenal glands, and hemorrhage by enlargement with characteristic intensity.

Treatment of Adrenal Insufficiency

In primary adrenal insufficiency, steroids from the G- and R-zone are replaced: aldosterone (Florinef, 50 to 100 μg/d) and cortisol (hydrocortisone 20 to 25 mg/d or prednisone 5 mg/d). In secondary adrenal insufficiency, steroidogenesis in the G-zone remains intact, so only cortisol requires replacement. Most clinicians double

Frequency	Symptoms	Signs
100%	Weakness Fatigue Anorexia	Weight loss
90%		Hyperpigmentation (primary adrenal insufficiency)
50%	Nausea Diarrhea	
10%	Pain	Adrenal calcification

FIGURE 21-9 Signs and symptoms of adrenal insufficiency.

the dose of glucocorticoids during mild stress and give hydrocortisone 300 mg/d in divided doses for significant stressors such as surgery.

HYPERCORTISOLISM

Overproduction of CRH or ACTH, excess adrenal glucocorticoid secretion, and exogenous intake cause hypercortisolism. Excess cortisol affects multiple systems including immune (suppression), dermatologic (thin, friable skin, wide purple striae, poor healing), vascular (vessel fragility, ecchymoses), adipose (increased fat with redistribution to upper back and central locations), muscle (wasting, proximal muscle weakness, heart failure), neurologic (peripheral neuropathy, autonomic dysregulation), bone (osteopenia or osteoporosis), renal (edema, HTN, calciuria), and metabolic (hyperglycemia and insulin resistance). Cortisol also has central nervous system actions, influencing pain perception and sense of well-being. Clinical presentation of hypercortisolism is variable, with no single feature common in all cases.

Multiple conditions are associated with high cortisol levels as outlined in Figure 21-11. These conditions present with different comorbidities and require different treatment. Determining the cause of hypercortisolism can be difficult because laboratory values and clinical findings often overlap between syndromes.

CUSHING'S SYNDROME

Cushing's syndrome describes the array of signs and symptoms (Fig. 21-11) resulting from excess glucocorticoid production or prolonged exogenous steroid use. The most common causes of Cushing's syndrome are ACTH-secreting pituitary adenoma known as Cushings's disease (68%), autonomous cortisol production from an adrenal tumor (17%), and ectopic ACTH or CRH production (15%).[10,11]

When Endogenous Cushing's Syndrome Is Confirmed

Distinguishing ACTH-dependent versus ACTH-independent hypercortisolism is necessary as this directs the clinician to the most likely cause of the disease. This determination can be made with a reliable two-site IRMA (immunoradiometric assay) assay for ACTH. One can presume that cortisol secretion is independent of ACTH if the serum cortisol is greater than 15 μg/dL with ACTH less than 5 pg/μL. If ACTH is greater than 15 pg/μL, cortisol secretion is considered ACTH dependent. ACTH values between 5 and 15 pg/μL usually indicate cortisol secretion is also ACTH independent. Imaging for primary adrenal disease with CT or MRI of the adrenals is the next procedure in ACTH-independent Cushing's syndrome. Adrenal adenomas are generally smaller than *carcinomas* and have lower unenhanced CT attenuation. MRI may provide even better differentiation between benign and malignant tumors.

Pituitary versus Ectopic ACTH Secretion

Most patients with ACTH-dependent Cushing's syndrome have pituitary adenomas or hyperplasia, but distinguishing between pituitary and ectopic sources of ACTH is essential. ACTH and urine free cortisol elevation are typically higher in ectopic ACTH syndrome than in Cushing's disease. Hypokalemia also suggests an ectopic source. There is overlap between these causes. ACTH-secreting

Stress

Infection

Severe obesity (visceral)
Polycystic ovary syndrome (up to 40% have slightly elevated urine cortisol)
Chronic alcoholism (cortisol normalizes with abstinence)
Depression (up to 80% have abnormal cortisol levels, disappears with remission)
Iatrogenic Cushing's (<1% inhaled, topical, oral glucocorticoid use)

Cushing's Syndrome	Symptoms of Cushing's Syndrome	
	HTN	(85–90%)
	Central obesity	(90%)
	Glucose intolerance	(80%)
	Plethoric faces	(80%)
	Purple striae	(65%)
	Hirsuitism	(65%)
	Abnormal menses	(60%)
	Muscle weakness	(60%)

FIGURE 21-11 Conditions associated with hypercortisolism. HTN, hypertension.

pituitary adenomas are relatively resistant to negative feedback regulation by glucocorticoids (dexamethasone), whereas most nonpituitary tumors causing ectopic ACTH syndrome are completely resistant to feedback suppression. The high-dose dexamethasone suppression test can be performed overnight or over 48 hours. The overnight test involves administration of 8 to 12 mg of dexamethasone at 11:00 PM followed by an 8:00 AM ACTH and cortisol measurement. The standard 2-day high-dose dexamethasone suppression test uses 2 mg of dexamethasone every 6 hours for eight doses with measurement of urine free cortisol or plasma cortisol. A 50% suppression from the baseline cortisol value is considered a positive test. In several studies, approximately 60% of patients with Cushing's disease exhibit greater than 90% suppression compared with none with ectopic disease. Ectopic ACTH secretion from carcinoid tumors might suppress with high-dose dexamethasone. Thus, the sensitivity was greater than 60% and the specificity was 100% for Cushing's disease. Pituitary gland stimulation with CRH can also be performed. *Scintigraphy* may be used for localization of neuroendocrine tumors.

Inferior Petrosal Sinus Sampling

The source of ACTH hypersecretion can be investigated by simultaneous sampling of blood from the inferior petrosal sinus and a peripheral vein both before and after stimulation of the pituitary gland with CRH. A petrosal sinus–to–peripheral blood ACTH ratio of greater than 2 to 3 is 97% sensitive and 100% specific for ACTH hypersecretion from the pituitary gland, or Cushing's disease.

Imaging with CT or MRI is used for localization of pituitary or ectopic ACTH-secreting tumors.

Patients with Cushing's syndrome share striking similarity to patients with type 1 diabetes. They have a fourfold increase in mortality even after successful therapy, primarily a result of cardiovascular disease. Because mineralocorticoid receptors are equally responsive to glucocorticoids, excess cortisol can promote HTN in association with left ventricular hypertrophy. Electrocardiogram abnormalities and loss of normal nocturnal fall in blood pressure are also seen. Untreated disease has a 5-year mortality rate of 50%.

Iatrogenic Cushing's syndrome is relatively common, but some sources may not be obvious. All glucocorticoids, including synthetic, inhaled, and topical, can inhibit ACTH secretion; therefore, plasma ACTH, serum cortisol, and cortisol excretion may all be low (unless cortisol or cortisone is used). In contrast, urine contamination with topical hydrocortisone (vulvovaginal or perineal use) can falsely elevate urine cortisol values. Relatively greater urinary than serum cortisol and cortisone values suggest that hydrocortisone is added to the urine. If suspected, synthetic glucocorticoids can be detected chromatographically.

Diagnosis of Cushing's Syndrome

Clinical symptoms are supported by laboratory findings of cortisol excess, loss of diurnal rhythm, and suppression resistance. Exogenous glucocorticoid administration must be excluded. A universal diagnostic algorithm for Cushing's syndrome has not been established for the following reasons: (1) ACTH and cortisol are secreted in bursts and excess secretion may occur episodically; (2) each patient has unique metabolism, metabolites, and metabolic clearance rates; (3) stimulation and suppression thresholds often vary (nonsuppressible lesions can occasionally be suppressed, and normal patients can display suppression resistance); and (4) compliance and accuracy issues regarding sample collection and processing are common. Standard assessment tests for diagnosing Cushing's syndrome are listed next.[12]

Document Cortisol Excess
Urine free cortisol (and/or metabolites) (Fig. 21-3). Urine cortisol is a sensitive indicator of endogenous cortisol production. When serum cortisol exceeds the binding capacity of its carrier protein, free cortisol levels rise rapidly, increasing the free cortisol filtered into the urine. This value may be erroneous with high urine volume (>3 L) because patients who drink more than 5 L/d will have a 64% increase in urine cortisol. In contrast, urine 17-hydroxycorticosteroid excretion occurs at a constant rate and is not affected by volume changes; however, the sensitivity and specificity of this method are poor.

A 24-hour urine free cortisol measured by tandem mass spectroscopy is the most sensitive (95% to 100%) and specific (98%) screen for excess cortisol production. A revised method, collecting overnight (10:00 PM to 8:00 AM) urine samples for cortisol factored by urinary creatinine, appears equally valid (specificity and sensitivity of 97% to 100%). In one large study, 21% to 47% of Cushing's syndrome patients had at least one normal 24-hour urine cortisol; therefore, patients with intermediate values should be reevaluated 2 to 3 months later.[12]

Random plasma cortisol levels are of little value for the diagnosis of Cushing's syndrome. Levels in normal people vary widely during the day and overlap with levels found in patients with Cushing's syndrome.

Baseline AM cortisol concentrations have no diagnostic value unless they are clearly above the normal range.

Determine if Diurnal Rhythm Is Lost (Late-Night Values Remain High)
Plasma cortisol is highest between 6:00 and 8:00 AM and 50% to 80% lower between 10:00 PM and 12:00 AM. Measuring late-night cortisol is justified by the fact that its normal evening nadir is lost in Cushing's syndrome and bilateral nodular hyperplasia but preserved in obese and depressed patients, two causes of pseudo-Cushing's.

Ideally, a blood sample (for cortisol and ACTH) is drawn between 11:00 PM and 12:00 AM. Samples are stabilized, stored, and sent to the laboratory if the previously determined urine cortisol is elevated. Late-evening saliva, serum free, or serum total cortisol values may be more reliable than urine cortisol for the diagnosis of Cushing's syndrome.

In two studies, a single midnight serum cortisol concentration (>7.5 µg/dL) was 90% to 96% sensitive and 100% specific for Cushing's syndrome.[12]

In another study of Cushing's syndrome patients (30 normal and 18 obese subjects), a single 11:00 PM salivary cortisol level, when combined with the 8:00 AM salivary cortisol concentration after a 1 mg overnight dexamethasone suppression test, had a sensitivity and specificity of 100%.[12]

Saliva cortisol is stable at room temperature for days and collection is noninvasive, can be performed at home, and has greater specificity (100%); however, it is less sensitive (92%) than serum or urine levels in detecting Cushing's syndrome. Midnight (12:00 AM) values less than 1.3 ng/mL determined by radioimmunoassay (RIA) or greater than 1.5 ng/mL by competitive protein-binding assay help exclude the diagnosis. Saliva measurements are useful in patients with suspected intermittent Cushing's syndrome for whom numerous samples need to be collected over extended periods.

Determine Loss of Normal Cortisol Suppression by Dexamethasone

Dexamethasone acts as an exogenous cortisol substitute, suppressing ACTH if the pituitary gland is normal and cortisol secretion if the adrenal gland is normal.

An overnight dexamethasone suppression test is commonly used to screen patients for autonomous overproduction of cortisol. Dexamethasone (1 mg) given at about 11:00 PM acts to suppress the early morning ACTH-stimulated rise in cortisol. Suppressed total cortisol less than 3.6 µg/dL measured between 8:00 and 9:00 AM is considered a negative test. Although it appears that

repeated ingestion of dexamethasone minimizes individual differences in drug clearance, the low-dose (1 mg) suppression test was 95% accurate and equally reliable as the standard 2-day, low-dose dexamethasone suppression (0.5 mg every 6 h to 2 d, with normal urine free cortisol <10 µg/dL on day 2) per a retrospective analysis of 426 Cushing's syndrome patients.[12] While the predictive value for a negative test nears 100%, false-positive results are common (up to 15%). Causes for this include testing errors, other cortisol suppression–resistant states (e.g., physical stress, anorexia nervosa, alcoholism, depression, acute illness, obesity, and renal insufficiency), and altered drug metabolism and drug interactions (e.g., dilantin, barbiturates, carbamazepine, and rifampin).

Except in rare cases, a normal (overnight or 2-day) dexamethasone suppression test virtually excludes the possibility of Cushing's syndrome. Although not required for diagnosis, measured changes in saliva cortisol (normal, <2 ng/mL) and ACTH after dexamethasone suppression can be complementary for a diagnosis.[13]

As in adrenal insufficiency, ACTH levels, both baseline and following low (1 mg) or high (8 mg) dexamethasone suppression, can help determine an underlying etiology of cortisol excess states. One study demonstrated that high-dose dexamethasone was only 57% specific for differentiating an ectopic from pituitary source of ACTH hypersecretion (Fig. 21-12).[12]

When Cushing's Syndrome Is Confirmed, CRH Stimulation Tests Help Determine ACTH Dependency

CRH stimulation is a newer and more helpful test for differentiating types of Cushing's syndrome (central disease versus ectopic ACTH disease). An 8:00 AM serum cortisol and ACTH level is drawn following CRH injection. At baseline, in ACTH-independent Cushing's syndrome, cortisol is high (>25 µg/dL) while ACTH is suppressed (<10 pg/mL), demonstrating that ACTH production is not driving excess cortisol production. In this case, an

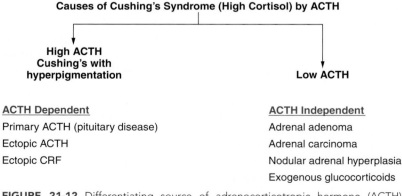

FIGURE 21-12 Differentiating source of adrenocorticotropic hormone (ACTH) secretion.

adrenal cause for excess cortisol is sought. In ACTH-dependent Cushing's syndrome, both cortisol (>25 μg/dL) and ACTH (>10 pg/mL) are elevated. Autonomous ACTH is from a pituitary or ectopic source.

To determine if ACTH excess results from a pituitary or ectopic source, a CRH-stimulated bilateral inferior petrosal sinus sampling and peripheral vein sampling are performed. The results are expressed in a ratio. A petrosal sinus ACTH–to–peripheral vein ACTH ratio greater than 3 is diagnostic for pituitary disease. A ratio less than 2.5 suggests an ectopic (nonpituitary) source of ACTH production.

Remission rates for pituitary microadenoma approximate 85%; rates for invasive adenomas are less than 50% when resected. With additional treatment (pituitary irradiation), remission rates of invasive adenomas may slowly reach 85%.

The most common tumors producing ectopic ACTH are small cell lung carcinomas and bronchial carcinoids. For ectopic ACTH, localization and surgical removal of autonomous ACTH-producing lesions is attempted. Other treatment options include bilateral adrenalectomy and medications to inhibit adrenal enzymes in an effort to reduce cortisol levels.

Localization Procedures

- Adrenal Cushing's syndrome
  - Adrenal CT may distinguish tumor from hyperplasia [R-zone DHEA(S) normal with F-zone adrenal adenomas]

- Adrenal MRI T2-weighted image helps distinguish carcinoma. Cancer often involves other adrenal layers with the R-zone DHEA(S) being high in carcinoma; immunohistochemical markers, *p53*, and MIB-1 are also positive in carcinomas.
- Pituitary Cushing's syndrome—Cushing's disease
  - Pituitary MRI (detects 85% of microadenomas)
- Ectopic Cushing's syndrome—majority are intrathoracic
  - Chest CT (e.g., bronchial carcinoid, small cell lung carcinoma, and medullary thyroid carcinoma)

Algorithm for Suspected Cushing's Syndrome

DAY 1

8:00 AM: Completely empty bladder and start baseline urine collection.
11:00 PM: Collect saliva sample for cortisol level; ingest dexamethasone (1 mg); empty bladder; end baseline urine collection.
Optional extended workups: Begin overnight dexamethasone-suppressed urine collection.

DAY 2

8:00 AM: Empty bladder (postsuppression urine cortisol complete); venous blood or saliva for cortisol; ACTH; dexamethasone (compliance); hold samples until needed.

See flowcharting interpretation of Cushing's syndrome workup (Fig. 21-13).

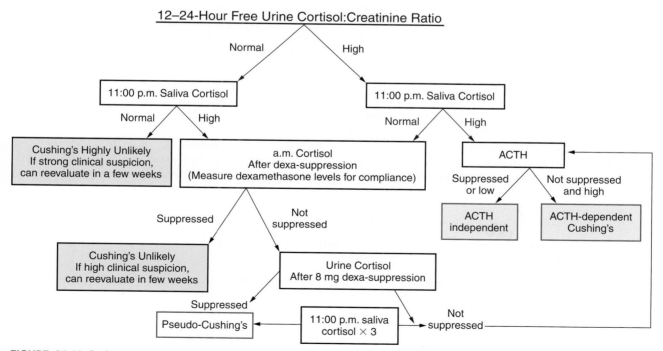

FIGURE 21-13 Cushing's syndrome workup. Note that dexamethasone serum levels (for standard test, 2 ng/mL; suppression test, 6.5 ng/mL) can be drawn at 8:00 AM (or 6 h after the last dose) to help clarify or determine compliance. Normal dexamethasone saliva levels have not been determined. ACTH, adrenocorticotropic hormone.

Treatment

Options for primary (adrenal cortisol overproduction) and secondary (pituitary or ectopic ACTH overproduction) Cushing's syndrome are similar: surgery, radiation, and/or medications to suppress adrenal cortisol production or actions. Treatment strategies vary with clinical situations.

Lifelong replacement of glucocorticoids and mineralocorticoids (Florinef) is necessary in patients with bilateral adrenalectomy. Any patient undergoing bilateral adrenalectomy as a result of an ACTH-producing pituitary tumor should be routinely screened and closely followed for symptoms of increasing mass lesion of the pituitary gland (Nelson's syndrome). Finally, Cushing's syndrome can recur in adrenal rests; therefore, periodic, lifetime screening for adrenal overproduction is warranted in these patients.

ADRENAL ANDROGENS

Androgens are produced as by-products of cortisol synthesis that are regulated by ACTH. Although prolactin, pro-opiomelanocortin peptides, and T lymphocytes are known stimulators of androgens, regulatory mechanisms of R-zone biosynthesis remain uncertain (Fig. 21-14). R-cells primarily produce DHEA and multiple 19-carbon steroids (androgens and estrogens) from 17α-hydroxylated pregnenolone and progesterone. DHEA is sulfated to DHEAS by sulfotransferase, an adrenal enzyme, and secreted daily (Fig. 21-1).

Both DHEA and DHEAS are precursors to more active androgens (e.g., androstenedione, testosterone, and 5-dihydrotestosterone) and estrogens (e.g., estradiol and estrone). Although DHEA and DHEAS have minimal androgenic activity, adverse effects are caused by conversion to active androgens in the adrenal and peripheral tissue (e.g. hair follicles, sebaceous glands, genitalia, adipose, and prostate tissue). Although men derive less than 5% of their testosterone from adrenal or peripheral sources, women rely on the adrenals for 40% to 65% of their daily testosterone production from precursor.[14]

Although observational data demonstrate adrenal androgen production increases in both genders in late childhood and correlates with the onset of pubic hair (adrenarche), it peaks in young adults and progressively declines with age.

Androgen Excess

Androgen excess causes ambiguous genitalia in infant girls and precocious puberty in children of both sexes. Androgens stimulate organ development, linear growth, and epiphyseal fusion. Virilization in boys includes penile enlargement, androgen-dependent hair growth, and other secondary sexual characteristics. Girls develop hirsutism, acne, and clitorimegaly. Untimely overproduction can cause short stature by leading to early epiphyseal fusion.

In women, androgen overproduction can cause infertility, with masculinizing effects (e.g., hirsutism, acne, male pattern baldness, menstrual irregularities, and virility).

In men, excess adrenal androgens converted to estrogen can also cause infertility with feminizing effects and inhibition of pituitary gonadotropins, which lowers testicular testosterone production. Despite overall adrenal androgen excess, males can experience hypogonadal symptoms including loss of muscle mass and decreased hair growth, testes size, testicular testosterone production, and spermatogenesis.

Diagnosis of Excess Androgen Production

Less than 10% of DHEAS and DHEA are produced by the gonads; therefore, high DHEAS and DHEA production strongly suggests adrenal hyperandrogenism, whereas elevated testosterone values are seen with either adrenal or gonadal hyperandrogenism.

Plasma DHEAS, DHEA, or urinary 17-ketosteroids can identify patients with adrenal causes of pathologic masculinization (females) and feminization (males).

Treatment for Adrenal Androgen Overproduction

Similar to the previously described disorders of overproduction, differentiation between ACTH-dependent and ACTH-independent secretion is assessed

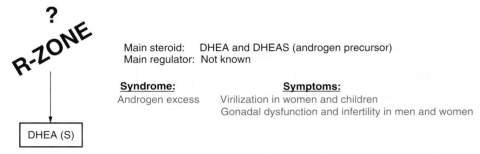

FIGURE 21-14 R-zone function and pathology. Manifestations of adrenal hyperandrogenism vary with age, onset, and gender. DHEA, dehydroepiandrosterone; DHEAS, dehydroepiandrosterone sulfate.

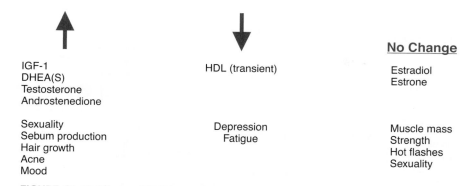

FIGURE 21-15 Effects of DHEA supplementation. DHEA, dehydroepiandrosterone; IGF-1, insulin growth factor 1; HDL, high-density lipoprotein.

by dexamethasone suppression tests followed by imaging studies (CT, MRI). Adenomas and carcinomas are surgically removed. Glucocorticoid-suppressible causes are treated accordingly. Exogenous sources are discontinued and other nonadrenal conditions are treated. Drugs with antiandrogenic properties (e.g., minoxidil, spironolactone, birth control pills) are occasionally used.

Exogenous DHEA is a popular nutritional supplement with numerous purported properties (only a few studied), including vasodilatory, anti-inflammatory, antiaging, and antiatherosclerosis.

The clinical relevance of DHEA(S) interactions with nonandrogen/estrogen receptors remains unknown. DHEA (4 mg/d) and DHEAS (7 to 15 mg/d) are secreted as the major components of adrenal androgens. There is no evidence that this molecule is required for health or that it contributes to disease. Steroid receptors for DHEA have not been clearly identified. DHEA actions are attributed to its downstream products, testosterone and estrogen.

In normal and compromised patients (e.g., adrenal insufficiency, glucocorticoid therapy, depression, older persons, and trained athletes), DHEA can increase the sense of well-being and raises or lowers a variety of serum markers (Fig. 21-15), although the changes are small. Supplementation (50 to 100 mg/d) in some androgen-deficient patients (e.g., those with adrenal insufficiency, ACTH deficiency, and glucocorticoid therapy) may help ameliorate adverse effects of deficiency and may inhibit glucocorticoid-induced bone loss. However, DHEA can cause adverse androgenic effects in women, and the long-term consequences of supplementation remain unknown.

THE ADRENAL MEDULLA

The adrenal medulla functions as an atypical sympathetic ganglion. In response to sympathetic stimulation, the medulla secretes catecholamines directly into the circulation in lieu of transmitting messages via efferent axons. Medullary catecholamine products serve as first

responders to stress by acting within seconds (cortisol takes 20 min) to promote the fight-or-flight response, which increases cardiac output and blood pressure, diverts blood toward muscle and brain, and mobilizes fuel from storage.

Development

Sympathetic cells arise from primordial neural crest stem cells (sympathogonia), which migrate out of the central nervous system to a space behind the aorta where they differentiate into sympathoblasts (sympathetic ganglion cells) or pheochromoblasts (medulla chromaffin cells). Tumors that arise from either cell line share similar histologic and biochemical properties. Malignant neuroblastomas and benign ganglioneuromas arise from sympathoblasts, secrete homovanillic acid and are rarely seen after adolescence. In contrast, tumors of chromaffin cells (pheochromocytomas) maintain the capacity to synthesize and store catecholamines (norepinephrine [NE] and EPI) throughout life.[15]

Biosynthesis and Storage of Catecholamines

NE and EPI biosynthesis begins with the sequential conversion of phenylalanine substrates in a tightly regulated, compartmentalized manner. All reactions take place in the cytoplasm, except for the production of NE, which occurs within lipid vesicles or outer mitochondrial membranes, as illustrated in Figure 21-16.

In sympathetic neurons, cytoplasmic dopamine is sequestered into vesicles, converted into NE, and stored until nerve stimulation causes its release.

In medulla chromaffin cells, NE can passively diffuse into the cytosol. In the cytosol, NE is converted into EPI by a cortisol-dependent enzyme called phenylethanolamine N-methyltransferase. Any form of stress that increases cortisol levels stimulates EPI production. Free cytosolic EPI (like dopamine) is actively transported into secretory vesicles by vesicular monoamine transporters (VMATs) in pheochromocytes. The ratio of NE to EPI

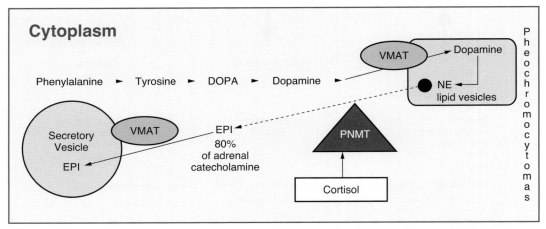

FIGURE 21-16 Biosynthesis and storage of catecholamines. VMAT, vesicular monoamine transporter; NE, norepinephrine; EPI, epinephrine; PNMT, phenylethanolamine N-methyltransferase.

in the serum is normally 9:1 (98% from postganglionic neurons, 2% from the medulla). In adrenal insufficiency (low cortisol), that ratio increases to 45:1 in females and 24:1 in males.

Catecholamine Degradation

All catecholamines are rapidly eliminated from target cells and the circulation by three mechanisms:

1. Reuptake into secretory vesicles
2. Uptake in nonneuronal cells (mostly liver)
3. Degradation

Degradation relies on two enzymes—catechol methyltransferase (in nonneuronal tissues) and monoamine oxidase (MAO) (within neurons)—to produce metabolites (metanephrines and vanillylmandelic acid [VMA]) from free catecholamines. Metabolites and free catecholamines are eliminated by direct filtration into the urine and excreted as free NE (5%), conjugated NE (8%), metanephrines (20%), and VMA (30%) (Fig. 21-17).

Urine and Plasma Catecholamine Measurements

Catecholamines are hydrophilic, circulate in low levels (50% albumin bound), have short half-lives (seconds to 2 min), and produce wide, rapidly fluctuating plasma levels that render accurate determination and interpretation technically challenging.

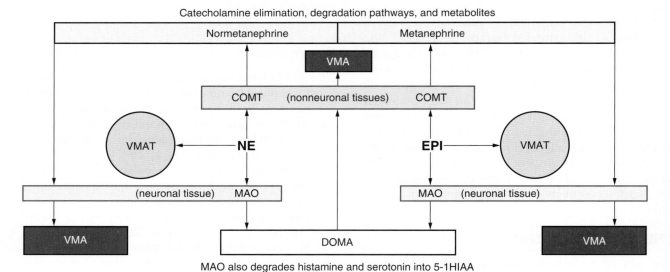

FIGURE 21-17 Catecholamine degradation. Free catecholamines (EPI and NE) are either sequestered into VMAT-containing vesicles or converted into metabolites, DOMA by neuronal MAOs and metanephrines by nonneuronal COMTs. These metabolites are ultimately degraded to VMA (DOMA by COMTs and metanephrines by MAOs) and excreted. EPI, epinephrine; NE, norepinephrine; VMAT, vesicular monoamine transporter; DOMA, 3,4-dihydroxymandelic acid; MAO, monoamine oxidase; COMT, catechol methyltransferases; VMA, vanillylmandelic acid.

Urine catecholamines (free NE and EPI) are assayed using liquid chromatography (LC), fluorometry, and LC-tandem mass spectrometry (LC-MS/MS). Twenty-four–hour urine catecholamine and metabolite levels are more reliable and are not altered by age or gender.

Most antihypertensive drugs and many other medications interfere with accurate catecholamine measurement by fluorometric assays. Substances causing autofluorescence (e.g., tetracyclines, ephedrine, α-methyldopa) can produce erroneous results when measured by fluorometric assays. Central α-antagonists (clonidine) and thiazides are preferred agents to control HTN during evaluation of conditions causing excessive sympathetic activation (high catecholamine states).

Causes of Sympathetic Hyperactivity

- Autonomic dysfunction
- Panic attack (emotions)
- Stress responses: hypoglycemia, injury, infarction, infection, psychosis, and seizures
- Drugs: decongestants, appetite suppressants, stimulants, bronchodilators, MAO inhibitors, thyroid hormone, cortisol, nicotine withdrawal, or short-acting sympathetic antagonists (clonidine or propranolol)
- Foods containing tyramine: imported beer, red wine, soy sauce, overripe/fermented foods, smoked or aged meats
- Pheochromocytoma (catecholamine-producing tumor).

Pheochromocytomas are rare (<0.1% of hypertensive patients), catecholamine-producing tumors arising from chromaffin tissue that cause HTN in association with nonspecific clinical symptoms mimicking anxiety. Symptoms include palpitations, diaphoresis, and headaches. In a retrospective study, 40% of patients evaluated for pheochromocytoma met the criteria for panic disorder, compared with 5% of control patients with HTN (Fig. 21-18).[16,17]

Patient presentation is highly variable. Pheochromocytoma symptoms are related to the type of catecholamines secreted by the tumor and the receptors they activate. Most patients have episodes of HTN, palpitations, and diaphoresis associated with other nonspecific symptoms. These episodes may be initiated by various stimuli including physical exertion, torso twisting, Valsalva, micturition, or coitus. Other individuals have sustained HTN (some refractory to treatment) and many have no symptoms. Rarely, patients with EPI or dopamine-secreting tumors may present with orthostatic hypotension. Additional signs may include pallor, increased erythrocyte sedimentation rate, dilated cardiomyopathy, and erythrocytosis as a result of overproduction of erythropoietin.

Mechanisms of catecholamine secretion by pheochromocytomas remain unclear (tumors are not innervated). Increased catecholamine synthesis, limited degradation capacity, and limited storage for excess NE and metabolites likely cause spillover into the blood, increasing circulating free NE and/or EPI along with other active peptides that cause symptoms. Because medullary catecholamines and adrenal cortical hormones serve similar functions that produce similar effects, a rare patient with clinical and biochemical evidence of catecholamine hypersecretion may have an adrenocortical adenoma or carcinoma rather than a medullary tumor causing the symptoms.

Diagnosis of Pheochromocytoma

The best test for diagnosing pheochromocytoma is measurement of fractionated metanephrines and catecholamines in a 24-hour urine collection. This yields a sensitivity of 98% and a specificity of 98%. Fractionated plasma free metanephrines have a high sensitivity (96% to 100%) but a poor specificity (85% to 89%), which is even lower (77%) in patients older than 60 years. Although the majority of patients with pheochromocytoma have obvious diagnostic abnormalities on most tests, others can produce confounding results. When one test is equivocal, a different test should be performed if clinical suspicion remains high.[18,19]

For a 24-hour urine collection, the following values are associated with the presence of a pheochromocytoma: NE > 170 μg/24 h, EPI > 35 μg/24 h, dopamine >700 μg/24 h, normetanephrine >900 μg/24 h, or metanephrine >400 μg/24 h.[20] Normal values of plasma-fractionated metanephrines vary according to the method of collection. For samples obtained following an overnight fast and 20 min after catheter insertion, the diagnostic cutoff is a metanephrine <0.3 nmol/L and a normetanephrine <0.66 nmol/L. In the nonfasting

10%
Incidentally discovered (imaging, surgery, autopsy)
Multiple
Extra-adrenal (chest, neck, abdomen, bladder)
Malignant (invasion, distant metastases)
Familial (Von Hippel-Lindau, MEN-II, parathyroid hyperplasia, medullary thyroid carcinoma, neurofibromatosis, paraganglioma)

90%
Intra-adrenal
Intra-abdominal (95%)
Single
Benign

FIGURE 21-18 Pheochromocytomas.

state, a sample obtained through standard venipuncture should be interpreted with cutoff values of <0.5 nmol/L for metanephrines and <0.9 nmol/L for normetanephrines.[20] A retrospective cohort study including 1,003 individuals referred for evaluation of pheochromocytoma found that plasma levels of metanephrines less than 62 ng/L (0.31 nmol/L) and of normetanephrines less than 112 ng/L (0.61 nmol/L) essentially exclude the diagnosis of pheochromoctyoma. Sensitivity is 99% and specificity is 89% using these values. In this study, plasma levels of metanephrines greater than 236 ng/L (1.2 nmol/L) or of normetanephrines greater than 400 ng/L (2.19 nmol/L) were associated with a zero false-positive rate.[21]

Plasma metanephrines, measured by high-performance LC or RIA, are often touted as the most specific and sensitive diagnostic test. Yet, investigators at the Mayo Clinic found that plasma metanephrines lack specificity (15% false-positive rate) and for this reason do not recommend it as a first-line test but reserve it for high-risk patients or patients who cannot collect an accurate 24-hour urine specimen. Urinary VMA has poor sensitivity and specificity. The higher specificity of 24-hour urine catecholamines and fractionated metanephrines makes it a better screening test in low-risk individuals.[20]

Chromogranin A is costored and secreted in quantum with catecholamines. Eighty percent of pheochromocytoma patients have increased plasma chromogranin levels. Serum chromogranin A is not routinely measured because it is less sensitive and specific for pheochromocytoma than are direct catecholamine and metabolite measurements. In combination, serum chromogranin A and plasma catecholamines are specific (95%) but less sensitive (88%), likely because of high dependence on renal function. If the glomerular filtration rate is less than 80 mL/min, test sensitivity drops to 70%. Combined, resting plasma catecholamines greater than 200 pg/mL and chromogranin A greater than 20 pg/mL have a positive predictive value of 97% when glomerular filtration rate is normal.

If results of the preceding tests are equivocal, a clonidine suppression test can be performed to separate patients with pheochromocytoma (low levels of biosynthetic activity) from those without pheochromocytoma who are experiencing similar symptoms secondary to increased sympathetic outflow. Clonidine, an antihypertensive agent, suppresses central sympathetic outflow.

The clonidine suppression test (92% accurate) determines if excess catecholamine production is suppressible. Because sympathetic activation is not responsible for secretion of catecholamines from pheochromocytomas, suppression of sympathetic activation via clonidine, through activation of central α2-receptors, will not lower NE levels in patients with pheochromocytoma.

After stopping antihypertensive drugs for at least 12 hours, total plasma catecholamines are measured. Clonidine (0.3 mg) is administered and repeat plasma catecholamine levels are obtained 3 hours later. Patients without pheochromocytoma will have a fall in plasma total catecholamines greater than 500 pg/mL (this is inaccurate in patients with normal catecholamine levels).[22]

Biochemical confirmation of pheochromocytoma should be followed by radiographic localization. Although any site containing paraganglionic tissue may be involved, the most common extra-adrenal locations are the superior and inferior para-aortic areas (75%), bladder (10%), thorax (10%), and head, neck, and pelvis (5%).

For localization of pheochromocytoma, either CT or MRI of the abdomen and adrenal glands is performed. On T2-weighted images, pheochromocytomas appear hyperintense, while other adrenal tumors look isointense compared with the liver. Either test detects most sporadic tumors with 98% to 100% sensitivity and 70% specificity. The lower specificity is due to relatively higher prevalence of adrenal incidentalomas. ^{123}I-labeled meta-iodo-benzylguanidine (MIBG) (an NE analogue that concentrates in the adrenal and pheochromocytoma via VMAT) scintigraphy can be performed and is 100% specific for pheochromocytoma but not sensitive enough for routine screening. Positron emission tomographic scanning with ^{18}F-fluorodeoxyglucose, ^{11}C-hydroxyephedrine, or 6-[^{18}F]fluorodopamine may be helpful in identifying sites of metastatic disease.[23]

Treatment of Pheochromocytoma

Once pheochromocytoma is diagnosed, all patients are surgical candidates following appropriate medical preparation. Removal is a high-risk procedure. In one of the largest surgical series (147 pheochromocytoma patients) at one institution (1975 to 1997), overall perioperative mortality and morbidity rates were 2.4%.[18] Patients with severe preoperative HTN or highly secretory tumors or those undergoing repeat intervention were at highest risk for complications. Catecholamines fall to normal within 1 week of resection.

Although perioperative α-blockade is widely recommended, fewer perioperative complications were observed in those not given α-blockers (study of 113 pheochromocytoma patients undergoing resection). A second regimen proposed by the Cleveland Clinic resulted in successful use of a calcium channel blocker for blood pressure control.

Outcome and Prognosis

Surgical removal of a pheochromocytoma is the primary therapy; nevertheless, excision does not necessarily lead to long-term cure of pheochromocytoma or HTN (even in patients with benign tumors). Patients with familial pheochromocytomas, right adrenal tumors,

Incidentaloma Function Evaluation		
	Clinical Features	Screening Tests Negative Results
Pheochromocytoma	**HTN** (paroxysmal) with spells (sweating, HA, or palpitations)	24-hour urine metanephrines <1 μg or 5.5 μmol/mg creatine
Cushing's syndrome	**HTN**, obesity (truncal) weakness	1 mg bedtime dexamethasone 8 AM cortisol < 3.6 μg/dL, or 24-hour urine free cortisol normal
Primary aldosteronism	**HTN**, hypokalemia, weakness	Serum potassium, *if low* urine K^+ excretion (<30 mmol)
Adrenocarcinoma	Virilization (+ above)	Plasma renin:aldosterone ratio < 30 Plasma DHEAS (<9.2 μmol/L) Urine 17-ketosteroid < 20 mg

FIGURE 21-19 Brief functional screen for adrenal masses. HTN, hypertension; HA, hyperaldosteronism; DHEAS, dehydroepiandrosterone sulfate.

and extra-adrenal tumors are more likely to have recurrence. In one retrospective series of 176 patients, pheochromocytoma recurred in 16% (52% of those were malignant).[24,25] Long-term monitoring is indicated in all patients, even those who are apparently cured.

ADRENAL "INCIDENTALOMA"

Given the frequent use of CT, MRI, and ultrasound imaging of the abdomen for reasons unrelated to the adrenal glands, many adrenal masses, typically greater than 1 cm in diameter, are found incidentally and are thus termed "incidentalomas." Autopsy studies report a frequency of adrenal adenomas at about 6%, and the prevalence increases with age.[26,27] Although most of these lesions are nonfunctioning and benign, all should be assessed for malignancy or hypersecretion.[28] Surgery is considered if the adrenal mass is cancerous; is autonomously secreting cortisol, aldosterone, or catecholamines; is 4 cm or greater in diameter; or is increasing in size on serial examinations.[29]

Figure 21-19 illustrates a brief functional screen for adrenal masses, which assesses the function of all adrenal layers and serves as a clinical summary.

CASE STUDIES

Hypertension is common and most often presents as an independent medical condition. Occasionally, hypertension is a result of an underlying illness and requires different treatment. Because adrenal function is critical for (1) blood pressure, (2) potassium, and (3) glucose homeostasis, an adrenal etiology should be considered in all patients with blood pressure problems accompanied by electrolyte abnormalities, unexplained change in weight, failure to thrive, inappropriate virilization, and anxiety periods.

Eight different clinical scenarios are presented below. Each presentation is associated with a different diagnosis and treatment. A discussion of adrenal causes, diagnoses, and treatments for each is found within the chapter. Each numbered case study completes the following opening statement: A 22-year-old woman (previously adopted, not currently taking medications, negative medical history) presents with …

CASE STUDY 21-1

… hypertension, with weakness and hypokalemia. The patient also has a high urine potassium excretion without diuretics.

Question

1. What is the diagnosis?

CASE STUDY 21-2

… hypertension, with weakness and rapid onset of obesity. This patient also exhibits central fat pads, buffalo hump, plethora, thin skin, purple striae, easy bruising, osteoporosis, hyperglycemia/insulin resistance, and recurrent infections.

Question

1. What is the diagnosis?

CASE STUDY 21-3

… hypertension, with weakness, irregular menses, and hypokalemia. Her young age, borderline low cortisol, and low androgens also are significant.

Question

1. What is the diagnosis?

CASE STUDY 21-4

… hypertension, with periods of panic attacks and hot flashes. She also presents with headache, hyperglycemia, hyperthyroidism, and gastrointestinal complaints.

Question

1. What is the diagnosis?

CASE STUDY 21-5

… hypertension, with virilization. This young woman presents with irregular menses diagnosed with polycystic ovary syndrome. She has a borderline low cortisol and elevated 17-OH progesterone.

Question

1. What is the diagnosis?

CASE STUDY 21-6

… hypertension and hyperkalemia. She has normal renal function (low urine potassium⁺) and metabolic acidosis.

Question

1. What is the diagnosis?

CASE STUDY 21-7

… hypotension, failure to thrive, weight loss, and weakness. Her laboratory results reveal hyperkalemia, fasting hypoglycemia, and metabolic acidosis.

Question

1. What is the diagnosis?

CASE STUDY 21-8

… new virilization and hirsutism. Laboratory results show increased IGF-1 (insulin growth factor 1), DHEA(S), and testosterone levels. She is a health food enthusiast who experiments with nutritional supplements.

Question

1. What is the diagnosis?

For additional student resources please visit thePoint at http://thepoint.lww.com. **thePoint**

QUESTIONS

1. When considering an endocrine cause for a patient's hypertension, the _____ _____ is the usual suspect.

2. When hypertension results from an endocrine disorder, what hormonal state is usually found: hormone underproduction or overproduction?

3. True or false? Major warning signs of adrenal disease include abnormal blood pressure, abnormal electrolytes (potassium, acid–base status, urine dilution), and unexplained weight change.

4. _____ is the common substrate from which all adrenal steroids are produced.

5. True or false? When produced, free catecholamines (NE and EPI) are short-lived. They

are best measured in the urine, though catecholamine metabolites are best measured in the serum.

6. _____ is responsible for epinephrine production.

7. A primary hyperaldosteronemic state is characterized by:
   a. A urine potassium of 35 mmol/d.
   b. A urine potassium of 21 mmol/d.
   c. A spot urine test where the sodium levels are greater than potassium levels.
   d. Within 3 hours of taking 50 mg of captopril, plasma aldosterone was low.
   e. All of the above are characteristic of hypoaldosteronism.

8. During a low dose (1 mg) dexamethasone suppression test, total cortisol levels measured in a patient at 8:35 am was 2.8 μg/dL. How is this interpreted?
   a. The patient is normal.
   b. The patient has Cushings' syndrome.
   c. The patient has a nonpituitary tumor causing ectopic ACTH syndrome.
   d. The patient has an ACTH-secreting pituitary adenoma.

9. The most biologically active androgen in this list is:
   a. DHEA
   b. DHEAS
   c. LH
   d. FSH
   e. Estrone

10. Which amino acid is needed for the biosynthesis of norepinephrine and epinephrine?
    a. Alanine
    b. Phenylalanine
    c. Isoleucine
    d. Leucine
    e. Serine

11. Which of the following describes catecholamines?
    a. Hydrophobic
    b. Degraded rapidly in nonneuronal cells by monamine reductase
    c. Have long half-lives
    d. Circulating blood catecholamines are 99% bound to albumin.
    e. None of the above accurately describes catecholamines.

12. The collection of a 24-hour urine is used for measuring:
    a. Creatinine clearance
    b. Norepinephrine
    c. Dopamine
    d. All of the above may be measured in a 24-hour urine
    e. All but one of the above may be measured in a 24-hour urine

REFERENCES

1. Kacsoh D. The adrenal gland. In: Dolan J, ed. *Endocrine Physiology.* New York, NY: McGraw-Hill; 2000:360-448.
2. Roman S, Wu L. Surgical anatomy of the adrenal glands. www.UpToDate.com, online 19.3, 1/12.
3. Miller W. The adrenal cortex. In: Felig P, ed. *Endocrinology and Metabolism.* New York, NY: McGraw-Hill; 2001:387-493.
4. Lacroix A. The adrenal cortex: basic concepts and diagnostic procedures. In: Pinchera A, et al., eds. *Endocrinology and Metabolism.* London: McGraw-Hill; 2001:285-297.
5. Merke D, Bornstein S. Congenital hyperplasia. *Lancet.* 2005;365:2125-2136.
6. Levine L. Congenital adrenal hyperplasia. In: Lavin M, ed. *Manual of Endocrinology and Metabolism.* Philadelphia, PA: Lippincott Williams & Wilkins; 2002:147-163.
7. Stern N. The adrenal cortex and mineralocorticoid hypertension. In: Lavin M, ed. *Manual of Endocrinology and Metabolism.* Philadelphia, PA: Lippincott Williams & Wilkins; 2002:115-139.
8. Kaplan N. Primary aldosteronism. In: Pine J, ed. *Clinical Hypertension.* Baltimore, MD: Lippincott Williams & Wilkins; 1998:365-383.
9. Thomopoulos P. Adrenocortical insufficiency. In: Jeffers D, ed. *Endocrinology and Metabolism.* London: McGraw-Hill; 2001:297-305.
10. Bertagna X. Cushing's syndrome. In Pinchera A, et al., eds. *Endocrinology and Metabolism.* London: McGraw-Hill; 2001:311-323.
11. Besser G. Cushing's syndrome. *J Clin Endocrinol Metab.* 1972;1:451.
12. Nieman L. Establishing the diagnosis of Cushing's syndrome. www.UpToDate.com, online 19.3, 1/12.
13. Castro M, Elias PC, Quidute AR, Halah FP, Moreira AC. Outpatient screening for Cushing's syndrome: sensitivity of the combination of circadian rhythm and overnight dexamethasone suppression salivary cortisol tests. *J Clin Endocrinol Metab.* 1999;84:878.
14. Chrovsos G. Dehydroepiandrosterone and its sulfate. www.UpToDate.com, online 12.1, 4/03.
15. Bravo E. The adrenal medulla: basic concepts. In: Pinchera A, et al., eds. *Endocrinology and Metabolism.* London: McGraw-Hill; 2001:337-341.

16. Kaplan N. Pheochromocytoma. In: Pine J, ed. *Clinical Hypertension.* Baltimore, MD: Lippincott Williams & Wilkins; 1998:345-365.
17. Sowers K. Pheochromocytomas. In: Lavin M, ed. *Manual of Endocrinology and Metabolism.* Philadelphia, PA: Lippincott Williams & Wilkins; 2002:139-145.
18. Bravo E. Diagnosis and management of pheochromocytoma. In: Pinchera A, et al., eds. *Endocrinology and Metabolism.* London: McGraw-Hill; 2001:341-349.
19. Fogarty J, Engel C, Russo J, Simon G, Katon W. Hypertension and pheochromocytoma testing: the association with anxiety disorders. *Arch Fam Med.* 1994;3:55-60.
20. Young W, Kaplan N. Clinical presentation and diagnosis of pheochromocytoma. www.UpToDate.com, online 19.3, 1/12.
21. Lenders J, Pacak K, Walther MW, et al. Biochemical diagnosis of pheochromocytoma. *JAMA.* 2002;287:1427-1434.
22. Sjoberg R, Kidd G. The clonidine suppression test for pheochromocytoma: a review of its utility and pitfalls. *Arch Intern Med.* 1992;152:1193.
23. Pacak K, Eisenhofer G, Carrasquillo J, et al. 6-[^{18}F]fluorodopamine positron emission tomographic (PET) scanning for diagnostic localization of pheochromocytoma. *Hypertension.* 2001;38:6-8.
24. Young WF, Kaplan NM, Kebebew E. Treatment of pheochromocytoma in adults. www.UpToDate.com, online 19.3, 1/12.
25. Amar L, Servais A, Gimenez-Roqueplo A, Zinzindohoue F, Chatellier G, Plouin P. Year of diagnosis, features at presentation, and risk of recurrence in patients with pheochromocytoma or secreting paraganglioma. *J Clin Endocrinol Metab.* 2005;90:2110-2116.
26. Young WF Jr. Management approaches to adrenal incidentalomas: a view from Rochester, Minnesota. *Endocrinol Metab Clin North Am.* 2000;29:159-185.
27. Kloos RT, Gross MD, Francis IR, Korobkin M, Shapiro B. Incidentally discovered adrenal masses. *Endocr Rev.* 1995;16:460-484.
28. Lutton J. The incidentally discovered adrenal mass. In: Pinchera A, et al., eds. *Endocrinology and Metabolism.* London: McGraw-Hill; 2001:323-329.
29. Young WF Jr. The incidentally discovered adrenal mass. *N Engl J Med.* 2007;356:601-610.

Gonadal Function

MAHIMA GULATI, A. WAYNE MEIKLE

CHAPTER

22

CHAPTER OUTLINE

Chapter Objectives

Upon completion of this chapter, the clinical laboratorian should be able to do the following:

• Discuss the biosynthesis, secretion, transport, and action of the sex steroids and gonadotropins.
• Identify the location of the pituitary, ovaries, and testes.
• Describe the hypothalamic–pituitary–ovarian and hypothalamic–pituitary–testicular axes and how they regulate sex steroid and gonadotropin hormone production.

• Explain the principles of each diagnostic test for pituitary–gonadal axes dysfunction.
• Correlate laboratory information with regard to suspected gonadal disorders, given a patient's clinical data.
• Describe the appropriate laboratory testing protocol to effectively evaluate or monitor patients with suspected gonadal disease.

KEY TERMS

Amenorrhea
Androgen
Corpus luteum
Follicle-stimulating hormone
Follicular phase
Graafian follicle
Gynecomastia
Hirsutism

Hypogonadism
Inhibin
Leydig cell
Luteal phase
Luteinizing hormone
Ovulation
Sertoli cell
Virilization

THE TESTES

By the sixth week of development in both sexes, the primordial germ cells have migrated from their extraembryonic location to the gonadal ridges, where they are surrounded by the sex cords to form a pair of primitive gonads. Whether chromosomally 46 XX or 46 XY, the developing gonad at this stage of development is bipotential.

The ovarian pathway is followed unless a gene on the short arm of the Y chromosome, designated TDF (testis-determined factor), acts as a switch, diverting development into the male pathway. In the presence of the Y chromosome, the medullary tissue forms typical testes with seminiferous tubules and Leydig cells, which under the stimulation of human chorionic gonadotropin (hCG) from the placenta become capable of androgen secretion.

The spermatogonia, derived from the primordial germ cells by 200 or more successive mitoses, form the walls of the seminiferous tubules together with supporting Sertoli cells.

While the primordial germ cells are migrating to the genital ridges, thickenings in the ridges indicate the developing genital ducts and the mesonephric (formerly called Wolffian) and paramesonephric (formerly called Müllerian) ducts. In the male, the Leydig cells of the fetal testes produce androgen, which stimulates the mesonephric ducts to form the male genital ducts, and the Sertoli cells produce a hormone that suppresses formation of the paramesonephric ducts. In the female (or in an embryo with no gonads), the mesonephric ducts regress, and the paramesonephric ducts develop into the female duct system. In the early embryo, the external genitalia consist of a genital tubercle, paired labioscrotal swellings, and paired urethral folds. From this undifferentiated state, male external genitalia develop under the influence of androgens or, in the absence of a testis, female external genitalia are formed regardless of whether an ovary is present.

There are three important steps in sexual differentiation and the development of the normal male phenotype. The first is the differentiation of bipotential gonad primordia (identical in both XX and XY fetuses) into testes that secrete testosterone. The second is the development of the internal reproductive tract. In male fetuses, this requires the presence of anti-Müllerian hormone (AMH) that causes involution of the Müllerian ducts, the anlage for the female type reproductive tract. The third is the development of the external genitalia that requires testosterone and, in some target tissues, its more potent metabolite 5α-dihydrotestosterone (DHT).

The genes involved in gonadal differentiation have been determined. To date, three genes have been identified in the formation of the bipotential gonad. WT1[1] and LIM1[2] code for zinc-finger DNA binding proteins and are expressed early in gonadal development. FTZ-F1 codes for an orphan nuclear hormone receptor, steroidogenic factor-1 (SF-1).[2] Several functions have been ascribed to SF-1 including differentiation and maintenance of both gonadal and adrenal tissue, increasing the synthesis of testosterone and reducing its conversion to estradiol via the transcriptional regulation of the hydroxylases and P450 aromatase, respectively. It may also regulate transcription of the AMH[3] gene.

Functional Anatomy of the Male Reproductive Tract

Adult testes are paired, ovoid organs that hang from the inguinal canal by the spermatic cord, which comprises a neurovascular pedicle, vas deferens, and cremasteric muscle. The testes are located outside the body, encased by a muscular sac. Blood flow is governed by an intricate plexus of arterial and venous blood flow that, together with contraction of the dartos muscle in the scrotal sac, regulates the temperature of the testicles to 2°C below core body temperature. This important function is vital to uninterrupted sperm production. Also encased in the muscular sheath is the spermatic cord, which has the ability to retract the testicles into the inguinal canal in instances of threatened injury. The testes themselves are comprised of two anatomical units: a network of tubules, known as the seminiferous tubules, and an interstitium. The tubules contain germ cells and Sertoli cells and are responsible for sperm production. The testes serve dual functions, which include (1) production of sperm and (2) production of reproductive steroid hormones.[4] In the embryonic stage, the dominant male sex hormone, testosterone (T), aids in development and differentiation of the primordial gonads.

Puberty marks the transition from a non-reproductive state into a reproductive state and is associated with adrenarche with increase in adrenal androgen and gonadarche. Tanner staging of the pubertal and axillary hair changes and genitalia are used in children to mark pubertal changes, which are characterized by growth spurt, increased muscle mass, psychological changes, and male pattern hair growth. The earliest sign of puberty in boys is testicular enlargement that results from rising luteinizing hormone (LH) and follicle-stimulating hormone (FSH). After puberty, throughout adulthood, and until late in old age, testosterone helps with sperm production and maintains secondary sexual characteristics.

The sperm move sequentially through the tubuli recti; rete testes; ductuli efferentes testes; the head, body, and tail of the epididymis; and, finally, into the vas deferens. Various secretory products of the seminal vesicles and prostate mix with sperm to form the final product: semen. Seminal vesicle secretions are rich in vitamin C and fructose, important for the preservation of motility of the sperm.

Physiology of the Testicles

Spermatogenesis
Sperm are formed from stem cells called *spermatogonia*. The spermatogonia undergo mitosis and meiosis; finally, the haploid cells transform to form mature sperm. The mature sperm has a head, body, and tail, which enables it to swim for the purpose of forming a zygote with the haploid ovum. Certain spermatogonia stagger division so that sperm production is uninterrupted and continuous. The Sertoli cells are polyfunctional cells that aid in the development and maturation of sperm.[5]

Hormonogenesis
Testosterone, the predominant hormone secreted by the testes, is controlled primarily by two pituitary hormones: FSH and LH.[6] Because these hormones were

first described in women, they are named in reference to the menstrual cycle. Both hormones are produced by a single group of cells in the pituitary called *gonadotrophs*. FSH acts primarily on germinal stem cells[7] and LH acts primarily on the Leydig cells[6]—located in the testicular insterstitium—that synthesize testosterone. Gonadotropins (LH and FSH) are glycoproteins and share an alpha subunit with thyroid-stimulating hormone (TSH) and hCG. The beta subunit confers biological specificity for them.

Hormonal Control of Testicular Function

The hypothalamus, located in the brain, generates a hormone called gonadotropin-releasing hormone (GnRH) in a pulsatile fashion. GnRH is synthesized in neurons situated in the arcuate nucleus and other nuclei of the hypothalamus and is released into the portal hypophyseal system that, in turn, determines the production of LH and FSH from the pituitary gland. Impaired pulse generation of GnRH leads to inadequate production of LH and FSH, resulting in hypogonadism.[8] The first, and rate-limiting, step in the testicular steroidogenesis is the conversion of cholesterol to pregnenolone. This cholesterol is either trapped by endocytosis from the blood lipoproteins or synthesized within the Leydig cells. The LH binds to the glycoprotein receptor in the cell wall and induces intracellular cyclic AMP production that, in turn, activates protein kinase A, which catalyzes protein phosphorylation. This latter step induces testosterone synthesis. The testicular steroidogenesis pathway is similar to the pathway in the adrenal cortex and they share the same enzymatic systems. Testosterone is the principal androgen hormone in the blood, and after puberty the testes secrete 4 to 10 mg daily and less than 5% is derived from adrenal precursors such as dehydroepiandrosterone (DHEA) and androstenedione. It is largely bound, with 2% to 3% free. About 50% of testosterone is bound to albumin and about 45% is bound to sex hormone–binding globulin (SHBG). The concentration of binding protein determines the level of total testosterone but not the free testosterone levels during laboratory estimation. Testosterone and inhibin are the two hormones secreted by the testes that provide feedback control to the hypothalamus and pituitary. Leydig cell steroidogenesis of testosterone is primarily controlled by LH secretion, with negative feedback of testosterone and estradiol on the hypothalamic–pituitary axis. FSH acts on Sertoli cells to stimulate protein synthesis, inhibin, and androgen-binding protein. The actions of both testosterone and FSH on Sertoli cells are synergistic, permitting completion of spermatogenesis. FSH stimulates production of an androgen receptor that makes the Sertoli cell responsive to androgen and in turn androgens stimulate synthesis of FSH receptors. Feedback on FSH is attributed to inhibin.

Testosterone concentration fluctuates in a circadian fashion, reflecting the parallel rhythms of LH and FSH levels. This fact should be considered when interpreting serum levels of testosterone: the highest level is found at about 6 am and correlates with most laboratory normal ranges, and the lowest level is found at about 12 am.

Cellular Mechanism of Testosterone Action

Testosterone enters the cell and converts to DHT in cells rich in 5α-reductase, such as some hair follicles and prostate. DHT and testosterone complex with an intracellular receptor protein and this complex binds to the nuclear receptor, effecting protein synthesis and cell growth.

Physiologic Actions of Testosterone

Prenatal Development

Early in development, embryos have primordial components of the genital tracts of both sexes. The primitive gonads become distinguishable at about the seventh week of embryonic stage. Both chorionic gonadotropins and fetal LH stimulate production of testosterone by the fetal Leydig cells. In the fetus, the hypothalamo-hypophyseal vascular connections are responsible for LH release by hypothalamic GnRH and are established between 11 and 12 weeks after conception, which is 3 weeks after testosterone production by the Leydig cells of the testis. hCG, which has LH-like action, made by the placenta, accounts for this gap in stimulation of testosterone production by the fetal testes. Exposure of testosterone to the Wolffian duct leads to differentiation of the various components of the male genital tract. Sertoli cells produce AMH, which aids in regression of the female primordial genital tract. The scrotal skin is rich in 5α-reductase, which converts testosterone to DHT. Fetal exposure to drugs that block this enzyme and DHT formation leads to feminization of the genitalia of the male fetus.

Postnatal Development

Testicular function is reactivated during puberty after a period of quiescence to produce testosterone that results in development of secondary sex hair (face, chest, axilla, and pubis), enhanced linear skeletal growth, development of internal and external genitalia, increased upper body musculature, and development of larynx and vocal cords with deepening of the voice.[10-12] Possible mood changes and aggression are undesired effects that may occur during puberty. The linear growth effects of testosterone are finite, with epiphyseal closure when genetically determined height is achieved. Hypogonadism during puberty leads to imprecise closure of growth plates, leading to excessive height, long limbs, and disproportionate upper and lower body segments. Male secondary sexual characteristics can be staged by a system of development devised by Marshall and Tanner (Table 22-1).

TABLE 22-1	TANNER STAGING OF GENITAL AND PUBIC HAIR DEVELOPMENT IN MALES

STAGES OF GENITAL DEVELOPMENT

1. Prepubertal
2. Enlargement of scrotum and testes
3. Increased length of penis, further enlargement of testes
4. Enlargement of testes, scrotum, and penis with growth of glans; darkening of scrotal skin
5. Mature genitalia

STAGES OF PUBIC HAIR DEVELOPMENT

1. Lanugo-type hair (prepubertal)
2. Dark terminal hair at base of penis
3. Darker terminal hair spreading over junction of pubes
4. Terminal hair covering pubic region, no spread to medial thighs
5. Mature stage with horizontal distribution of terminal hair to inner thighs

Effect on Spermatogenesis

Stimulation of Leydig cells induces production of testosterone. Testosterone, acting with FSH, has paracrine effects on the seminiferous and Sertoli cells, inducing spermatogenesis. Exogenous overuse or abuse of testosterone, such as occurs with some athletes, will reduce the high intratesticular concentration of testosterone, leading to reduction of sperm production.

Effect on Secondary Sexual Effects

Testosterone has growth-promoting effects on various target tissues. The secondary sex characteristics that develop during puberty are maintained into late adulthood by testosterone.[12] The prostate enlarges progressively during adulthood, while exposure of scalp hair results in regression of the hair follicles (temporal hairline recession). Failure to develop secondary sexual characteristics should prompt evaluation for hypogonadism or constitutional delay in boys. Loss of secondary sexual characteristics might occur gradually and should prompt evaluation for hypogonadism because, among other effects, low testosterone levels lead to loss of bone mass and development of osteoporosis in males at any age.

Disorders of Sexual Development and Testicular Hypofunction

Pubertal development could be premature (precocious) or delayed, even if development is normal at birth.[13,14] Precocious sexual development results from the premature exposure of sex steroids, which might arise from early gonadotropin secretion or production

by the adrenal glands or testes. Detailed descriptions of the sequence of hormonal pubertal abnormalities of hair, genitals, and breasts are beyond the scope of this text. The differential diagnosis of hypogonadism includes a diverse group of disorders affecting the testicles and the hypothalamic–pituitary regulation of the testes outlined in Box 22-1. Certain important disorders are explained in the following section.

Hypergonadotropic Hypogonadism

Hypergonadotropic hypogonadism incorporates a group of disorders characterized by low testosterone, elevated FSH or LH, and impaired sperm production.

Klinefelter's Syndrome

Klinefelter's syndrome occurs in about 1 of 400 men and is caused by the presence of an extra chromosome. The most

BOX 22-1 CAUSES OF DELAYED PUBERTY

- Delayed puberty or hypogonadism, with increased gonadotropins (FSH and/or LH)
  - Klinefelter's syndrome
  - Bilateral gonadal failure
  - Primary testicular failure
  - Anorchia
  - Vanishing testicles
  - Chemotherapeutic agents
  - Irradiation
  - Trauma
  - Infection (mumps orchitis)
- Delayed puberty with normal or low FSH and/or LH
  - Constitutional delayed puberty[15]
  - Hypothalamic dysfunction
  - Malnutrition
  - Chronic systemic illness
  - Severe obesity
  - Central nervous system tumors
  - Hypopituitarism
  - Panhypopituitarism
  - Kallmann's syndrome (anosmia, cleft palate, and reduced FSH and LH levels)
  - Isolated GH deficiency
  - Hyperprolactinemia (prolactinoma or drug induced)
  - Hypothyroidism
- Miscellaneous
  - Prader-Willi syndrome
  - Laurence-Moon syndrome
  - LEOPARD syndrome
  - Bloom syndrome
  - Germ cell neoplasia
  - Male pseudohermaphroditism
  - Ataxia-telangiectasia
  - Steroidogenic enzyme defects

common karyotype is 47,XXY.[11] Men with this disorder have small (<2.5 cm), firm testicles. Gynecomastia (enlargement of the male breast) is commonly present at the time of diagnosis. Due to reduced production of testosterone, LH levels are elevated. Due to deficient seminiferous tubule mass, FSH is elevated from underproduction of inhibin.[16] These men also have azoospermia and resultant sterility. Men with *mosaicism* may produce some sperm and pregnancies have been reported with such men. Elevated levels of FSH and LH induce increased aromatase activity, resulting in elevated estrogen levels. Men with Klinefelter's syndrome may have reduced bone density and breast cancer risk comparable to women.

Testicular Feminization Syndrome

Testicular feminization syndrome is the most severe form of androgen resistance syndrome, resulting from mutations of the androgen receptor and impaired androgen actions in target tissues. As a result of the lack of androgen and unopposed estrogen effects, the physical development pursues the female phenotype, with fully developed breast and female distribution of fat and hair. Most present for evaluation of primary amenorrhea, at which time the lack of female internal genitalia becomes apparent. The testicles are often undescended, and failure to promptly remove these organs is essential to abort malignant transformation. Biochemical evaluation reveals normal or elevated serum concentrations of testosterone with elevated FSH and LH levels. There is no utility or response to administration of exogenous testosterone. They are reared as girls. There is a wide variation in androgen insensitivity and in corresponding clinical deficits in male sexual development.

5α-Reductase Deficiency

Deficiency of 5α-reductase is a rare cause of androgen insensitivity and results in a mutation encoding the type 2 isoenzyme, maps to chromosome 2p23, and is expressed in XY males. A reduction in levels of the enzyme 5α-reductase results in decreased DHT concentrations. Physical development is similar to the female phenotype until puberty when the Wolffian ducts virilize in response to testosterone. The female internal genitalia are absent and the male internal genitalia are well developed (epididymis, vas deferens, and seminal vesicle) in response to testosterone. DHT is essential for the development of the prostate and external genitalia during embryonic virilization.

Myotonic Dystrophy

Myotonic dystrophy is inherited in an autosomal dominant fashion and presents with primary hypogonadism, frontal balding, diabetes, and muscle weakness, atrophy, and dystonia (an inability of the muscle to relax adequately after contraction). Testicular failure typically presents in the fourth decade of life; however, puberty progresses normally and male secondary sexual characteristics, height, bone growth, etc., are attained normally during pubertal course of development. Primary hypogonadism occurs with primarily germ cell compartment failure (i.e., oligozoospermia and infertility), with elevated serum FSH. In later stages, failure of Leydig cell compartment resulting in low serum testosterone, elevated LH concentrations, and testicular atrophy occurs. Testicular failure happens more commonly in DM1 (type 1 myotonic dystrophy) than in DM2.

Testicular Injury and Infection

Postpubertal mumps infection can result in mumps orchitis and permanent testicular injury. Testicular damage due to viral orchitis and HIV infection has also been reported. Radiation and chemotherapy for cancer can also result in long-term damage.

Sertoli Cell–Only Syndrome

Sertoli cell–only syndrome is characterized by a lack of germ cells. Men present with small testes, high FSH levels, azoospermia, and normal testosterone levels. Testicular biopsy is the only procedure to confirm this diagnosis.

Hypogonadotropic Hypogonadism

The hallmark of disorders of hypogonadotropic hypogonadism is the occurrence of low testosterone levels together with low or inappropriately normal FSH or LH levels.

Kallmann's Syndrome

The impaired secretion of GnRH has been elucidated in the X-linked form of congenital GnRH deficiency, which results from impaired migration of GnRH neurons and olfactory nerves to the ventral hypothalamus during embryogenesis. Proper migration of these neurons is dependent on the correct expression of anosmin, a 680–amino acid neural cell adhesion molecule–like protein, which is the product of the KAL1 gene.

Mutations in the KAL1 gene (a gene found on the X chromosome) occur less often in sporadic cases (<10%). In general, the clinical phenotypes of idiopathic hypogonadotropic hypogonadism (IHH) subjects with KAL1 mutations are characterized with a high incidence of microphallus, cryptorchidism, and small testes. X-linked KAL mutations have never been observed in families with normosmic IHH (nIHH) or in families with both anosmic and nonanosmic individuals.[17,18]

Kallmann's syndrome is a result of an inherited, X-linked recessive trait that manifests as hypogonadism during puberty. The frequency of this syndrome is 1 of 10,000 males. Certain men also have red-green color blindness, congenital deafness, or cerebellar dysfunction.

Hyperprolactinemia

Prolactin elevation resulting from any cause (drug-induced or prolactin-producing tumors of the pituitary) can result in hypogonadotropic hypogonadism[19,20] due to impairment of pulsatile secretion of FSH and LH, because of incompletely understood mechanisms (may involve disruption of GnRH pulsatile secretion).

Type 2 Diabetes

Type 2 diabetes is also associated with hypogonadotropic hypogonadism in at least 25% of men.[22] It is characterized by low free or total serum concentrations of testosterone and inappropriately low LH.[21] The mechanism underlying this seems to be a combination of both insulin resistance (insulin action seems to be important for LH release by gonadotropes) and inflammation (hypogonadism in type 2 diabetic males was seen to be associated with high C-reactive protein levels, an inflammatory marker).[22]

Age

There is a gradual reduction in testosterone after age 30, with an average decline of about 110 ng/dL every decade. The Baltimore Longitudinal Study of Aging revealed "hypogonadism" (reduced total testosterone concentrations) of 19% at age 60, 28% at age 70, and 49% at age 80,[23] with free testosterone concentrations much lower in these men. Age is also associated with elevation of SHBG by about 1% per year. Similar findings emerged from the Massachusetts Male Aging Study, which showed 1.6%/year decline in total testosterone levels; and 2% to 3%/year decline in bioavailable testosterone (free and albumin-bound testosterone) levels.[24]

Total testosterone levels may be normal in aging men but the free (unbound) concentrations of testosterone are more reliable indicators of biochemical reduction. The associated features of reduced secondary sex hair growth, loss of muscle bulk and strength, and loss of bone density are corroborative evidence indicative of the lack of tissue effects of testosterone. Testosterone deficiency is a constellation of clinical features of hypogonadism combined with low serum testosterone concentrations. The combination of biochemical and clinical evidence of testosterone should prompt consideration of testosterone replacement in older men.

Pituitary Disease

Acquired hypogonadism can follow injury to the pituitary as a result of tumors, surgical trauma, vascular injury, autoimmune hypophysitis, or granulomatous or metastatic disease. Hemochromatosis is a rare cause of pituitary dysfunction.

Diagnosis of Hypogonadism

Both clinical and biochemical features must be met (Fig. 22-1) to make the diagnosis of hypogonadism.

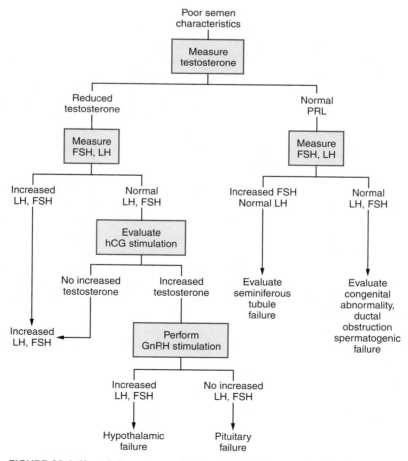

FIGURE 22-1 Clinical diagnostic evaluation of male hypogonadism. PRL, prolactin; FSH, follicle-stimulating hormone; LH, luteinizing hormone; hCG, human chorionic gonadotropin; GnRH, gonadotropin-releasing hormone.

Testosterone concentrations have a circadian rhythm and the time of sampling must be considered. Morning samples between 8 and 10 am are recommended to match values from reference interval studies. Multiple estimation of free and bound testosterone levels should be done on different days before a diagnosis of testosterone deficiency is confirmed.[25] The distinction between primary (disease or destruction of the testes) versus secondary (disease or destruction of the pituitary) or tertiary (hypothalamic) is relatively easy to make. FSH and/or LH[26] values are elevated in primary hypogonadism and are inappropriately normal or low with secondary or tertiary etiologies. Pituitary MRI should be done in secondary hypogonadism in young individuals. Older individuals often have secondary or tertiary (hypothalamic) dysfunction as a result of reduced hypothalamic pulse generator frequency, resulting in low or inappropriately normal FSH and/or LH levels.[27] Clinical signs and symptoms of hypogonadism (e.g., loss of secondary sexual characteristics and osteoporosis) should be corroborated with low testosterone levels, particularly when testosterone replacement therapy is considered.[25]

Testosterone Replacement Therapy

The following principles should guide testosterone therapy: Testosterone should be administered **only to a man who is hypogonadal**, as evidenced by clinical symptoms and signs consistent with androgen deficiency and a distinctly subnormal serum testosterone concentration. Treating symptoms of hypogonadism without corroborating biochemical evidence of testosterone deficiency is not recommended. Restoring testosterone to mid-normal concentrations can be achieved satisfactorily whether the testosterone deficiency is due to primary or secondary hypogonadism.

The currently available modes[28] of testosterone administration in the United States are as follows:

1. **Parenteral testosterone.** This is the most widely available and cost-effective mode of administration. The cypionate and enanthate esters of testosterone are available for intramuscular injection. The peak level is achieved in 72 hours and the effect lasts for a period of 1 to 2 weeks. Weekly administration provides for a lower peak and less fluctuation within the normal range of testosterone levels. Usual dosing is 50 to 100 mg weekly or 200 to 250 mg once every 2 weeks. Testosterone dose should be based on lean body mass, not on body weight, and is best reached by administering a standard dose of testosterone, with minor dose escalations based on serum testosterone levels measured midpoint between two injections. The goal is to maintain this mid-dose level at midpoint of the normal ranges.
2. **Transdermal testosterone patch therapy.** This mode of administration provides more physiologic levels of testosterone. The patch is permeability enhanced to aid in the absorption of testosterone through normal skin. Local skin irritation can occur and often limits the patch use.
3. **Testosterone gel.** This hydroalcoholic gel preparation is applied to nongenital skin once daily. The absorption is gradual and provides blood levels of testosterone in the normal range for 24 hours. The main concern with this preparation is potential transmission to female partners or children on close skin contact.
4. **Testosterone buccal pellet.** This plastic tablet is placed along the gum line twice daily. Local discomfort and the need for twice-daily dosing sometimes limit use.
5. **Testosterone pellet.** A subcutaneous testosterone pellet (Testopel) is now available. The manufacturer recommends three to six 75 mg testosterone pellets every 3 to 6 months. Pellets are implanted into the subdermal fat of the buttocks, lower abdominal wall, or thigh with a trocar under sterile conditions using a local anesthetic. There are adverse events including pellet extrusion, infection, and fibrosis. Because of limited data on the serum testosterone concentrations during treatment, we do not routinely recommend this preparation.

Complications of testosterone replacement are acne, polycythemia, prostate enlargement, possible growth-promoting effect on undiagnosed prostate cancer, worsening of obstructive sleep apnea, peripheral edema, and gynecomastia.

Oral alkylated androgens are not recommended due to adverse effects of decreased high-density lipoprotein,[29] increase in low-density lipoprotein (LDL), and also incidence of cholestatic jaundice and peliosis hepatis.

Monitoring Testosterone Replacement Therapy

Prostate-specific antigen (PSA), blood counts (for hematocrit), and lipid levels should be checked 3 to 6 months after initiation of testosterone replacement and at least yearly thereafter. Routine clinical evaluation for leg edema, worsening of sleep apnea, and prostate enlargement is also recommended. Pharmacologic use of testosterone may also reduce sperm count by reducing the intratesticular testosterone concentration that is manyfold higher than serum concentrations. If PSA elevation is noted after testosterone replacement, prostate evaluation with possible biopsy is recommended. Prostatic carcinoma is a contraindication to testosterone replacement.

THE OVARIES

Early Ovarian Development

If no Y chromosome or TDF is present, the gonad, by default, forms an ovary; the cortex develops, the medulla regresses, and oogonia begin to develop within follicles. The oogonia are derived from the primitive germ cells by a series of about 30 mitoses, far fewer than the number required for spermatogenesis. Beginning at about the end of the third month, the oogonia enter meiosis I, but this process is arrested at a stage called dictyotene, in which the cell remains until ovulation occurs many years later (this cell is called "primary oocyte"). Many of the oogonia degenerate before birth, and only about 400 mature into ova during the 30 years or so of sexual maturity of the female. It is evident that the gonads are paired bilateral structures; in very rare circumstances the developmental processes may be different on either side. Estrogen formation in the fetal ovary begins in early development despite primordial follicles not having begun forming until the second trimester of pregnancy (at 16 weeks of gestation). The gonadotropins from the pituitary gradually take over the role of maternal placental hCG, and fetal pituitary LH and FSH peak near mid-gestation and then fall to low concentrations at birth. Postpartum, a smaller peak of LH and FSH occur, which stimulates steroid secretion leading to neonatal milk production from the breast.

Pubertal Changes of Ovarian Function

The onset of puberty is characterized by increasing secretion of LH and FSH that stimulates gonadal activity and is driven by increased activity of the hypothalamic GnRH neurons. In the ovary both LH and FSH are involved in the control of steroidogenesis, and there are numerous isoforms of circulating LH and FSH and their biological potency depends on the degree of glycosylation, which is associated with differences in assays for LH and FSH. The genes coding LH and FSH receptors are on chromosome 2p21. Inactivating mutations of the β-chain of the LH receptor have been described. Before the onset of puberty, both LH and FSH are secreted in small amounts, but as puberty approaches the amplitude of LH and FSH pulsatile secretions increases and the nocturnal rise in LH secretion increases. The nocturnal rise disappears with adulthood.

The ovaries are paired organs that, like the male gonads, perform the dual functions of gamete (ovum) and steroid hormone production.[30-32] Unlike in the male, the primordial reproductive cells in the female typically produce a solitary gamete. Ovarian and menstrual events are carefully synchronized by a complex interplay of hormones among the hypothalamus, pituitary, and ovaries to prepare the uterus for implantation of an embryo. In the absence of implantation, the uterine lining is shed, resulting in menses.[33,34]

The length of the menstrual cycle is the time between any two consecutive cycles. The typical duration is 28 (±3) days, with average menstrual flow about 2 to 4 days.[34]

Functional Anatomy of the Ovaries

The ovaries are oval organs that lie in the pelvic fossa, formed by the posterior and lateral pelvic wall, and attach to the posterior surface of the broad ligament by the peritoneal fold, otherwise known as the mesovarium. They are positioned near the fimbrial end of the fallopian tubes, which are connected to the uterine cavity. An adult ovary averages 2 to 5 cm in length, weighs an average of 14 g, and typically contains 2 to 4 million primordial follicles.[35] These primordial follicles are present at birth; however, maturation is blocked until puberty. Following the onset of puberty, each ovarian cycle is marked by recruitment of a few primordial follicles for maturation. Typically, all but one of these follicles will then atrophy, in a process termed the follicular phase.

The single remaining follicle—known as the Graafian follicle—is composed of an outer and inner layer (the theca externa and theca interna, respectively) encasing a central fluid-filled cavity and a layer of cells known as the granulosa layer.[36-38] The maturing ovum attaches to the inside of the follicle via cells derived from granulosa cells, called *cumulus cells*. During the luteal phase of the ovarian cycle, the Graafian follicle releases its ovum in response to ovarian stimulation by LH. When the ovum is extruded, the Graafian follicle undergoes a morphologic change with hypertrophy of the theca and granulosa cells to become the corpus luteum. This process is called *luteinization*. The corpus luteum is rich in cholesterol and acts as a substrate for continued production of progesterone and estrogen, maintaining the endometrium for conception. If conception or implantation fails to occur, the endometrium is shed and the corpus luteum atrophies to an atretic follicle.

Hormonal Production by the Ovaries

As in the adrenal glands and the testes, the steroidogenic pathway and synthetic enzymes are present in the ovaries. Cholesterol is either synthesized from acetate or actively transported from the LDL particle in blood and then used as a substrate for hormonal production.[39]

Estrogen

Naturally synthesized estrogens are carbon-18 compounds. The principal estrogen produced in the ovary is estradiol. Estrone and estriol are primarily metabolites of intraovarian and extraglandular conversion. Estrogens promote breast, uterine, and vaginal development and also affect the skin, vascular smooth muscles, bone cells, and the central nervous system.[40] The lack of estrogen that naturally occurs with the onset of menopause leads to atrophic changes in these organs.[41] During the reproductive period, it is estrogen that is responsible for follicular phase changes in the uterus, with deficiency resulting in irregular and incomplete development of the endometrium.

Progesterone

Progesterone is a carbon-21 compound within the steroid family and is produced by the corpus luteum.

Progesterone induces the secretory activity of those endometrial glands that have been primed by estrogen, readying the endometrium for embryo implantation. Other effects include thickening of the cervical mucus, reduction of uterine contractions, and thermogenic effect, in which basal body temperature rises after ovulation. This effect is of clinical use in marking the occurrence of ovulation. Progesterone is the dominant hormone responsible for the luteal phase, and deficiency results in failure of implantation of the embryo.[42]

Androgens

Ovaries produce the androgens androstenedione, dehydroandrostenedione, testosterone, and DHT, all of which are carbon-19 compounds. Excess production of ovarian androgens in women leads to excess hair growth (hirsutism), loss of female characteristics, and—in severe cases—development of overt male secondary sexual features (masculinization or virilization).[42-44] Unlike estrogen, which is not produced in the ovary after menopause, ovarian androgen synthesis continues well into advanced age.[45]

Others

Inhibins A and B, which are produced by the ovaries, are hormones that inhibit FSH production.[46] Activin is a hormone that enhances FSH secretion and induces steroidogenesis.[46] Folliculostatin, relaxin,[47] follicle regulatory protein, oocyte maturation factor, and meiosis-inducing substance are hormones that appear to have important, yet not clearly characterized, functions.

The Menstrual Cycle

By convention, the menstrual cycle is considered to start on the first day of menses (day 1). The menstrual cycle consists of two phases of parallel events occurring at the ovaries and endometrium. Within the ovaries, these events are known as the follicular and luteal phases, while the concurrent endometrial events are known as the proliferative and secretory phases.[48]

The Follicular Phase

The follicular phase begins with the onset of menses and ends on the day of LH surge. Early in the follicular phase, the ovary secretes very little estrogen or progesterone. A rise in FSH, however, stimulates estrogen production. The estrogen secreted by the developing follicle within the ovary stimulates uterine epithelial cells, blood vessel growth, and endometrial gland development to increase the thickness of the endometrium. The intense secretory capacity of the uterine glands aids the implantation of the embryo.

The Luteal Phase

Estrogen levels peak 1 day before ovulation, at which point a positive feedback system results in an LH surge. The start of the luteal phase is marked by the extrusion of the ovum approximately 36 hours after this LH surge, with subsequent luteinization of the Graafian follicle to form the corpus luteum. The corpus luteum secretes progesterone to aid in the implantation of the embryo. In the absence of fertilization, with a gradual decline in the production of progesterone and estrogen by the corpus luteum there is a loss of endometrial blood supply; this results in shedding of the endometrium approximately 14 days after ovulation occurred. The typical duration of menstrual bleeding is 3 to 5 days, with blood loss averaging 50 mL. Onset of menses marks the end of the luteal phase.

Hormonal Control of Ovulation

The central control of FSH and LH secretion resides in the GnRH pulse generator of the arcuate nuclei and medial preoptic nuclei of the hypothalamus.[48] Positive and negative feedback responses exist among estrogen, progesterone, LH, and FSH production. It is because of the lack of estrogen after menopause that both FSH and LH levels rise.[49] During reproductive years, FSH levels are elevated early in the follicular phase. A midcycle surge in LH production stimulates a series of events that culminate in ovulation, with FSH levels falling after this event. Any injury to the hypothalamus or the presence of either psychosocial or physical stressors leads to changes in these hormonal cues and results in anovulation and amenorrhea.[50]

CASE STUDY 22-1

A 39-year-old woman presented with hot flashes and irregular menstrual cycles for 6 months. Clinical examination did not reveal abnormality. Laboratory evaluation reveals the following: CBC, normal; blood glucose, 89 mg/dL; TSH, 1.5 mIU/L; FSH, 128 IU/L; and LH, 30 IU/L.

This clinical situation is consistent with one of the following:

1. PCOS

2. Prolactinoma

3. Pituitary tumor

4. Menopause

5. Hypothalamic hormone deficiency

Pubertal Development in the Female

As with males, puberty in females consists of a sequence of hormonally mediated events resulting in the development of secondary sexual characteristics and attainment of final adult height. Thelarche (development of breast tissue) is typically the earliest sign of sexual development, followed by development of pubic hair. Menarche, or initiation of menses, occurs an average of 2 to 3 years after the onset of puberty.

Precocious Sexual Development

Precocious sexual development occurs in response to premature exposure of tissues to sex steroids from any source and is distinguished from precious puberty, which can be arrested by suppression of GnRH with analogs of GnRH that will suppress LH. If untreated, precious puberty or sexual development can lead to short stature. Premature breast development is characterized by isolated breast development and occurs in response to earlier estrogen secretion, albeit at low circulating concentrations. Premature adrenarche may occur between 4 and 8 years of age and is characterized by pubic hair growth and most commonly precious puberty does not ensue. Gonadotropins and gonadal steroid secretion help differentiate between them. DHEA and dehydroepiandrosterone sulfate (DHEAS) are elevated for age, but match the child's bone age.

In girls with delayed puberty, sex steroids and gonadotropins are low, but they continue growing and may be tall because growth hormone (GH) and other pituitary hormones are unaffected unless pituitary or hypothalamic dysfunction is present.

Devised by Marshall and Tanner as a way to determine pubertal staging, the Tanner staging system, outlined in Table 22-2, is used to monitor and assess the growth stages of breast and pubic hair.[51]

Menstrual Cycle Abnormalities

The menstrual cycle ranges from 25 to 35 days, with an average 28-day duration. The average age of menopause in the United States is between 45 and 55 years, with the median at 53 years.[49]

Amenorrhea is defined as the absence of menses. *Primary amenorrhea* is used to describe a woman who has never menstruated by age 16 years, while *secondary amenorrhea* is used to describe a woman who has had at least one menstrual cycle followed by absence of menses for a minimum of 3 to 6 months.[50] Frequency of the different etiologies for amenorrhea, both primary and secondary, is listed in Table 22-3.

Oligomenorrhea refers to infrequent irregular menstrual bleeding, with cycle lengths in excess of 35 to 40 days. Uterine bleeding in excess of 7 days is dysfunctional and is termed *menorrhagia*. In a patient with infertility, the diagnosis of inadequate luteal phase is made when the luteal phase is less than 10 days or when an endometrial biopsy indicates the progression of endometrial changes is delayed or out of phase, resulting in implantation

TABLE 22-2 TANNER STAGING OF BREAST AND PUBIC HAIR DEVELOPMENT IN FEMALES

STAGES OF BREAST DEVELOPMENT
1. Prepubertal
2. Elevation of breast bud and papilla, areolar enlargement
3. Elevation of breast tissue and papilla
4. Elevation of areola and papilla in secondary mound above the level of the breast
5. Mature stage: recession of areola into the breast with projection of papilla only

STAGES OF PUBIC HAIR DEVELOPMENT
1. Lanugo-type hair (prepubertal)
2. Dark terminal hair on labia majora
3. Terminal hair covering labia majora and spreading to the mons pubis
4. Terminal hair fully covering the labia majora and mons pubis
5. Terminal hair covering the labia majora, mons pubis, and inner thighs

failure.[52] The multiple causes of male and female infertility are shown in Table 22-4.

The principles underlying the evaluation of disorders of normal menstrual functions, as outlined by the World Health Organization, are the same for ovarian and pituitary dysfunction (Box 22-2). A diagnostic approach to secondary amenorrhea is outlined in Figure 22-2.

Hypogonadotropic Hypogonadism
Hypogonadotropic hypogonadism, or gonadotropin (FSH and LH) deficiency resulting in decreased sex steroid production, is a common cause of secondary amenorrhea. There are many physiologic and pathologic causes of hypogonadotropic hypogonadism, including

TABLE 22-3 ETIOLOGIES OF AMENORRHEA

	PRIMARY (%)	SECONDARY (%)
Hypothalamus	27	38
Pituitary	2	15
Polycystic ovarian syndrome	7	30
Ovary	43	12
Uterus/outflow	19	7

TABLE 22-4	CAUSES OF INFERTILITY	
TARGET	**RESULT**	**CAUSE**
FEMALE		
Hypothalamus	Decreased GnRH	Drugs
		Increased stress
		Diet
Pituitary	Decreased FSH, LH	Destructive tumor or vesicular lesion
Ovaries	Decreased estradiol or progesterone	Organ failure
		Organ dysgenesis
		Antiovarian antibodies
		Malnourishment, very low weight, metabolic disease
Fallopian tubes and uterus	Inadequate endometrium	Low progesterone output
	Tubal scarring and closure	Pelvic inflammatory disease
	Decreased cervical mucus	Cervical infections
Conception	Immobilization and destruction of sperm	Antisperm antibodies
MALE		
Hypothalamus and pituitary	Oligospermia to azoospermia (no sperm)	Primary defects in hypothalamic or pituitary glands
		Exogenous androgens
		Testicular dysfunction
Testes	Oligospermia to azoospermia	Orchitis
	Delayed or deficient sexual maturity	Testicular infections (mumps)
	Decreased testosterone	Alcoholism/substance abuse
		Chromosomal defects
Prostate	Decreased seminal fluid	Infections of prostate or seminal vesicles
Urethrogenital tract	Retrograde or absent ejaculation	Physical abnormalities
		Chronic diabetes

GnRH, gonadotropin-releasing hormone; FSH, follicle-stimulating hormone; LH, luteinizing hormone.

weight loss as associated with anorexia nervosa or various disease processes, intense physical exercise (commonly termed *runner's amenorrhea*), and pituitary tumors that disrupt secretion of FSH or LH.[50] Prolactin production by prolactinomas can have similar effects. Any secondary cause of chronic hypogonadism can induce pathologic bone loss, resulting in osteopenia or, if severe, osteoporosis.

BOX 22-2 CLASSIFICATION OF AMENORRHEA BY WORLD HEALTH ORGANIZATION (WHO) GUIDELINES

- Type 1. Hypothalamic hypogonadism (low or normal FSH and/or LH)
  - Hypothalamic amenorrhea (anorexia nervosa, idiopathic, exercise induced)
  - Kallmann's syndrome
  - Isolated gonadotropin deficiency
- Type 2. Estrogenic chronic anovulation (normal FSH and LH)
- Polycystic ovarian syndrome (LH > FSH in some patients 2:1 or greater)
- Hyperthecosis
- Type 3. Hyperthalamic hypogonadism (elevated FSH and/or LSH)
  - Premature ovarian failure
  - Turner's syndrome

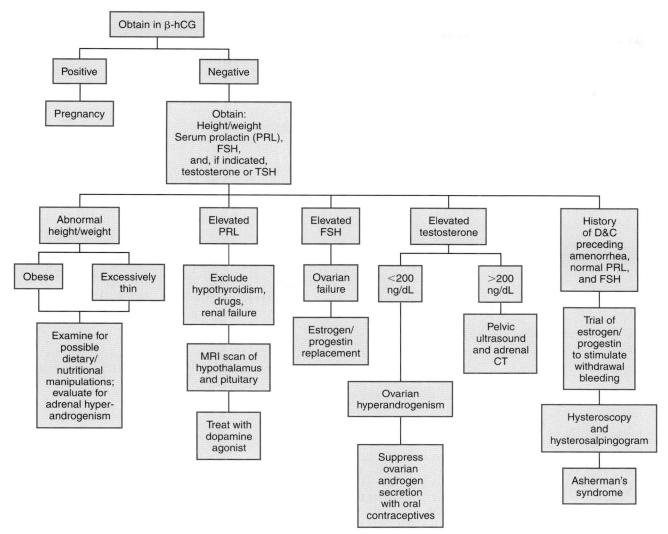

FIGURE 22-2 Diagnostic approach to secondary amenorrhea. FSH, follicle-stimulating hormone; TSH, thyroid-stimulating hormone; hCG, human chorionic gonadotropin.

CASE STUDY 22-2

A 49-year-old woman presented with increased hair growth for the past 6 months that started abruptly; she had male pattern hair loss, as well. On examination, she had temporal loss of hair and clitorimegaly. Laboratory evaluation revealed the following: testosterone, 360 ng/dL; FSH, 12 IU/L; LH, 9 IU/L; and a normal prolactin level.

The next step in the evaluation is one of the following:

1. DHEAS level
2. Repeat FSH and LH levels
3. Fasting blood sugar level
4. Fasting lipid level
5. Computed tomography of adrenal and ovaries

Hypergonadotropic Hypogonadism

Hypergonadotropic hypogonadism is characterized by ovarian failure resulting in elevation of FSH concentrations, with or without LH elevations. Ovarian failure occurs naturally between 45 and 55 years of age in American women. When the depletion of oocytes and follicles occurs at the expected time, it is termed *menopause*. Menopause is a natural, inevitable event that results in elevation of FSH and LH levels, with low levels of estrogen.[49]

Premature ovarian failure is defined as primary hypogonadism in a woman before the age of 40 and can be a result of congenital chromosomal abnormality (e.g., Turner's syndrome[53]) or premature menopause.[54] Patients with Turner's syndrome do not complain of the same hot flashes experienced by patients with secondary hypergonadotropic hypogonadism. Premature menopause can occur in isolation or in association with other endocrine gland failure such as hypoparathyroidism, hypothyroidism, or hypoadrenalism.[54]

CASE STUDY 22-3

A 24-year-old man presented with a history of hay fever, which had been treated with antihistamines. He relates diminished smell. He continues to grow slowly and pubertal development has been slow. The man denies erections or nocturnal emissions.

Management

Testosterone replacement therapy

Sexual maturity

Later desired fertility

GnRH pulsatile therapy produced a normal sperm count in 4 months and the man's wife became pregnant.

Questions

1. What is the level of the defect?

2. What is the significance of the body measurements?

3. What are the diagnostic considerations?

4. What test(s) might be obtained to make the diagnosis?

5. What constitutes normal fertility?

6. How will you counsel this man when he asks if he can have children?

PE	EUNUCHOIDAL MAN, APPEARING YOUNGER THAN AGE
Height	72 in.
Arm span	75 in.
Weight	180 lb
Blood pressure	130/82 mm Hg
Hair	Spare facial, axillary, and pubic
Genitalia	Penis, 3.1 cm (small)
Testes	Soft, 1 cm × 1.5 cm × 1.5 cm (normal, >4.5 cm × 3 cm × 3 cm)

GnRH STIMULATION

TIME (MINUTES)	LH	NORMAL
0, GnRH	<2 mU/mL	Pre-, <5
		Adult, 3–18
15	<2	Post-, 2.5 times baseline at some point
30	3	
45	<2	
60	3	

AFTER GnRH PRIMING

TIME (MINUTES)	LH	NORMAL
0	<2 mU/mL	Pre-, <5
		Adult, 3–18
15	10	LH rise greater than 2.5 times baseline
30	12	
45	16	
60	12	

LABORATORY VALUES

Testosterone	157 ng/dL (normal, prepubertal <100; adult, 300–1,000)
LH	<2 mU/mL (normal, prepubertal <5; adult, 3–18)
Prolactin	6 ng/mL (normal, 5–25)
TSH	1.2 mU/mL (normal, 0.3–5.0)

Polycystic Ovary Syndrome

This common disorder can present in many ways: infertility, hirsutism, chronic anovulation, glucose intolerance, hyperlipidemia or dyslipidemia, and hypertension.[42-44] The onset is often perimenarcheal, chronic, and notable for its slow progression. Investigations for this disorder involve estimation of free testosterone, SHBG, FSH, LH, fasting glucose, insulin, and lipid levels. Ovarian ultrasound reveals multiple cysts in many patients (about 30% of patients do not have ovarian cysts). Most patients with this disorder are overweight; however, patients with polycystic ovary syndrome (PCOS) of eastern Asian or South American descent are of normal weight. Most symptoms and laboratory abnormalities are reversed with weight loss and increased physical activity. The drug Glucophage (metformin), commonly used for the treatment of diabetes, is useful in this condition, even in the absence of diabetes. Although not U.S. Food and

BOX 22-3 CLASSIFICATION OF HIRSUTISM[43]

Functional (normal androgen levels with excess hair growth) or true androgen excess (elevated androgens)
Ovarian (LH mediated) or adrenal (adrenocorticotropin hormone mediated)
Peripheral conversion of androgens (obesity)
Tumoral hyperandrogenism (ovarian, adrenal)
Chorionic gonadotropin mediated

TABLE 22-5 CAUSES OF HIRSUTISM

COMMON
Idiopathic
Polycystic ovary syndrome
UNCOMMON
Drugs: danazol, oral contraceptives with androgenic progestins
Congenital adrenal hyperplasia
Hyperprolactinemia
Cushing syndrome
Adrenal tumors
Ovarian tumors

Drug Administration approved for this use, it reportedly normalizes menstrual cycles and improves conception rates.[55]

Hirsutism

Hirsutism is abnormal, abundant, androgen-sensitive terminal hair growth in areas in which terminal hair follicles are sparsely distributed or not normally found in women. Most commonly, hirsutism is idiopathic[56] in etiology (60% of cases), with PCOS the next most common cause (35%) (Box 22-3). Typical causes of hirsutism are listed in Table 22-5.[43]

Hirsutism should only be considered in the context of a woman's ethnic origin. Women of Italian, eastern European, eastern Indian, and Irish descent possess more androgen-sensitive terminal hair than do most northern European women, making a careful elicitation of ethnic background important prior to initiation of an extensive laboratory evaluation in a woman born in the United States. It is estimated that about 5% to 10% of American women have hirsutism, which can be quantified using a measurement technique known as the Ferriman-Gallwey Scale that identifies nine areas (lip, chin, sideburn region, neck, chest, abdomen, upper and lower back, and thigh) for assessment and allots points on a scale of 1 to 4 based on hair thickness and pigmentation. A score of higher than 8 is consistent with a diagnosis of hirsutism.[57] Hormonal abnormalities associated with hirsutism are summarized in Table 22-6.

Estrogen Replacement Therapy

Estrogen replacement remains a contentious issue. The Women's Health Initiative study enrolled 16,608 postmenopausal women who were placed on conventional hormone replacement combinations. The study showed an increased incidence of invasive breast cancer (hazard ratio, 1.26) and venous clot formation and no benefit in cognitive decline or coronary artery disease. Conversely, reductions in bone loss, colon polyp formation, and menopausal symptoms (hot flashes and vaginal dryness) were noted. Currently, estrogen replacement remains a treatment option in select women after careful risk counseling.[58-60]

TABLE 22-6 ANDROGEN LEVELS IN HIRSUTISM AND VIRILIZATION

	ANALYTE		
CONDITION	TOTAL TESTOSTERONE	FREE TESTOSTERONE	DEHYDROEPIANDROSTERONE SULFATE
Idiopathic hirsutism	↑	↑↑↑	↑
Polycystic ovary syndrome	↑	↑↑	↑
Congenital adrenal hyperplasia	↑↑	↑↑	↑↑↑
VIRILIZING TUMORS			
Ovarian	↑↑↑	↑↑↑	↑
Adrenal	↑↑	↑↑	↑↑↑

Modified from Demers LM. *Hirsutism and Virilization, News and Views.* Washington, D.C.: American Association for Clinical Chemistry; 1989.

CASE STUDY 22-4

A school physical examination of a 17-year-old boy showed less pubic and axillary hair than those of peers, penis and scrotum that were smaller, breast tissue since age 13, no erections or nocturnal emissions, and no adolescent growth spurt. Sleeve and pant lengths increased every 4 to 6 months.

Questions

1. At what level is the defect in this case?

2. What diagnostic possibilities would explain the endocrine data?

3. What treatment(s) would be available to

   a. Treat his androgen deficiency?

   b. Allow him to father children if he wanted fertility?

4. His appearance shows the defect occurred

   a. Prior to birth (during fetal life)

   b. After birth (postnatal)

PE

Height	73 in.
Arm span	74 in.
Weight	148 lb
BP	110/70 mm Hg
Pulse	69 bpm
Hair	Scant axillary and pubic
Breasts	Moderate gynecomastia, 3 cm
Genitalia	Penis, 4.5 cm
Testes	1.5 × 1 × 1 cm, bilaterally (normal, >4.5 × 3 × 3 cm)

LABORATORY

Testosterone, total	115 ng/dL (normal, 300–1,000)
LH	42 mU/mL (normal, adult, 3–18)
Karyotype	47,XXY

For additional student resources please visit thePoint at http://thepoint.lww.com. **thePoint**

QUESTIONS

1. If serum levels of estradiol do not increase after injection of hCG, the patient has
   a. Primary ovarian failure
   b. Pituitary failure
   c. Tertiary ovarian failure
   d. Secondary ovarian failure

2. If a patient had a luteal phase defect, which hormone would most likely be deficient?
   a. Progesterone
   b. Estrogen
   c. hCG
   d. FSH
   e. Prolactin

3. Which of the following is the precursor for estradiol formation in the placenta?
   a. Fetal adrenal DHEAS
   b. Maternal testosterone
   c. Maternal progesterone
   d. Placental hCG
   e. Fetal adrenal cholesterol

4. Which of the following target tissues is incapable of producing steroidal hormones?
   a. Adrenal medulla
   b. Placenta
   c. Ovary
   d. Testis
   e. Adrenal cortex

5. The parent substance in the biosynthesis of androgens and estrogens is
   a. Cholesterol
   b. Cortisol
   c. Catecholamines
   d. Progesterone

6. The biologically most active, naturally occurring androgen is
   a. DHEA
   b. Androstenedione
   c. Epiandrosterone
   d. Testosterone

7. For the past 3 weeks, serum estriol levels in a pregnant woman have been steadily increasing. This is consistent with
   a. A normal pregnancy
   b. Hemolytic disease of the newborn
   c. Fetal death
   d. Congenital cytomegalovirus infection

8. Which of the following is secreted by the placenta and used for the early detection of pregnancy?
   a. hCG
   b. FSH
   c. LH
   d. Progesterone

9. Chronic fetal metabolic distress is demonstrated by
   a. Decreased urinary estriol excretion and decreased maternal serum estriol
   b. Decreased estrogen in maternal plasma and increased estriol in amniotic fluid
   c. Increased estradiol in maternal plasma, with a corresponding increase of estriol in amniotic fluid
   d. Increased urinary estriol excretion and increased maternal serum estriol

10. Androgen secretion by the testes is stimulated by
    a. LH
    b. FSH
    c. Testosterone
    d. Gonadotropins

11. A deficiency in estrogen during the follicular phase will result in:
    a. A failure of embryo implantation.
    b. An increased length of the menstrual cycle.
    c. A lack of Graafian follicle release from the ovary.
    d. An incomplete development of the endometrium.

12. Which hormone is responsible for an increase in body temperature at the time of ovulation?
    a. Progesterone
    b. Estrogen
    c. LH
    d. FSH
    e. Estradiol

13. A midcycle LH surge will stimulate which series of events?
    a. An increase in FSH
    b. A decrease in FSH
    c. Anovulation
    d. Amenorrhea
    e. A decrease in progesterone production

REFERENCES

1. Gao F, Maiti S, Huff V. The Wilms tumor gene, Wt1, is required for Sox9 expression and maintenance of tubular architecture in the developing testis. *Proc Natl Acad Sci U S A.* August 2006;103(32):11987-11992.
2. Sinisi AA, Pasquali D, Notaro A, Bellastella A. Sexual differentiation. *J Endocrinol Invest.* 2003;26(3 suppl):23-28.
3. Dewing P, Bernard P, Vilain E. Disorders of gonadal development. *Semin Reprod Med.* 2002;20:189-198.
4. Durlinger AL, Visser JA, Themmen AP. Regulation of ovarian function: the role of anti-Mullerian hormone. *Reproduction.* November 2002;124:601-609.
5. Sharpe RM, McKinnell C, Kivlin C, Fisher JS. Proliferation and functional maturation of Sertoli cells, and their relevance to disorders of testis function in adulthood. *Reproduction.* 2003;125:769-784.
6. SvechnikovK, Landreh L, Weisser J, et al. Origin, development and regulation of human Leydig cells. *Horm Res Paediatr.* 2010;73: 93-101.
7. Rey RA, Grinspon RP. Normal male sexual differentiation and aetiology of disorders of sex development. *Best Pract Res Clin Endocrinol Metab.* 2011;25(2):221-238.
8. Campbell RE, Suter KJ. Redefining the gonadotropin-releasing hormone neurone dendrite. *J Neuroendocrinol.* 2010;22(7):650-658.
9. Grover A, Smith CE, Gregory M, Cyr DG, Sairam MR, Hermo L. Effects of FSH receptor deletion on epididymal tubules and sperm morphology, numbers, and motility. *Mol Reprod Dev.* October 2005;72(2):135-144.
10. Labrie F. Extragonadal synthesis of sex steroids: intracrinology. *Ann Endocrinol (Paris).* 2003;64:95-107.
11. Hiort O, Holterhus PM. Androgen insensitivity and male infertility. *Int J Androl.* 2003;26:16-20.
12. Lee DK, Chang C. Molecular communication between androgen receptor and general transcription machinery. *J Steroid Biochem Mol Biol.* 2003;84:41-49.
13. Sultan C, Gobinet J, Terouanne B, et al. The androgen receptor: molecular pathology. *J Soc Biol.* 2002;196:223-240.
14. Sultan C, Lumbroso S, Paris F, et al. Disorders of androgen action. *Semin Reprod Med.* 2002;20:217-228.
15. Segal TY, Mehta A, Anazodo A, Hindmarsh PC, Dattani MT. Role of gonadotropin-releasing hormone and human chorionic gonadotropin stimulation tests in differentiating patients with hypogonadotropic hypogonadism from those with constitutional delay of growth and puberty. *J Clin Endocrinol Metab.* March 2009;94(3):780-785.
16. Tong S, Wallace EM, Burger HG. Inhibins and activins: clinical advances in reproductive medicine. *Clin Endocrinol (Oxf).* 2003;58:115-127.
17. Cheng CK, Leung PCK. Molecular biology of gonadotropin-releasing hormone (GnRH)-I, GnRH-II, and their receptors in humans. *Endocr Rev.* 2005;26(2):283-306.
18. Seminara SB, Hayes FJ, Crowley WF Jr. Gonadotropin-releasing hormone deficiency in the human (idiopathic hypogonadotropic hypogonadism and Kallmann's syndrome): pathophysiological and genetic considerations. *Endocr Rev.* 1998;19:521-539.
19. De Rosa M, Zarrilli S, Di Sarno A, et al. Hyperprolactinemia in men: clinical and biochemical features and response to treatment. *Endocrine.* 2003;20:75-82.
20. Heaton JP, Morales A. Endocrine causes of impotence (nondiabetes). *Urol Clin North Am.* 2003;30:73-81.
21. Dhindsa S, Prabhakar S, Sethi M, et al. Frequent occurrence of hypogonadotropic hypogonadism in type 2 diabetes. *J Clin Endocrinol Metab.* 2004;89(11):5462-5468.

22. Dandona P, Dhindsa S. Update: hypogonadotropic hypogonadism in type 2 diabetes and obesity. *J Clin Endocrinol Metab.* 2011;96(9): 2643-2651.

23. Harman SM, Metter EJ, Tobin JD, et al. Longitudinal effects of aging on serum total and free testosterone levels in healthy men. Baltimore Longitudinal Study of Aging. *J Clin Endocrinol Metab.* 2001;86:724-731.

24. Feldman HA, Longcope C, Derby CA, et al. Age trends in the level of serum testosterone and other hormones in middle-aged men: longitudinal results from the Massachusetts Male Aging Study. *J Clin Endocrinol Metab.* 2002;87(2):589-598.

25. Bhasin S, Snyder PJ, Montori VM, et al. Testosterone therapy in adult men with androgen deficiency syndromes: an Endocrine Society clinical practice guideline. *J Clin Endocrinol Metab.* 2006;91(6):1995-2010.

26. Dandona P, Rosenberg MT. A practical guide to male hypogonadism in the primary care setting. *Int J Clin Pract.* 2010;64(6): 682-696.

27. Testosterone for 'late-onset hypogonadism' in men? *Drug Ther Bull.* 2010;48:69-72.

28. Srinivas-Shankar U, Wu FC. Drug insight: testosterone preparations. *Nat Rev Urol.* 2006;3:653-665.

29. Friedl KE, Hannan CJ Jr, Jones RE, Plymate SR. High-density lipoprotein cholesterol is not decreased if an aromatizable androgen is administered. *Metabolism.* 1990;39:69-74.

30. McGee EA, Hsueh AJW. Initial and cyclic recruitment of ovarian follicles. *Endocr Rev.* 2000;21(2):200-214.

31. Sherman BM, West JH, Korenman SG. The menopausal transition: analysis of LH, FSH, estradiol, and progesterone concentrations during menstrual cycles of older women. *J Clin Endocrinol Metab.* 1976;42:629-636.

32. Jost A, Vigier B, Prepin J, Perchellet JP. Studies on sex differentiation in mammals. *Recent Prog Horm Res.* 1973;29:1-41.

33. Messinis IE. Ovarian feedback, mechanism of action and possible clinical implications. *Hum Reprod Update.* 2006;12(5):557-571.

34. Filicori M, Santoro N, Merriam GR, Crowley WF Jr. Characterization of the physiological pattern of episodic gonadotropin secretion throughout the human menstrual cycle. *J Clin Endocrinol Metab.* 1986;62:1136-1144.

35. Badouraki M, Christoforidis A, Economou I, Dimitriadis AS, Katzos G. Sonographic assessment of uterine and ovarian development in normal girls aged 1 to 12 years. *J Clin Ultrasound.* 2008;36(9):539-544.

36. Canipari R, Cellini V, Cecconi S. The ovary feels fine when paracrine and autocrine networks cooperate with gonadotropins in the regulation of folliculogenesis. *Curr Pharm Des.* 2012;18(3):245-255.

37. Peters H, Byskov AG, Grinsted J. Follicular growth in fetal and prepubertal ovaries of humans and other primates. *Clin Endocrinol Metab.* 1978;7:469-485.

38. Gougeon A. Dynamics of follicular growth in the human: a model from preliminary results. *Hum Reprod.* 1986;1:81-87.

39. Fakheri RJ, Javitt NB. Autoregulation of cholesterol synthesis: physiologic and pathophysiologic consequences. *Steroids.* 2011;76(3):211-215.

40. Poutanen M. Understanding the diversity of sex steroid action. *J Endocrinol.* 2012;212:1-2.

41. te Velde ER, Pearson PL. The variability of female reproductive ageing. *Hum Reprod Update.* 2002;8(2):141-154.

42. Carmina E, Campagna AM, Lobo RA. A 20-year follow-up of young women with polycystic ovary syndrome. *Obstet Gynecol.* 2012;119(2):263-269.

43. Escobar-Morreale HF, Carmina E, Dewailly D, et al. Epidemiology, diagnosis and management of hirsutism: a consensus statement by the Androgen Excess and Polycystic Ovary Syndrome Society. *Hum Reprod Update.* 2012;18(2):146-170.

44. Panidis D, Tziomalos K, Misichronis G, et al. Insulin resistance and endocrine characteristics of the different phenotypes of polycystic ovary syndrome: a prospective study. *Hum Reprod.* 2012;27(2):541-549.

45. Sarfati J, Bachelot A, Coussieu C, Meduri G, Touraine P; Study Group Hyperandrogenism in Postmenopausal Women. Impact of clinical, hormonal, radiological, and immunohistochemical studies on the diagnosis of postmenopausal hyperandrogenism. *Eur J Endocrinol.* 2011;165:779-788.

46. Robertson DM. Inhibins and activins in blood: predictors of female reproductive health? *Mol Cell Endocrinol.* June 2011. [Epub ahead of print].

47. Sherwood OD. Relaxin's physiological roles and other diverse actions. *Endocr Rev.* 2004;25(2):205-234.

48. Jabbour HN, Kelly RW, Fraser HM, Critchley HO. Endocrine regulation of menstruation. *Endocr Rev.* 2006;27(1):17-46.

49. Broekmans FJ, Soules MR, Fauser BC. Ovarian aging: mechanisms and clinical consequences. *Endocr Rev.* 2009;30(5):465-493.

50. Santoro N. Update in hyper- and hypogonadotropic amenorrhea. *J Clin Endocrinol Metab.* 2011;96(11):3281-3288.

51. Marshall WA, Tanner JM. Variations in pattern of pubertal changes in girls. *Arch Dis Child.* 1969;44:291-303.

52. Lessey BA. Assessment of endometrial receptivity. *Fertil Steril.* 2011;96:522-529.

53. Elsheikh M, Dunger DB, Conway GS, Wass JA. Turner's syndrome in adulthood. *Endocr Rev.* February 2002;23(1):120-140.

54. Hoek A, Schoemaker J, Drexhage HA. Premature ovarian failure and ovarian autoimmunity. *Endocr Rev.* 1997;18(1):107-134.

55. Palomba S, Falbo A, Zullo F, Orio F Jr. Evidence-based and potential benefits of metformin in the polycystic ovary syndrome: a comprehensive review. *Endocr Rev.* 2009;30(1):1-50.

56. Azziz R, Carmina E, Sawaya ME. Idiopathic hirsutism. *Endocr Rev.* 2000;21(4):347-362.

57. Cook H, Brennan K, Azziz R. Reanalyzing the modified Ferriman-Gallwey score: is there a simpler method for assessing the extent of hirsutism? *Fertil Steril.* 2011;96(5):1266-1270.

58. Chlebowski RT, Wactawski-Wende J, Ritenbaugh C, et al.; Women's Health Initiative Investigators. Estrogen plus progestin and colorectal cancer in postmenopausal women. *N Engl J Med.* 2004;350(10):991-1004.

59. Manson JE, Hsia J, Johnson KC, et al.; Women's Health Initiative Investigators. Estrogen plus progestin and the risk of coronary heart disease. *N Engl J Med.* 2003;349(6):523-534.

60. Hays J, Ockene JK, Brunner RL, et al.; Women's Health Initiative Investigators. Effects of estrogen plus progestin on health-related quality of life. *N Engl J Med.* 2003;348(19):1839-1854.

The Thyroid Gland

MARISSA GROTZKE

CHAPTER OUTLINE

Chapter Objectives

Upon completion of this chapter, the clinical laboratorian should be able to do the following:

- Discuss the biosynthesis, secretion, transport, and action of the thyroid hormones.
- Know the location of the thyroid gland.
- Describe the hypothalamic–pituitary–thyroid axis and how it regulates thyroid hormone production.
- Explain the principles of each thyroid function test discussed.
- Correlate laboratory information with regard to suspected thyroid disorders, given a patient's clinical data.
- Describe the appropriate laboratory thyroid function testing protocol to use to effectively evaluate or monitor patients with suspected thyroid disease.

KEY TERMS

Chronic lymphocytic thyroiditis
Follicular cells
Free T_3
Free T_4
Graves' disease
Hashimoto's thyroiditis
Hyperthyroidism
Hypothalamic–pituitary–thyroid axis
Hypothyroidism
Parathyroid glands
Subacute thyroiditis
Subclinical hyperthyroidism
Subclinical hypothyroidism
Thyroglobulin
Thyroid peroxidase (TPO)
Thyrotoxicosis
Thyrotropin-releasing hormone (TRH)
Thyroxine (T_4)
Thyroxine-binding globulin (TBG)
Thyroxine-binding prealbumin (TBPA)
Triiodothyronine (T_3)
TSH receptor antibodies

THE THYROID

The thyroid gland is responsible for the production of two hormones: thyroid hormone and calcitonin. Calcitonin is secreted by parafollicular C cells and is involved in calcium homeostasis. Thyroid hormone is critical in regulating body metabolism, neurologic development, and numerous other body functions. Clinically, conditions affecting thyroid hormone levels are much more common than those affecting calcitonin and are the major focus of this chapter.

Thyroid Anatomy and Development

The thyroid gland is positioned in the lower anterior neck and is shaped like a butterfly. It is made up of two lobes that rest on each side of the trachea, with a band of thyroid tissue—called the isthmus—running anterior to the trachea and bridging the lobes. Posterior to the thyroid gland are the parathyroid glands that regulate serum calcium levels and the recurrent laryngeal nerves that innervate the vocal cords. These posterior structures become important during thyroid surgery, when care must be exercised to avoid injury that could lead to hypocalcemia or permanent hoarse voice.

The fetal thyroid develops from an outpouching of the foregut at the base of the tongue and migrates to its normal location over the thyroid cartilage in the first 4 to 8 weeks of gestation. By week 11 of gestation, the thyroid gland begins to produce measurable amounts of thyroid hormone.[1] Thyroid hormone is critical to neurologic development of the fetus. Iodine is an essential component of thyroid hormone. In parts of the world where severe iodine deficiency exists, neither the mother nor the fetus can produce thyroid hormone and both develop hypothyroidism. The impact is most severe on the fetus because hypothyroidism leads to mental retardation and cretinism. In areas where iodine deficiency is not an issue, other problems can occur with thyroid development. Congenital hypothyroidism occurs in 1 of 4,000 live births.[2] If the mother has normal thyroid function, the fetus will be protected during development by small amounts of maternal thyroid hormone crossing the placenta. Immediately postpartum, however, these newborns require initiation of appropriate doses of thyroid hormone or their neurologic development will be significantly impaired. In the developed world, screening tests are performed on all newborns to diagnose congenital hypothyroidism and prevent catastrophic complications by the timely institution of thyroid hormone therapy.

Thyroid Hormone Synthesis

Thyroid hormone is made primarily of the trace element iodine, making iodine metabolism a key determinant in thyroid function.[1] Iodine is found in seafood, dairy products, iodine-enriched breads, and vitamins. Significantly, iodine is used in high concentrations in the contrast medium used in computed tomography (CT) scans and to visualize arteries during heart catheterization. It is also present in amiodarone, a medication used to treat certain heart conditions. The recommended minimum daily intake of iodine is 150 μg, although most individuals in developed countries ingest far more than this amount. In the United States, the average adult daily intake of iodine has decreased since the 1970s but remains sufficient at an estimated range between 240 and 740 μg.[3] If iodine intake drops below 50 μg daily, the thyroid gland is unable to manufacture adequate amounts of thyroid hormone and thyroid hormone deficiency—hypothyroidism—results.[4]

Thyroid cells are organized into follicles. Follicles are spheres of thyroid cells surrounding a core of a viscous substance termed *colloid*. The major component of colloid is thyroglobulin, a glycoprotein manufactured exclusively by thyroid follicular cells. Thyroglobulin is rich in the amino acid tyrosine. Some of these tyrosyl residues can be iodinated, producing the building blocks of thyroid hormone. On the outer side of the follicle, iodine is actively transported into the thyroid cell by the Na^+/I^- symporter located on the basement membrane. Inside the thyroid cell, iodide diffuses across the cell to the apical side of the follicle, which abuts the core of colloid. Here, catalyzed by a membrane-bound enzyme called thyroid peroxidase (TPO), concentrated iodide is oxidized and bound with tyrosyl residues on thyroglobulin. This results in production of monoiodothyronine (MIT) and diiodothyronine (DIT). This same enzyme also aids in the coupling of two tyrosyl residues to form triiodothyronine (T_3) (one MIT residue + one DIT residue) or thyroxine (T_4) (two DIT residues). These are the two active forms of thyroid hormone. This thyroglobulin matrix, with branches now holding T_4 and T_3, is stored in the core of the thyroid follicle. *Thyroid-stimulating hormone (TSH)* signals the follicular cell to ingest a microscopic droplet of colloid by endocytosis. Inside the follicular cell, these droplets are digested by intracellular lysosomes into T_4, T_3, and other products. T_4 and T_3 are then secreted by the thyroid cell into the circulation (Fig. 23-1).

The activity of thyroid hormone is dependent on the location and number of iodine atoms. Approximately 80% of T_4 is metabolized into either T_3 (35%) or reverse T_3 (rT_3) (45%). Outer ring deiodination of T_4 (5'-deiodination) leads to the production of 3,5,3'-triiodothyronine (T_3). T_3 is three to eight times more metabolically active than T_4 and often considered to be the active form of thyroid hormone, while T_4 is the "pre" hormone (with thyroglobulin being the "prohormone"). In addition to its "pre" hormone activity, however, inner ring deiodination of T_4 results in the production of metabolically inactive rT_3 (Fig. 23-2).

There are three forms of iodothyronine 5'-deiodinase. Type 1 iodothyronine 5'-deiodinase, the most abundant form, is found mostly in the liver and kidney and is responsible for the largest contribution to the circulating T_3 pool. Certain drugs (e.g., propylthiouracil [PTU], glucocorticoids, and propranolol) can slow the activity of this deiodinase and are used in the treatment of severe hyperthyroidism. Type 2 iodothyronine 5'-deiodinase is found in the brain and pituitary gland. Its function is to maintain constant levels of T_3 in the central nervous system. Its activity is decreased when levels of circulating T_4 are high and increased when levels are low. Activity of the deiodination enzymes gives another level of control on thyroid hormone activity beyond hypothalamic–pituitary control through thyrotropin-releasing hormone (TRH) and TSH (Fig. 23-2).[1]

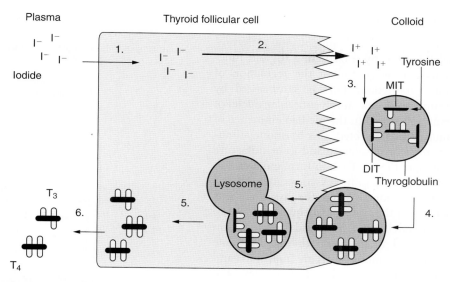

FIGURE 23-1 Biosynthesis of thyroid hormone. Thyroid hormone synthesis includes the following steps: (1) iodide (I⁻) trapping by thyroid follicular cells; (2) diffusion of iodide to the apex of the cell and transport into the colloid; (3) oxidation of inorganic iodide to iodine and incorporation of iodine into tyrosine residues within thyroglobulin molecules in the colloid; (4) combination of two diiodotyrosine (DIT) molecules to form tetraiodothyronine (thyroxine, T_4) or of monoiodotyrosine (MIT) with DIT to form triiodothyronine (T_3); (5) uptake of thyroglobulin from the colloid into the follicular cell by endocytosis, fusion of the thyroglobulin with a lysosome, and proteolysis and release of T_4 and T_3; and (6) release of T_4 and T_3 into the circulation.

Protein Binding of Thyroid Hormone

When released into the circulation, only 0.04% of T_4 and 0.4% of T_3 are unbound by proteins and available for hormonal activity. The three major binding proteins, in order of significance, are thyroxine-binding globulin (TBG), thyroxine-binding prealbumin, and albumin. The quantity of T_4 and T_3 in the circulation can be significantly affected by the amount of binding protein available for carrying these hormones. For example, high estrogen levels during pregnancy lead to increased thyroxine-binding protein production by the liver. High TBG levels result in higher levels of bound thyroid hormones, leading to high levels of total T_3 and total T_4. In euthyroid individuals, levels of the active free thyroid hormone remain in the normal range. In some instances, however, measurement of free T_4 and free T_3 may be necessary to eliminate any confusion caused by abnormal binding protein levels.

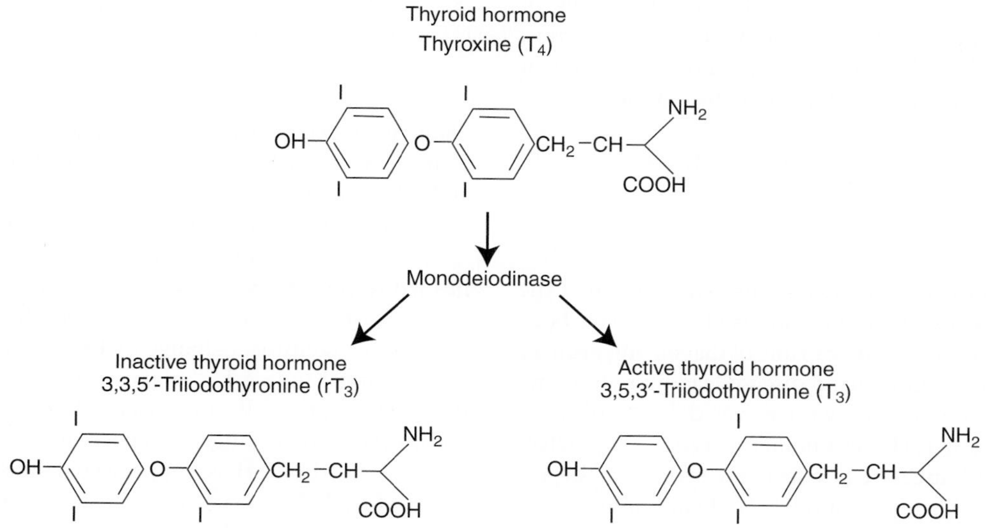

Thyroid hormone
Thyroxine (T_4)

Monodeiodinase

Inactive thyroid hormone
3,3,5'-Triiodothyronine (rT_3)

Active thyroid hormone
3,5,3'-Triiodothyronine (T_3)

FIGURE 23-2 Metabolism of thyroxine.

Control of Thyroid Function

Understanding of the hypothalamic–pituitary–thyroid axis is essential for correctly interpreting thyroid function testing. This axis is central in the regulation of thyroid hormone production. TRH is synthesized by neurons in the supraoptic and supraventricular nuclei of the hypothalamus and stored in the median eminence of the hypothalamus. When secreted, this hormone stimulates cells in the anterior pituitary gland to manufacture and release *thyrotropin (TSH)*. TSH, in turn, circulates to the thyroid gland and leads to increased production and release of thyroid hormone. When the hypothalamus and pituitary sense that there is an inadequate amount of thyroid hormone in circulation, TRH and TSH secretion increases and will lead to increased thyroid hormone production. If thyroid hormone levels are high, TRH and TSH release will be inhibited, leading to lower levels of thyroid hormone production and vice versa if thyroid hormone levels are low. This feedback loop requires a normally functioning hypothalamus, pituitary, and thyroid gland, as well as an absence of any interfering agents or agents that mimic TSH action (Fig. 23-3).

Actions of Thyroid Hormone

Once released from the thyroid gland, thyroid hormone circulates in the bloodstream where free T_4 and T_3 are available to travel across the cell membrane. In the cytoplasm, T_4 is deiodinated into T_3, the active form of thyroid hormone. T_3 combines with its nuclear receptor on thyroid hormone–responsive genes, leading to the production of messenger RNA that, in turn, leads to the production of proteins that influence metabolism and development. Effects of thyroid hormone include tissue growth, brain maturation, increased heat production, increased oxygen consumption, and an increased number of β-adrenergic receptors. Clinically, individuals who have excess thyroid hormone (thyrotoxicosis) will have symptoms of increased metabolism such as tachycardia and tremor, while individuals with hypothyroidism note symptoms of lowered metabolism like edema and constipation.

TESTS FOR THYROID EVALUATION

Blood Tests

Thyroid-Stimulating Hormone

The most useful test for assessing thyroid function is the TSH. Over the years, three generations of assays have been developed. All the assays are capable of diagnosing primary hypothyroidism (thyroid gland disease leading to low thyroid hormone production) with elevated levels of TSH. Second-generation TSH immunometric assays, with detection limits of 0.1 mU/L, can effectively screen for hyperthyroidism, but third-generation TSH chemiluminometric assays, with detection limits of 0.01 mU/L, are less likely to give false-negative results and can more accurately

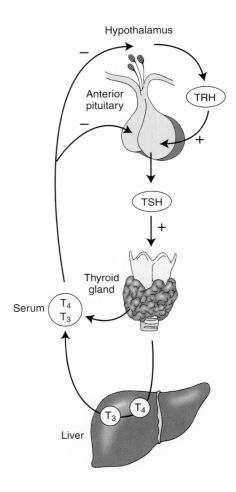

FIGURE 23-3 Hypothalamic–pituitary–thyroid axis. Thyrotropin-releasing hormone (TRH) stimulates the production and release of thyrotropin (TSH). TSH stimulates the thyroid gland to synthesize and secrete thyroid hormone. T_4 that is released by the thyroid gland is mostly converted to T_3 by the liver and kidney. T_3 and T_4 feedback inhibit TSH release directly through action at the pituitary and indirectly by decreasing TRH release from the hypothalamus. (Adapted from Surks MI, Sievert R. Drugs and thyroid function. *N Engl J Med.* 1995;333:1688.)

distinguish between euthyroidism and hyperthyroidism. Third-generation TSH assays are routinely used to monitor and adjust thyroid hormone replacement therapy as well as screen for both hyperthyroidism and hypothyroidism.[5]

The sensitivity of the third-generation TSH assays has led to the ability to detect what is termed subclinical disease—or a mild degree of thyroid dysfunction—due to the large reciprocal change in TSH levels seen for even small changes in free T_4.[6] In subclinical hypothyroidism, the TSH is minimally increased while the free T_4 stays within the normal range. Likewise, in subclinical hyperthyroidism, the TSH is suppressed while the free T_4 is normal (Table 23-1). The clinical significance of subclinical disease and thresholds for treatment remain somewhat unclear and are a continued topic of investigation.

TABLE 23-1	INTERPRETATION OF THYROID TESTS		
	LOW FREE T_4	**NORMAL FREE T_4**	**HIGH FREE T_4**
Low TSH	Secondary hypothyroidism	Subclinical hyperthyroidism	Hyperthyroidism
	Severe nonthyroidal illness	Nonthyroidal illness	
Normal TSH	Secondary hypothyroidism	Normal	Artifact
	Severe nonthyroidal illness		Pituitary hyperthyroidism
			Laboratory draw within 6 h of thyroxine dose
High TSH	Primary hypothyroidism	Subclinical hypothyroidism	Test artifact
			Pituitary hyperthyroidism
			Thyroid hormone resistance

TSH, thyroid-stimulating hormone.

Serum T_4 and T_3

Serum total T_4 and T_3 levels are usually measured by radioimmunoassay (RIA), chemiluminometric assay, or similar immunometric technique. Because more than 99.9% of thyroid hormone is protein bound, alterations in thyroid hormone–binding proteins, unrelated to thyroid disease, frequently lead to total T_4 and T_3 levels outside of the normal range. Because of this, assays have been developed to measure free T_4 and T_3, the biologically active forms of thyroid hormone, and free T_4 kits have replaced total T_4 determinations at the clinical level, secondary to ease of interpretation and lower processing cost.[7] Currently available assay kits for measuring free T_4 levels are not error proof, though, and can still be affected by some binding protein abnormalities.[8] When this is suspected, measurement of free T_4 levels is performed by dialysis. Kits that estimate free T_3 levels also have theoretical advantages; however, actual clinical utility is yet to be clearly defined.

Thyroglobulin

Thyroglobulin is a protein synthesized and secreted exclusively by thyroid follicular cells. This prohormone in the circulation is proof of the presence of thyroid tissue, either benign or malignant. This fact makes thyroglobulin an ideal tumor marker for thyroid cancer patients. Patients with well-differentiated thyroid cancer who have been treated successfully with surgery and radioactive iodine ablation should have undetectable thyroglobulin levels.

Thyroglobulin is currently measured by double-antibody RIA, enzyme-linked immunoassay, immunoradiometric assay, and immunochemiluminescent assay methods. The accuracy of the thyroglobulin assay is primarily dependent on the specificity of the antibody used and the absence of antithyroglobulin autoantibodies.

Even with modern assays, antithyroglobulin autoantibodies interfere with measurements and lead to unreliable thyroglobulin results. For this reason, it is critically important to screen for autoantibodies whenever thyroglobulin is being measured. If antibodies are present, the value of the thyroglobulin assay is marginal. Approximately 25% of patients with well-differentiated thyroid cancer will have antithyroglobulin autoantibodies. This is approximately twice as high as in the general population. If a patient with well-differentiated thyroid cancer and antithyroglobulin autoantibodies has been successfully treated with surgery and radioactive iodine ablation, autoantibodies should disappear over time.[5]

Thyroid Autoimmunity

Many diseases of the thyroid gland are related to autoimmune processes. In autoimmune thyroid disease, antibodies are directed at thyroid tissue with variable responses. The most common cause of hyperthyroidism is an autoimmune disorder called Graves' disease. The antibody in this condition is directed at the TSH receptor and stimulates the receptor, leading to growth of the thyroid gland and production of excessive amounts of thyroid hormone. This condition can be diagnosed with tests that detect antibodies to the TSH receptor. Thyroid-stimulating antibodies (TRAb, thyroid-stimulating immunoglobulin [TSI]) are tested using a bioassay to determine the presence of autoimmune hyperthyroidism. Tests for TSH receptor antibodies (TRAb, TSHRAb) can detect antibodies directed against the TSH receptor whether they act to stimulate or block the TSH receptor. Both stimulating and blocking antibody assays will be positive in 70% to 100% of patients with Graves' disease. Chronic lymphocytic thyroiditis—commonly known as Hashimoto's thyroiditis—is at the other end of the autoimmune continuum. This is the most common

TABLE 23-2	PREVALENCE OF THYROID AUTOANTIBODIES		
ANTIBODY	**GENERAL POPULATION**	**GRAVES' DISEASE**	**AUTOIMMUNE HYPOTHYROIDISM**
Antithyroglobulin	3%	12–30%	35–60%
Thyroid peroxidase (previously antimicrosomal)	10–15%	45–80%	80–99%
Anti-TSH receptor	1–2%	70–100%	6–60%

TSH, thyroid-stimulating hormone.

cause of hypothyroidism in the developed world. In this condition, antibodies lead to decreased thyroid hormone production by the thyroid gland. The best test for this condition is the TPO antibody, which is present in 10% to 15% of the general population and 80% to 99% of patients with autoimmune hypothyroidism (Table 23-2).

OTHER TOOLS FOR THYROID EVALUATION

Nuclear Medicine Evaluation

Radioactive iodine is useful in assessing the metabolic activity of thyroid tissue and assisting in the evaluation and treatment of thyroid cancer. When radioactive iodine is given orally, a percentage of the dose is taken up by the thyroid gland. This percentage is called the radioactive iodine uptake (RAIU). High uptake suggests that the gland is metabolically active and producing significant amounts of thyroid hormone. Low uptake suggests that the gland is metabolically inactive. Because TSH stimulates iodine uptake by the thyroid gland, it is important to interpret the scan in conjunction with an assessment of TSH levels. An undetectably low TSH should turn off the thyroid gland's uptake of iodine. If the uptake is high despite an undetectable TSH, the thyroid must be acting either autonomously without regard to the hypothalamus–pituitary–thyroid feedback system or through a TSH surrogate. Such is the case with Graves' disease, where an immunoglobulin activates the TSH receptor on the thyroid gland, leading to high rates of thyroid hormone production and a high RAIU. The high level of thyroid hormone in the circulation feeds back on the pituitary and hypothalamus, turning off TSH, but this has no effect on the levels of TSI (the TSH surrogate). Conversely, if the RAIU is low in the presences of an undetectable TSH, the differential diagnosis includes excess exogenous thyroid hormone ingestion, high iodine intake, or a condition in which stored thyroid hormone is leaking from the thyroid gland (typically in a setting known as subacute thyroiditis).

Radioactive iodine can also be useful in the evaluation of thyroid nodules in the presence of a low or unde-

tectable TSH. Thyroid nodules that take up significant amounts of radioactive iodine on thyroid scans—termed "hot" nodules—are unlikely to be thyroid cancer. The converse, however, does not hold true as nodules that show little or no radioiodine uptake—indeterminate or "cold" nodules, respectively—may be cancerous, but the majority of such nodules are benign.

Thyroid Ultrasound

The significance of thyroid ultrasound in the assessment of thyroid anatomy and characterization of palpable thyroid abnormalities has progressively increased in the last several years. Thyroid ultrasounds are capable of detecting even thyroid nodules of such a small size as to be of unclear or even no clinical significance; depending upon age, in up to 50% of clinically normal thyroid glands, small <1cm) thyroid nodules can be seen.[9]

Fine-Needle Aspiration

Thyroid fine-needle aspiration (FNA) biopsy is often the first step and the most accurate tool in the evaluation of thyroid nodules. The routine use of FNA biopsy allows prompt identification and treatment of thyroid malignancies and avoids unnecessary surgery in most individuals with benign thyroid lesions. In this procedure, a small-gauge needle is inserted into the nodule

CASE STUDY 23-1

A 24-year-old woman presents 2 months' postpartum with symptoms of hyperthyroidism. She does not have evidence of Graves' ophthalmopathy. Her TSH level is undetectable, and free T_4 is two times the upper limit of normal.

Questions

1. What are possible causes for her thyrotoxicosis?

2. What tests would be useful to sort out the cause of her thyrotoxicosis?

BOX 23-1 SIGNS AND SYMPTOMS OF HYPOTHYROIDISM

Signs

- Delayed relaxation phase of deep tendon reflex testing
- Bradycardia
- Diastolic hypertension
- Coarsened skin, yellowing of skin (carotenemia)
- Periorbital edema
- Thinning of eyebrows/loss of lateral aspect of brows
- Slowed movements/speech
- Pleural/pericardial effusion
- Ascites

Symptoms

- Cold intolerance
- Depression
- Mental retardation (infants), slowed cognition
- Menorrhagia
- Growth failure (children)
- Pubertal delay
- Dry skin
- Edema
- Constipation
- Hoarseness
- Dyspnea on exertion

and cells are aspirated for cytologic evaluation. The procedure can be performed using palpation if the nodule is palpable, or with the assistance of ultrasound imaging in cases of nonpalpable nodules. FNA biopsy results are reported according to six categories: nondiagnostic, malignant, suspicious for malignancy, indeterminate or suspicious for neoplasm, follicular lesion of undetermined significance, and benign. These categories dictate subsequent treatment, ranging from routine ultrasound monitoring to surgical excision.[10]

DISORDERS OF THE THYROID

Hypothyroidism

Hypothyroidism—defined as a low free T_4 level with a normal or high TSH—is one of the most common disorders of the thyroid gland, occurring in 5% to 15% of women over the age of 65. Symptoms of hypothyroidism vary, depending on the degree of hypothyroidism and the rapidity of its onset (Box 23-1). When thyroid hormone is significantly decreased, symptoms of cold intolerance, fatigue, dry skin, constipation, hoarseness, dyspnea on exertion, cognitive dysfunction, hair loss, and weight gain have been reported. On physical examination, those with severe hypothyroidism may have low body temperature, slowed movements, bradycardia, delay in the relaxation phase of deep tendon reflexes, yellow discoloration of the skin (from hypercarotenemia), hair loss, diastolic hypertension, pleural and pericardial effusions, menstrual irregularities, and periorbital edema.

Because of the diffuse distribution of thyroid hormone receptors and many metabolic effects of thyroid hormone, hypothyroidism can lead to a variety of other abnormalities. Hyponatremia can occur due to inappropriate levels of antidiuretic hormone, and significant degrees of hypothyroidism can also lead to myopathy and elevated levels of creatine kinase (CK).[11,12] Anemia can also be

seen, either as a result of a decreased demand for oxygen-carrying capacity or through an associated autoimmune pernicious anemia.[13] Hypothyroidism may also lead to hyperlipidemia, most notably when the TSH is greater than 10 mU/L.[14] One study documented more than half of those with hypothyroidism who were studied had hypercholesterolemia, while another study showed 4.2% of patients with hyperlipidemia had hypothyroidism.[15] In the presence of these clinical abnormalities (hyponatremia, unexplained elevation of CK, anemia, or hyperlipidemia), evaluation for hypothyroidism as a potential secondary cause should be considered.

Hypothyroidism can be divided into primary, secondary, or tertiary disease, depending on the location of the defect (Box 23-2). The most common cause of hypothyroidism in developed countries is chronic lymphocytic thyroiditis, or Hashimoto's thyroiditis. This disorder is an autoimmune disease targeting the thyroid gland, often associated with an enlarged gland, or goiter. TPO antibody testing is positive in 80% to 99% of patients with chronic lymphocytic thyroiditis. Other common causes of hypothyroidism include iodine deficiency, thyroid surgery, and radioactive iodine treatment (Table 23-3). Occasionally, individuals will experience transient hypothyroidism associated with inflammation of the thyroid gland. Examples of transient hypothyroidism include recovery from non-

BOX 23-2 TYPES OF HYPOTHYROIDISM

Primary
Thyroid gland dysfunction

Secondary
Pituitary dysfunction

Tertiary
Hypothalamic dysfunction

TABLE 23-3	CAUSES OF HYPOTHYROIDISM	
	CONDITION	**COMMENTS**
Primary	Chronic lymphocytic thyroiditis (Hashimoto's thyroiditis)	TPOAb or TgAb positive in 80–99% of cases
	Treatment for toxic goiter—subtotal thyroidectomy or radioactive iodine	History and physical examination (neck scar) are key to diagnosis
	Excessive iodine intake	History and urinary iodine measurement useful
	Subacute thyroiditis	Usually transient
Secondary	Hypopituitarism	Caused by adenoma, radiation therapy, or destruction of pituitary
Tertiary	Hypothalamic dysfunction	Rare

TgAb, thyroglobulin antibodies; TPOAb, thyroid peroxidase antibodies.

thyroidal illness and the hypothyroid phase of any of the forms of subacute thyroiditis (painful thyroiditis, postpartum thyroiditis, and painless thyroiditis).

American Thyroid Association Guidelines for Hypothyroidism Screening[16,17]
Measurement of TSH

- At age 35
- Every 5 years after the age of 35
- More frequently with risk factors or symptoms: goiter, family history, lithium use, amiodarone use

Hypothyroidism is treated with thyroid hormone replacement therapy. Levothyroxine (T_4) is the treatment of choice. In primary hypothyroidism, the goal of therapy is to achieve a normal TSH level. If hypothyroidism is secondary or tertiary in origin, TSH levels will not be useful in managing the condition and a midnormal free T_4 level becomes the target of therapy. Levothyroxine has a half-life of approximately 7 days. When doses of thyroid hormone are changed, it is important to wait at least five half-lives before rechecking thyroid function tests in order to achieve a new steady state.

Thyrotoxicosis

Thyrotoxicosis is a constellation of findings that result when peripheral tissues are presented with, and respond to, an excess of thyroid hormone. Thyrotoxicosis can be the result of excessive thyroid hormone ingestion, leakage of stored thyroid hormone from storage in the thyroid follicles, or excessive thyroid gland production of thyroid hormone. The latter form of thyrotoxicosis is called hyperthyroidism. The manifestations of thyrotoxicosis vary, depending on the degree of thyroid hormone elevation and the status of the affected individual. Symptoms typically include anxiety, emotional lability, weakness, tremor, palpitations, heat intolerance, increased perspiration, and weight loss despite a normal or increased appetite (Box 23-3).

BOX 23-3 SIGNS AND SYMPTOMS OF THYROTOXICOSIS

Signs
- Tachycardia
- Tremor
- Warm, moist, flushed, smooth skin
- Lid lag, widened palpebral fissures
- Ophthalmopathy (Graves' disease)
- Goiter
- Brisk deep tendon reflexes
- Muscle wasting and weakness
- Dermopathy/pretibial myxedema (Graves' disease)
- Osteopenia, osteoporosis

Symptoms
- Nervousness, irritability, anxiety
- Tremor
- Palpitations
- Fatigue, weakness, decreased exercise tolerance
- Weight loss
- Heat intolerance
- Hyperdefecation
- Menstrual changes (oligomenorrhea)
- Prominence of eyes

Graves' Disease

Graves' disease is the most common cause of thyrotoxicosis. It is an autoimmune disease in which antibodies are produced that activate the TSH receptor. Features of Graves' disease include thyrotoxicosis, goiter, ophthalmopathy (eye changes associated with inflammation and infiltration of periorbital tissue) and dermopathy (skin changes in the lower extremities that have an orange peel texture). There is a strong familial disposition to Graves' disease: 15% of patients will have a close relative with this condition. Women are five times more likely than men to develop this condition. Laboratory testing will usually document a high free T_4 and/or T_3 level with a low or undetectable TSH. TSIs and TSH receptor antibodies are usually positive in this condition. RAIU will be elevated, and the thyroid scan will show diffuse uptake (Table 23-4). Graves' ophthalmopathy can be of particular concern.[18] Approximately 20% to 25% of patients with Graves' hyperthyroidism have clinically obvious Graves' ophthalmopathy. With more sensitive testing, such as orbital CT scanning or magnetic resonance imaging, most patients with Graves' hyperthyroidism will be shown to have ophthalmopathy.[19] The findings in Graves' ophthalmopathy can include orbital soft tissue swelling, injection of the conjunctivae, proptosis (forward protrusion of the eye, secondary to infiltration of retroorbital muscles and fat), double vision (secondary to orbital muscle involvement and fibrosis), and corneal disease (often related to difficulty closing the eyelids). Treatment of Graves' ophthalmopathy is controversial. Occasionally, patients

require surgical decompression of the orbits to prevent optic nerve injury and blindness

Thyroid disease associated with Graves' disease is treated with medication, radioactive iodine, or surgery. Initially, many thyrotoxic patients require β-blockers to control symptoms of adrenergic excess, such as tremor and tachycardia. PTU or methimazole (MMI) can be added to inhibit thyroid hormone biosynthesis and secretion.[20] The antithyroid medications, as they are known, carry a significant risk profile that includes rash, hepatotoxicity, agranulocytosis, and aplastic anemia. These medications may have immunomodulatory effects on the underlying autoimmune disease, helping promote remission of the condition after several months of therapy. Long-term remission rates vary but generally run between 20% and 50% in the United States. Women are more likely to achieve remission than men. Likewise, patients with small goiters and mild hyperthyroidism are more likely to achieve remissions. Low dietary iodine increases the chance of staying in long-term remission. Patients experiencing such a remission do not require therapy with thyroid hormone replacement.

When radioactive iodine or surgery is used, the goal is to destroy or remove enough thyroid tissue so that the patient becomes hypothyroid. Subsequent lifelong treatment with thyroid hormone replacement therapy is usually required. Radioactive iodine therapy has been used for the treatment of Graves' disease for more than 50 years and is both safe and effective. Surgery is associated with risk of recurrent laryngeal nerve injury, leading

TABLE 23-4 DISORDERS ASSOCIATED WITH THYROTOXICOSIS

	CONDITION	PATHOGENIC MECHANISM	TSH LEVEL	RAIU	OTHER TESTS
Hyperthyroidism	Graves' disease	TSHRAb	↓	↑	TRAb positive; TSI positive
	Toxic adenoma	Benign nodule	↓	↑	Seen on thyroid scan
	Toxic multinodular goiter	Foci of functional autonomy	↓	↑	Seen on thyroid scan
	TSH-secreting tumor	Benign pituitary tumor	Normal/↑	↑	Pituitary MRI
Nonhyperthyroidism	Painful thyroiditis	Leakage of thyroid hormone	↓	↓	Tg inappropriately high
	Postpartum thyroiditis	Leakage of thyroid hormone	↓	↓	TPOAb often high
	Exogenous hormone	Medication	↓	↓	
	Ectopic thyroid tissue	Metastatic thyroid cancer; struma ovarii	↓	↓	Distant metastases seen on thyroid scan

TSH, thyroid-stimulating hormone; RAIU, radioactive iodine uptake; Tg, thyroglobulin; TSHRAb, TSH receptor antibodies; TSI, thyroid-stimulating immunoglobulins; MRI, magnetic resonance imaging; TPOAb, thyroid peroxidase antibodies.

CASE STUDY 23-2

A 67-year-old woman is referred for treatment of hyperlipidemia. Her cholesterol and triglycerides are high, despite treatment with lipid-lowering medication. She is noted to have hair loss (wearing a wig) and hoarseness to her voice. She complains of cold intolerance and fatigue.

Questions

1. What testing would be helpful to screen for thyroid disease?

2. What treatment might she require?

3. What other laboratory abnormalities are commonly seen in hypothyroid patients other than hyperlipidemia and abnormal thyroid function tests?

to permanent hoarseness, and injury to the parathyroid glands, causing hypoparathyroidism leading to hypocalcemia.

Because of their comparative risks for adverse events, radioactive iodine is generally the preferred treatment modality in the United States. Antithyroid medications are typically used either because of patient preference or during pregnancy and breastfeeding. There are two situations in Graves' disease in which surgery is preferred to other forms of therapy. If there is concern that the patient may have thyroid cancer in addition to Graves' disease, surgery is the best way to ensure removal of the potential cancer. In patients with severe ophthalmopathy, some experts in Graves' disease management prefer surgery because of concern that radioactive iodine treatment may cause an acute flaring of associated eye problems.

Toxic Adenoma and Multinodular Goiter

Toxic adenomas and multinodular goiter are two relatively common causes of hyperthyroidism. These conditions are caused by autonomously functioning thyroid tissue. In these instances, neither TSH nor TSH receptor–stimulating immunoglobulin is required to stimulate thyroid hormone production. In some toxic nodules, receptor mutations have been identified. These mutations have the same effect as chronic stimulation of the TSH receptor on thyroid hormone production. Clinically, toxic adenomas present in patients with hyperthyroidism and a palpable thyroid nodule. On a thyroid scan, the nodules are "hot"—that is, they avidly take up radioactive iodine. The RAIU is also inappropriately high for the suppressed level of TSH. In toxic multinodular goiter, there are multiple areas within the thyroid gland that are autonomously

producing thyroid hormone (Table 23-4). Treatment for these two conditions involves surgery, radioactive iodine, or medication (PTU or MMI). Although the medications can block thyroid hormone production, they are not expected to lead to remission in these two conditions. Often, the toxic nodules produce so much thyroid hormone that the rest of the thyroid gland is suppressed and metabolically inactive. When radioactive iodine is given, it tends to destroy only the hyperactive (autonomous) portions of the thyroid gland, leaving normal (suppressed) thyroid tissue undamaged. Because the normal thyroid tissue is hypofunctioning and takes up little of the radioactive iodine, when treatment is given the patient may be left with normal thyroid function without the need for thyroid hormone replacement therapy.

DRUG-INDUCED THYROID DYSFUNCTION

Amiodarone-Induced Thyroid Disease

Several drugs other than PTU and MMI can affect thyroid function. Amiodarone, a drug used to treat cardiac arrhythmias, is a fat-soluble drug with a long half-life (50 days) in the body that interferes with normal thyroid function.[21] The fact that 37% of the molecular weight of amiodarone is iodine accounts for a significant part of the thyroid dysfunction seen. Iodine, when given in large doses, leads to acute inhibition of thyroid hormone production. This is called the Wolff-Chaikoff effect. Amiodarone also blocks T_4-to-T_3 conversion. The combination of these two actions leads to hypothyroidism in 8% to 20% of patients on chronic amiodarone therapy. Amiodarone can also lead to hyperthyroidism in 3% of patients treated chronically with this medication. Certain patients develop hyperthyroidism as they escape the Wolff-Chaikoff effect and use the excess iodine for thyroid hormone production. Others develop hyperthyroidism if the medication leads to inflammation of the thyroid gland (subacute thyroiditis) and subsequent leakage of stored thyroid hormone into the circulation.

Subacute Thyroiditis

Several conditions occur that lead to transient changes in thyroid hormone levels.[22] These conditions are associated with inflammation of the thyroid gland, leakage of stored thyroid hormone, and then repair of the gland. Although nomenclature varies between authors, grouping together postpartum thyroiditis, painless thyroiditis, and painful thyroiditis as forms of subacute thyroiditis is one of the simplest classification schemes. These conditions are often associated with a thyrotoxic phase when thyroid hormone is leaking into the circulation, a hypothyroid phase when the thyroid gland is repairing itself, and a euthyroid phase when the gland is repaired. These phases can last from weeks to months.

Postpartum thyroiditis is the most common form of subacute thyroiditis. It occurs in 3% to 16% of women in the postpartum period.[23] It is strongly associated with the presence of TPO antibodies and chronic lymphocytic thyroiditis. Patients may experience a period of thyrotoxicosis followed by hypothyroidism or simply hypothyroidism or hyperthyroidism. Thyroid hormone levels usually return to normal after several months; however, by 4 years' postpartum, 25% to 50% of patients have persistent hypothyroidism, goiter, or both.[24] During the thyrotoxic phase, beta-blockers can be used if treatment is necessary. During the hypothyroid phase, thyroid hormone replacement therapy can be given if symptoms require, usually for 3 to 6 months, unless permanent hypothyroidism evolves. The thyrotoxic phase of this condition, as well as other forms of subacute thyroiditis, can be distinguished from Graves' disease by a low RAIU and an absence of TSI or TSH receptor antibodies (Table 23-4). Painless thyroiditis or subacute lymphocytic thyroiditis shares many characteristics of postpartum thyroiditis, except that there is no associated pregnancy.

Painful thyroiditis, also called *subacute granulomatous thyroiditis*, *subacute nonsuppurative thyroiditis*, or *de Quervain's thyroiditis*, is characterized by neck pain, low-grade fever, myalgia, a tender diffuse goiter, and swings in thyroid function tests (as discussed earlier). Viral infections are felt to trigger this condition. TPO antibodies are usually absent; erythrocyte sedimentation rate and thyroglobulin levels are often elevated.

NONTHYROIDAL ILLNESS

Hospitalized patients, especially critically ill patients, often have abnormalities in their thyroid function tests. Typically, the laboratory pattern is one of low total T_4, free T_4, and (sometimes) TSH. Because illness decreases 5′-monodeiodinase activity, less T_4 is converted to active T_3. This leads to decreased levels of T_3 and higher levels of rT_3. There also seems to be an element of central hypothyroidism and thyroid hormone–binding changes associated with severe illness. It is believed that many of these changes are an appropriate adaptation to illness. Thyroid hormone replacement therapy is not indicated.

THYROID NODULES

Thyroid nodules are common. Clinically apparent thyroid nodules are present in 6.4% of adult women and 1.5% of adult men, according to the Framingham data.[25] Thyroid ultrasound finds unsuspected thyroid nodules in 20% to 45% of women and 17% to 25% of men.[26] The major concern with thyroid nodules is that they may represent a thyroid cancer. Fortunately, only 5% to 9% of thyroid nodules prove to be thyroid cancer. FNA of these nodules, with cytologic examination of the aspirate, has become a routine practice to help distinguish the nodules that require surgical removal from those that do not.[27]

For additional student resources please visit thePoint at http://thepoint.lww.com.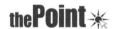

QUESTIONS

1. All of the following statements about iodine are true EXCEPT
   a. Radioactive iodine treatment of Graves' disease is effective in less than 40% of patients treated with this agent.
   b. Iodine deficiency is one of the most common causes of hypothyroidism in the world.
   c. T_4 has 4 iodine molecules.
   d. RAIU is often useful in determining the cause of thyrotoxicosis.

2. The fetus
   a. Is dependent on thyroid hormone for normal neurologic development
   b. Does not develop a thyroid gland until the third trimester
   c. Is not susceptible to damage from radioactive iodine therapy given to the mother
   d. Will be born with hypothyroidism in approximately 1 of 400 births in developed countries

3. The thyroid gland
   a. Depends on TPO to permit iodination of the tyrosyl residues to make MIT and DIT
   b. Is an ineffective iodine trap
   c. Depends on TPO to permit the joining of two DIT residues to form T_3
   d. Usually functions independent of TSH levels

4. The thyroid gland produces all of the following EXCEPT
   a. TSH
   b. Thyroglobulin
   c. T_3
   d. T_4

5. Hypothyroidism is generally associated with all of the following EXCEPT
   a. TSH receptor antibodies
   b. Depression
   c. An elevation of TSH levels
   d. TPO antibodies

6. A 34-year-old woman presents with goiter, tachycardia, and weight loss of 2 months duration. TSH is undetectable and free T_4 is high. All of the following tests are useful in diagnosing the cause of the hyperthyroidism EXCEPT
   a. FNA biopsy of the thyroid gland
   b. TSH receptor antibodies
   c. RAIU
   d. TSH

7. A 65-year-old woman presents with fatigue, hypothermia, pericardial effusions, and hair loss. Her thyroid function tests show a significantly elevated TSH and a low free T_4. All of the following laboratory test abnormalities may be associated with her underlying condition EXCEPT
   a. Elevated WBC
   b. An elevated cholesterol level
   c. Anemia
   d. Elevated CPK levels

8. A 26-year-old man presents with a 3-cm, right lobe, thyroid nodule and a normal TSH. What is the next test that should be performed?
   a. FNA of the nodule
   b. Free T_4 level
   c. Thyroid ultrasound
   d. Thyroid scan

9. The following are treatment options for hyperthyroidism associated with Graves' disease EXCEPT
   a. Thyroid hormone
   b. PTU
   c. Beta-blockers
   d. Radioactive iodine

10. All of the following abnormalities might be expected in a severely ill patient EXCEPT
    a. Low rT_3
    b. Low T_4
    c. Low T_3
    d. Low TSH

11. Of the following thyroid hormones, which is considered the most biologically active?
    a. T_3 bound to TBG
    b. T_4 bound to TBG
    c. Free T_4
    d. Free T_3
    e. rT_3

12. The primary serum test to screen for thyroid disease is:
    a. Free T_4
    b. rT_3
    c. Total T_4
    d. Autoimmune antibodies to thyroid tissue
    e. TSH

13. Of the following, which will MOST likely interfere with quantitation of thyroglobulin?
    a. Antithyroglobulin autoantibodies
    b. Thyroid-stimulating antibodies
    c. TSH receptor antibodies
    d. Thyroid peroxidase antibodies

REFERENCES

1. Greenspan FS. The thyroid gland. In: Greenspan FS, Strewler GJ, eds. *Basic & Clinical Endocrinology*. 5th ed. New York, NY: Appleton & Lange; 1997;192-262.
2. Lavin L. *Manual of Endocrinology*. 2nd ed. Boston, MA: Little, Brown & Co; 1994:395.
3. Caldwell KL, Makhmudov A, Ely E, Jones RL, Wang RY. Iodine status of the U.S. populations, national health and nutrition examination survey, 2005-2006 and 2007-2008. *Thyroid*. 2001;21:419-427.
4. Kopp P. Thyroid hormone synthesis. In: Braverman LE, Utiger RD, eds. *The Thyroid: Fundamental and Clinical Text*. 9th ed. Philadelphia, PA: Williams and Wilkins; 2005;52-76.
5. Ross DS, Ardisson LJ, Meskell MJ. Measurement of thyrotropin in clinical and subclinical hyperthyroidism using a new chemiluminescent assay. *J Clin Endocrinol Metab*. 1989;69(3):684.
6. Spencer CA, LoPresiti JS, Patel A, et al. Applications of a new chemiluminometric thyrotropin assay to subnormal measurement. *J Clin Endocrinol Metab*. 1990;70:453-460.
7. Ekins R. The free hormone hypothesis and measurement of free hormones [editorial]. *Clin Chem*. 1992;38:1289-1293.
8. Wong TK, Pekary AE, Hoo GS, et al. Comparison of methods for measuring free thyroxine in nonthyroidal illness. *Clin Chem*. 1992;38:720-724.
9. Tan GH, Gharib H. Thyroid incidentalomas: management approaches to nonpalpable nodules discovered incidentally on thyroid imaging. *Ann Intern Med*. 1997;126:226.
10. Cooper DS, Doherty GM, Haugen BR, et al. American Thyroid Association (ATA) Guidelines Taskforce on Thyroid Nodules and Differentiated Thyroid Cancer. Revised American Thyroid Association Management guidelines for patients with thyroid nodules and differentiated thyroid cancer. *Thyroid*. 2009;19(11):1173-1174.
11. Skowsky WR, Kikuchi TA. The role of vasopressin in the impaired water excretion of myxedema. *Am J Med*. 1987;64:613-621.
12. Khaleeli AA, Gohil K, McPhail G, et al. Muscle morphology and metabolism in hypothyroid myopathy: effects of treatment. *J Clin Pathol*. 1983;36:519-526.
13. Green ST, Ng JP. Hypothyroidism and anaemia. *Biomed Pharmacother*. 1986;40:326-331.
14. Diekman T, Lansberg PJ, Kastelein JJ, Wiersinga WM. Prevalence and correction of hypothyroidism in a large cohort of patients referred for dyslipidemia. *Arch Intern Med*. 1995;155:1490-1495.

15. O'Brien T, Dinneen SF, O'Brien PC, Palumbo PJ. Hyperlipidemia in patients with primary and secondary hypothyroidism. *Mayo Clin Proc.* 1993;68:860-866.

16. American College of Physicians. Clinical Guideline, part 1. Screening for thyroid disease. *Ann Intern Med.* 1998;129:141-143.

17. Ladenson PW, Singer PA, Ain KB, et al. American Thyroid Association guidelines for detection of thyroid dysfunction. *Arch Intern Med.* 2000;160:1573-1575.

18. Burch HB, Wartofsky L. Graves' ophthalmopathy: current concepts regarding pathogenesis and management. *Endocr Rev.* 1993;14:747-793.

19. Villadolid MC, Yokoyama N, Izumi M, et al. Untreated Graves' disease patients without clinical ophthalmopathy demonstrate a high frequency of extraocular muscle (EOM) enlargement by magnetic resonance. *J Clin Endocrinol Metab.* 1995;80:2830-2833.

20. Solomon BL, Evaul JE, Burman KD, Wartofsky L. Remission rates with antithyroid drug therapy: continuing influence of iodine intake? *Ann Intern Med.* 1987;107:510-512.

21. Nademanee K, Singh BN, Callahan B, et al. Amiodarone, thyroid hormone indexes, and altered thyroid function: long-term serial effects in patients with cardiac arrhythmias. *Am J Cardiol.* 1986;58:981-986.

22. Pearce EN, Farwell AP, Braverman LE. Thyroiditis. *N Engl J Med.* 2003;348(26):2646-2655.

23. Gerstein HC. How common is postpartum thyroiditis? A methodologic overview of the literature. *Arch Intern Med.* 1990;150:1397-1400.

24. Othman S, Phillips DI, Parkes AB, et al. A long-term follow-up of postpartum thyroiditis. *Clin Endocrinol (Oxf).* 1990;32:559-564.

25. Vander JB, Gaston EA, Dawber TG. The significance of nontoxic thyroid nodules. *Ann Intern Med.* 1968;69:537.

26. Brander A, Viikinkoski P, Nickels J, et al. Thyroid gland: US screening in a random adult population. *Radiology.* 1991;181:683.

27. Ezzat S, Sarti DA, Cain DR, et al. Thyroid incidentalomas: prevalence by palpation and ultrasonography. *Arch Intern Med.* 1994;154:1838.

28. Gharif H. Changing concepts in the diagnosis and management of thyroid nodules. *Endocrinol Metab Clin North Am.* 1997;26:777.

Calcium Homeostasis and Hormonal Regulation

CHAPTER 24

JOSEPHINE ABRAHAM, DEV ABRAHAM

CHAPTER OUTLINE

Chapter Objectives

Upon completion of this chapter, the clinical laboratorian should be able to do the following:

• Describe the endocrine and organ physiology of calcium metabolism.

• Discuss the laboratory tools used to evaluate calcium metabolism.

• Apply the laboratory tools to clinical disease states of calcium metabolism.

KEY TERMS

1,25-Dihydroxy vitamin D
25-Hydroxy vitamin D
Bisphosphonates
Bone turnover
Calcium-sensing receptor
Cinacalcet
Cortical bone
Dual-energy x-ray absorptiometry
Hypercalcemia
Hypocalcemia

Lithium
Osteoblast
Osteoclast
Osteomalacia
Osteoporosis
Parathyroid hormone
Parathyroid hormone–related protein
Rickets
Teriparatide
Thiazide diuretics
Trabecular bone
Vitamin D

CALCIUM HOMEOSTASIS

Serum calcium level is maintained at a constant level for the optimal excitability of neural and muscular tissue and the coordinated functioning of various organ systems in the human body. In this chapter, the control of blood calcium and how disorders of these systems can cause bone disease will be reviewed. A preview of organs and organ systems involved is as described in Figure 24-1.

An adult human body contains 1,000 g of calcium.[1] About 99% of this is in the form of hydroxyapatite salt (provides structural rigidity along with collagen matrix) and the remainder (1%) is in the extra-cellular fluids and regulates various biochemical events. In the blood, calcium exists in ionized (50%), protein bound (40% to plasma proteins), and complexed (10% to citrate and phosphate) forms. The pH of blood influences binding with proteins

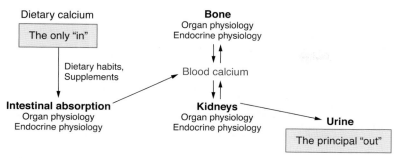

FIGURE 24-1 Calcium homeostasis. Tissue and organs involved in calcium homeostasis (gut, skeleton, and kidneys) and how they relate to blood calcium. Also shown is the means of getting calcium de novo into the system (GI absorption) and elimination of calcium from the system (renal excretion) under normal physiologic conditions.

(binding increases with high pH and decreases with low pH). The ionized calcium is the only relevant fraction from the cellular function standpoint. The principal organs involved in calcium homeostasis are the skin, liver, small intestine, skeleton, parathyroid glands, and kidneys. Diet is the only source of calcium. The skeleton acts as a mineral repository, releasing calcium into blood on demand, especially during times of poor intake. During prolonged low oral intake or malabsorption, the blood levels are maintained at near-normal levels at the expense of the skeletal stores. The human skeleton also plays vital roles involving ambulation and protection of vital organs (brain and thoracic viscera). The only significant loss of calcium from the body is into urine.

HORMONAL REGULATION OF CALCIUM METABOLISM

Vitamin D and parathyroid hormone (PTH) are the two most important hormones that regulate calcium and phosphate homeostasis. No clear role for calcitonin has been established in healthy humans.

Vitamin D

Vitamin D is a steroid hormone that is synthesized in the skin following exposure to UVB rays from the sun.

Following the photo-biosynthesis of vitamin D from cholesterol, it undergoes further hydroxylation in the liver and kidneys (Fig. 24-2).[2]

The hepatic enzyme, 25-hydroxylase, metabolizes vitamin D_3 to 25-hydroxy vitamin D_3. Serum 25-hydroxy vitamin D estimation is the best indicator of body stores; therefore, low 25-hydroxy vitamin D levels in the blood imply deficiency. The renal 1α-hydroxylase, under PTH regulation, completes the formation of the active metabolite, 1,25-dihydroxy vitamin D (1,25($OH)_2$D).

Endogenous synthesis of vitamin D is influenced by the amount of sun exposure, available sunlight (less in northern latitudes), skin covering (clothing and sun block), and age of the individual. Older individuals have less effective photo-biosynthesis of vitamin D.

Vitamin D_3 (cholecalciferol) is scarcely found in nature. The major dietary sources are internal organs such as liver and sea food. Vitamin D_2 (ergocalciferol) is found in edible mushrooms. Commercially available milk is fortified with vitamin D_3. Breast-fed infants are at risk for vitamin D deficiency, since breast milk is a poor source of vitamin D. Multivitamins contain 400 units of vitamin D_3, about the same amount found in a quart of vitamin D—fortified milk.

Vitamin D is a steroid hormone derived from cholesterol. The same cholesterol biosynthetic pathway that

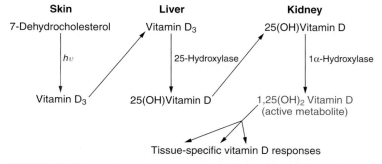

FIGURE 24-2 Vitamin D synthesis. Tissues involved in the synthesis of vitamin D and the steps that each tissue is responsible for. Also shown are enzymes responsible for the two enzymatically mediated steps (hepatic 25-hydroxylation and renal 1α-hydroxylation). The product of this pathway, 1,25($OH)_2$D, is responsible for the tissue-specific effects of vitamin D.

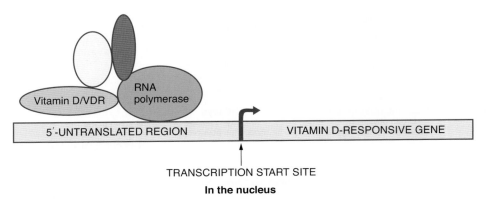

TRANSCRIPTION START SITE

In the nucleus

FIGURE 24-3 Vitamin D mechanism of action. DNA binding and interaction with other components of the transcriptional machinery of the vitamin D–vitamin D receptor complex are shown. Note the striking evolutionary similarity between this mechanism and that of other steroid and thyroid hormones. As prime examples, vitamin D inhibits transcription of the *PTH* gene in parathyroid tissue and stimulates transcription of the calcium transporter in the intestinal brush border epithelium.

provides the precursors for vitamin D also provides the precursors for other steroid hormones from the adrenal gland and gonads. The steroid receptor supergene family of nuclear receptors carry out its physiologic regulation by directing transcription of specific vitamin D–responsive genes. $1,25(OH)_2D$ is the natural ligand for the vitamin D receptor. Synthetic analogs of vitamin D such as paricalcitol bind to vitamin D receptors with very high affinity and are used to treat secondary hyperparathyroidism due to chronic renal failure.

The $1,25(OH)_2D$–vitamin D receptor complex binds to the vitamin D response element upstream (5′) of the transcription start site of vitamin D genes and induces gene transcription (Fig. 24-3).

Activated vitamin D, $1,25(OH)_2D$, induces active absorption of calcium in the small bowel cells, which is the dominant mechanism of calcium absorption in humans. Only about 5% to 10% of calcium is absorbed passively.[3,4] The lack of active intestinal absorption of calcium induced by activated vitamin D, $1,25(OH)_2D$, results in hypocalcemia. Even though activated $1,25(OH)_2D$ also stimulates absorption of phosphate, a larger fraction of phosphate absorption occurs passively and is much less dependent upon normal $1,25(OH)_2D$ levels. This mechanism is illustrated in chronic renal failure patients.

In the bone, $1,25(OH)_2D$ stimulates differentiation of osteoclast precursors to osteoclasts. $1,25(OH)_2D$ also stimulates osteoblasts to influence osteoclasts to mobilize bone calcium. $1,25(OH)_2D$ does not directly affect *mature* osteoclast function. $1,25(OH)_2D$ plays an important role in the mineralization of bone, and abnormal bone results when vitamin D is deficient (e.g., celiac sprue) or its metabolism is defective (e.g., renal failure).

As noted earlier, $1,25(OH)_2D$ increases blood calcium by augmenting intestinal absorption of calcium. Blood calcium feeds back to parathyroid glands and regulates the synthesis and secretion of PTH. Also, $1,25(OH)_2D$ has direct control over the *PTH* secretion, and high levels reduce secretion of PTH. Elevated serum phosphate levels reduce $1,25(OH)_2D$ formation (Fig. 24-4).

Parathyroid Hormone

PTH is secreted from four parathyroid glands that are located adjacent to the thyroid gland. The parathyroid glands were first described in 1852 by Sir. Richard Owen,[5] when he performed postmortem dissection on an Indian Rhinoceros that had died in London Zoo. Normal parathyroid glands are ovoid or bean shaped and measure approximately 3 mm in size. The superior parathyroid glands are smaller than the inferior pair. The parathyroid

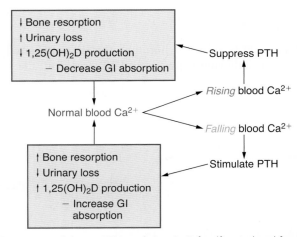

FIGURE 24-4 Calcium, PTH, and vitamin D feedforward and feedback loops. The endocrine response to shifts in blood calcium (rising or falling) is shown. A concerted hormone response, mediated at the organ level by the organs shown in Figure 24-1, helps restore blood calcium toward normal.

glands have an anatomically distinct vascular supply from that of the thyroid gland and are enveloped in a pad of anatomically distinct fibro-fatty capsule.[6]

One human postmortem examination study revealed that four glands are found in 91% of the subjects, three glands in 5%, and five glands in 4%.[7] The locations of parathyroid glands vary widely due to the embryonic origination from the third and fourth pharyngeal pouches with eventual migration to the lower neck. The superior parathyroid glands develop in the fourth pharyngeal pouch and migrate caudally along with the ultimobranchial bodies, which give rise to parafollicular (C) cells of the thyroid gland. The superior pair is commonly located along the upper two-thirds of the posterior margin of the thyroid lobe. The superior parathyroid glands are relatively constant in their location along the posterior margin of the thyroid gland. The third bronchial pouches give rise to the inferior pair and the thymus gland, and together they migrate to the lower neck; in some individuals the inferior parathyroid glands can migrate into the thorax.

The parathyroid glands have specialized calcium-sensing receptors (CSRs) that respond to rising or falling calcium levels by increasing or decreasing PTH secretion, respectively. The primary targets for the PTH are the bone and kidneys. PTH mobilizes calcium from bone by increasing bone resorption. PTH has three effects on the kidneys:

1. Increase the reabsorption of renal tubular calcium
2. Increase phosphate excretion
3. Enhance 1α-hydroxylation of 25-hydroxy vitamin D

Activated $1,25(OH)_2D$ promotes meal-related intestinal absorption of calcium. In summary, low blood calcium is sensed by the parathyroid CSR, which in turn secretes PTH and sets into motion a cascade of events aimed at restoring normal blood calcium levels.

The multiple actions of PTH described above are mediated via PTH receptor, located on the cell membrane of target tissues. This receptor activates adenylate cyclase and the "second messenger" pathway involving cyclic AMP (cAMP), which modulates protein phosphorylation.

ORGAN SYSTEM REGULATION OF CALCIUM METABOLISM

The three organ systems that regulate calcium metabolism are the gastrointestinal (GI) tract, the kidneys, and bone.

GI Regulation

Normal intestinal function is required for calcium absorption. Interruptions in intestinal function, as may be seen with short bowel syndromes (following resection), gastric weight loss surgeries, intestinal mucosal disease (celiac disease), genetic defects, and bowel fistula, etc., may affect calcium absorption. Adequate dietary calcium intake, the availability of normal amounts of vitamin D, and metabolism are all necessary for optimal calcium absorption. $1,25(OH)_2D$ controls calcium absorption from the small bowel. Dietary phosphate can bind dietary calcium in the intestinal lumen, forming the insoluble and nonabsorbable precipitate, calcium phosphate. The insolubility of calcium phosphate is the basis for the use of calcium carbonate as a "phosphate binder" in patients with renal failure. Likewise, a diet rich in phosphate will tend to inhibit calcium absorption by the same mechanism.

Role of Kidneys

The kidneys play an essential role in calcium metabolism. This is exemplified in subjects who develop renal failure, leading to markedly disordered calcium and phosphate metabolism.[8] Impaired hydroxylation of 25-hydroxy vitamin D to form the active $1,25(OH)_2D$ results in poor calcium absorption from the gut. Diseased kidneys fail to excrete phosphate, leading to elevated serum phosphate levels. Hyperphosphatemia is a powerful stimulus for PTH and fibroblast growth factor 23 (FGF 23) secretion. FGF 23 is a powerful phosphaturic hormone. Serum PTH levels can be elevated into the thousands in chronic renal failure patients. Once a critical calcium/phosphate product is reached, precipitation of these minerals occurs within the tissues, leading to devastating consequences.

In physiological state, PTH increases renal tubular reabsorption of calcium, thereby reducing renal loss. Hypercalcemia, whether as a result of autonomous overproduction of PTH, termed *primary hyperparathyroidism (PHPT)*, or from other causes, greatly increases the filtered load of calcium. Even though PTH stimulates tubular reabsorption of calcium, this process is overwhelmed, and the *net* calcium excretion is increased compared with normal state. This is the fundamental mechanism by which PHPT subjects form calcium kidney stones. See Figure 24-5 for organ system integration of calcium homeostasis.

Bone Physiology

Bone contains about 1 kg of calcium and serves as a repository for calcium, phosphate, and magnesium. Bone turnover or "remodeling" is a regulated and coupled process of simultaneous bone formation and breakdown that occurs to varying degrees throughout the life and at multiple sites in the skeleton. The process of "coupling" ensures that neither resorption nor formation occurs in excess compared to the other, thereby preventing imbalance between formation and loss of bone. Too much resorption results in weaker bones and too much bone formation can obliterate

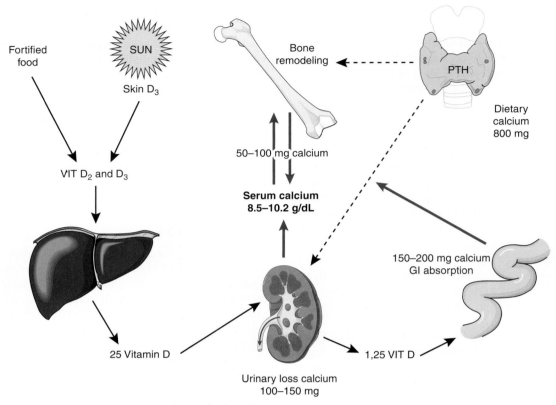

FIGURE 24-5 Organ system integration of calcium homeostasis.

the marrow space. Bone formation is mediated by osteoblasts, and bone breakdown, or resorption, is mediated by osteoclasts (a cell in the monocyte/macrophage lineage). Interestingly, although osteoclasts are required to mobilize calcium from bone, they do not appear to express receptors for either $1,25(OH)_2D$ or for PTH. Rather, these hormones act directly on osteoblasts, which in turn produce a complex array of hormones, which regulate the osteoclast activity, either activating or deactivating them. When the net rates of osteoblast-mediated bone formation and osteoclast-mediated bone resorption are mismatched, or uncoupled, such that resorption exceeds formation, bone mass will ultimately decrease. Decreased bone mass translates clinically into an increased risk of fracture, as seen in osteoporosis. As bones turn over several proteins are released into the blood and eventually excreted in the urine, collectively called as bone turnover markers.[9] Bone turnover markers are useful in the monitoring of clinical response to osteoporosis therapies and for predicting fracture risks.

Resorption markers include the following:

- Hydroxyproline
- N telopeptides
- C telopeptides
- Cross-links

- TRAP (tartrate-resistant acid phosphatase)

Formation markers include the following:

- BSAP (bone-specific alkaline phosphatase
- Osteocalcin
- Procollagen N-terminal extension peptides

There are two main types of bones found in the skeleton: cortical bone and trabecular bone. Cortical bone is the predominant bone type found in the shaft of long bones, such as the femur. Cortical bone is very strong, yet light in weight, and is therefore well suited for the mechanical needs of the extremities. Trabecular bone is the primary bone type found in the axial skeleton, such as the vertebrae. It consists of numerous cross-hair or honey-comb–type connections called *trabeculae*. These interconnected trabeculae give this type of bone considerable strength for weight bearing. Although the femur is primarily cortical bone and the vertebrae is primarily trabecular bone, sites such as the femoral trochanter and proximal humerus are a mixture of both cortical and trabecular bones. The ends of long bones contain more trabecular bone. The shafts of long bones are predominantly cortical. Certain disease states induce preferential bone loss in specific bone types. Cortical bone is preferentially lost in PHPT and trabecular bone is mostly lost in post menopausal osteoporosis. In most conditions bone loss is diffuse.

In summary, normal calcium homeostasis is achieved by a complex and regulated interplay between vitamin D, PTH, and the target organs. Defects in the function and formation of hormones or organ system disorders can induce disease states, which will be reviewed in the rest of this chapter.

HYPERCALCEMIA

Hypercalcemia results when blood calcium levels in a subject are above the expected normal range of a healthy population. Patients with low serum albumin would be expected to have low total calcium and normal ionized calcium; the opposite is true for patients with high serum albumin. Ionized calcium best correlates with the biological activity of calcium, as well as with symptoms of hypercalcemia or hypocalcemia, and thus the direct measurement of ionized calcium may often be more valuable clinically. The binding of calcium to proteins should be taken into consideration during assessment of blood calcium levels.

The duration and the level of calcium elevation determine the severity of symptoms and the degree of end-organ damage. Some common symptoms of acute severe hypercalcemia include lethargy, stupor, and coma. Patients with chronic mild hypercalcemia are symptom free. Moderate calcium elevation is associated with intellectual weariness, personality changes, nausea, anorexia, polyuria, kidney stones, hypertension, and electrocardiogram (ECG) changes. In the outpatients setting, PHPT is the commonest cause for hypercalcemia.

Cancer-mediated hypercalcemia often presents with profound central nervous system (CNS) symptoms due to rapid and significant calcium elevation at the time of diagnosis.

Causes of Hypercalcemia

1. **Disorders of parathyroid glands and CSRs:**

   - PHPT (autonomous overproduction of PTH): adenoma (>80%), hyperplasia (5% to 10%), carcinoma (<1%), and familial syndromes (MEN 1, MEN 2a, and PHPT-jaw tumor syndrome).
   - Secondary and tertiary hyperparathyroidism: In chronic renal failure patients, the sustained hypocalcemic–hyperphosphatemic stimuli result in parathyroid hyperplasia, leading to sustained and autonomous overproduction of PTH with ensuing hypercalcemia.
   - CSR abnormalities (extracellular calcium levels are sensed aberrantly resulting in hypercalcemia): familial hypocalciuric hypercalcemia (FHH) (inactivating mutation of CSR), calcium receptor antibodies, and lithium carbonate.

   - Other endocrine disorders: adrenal insufficiency, hyperthyroidism, pheochromocytomas, VIPoma.

2. **Cancer-mediated hypercalcemia (paraneoplastic hypercalcemia):**

   - PTHrP production by tumors: Upper GI adenocarcinomas, squamous cell carcinomas of head and neck and lung, renal cell carcinoma, ovarian carcinoma, HTLV 1 lymphoma, adrenal cancer, carcinoid tumor, islet cell cancer, and pheochromocytoma. Prostate and colonic cancers rarely produce PTHrP.
   - 1,25 Hydroxylation of 25-hydroxy vitamin D: Various cell types of lymphomas.
   - Cytokine production by tumor cells leads to activation of bone resorption (myeloma and diffuse bone metastasis): Cytokines such as macrophage inflammatory protein 1 alpha, tumor necrosis factor alpha, prostaglandins, and IL-6 which activate osteoclasts through RANK (receptor activator of nuclear factor kappa B).

3. **Granulomatous diseases:** Sarcoidosis, tuberculosis, leprosy, fungal infections, Crohn disease (granulomas express the hydroxylation enzyme that is required to convert 25-hydroxy vitamin D to active $1,25(OH)_2D$).

4. **Medications:** Hydrochlorothiazide (HCTZ), lithium, vitamin A and/or D toxicity, oral calcium excess (milk alkali syndrome [MAS]), tamoxifen, aminophylline toxicity.

5. **Miscellaneous:** William's syndrome, chronic immobilization.

The signs and symptoms of hypercalcemia are highly variable and depend upon the rapidity of onset and severity of hypercalcemia. Clinically, the signs and symptoms also vary from patient to patient and comorbid conditions may also influence the development of symptoms. The signs and symptoms are best described by organ systems:

CNS: Impairment of CNS function, including lethargy, decreased alertness, depression, confusion, forgetfulness, obtundation, and coma.
GI: Patients may experience anorexia, constipation, peptic ulcers, and nausea and vomiting.
Renal: Hypercalciuria leading to kidney stone formation and calcification of renal tubules resulting in nephrogenic diabetes insipidus.
Skeletal: Increased bone resorption and demineralization leading to fractures.
Cardiovascular: Hypercalcemia may cause or exacerbate hypertension. The following ECG changes are seen in hypercalcemia: Increased PR interval, wide QRS complex, and short QT syndrome.

Primary Hyperparathyroidism

PHPT is the commonest cause of hypercalcemia, with an incidence of 1 in 500 to 1,000 in the general population. Women are affected threefold more commonly than men. The hallmark of this disorder is the autonomous overproduction of PTH, most commonly by a single adenoma in one of the parathyroid glands (>80%), less commonly by multiple gland hyperplasia (~5% to 10%), and very rarely by parathyroid cancer. Parathyroid carcinoma occurs more commonly in a familial syndrome called the hyperparathyroidism-jaw tumor syndrome. PHPT is also encountered in multiple endocrine neoplasia types 1 and 2 (MEN 1 and 2a). The apparent increase in the incidence of PHPT was traced to the introduction and wide availability of multichannel analyzers in the 1970s. The incidence of PHPT increased from 7.8 cases per 100,000 to 51 cases per 100,000 in Olmsted County, Minnesota, USA, following the introduction of routine calcium testing.[10] Fuller Albright's description of the disease in the 1930s was notable for advanced bone and end-stage kidney disease at the time of diagnosis.[11] This presentation is almost never seen now. The fortuitous detection of a large proportion of the prevalent subclinical PHPT subjects, along with early intervention and treatment, has changed the clinical presentation of PHPT. In countries where multi-channel analyzers are not available, the disease presentation is severe and with catastrophic renal and skeletal consequences, similar to how it was in the USA in the early 1900s.

The diagnosis of PHPT is made by biochemical testing, and elevated serum calcium (or ionized calcium) level with inappropriately normal or elevated PTH level confirms the diagnosis. The biochemical differential diagnosis of hypercalcemia is listed in Table 24-1.

PTH Assays

PTH is a polypeptide hormone with C-terminal and amino (N)-terminal ends composed of 84 amino acid residues. PTH 1 to 84 refer to the entire hormone sequence. n-Truncated PTH (7 to 84 PTH) are deficient in the first few residues of the n-terminal end and hence biologically inactive. The integrity of 1 to 11 amino acid residues in the N-terminal end of PTH is required for the biologic activity of PTH. PTH assays use two antibodies that bind to specific sites (one on each of the C- and N-terminal ends), which enable precise detection of

---

CASE STUDY 24-1

A 40-year-old woman presents to her physician complaining of marked left flank pain that began the previous night. She reports that the pain is worse than that of giving birth. She also reports blood in her urine earlier on the day she came to see her doctor. She has felt more fatigued, and as if her concentration has not been as good as normal for the last year or so, and she feels more forgetful. She has no significant past medical history. She is taking no medications. Family history contributes no pertinent information. On physical examination, she appears to be in extreme pain. There is marked tenderness on very gentle percussion over the left costovertebral angle. Labs are drawn and are notable for calcium 11.2 mg/dL (normal, 8.5 to 10.2 mg/dL), albumin 3.8 g/dL (normal, 3.5 to 4.8 g/dL), and intact PTH 162 pg/mL (normal, 11 to 54 pg/mL). Renal function is normal (BUN 25 mg/dL and creatinine 0.9 mg/dL). Urine analysis is notable for blood and >50 red blood cells per high-power field. This prompts a 24-hour urine collection, which reveals calcium elevated at 483 mg per 24 hour (normal, 100 to 250 mg per 24 hour).

Questions

1. Which laboratory results are abnormal?

2. What is the presumptive diagnosis for this patient? The differential diagnosis?

3. What treatment is indicated for this disease?

TABLE 24-1	BIOCHEMICAL DIFFERENTIAL DIAGNOSIS OF HYPERCALCEMIA					
CAUSES	Sr CA	Sr PO4	PTH	PTHrP	1,25 VIT D	URINE CALCIUM
PHPT	↑	↓	↑→	↓	↑	↑↑
Cancer PTHrP	↑↑	↓	↓	↑	↓	↑↑
CRF–3HPT Creatinine ↑	↑↓	↑↑	↑↑	↓	↓	↓
FHH Mg ↑	↑	→	↑→	↓	→	↓↓
Milk alk Vit D	↑	↑↓	↓	↓	↑	↑

PTH, parathyroid hormone; PTHrP, parathyroid hormone–related protein; PHPT, primary hyperparathyroidism; CRF, chronic renal failure; HPT, hyperparathyroidism; FHH, familial hypocalciuric hypercalcemia; milk alk Vit D, milk alkali vitamin D.

intact PTH. A few commonly available assays include the following:

- Intact PTH: measures 7 to 84 PTH and 1 to 84 PTH
- Bioactive PTH: measures 1 to 84 PTH
- CAP assay: cAMP inducible PTH. This assay detects biologically active PTH by its ability to induce formation of cAMP.
- PRHrP assays and PTH assays are exclusive to each other, by design. There is no cross-reactivity. Therefore, PTH levels are low in subjects with cancers producing PTHrP.
- PTH can also be estimated in needle biopsy specimens obtained from parathyroid tumors. Hook effect has not been observed despite massive elevation of PTH levels in these specimens obtained by direct puncture of enlarged parathyroid glands.[12]

Biochemical Findings in PHPT

1. Hypercalcemia
2. Hypophosphatemia: PTH induces phosphaturia.
3. Elevated PTH relative to serum calcium (inappropriately normal PTH in the face of hypercalcemia)
4. Low-normal 25-OH-D and high normal or elevated (30%) $1,25(OH)_2D$ due to PTH-enhancing renal hydroxylation
5. Urinary calcium excretion is elevated.
6. Metabolic hyperchloremic acidosis (chloride is exchanged for phosphate)
7. Elevated serum alkaline phosphatase in severe disease

Management of PHPT

Surgical resection of the affected gland(s) results in cure. Only about 30% of patients with PHPT need surgery at the time of diagnosis. Therefore, the following consensus criteria were generated by a panel of experts, and some changes to these criteria were adopted later:

1. Serum calcium levels >11.5 mg/dL on at least two determinations
2. Urinary calcium level of >400 mg in 24 hours or urine random calcium to creatinine ratio of ≥0.4 on two determinations. Newer recommendations removed this criterion.
3. Creatinine clearance that has dropped >30% (unexplained by other reasons) corrected for age and sex
4. Loss of bone density greater than −2.5 standard deviations (SDs) below young normal (T-score); cortical bone is preferentially lost in PHPT (e.g., wrist and hips)
5. Age <50 years

Surgical management of PHPT involves neck exploration with removal of the abnormal gland. Minimally invasive surgery (MIS) utilizes pre-surgical imaging to locate the abnormal gland, thereby guiding the surgeon

PHPT: Important Points

Insidious onset and gradual progression
Kidney stones in 20% to 30%
Bone loss—cortical > trabecular bone
Surgery is the only definitive management
Single gland tumor is common (85%)

to the diseased gland. MIS results in smaller incision and shorter recuperation times when compared with traditional exploration. Technetium 99m sestamibi scan (Parathyroid adenomas are rich in mitochondria, which trap this isotope. This scan is also used in cardiac imaging. The heart is another mitochondria-rich organ.) and high-resolution neck ultrasound are the two commonly used imaging tools. Also, with the availability of rapid PTH, once the adenoma is removed, PTH levels plummet (the half-life of PTH is <5 min), which enables biochemical confirmation of adenoma removal.

Medical management of PHPT is practiced in poor surgical candidates and those with mild disease. Bisphosphonates, selective estrogen receptor modulators (SERMs), and estrogen are all useful to varying degrees in any given patient. Allosteric calcium receptor modulator such as cinacalcet that binds to CaSR is used for controlling calcium levels in select patients with PHPT.

Familial Hypocalciuric Hypercalcemia

Familial hypocalciuric hypercalcemia (FHH) is a benign condition that results from germline mutation involving the CSR.[13,14] These inactivating mutations affecting the CSR upset their operating set point ranges (Fig. 24-6). Unlike in PHPT, the PTH production and calcium elevation in this condition are not progressive and result in stable mild hypercalcemia since birth. The hallmarks of this disorder include mild hypercalcemia, hypocalciuria (renal tubular cell calcium sensing is upset resulting in urine 24 hour calcium levels of <100 mg/d), mild PTH elevation (the parathyroid cellular calcium sensing is also abnormal), and mild elevation of magnesium. The hallmark is low urinary calcium excretion. Urinary fractional excretion in this condition is <1%, i.e., <0.01. Magnesium levels are mildly elevated. Inheritance is autosomal dominant with 100% penetrance among carriers, resulting in multiple members in the family being affected.

The following are the salient clinical and diagnostic features:

1. Serum calcium is elevated (mild to moderate elevation).
2. Serum magnesium is mildly elevated.
3. PTH is mildly elevated.

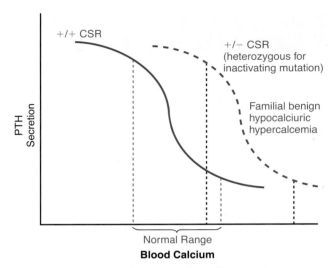

FIGURE 24-6 *Calcium-sensing receptor: effect on PTH secretion. Shown is the response of parathyroid tissue (as demonstrated by PTH secretion) to blood calcium. The* set point *is determined by the parathyroid response mediated by the transmembrane calcium-sensing receptor. The* normal curve *is for heterozygosity for the "wild-type" calcium-sensing receptor (+/+). The* right-shifted curve *is shown for the case where there is heterozygosity for the receptor (familial benign hypocalciuric hypercalcemia): one wild-type copy of the gene and one inactivating mutation (+/–).*

4. Urine calcium levels are typically <100 mg in 24 hours, with fractional excretion of urine calcium of <1% (i.e., ≤0.01 is highly suggestive of a diagnosis of FHH).
5. Mutant CSR can be demonstrated.
6. End-organ dysfunction (bone and kidney) is uncommon; therefore, surgery should not be performed.

Antibodies to the CSR upset the set point and induce hypercalcemia; these patients have normal calcium receptors. Surgical removal of parathyroid gland(s) should not be performed in these patients. Hence, it is very important to differentiate this disorder from PHPT to avoid unnecessary and ineffective surgeries.

Hyperthyroidism

Due to the direct effects of thyroxine on the bones, there is increased resorption and hypercalcemia. PTH levels are low.

FHH: Important Points

Low urine calcium
No end-organ damage
Multiple family members are affected
Mild elevation of magnesium
Surgery is ineffective and should not be performed

Addison's Disease

Hypercalcemia is commonly seen in patients presenting with Addisonian crisis. PTH levels are low. It gets corrected promptly with fluid and steroid replacement. It is thought to be a result of hypovolemia and dehydration. The exact mechanism is truly unknown.

Milk Alkali Syndrome

This syndrome in its classic form, described in the 1930s, follows the oral administration of very high (>20 g) amount of calcium and large amounts of milk to control gastric acid levels in patients with peptic ulcer disease. The hallmark of this disorder includes hypercalcemia, alkalosis, and renal impairment. Serum phosphate is often elevated. It is very rare to see the typical form of MAS now because of the use of proton pump inhibitors and H_2 blockers.

The reappearance of MAS in the 1990s follows the supplementation with lower amounts (even 1.5 to 2 g) of calcium carbonate for the treatment of osteoporosis in elderly patients with renal insufficiency. The presenting features are hypercalcemia, alkalosis, dehydration, and renal impairment with mental status changes. Serum phosphate level is low (administered salt is carbonate or citrate). Therapy includes intravenous and oral hydration and cessation of excessive calcium supplementation.

Medications That Cause Hypercalcemia

HCTZ and lithium are the commonest of drugs that induce hypercalcemia. HCTZ enhances distal tubular calcium absorption. Lithium affects the formation of intracellular inositol triphosphate, thereby upsetting the CSR function (similar to FHH).

Hypervitaminosis D is a condition that may result from excessive intake of vitamin D. It may also result from aberrant production of $1,25(OH)_2D$ as a result of extrarenal 1α-hydroxylation of 25-hydroxy vitamin D. Granulomatous diseases such as sarcoidosis and tuberculosis and certain lymphomas are capable of this effect. The granulomas or lymphoid tissue that hydroxylates vitamin D is autonomous and this is not regulated by the normal feedback mechanism; therefore, calcium elevation can be significant. Hypercalcemia results from increased GI absorption of calcium, without increase in bone resorption; therefore, bisphosphonates are not useful to control blood calcium levels. Also, the normal parathyroid glands respond to the elevation of calcium with reduction of PTH production, resulting in low PTH levels. These subjects also have elevated urine calcium levels.[14]

A variety of cancers may lead to hypercalcemia as a result of production and release of cytokines or PTH-like substances. These tumor-produced humoral substances are not responsive to negative feedback by calcium; therefore, these subjects can have massive elevation of serum calcium levels with low serum PTH levels.[14]

Parathyroid hormone–related protein (PTHrP) is a substance secreted by cancers that shares structural similarities to the N-terminal portion of human PTH molecule. Therefore, it retains functional features of PTH, with some critical differences. Both PTH and PTHrP bind to the same receptor in the kidney and bone as well as a variety of other tissues. In humans, PTHrP functions in the paracrine regulation of cartilage, skin, brain, and lactating breast tissue. In healthy humans, circulating levels of PTHrP are very low or immeasurable. Normal lactating breast tissue is capable of producing PTHrP, which can result in hypercalcemia and resolves following stopping breast-feeding. In most clinical situations of hypercalcemia due to PTHrP secretion, an underlying cancer is the root cause.[15] PTHrP can be secreted by a variety of cancers as described earlier in this chapter. The secretion is not regulated by even very high blood calcium levels, which results in severe hypercalcemia (Fig. 24-7). When humoral hypercalcemia of malignancy is suspected, PTHrP can be measured by specific immunoassay. Also, the intact PTH assay does not cross-react with circulating PTHrP. Normal parathyroid glands sense the elevated calcium levels and markedly reduce the secretion of PTH; therefore, PTH is very low. One salient difference in the biological functions between PTH and PTHrP is the inability of the latter to facilitate renal hydroxylation of 25-hydroxy vitamin D. This dichotomy in function between these otherwise functionally similar protein hormones remains unexplained.

There are a variety of medications that can cause hypercalcemia. Thiazide diuretics are used in the treatment of hypertension. This agent reduces the renal excretion of calcium, leading to calcium retention and hypercalcemia. At doses routinely used to treat hypertension, hypercalcemia is uncommon in subjects with normal calcium axis. However, when thiazide diuretics are used in subjects with other conditions associated with hypercalcemia such as PHPT, hypercalcemia can be worsened. In patients with subclinical PHPT, hypercalcemia can be precipitated by thiazide diuretics, leading to "unmasking" of PHPT.

Lithium carbonate, when used to treat bipolar disorder, can cause hypercalcemia. Lithium reduces intracellular formation of inositol triphosphate levels altering the "set point" of CSRs, a mechanism similar to FHH mentioned earlier.

High doses of vitamin A, or vitamin A analogs/metabolites in the retinoic acid family, may cause hypercalcemia. Vitamin A is believed to activate osteoclasts and enhance bone resorption, elevating blood calcium. In this condition, both PTH and $1,25(OH)_2D$ are suppressed.

CASE STUDY 24-2

A 58-year-old man has been a smoker since childhood. He has been smoking three packs per day since he can remember but insists his cigarettes "don't hurt me none, doc." He has been feeling ill recently, however, with loss of appetite, malaise, and weight loss. His mental ability has been dulled recently, and he can't remember from "one minute to the next" especially notable during his work as a cowboy. His cigarettes have not been as enjoyable for him as they used to be. His baseline cough has worsened, and he has noticed blood streaking his sputum when he clears sputum from his throat. He has no significant past medical history other than his tobacco abuse. He takes no medications. His family history is only notable for his father dying of lung cancer at age 63 and his mother dying of emphysema at age 68. On physical examination, he is a thin man who looks much older than his chronologic age and appears unwell. When he produces some sputum at the physician's request, it does indeed have a pink tinge and is streaked with blood. Chest examination reveals some scattered wheezing and some rales in the right upper lung region. He is diffusely weak on muscle strength testing. Labs are notable for calcium 16.8 mg/dL (normal, 8.5 to 10.2 mg/dL), albumin 3.4 (normal, 3.5 to 4.8 g/dL), BUN 27 mg/dL, and creatinine 1.3 mg/dL. Chest radiograph reveals a 3-cm proximal right hilar mass with distal streaking. Further testing is prompted and reveals a PTH of <1 pg/mL (normal, 11 to 54 pg/mL), and PTHrP elevated at 18.3 pmol/L (normal 0.0 to 1.5 pmol/L).

Questions

1. Do you think this patient's smoking is related to his hypercalcemia?

2. What other laboratory results are abnormal?

3. What is this patient's diagnosis? His prognosis?

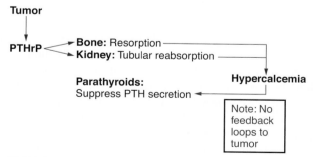

FIGURE 24-7 PTHrP endocrine pathophysiology. This demonstrates the effect of tumors that overproduce PTHrP. The pathophysiologic effect is via the same organ systems used by PTH to increase blood calcium. The difference between PTH and PTHrP is that PTH is subject to feedback regulation, whereas PTHrP is not subject to any feedback regulation by calcium (compare with Fig. 24-4).

HYPOCALCEMIA

Hypocalcemia refers to low blood calcium levels. It can result from a wide variety of conditions, from organ system dysfunction to lack of hormone effect to acid–base disturbances. The signs and symptoms of hypocalcemia are described below:

Neuromuscular: Tetany (involuntary muscle contraction) affecting primarily the muscles in the hands, feet, legs, and back may be seen. Percussion on cranial nerve VII (facial nerve) just anterior to the ear may elicit twitching in the ipsilateral corner of the mouth (Chvostek's sign). Numbness and tingling in the face, hands, and feet may be seen. Inflation of a blood pressure cuff to 20 mm Hg above the patient's systolic blood pressure to induce a state of ischemia in the arm (metabolic acidosis) may cause spasm in the muscles of the wrist and hand (Trousseau's sign).

CNS: Irritability, seizures, personality changes, and impaired intellectual functioning may be seen.

Cardiovascular: Calcium plays a crucial role not only in the slow inward calcium current of the QRS complex of ventricular depolarization but also in electromechanical coupling. In hypocalcemia, QT prolongation may be seen on the ECG. In the extreme, electromechanical dissociation may be seen. Cardiac contractile dysfunction is rare but in the extreme can result in congestive heart failure. Cardiac dysfunction from hypocalcemia should be treated with emergent intravenous calcium.

Causes of Hypocalcemia

1. Endocrine causes: hypoparathyroidism (lack of PTH)

   - Postoperative
   - Autoimmune (isolated or part of polyglandular autoimmune syndrome)
   - Congenital (mutations of CSR, PTH, and parathyroid aplasia)
   - Pseudohypoparathyroidism, types 1a, 1b, and 2

2. Deficiency of vitamin D: malnutrition, malabsorption due to celiac sprue, weight loss, gastric surgeries, short bowel syndrome, abdominal irradiation, pancreatic disease, liver disease, and renal disease

3. Hypomagnesemia: magnesium depletion leads to lack of PTH synthesis and release

The causes of hypocalcemia will be discussed in the setting of both endocrine and organ system dysfunction. However, one key concept should be emphasized when considering hypocalcemia: when functioning properly, the parathyroid glands will not only correct falling blood calcium but also *prevent* it, by increasing PTH secretion.

CASE STUDY 24-3

A 26-year-old man presents to his physician 3 weeks after having his thyroid surgically removed for thyroid cancer. His doctor is certain that she "got it all." However, since the time he went home from the hospital, he has noticed painful, involuntary muscle cramping. He also feels numbness and tingling around his mouth and in his hands and feet. His girlfriend says he has been irritable for the last couple of weeks. His past medical history is notable only for the recent diagnosis of thyroid cancer, and its resection 3 weeks prior to this visit. His only medication is levothyroxine. Family history contributes no relevant information. On physical examination, he has a well-healing thyroidectomy scar. Tapping on the face interior to the ears causes twitching in the ipsilateral corner of the mouth (Chvostek's sign). There are no palpable masses in the thyroid bed. A blood pressure cuff inflated above the systolic pressure induces involuntary muscle contracture in the ipsilateral hand after 60 seconds (Trousseau's sign). Labs are notable for calcium 5.6 mg/dL (normal, 8.5 to 10.2 mg/dL), albumin 4.1 g/dL, BUN 20 mg/dL, and creatinine 1.0 mg/dL. PTH is undetectable at <1 pg/mL.

Questions

1. Which laboratory results are abnormal?

2. What condition is he experiencing since his thyroidectomy?

3. What is the cause of this symptomatic condition?

4. What is the treatment for this patient, in addition to thyroxine medication?

The compensatory rise in PTH secretion, in response to factors that would lower blood calcium, is known as *secondary hyperparathyroidism*. Thus, an individual may have an elevated PTH level—for example, in response to low 25-hydroxy vitamin D—and thus maintain normocalcemia. Secondary hyperparathyroidism is notable for the normal response of parathyroid glands with appropriate and vigorous secretion of PTH. The biochemical constellation includes low blood calcium, elevated PTH, low serum phosphate, elevated alkaline phosphatase, hypocalciuria, phosphaturia, and vitamin D deficiency or lack of vitamin D effect.[16] Treatment of secondary hyperparathyroidism is directed toward correcting the process inducing hypocalcemia and/or vitamin D deficiency.[17]

Endocrine Causes of Hypocalcemia

Because proper PTH secretion and action are necessary to maintain normocalcemia, any inadequacy of parathyroid gland function will cause hypocalcemia. The most common cause of hypoparathyroidism is neck surgery, especially, after thyroidectomy with lymph node dissection. This results from accidental removal of these glands due to their small size. The most common outcome is temporary hypoparathyroidism following surgery, due to damage of the delicate parathyroid blood supply which results in full recovery in most subjects. Parathyroid glands can be reimplanted into pouches created in skeletal muscles (deltoid, sternomastoid, or fore-arm muscles). Parathyroid glands also survive careful cryopreservation and re-implantation back into its original owner. Additional causes of hypoparathyroidism include autoimmune destruction of parathyroid tissue. This condition is often associated with other autoimmune diseases such as type 1 diabetes, Hashimoto's thyroiditis, and Addison's disease. Magnesium deficiency can inhibit the secretion of PTH and also blunt its actions on target tissues. Following the correction of hypomagnesemia, PTH secretion and function is re-established. Depending on the cause, hypoparathyroidism can usually be treated with relatively high doses of vitamin D and calcium. In the absence of PTH, even the small fraction of passively absorbed calcium may simply be excreted in the urine. Hypercalciuria increases the risk of development of kidney stones in these subjects. The use of HCTZ reduces urine calcium losses and elevates serum calcium levels in PTH-deficient subjects.

Pseudohypoparathyroidism is a heritable disorder resulting in a lack of responsiveness to PTH in the target tissue. This results from uncoupling of the PTH receptor from adenylate cyclase, due to a mutant stimulatory G protein (G_s). PTH binds its receptor but cannot activate the second messenger, cAMP, and thus there is no response. Hypocalcemia develops, although unlike other forms of hypoparathyroidism mentioned, those with pseudohypoparathyroidism have markedly elevated levels of PTH. This is an example of a hormone resistance syndrome. Treatment is with calcium and vitamin D supplementation.

Hypovitaminosis D describes a collection of conditions, including low vitamin D availability, defective metabolism of vitamin D, or mutations in the vitamin D receptor, all of which predispose to hypocalcemia.

Organ System Causes of Hypocalcemia

A variety of intestinal disorders can result in malabsorption of calcium or vitamin D resulting in hypocalcemia. Causes include short bowel syndrome, abdominal irradiation, weight loss surgeries, celiac sprue, and bowel fistulation. Treatment end points are normalization of urine calcium excretion and normalization of PTH.

METABOLIC BONE DISEASES

A variety of disease states can affect skeletal architecture, strength, and integrity. Only rickets, osteomalacia, and osteoporosis are described here.

Rickets and Osteomalacia

Rickets and osteomalacia are diseases caused by abnormal mineralization of bone. They result from vitamin D deficiency. *Rickets* refers to the disease state affecting growing bones (in children); therefore, permanent skeletal deformity can be seen. *Osteomalacia* refers to the abnormal mineralization of bone in adults, or after completion of skeletal maturation. Rickets is associated with bony deformities because of bending of long bones under weight loading and effects of gravity. Bone deformity is not seen in adults. Both conditions are associated with similar biochemical findings of secondary hyperparathyroidism. Fractures may result in either case because of poor bone structure. Hypocalcemia may be seen when the response of secondary hyperparathyroidism is inadequate to counteract the threat of hypocalcemia posed by the vitamin D deficiency. Because of vitamin D fortification of milk—and public awareness—both conditions are in this era quite uncommon. However, those of any age who live indoors, with minimal or no sun exposure,

---

CASE STUDY 24-4

An 82-year-old woman living in a nursing home feels unsteady on her feet and does not wander outside anymore. She has lactose intolerance and has never been able to drink milk. She does not take any dietary supplements. She says, "I feel my age, doc," but otherwise has no specific complaints. On her annual laboratory assessment, her calcium level is found to be slightly low at 8.2 mg/dL (normal, 8.5 to 10.2 mg/dL) with albumin 3.5 g/dL (normal, 3.5 to 4.8 g/dL), BUN 28 mg/dL, and creatinine 1.1 mg/dL. This prompts further evaluation, which reveals PTH elevated at 181 pg/mL and 25-hydroxy vitamin D low at 6 ng/mL (normal, 20 to 50 ng/mL)[4]

Questions

1. What diagnostic possibility is suggested from the initial laboratory results of her annual assessment?

2. This patient's differential diagnosis includes two diseases. What are they?

3. Is her renal function related to either of these two diseases?

4. How should this patient be treated?

or who lack dietary vitamin D, are at risk for developing this condition. As mentioned in the discussion on vitamin D physiology, adequacy of vitamin D in the body can be assessed by measuring the blood level of 25-hydroxy vitamin D. Because secondary hyperparathyroidism is also expected in the setting of rickets or osteomalacia, PTH and calcium should be obtained to further confirm the suspected diagnosis.

Rickets can, however, develop under conditions of adequate amounts of vitamin D. This unique situation may develop from genetic defects in vitamin D metabolism or in the vitamin D receptor. Although 25-hydroxy vitamin D level is often normal, $1,25(OH)_2D$ level may be low, normal, or high depending on the genetic defect. Defects in vitamin D metabolism are best treated by supplying the metabolically active compound, $1,25(OH)_2D$ (calcitriol). A wide variety of vitamin D receptor defects have been described, including abnormal ligand binding, abnormal DNA binding, and abnormal transactivation of transcriptional machinery at the regulatory site of vitamin D–responsive genes. The type of defect present determines how well the patient will respond to pharmacologic doses of calcitriol.

Osteoporosis

Osteoporosis is the most prevalent metabolic bone disease in adults. Osteoporosis affects an estimated 20 to 25 million Americans with an estimated 4:1 female:male predominance. It is believed to cause approximately 1.5 million fractures annually in the United States. A recent study estimates that 4.5 million women, aged >50 years, have osteoporosis of the hip.[18] The most devastating consequence of osteoporosis is a hip fracture. While as many as half of vertebral compressions may be asymptomatic, a hip fracture carries with it a significant morbidity as well as an increased mortality. Most hip fractures require surgery at the very least. Mortality from hip fracture is increased by about 20% in the first year following the fracture, and it is estimated that the number of deaths related to hip fracture are now on par with those from breast cancer.

Multiple additional conditions have been identified as significant risk factors for reduced bone mass and a consequent increased risk of fracture, although risk factor assessment alone is generally not sufficient to characterize or quantify bone mass and diagnose osteoporosis. The following are validated risk factors for the prediction of fracture, independent of formal bone density evaluation: decreased bone mass due to previous fracture, advanced age, family history of osteoporosis or fracture, body weight less than 127 lb, long-term glucocorticoid therapy, cigarette smoking, or excess alcohol intake. Other conditions known to also alter calcium metabolism and increase fracture risk include Cushing's syndrome, hyperparathyroidism, disorders of vitamin D

CASE STUDY 24-5

A 6-year-old girl is brought to a pediatrician by her parents who report that her height is not progressing as they think it should (or like it did for her 8-year-old sister) and her legs look bowed. The patient drinks milk, and other than her shorter stature and bowed legs, she has the normal characteristics of her 6-year-old friends. She takes no medications. Family history is notable for some cousins on the father's side with a similar problem back in the Appalachian Hill country along Virginia/Tennessee border where the family hails from. The pediatrician obtains lab studies that are notable for a calcium level of 7.2 mg/dL (normal, 8.5 to 10.2 mg/dL) with albumin 4.1 g/dL (normal, 3.5 to 4.8 g/dL). Lower extremity radiographs show bowing of the long bones and generalized demineralization. This prompts the measurement of several other laboratory tests, which reveal intact PTH elevated at 866 pg/mL (normal, 11 to 54 pg/mL), 25-hydroxy vitamin D normal at 35 ng/mL (normal, 20 to 57 ng/mL), and $1,25(OH)_2D$ undetectable at <1 pg/mL (normal, 20 to 75 pg/mL).

Questions

1. What condition do the preliminary lab tests indicate?

2. What is the significance of 25-hydroxy vitamin D and $1,25(OH)_2D$ levels in the follow-up laboratory tests?

3. Describe the inborn error of metabolism with this patient.

4. What secondary condition will recur if vitamin D treatment is discontinued later in her life?

metabolism, hyperthyroidism, and certain malignancies (mast cell disease). Several medications have negative effects on the skeleton, leading to low bone mass and increase in the risk of fractures. The most notable are the glucocorticoids. They are widely used to treat a variety of inflammatory conditions such as asthma, rheumatoid arthritis, and lupus, as well as to prevent rejection after organ transplantation. First, they limit bone formation by inhibiting the action of osteoblasts while also inducing osteoblast apoptosis. They also increase the bone breakdown by stimulating the formation and action of osteoclasts. Therefore, the net loss of bone mass is compounded. "Glucocorticoid-induced osteoporosis" is a major source of morbidity associated with pharmacologic doses of glucocorticoids. Two bisphosphonates, alendronate and risedronate, are approved by the Food and Drug Administration (FDA) for the treatment of

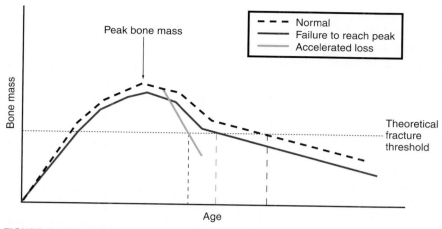

FIGURE 24-8 Bone mass as a function of age; perturbations that can affect bone mass. Shown is the accrual of bone mass with age to a peak that occurs in the mid-twenties to early thirties (for both sexes) and the bone loss that occurs throughout life after the peak. Fracture risk increases as bone mass is lost. The "theoretical fracture threshold" is an artificial notion but may be useful in demonstrating that at a given degree of trauma (varying from the simple act of weightbearing to increasing levels of impact) factors that are associated with low bone mass increase fracture risk and that the age that fracture risk is reached is relatively lower if the lower bone mass is reached earlier.

glucocorticoid-induced bone loss. Other medications that induce low bone mass include anticonvulsants (particularly phenytoin) and cyclosporin A.

Diagnosis of Osteoporosis

Several laboratory tests are available and useful for the evaluation of a subject with osteoporosis and other bone disorders. There are no specific laboratory tests that can be used to diagnose osteoporosis. The vast majority of osteoporotic subjects will have normal biochemical tests. The diagnosis rests on clinical risk factors and dual-energy x-ray absorptiometry (DEXA) scan. In 2008, the WHO created a well-validated fracture assessment tool, which enables clinicians to identify a given individual's 10-year fracture risk based on simple data, even in the absence of DEXA scan results. The hallmark of osteoporosis is skeletal fragility; therefore, it can be diagnosed without any additional testing when a fracture occurs at an inappropriate degree of trauma or following trivial trauma or no trauma at all. This is termed a *fragility* fracture (Fig. 24-8). The occurrence of one fragility fracture predicts further fragility fractures. Currently, osteoporosis is also diagnosed based upon calculated bone density using DEXA of the lumbar spine and the hip. This imaging technique, commonly referred to as bone mineral densitometry, measures grams of calcium per square centimeter of cross-sectional area of bone (g/cm^2). Density is mass/volume, or g/cm^3, so the term bone *density* is a misnomer. Peak bone mass usually occurs at about the age of 30 years for both men and women and is associated with the lowest risk of fracture. The bone "density," as calculated by DEXA, is then compared with that expected in a healthy 30-year-old individual of the

same race and gender. This is reported as SDs above or below the mean peak bone mass using a "T-score." A positive or "+" T-score equates to above the average peak bone mass and negative or "−" is for below the average peak bone mass. Normal bone density is defined as 1 SD from the mean, or a T-score between −1.0 and +1.0. Osteoporosis is defined as a T-score of −2.5 or below. An intermediate between normal and osteoporosis, termed *osteopenia*, is diagnosed as a T-score between −1.0 and −2.5. In summary, osteoporosis is diagnosed by either the occurrence of a fragility fracture or a T-score of −2.5 or below by DEXA imaging.

Treatment of Osteoporosis

Treatment of osteoporosis is directed at prevention of the primary consequence of this disease: fracture. All treatment plans should include modification of preventable risk factors such as smoking and alcohol consumption. They should also include an evaluation of fall risk and consideration of walkers, hand rails, night lights, hip pads, etc. Further, all patients with osteoporosis—or those at high risk for developing osteoporosis—should have adequate dietary calcium (usually 1,200 to 1,500 mg daily) and vitamin D (usually 400 to 800 IU daily). The most commonly used medications for the prevention and treatment of osteoporosis are the antiresorptive agents. Examples of commonly used bisphosphonates include alendronate, risedronate, ibandronate, and zoledronate. The bisphosphonate agents have unusual side effects. They can cause upper GI ulceration if the pill gets retained in the esophagus; therefore, patients are instructed to stay upright after swallowing the pills with water, to prevent retention. Chronic use is associated with osteonecrosis of the jaw and low bone turnover fracture of the thigh bone.[19,20] The most commonly used SERM is raloxifene. Testosterone is commonly used in males with hypogonadism and estrogen ± progestin in women. Teriparatide is an anabolic agent, one which forms bone, rather than blocks resorption, unlike bisphosphonates. It is very effective for the treatment of those with osteoporosis. Teriparatide stimulates the formation of both cortical and trabecular bones without increasing the bone resorption. Furthermore, it can be used sequentially with an antiresorptive drug, which can further potentiate the positive effects on the skeleton. Because it is a peptide hormone, it requires subcutaneous injections. Currently, it is only approved for the treatment of severe osteoporosis, and its use for the treatment of hypoparathyroidism is being evaluated. This agent is used for a period of 2 years. A unique side effect in experimental animals is the formation of bone tumor, which has not been observed in human subjects.

CASE STUDY 24-6

A 74-year-old woman slipped while mopping the kitchen floor, fell, and sustained a hip fracture. The hip fracture was treated with open reduction and internal fixation. After discharge from the hospital, she presents to her physician and asks if she has osteoporosis and, if so, what should be done. She only drinks milk on her cereal and takes no dietary supplements of calcium or vitamin D. She has asthma and has been treated with prednisone bursts and tapers about six times in her life (as best she can recall). She went through menopause at age 49 and never took hormone replacement. Other than her hip, she reports no other fractures in adulthood but does report that she thinks she has lost about 2.5 in. in height. She thinks her mom had osteoporosis, because she had a "dowager's hump." The physician orders bone densitometry, which shows posteroanterior spine T-score −3.8 and hip T-score −3.1 (done on the nonfractured hip!). Labs revealed normal calcium and albumin, renal function, thyroid function, albumin, and CBC. Alkaline phosphatase is slightly elevated, but she has a recent fracture.

Questions

1. What is this patient's diagnosis?

2. Name four or five risk factors for this diagnosis.

3. In addition to adequate calcium and vitamin D supplements, this patient would be a candidate for which new therapeutic drug?

SECONDARY HYPERPARATHYROIDISM IN RENAL FAILURE

The kidney's central role in the regulation of bone and mineral metabolism was discussed earlier. Chronic kidney disease (CKD) results in striking bone mineral and skeletal changes. The diseased kidneys fail to excrete phosphate; this along with the impaired formation of $1,25(OH)_2D$ leads to a vicious cycle of events resulting in parathyroid gland stimulation and hyperplasia. The bone mineral metabolic changes are progressive and proportional to the severity of renal dysfunction and eventually ubiquitous in patients with end-stage renal disease. In severe cases, the ensuing parathyroid hyperplasia results in autonomy of the parathyroid gland leading to hypercalcemia; this is also referred to as tertiary hyperparathyroidism. The difference between secondary and tertiary hyperparathyroidism is the development of sustained hypercalcemia. Patients who develop transient, iatrogenic hypercalcemia encountered in a renal failure patient should not be given the diagnosis of tertiary hyperparathyroidism. The term tertiary is not widely used nowadays. In early stages of CKD, in response to low blood calcium and elevation of phosphate levels, compensatory elevation of PTH and FGF 23 maintains near-normal calcium and phosphorus levels.[21] As kidney disease becomes severe, the compensatory mechanisms are overwhelmed, leading to permanent abnormalities of calcium, phosphorus, PTH, vitamin D, bone mineralization, and vascular and soft tissue calcification. These biochemical changes completely resolve following renal transplantation. Renal replacement therapies such as hemodialysis and peritoneal dialysis only induce partial correction of these changes.

One of the earliest changes in CKD is reduction of urinary phosphorus excretion, leading to an increase in serum phosphorus levels. Compensatory increase in the phosphaturic hormones such as FGF 23 and PTH helps maintain near-normal serum phosphate levels for a period. When renal function declines to lower than 30 mL/min, hyperphosphatemia is observed. Hyperphosphatemia also stimulates PTH secretion and inhibits $1,25(OH)_2D$ production. Low $1,25(OH)_2D$ leads to poor GI absorption of calcium. Hyperphosphatemia and elevation of FGF 23 levels are independent predictors of survival; higher levels are associated with poorer outcomes.[21] Hyperphosphatemia is treated with a combination of dietary restriction of phosphorus and oral phosphate binders. Commonly used phosphate binders include calcium carbonate, calcium acetate, and noncalcium binders including sevelamar and lanthanum. Patients with CKD have low blood calcium levels. The imbalance in calcium and phosphate levels results in extracellular deposition of calcium resulting in vascular and tissue calcification, a condition called calciphylaxis, which results in increased mortality.

Most patients with CKD have low $1,25(OH)_2D$ levels. As phosphorus levels increase, FGF 23 levels increase as a compensatory mechanism, which in turn inhibits 1α-hydroxylation of 25-hydroxy vitamin D. The decreased $1,25(OH)_2D$ leads to impaired calcium absorption and the lower calcium levels stimulate PTH release. This triggers a cascade of bone mineral metabolic events leading to poor bone mineralization.

PTH is secreted in response to hypocalcemia, hyperphosphatemia, and/or low $1,25(OH)_2D$ levels. PTH levels trend up with increasing severity of renal disease. Secondary hyperparathyroidism is treated with vitamin D analogues such as calcitriol, doxercalciferol, and paricalcitol.[22] Calcimimetics are allosteric activators of the extracellular CSR, sensitizing the parathyroid gland to extracellular calcium and decreasing PTH secretion independent of vitamin D. Calcimimetics such as cinacalcet have been shown to decrease PTH, calcium, and phosphorus.[23]

For additional student resources please visit thePoint at http://thepoint.lww.com. **the Point** ✳

QUESTIONS

1. True or false? PTH and $1,25(OH)_2D$ (vitamin D) are the principal hormones involved in the normal physiologic regulation of calcium homeostasis.

2. The primary organs involved in the maintenance of calcium homeostasis are the intestine, _____, and kidney.

3. Skin, _____, and kidneys are involved in the production of the active metabolite of vitamin D.

4. True or false? Cod liver oil (ugh!) is a source of vitamin D.

5. True or false? $1,25(OH)_2D$ is the best blood test for determining adequacy of vitamin D stores in the body.

6. True or false? PTHrP is produced by some cancers and often leads to cancer-associated hypercalcemia.

7. True or false? $1,25(OH)_2D$, due to 1-hydroxylase activity in macrophages, may be produced to excess in granulomatous diseases and lymphoid disorders, leading to hypercalcemia.

8. In PHPT, the defect primarily lies in _____. In secondary hyperparathyroidism, the defect primarily lies with the threat of _____ to the body.

9. Development of _____ _____ is the primary complication of hypercalciuria (increased urinary excretion of calcium).

10. _____ _____ is the most common cause of hypoparathyroidism.

11. _____ is a type of bone most rapidly lost in response to hypogonadism and glucocorticoid therapy.

12. _____ cells in bone are responsible for bone resorption, and _____ cells are responsible for bone formation.

13. _____ is the most prevalent metabolic bone disease in the United States.

14. True or false? Hormone replacement does not inhibit bone resorption in osteoporotic patients.

15. True or false? Teriparatide is the only drug currently approved by the FDA for the treatment of osteoporosis that directly stimulates bone formation (i.e., it is not an antiresorptive drug).

REFERENCES

1. Neer R, Berman M, Fisher L, Rosenberg LE. Multicompartmental analysis of calcium kinetics in normal adult males. *J Clin Invest.* 1967;46:1364-1379.
2. Norman AW, Roth J, Orci L. The vitamin D endocrine system: steroid metabolism, hormone receptors and biological response. *Endocrine Rev.* 1982;3:331-366.
3. Sheikh MD, Ramirez A, Emmett M, et al. Role of vitamin D dependent and vitamin D independent mechanisms in absorption of food calcium. *J Clin Invest.* 1988;81:126-132.
4. Gallagher JC, Riggs BL, Eisman J, et al. Intestinal calcium absorption and serum vitamin D metabolites in normal subjects and osteoporotic patients. *J Clin Invest.* 1979;64:729-736.
5. Owen R. On the anatomy of the Indian Rhinoceros (Rh. Unicornis L.). *Trans Zool Soc Lond.* 1862;4:31-58.
6. Gilmore JR. The gross anatomy of parathyroid glands. *J Pathol.* 1938;46:133.
7. Alveryd A. Parathyroid glands in thyroid surgery. *Acta Chir Scand.* 1968;389:1.
8. Block GA, Klassen PS, Lazarus JM, Ofsthun N, Lowrie EG, Chertow GM. Mineral metabolism, mortality, and morbidity in maintenance hemodialysis. *J Am Soc Nephrol.* 2004;15(8):2208-2218.
9. Sakou T. Bone morphogenic proteins: from basic studies to clinical approaches. *Bone.* 1998;22:591-603.
10. Heath H, Hodgson SR, Kennedy MA. Primary hyperparathyroidism: incidence, morbidity and economic impact in a community. *N Eng J Med.* 1980;302:189-193.

11. Albright E, Reifenstein EC. *The Parathyroid Glands and Metabolic Bone Disease.* Baltimore, MD: Williams and Wilkins; 1948.

12. Abraham D, Sharma PK, Bentz J, Gault PM, Neumayer L, McClain DA. The utility of ultrasound guided FNA of parathyroid adenomas for pre-operative localization prior to minimally invasive parathyroidectomy. *Endocr Pract.* July-August 2007; 13(4):333-337.

13. Brown EM, Gamba G, Rccardi D, et al. Cloning and characterization of an extracellular calcium sensing receptor from bovine parathyroid. *Nature.* 1993;366:575.

14. Hendy GN, D'Souza-Li L, Yang B, et al. Mutations of the calcium-sensing receptor (CASR) in familial hypocalciuric hypercalcemia, neonatal severe hyperparathyroidism, and autosomal dominant hypocalcemia. *Hum Mutat.* 2000;16:281.

15. Stewart AF, Horst F, Deftos LJ, et al. Biochemical evaluation of patients with cancer-associated hypercalcemia: evidence for humoral and non-humoral groups. *N Eng J Med.* 1980;303: 1377-1383.

16. Lips, P, van Schoor, NM, Bravenboer, N. Vitamin D-related disorders. In: Rosen CJ, ed. *Primer on the Metabolic Bone Diseases and Disorders of Mineral Metabolism.* 7th ed. Washington, DC: American Society of Bone and Mineral Research; 2008:329.

17. Holick MF, Binkley NC, Bischoff-Ferrari HA, et al. Evaluation, treatment, and prevention of vitamin D deficiency: an Endocrine Society clinical practice guideline. *J Clin Endocrinol Metab.* 2011;96:1911.

18. Looker AC, Melton LJ 3rd, Harris TB, Borrud LG, Shepherd JA. Prevalence and trends in low femur bone density among older US adults: NHANES 2005-2006 compared with NHANES III. *J Bone Miner Res.* January 2010;25(1):64-71.

19. Watts NB, Diab DL. Long-term use of bisphosphonates in osteoporosis. *J Clin Endocrinol Metab.* 2010;95:1555.

20. Neer RM, Arnaud CD, Zanchetta JR, et al. Effect of parathyroid hormone (1-34) on fractures and bone mineral density in postmenopausal women with osteoporosis. *N Engl J Med.* 2001;344:1434-1441.

21. Gutierrez OM, Mannstadt M, Isakova T, et al. Fibroblast growth factor 23 and mortality among patients undergoing hemodialysis. *N Engl J Med.* 2008;359(6):584-592.

22. Sprague SM, Coyne D. Control of secondary hyperparathyroidism by vitamin D receptor agonists in chronic kidney disease. *Clin J Am Soc Nephrol.* 2010;5(3):512-518.

23. Block GA, Martin KJ, de Francisco AL, et al. Cinacalcet for secondary hyperparathyroidism in patients receiving hemodialysis. *N Engl J Med.* 2004;350(15):1516-1525.

Liver Function

JANELLE M. CHIASERA, XIN XU

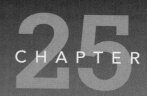

CHAPTER OUTLINE

Chapter Objectives

Upon completion of this chapter, the clinical laboratorian will be able to do the following:

- Diagram the anatomy of the liver.
- Explain the following functions of the liver: bile secretion, synthetic activity, and detoxification.
- List two important cell types associated with the liver and state the function of each.
- Define jaundice and classify the three different types of jaundice.
- Discuss the basic disorders of the liver and which laboratory tests may be performed to diagnose them.
- Evaluate liver-related data and correlate that data with normal or pathology states.
- Compare and contrast how total and direct bilirubin measurements are performed.
- List the enzymes most commonly used to assess hepatocellular and hepatobiliary disorders.
- Describe the various types of hepatitis to include cause, transmission, occurrence, alternate name, physiology, diagnosis, and treatment.

KEY TERMS

Bile
Bilirubin
Cirrhosis
Conjugated bilirubin
Hepatitis
Hepatoma

Icterus
Kupffer cells
Lobule
Posthepatic
Prehepatic
Sinusoids
Urobilinogen

The liver is a very large and complex organ responsible for performing vital tasks that impact all body systems. Its complex functions include metabolism of carbohydrates, lipids, proteins, and bilirubin; detoxification of harmful substances; storage of essential compounds; and excretion of substances to prevent harm. The liver is unique in the sense that it is a relatively resilient organ that can regenerate cells that have been destroyed by some short-term injury or disease or have been removed. However, if the liver is damaged repeatedly over a long period of time, it may undergo irreversible changes that permanently interfere with its essential functions. If the liver becomes completely nonfunctional for any reason, death will occur within approximately 24 hours due to hypoglycemia. This chapter focuses on the normal structure and function of the liver, the pathology associated with it, and the laboratory tests used to aid in the diagnosis of liver disorders.

ANATOMY

Gross Anatomy

Understanding the function and dysfunction of the liver depends on understanding its gross and microscopic structure. The liver is a large and complex organ weighing approximately 1.2 to 1.5 kg in the healthy adult. It is located beneath and attached to the diaphragm, is protected by the lower rib cage, and is held in place by ligamentous attachments. Despite the functional complexity of the liver, it is relatively simple in structure. It is divided unequally into two lobes by the falciform ligament. The right lobe is approximately six times larger than the left lobe. The lobes are functionally insignificant; however, communication flows freely between all areas of the liver (Fig. 25-1).

Unlike most organs, which have a single blood supply, the liver is an extremely vascular organ that receives its blood supply from two sources: the hepatic artery and the portal vein. The hepatic artery, a branch of the aorta, supplies oxygen-rich blood from the heart to the liver and is responsible for providing approximately 25% of the total blood supply to the liver. The portal vein supplies nutrient-rich blood (collected as food is digested) from the digestive tract, and it is responsible for providing approximately 75% of the total blood supply to the liver. The two blood supplies eventually merge into the hepatic sinusoid, which is lined with hepatocytes capable of removing potentially toxic substances from the blood. From the sinusoid, blood flows to the central canal (central vein) of each lobule. It is through the central canal

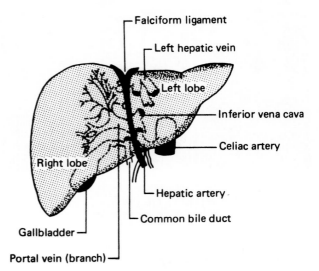

FIGURE 25-2 Blood supply to the liver.

that blood leaves the liver. Approximately 1,500 mL of blood passes through the liver per minute. The liver is drained by a collecting system of veins that empties into the hepatic veins and ultimately into the inferior vena cava (Fig. 25-2).

The excretory system of the liver begins at the bile canaliculi. The bile canaliculi are small spaces between the hepatocytes that form intrahepatic ducts, where excretory products of the cell can drain. The intrahepatic ducts join to form the right and left hepatic ducts, which drain the secretions from the liver. The right and left hepatic ducts merge to form the common hepatic duct, which is eventually joined with the cystic duct of the gallbladder to form the common bile duct. Combined digestive secretions are then expelled into the duodenum (Fig. 25-3).

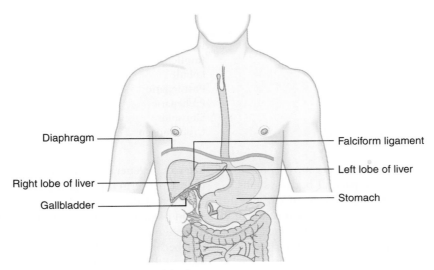

FIGURE 25-1 Gross anatomy of the liver.

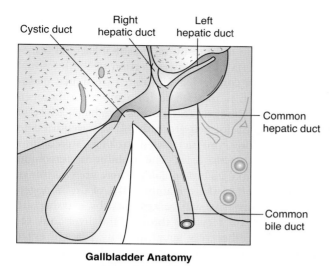

Gallbladder Anatomy

FIGURE 25-3 Excretory system of the liver.

Microscopic Anatomy

The liver is divided into microscopic units called lobules. The lobules are the functional units of the liver; they are responsible for all metabolic and excretory functions performed by the liver. Each lobule is roughly a six-sided structure with a centrally located vein (called the *central vein*) with portal triads at each of the corners. Each portal triad contains a hepatic artery, a portal vein, and a bile duct surrounded by connective tissue. The liver contains two major cell types: hepatocytes and Kupffer cells. The hepatocytes, making up approximately 80% of the volume of the organ, are large cells that radiate outward from the central vein in plates to the periphery of the lobule. These cells perform the major functions

associated with the liver and are responsible for the regenerative properties of the liver. Kupffer cells are macrophages that line the **sinusoids** of the liver and act as active phagocytes capable of engulfing bacteria, debris, toxins, and other substances flowing through the sinusoids (Fig. 25-4).

BIOCHEMICAL FUNCTIONS

The liver performs four major functions: excretion/secretion, metabolism, detoxification, and storage. The liver is so important that if the liver becomes nonfunctional, death will occur within 24 hours due to hypoglycemia. Although the liver is responsible for a number of functions, this chapter focuses on the four major functions mentioned previously.

Excretory and Secretory

One of the most important functions of the liver is the processing and excretion of endogenous and exogenous substances into the bile or urine such as the major heme waste product, bilirubin. The liver is the only organ that has the capacity to rid the body of heme waste products. Bile is made up of bile acids or salts, bile pigments, cholesterol, and other substances extracted from the blood. The body produces approximately 3 L of bile per day and excretes 1 L of what is produced. Bilirubin is the principal pigment in bile, and it is derived from the breakdown of red blood cells. Approximately 126 days after the emergence from the reticuloendothelial tissue, red blood cells are phagocytized and hemoglobin is released. Hemoglobin is degraded to heme, globin, and iron. The iron is bound by transferrin and is returned to iron

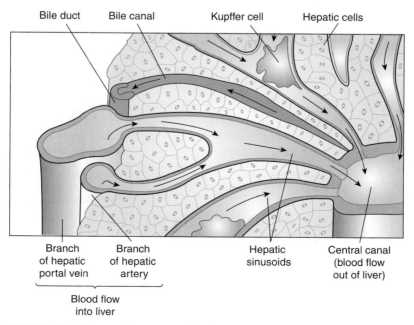

FIGURE 25-4 Microscopic anatomy of the liver.

stores in the liver or bone marrow for reuse. The globin is degraded to its constituent amino acids, which are reused by the body. The heme portion of hemoglobin is converted to bilirubin in 2 to 3 hours. Bilirubin is bound by albumin and transported to the liver. This form of bilirubin is referred to as *unconjugated* or *indirect bilirubin*. This form of bilirubin is insoluble in water and cannot be removed from the body until it has been conjugated by the liver. Once at the liver cell, unconjugated bilirubin flows into the sinusoidal spaces and is released from albumin so it can be picked up by a carrier protein called *ligandin*. Ligandin, which is located in the hepatocyte, is responsible for transporting unconjugated bilirubin to the endoplasmic reticulum, where it may be rapidly conjugated. The conjugation (esterification) of bilirubin occurs in the presence of the enzyme uridyldiphosphate glucuronyl transferase (UDPGT), which transfers a glucuronic acid molecule to each of the two propionic acid side chains of bilirubin to form bilirubin diglucuronide, also known as conjugated bilirubin. This form of bilirubin is water soluble and is able to be secreted from the hepatocyte into the bile canaliculi. Once in the hepatic

duct, it combines with secretions from the gallbladder through the cystic duct and is expelled through the common bile duct to the intestines. Intestinal bacteria (especially the bacteria in the lower portion of the intestinal tract) work on conjugated bilirubin to produce mesobilirubin, which is reduced to form mesobilirubinogen and then urobilinogen (a colorless product). Most of the urobilinogen formed (roughly 80%) is oxidized to an orange-colored product called *urobilin* (stercobilin) and is excreted in the feces. The urobilin or stercobilin is what gives stool its brown color. There are two things that can happen to the remaining 20% of urobilinogen formed. The majority will be absorbed by extrahepatic circulation to be recycled through the liver and re-excreted. The other very small quantity left will enter systemic circulation and will subsequently be filtered by the kidney and excreted in the urine (Fig. 25-5).[1]

Approximately 200 to 300 mg of bilirubin is produced per day, and it takes a normally functioning liver to process the bilirubin and eliminate it from the body. This, as stated earlier, requires that bilirubin be conjugated. Almost all the bilirubin formed is eliminated in

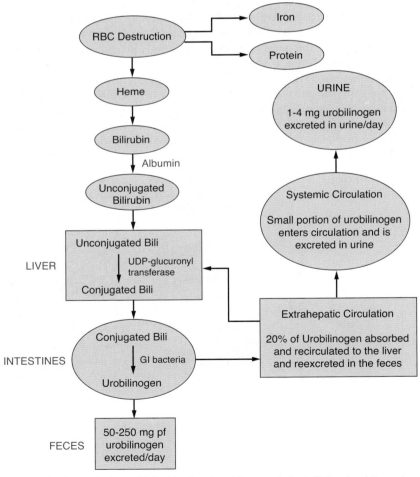

FIGURE 25-5 Metabolism of bilirubin. Reprinted by permission of Waveland Press, Inc. from Anderson SC, Cockayne S. *Clinical Chemistry/Concepts and Applications/2003.* Long Grove, IL: Waveland Press, Inc.; 2007. All rights reserved.

the feces, and a small amount of the colorless product, urobilinogen, is excreted in the urine. The healthy adult has very low levels of total bilirubin (0.2 to 1.0 mg/dL) in the serum, and of this amount, the majority is in the unconjugated form.[2]

Metabolism

The liver has extensive metabolic capacity; it is responsible for metabolizing many biological compounds including carbohydrates, lipids, and proteins.

The metabolism of carbohydrates is one of the most important functions of the liver. When carbohydrates are ingested and absorbed, the liver can do three things: (1) use the glucose for its own cellular energy requirements, (2) circulate the glucose for use at the peripheral tissues, or (3) store glucose as glycogen (principal storage form of glucose) within the liver itself or within other tissues. The liver is the major player in maintaining stable glucose concentrations due to its ability to store glucose as glycogen (glycogenesis) and degrade glycogen (glycogenolysis) depending on the body's needs. Under conditions of stress or in a fasting state when there is an increased requirement for glucose, the liver will break down stored glycogen (glycogenolysis) and when the supply of glycogen becomes depleted, the liver will create glucose from nonsugar carbon substrates like pyruvate, lactate, and amino acids (*gluconeogenesis*).

Lipids are metabolized in the liver under normal circumstances when nutrition is adequate and the demand for glucose is being met. The liver is responsible for metabolizing both lipids and the lipoproteins and is responsible for gathering free fatty acids from the diet, and those produced by the liver itself, and breaking them down to produce acetyl-CoA. Acetyl-CoA can then enter several pathways to form triglycerides, phospholipids, or cholesterol. Despite popular belief, the greatest source of cholesterol in the body comes from what is produced by the liver, not from dietary sources. In fact, approximately 70% of the daily production of cholesterol (roughly 1.5 to 2.0 g) is produced by the liver.[3] A more thorough discussion of lipid metabolism may be found in Chapter 15.

Almost all proteins are synthesized by the liver except for the immunoglobulins and adult hemoglobin. The liver plays an essential role in the development of hemoglobin in infants. One of the most important proteins synthesized by the liver is albumin, which carries with it a wide range of important functions. The liver is also responsible for synthesizing the positive and negative acute-phase reactants and coagulation proteins, and it also serves to store a pool of amino acids through protein degradation. The most critical aspect of protein metabolism includes transamination and deamination of amino acids. Transamination (via a transaminase) results in the exchange of an amino group on one acid with a ketone group on another acid. After transamination, deamination degrades them to produce ammonium ions that are

CASE STUDY 25-1

The following laboratory test results were obtained in a patient with severe jaundice, right upper quadrant abdominal pain, fever, and chills (Case Study Table 25-1.1).

Questions

1. What is the most likely cause of jaundice in the patient?

CASE STUDY TABLE 25-1.1
LABORATORY RESULTS

Serum alkaline phosphatase	Four times normal
Serum cholesterol	Increased
AST (SGOT)	Normal or slightly increased
5′-Nucleotidase	Increased
Total serum bilirubin	25 mg/dL
Conjugated bilirubin	19 mg/dL
Prothrombin time	Prolonged but improves with a vitamin K injection

consumed in the synthesis of urea and urea is excreted by the kidneys.

Although it would seem logical that any damage to the liver would result in a loss of synthetic and metabolic functions of the liver, that is not the case. The liver must be extensively impaired before it loses its ability to perform these essential functions.

Detoxification and Drug Metabolism

The liver serves as a gatekeeper between substances absorbed by the gastrointestinal tract and those released into systemic circulation. Every substance that is absorbed in the gastrointestinal tract must first pass through the liver; this is referred to as *first pass*. This is an important function of the liver because it can allow important substances to reach the systemic circulation and can serve as a barrier to prevent toxic or harmful substances from reaching systemic circulation. The body has two mechanisms for detoxification of foreign materials (drugs and poisons) and metabolic products (bilirubin and ammonia). It may either bind the material reversibly so as to inactivate the compound or it may chemically modify the compound so it can be excreted. The most important mechanism is the drug-metabolizing system of the liver. This system is responsible for the detoxification of many drugs through oxidation, reduction, hydrolysis, hydroxylation, carboxylation, and demethylation. Many of these take place in the liver microsomes via the cytochrome P-450 isoenzymes.

LIVER FUNCTION ALTERATIONS DURING DISEASE

Jaundice

The word *jaundice* comes from the French word *jaune*, which means "yellow," and it is one of the oldest known pathologic conditions reported, having been described by Hippocratic physicians.[4] Jaundice, or icterus, is used to describe the yellow discoloration of the skin, eyes, and mucous membranes most often resulting from the retention of bilirubin; however, it may also occur due to the retention of other substances. Although the upper limit of normal for total bilirubin is 1.0 to 1.5 mg/dL, jaundice is usually not noticeable to the naked eye (known as *overt jaundice*) until bilirubin levels reach 3.0 to 5.0 mg/dL. Although the terms *jaundice* and *icterus* are used interchangeably, the term *icterus* is most commonly used in the clinical laboratory to refer to a serum or plasma sample with a yellow discoloration due to an elevated bilirubin level. Jaundice is most commonly classified based on the site of the disorder: prehepatic, hepatic, and posthepatic jaundice. This classification is important because knowing the classification of jaundice will aid health-care providers in formulating an appropriate treatment or management plan. *Prehepatic* and *posthepatic jaundice*, as the names imply, are caused by abnormalities outside the liver, either before, as in "prehepatic," or after, as in "posthepatic." In these conditions, liver function is normal or it may be functioning at a maximum to compensate for abnormalities occurring elsewhere. This is not the case with hepatic jaundice, where the jaundice is due to a problem with the liver itself—an intrinsic liver defect or disease.

Prehepatic jaundice occurs when the problem causing the jaundice occurs prior to liver metabolism. It is most commonly caused by an increased amount of bilirubin being presented to the liver such as that seen in acute and chronic hemolytic anemias. Hemolytic anemia causes an increased amount of red blood cell destruction and the subsequent release of increased amounts of bilirubin presented to the liver for processing. The liver responds by functioning at maximum capacity; therefore, people with prehepatic jaundice rarely have bilirubin levels that exceed 5.0 mg/dL because the liver is capable of handling the overload. This type of jaundice may also be referred to as *unconjugated hyperbilirubinemia* because the fraction of bilirubin increased in people with prehepatic jaundice is the unconjugated fraction. This fraction of bilirubin (unconjugated bilirubin) is not water soluble, is bound to albumin, is not filtered by the kidneys, and is not seen in the urine.

Hepatic jaundice occurs when the primary problem causing the jaundice resides in the liver (intrinsic liver defect or disease). This intrinsic liver defect or disease can be due to disorders of bilirubin metabolism and transport defects (Crigler-Najjar syndrome, Dubin-Johnson syndrome, Gilbert's disease, and neonatal physiologic

jaundice of the newborn) or due to diseases resulting in hepatocellular injury or destruction. Gilbert's disease, Crigler-Najjar syndrome, and physiologic jaundice of the newborn are hepatic causes of jaundice that result in elevations in unconjugated bilirubin. Conditions such as Dubin-Johnson and Rotor syndrome are hepatic causes of jaundice that result in elevations in conjugated bilirubin.

Gilbert's syndrome, first described in the early twentieth century, is a benign autosomal recessive hereditary disorder that affects approximately 5% of the U.S. population.[5] Gilbert's syndrome results from a genetic mutation in the gene (UGT1A1) that produces UDPGT, one of the enzymes important for bilirubin metabolism. The UGT1A1 gene is located on chromosome 2, and other mutations of this same gene produce Crigler-Najjar syndrome, a more severe and dangerous form of hyperbilirubinemia.[6]

Of the many causes of jaundice, Gilbert's syndrome is the most common cause, and interestingly, it carries no morbidity or mortality in the majority of those affected and carries generally no clinical consequences. It is characterized by intermittent unconjugated hyperbilirubinemia, underlying liver disease due to a defective conjugation system in the absence of hemolysis. The hyperbilirubinemia usually manifests during adolescence or early adulthood. Total serum bilirubin usually fluctuates between 1.5 and 3.0 mg/dL, and it rarely exceeds 4.5 mg/dL. The molecular basis of Gilbert's syndrome (in whites) is related to the UDPGT superfamily, which is responsible for encoding enzymes that catalyze the conjugation of bilirubin. The UGT1A1 (the hepatic 1A1 isoform of UDPGT) contributes substantially to the process of conjugating bilirubin. The UGT1A1 promoter contains the sequence (TA)6TAA. The insertion of an extra TA in the sequence, as seen in Gilbert's syndrome, reduces the expression of the *UGT1A1* gene to 20% to 30% of normal values. That is, the liver's conjugation system in Gilbert's syndrome is working at approximately 30% of normal.[7,8]

Crigler-Najjar syndrome was first described by Crigler and Najjar in 1952 as a syndrome of chronic nonhemolytic unconjugated hyperbilirubinemia.[9] Crigler-Najjar syndrome, like Gilbert's syndrome, is an inherited disorder of bilirubin metabolism resulting from a molecular defect within the gene involved with bilirubin conjugation. Crigler-Najjar syndrome may be divided into two types: type 1, where there is a complete absence of enzymatic bilirubin conjugation, and type II, where there is a mutation causing a severe deficiency of the enzyme responsible for bilirubin conjugation. Unlike Gilbert's syndrome, Crigler-Najjar syndrome is rare and is a more serious disorder that may result in death.[10]

While Gilbert's disease and Crigler-Najjar syndrome are characterized as primarily unconjugated hyperbilirubinemias, Dubin-Johnson syndrome and Rotor syndrome are characterized as conjugated hyperbilirubinemias. Dubin-Johnson syndrome is a rare autosomal recessive inherited disorder caused by a deficiency of the canalicular multidrug resistance/multispecific organic anionic transporter protein (MDR2/cMOAT). In other words, the liver's ability to uptake and conjugate bilirubin is functional; however, the removal of conjugated bilirubin from the liver cell and the excretion into the bile are defective. This results in accumulation of conjugated and, to some extent, unconjugated bilirubin in the blood, leading to hyperbilirubinemia and bilirubinuria. Dubin-Johnson is a condition that is obstructive in nature, so much of the conjugated bilirubin circulates bound to albumin. This type of bilirubin (conjugated bilirubin bound to albumin) is referred to as *delta bilirubin*. An increase in delta bilirubin poses a problem in laboratory evaluation because the delta bilirubin fraction reacts as conjugated bilirubin in the laboratory method to measure conjugated or direct bilirubin. A distinguishing feature of Dubin-Johnson syndrome is the appearance of dark-stained granules (thought to be pigmented lysosomes) on a liver biopsy sample. Usually, the total bilirubin concentration remains between 2 and 5 mg/dL, with more than 50% due to the conjugated fraction. This syndrome is relatively mild in nature with an excellent prognosis. People with Dubin-Johnson syndrome have a normal life expectancy, so no treatment is necessary.[11,12]

Rotor syndrome is clinically similar to Dubin-Johnson syndrome but the defect causing Rotor syndrome is not known.[13] It is hypothesized to be due to a reduction in the concentration or activity of intracellular binding proteins such as ligandin. Unlike in Dubin-Johnson syndrome, a liver biopsy does not show dark pigmented granules. Rotor syndrome is seen less commonly than Dubin-Johnson syndrome; it is a relatively benign condition and carries an excellent prognosis, and therefore treatment is not warranted. However, an accurate diagnosis is required to aid in distinguishing it from more serious liver diseases that require treatment.

Physiologic jaundice of the newborn is a result of a deficiency in the enzyme glucuronyl transferase, one of the last liver functions to be activated in prenatal life since bilirubin processing is handled by the mother of the fetus. Premature infants may be born without glucuronyl transferase, the enzyme responsible for bilirubin conjugation. This deficiency results in the rapid buildup of unconjugated bilirubin, which can be life threatening. When this type of bilirubin builds up in the neonate, it cannot be processed and it is deposited in the nuclei of brain and degenerate nerve cells, causing kernicterus. Kernicterus often results in cell damage and death in the newborn, and this condition will continue until glucuronyl transferase is produced. Infants with this type of jaundice are usually treated with ultraviolet radiation to destroy the bilirubin as it passes through the capillaries of the skin. In extreme cases, some infants require an exchange transfusion. Because this condition is so serious, bilirubin levels are carefully and frequently monitored so the dangerously high levels of unconjugated bilirubin (approximately 20 mg/dL) can be detected and treated.[14]

Posthepatic jaundice results from biliary obstructive disease, usually from physical obstructions (gallstones or tumors) that prevent the flow of conjugated bilirubin into the bile canaliculi. Since the liver cell itself is functioning, bilirubin is effectively conjugated; however, it is unable to be properly excreted from the liver. Since bile is not being brought to the intestines, stool loses its source of normal pigmentation and becomes clay-colored. The laboratory findings for bilirubin and its metabolites in the above-mentioned types of jaundice are summarized in Table 25-1. Mechanisms of hyperbilirubinemia may be found in Figure 25-6.

TABLE 25-1	CHANGES IN CONCENTRATION OF BILIRUBIN IN THOSE WITH JAUNDICE		
	SERUM		
TYPE OF JAUNDICE	**TOTAL BILIRUBIN**	**CONJUGATED BILIRUBIN**	**UNCONJUGATED BILIRUBIN**
Prehepatic	↑	↔	↑
Hepatic			
• Gilbert's disease	↑	↔	↑
• Crigler-Najjar syndrome	↑	↓	↑
• Dubin-Johnson	↑	↑	↔
• Rotor syndrome	↑	↑	↔
• Jaundice of newborn	↑	↔	↑
Posthepatic	↑	↑	↑

Adapted from Table 27-3 of Kaplan LA, Pesce AJ, Kazmierczak S. *Clinical Chemistry: Theory, Analysis, Correlation.* 4th ed. St. Louis, MO: Mosby; 2003.

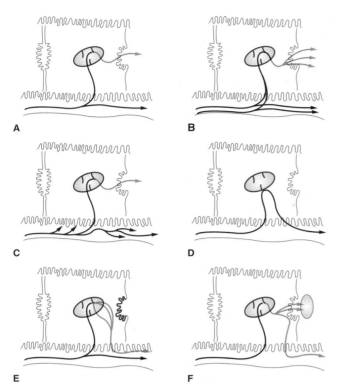

FIGURE 25-6 Mechanisms of hyperbilirubinemia. (A) Normal bilirubin metabolism, (B) hemolytic jaundice, (C) Gilbert's disease, (D) physiologic jaundice, (E) Dubin-Johnson syndrome, and (F) intrahepatic or extrahepatic obstruction. (Adapted from Kaplan LA, Pesce AJ, Kazmierczak S. *Clinical Chemistry: Theory, Analysis, Correlation.* 4th ed. St. Louis, MO: Mosby; 2003:449.)

Cirrhosis

Cirrhosis is a clinical condition in which scar tissue replaces normal, healthy liver tissue. As the scar tissue replaces the normal liver tissue, it blocks the flow of blood through the organ and prevents the liver from functioning properly. Cirrhosis rarely causes signs and symptoms in its early stages, but as liver function deteriorates, the signs and symptoms appear, including fatigue, nausea, unintended weight loss, jaundice, bleeding from the gastrointestinal tract, intense itching, and swelling in the legs and abdomen. Although some patients with cirrhosis may have prolonged survival, they generally have a poor prognosis. Cirrhosis was the twelfth leading cause of death by disease in 2010, killing just over 31,000 people.[15] In the United States, the most common cause of cirrhosis is chronic alcoholism. Other causes of cirrhosis include chronic hepatitis B (HBV), C (HCV), and D virus (HDV) infection, autoimmune hepatitis, inherited disorders (e.g., α1-antitrypsin deficiency, Wilson disease, hemochromatosis, and galactosemia), nonalcoholic steatohepatitis, blocked bile ducts, drugs, toxins, and infections.

Liver damage from cirrhosis cannot easily be reversed, but treatment can stop or delay further progression of the disorder. Treatment depends on the cause of cirrhosis and any complications a person is experiencing. For example, cirrhosis caused by alcohol abuse is treated by abstaining from alcohol. Treatment for hepatitis-related cirrhosis involves medications used to treat the different types of hepatitis, such as interferon for viral hepatitis and corticosteroids for autoimmune hepatitis.

Tumors

Cancers of the liver are classified as primary or metastatic. Primary liver cancer is cancer that begins in the liver cells while metastatic cancer occurs when tumors from other parts of the body spread (metastasize) to the liver. Metastatic liver cancer is much more common than primary liver cancer; 90% to 95% of all hepatic malignancies are classified as metastatic. Cancers that commonly spread to the liver include colon, lung, and breast cancer. Tumors of the liver may also be classified as benign or malignant. The common benign tumors of the liver include hepatocellular adenoma (a condition occurring almost exclusively in females of child-bearing age) and hemangiomas (masses of blood vessels with no known etiology). Malignant tumors of the liver include hepatocellular carcinoma (HCC) (also known as hepatocarcinoma, and hepatoma) and bile duct carcinoma. Of those, HCC is the most common malignant tumor of the liver. Hepatoblastoma is an uncommon hepatic malignancy of children.

HCC has become increasingly important in the United States. Approximately 85% of the new cases of this liver cancer occur in developing countries, with the highest incidence of HCC reported in regions where HBV is endemic such as Southeast Asia and sub-Saharan Africa. Approximately 500,000 people are diagnosed annually with HCC worldwide, of which 28,000 new cases and 20,000 deaths were reported in the United States in 2012.[16,17] It is estimated that in the United States, chronic HBV and HCV infections account for approximately 30% and 40% of cases of HCC.[18]

Approximately 80% of cases worldwide are attributable to HBV and HCV; however, the mechanism by which the infection leads to HCC is not well established. While surgical resection of HCC is sometimes possible, currently, orthotopic liver transplantation in people with HCC with underlying cirrhosis who meet the Milan criteria (single tumor ≤5 cm in size or ≤3 tumors each ≤3 cm in size, and no macrovascular invasion) is also available for HCC. The estimated 4-year survival rate is 85% and the recurrence-free survival rate is 92%.[19]

Whether primary or metastatic, any malignant tumor in the liver is a serious finding and carries a poor prognosis, with survival times measured in months.

Reye Syndrome

Reye syndrome is a term used to describe a group of disorders caused by infectious, metabolic, toxic, or drug-induced disease found almost exclusively in children, although adult cases of Reye syndrome have been reported.[20] Although the precise cause of Reye syndrome is unknown, it is often preceded by a viral syndrome such as varicella, gastroenteritis, or an upper respiratory tract infection such as influenza.[21-23] Although not described as the precise cause of Reye syndrome, studies have demonstrated a strong epidemiologic association between the ingestion of aspirin during a viral syndrome and the subsequent development of Reye syndrome.[24,25] As a result, the Centers for Disease Control and Prevention (CDC) cautioned physicians and parents to avoid salicylate use in children with a viral syndrome, and the U.S. Surgeon General mandated that a warning label be added to all aspirin-containing medications, beginning in 1986.[26,27] Reye syndrome is an acute illness characterized by noninflammatory encephalopathy and fatty degeneration of the liver, with a clinical presentation of profuse vomiting accompanied with varying degrees of neurologic impairment such as fluctuating personality changes and deterioration in consciousness. The encephalopathy is characterized by a progression from mild confusion (stage 1) through progressive loss of neurologic function to loss of brain stem reflexes (stage 5). The degeneration of the liver is characterized by a mild hyperbilirubinemia and threefold increases in ammonia and the aminotransferases (aspartate aminotransferase [AST] and alanine aminotransferase [ALT]). Without treatment, rapid clinical deterioration leading to death may occur.[28,29]

Drug- and Alcohol-Related Disorders

Drug-induced liver disease is a major problem in the United States, accounting for one-third to one-half of all reported cases of acute liver failure. The liver is a primary target organ for adverse drug reactions because it plays a central role in drug metabolism. Many drugs are known to cause liver damage, ranging from very mild transient forms to fulminant liver failure. Drugs can cause liver injury by a variety of mechanisms, but the most common mechanism of toxicity is via an immune-mediated injury to the hepatocytes.[30] In this type of mechanism, the drug induces an adverse immune response directed against the liver itself and results in hepatic and/or cholestatic disease.[31]

Of all the drugs associated with hepatic toxicity, the most important is ethanol. In very small amounts, ethanol causes very mild, transient, and unnoticed injury to the liver; however, with heavier and prolonged consumption, it can lead to alcoholic cirrhosis. While the exact amount of alcohol needed to cause cirrhosis is unknown, a small minority of people with alcoholism develop this condition.[32] Approximately 90% of the alcohol absorbed from the stomach and small intestines is transported to the liver for metabolism. Within the liver, the elimination of alcohol requires the enzymes alcohol dehydrogenase and acetaldehyde dehydrogenase to convert alcohol to acetaldehyde and subsequently to acetate. The acetate can then be oxidized to water and carbon dioxide, or it may enter the citric acid cycle.

Long-term excessive consumption of alcohol can result in a spectrum of liver abnormalities that may range from alcoholic fatty liver with inflammation (steatohepatitis) to scar tissue formation, as in hepatic fibrosis, to the destruction of normal liver structure seen in hepatic cirrhosis. Alcohol-induced liver injury may be categorized into three stages: alcoholic fatty liver, alcoholic hepatitis, and alcoholic cirrhosis. The risk for the development of cirrhosis increases proportionally with the consumption of more than 30 g (the equivalent of 3 to 4 drinks) of alcohol per day, with the highest degree of risk seen with the consumption of greater than 120 g (the equivalent of 12 to 16 drinks) per day.[33]

Alcoholic fatty liver represents the mildest category where very few changes in liver function are measurable. This stage is characterized by slight elevations in AST, ALT, and γ-glutamyltransferase (GGT), and on biopsy, fatty infiltrates are noted in the vacuoles of the liver. This stage tends to affect young to middle-aged people with a history of moderate alcohol consumption. A complete recovery within 1 month is seen when the drug is removed. Alcoholic hepatitis presents with common signs and symptoms including fever, ascites, proximal muscle loss, and far more laboratory evidence of liver damage such as moderately elevated AST, ALT, GGT, and alkaline phosphatase (ALP) and elevations in total bilirubin greater than 5 mg/dL. The elevations in AST are more than twice the upper reference of normal but rarely exceed 300 IU/mL. The elevations in ALT are comparatively lower than AST, resulting in an AST/ALT ratio (De Ritis ratio) greater than 2. Serum proteins, especially albumin, are decreased and the international normalized ratio (INR, which is a ratio of coagulation time in the patient compared with a normal coagulation time) is elevated. Prognosis is dependent on the type and severity of damage to the liver and when serum creatinine levels begin to increase, it is a threatening sign which may precede the onset of hepatorenal syndrome and death.[34] There are a variety of scoring systems that have been used to assess the severity of alcoholic hepatitis and to guide treatment including the Maddrey's discriminant function,[35] the Glasgow score,[36] and the Model for End-Stage Liver Disease (MELD) score.[37] All three scoring systems use bilirubin, INR, creatinine, age, white cell counts, blood urea nitrogen, and albumin levels to stage and guide treatment. The last and most severe stage is alcoholic cirrhosis. The prognosis associated with alcoholic cirrhosis is dependent on the nature and severity of associated conditions such as a gastrointestinal bleeding or ascites; however, the 5-year survival rate is 60% in those who abstain from alcohol and 30% in those who continue to drink. This condition appears to be more common in males than in females, and the symptoms tend to be nonspecific and include weight loss, weakness, hepatomegaly, splenomegaly, jaundice, ascites, fever, malnutrition, and edema. Laboratory abnormalities include increased liver function tests (AST, ALT, GGT, ALP, and total bilirubin), decreased albumin, and a prolonged prothrombin time. A liver biopsy is the only method by which a definitive diagnosis may be made.[38]

Other drugs, including tranquilizers, some antibiotics, antineoplastic agents, lipid-lowering medication, and anti-inflammatory drugs, may cause liver injury ranging from mild damage to massive hepatic failure and cirrhosis. One of the most common drugs associated with serious hepatic injury is acetaminophen. When acetaminophen is taken in massive doses, it is virtually certain to produce fatal hepatic necrosis unless rapid treatment is initiated.

CASE STUDY 25-2

The following laboratory test results were found in a patient with mild weight loss and nausea and vomiting, who later developed jaundice and an enlarged liver (Case Study Table 25-2.1)

Questions

1. What disease process is most likely in this patient?

CASE STUDY TABLE 25-2.1
LABORATORY RESULTS

Total serum bilirubin	20 mg/dL
Conjugated bilirubin	10 mg/dL
Alkaline phosphatase	Mildly elevated
AST (SGOT)	Significantly elevated
ALT (SGPT)	Moderately elevated
Albumin	Decreased
γ-Globulin	Increased

ASSESSMENT OF LIVER FUNCTION/LIVER FUNCTION TESTS

Bilirubin

Analysis of Bilirubin: A Brief Review
The reaction of bilirubin with a diazotized sulfanilic acid solution to form a colored product was first described by Ehrlich in 1883 using urine samples. Since then, this type of reaction (bilirubin with a diazotized sulfanilic acid solution) has been referred to as the classic *diazo reaction*, a reaction on which all commonly used methods today are based. In 1913, van den Bergh found that the diazo reaction may be applied to serum samples but only in the presence of an accelerator (solubilizer). However, this methodology had errors associated with it. It was not until 1937 that Malloy and Evelyn developed the first clinically useful methodology for the quantitation of bilirubin in serum samples using the classic diazo reaction with a 50% methanol solution as an accelerator. In 1938, Jendrassik and Grof described a method using the diazo reaction with caffeine-benzoate-acetate as an accelerator. Today, all commonly used methods for measuring bilirubin and its fractions are modifications of the technique described by Malloy and Evelyn. Total bilirubin and conjugated bilirubin (direct bilirubin) are measured and unconjugated bilirubin (indirect bilirubin) is determined by subtracting conjugated bilirubin from total bilirubin (refer Fig. 25-7).

Bilirubin has also been quantified using bilirubinometry in the neonatal population. This methodology is only useful in the neonatal population because of the presence of carotenoid compounds in adult serum that causes strong positive interference in the adult population. Bilirubinometry involves the measurement of reflected light from the skin using two wavelengths that provide a numerical index based on spectral reflectance. Newer-generation bilirubinometers use microspectrophotometers that determine the optical densities of bilirubin, hemoglobin, and melanin in the subcutaneous layers of the infant's skin. Mathematical isolation of hemoglobin and melanin allows measurement of the optical density created by bilirubin.[39]

When using the several methods described earlier, two of the three fractions of bilirubin were identified: conjugated (direct) and unconjugated (indirect) bilirubin. Unconjugated (indirect) bilirubin is a nonpolar and water-insoluble substance that is found in plasma bound to albumin. Because of these characteristics, unconjugated

Bilirubin + diazotized sulfanilic acid + accelerator ⟶ 2 azobilirubin (Total bilirubin)

Bilirubin + diazotized sulfanilic acid ⟶ 2 azobilirubin (Conjugated bilirubin)

Total bilirubin − Conjugated bilirubin = Unconjugated bilirubin (Indirect bilirubin)

FIGURE 25-7 Methods to measure different fractions of bilirubin.

bilirubin will only react with the diazotized sulfanilic acid solution (diazo reagent) in the presence of an accelerator (solubilizer). Conjugated (direct) bilirubin is a polar and water-soluble compound that is found in plasma in the free state (not bound to any protein). This type of bilirubin will react with the diazotized sulfanilic acid solution directly (without an accelerator). Thus, conjugated and unconjugated bilirubin fractions have historically been differentiated by solubility of the fractions. Conjugated bilirubin reacts in the absence of an accelerator, whereas unconjugated bilirubin requires an accelerator. While for many years bilirubin results were reported as direct and indirect, this terminology is now outdated. Direct and indirect bilirubin results should be reported as conjugated and unconjugated, respectively.[40]

The third fraction of bilirubin is referred to as "delta" bilirubin. Delta bilirubin is conjugated bilirubin that is covalently bound to albumin. This fraction of bilirubin is seen only when there is significant hepatic obstruction. Because the molecule is attached to albumin, it is too large to be filtered by the glomerulus and excreted in the urine. This fraction of bilirubin, when present, will react in most laboratory methods as conjugated bilirubin. Thus, total bilirubin is made up of three fractions: conjugated, unconjugated, and delta bilirubin. The three fractions together are known as *total bilirubin*.

Specimen Collection and Storage

Total bilirubin methods using a diazotized sulfanilic acid solution may be performed on either serum or plasma. Serum, however, is preferred for the Malloy-Evelyn procedure because the addition of the alcohol in the analysis can precipitate proteins and cause interference with the method. A fasting sample is preferred as the presence of lipemia will increase measured bilirubin concentrations. Hemolyzed samples should be avoided as they may decrease the reaction of bilirubin with the diazo reagent. Bilirubin is very sensitive to and is destroyed by light; therefore, specimens should be protected from light. If left unprotected from light, bilirubin values may reduce by 30% to 50% per hour. If serum or plasma is separated from the cells and stored in the dark, it is stable for 2 days at room temperature, 1 week at 4°C, and indefinitely at −20°C.[41]

Methods

There is no preferred reference method or standardization of bilirubin analysis; however, the American Association for Clinical Chemistry and the National Bureau of Standards have published a candidate reference method for total bilirubin, a modified Jendrassik-Grof procedure using caffeine-benzoate as a solubilizer.[42] Because they both have acceptable precision and are adapted to many automated instruments, the Jendrassik-Grof or Malloy-Evelyn procedure is the most frequently used method

to measure bilirubin. The Jendrassik-Grof method is slightly more complex, but it has the following advantages over the Malloy-Evelyn method:

- Not affected by pH changes
- Insensitive to a 50-fold variation in protein concentration of the sample
- Maintains optical sensitivity even at low bilirubin concentrations
- Has minimal turbidity and a relatively constant serum blank
- Is not affected by hemoglobin up to 750 mg/dL

Because this chapter does not allow for a detailed description of all previously mentioned bilirubin test methodologies, only the most widely used principles for measuring bilirubin in the adult and pediatric population are covered.[43-45]

Malloy-Evelyn Procedure

Bilirubin pigments in serum or plasma are reacted with a diazo reagent. The diazotized sulfanilic acid reacts at the central methylene carbon of bilirubin to split the molecule forming two molecules of azobilirubin. This method is typically performed at pH 1.2 where the azobilirubin produced is red-purple in color with a maximal absorption of 560 nm. The most commonly used accelerator to solubilize unconjugated bilirubin is methanol, although other chemicals have been used.[46]

Jendrassik-Grof Method for Total and Conjugated Bilirubin Determination

Principle

Bilirubin pigments in serum or plasma are reacted with a diazo reagent (sulfanilic acid in hydrochloric acid and sodium nitrite), resulting in the production of the purple product azobilirubin. The product azobilirubin may be measured spectrophotometrically. The individual fractions of bilirubin are determined by taking two aliquots of sample and reacting one aliquot with the diazo reagent only and the other aliquot with the diazo reagent and an accelerator (caffeine-benzoate). The addition of caffeine-benzoate will solubilize the water-insoluble fraction of bilirubin and will yield a total bilirubin value (all fractions). The reaction without the accelerator will yield conjugated bilirubin only. After a short period of time, the reaction of the aliquots with the diazo reagent is terminated by the addition of ascorbic acid. The ascorbic acid destroys the excess diazo reagent. The solution is then alkalinized using an alkaline tartrate solution, which shifts the absorbance spectrum of the azobilirubin to a more intense blue color that is less subject to interfering substances in the sample. The final blue product is measured at 600 nm, with the intensity of color produced directly proportional to bilirubin concentration. Indirect (unconjugated) bilirubin may be calculated by subtracting the conjugated bilirubin concentration from the total bilirubin concentration.

Comments and Sources of Error
Instruments should be frequently standardized to maintain reliable bilirubin results, and careful preparation of bilirubin standards is critical as these are subject to deterioration from exposure to light. Hemolysis and lipemia should be avoided as they will alter bilirubin concentrations. Serious loss of bilirubin occurs after exposure to fluorescent and indirect and direct sunlight; therefore, it is imperative that exposure of samples and standards to light be kept to a minimum. Specimens and standards should be refrigerated in the dark until testing can be performed.

Reference Range
See Table 25-2.

Urobilinogen in Urine and Feces

Urobilinogen is a colorless end product of bilirubin metabolism that is oxidized by intestinal bacteria to the brown pigment urobilin. In the normal individual, part of the urobilinogen is excreted in feces, and the remainder is reabsorbed into the portal blood and returned to the liver. A small portion that is not taken up by the hepatocytes is excreted by the kidney as urobilinogen. Increased levels of urinary urobilinogen are found in hemolytic disease and in defective liver cell function, such as that seen in hepatitis. Absence of urobilinogen from the urine and stool is most often seen with complete biliary obstruction. Fecal urobilinogen is also decreased in biliary obstruction, as well as in HCC.[47]

Most quantitative methods for urobilinogen are based on a reaction first described by Ehrlich in 1901: the reaction of urobilinogen with *p*-dimethylaminobenzaldehyde (Ehrlich's reagent) to form a red color. Many modifications of this procedure have been made over the years to improve specificity. However, because the modifications did not completely recover urobilinogen from the urine, most laboratories use the less laborious, more rapid, semiquantitative method described next.

Determination of Urine Urobilinogen (Semiquantitative)

Principle
Urobilinogen reacts with *p*-dimethylaminobenzaldehyde (Ehrlich's reagent) to form a red color, which is then measured spectrophotometrically. Ascorbic acid is added as a reducing agent to maintain urobilinogen in the reduced state. The use of saturated sodium acetate stops the reaction and minimizes the combination of other chromogens with the Ehrlich's reagent.[48]

Specimen
A *fresh* 2-hour urine specimen is collected. This specimen should be kept cool and protected from light.

Comments and Sources of Error

1. The results of this test are reported in Ehrlich units rather than in milligrams of urobilinogen because substances other than urobilinogen account for some of the final color development.
2. Compounds, other than urobilinogen, that may be present in the urine and react with Ehrlich's reagent include porphobilinogen, sulfonamides, procaine, and 5-hydroxyindoleacetic acid. Bilirubin will form a green color and, therefore, must be removed, as previously described.
3. Fresh urine is necessary, and the test must be performed without delay to prevent oxidation of urobilinogen to urobilin. Similarly, the spectrophotometric readings should be made within 5 minutes after color production because the urobilinogen-aldehyde color slowly decreases in intensity.

TABLE 25-2	REFERENCE RANGES FOR BILIRUBIN IN ADULTS AND INFANTS	
POPULATION	**TYPE OF BILIRUBIN**	**REFERENCE RANGE**
Adults	Conjugated bilirubin	0.0–0.2 mg/dL (0–3 µmol/L)
	Unconjugated bilirubin	0.2–0.8 mg/dL (3–14 µmol/L)
	Total bilirubin	0.2–1.0 mg/dL (3–17 µmol/L)
Premature infants	Total bilirubin at 24 h	1–6 mg/dL (17–103 µmol/L)
	Total bilirubin at 48 h	6–8 mg/dL (103–137 µmol/L)
	Total bilirubin 3–5 d	10–12 mg/dL (171–205 µmol/L)
Full-term infants	Total bilirubin at 24 h	2–6 mg/dL (34–103 µmol/L)
	Total bilirubin at 48 h	6–7 mg/dL (103–120 µmol/L)
	Total bilirubin 3–5 d	4–6 mg/dL (68–103 µmol/L)

Reference Range

Urine urobilinogen, 0.1 to 1.0 Ehrlich units every 2 hours or 0.5 to 4.0 Ehrlich units per day (0.86 to 8 mmol/d); 1 Ehrlich unit is equivalent to approximately 1 mg of urobilinogen.

Fecal Urobilinogen

Visual inspection of the feces is usually sufficient to detect decreased urobilinogen. However, the semiquantitative determination of fecal urobilinogen is available and involves the same principle described earlier for the urine. It is carried out in an aqueous extract of fresh feces, and any urobilin present is reduced to urobilinogen by treatment with alkaline ferrous hydroxide before Ehrlich's reagent is added. A range of 75 to 275 Ehrlich units per 100 g of fresh feces or 75 to 400 Ehrlich units per 24-hour specimen is considered a normal reference range.[48]

Serum Bile Acids

Serum bile acid analysis is rarely performed because the methods required are very complex. These involve extraction with organic solvents, partition chromatography, gas chromatography–mass spectrometry, spectrophotometry, ultraviolet light absorption, fluorescence, radioimmunoassay, and enzyme immunoassay (EIA) methods. Although serum bile acid levels are elevated in liver disease, the total concentration is extremely variable and adds no diagnostic value to other tests of liver function. The variability of the type of bile acids present in serum, together with their existence in different conjugated forms, suggests that more relevant information of liver dysfunction may be gained by examining patterns of individual bile acids and their state of conjugation. For example, it has been suggested that the ratio of the trihydroxy to dihydroxy bile acids in serum will differentiate patients with obstructive jaundice from those with hepatocellular injury and that the diagnosis of primary biliary cirrhosis and extrahepatic cholestasis can be made on the basis of the ratio of the cholic to chenodeoxycholic acids. However, the high cost of these tests, the time required to do them, and the current controversy concerning their clinical usefulness render this approach unsatisfactory for routine use.[49,50]

Enzymes

Liver enzymes play an important role in the assessment of liver function because injury to the liver resulting in cytolysis or necrosis will cause the release of enzymes into circulation. Enzymes also play an important role in differentiating hepatocellular (functional) from obstructive (mechanical) liver disease, which is an important clinical distinction because failure to identify an obstruction will result in liver failure if the obstruction is not rapidly treated. Although many enzymes have been identified as useful in the assessment of liver function, the most clinically useful include the aminotransferases (ALT and AST), the phosphatases (ALP and 5'-neucleotidase), GGT, and lactate dehydrogenase (LD).

The methods used to measure these enzymes, the normal reference ranges, and other general aspects of enzymology are discussed in Chapter 13. Discussion in this chapter focuses on the characteristic changes in serum enzyme levels seen in various hepatic disorders. It is important to note that the diagnosis of disease depends on a combination of patient history, physical examination, laboratory testing, and sometimes radiologic studies and biopsy and therefore abnormalities in liver enzymes alone are not diagnostic in and of themselves.[51,52]

Aminotransferases

The two most common aminotransferases measured in the clinical laboratory are AST (formerly referred to as serum glutamic oxaloacetic transaminase [SGOT]) and ALT (formerly referred to as serum glutamic pyruvic transaminase [SGPT]). The aminotransferases are responsible for catalyzing the conversion of aspartate and alanine to oxaloacetate and pyruvate, respectively. In the absence of acute necrosis or ischemia of other organs, these enzymes are most useful in the detection of hepatocellular (functional) damage to the liver. ALT is found mainly in the liver (lesser amounts in skeletal muscle and kidney), whereas AST is widely distributed in equal amounts in the heart, skeletal muscle, and liver, making ALT a more "liver-specific" marker than AST. Regardless, the serum activity of both transaminases rises rapidly in almost all diseases of the liver and may remain elevated for up to 2 to 6 weeks. The highest levels of AST and ALT are found in acute conditions such as viral hepatitis, drug- and toxin-induced liver necrosis, and hepatic ischemia. The increase in ALT activity is usually greater than that for AST. Only moderate increases are found in less severe conditions. AST and ALT are found to be normal or only mildly elevated in cases of obstructive liver damage. Because AST and ALT are present in other tissues besides the liver, elevations in these enzymes may be a result of other organ dysfunction or failure such as acute myocardial infarction, renal infarction, progressive muscular dystrophy, and those conditions that result in secondary liver disease such as infectious mononucleosis, diabetic ketoacidosis, and hyperthyroidism. It is often helpful to conduct serial determinations of aminotransferases when following the course of a patient with acute or chronic hepatitis, and caution should be used in interpreting abnormal levels because serum transaminases may actually decrease in some patients with severe acute hepatitis, owing to the exhaustive release of hepatocellular enzymes.[51,52]

Phosphatases
Alkaline Phosphatase
The ALP family of enzymes are zinc metalloenzymes that are widely distributed in all tissues; however, highest activity is seen in the liver, bone, intestine, kidney, and

placenta. The clinical utility of ALP lies in its ability to differentiate hepatobiliary disease from osteogenic bone disease. In the liver, the enzyme is localized to the microvilli of the bile canaliculi, and therefore it serves as a marker of extrahepatic biliary obstruction, such as a stone in the common bile duct, or in intrahepatic cholestasis, such as drug cholestasis or primary biliary cirrhosis. ALP is found in very high concentrations in cases of extrahepatic obstruction with only slight to moderate increases seen in those with hepatocellular disorders such as hepatitis and cirrhosis. Because bone is also a source of ALP, it may be elevated in bone-related disorders such as Paget's disease, bony metastases, diseases associated with an increase in osteoblastic activity, and rapid bone growth during puberty. ALP is also found elevated in pregnancy due to its release from the placenta, where it may remain elevated up to several weeks postdelivery. As a result, interpretation of ALP concentrations is difficult because enzyme activity of ALP can increase in the absence of liver damage.[51,52]

5′-Nucleotidase
5′-Nucleotidase (5NT) is a phosphatase that is responsible for catalyzing the hydrolysis of nucleoside-5′-phosphate esters. Although 5NT is found in a wide variety of cells, serum levels become significantly elevated in hepatobiliary disease. There is no bone source of 5NT, so it is useful in differentiating ALP elevations due to the liver from other conditions where ALP may be seen in increased concentrations (bone diseases, pregnancy, and childhood growth). Levels of both 5NT and ALP are elevated in liver disease, whereas in primary bone disease, ALP level is elevated, but the 5NT level is usually normal or only slightly elevated. This enzyme is much more sensitive to metastatic liver disease than is ALP because, unlike ALP, its level is not significantly elevated in other conditions, such as in pregnancy or during childhood. In addition, some increase in enzyme activity may be noted after abdominal surgery.[51-54]

γ-Glutamyltransferase
GGT is a membrane-localized enzyme found in high concentrations in the kidney, liver, pancreas, intestine, and prostate but not in bone. Similar to the clinical utility of 5NT (see earlier), GGT plays a role in differentiating the cause of elevated levels of ALP as the highest levels of GGT are seen in biliary obstruction. GGT is a hepatic microsomal enzyme; therefore, ingestion of alcohol or certain drugs (barbiturates, tricyclic antidepressants, and anticonvulsants) elevates GGT. It is a sensitive test for cholestasis caused by chronic alcohol or drug ingestion. Measurement of this enzyme is also useful if jaundice is absent for the confirmation of hepatic neoplasms.[51-55]

Lactate Dehydrogenase
LD is an enzyme with a very wide distribution throughout the body. It is released into circulation when cells of the body are damaged or destroyed, serving as a general, nonspecific marker of cellular injury. Moderate elevations of total serum LD levels are common in acute viral hepatitis and in cirrhosis, whereas biliary tract disease may produce only slight elevations. High serum levels may be found in metastatic carcinoma of the liver. As a result of its wide distribution, LD measurements provide no additional clinical information above that which is provided by the previously mentioned enzymes. However, fractionation of LD into its five tissue-specific isoenzymes may give useful information about the site of origin of the LD elevation.

Tests Measuring Hepatic Synthetic Ability

A healthy functioning liver is required for the synthesis of serum proteins (except the immunoglobulins). The measurement of serum proteins, therefore, can be used to assess the synthetic ability of the liver. Although these tests are not sensitive to minimal liver damage, they may be useful in quantitating the severity of hepatic dysfunction.

A decreased serum albumin may be a result of decreased liver protein synthesis, and the albumin level correlates well with the severity of functional impairment and is found more often in chronic rather than in acute liver disease. The serum α-globulins also tend to decrease with chronic liver disease. However, a low or absent α-globulin suggests α-antitrypsin deficiency as the cause of the chronic liver disease. Serum γ-globulin levels are transiently increased in acute liver disease and remain elevated in chronic liver disease. The highest elevations are found in chronic active hepatitis and postnecrotic cirrhosis. In particular, immunoglobulin G (IgG) and IgM levels are more consistently elevated in chronic active hepatitis; IgM, in primary biliary cirrhosis; and IgA, in alcoholic cirrhosis.

Prothrombin time is commonly increased in liver disease because the liver is unable to manufacture adequate amounts of clotting factor or because the disruption of bile flow results in inadequate absorption of vitamin K from the intestine. However, a prothrombin time is not routinely used to aid in the diagnosis of liver disease. Rather, serial measurements of prothrombin times may be useful in following the progression of disease and the assessment of the risk of bleeding. A marked prolongation of the prothrombin time indicates severe diffuse liver disease and a poor prognosis.

Tests Measuring Nitrogen Metabolism

The liver plays a major role in removing ammonia from the bloodstream and converting it to urea so that it can be removed by the kidneys. A plasma ammonia level, therefore, is a reflection of the liver's ability to perform this conversion. In liver failure, ammonia and other toxins increase in the bloodstream and may ultimately cause hepatic coma. In this condition, the patient becomes increasingly disoriented and gradually lapses into unconsciousness. The cause of hepatic coma is not fully known, although ammonia is presumed to play a major role. However, the correlation between blood ammonia levels and the severity of the hepatic coma is poor. Therefore, ammonia levels are most useful when multiple measurements are made over time.

The most common laboratory determination of ammonia concentrations is based on the following reaction:

$$NH_4^+ + \alpha\text{-ketoglutaric acid} + NADH \xrightarrow{\text{Glutamate dehydrog}} \text{glutamic acid} + NAD^+ \quad \text{(Eq. 25-1)}$$

The resulting decrease in absorbance at 340 nm is measured and is proportional to ammonia concentration. The sample of choice is plasma collected in ethylenediaminetetraacetic acid (EDTA), lithium heparin, or potassium oxalate, and the samples should be immediately placed on ice to prevent metabolism of other nitrogenous compounds to ammonia in the sample, leading to false elevations in ammonia. If analysis cannot be performed immediately, the plasma should be removed and placed on ice or frozen. Frozen (−70°C) samples are stable for several days. Hemolyzed samples should be rejected for analysis as red blood cells have a concentration of ammonia two to three times higher than that of plasma.[56] Lipemic samples and those with high bilirubin concentrations may be unsuitable for analysis in some systems. The glutaminase activity of γ-glutamyl transferase is a major contributor to the endogenous production of ammonia; therefore, concentrations may be artifactually increased in samples with raised γ-glutamyl transferase activity.[57]

Hepatitis

Hepatitis implies injury to the liver characterized by the presence of inflammation in the liver tissue. Infectious causes for the inflammation of liver include viral, bacterial, and parasitic infections, as well as noninfectious causes, such as radiation, drugs, chemicals, and autoimmune diseases and toxins. Viral infections account for the majority of hepatitis cases observed in the clinical setting. Major hepatitis subtypes include HAV, HBV, HCV, HDV, and HEV. Infections with these viruses can lead to the onset of acute disease with symptoms, including jaundice, dark urine, fatigue, nausea, vomiting, and abdominal pain. Some subtypes, such as HBV and HCV, can lead to the prolonged elevation of serum transaminase level (longer than 6 months), a condition termed *chronic hepatitis*. Routes of transmission vary from one viral subtype to another. HAV and HEV are typically caused by ingestion of contaminated food or water. HBV, HCV, and HDV usually occur as a result of parenteral contact with infected body fluids (e.g., from blood transfusions or invasive medical procedures using contaminated equipment) and sexual contact. Refer Table 25-3 for a list of hepatitis viruses.

Hepatitis A

HAV, also known as infectious hepatitis or short-incubation hepatitis, is the most common form of viral hepatitis worldwide. It is caused by a nonenveloped RNA virus of the Picornavirus family. Tens of millions of HAV infections occur annually, with the most common reported source of infection in the household occurring via contaminated or improperly handled food.[58] Because HAV is excreted in bile and shed in the feces, which can contain up to 10^9 infectious virions per gram, the fecal–oral route is the primary means of HAV transmission.[59,60] Patients with HAV infection present with symptoms of fever, malaise, anorexia, nausea, abdominal discomfort, dark urine, and jaundice. Symptoms are generally self-limited and resolve within 3 weeks. However, in rare instances, patients develop fulminant liver failure. Chronic infection with HAV is not found and there is no evidence of a carrier state or long-term sequelae in humans.[58]

Clinical markers for the diagnosis and the progression of HAV infection are measured through the presence of serologic antibodies. IgM antibodies to HAV (IgM anti-HAV) are detectable at or prior to the onset of clinical illness and decline in 3 to 6 months, when it becomes undetectable by commercially available diagnostic tests.[61] IgG antibodies to HAV (IgG anti-HAV) appear soon after IgM, persist for years after infection, and confer lifelong immunity.[62] IgM anti-HAV has been used as the primary marker of acute infection.[63] The presence of elevated titers of IgG anti-HAV in the absence of IgM indicates a past infection. Another reliable method to detect acute infection in patients is assaying for the presence of viral antigen, which is shed in the feces.

TABLE 25-3 THE HEPATITIS VIRUSES

	NUCLEOTIDE	INCUBATION PERIOD	PRIMARY MODE OF TRANSMISSION	VACCINE	CHRONIC INFECTION	SEROLOGIC DIAGNOSIS AVAILABLE
Hepatitis A	RNA	2–6 wk	Fecal–oral	Yes	No	Yes
Hepatitis B	DNA	8–26 wk	Parenteral, sexual	Yes	Yes	Yes
Hepatitis C	RNA	2–15 wk	Parenteral, sexual	No	Yes	Yes
Hepatitis D	RNA	—	Parenteral, sexual	Yes	Yes	Yes
Hepatitis E	RNA	3–6 wk	Fecal–oral	No	?	Yes

However, the antigen is no longer present soon after liver enzymes have reached their peak levels. Another method of detecting HAV infection is amplification of viral RNA by reverse transcription–polymerase chain reaction (RT-PCR). Nucleic acid detection techniques are more sensitive than immunoassays for viral antigen to detect HAV in samples of different origins (e.g., clinical specimens, environmental samples, or food). Because of the high proportion of asymptomatic HAV infections, nucleic acid amplification techniques are useful to determine the extent to which unidentified infection occurs.[64]

The availability of vaccines to provide long-term immunity against HAV infection has the potential to significantly reduce the incidence of disease and possibly eliminate the transmission of this virus worldwide.[65-68] In 2006, following the approval of the HAV vaccine for children in the United States, the U.S. Food and Drug Administration (FDA)/CDC recommended that all children receive the HAV vaccine as early as age 12 to 23 months.[69] The use of this vaccine has significantly reduced the incidence of HAV in the United States and has therefore changed the epidemiology of this infection.

Hepatitis B

Known as *serum hepatitis* or *long-incubation hepatitis*, HBV can cause both acute and chronic hepatitis and is the most ubiquitous of the hepatitis viruses. Two billion individuals are infected globally and between 350 and 400 million persons are carriers of the virus. In the United States, 1 million infected individuals are estimated to be chronic carriers of the virus.[58] The highest incidence of acute HBV was among adults aged 25 to 45 years.[70] HBV is comparatively stable in the environment and remains viable for longer than 7 days on environmental surfaces at room temperature.[71] It is detected in virtually all body fluids, including blood, feces, urine, saliva, semen, tears, and breast milk; the three major routes of transmission are parenteral, perinatal, and sexual. Persons at high risk for infection in the United States include persons who engage in the sharing of body fluids, such as high-risk sexual behaviors (e.g., prostitution and male homosexuality) and the sharing of drug injection needles. Children born to mothers who are hepatitis B surface antigen (HBsAg) positive at the time of delivery, immigrants from endemic areas, and sexual partners and household contacts of patients who have HBV are high-risk groups for HBV infection. Although transmission of HBV by blood transfusion occurs, effective screening tests now make this transmission route rare. Health-care workers, including laboratory personnel, may be at increased risk for developing HBV, depending on their degree of exposure to blood and body fluids.[72]

Serologic Markers of HBV Infection

HBV is a 42-nm DNA virus classified in the Hepadnaviridae family. The liver is the primary site of HBV replication. Following an HBV infection, the core of the antigen is synthesized in the nuclei of hepatocytes and then passed into the cytoplasm of the liver cell, where it is surrounded by the protein coat. An antigen present in the core of the virus (HBcAg) and a surface antigen present on the surface protein (HBsAg) have been identified by serologic studies. Another antigen, called the e antigen (HBeAg), has also been identified.[73]

Hepatitis B Surface Antigen

Previously known as the Australia antigen and hepatitis-associated antigen, HBsAg is the antigen for which routine testing is performed on all donated units of blood. HBsAg is a useful serologic marker in patients before the onset of clinical symptoms because it is present during the prodrome of acute HBV. HBsAg is not infectious; however, its presence in the serum may indicate the presence of the hepatitis virus. Therefore, persons who chronically carry HBsAg in their serum must be considered potentially infectious because the presence of the intact virus cannot be excluded. HBsAg is the only serologic marker detected during the first 3 to 5 weeks after infection in newly infected patients. The average time from exposure to detection of HBsAg is 30 days (range 6 to 60 days).[74-76] Highly sensitive single-sample nucleic acid tests can detect HBV DNA in the serum of an infected person 10 to 20 days before detection of HBsAg.[76] HBsAg positivity has been reported for up to 18 days after HBV vaccination and is clinically insignificant.[78,79] Patients who achieve complete viral clearance develop the antibody to the HBsAg, following the disappearance of the HBsAg (Fig. 25-8). The presence of anti-HBs antibody in patients is frequently observed in the general population, suggestive of past infection. Patients who have developed the antibody to the HBsAg are not susceptible to future reinfection with HBV.[72]

Hepatitis B Core Antigen

HBcAg has not been demonstrated to be present in the plasma of hepatitis victims or blood donors. This antigen is present only in the nuclei of hepatocytes during an acute infection with HBV. The antibody to the core antigen, anti-HBc, usually develops earlier in the course of infection than the antibody to the surface antigen (Fig. 25-8). A test for the IgM antibody to HBcAg was recently developed as a serologic marker for clinical use. The presence of this IgM antibody is specific for acute HBV infection. In patients who have chronic HBV infection, the IgM anti-HBc antibody titer can persist during chronic viral replication at low levels that typically are not detectable by assays used in the United States. However, persons with exacerbation of chronic infection can test positive for IgM anti-HBc.[79] Another marker for acute infection is a viral DNA-dependent DNA polymerase that is closely associated with the presence of the core antigen. This viral enzyme is required for viral replication and is detectable in serum early in the course of viral hepatitis, during the phase of active viral replication.[80]

Sequence of HBV Markers

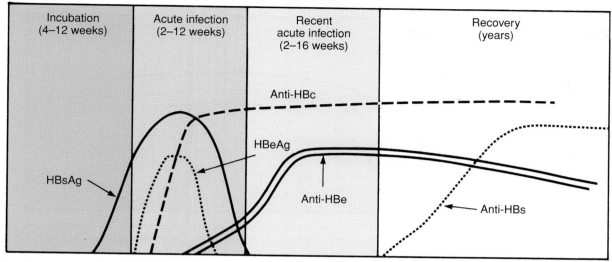

FIGURE 25-8 Serology of hepatitis B infection with recovery.

CASE STUDY 25-3

The following laboratory results were obtained from a 19-year-old college student who consulted the Student Health Service because of fatigue and lack of appetite. She adds that she recently noted that her sclera appears somewhat yellowish and that her urine has become dark (Case Study Table 25-3.1).

Questions

1. What is the most likely diagnosis?

2. What additional factors in the patient's history should be sought?

3. What is the prognosis?

CASE STUDY TABLE 25-3.1
LABORATORY RESULTS

ALT (SGPT)	Elevated
AST (SGOT)	Elevated
Alkaline phosphatase	Minimally elevated
Lactate dehydrogenase	Elevated
Serum bilirubin	5 mg/dL
Urine bilirubin	Increased
Hepatitis A antibody (IgG)	Negative
Hepatitis A antibody (IgM)	Positive
Hepatitis B surface antigen	Negative
Hepatitis B surface antibody	Negative
Hepatitis C antibody	Negative

Hepatitis B e Antigen

The e antigen, an antigen closely associated with the core of the viral particle, is detected in the serum of persons with acute or chronic HBV infection. The presence of the e antigen appears to correlate well with both the number of infectious virus particles and the degree of infectivity of HBsAg-positive sera. The presence of HBeAg in HBsAg carriers is an unfavorable prognostic sign and predicts a severe course and chronic liver disease. Conversely, the presence of anti-HBe antibody in carriers indicates a low infectivity of the serum (Fig. 25-9). The e antigen is detected in serum only when surface antigen is present (Fig. 25-10).

The serologic markers of HBV infection typically used to differentiate among acute, resolving, and chronic infections are HBsAg, anti-HBc, and anti-HBs (Table 25-4). Persons who recover from natural infection typically will be positive for both anti-HBs and anti-HBc, whereas persons who respond to HBV vaccine have only anti-HBs. Persons who become chronically infected fail to develop antibody to the HBsAg, resulting in the persistent presence of HBsAg as well as the presence of anti-HBc in patient serum, typically for life.[81-84] HBeAg and anti-HBe screenings typically are used for the management of patients with chronic infection. Serologic assays are available commercially for all markers except HBcAg because no free HBcAg circulates in blood.[70]

Nucleic acid hybridization or PCR technique is used to detect HBV DNA in the blood and is another method used to measure disease progression. This technique provides a more sensitive measurement of infectivity and disease progression than serology. It may be used to monitor the effectiveness of antiviral therapy in patients

Sequence of HBV Surface Markers
Chronic Hepatitis

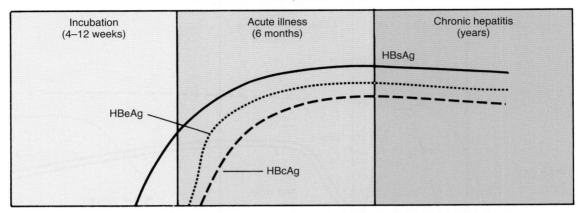

FIGURE 25-9 No antibody is formed against HBsAg. The persistence of HBeAg implies high infectivity and a generally poor prognosis. This patient would likely develop cirrhosis unless seroconversion occurs or treatment is given.

Sequence of HBV Surface Markers
Chronic Hepatitis

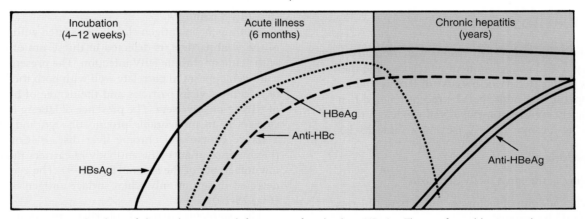

FIGURE 25-10 Serology of chronic hepatitis with formation of antibody to HBeAg. This is a favorable sign and suggests that the chronic hepatitis may resolve. Complete recovery would be heralded by the disappearance of HBsAg and formation of its corresponding antibody.

with chronic HBV infection, but it supplements rather than replaces current HBV serologic assays.[85-87]

Chronic Infection with HBV
Approximately 90% of patients infected with HBV recover within 6 months. Recovery is accompanied by the development of the antibody to the HBsAg. However, about 10% of patients progress to a chronic hepatitis infection. The likelihood of developing chronic HBV infection is higher in individuals infected perinatally (90%) and during childhood (20% to 30%), when the immune system is thought to be less developed and unable to achieve efficient viral clearance, than in adult immunocompetent subjects (<1%).[88] Approximately 25% of persons who were chronically infected since childhood and 15% of those who were chronically infected since adulthood die

prematurely from cirrhosis or liver cancer. In the majority of cases, patients remain asymptomatic until the onset of cirrhosis.[89]

Patients with chronic HBV display the characteristic serologic profile as shown in Figure 25-10. The presence of HBsAg in chronically infected patients is an indication that they are infectious and at risk for developing complications, including cirrhosis and HCC. The natural course of chronic HBV infection is divided into four phases based on the virus–host interaction: immune tolerance, immune clearance (HBeAg-positive chronic hepatitis), low or non-replication (inactive HBsAg carrier), and reactivation (HBeAg-negative chronic hepatitis).[90-92] Patients can be classified according to their serologic status as shown in Table 25-5.[88]

TABLE 25-4	TYPICAL INTERPRETATION OF SEROLOGIC TEST RESULTS FOR HEPATITIS B VIRUS INFECTION

		SEROLOGIC MARKER			
HBSAG[a]	TOTAL ANTI-HBC[b]	IGM[c] ANTI-HBC	ANTI-HBS[d]	INTERPRETATION
−[e]	−	−	−	Never infected
+[f,g]	−	−	−	Early acute infection; transient (up to 18 d) after vaccination
+	+	+	−	Acute infection
−	+	+	+ or −	Acute resolving infection
−	+	−	+	Recovered from past infection and immune
+	+	−	−	Chronic infection
−	+	−	−	False positive (i.e., susceptible); past infection, "low-level" chronic infection[h]; or passive transfer of anti-HBc to infant born to HBsAg-positive mother
−	−	−	+	Immune if concentration is ≥10 mIU/mL after vaccine series completion; passive transfer after hepatitis B immune globulin administration

[a]Hepatitis B surface antigen.
[b]Antibody to hepatitis B core antigen.
[c]Immunoglobulin M.
[d]Antibody to HBsAg.
[e]Negative test result.
[f]Positive test result.
[g]To ensure that an HBsAg-positive test result is not a false positive, samples with reactive HBsAg results should be tested with a licensed neutralizing confirmatory test if recommended in the manufacturer's package insert.
[h]Persons positive only for anti-HBc are unlikely to be infectious except under unusual circumstances in which they are the source for direct percutaneous exposure of susceptible recipients to large quantities of virus (e.g., blood transfusion or organ transplant).

HBV Treatment and Prevention

Persons who have chronic HBV infection require medical evaluation and regular monitoring.[93-95] The FDA has approved several drugs for the treatment of chronic HBV that can achieve sustained suppression of HBV replication and remission of liver disease in certain persons.[94]

HBV vaccination is the most effective measure to prevent HBV infection and therefore obviate its consequences, including cirrhosis of the liver, liver cancer, liver failure, and death. HBsAg is the antigen used for HBV vaccination.[96,97] The vaccine is highly effective in stimulating the production of hepatitis B surface antibody

TABLE 25-5	SEROLOGICAL PROFILES OF CHRONIC HEPATITIS B VIRUS INFECTION

PHASE	SERUM ALT	HBEAG	ANTI-HBE		HBV DNA	
					COPIES/ML	IU/ML
Immune tolerance	Normal or minimally	Positive	Negative	Very high levels	$10^8–10^{11}$ elevated	20 million–20 billion
HBeAg-positive chronic	Persistently elevated hepatitis	Positive	Negative	High levels	$10^6–10^{10}$	200,000–2 billion
HBeAg-negative chronic hepatitis	Elevated and often fluctuating	Negative	Positive	Moderate levels, often fluctuating	$10^4–10^8$	2,000–20 million
Inactive carrier	Normal	Negative	Positive	Low or no detectable levels	$<10^4$	<2,000

ALT, alanine aminotransferase; HBV, hepatitis B virus.

Adapted from Fattovich G, Bortolotti F, Donato F. Natural history of chronic hepatitis B: special emphasis on disease progression and prognostic factors. *J Hepatol.* 2008;48:335-352.

and thereby rendering the recipient immune. As a result of the national program of childhood immunization, by 2005, a 98% decline in HBV infection was reported among children aged 13 years or younger, as well as a 97% decline among adolescents aged 12 to 19 years.[58] In 2006, the Advisory Committee on Immunization Practices (ACIP) recommended universal HBV vaccination for all unvaccinated adults at risk for HBV infection and for all adults requesting protection from HBV infection. All health-care workers who handle blood products and are in close proximity to body fluids should have the hepatitis vaccine. The hepatitis B immune globulin (HBIG) provides passively acquired anti-HBs and temporary protection (i.e., 3 to 6 months) when administered in standard doses. HBIG typically is used as an adjunct to HBV vaccine for postexposure immunoprophylaxis to prevent HBV infection. For nonresponders to HBV vaccination, HBIG administered alone is the primary means of protection after an HBV exposure.[70]

Hepatitis C

HCV (originally "non-A non-B hepatitis") is caused by a virus with an RNA genome that is a member of the Flaviviridae family. HCV is transmitted parenterally. Although the sexual and fecal–oral routes as modes of transmission have been documented, the virus is transmitted primarily by blood transfusion of inappropriately screened blood products.[98-100] Approximately 3% of the world population is infected by the virus and most infections become chronic and may lead to cirrhosis, end-stage liver disease, HCC, and death. In the United States, HCV infection is present in about 1.6% of the noninstitutionalized population.[101] As many as 4 million Americans are chronically infected.[58] Clinically, acute HCV infection presents only mild infection and patients may remain completely asymptomatic. However, HCV infection has a high rate of progression to chronic hepatitis, cirrhosis, and liver carcinoma, making HCV a major cause of chronic hepatitis in the United States.[100,102] In addition, HCV infection is a leading cause of liver transplantation in this country.[103]

Laboratory Tests for Hepatitis C

The hepatitis C antibody is usually not detected in the first few months of infection but will almost always be present in the later stages. The antibody is not protective against reinfection and sometimes disappears several years following resolution of the infection. Laboratory testing for the diagnosis of HCV infection in the clinical setting is relatively straightforward. Currently, two laboratory tests are commonly used to diagnose HCV infection in clinical practice: anti-HCV detection by EIA and quantitative nucleic acid PCR assays for serum HCV RNA.[104-109] In clinical practice, the most common approach is initially to test a patient's serum for the presence of anti-HCV by EIA. If this test gives a positive result, the next step is

to test for serum HCV RNA by PCR.[106] The HCV antibody test is designed to detect antibodies generated in response to HCV infection.[106,108] Although a positive HCV antibody test result generally indicates that the patient has been exposed to the HCV virus, this test cannot determine whether the patient is currently infected with HCV or has recovered from HCV infection.[104,108] Some patients with a positive HCV antibody test result have spontaneously cleared HCV. These patients (anti-HCV positive but HCV RNA negative) are recommended to retake the test for HCV RNA on a second occasion, 3 to 6 months after the first HCV RNA test.[108]

Chronic HCV Infection

Most patients with HCV infection progress to chronic infection. Although patients with chronic HCV infection appear to be at high risk for liver cirrhosis, the role of HCV in the development of HCC is not clear. Most chronically infected patients are asymptomatic and manifest only mild elevations of liver function tests, especially transaminases. The degree of elevation in liver enzymes has little predictive value toward disease progression. About 80% of infected patients develop chronic hepatitis, although, in most cases, the disease does not progress. The percentage of patients progressing to liver cirrhosis varies widely in different studies but has been estimated to be as high as 40% after 40 years. Alcohol consumption concomitant with chronic HCV infection significantly increases the risk of cirrhosis. Liver biopsies are performed periodically in these patients, with the degree of inflammation and fibrosis correlating with the risk of cirrhosis.[110-113]

Patients with chronic HCV infection are usually treated with pegylated interferon and ribavirin. Therapeutic efficacy is monitored by using PCR to determine the number of viral copies in serum.[114] A prototypic envelope peptide-based vaccine has been reported to induce antibodies in human subjects, but there is no evidence for the presence of a neutralizing antibody against HCV.[115] Likely, an effective and safe vaccine against HCV will not be available soon.

Hepatitis D

HDV is a unique subviral satellite virus infection. It is a small, defective RNA-containing virus that cannot replicate independently but rather requires the HBsAg of HBV for replication. Therefore, it is incapable of causing any illness in patients who do not have HBV infection. Modes of transmission are generally similar to those of HBV. Approximately 5% of the global HBV carriers are coinfected with HDV, leading to a total of 10 to 15 million HDV carriers worldwide.[116,117] Each year, 7,500 new cases of HDV infections are estimated to occur in the United States.[118] Chronic HDV infection is estimated to be responsible for more than 1,000 deaths each year in the United States.[119]

HDV virions possess an outer envelope composed of HBsAg proteins and host membrane lipids and an inner nucleocapsid consisting of viral RNA and hepatitis delta antigen (HDAg). It is believed that HBsAg-mediated binding to a cellular receptor helps HDV penetrate the hepatocyte.[120] Nuclear localization signal domain on the HDAg facilitates transit of its genome into the nucleus, where viral replication takes place.[121] HDV infection can occur concurrently with HBV infection (coinfection) or in a patient with established HBV infection (super-infection) (Table 25-6). The rate of chronicity following coinfection with HBV and HDV is equal to that of HBV infection alone.[122] HDV superinfection is likely to become chronic simply because HBV infection is already chronic. In general, in the acute phase, HDV superin-fected carriers may develop severe hepatitis, and around 70% to 90% will progress to chronicity.[123]

The diagnosis of HDV relies on detection of anti-bodies against HDAg and serum HDV RNA, as well as HBV markers.[124] Clinical symptoms of HDV cannot be distinguished from those of other hepatic viruses. Accurate diagnosis is made by a negative test for IgM anti-HBc and confirmed by the detection of HDV mark-ers.[125] Widespread use of the HBV vaccine has resulted in a decline in the incidence of HDV.[126] Interferon-α is currently the therapy used for treating chronic HDV infection. Compared with chronic HBV or HCV, chronic HDV treatment requires a higher dosage and a longer duration of treatment, and posttreatment relapses are common.[125]

CASE STUDY 25-4

The following results were obtained in the patient from Case Study 25-2 (Case Study Table 25-4.1).

Questions

1. What is the most likely diagnosis?

2. What is the prognosis?

3. What complications may develop?

CASE STUDY TABLE 25-4.1 LABORATORY RESULTS

Hepatitis A antibody (IgG)	Positive
Hepatitis A antibody (IgM)	Negative
Hepatitis B surface antigen	Positive
Hepatitis B surface antibody	Negative
Hepatitis core antibody (IgM)	Positive
Hepatitis C antibody	Negative

TABLE 25-6	CLINICAL FEATURES OF HEPATITIS D VIRUS (HDV) COINFECTION AND SUPERINFECTION IN HEPATITIS B VIRUS (HBV)	
	COINFECTION	**SUPERINFECTION**
HBV infection	Acute	Chronic
Outcomes	Recovery with seroclearance	Usually persistent infection
Markers		
HBsAg	Positive, early and transient	Positive and persistent
IgM anti-HBc	Positive	Negative
Anti-HBs	Positive in recovery phase	Negative
HDV infection	Acute	Acute or chronic
Outcomes	Recovery with seroclearance	Usually persistent infection
Markers		
Serum HDAg[a]	Early and short-lived	Early and transient, undetectable later
Liver HDAg	Positive and transient	Positive, maybe negative in late stage
Serum HDV RNA	Positive, early and transient	Positive, early and persistent
Anti-HDV	Late acute phase, low titer	Rapidly increasing, high titers
IgM anti-HDV	Positive, transient, pentameric	Rapidly increasing, high titers, monomeric

IgM, immunoglobulin M; HDAg, hepatitis delta antigen.

[a]Using immunoblot assay, detection rate of serum HDAg may be comparable to Northern blot detection of HDV RNA using cDNA probe.

Adapted from Hsieh TH, Liu CJ, Chen DS, Chen PJ. Natural course and treatment of hepatitis D virus infection. *J Formos Med Assoc.* 2006;105:869-881.

Hepatitis E

The RNA-containing HEV, a nonenveloped RNA virus that is only 27 to 34 nm in diameter, is the sole member of the genus *Hepevirus* in the family Hepeviridae. After infection, the incubation period is short, generally between 21 and 42 days prior to the onset of symptoms. The virus may be detected in feces and bile by about 7 days after infection. HEV is transmitted primarily by the fecal–oral route, and waterborne epidemics are characteristic of HEV in many developing countries. However, in industrialized countries, several nonhuman mammals such as pigs, cows, and sheep are susceptible to infection with HEV, leading to the potential spread of the virus through zoonosis.[127] The clinical presentation of HEV is comparable to that of HAV. The severity of an HEV infection is generally greater than the severity of an HAV infection.[128] In general, HEV infection is mild, except in pregnant women, in whom it may be a devastating illness.[129]

Because cases of HEV are not clinically distinguishable from cases of other types of acute viral hepatitis, diagnosis is made by biochemical assessment of liver function. Acute HEV is diagnosed when the presence of IgM anti-HEV is detected.[128,130] The presence of a high or increasing anti-HEV IgG titer may support the diagnosis of acute HEV infection, and in such cases acute HEV can be presumed even in the absence of IgM anti-HEV.[131] EIA and immunochromatography are most convenient for the detection of IgM and/or IgG anti-HEV. Additional testing by RT-PCR has a limited confirmatory role. Acute-phase HEV RNA can be detected in feces by PCR in approximately 50% of cases. In most instances, there is a very good positive correlation between the results assayed by RT-PCR and EIA.[128] HEV should be suspected in outbreaks of waterborne hepatitis occurring in developing countries, especially if the disease is more severe in pregnant women, or if HAV has been excluded. If laboratory tests are not available, epidemiologic evidence can help in establishing a diagnosis.[132]

At present, no commercially available vaccines exist for the prevention of HEV. Experimental immune prophylaxis against HEV based on recombinant antigens appears to confer short-term protection and may be useful for pregnant women in endemic areas and travelers coming into these regions.

Other Forms of Hepatitis

Five forms of viral hepatitis (A, B, C, D, and E) are well recognized. The role of G viruses is currently unclear. Hepatitis F is an enteric agent that may be transmitted to primates. Again, more needs to be learned about this agent and its role, if any, in human disease. Other forms of viral hepatitis, such as TT virus and SEN virus, may exist. The GB group of flavo-like viruses, GBV-A, GBV-B, and GBV-C, are also associated with acute and chronic hepatitis. Little is known about these diseases, and no diagnostic tests for them are commercially available at this time.[133-136] Cytomegalovirus, Epstein-Barr virus, and probably several other agents can also cause hepatitis.

CASE STUDY 25-5

A 36-year-old man consulted his family physician because of liver function abnormalities, which had been noted initially during a preinsurance physical examination 6 months earlier. The following laboratory results were obtained, which were identical to those obtained 6 months ago (Case Study Table 25-5.1).

Questions

1. What is the most likely diagnosis?

2. What is the prognosis?

3. What complications may develop?

4. What additional tests should be done?

CASE STUDY TABLE 25-5.1
LABORATORY RESULTS

Hepatitis A antibody (IgG)	Positive
Hepatitis A antibody (IgM)	Negative
Hepatitis B surface antigen	Positive
Hepatitis B surface antibody	Negative
Hepatitis B core antibody (IgM)	Positive
Hepatitis C antibody	Negative

For additional student resources please visit thePoint at http://thepoint.lww.com.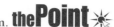

QUESTIONS

1. Which of the following enzymes would best aid in identifying hepatobiliary disease?
   a. Alkaline phosphatase (ALP)
   b. Aspartate aminotransferase (AST)
   c. Alanine aminotransferase (ALT)
   d. Ammonia

2. In which of the following types of cells does the conjugation of bilirubin take place?
   a. Hepatocytes
   b. Kupffer cells
   c. Macrophages
   d. Phagocytic cells

3. Which of the following enzymes is responsible for the conjugation of bilirubin?
   a. UDP-glucuronyl transferase
   b. Alkaline phosphatase
   c. Glutamate dehydrogenase
   d. Leucine aminopeptidase

4. Which of the following fractions of bilirubin is water soluble and reacts with a diazo reagent without the addition of an accelerator?
   a. Conjugated bilirubin
   b. Unconjugated bilirubin
   c. Total bilirubin
   d. Indirect bilirubin

5. Which form of hepatitis is caused by a DNA virus?
   a. Hepatitis B
   b. Hepatitis A
   c. Hepatitis C
   d. Hepatitis D

6. Which of the following enzymes is most useful in establishing the hepatic origin of an elevated serum alkaline phosphatase?
   a. 5′-Nucleotidase
   b. Alanine aminotransferase (ALT)
   c. Aspartate aminotransferase (AST)
   d. Lactate dehydrogenase

7. Hepatitis E is likely to cause serious consequences in
   a. Pregnant women
   b. Children
   c. Travelers in Third World countries
   d. Older people/

8. Worldwide, most primary malignant tumors of the liver are related to
   a. Alcoholism
   b. Gallstones
   c. Reye syndrome
   d. Malaria

9. The reagent *p*-dimethylaminobenzaldehyde is used to measure which of the following?
   a. Urobilinogen
   b. Total bilirubin
   c. Ammonia
   d. Alkaline phosphatase

10. Which of the following conditions would result in elevations in primarily conjugated bilirubin?
   a. Dubin-Johnson syndrome
   b. Physiologic jaundice of the newborn
   c. Crigler-Najjar syndrome
   d. Gilbert's syndrome

11. A urinalysis dipstick test indicated that urobilinogen was absent. Which condition does this support?
   a. Biliary obstruction
   b. Hepatitis A acute infection
   c. Defective liver cell function
   d. Hepatocellular disease
   e. This would support all of the above conditions

12. Measuring serum ammonia levels has the potential to be fraught with preanalytical errors that may interfere with achieving an accurate result. Of the following preanalytical steps, which is incorrect?
   a. After phlebotomy, the patient's blood should be immediately placed on ice.
   b. The blood should be collected in a red clot tube without anticoagulant.
   c. Hemolyzed samples should be rejected as this interferes by falsely increasing ammonia levels.
   d. Lipemia may also interfere with plasma ammonia measurements.
   e. All of the above are correct.

13. A patient presents with elevated levels of IgG anti-HAV while levels of IgM anti-HAV are nondetectable. This patient is likely to:
   a. Have an acute infection of HAV.
   b. Have a chronic infection of HAV.
   c. Have an immunity to HAV.
   d. Be a carrier of HAV.

REFERENCES

1. Wang X, Chowdhury JR, Chowdhury NR. Bilirubin metabolism: applied physiology. *Curr Paediatr.* 2006;16:70-74.
2. Ahlfors CE. Measurement of plasma unbound unconjugated bilirubin. *Anal Biochem.* 2000;279:130-135.
3. McNamara JR, Warnick GR, Wu LL. Lipids and lipoproteins. In: Bishop ML, Duben-Engellkirk JL, Fody EP, eds. *Clinical Chemistry: Principles, Procedures, Correlations.* Philadelphia, PA: Lippincott Williams & Wilkins; 2000:323.
4. Papavramidou N, Fee E, Christopoulou-Aletra H. Jaundice in the hippocratic corpus. *J Gastrointest Surg.* 2007;11: 1728-1731.
5. Pashankar D, Schreiber RA. Jaundice in older children and adolescents. *Pediatr Rev.* 2001;22:219-226.
6. Monaghan G, Ryan M, Seddon R, Hume R, Burchell B. Genetic variation in bilirubin UDP-glucuronosyltransferase gene promoter and Gilbert's syndrome. *Lancet.* 1996;347:578-581.
7. Black M, Billing BH. Hepatic bilirubin UDP-glucuronyl transferase activity in liver disease and Gilbert's syndrome. *N Engl J Med.* 1969;280:1266-1271.
8. Kaplan M, Hammerman C. Bilirubin and the genome: the hereditary basis of unconjugated neonatal hyperbilirubinemia. *Curr Pharmacogenomics.* 2005;3:21-42.
9. Crigler JF Jr, Najjar VA. Congenital familial nonhemolytic jaundice with kernicterus. *Pediatrics.* 1952;10:169-180.
10. Berk PD, Noyer C. The familial unconjugated hyperbilirubinemias. *Semin Liver Dis.* 1994;14:346-351.
11. Berk PD. Bilirubin metabolism and the hereditary hyperbilirubinemias. *Semin Liver Dis.* 1994;14:321-322.
12. Berk PD, Noyer C. The familial conjugated hyperbilirubinemias. *Semin Liver Dis.* 1994;14:386-394.
13. Zimniak P. Dubin-Johnson and Rotor syndromes: molecular basis and pathogenesis. *Semin Liver Dis.* 1993;13:248-260.
14. Dennery PA, Seidman DS, Stevenson DK. Neonatal hyperbilirubinemia. *N Engl J Med.* 2001;344:581-590.
15. Murphy SL, Xu J, Kochanek KD. Deaths: preliminary data for 2010. *Natl Vital Stat Rep.* 2012;60(4):1-69.
16. Ferlay J, Shin HR, Bray F, Forman D, Mathers C, Parkin DM. *GLOBOCAN 2008 v1.2, Cancer Incidence and Mortality Worldwide: IARC Cancer Base No. 10 [Internet].* Lyon, France: International Agency for Research on Cancer; 2010. http://globocan.iarc.fr. Accessed February 22, 2012.
17. El-Serag HB. Hepatocellular carcinoma. *N Engl J Med.* 2011; 365:1118-1127.
18. American Cancer Society. *Cancer Facts & Figures 2012.* Atlanta, GA: American Cancer Society; 2012. http://www.cancer.org/acs/groups/content/@epidemiologysurveilance/documents/document/acspc-031941.pdf. Accessed February 22, 2012.
19. Mazzaferro V, Regalia E, Doci R, et al. Liver transplantation for the treatment of small hepatocellular carcinomas in patients with cirrhosis. *N Engl J Med.* 1996;334:693-699.
20. Peters LJ, Wiener GJ, Gilliam J, et al. Reye's syndrome in adults. A case report and review of the literature. *Arch Intern Med.* 1986;146:2401-2403.
21. Preblud SR, Orenstein WA, Bart KJ. Varicella: clinical manifestations, epidemiology and health impact in children. *Pediatr Infect Dis.* 1984;3:505-509.
22. Edwards KM, Bennett SR, Garner WL, et al. Reye's syndrome associated with adenovirus infections in infants. *Am J Dis Child.* 1985;139:343-346.
23. Johnson GM, Scurletis TD, Carroll NB. A study of sixteen fatal cases of encephalitis. *N C Med J.* 1963;24:464-473.
24. Starko KM, Ray CG, Dominguez LB, et al. Reye's syndrome and salicylate use. *Pediatrics.* 1980;66:859-864.
25. Waldman RJ, Hall WN, McGee H, Van Amburg G. Aspirin as a risk factor in Reye's syndrome. *JAMA.* 1982;247:3089-3094.
26. Surgeon General's advisory on the use of salicylates and Reye syndrome. *MMWR Morb Mortal Wkly Rep.* 1982;31:289-290.
27. Davis DL, Buffler P. Reduction of deaths after drug labelling for risk of Reye's syndrome. *Lancet.* 1992;340:1042.
28. Daugherty CC, Gartside PS, Heubi JE, et al. A morphometric study of Reye's syndrome. Correlation of reduced mitochondrial numbers and increased mitochondrial size with clinical manifestations. *Am J Pathol.* 1987;129:313-326.
29. Belay ED, Bresee JS, Holman RC, et al. Reye's syndrome in the United States from 1981 through 1997. *N Engl J Med.* 1999;340:1377-1382.
30. Liu ZX, Kaplowitz N. Immune-mediated drug-induced liver disease. *Clin Liver Dis.* 2002;6:755-774.
31. Lieber CS. Alcohol and the liver: metabolism of alcohol and its role in hepatic and extrahepatic diseases. *Mt Sinai J Med.* 2000;67:84-94.
32. Bissell DM, Gores GJ, Laskin DL, Hoofnagle JH. Drug-induced liver injury: mechanisms and test systems. *Hepatology.* 2001;33:1009-1013.
33. Bellentani S, Saccoccio G, Costa G, et al. Drinking habits as cofactors of risk for alcohol induced liver damage. *Gut.* 1997;41:845-850.
34. Mutimer DJ, Burra P, Neuberger JM, et al. Managing severe alcoholic hepatitis complicated by renal failure. *Q J Med.* 1993;86: 649-656.
35. Maddrey WC, Boitnott JK, Bedine MS, Weber FL Jr, Mezey E, White RI Jr. Corticosteroid therapy of alcoholic hepatitis. *Gastroenterology.* 1978;75:193-199.
36. Forrest EH, Evans CD, Stewart S, et al. Analysis of factors predictive of mortality in alcoholic hepatitis and derivation and validation of the Glasgow alcoholic hepatitis score. *Gut.* 2005;54:1174-1179.
37. Dunn W, Jamil LH, Brown LS, et al. MELD accurately predicts mortality in patients with alcoholic hepatitis. *Hepatology.* 2005;41:353-358.
38. Nagata K, Suzuki H, Sakaguchi S. Common pathogenic mechanism in development progression of liver injury caused by non-alcoholic or alcoholic steatohepatitis. *J Toxicol Sci.* 2007;32:453-468.
39. Bertini G, Rubaltelli FF. Non-invasive bilirubinometry in neonatal jaundice. *Semin Neonatol.* 2002;7:129-133.
40. Lott JA, Doumas BT. "Direct" and total bilirubin tests: contemporary problems. *Clin Chem.* 1993;39:641-647.
41. Wilding P, Zilva JF, Wilde CE. Transport of specimens for clinical chemistry analysis. *Ann. Clin Biochem.* 1977;14:301-306.
42. Doumas BT, Kwok-Cheung PP, Perry BW, et al. Candidate reference method for determination of total bilirubin in serum: development and validation. *Clin Chem.* 1985;31:1779-1789.
43. Doumas BT, Wu TW. The measurement of bilirubin fractions in serum. *Crit Rev Clin Lab Sci.* 1991;28:415-445.
44. Ross JW, Miller WG, Myers GL, Praestgaard J. The accuracy of laboratory measurements in clinical chemistry: a study of 11 routine chemistry analytes in the College of American Pathologists Chemistry Survey with fresh frozen serum, definitive methods, and reference methods. *Arch Pathol Lab Med.* 1998;122:587-608.
45. Slaughter MR. Sensitivity of conventional methods for bilirubin measurements. *J Lab Clin Med.* 1996;127:233.
46. Malloy HT, Evelyn KA. The determination of bilirubin with the photoelectric colorimeter. *J Biol Chem.* 1937;119:481-490.
47. Hofmann AF. Bile acid secretion, bile flow and biliary lipid secretion in humans. *Hepatology.* 1990;12(3 pt 2):17S-22S.
48. Kotal P, Fevery J. Quantitation of urobilinogen in feces, urine, bile and serum by direct spectrophotometry of zinc complex. *Clin Chim Acta.* 1991;202:1-9.
49. Azer SA, Klaassen CD, Stacey NH. Biochemical assay of serum bile acids: methods and applications. *Br J Biomed Sci.* 1997;54:118-132.
50. Polkowska G, Polkowski W, Kudlicka A, et al. Range of serum bile acid concentrations in neonates, infants, older children, and in adults. *Med Sci Monit.* 2001;7(suppl 1):268-270.

51. Green RM, Flamm S. AGA technical review on the evaluation of liver chemistry tests. *Gastroenterology.* 2002;123:1367-1384.

52. American Gastroenterological Association medical position statement: evaluation of liver chemistry tests. *Gastroenterology.* 2002;123:1364-1366.

53. Pagani F, Panteghini M. 5′-Neucleotidase in the detection of increased activity of the liver form of alkaline phosphatase in serum. *Clin Chem.* 2001;47:2046-2048.

54. Sunderman FW. The clinical biochemistry of 5′-nucleotidase. *Ann Clin Lab Sci.* 1990;20:123-139.

55. Conigrave KM, Dengenhardt LJ, Whitfield JB. CDT, GGT and AST as markers of alcohol use: the WHO/ISBRA collaborative project. *Alcohol Clin Exp Res.* 2002;25:332-339.

56. Jay DW. Nonprotein nitrogen. In: Bishop ML, Duben-Englekirk JL, Fody EP, eds. *Clinical Chemistry: Principles, Procedures, Correlations.* Philadelphia, PA: Lippincott Williams & Wilkins; 2000:260-274.

57. da Fonseca-Wollheim F. Deamidation of glutamine by increased plasma gamma-glutamyltransferase is a source of rapid ammonia formation in blood and plasma specimens. *Clin Chem.* 1990;36:1479-1482.

58. Koff RS. Review article: vaccination and viral hepatitis—current status and future prospects. *Aliment Pharmacol Ther.* 2007;26:1285-1292.

59. Skinhoj P, Mathiesen LR, Kiryger P, Moller AM. Faecel excretion of hepatitis A virus in patients with symptomatic hepatitis A infection. *Scand J Gastroenterol.* 1981;16:1057-1059.

60. Tassopoulos NC, Papaevangelou GJ, Ticehurst JR, Purcell RH. Fecal excretion of Greek strains of hepatitis A virus in patients with hepatitis A and in experimentally infected chimpanzees. *J Infect Dis.* 1986;154:231-237.

61. Kao HW, Ashcavai M, Redeker AG. The persistence of hepatitis A IgM antibody after acute clinical hepatitis A. *Hepatology.* 1984;4:933-936.

62. Skinhoj P, Mikkelsen F, Hollinger FB. Hepatitis A in Greenland: importance of specific antibody testing in epidemiologic surveillance. *Am J Epidemiol.* 1977;105:140-147.

63. Cuthbert JA. Hepatitis A: old and new. *Clin Microbiol.* 2001;14:38-58.

64. Nainan OV, Xia G, Vaughan G, Margolis HS. Diagnosis of hepatitis A virus infection: a molecular approach. *Clin Microbiol Rev.* 2006;19:63-79.

65. Bell BP, Feinstone SM. Hepatitis A vaccine. In: Plotkin SA, Orenstein WA, Offit PA, eds. *Vaccine.* 4th ed. Philadelphia, PA: WB Saunders; 2004:269-297.

66. Centers for Disease Control and Prevention (CDC). Prevention of hepatitis A through active or passive immunization: recommendations of the Advisory Committee on Immunization Practices (ACIP). *MMWR Morb Mortal Wkly Rep.* 1999;48(RR-12):1-37.

67. Hollinger FB, Emerson SU. Hepatitis A virus. In: Knipe SM, Howley PM, eds. *Fields Virology.* 4th ed. New York, NY: Lippincott Williams & Wilkins; 2001:799-840.

68. Margolis HS. Viral hepatitis. In: Wallace RB, Doebbeling BN, eds. *Maxcy-Rosenau-Last Public Health and Preventive Medicine.* 14th ed. Stamford, CT: Appleton & Lange; 2000:174-188.

69. Centers for Disease Control and Prevention. Prevention of hepatitis A through active or passive immunization. Recommendations of the Advisory Committee on Immunization Practices (ACIP). *MMWR Morb Mortal Wkly Rep.* 2006;55(RR-07):1-23.

70. Centers for Disease Control and Prevention. A comprehensive immunization strategy to eliminate transmission of hepatitis B virus infection in the United States. Recommendations of the Advisory Committee on Immunization Practices (ACIP) Part II: immunization of adults. *MMWR Morb Mortal Wkly Rep.* 2006;55(RR-16):1-25.

71. Bond WW, Favero MS, Petersen NJ, et al. Survival of hepatitis B virus after drying and storage for one week. *Lancet.* 1981;1:550-551.

72. Davis GL. Hepatitis B: diagnosis and treatment. *South Med J.* 1997;90:866-870.

73. Neuschwander-Tetri BA. Common blood tests for liver disease. Which ones are most useful? *Postgrad Med.* 1995;98:49-56, 59, 63.

74. Krugman S, Overby LR, Mushahwar IK, et al. Viral hepatitis, type B. Studies on natural history and prevention re-examined. *N Engl J Med.* 1979;300:101-106.

75. Hoofnagle JH, DiBisceglie AM. Serologic diagnosis of acute and chronic viral hepatitis. *Semin Liver Dis.* 1991;11:73-83.

76. Biswas R, Tabor E, Hsia CC, et al. Comparative sensitivity of HBV NATs and HBsAg assays for detection of acute HBV infection. *Transfusion.* 2003;43:788-798.

77. Kloster B, Kramer R, Eastlund T, et al. Hepatitis B surface antigenemia in blood donors following vaccination. *Transfusion.* 1995;35:475-477.

78. Lunn ER, Hoggarth BJ, Cook WJ. Prolonged hepatitis B surface antigenemia after vaccination. *Pediatrics.* 2000;105:E81.

79. Kao JH, Chen PJ, Lai MY, Chen DS. Acute exacerbations of chronic hepatitis B are rarely associated with superinfection of hepatitis B virus. *Hepatology.* 2001;34(4 pt 1):817-823.

80. Kurstak C, Kurstak E, Hossain A. Progress in diagnosis of viral hepatitis A, B, C, D and E. *Acta Virol.* 1996;40:107-115.

81. Alward WL, McMahon BJ, Hall DB, et al. The long-term serological course of asymptomatic hepatitis B virus carriers and the development of primary hepatocellular carcinoma. *J Infect Dis.* 1985;151:604-609.

82. Liaw YF, Sheen IS, Chen TJ, et al. Incidence, determinants and significance of delayed clearance of serum HBsAg in chronic hepatitis B virus infection: a prospective study. *Hepatology.* 1991;13:627-631.

83. Adachi H, Kaneko S, Matsushita E, et al. Clearance of HBsAg in seven patients with chronic hepatitis B. *Hepatology.* 1992;16:1334-1337.

84. McMahon BJ, Holck P, Bulkow L, Snowball M. Serologic and clinical outcomes of 1536 Alaska Natives chronically infected with hepatitis B virus. *Ann Intern Med.* 2001;135:759-768.

85. Jalava T, Ranki M, Bengtström M, et al. A rapid and quantitative solution hybridization method for detection of HBV DNA in serum. *J Virol Methods.* 1992;36:171-180.

86. Malavé Lara C, Gorriño MT, Campelo C, et al. Detection of hepatitis B virus DNA in chronic carriers by the polymerase chain reaction. *Eur J Clin Microbiol Infect Dis.* 1992;11:740-744.

87. Aspinall S, Steele AD, Peenze I, Mphahlele MJ. Detection and quantitation of hepatitis B virus DNA: comparison of two commercial hybridization assays with polymerase chain reaction. *J Viral Hepatol.* 1995;2:107-111.

88. Fattovich G, Bortolotti F, Donato F. Natural history of chronic hepatitis B: special emphasis on disease progression and prognostic factors. *J Hepatol.* 2008;48:335-352.

89. Hadziyannis S, Papatheodoridis GV. Hepatitis B e antigen-negative chronic hepatitis: natural history and treatment. *Semin Liver Dis.* 2006;26:130-141.

90. EASL International Consensus Conference on Hepatitis B. Consensus statement. *J Hepatol.* 2003;38:533-540.

91. Perz JF, Armstrong GL, Farrington LA, et al. The contribution of hepatitis B virus and hepatitis C virus infections to cirrhosis and primary liver cancer worldwide. *J Hepatol.* 2006;45:529-538.

92. Lok ASF, McMahon BJ. Chronic hepatitis B. *Hepatology.* 2007;45:507-539.

93. Lok AS, McMahon BJ, Practice Guidelines Committee, American Association for the Study of Liver Disease (AASLD). Chronic hepatitis B. *Hepatology.* 2001;34:1225-1241.

94. Lok AS, McMahon BJ, Practice Guidelines Committee, American Association for the Study of Liver Disease (AASLD). Chronic hepatitis B: update of recommendations. *Hepatology.* 2004;39:857-861.

95. Bruix J, Sherman M, Practice Guidelines Committee, American Association for the Study of Liver Disease (AASLD). Management of hepatocellular carcinoma. *Hepatology*. 2005;42:1208-1236.

96. Purcell RH, Gerin JL. Hepatitis B subunit vaccine: a preliminary report of safety and efficacy tests in chimpanzees. *Am J Med Sci*. 1975;270:395-399.

97. Hilleman MR, McAleer WJ, Buynak EB, McLean AA. Quality and safety of human hepatitis B vaccine. *Dev Biol Stand*. 1983;54:3-12.

98. Alter MJ, Margolis HS, Krawczynski K, et al. The natural history of community-acquired hepatitis C in the United States. *N Engl J Med*. 1992;327:1899-1905.

99. Yen T, Keeffe EB, Ahmed A. The epidemiology of hepatitis C virus infections. *J Clin Gastroenterol*. 2003;36:47-53.

100. Koerner K, Cardoso M, Dengler T, et al. Estimated risk of transmission of hepatitis C virus by blood transfusion. *Vox Sang*. 1998;74:213-216.

101. Armstrong GL, Wasley A, Simard EP, et al. The prevalence of hepatitis C virus infection in the United States, 1999 through 2002. *Ann Intern Med*. 2006;144:705-714.

102. Holland PV. Post-transfusion hepatitis: current risks and causes. *Vox Sang*. 1998;74(suppl 2):135-141.

103. Rustgi VK. The epidemiology of hepatitis C infection in the United States. *J Gastroenterol*. 2007;42:513-521.

104. Strader DB, Wright T, Thomas DL, Seeff LB. American Association for the Study of Liver Diseases practice guideline: diagnosis, management, and treatment of hepatitis C. *Hepatology*. 2004;39:1147-1171.

105. Dal Molin G, Tiribelli C, Campello C. A rational use of laboratory tests in the diagnosis and management of hepatitis C virus infection. *Ann Hepatol*. 2003;2:76-83.

106. Pawlotsky J-M. Diagnostic testing in hepatitis C virus infection: viral kinetics and genomics. *Semin Liver Dis*. 2003;23(suppl 1):3-11.

107. Pawlotsky JM, Lonjon I, Hezode C, et al. What strategy should be used for diagnosis of hepatitis C virus infection in clinical laboratories? *Hepatology*. 1998;27:1700-1702.

108. Alter MJ, Kuhnert WL, Finelli L. Guidelines for laboratory testing and result reporting of antibody to hepatitis C virus. *MMWR Recomm Rep*. 2003;52(RR-03):1-16.

109. CDC. Recommendations for prevention and control of hepatitis C virus (HCV) infection and HCV-related chronic disease. *MMWR Recomm Rep*. 1998;47(RR-19):1-39.

110. Corrao G, Arico S. Independent and combined action of hepatitis C virus infection and alcohol consumption on the risk of symptomatic liver cirrhosis. *Hepatology*. 1994;20:1115-1120.

111. Seeff LB. The natural history of chronic hepatitis C virus infection. *Clin Liver Dis*. 1997;1:587-602.

112. Poynard T, Ratziu V, Charlotte F, et al. Rates and risk factors of liver fibrosis progression in patients with chronic hepatitis C. *J Hepatol*. 2001;34:730-739.

113. Forns X, Ampurdanès S, Sanchez-Tapias JM, et al. Long-term follow-up of chronic hepatitis C in patients diagnosed at a tertiary-care center. *J Hepatol*. 2001;35:265-271.

114. Mast EE, Kuramoto IK, Favorov MO, et al. Prevalence of and risk factors for antibody to hepatitis E virus seroreactivity among blood donors in Northern California. *J Infect Dis*. 1997;176:34-40.

115. Di Bisceglie AM, Frey S, Gorse GJ. A phase I safety and immunogenicity trial of a novel E1E2/MF59C.1 hepatitis C vaccine candidate in healthy HCV-negative adults [abstract]. *Hepatology*. 2005;42(suppl 1):750A.

116. Hadziyannis SJ. Decreasing prevalence of hepatitis D virus infection. *J Gastroenterol Hepatol*. 1997;12:745-746.

117. Farci P. Delta hepatitis: an update. *J Hepatol*. 2003;39(suppl 1):S212-S219.

118. Centers for Disease Control and Prevention. Hepatitis surveillance report. *MMWR Morb Mortal Wkly Rep*. 1990;53:23.

119. di Bisceglie AM. Interferon therapy for chronic viral hepatitis. *N Engl J Med*. 1994;330:137-138.

120. Sureau C, Moriarty AM, Thornton GB, et al. Production of infectious hepatitis delta virus in vitro and neutralization with antibodies directed against hepatitis B virus pre-S antigens. *J Virol*. 1992;66:1241-1245.

121. Taylor JM. The structure and replication of hepatitis delta virus. *Annu Rev Microbiol*. 1992;46:253-276.

122. Caredda F, d'Arminio Monforte A, Rossi E, et al. Prospective study of epidemic delta infection in drug addicts. *Prog Clin Biol Res*. 1983;143:245-250.

123. Wu JC, Chen TZ, Huang YS, et al. Natural history of hepatitis D viral superinfection: significance of viremia detected by polymerase chain reaction. *Gastroenterology*. 1995;108:796-802.

124. Macagno S, Smedile A, Caredda F, et al. Monomeric (7S) immunoglobulin M antibodies to hepatitis delta virus in hepatitis type D. *Gastroenterology*. 1990;98:1582-1586.

125. Hsieh TH, Liu CJ, Chen DS, Chen PJ. Natural course and treatment of hepatitis D virus infection. *J Formos Med Assoc*. 2006;105:869-881.

126. Mele A, Mariano A, Tosti ME, et al. Acute hepatitis delta virus infection in Italy: incidence and risk factors after the introduction of the universal anti-hepatitis B vaccination campaign. *Clin Infect Dis*. 2007;44:e17-e24.

127. Okamoto H. Genetic variability and evolution of hepatitis E virus. *Virus Res*. 2007;127:216-228.

128. Purcell RH. Hepatitis E virus. In: Fields BN, Knipe DM, Howley PM, eds. *Fields Virology*. 3rd ed. Philadelphia, PA: Lippincott-Raven; 1996:2831-2843.

129. Khuroo MS, Teli MR, Skidmore S, et al. Incidence and severity of viral hepatitis in pregnancy. *Am J Med*. 1981;70:252-255.

130. Ticehurst JR. Hepatitis E virus. In: Murray PR, Baron EJ, Pfaller MA, et al., eds. *Manual of Clinical Microbiology*. 7th ed. Washington, DC: American Society for Microbiology Press; 1999:1053-1069.

131. Panda SK, Thakral D, Rehman S. Hepatitis E virus. *Rev Med Virol*. 2007;17:151-180.

132. Harrison TJ. Hepatitis E virus: an update. *Liver*. 1999;19:171-176.

133. Frider B, Sookoian S, Castaño G, et al. Detection of hepatitis G virus RNA in patients with acute non-A-E hepatitis. *J Viral Hepat*. 1998;5:161-164.

134. Loya F. Does the hepatitis G virus cause hepatitis? *Tex Med*. 1996;92:68-73.

135. Doo EC, Lian TJ, Shiffs ER, et al. The hepatitis viruses. In: Schiff ER, Sorrell MF, Maddrey WC, eds. *Schiff's Diseases of the Liver*. Philadelphia, PA: Lippincott Williams & Wilkins; 2003:917-940.

136. Alter HJ, Umemura T, Tanaka Y. Putative new hepatitis virus. In: Schiff ER, Sorrell MF, Maddrey WC, eds. *Schiff's Diseases of the Liver*. Philadelphia, PA: Lippincott Williams & Wilkins; 2003:891-905.

Laboratory Markers of Cardiac Damage and Function

MICHAEL DURANDO, BRIAN C. JENSEN, MONTE S. WILLIS

CHAPTER 26

CHAPTER OUTLINE

Chapter Objectives

Upon completion of this chapter, the clinical laboratorian should be able to do the following:

- Diagram the anatomy of the heart.
- Explain the origin of general symptoms of cardiac disease.
- Discuss the etiology and physiologic effects of the following cardiac conditions:
  - Congenital heart disease
  - Hypertensive heart disease
  - Infectious heart diseases
  - Coronary heart disease
  - Congestive heart failure

- Identify risk factors for coronary heart disease.
- List features of an ideal cardiac marker.
- List and briefly describe three novel markers of inflammation currently under investigation.
- Compare and contrast the specificity and sensitivity of the most commonly used serum cardiac markers.
- Assess the clinical utility of the various cardiac markers to assess myocardial infarction.
- Analyze the role of the clinical laboratory in the assessment of a patient with cardiac disease.

KEY TERMS

Acute coronary syndromes
Angina pectoris
Arrhythmias
Atherosclerosis
Cardiac markers
CK-MB
Congestive heart failure
Creatine kinase (CK)

D-Dimer
Heart-type fatty acid–binding protein
Homocysteine
Ischemia-modified albumin
Myocardial infarction
Myocarditis
Myoglobin
Troponin I (TnI)
Troponin T (TnT)

Cardiovascular disease (CVD) commonly occurs in the general population and affects the majority of people older than 60 years. This includes four major types of CVD based on the location in which it occurs: (1) coronary heart disease (CHD); (2) cerebrovascular disease; (3) peripheral arterial disease; and (4) aortic atherosclerotic disease. CHD manifests as myocardial infarction (MI) (heart attack), angina pectoris (chest pain), heart failure, and sudden cardiac death. Cerebrovascular disease manifests as a stroke or transient ischemic attack (short, "reversible strokes"), while peripheral arterial disease manifests by intermittent claudication (acute localized pain to the arms and legs). Aortic atherosclerosis manifests as aneurysms (abnormal widening of an artery) or dissection (tears in thoracic or abdominal aorta), which are acute life-threatening events. There are common themes in the pathogenesis of these CVDs, including the presence of atherosclerosis, which increases the likelihood of ischemia (lack of blood supply) localized to different parts of the body. CHD, in which atherosclerosis and ischemia are localized to the vasculature of the heart, accounts for one-third of the total cases of CVD. The critical role of laboratory testing in diagnosing CHD will be the focus of this chapter.

One of the most common reasons people go to the emergency department is for the acute onset of chest pain. While nearly 7 million people end up in emergency departments for this reason, only 15% to 25% of them actually have acute coronary syndrome (ACS) resulting from CHD.[1,2] There are a number of non-cardiac reasons for having chest pain, including common maladies such as esophageal reflux ("heart burn") due to stomach acid moving retrograde into the esophagus. It is critical to differentiate cardiac from non-cardiac causes, but differentiating patients with ACS or other life-threatening conditions from patients with non–life-threatening diseases from non-cardiac causes is challenging. This is evidenced by the fact that the diagnosis of ACS is missed in ~2% of patients, which results in substantial morbidity and mortality.[2] Several advances in risk-stratifying patients with chest pain have been made, including better laboratory markers of cardiac injury,[3] which allows for rapid identification of those patients whose chest pain is due to CHD. Such patients benefit from rapid initiation of therapy directed at ACS. Patients without elevated cardiac markers are typically at lower risk and may undergo further evaluation of the cause of their symptoms, including through radionuclide imaging and computed tomography (CT).

The lack of an adequate blood supply to the heart leads to ischemia. Since the heart depends upon a constant supply of oxygen and nutrients supplied by the coronary arteries, any disruption in the balance of oxygen supply and cardiac demand puts the heart at serious risk. Adequate supply of blood to the heart is compromised by a number of factors, most commonly the formation of a thrombus in the context of underlying atherosclerosis, which is the underlying cause for myocardial infarction (narrowing of the coronary arteries). Atherosclerosis is a chronic process involving damage to the endothelium and the buildup of cholesterol-rich lesions that threaten to occlude the vasculature.

CARDIAC ISCHEMIA, ANGINA, AND HEART ATTACKS

Cardiac ischemia can lead to activity-related chest pain (stable angina) or an ACS. Stable angina predictably occurs with a given amount of activity and resolves with rest, whereas ACS frequently occurs unpredictably and does not respond to cessation of activity. ACS is further classified as unstable angina or the more severe acute MI, also known as a heart attack. Cardiac biomarkers are normal in the setting of unstable angina, but elevated in MI. The "classic" manifestation of cardiac ischemia is angina, described as a squeezing of the chest, heavy chest pressure, a burning feeling, or difficulty breathing.[4] This "classic" manifestation often radiates to the left shoulder, neck, or arm and typically increases in intensity over a period of minutes and gets worse with either physical or psychological stress. However, the symptoms often arise in the absence of situations that precipitate it. Non-classic symptoms, more commonly experienced by women, include a more stabbing, pulsating, or sharp chest pain rather than the typical vise-like pressure, nausea, shortness of breath, or abdominal pain.[5-7] In addition to these heart-related symptoms, the American Heart Association (AHA) and the American College of Cardiology (ACC) have also defined chest-related symptoms that are not indicative of cardiac involvement (see Table 26-1).

Guidelines from the ACC and the AHA recommend that patients be evaluated in person at an emergency department or a specialized chest pain unit when patients experience chest discomfort at rest for longer than 20 minutes.[8] Patients with syncope (loss of consciousness), near syncope, or hemodynamic instability (e.g., changes in blood pressure) in the setting of chest pain should also be evaluated.[8] If a patient does not need immediate intervention because of circulatory collapse (i.e., they are conscious), a history is taken to evaluate the chest pain for its likelihood

TABLE 26-1	SYMPTOMS NOT RELATED TO CARDIAC ISCHEMIA-INDUCED ANGINA (CHEST PAIN)[8]
Pleuritic pain (sharp/knife-like pain brought on by respiratory movements/cough)	
Primary/sole location in the abdomen	
Pain localized at the tip of one finger, particularly over the apex of the heart	
Pain reproducible by the movement/palpitation of the arms or chest wall	
Constant pain that lasts for many hours	
Very brief episodic pain for a few seconds or less	
Pain radiating to the lower extremities	

of being an MI. Risk factors for atherosclerosis should also be solicited, including advanced age, male gender, diabetes, and any previous history of MI. Younger patients with a low risk of ACS should be carefully screened for cocaine use, as it can cause vascular spasm of the coronary arteries, resulting in ischemia and chest pain.[8]

Patients with chest pain are initially evaluated by a physical examination, an electrocardiogram (ECG), a chest x-ray, and the detection of biomarkers by laboratory tests. The physical examination identifies possible causes of precipitating myocardial ischemia (high blood pressure, pulmonary disease, and heart failure or cardiac valve disease)[8] and may identify a non-cardiac cause for the symptom. An ECG should be obtained within the first 10 minutes after presentation for further risk stratification. The presence of new or transient changes (>1 mm) in the ST-segment of the ECG is strongly suggestive of acute ischemia.[8] Less specific ST-segment changes or T wave abnormalities can also be helpful in risk-stratifying patients.[8] A normal ECG, however, does not rule out the presence of ACS. Chest radiography can also assist in the evaluation of a patient with chest pain by identifying a non-cardiac source of the pain (e.g., pneumonia, pneumothorax, and aortic dissection) or sequelae of underlying cardiac causes (e.g., pulmonary edema caused by cardiac dysfunction).[8]

The use of biomarkers is critical in the evaluation of acute chest pain to identify angina (chest pain) as an MI (heart attack). Universal definitions of MI were recently published in 2008 outlining the consensus reached by the joint European Society of Cardiology/ACC/AHA/World Health Federation Task Force (see Table 26-2). These

CASE STUDY 26-1

A 15-month-old girl with a heart murmur since birth was evaluated for repeated pulmonary infections, failure to grow, cyanosis, and mild clubbing of fingers and toes. She had been on digitalis therapy by the referring physician. The radiograph showed a moderately enlarged heart and an enlarged pulmonary artery. Pertinent laboratory data were obtained.

Total protein (6.0–8.3 g/dL)	5.4
Albumin (3.5–5.2 g/dL)	3.0
Hemoglobin (14–18 g/dL)	19.2
Hematocrit (40–54%)	59
Erythrocyte count (4.3–5.7 × 10^6/mm^3)	6.4

A cardiac catheterization was performed, and a large ventricular septal defect was found.

Questions

1. How does this congenital defect affect the body's circulation?

2. Why are the red cell measurements increased in this patient?

3. What treatment will be suggested for this patient?

4. What is this patient's prognosis?

TABLE 26-2	UNIVERSAL DEFINITION OF MYOCARDIAL INFARCTION RELEASED BY THE JOINT EUROPEAN SOCIETY OF CARDIOLOGY/AMERICAN COLLEGE OF CARDIOLOGY/ AMERICAN HEART ASSOCIATION/WORLD HEALTH FEDERATION TASK FORCE (2007)[9]

ANY ONE OF THE FOLLOWING:

1. Typical rise and fall of troponin with at least one value above the 99th percentile of the URL, plus one of the following:
   a. Ischemic symptoms
   b. Development of pathologic Q waves on ECG
   c. ECG changes indicative of ischemia (ST-segment changes)
   d. Coronary artery intervention

2. Sudden, unexplained cardiac death before blood samples can be obtained or before biomarkers can appear in the blood, and accompanied by evidence of symptoms, ECG, coronary angiogram, or autopsy

3. For PCI[a] patients with normal baseline troponin levels, troponin >99th percentile of URL[c] are indicative of peri-procedural myocardial necrosis

4. For CABG[b] patients with normal baseline, troponin >99th percentile of URL[c] is indicative of peri-procedural myocardial necrosis

5. Pathologic findings of an acute MI

ECG, electrocardiogram.
[a]PCI, percutaneous coronary intervention (also known as "coronary angioplasty" or "angioplasty").
[b]CABG, coronary artery bypass graft (also known as "bypass surgery").
[c]URL, upper reference limit.

TABLE 26-3	CLASSIFICATION OF MYOCARDIAL INFARCTION ACCORDING TO THE UNIVERSAL DEFINITION OF MYOCARDIAL INFARCTION RELEASED BY THE JOINT EUROPEAN SOCIETY OF CARDIOLOGY/AMERICAN COLLEGE OF CARDIOLOGY/AMERICAN HEART ASSOCIATION/WORLD HEALTH FEDERATION TASK FORCE (2007)[9]
Type 1:	Spontaneous MI related to ischemia due to a primary coronary event such as plaque erosion and/or rupture, fissuring, or dissection.
Type 2:	MI secondary to ischemia due to either increased oxygen demand or decreased supply, e.g., coronary artery spasm, coronary embolism, anemia, **arrhythmias**, hypertension, and hypotension.
Type 3:	Sudden unexpected cardiac death, including cardiac arrest, often with symptoms suggestive of MI, accompanied by presumably new ST elevation, or new LBBB[a] or evidence of fresh thrombus in a coronary artery by angiography and/or at autopsy, but death occurring before blood samples could be obtained, or at a time before the appearance of cardiac biomarkers in the blood.
Type 4a:	MI associated with PCI[b].
Type 4b:	MI associated with stent thrombosis as documented by angiography or at autopsy.
Type 5:	MI associated with CABG[c].

MI, myocardial infarction.
[a]LBBB, left bundle branch block.
[b]PCI, percutaneous coronary intervention (also known as "coronary angioplasty" or "angioplasty").
[c]CABG, coronary artery bypass graft (also known as "bypass surgery").

guidelines emphasized the use of the term MI only in the setting of myocardial ischemia and not as a result of any other cause[9] and designated several types of MI (Table 26-3). It also emphasized the role of troponin testing in the diagnosis of MI and recommended a more stringent cutoff value (99th percentile of upper range limit). The use of cardiac imaging was also included in the criteria to help aid in the classification of the different classes of MI.

THE PATHOPHYSIOLOGY OF ATHEROSCLEROSIS, THE DISEASE PROCESS UNDERLYING MI

Atherosclerosis is a chronic disease process that occurs over a number of years and contributes to approximately 50% of all deaths in modern Western societies.[10] Evidence of atherosclerosis can often be found in the human aorta before the age of 10,[11] but atherosclerosis becomes pathologic with the development of atherosclerotic plaques (atheromas), which predispose the vasculature to thrombosis, leading to organ ischemia and infarction (Fig. 26-1). The pathophysiology of atherosclerosis is gradual and complicated, involving a progressive accumulation of lipids, smooth muscle cells, macrophages, and connective tissue within the intima of large- and medium-sized arteries, ultimately causing luminal narrowing and decreased perfusion (Fig. 26-1). Although the exact etiology of atherosclerosis remains unclear, the *reaction to injury* hypothesis is strongly favored by current evidence, proposing that atherosclerosis is due to a chronic inflammatory response to an accumulation of subtle vascular wall injuries.[12]

Pathohistological evidence from human and experimental studies demonstrates that endothelial and

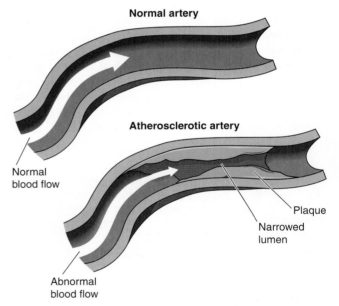

FIGURE 26-1 Comparison of normal and atherosclerotic arteries. Narrowing the arterial lumen due to atherosclerotic plaque leads to abnormal blood flow, contributing to progression of atherosclerosis (adapted from NHLBI Atherosclerosis homepage, http://www.nhlbi.nih.gov/health/health-topics/topics/atherosclerosis/).

inflammatory cells interact with chemical and inflammatory mediators to promote the development of atherosclerotic plaques. This process begins with vascular injury, which is initiated when endothelial cells are damaged or rendered dysfunctional by vascular abnormalities, such as turbulent blood flow, hyperlipidemia, and hyperhomocysteinemia. A damaged vascular endothelium has an increased permeability to circulating lipids, so having high cholesterol (hyperlipidemia) in the wake of a damaged endothelium favors the accumulation of lipoproteins, predominantly low-density lipoprotein (LDL) and very low density lipoprotein (VLDL), within the arterial intima (Fig. 26-1).[13] In addition, apoB-containing LDL has high affinity for arterial wall proteoglycans.[14] Retention of lipids in arterial walls due to hypercholesterolemia and/or elevated levels of apoB-containing lipoproteins is thus a crucial step in the pathogenesis of atherosclerotic lesions. The central role of cholesterol accumulation (i.e., LDL and VLDL) in the progression of atherosclerosis is the reason treating high cholesterol is such a priority in preventing and attenuating heart disease.

Once lesion initiation has begun, LDL deposited within the intima is oxidized by endothelial cells, lipoxygenase, and free radicals generated by the auto-oxidation of homocysteine.[11] The formation of oxidized LDL is central to lesion progression. Oxidized LDL is toxic to endothelial cells, causing additional intimal damage and subsequent retention of cholesterol-rich lipoproteins, and it elicits an inflammatory response that releases pro-inflammatory cytokines and recruits inflammatory cells to the early lesion. Among the earliest recruited leukocytes are neutrophils and monocytes, which play critical roles in early atherogenesis by maintaining a pro-inflammatory state around the initial lesion (Fig. 26-2).[10]

Maturation of monocytes into activated macrophages is a key step in lesion progression. Macrophage scavenger receptors recognize oxidized LDL, but not native LDL, and activated macrophages rapidly phagocytose cholesterol-rich lipoproteins that have been oxidized within the vessel wall (Fig. 26-2).[11] Excessive uptake of oxidized LDL transforms macrophages into bloated, cholesterol-filled cells called *foam cells*.[15] Filled with cytoplasmic lipid droplets, foam cells exhibit a variety of functions that both promote lesion progression, including the production of pro-inflammatory signals, and counter lesion progression, such as the secretion of HDL (Fig. 26-2). Foam cells also display numerous metabolic abnormalities, including activation of inflammasomes and the NF-κB pathway, and it is generally agreed that foam cells play a harmful role in lesion progression.[15] In addition, rupture of foam cells and release of their contents cause further damage to the vascular endothelium, stimulating more inflammation. Intimal deposition and subsequent oxidation of LDL and its effects on monocyte differentiation are thus of key importance in the early development of an atherosclerotic lesion.

As the cycle of endothelial cell damage progresses, additional cell types are recruited to the plaque, in particular T and B lymphocytes and macrophages (Fig. 26-3). These cells are activated by a stream of cytokines, such as interleukin (IL)-1 and tumor necrosis factor-α, that are released by endothelial cells within the plaque.[16]

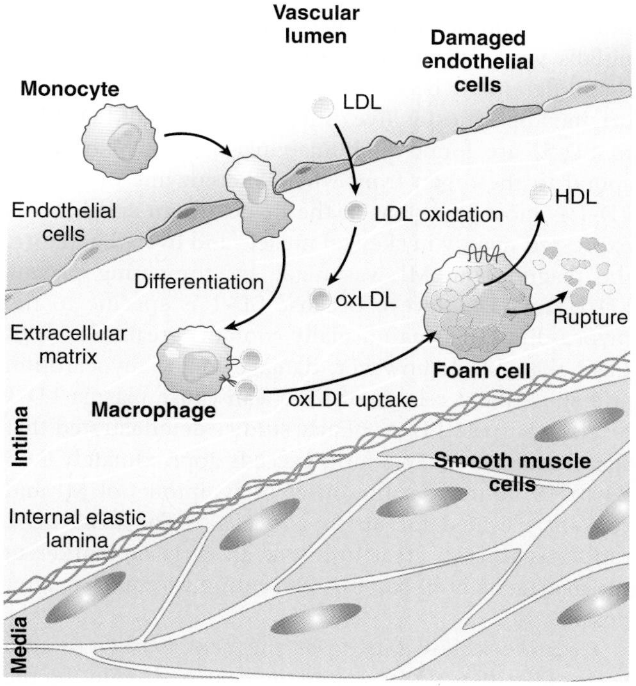

FIGURE 26-2 LDL deposition and oxidation within the vessel wall leads to monocyte recruitment and differentiation into activated macrophages that phagocytose oxidized LDL (oxLDL) to become foam cells. Foam cells release HDL and pro-inflammatory mediators and their rupture contributes to lesion progression. Adapted from Glass and Witztum.[10]

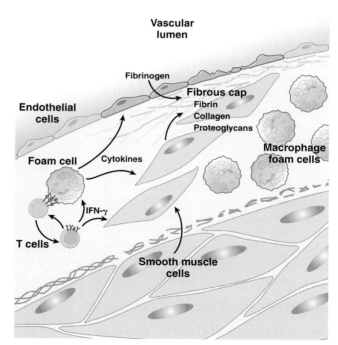

FIGURE 26-3 T cells and foam cells maintain a pro-inflammatory state that induces the migration of smooth muscle cells into the intima, where they secrete collagen, proteoglycans, and fibrin that form a fibrous cap around the atheroma. Adapted from Glass and Witztum.[10]

Interactions between T cells and foam cells promote a chronic inflammatory state and help recruit smooth muscle cells into the intima (Fig. 26-3).[10] Additionally, growth factors, such as platelet-derived growth factor, fibroblast growth factor, and tissue growth factor-α, are released by lymphocytes and endothelial cells, further stimulating smooth muscle cell migration and activation.[16]

Once smooth muscle cells migrate into the core of the atheroma, they proliferate and deposit extracellular matrix components that give stability and strength to the plaque.[10] Cytokines released from T cells, such as interferon-γ, exert a number of both pro- and anti-atherogenic effects on macrophages and smooth muscle cells, but the net effect of this cytokine release is pro-inflammatory and pro-atherogenic. Smooth muscle cells are induced to secrete collagen, elastin, and proteoglycans that form a fibrous backbone and outer shell that fix the plaque firmly in the vessel wall (Fig. 26-3). As the atheroma grows, its core becomes increasingly isolated from surrounding blood supply, leading to hypoxia that stimulates release of pro-angiogenic cytokines. This causes aberrant neovascularization around the periphery of the plaque, which predisposes to hemorrhage and deposition of erythrocyte components, such as hemosiderin and lipids, within the plaque core.[17] Microvasculature hemorrhage and subsequent deposition of additional debris provokes further inflammation, leukocyte recruitment, and remodeling of the plaque.

The steps described above—beginning with lipid and cellular infiltration following vascular injury and progressing to chronic inflammation and fibrosis—continue in a feed-forward cycle that ultimately culminates in complete vessel occlusion, thrombosis, plaque rupture, or some combination of the three. Each of these possible outcomes predisposes to organ ischemia. In the context of the heart, coronary artery ischemia and resultant hypoxia pose an immediate risk of cellular injury due to the high metabolic activity and oxygen demand of the myocardium. The ultimate outcome of such injury is ischemic heart disease, varying in severity from angina to MI, the symptoms of which are dependent on the extent of coronary artery atherosclerosis. The most common locations for symptomatic cardiac atheroma formation are the proximal left anterior descending, the proximal left main coronary, and the entire right coronary arteries. Coronary atherosclerosis typically becomes symptomatic only after atherosclerotic plaques obstruct approximately 75% (or >50% in the left main) of the cross-sectional area of the vessel.[10]

MARKERS OF CARDIAC DAMAGE

Initial Markers of Cardiac Damage

The first biochemical markers of cardiac damage were discovered in 1954 when Karmen et al.[18] hypothesized that "destruction of cardiac muscle, reported rich in transaminase activity, might result in a release of this enzyme into the blood stream and might thus increase the serum transaminase activity." Today, serum biomarkers have become the centerpiece of evaluation and management of patients presenting with chest pain. The underlying principle behind serum biomarkers of cardiac damage relies on the fact that cell death releases intracellular proteins from the myocardium into the circulation. Detection of cardiac proteins in plasma provides insight into the occurrence, extent, and timing of MI, all of which are critical for proper medical management.

The first cardiac markers to be used extensively in clinical practice were glutamic oxaloacetic transaminase, lactic dehydrogenase, and malic dehydrogenase. The first, glutamic oxaloacetic transaminase, now known as aspartate transaminase (AST), became widely used in the diagnosis of MI shortly after its discovery as a serum marker by Ladue et al. in 1954.[19] But because of the high false-negative rate of AST, the labor-intensive nature of the AST assay, and the short window of AST elevation, AST was soon replaced by lactate dehydrogenase (LD) as the marker of choice.[20]

Compared with AST, LD was found to be a more sensitive marker of MI that remains elevated for significantly longer post-MI, up to 2 weeks. But LD is involved in NADH-dependent reactions in the glycolytic pathway, which takes place in nearly all cells in the body, and its specificity to cardiac muscle is thus quite low. Early researchers observed that serum LD levels were elevated in other conditions such as cancer and anemia.[20] These pitfalls were overcome to some extent through assays that differentiate between LD of cardiac and non-cardiac origin.[21] Specifically, five different isoforms of LD (LD-1 to LD-5) are found in human plasma,[22] which correspond to the organ from where the enzyme originates. LD-1 is most abundant in the myocardium and LD-5 is expressed mainly in skeletal muscle and liver. Therefore, the diagnosis of MI was made by comparing plasma LD-1 and LD-2 levels. Because LD-1 is specific to the myocardium, plasma normally contains greater levels of LD-2 than LD-1; however, damage to the myocardium and subsequent release of LD-1 can cause plasma LD-1 levels to surpass LD-2.[23] Early studies demonstrated that the plasma LD-1:LD-2 ratio exceeds approximately 0.75 24 to 48 hours past the onset of symptoms of MI and remains elevated for up to 2 weeks.[23] The LD-1:LD-2 ratio was thus of great utility as an early biomarker in the management of patients presenting several days after possible MI.

Creatine kinase (CK) was the next marker to gain favor. Like LD, CK is found in nearly all cells in the body, but unlike LD, CK catalyzes a reaction important for high-energy phosphate production (the conversion of creatine to creatine phosphate), which is greatly upregulated in the muscle cells and brain. High levels of

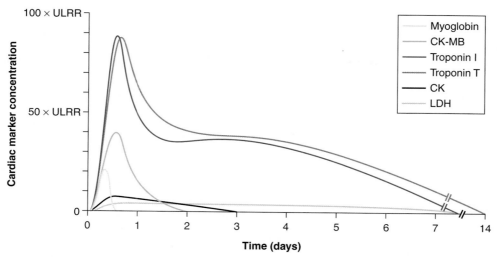

FIGURE 26-4 Temporal elevations of important markers of myocardial damage post-MI. ULRR, upper limit of reference range. Adapted from French and White.[26]

CK are thus found in all muscle cells, in particular striated muscle. Damage to the muscle or brain results in rapidly detectable increases in plasma CK, which can be readily detected in plasma with a high sensitivity at short times after muscle injury. After the discovery in 1960 of elevated levels of plasma CK post-MI,[24] CK became an important marker of cardiac damage. In a typical patient with acute MI, serum CK levels were found to exceed the normal range within 6 to 8 hours, to reach a peak of two- to ten-fold normal by 24 hours, and then decline to the normal range after 3 to 4 days (Fig. 26-4).[25] A CK plasma concentration greater than two times normal was shown to correlate with MI,[27] and an elevation in serum CK, together with elevated AST and LD, was used as the primary means of enzymatic detection of MI for many years.

Unfortunately, the ubiquitous expression of CK in all striated muscle was a problem for specificity of CK as a marker for MI, in spite of its high sensitivity. CK elevations were readily detected in conditions such as stroke, pulmonary disease, and chronic alcoholism and after strenuous exercise.[28] This obstacle was initially overcome through the discovery that CK exists in three cytoplasmic isoenzymes. The cytoplasmic isoenzymes are dimers composed of combinations of M and B subunits (where M is for muscle and B is for brain). Dimers of 2 M subunits are called CK-MM, 2 B subunits as CK-BB, and 1 M and 1 B subunit as creatine kinase MB (CK-MB). Elevated plasma levels of CK-MM or CK-BB can be found after injury to the muscle or brain, respectively. After it was found that 15% to 30% of CK in the myocardium is MB, compared with 1% to 3% in normal striated muscle, detection of elevated CK-MB was shown to be highly specific to myocardial damage.[29] Additionally, elevations in serum CK-MB could be detected at 4 to 6 hours after the onset of MI symptoms, significantly less than the 24 to 48 hours necessary

to detect peak LD plasma levels (Fig. 26-4). Like its rapid rise post-MI, CK-MB levels quickly drop to baseline levels by 2 to 4 days post-MI, compared with 10 to 14 days for LD.[30] Because of its higher specificity and its rapid elevation post-MI, CK-MB was long considered the most reliable serum marker of MI and is still widely used today.[31,32]

Use of these three markers—AST, LD, and CK—was the cornerstone of post-MI management for several decades. Each had its individual applications: CK for the early presentation, LD for the late presentation, and AST for the intermediate.[33] But their lack of specificity to the myocardium and to myocardial injury fueled the search for better markers. Extensive research in the 1970s led to the discovery that muscle cells express structural and regulatory proteins, such as troponin and tropomyosin, in a pattern that is tissue-specific.[32] The subsequent development of rapid and sensitive techniques for detection of the tissue-specific forms of troponin quickly made troponin a promising marker of cardiac injury.[34]

Cardiac Troponins

Troponin is a complex of three proteins that regulate the calcium-dependent interactions of myosin heads with actin filaments during striated muscle contraction. Troponin T (TnT) binds the troponin complex to tropomyosin, troponin I (TnI) inhibits the binding of actin and myosin, and troponin C (TnC) binds to calcium to reverse the inhibitory activity of TnI.[35] The troponin complex is responsible for transmitting the calcium signal that triggers muscle contraction (Fig. 26-5). Several properties of troponin made it attractive as a marker of myocardial damage.

In contrast to other cardiac markers, troponins were found to have tissue-specific isoforms that could be used

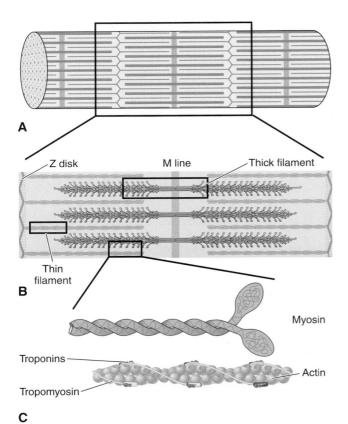

FIGURE 26-5 Regulatory proteins in the contractile apparatus of striated muscle. Striated muscle is composed of bundles of myofibril-containing fibers, made up of repeating units of cross-striations called sarcomeres **(A)**. The sarcomere is composed of thick and thin myofilaments, which tether the Z-disk to the M line **(B)**. Thick filaments are composed primarily of large molecules of myosin, which have a rod-like tail region and a protruding head region **(C)**. Thin filaments are composed of actin, which plays a structural role, and troponin and tropomyosin, which line actin filaments and regulate calcium-dependent interactions with myosin on thick filaments to stimulate contraction.

to detect damage to the heart. Although the same isoform of TnC is expressed in slow-twitch (type 2) and cardiac muscle, unique isoforms of TnI and TnT are expressed in fast-twitch (type 1), slow-twitch, and cardiac muscle.[35] Each TnI, TnT, and TnC isoform is encoded by a separate gene and expressed in a muscle-type–specific manner.[36] This allows for highly specific detection of troponin of cardiac origin (e.g., cardiac TnI [cTnI]). Further increasing the sensitivity of troponin detection was the demonstration that cardiac troponins are very tightly complexed to the contractile apparatus, such that circulating levels of cardiac troponins are normally extremely low.[35] Early studies demonstrated that normal levels of circulating cTnI are below 10 ng/mL, but patients with acute MI can have serum cTnI levels well over 100 ng/mL,[37] demonstrating the specificity of cardiac troponins as indicators of myocardial cell damage.

The development of sensitive detection methods was the next step toward integrating cardiac troponins into the diagnostic workup of MI. Because the skeletal and cardiac isoforms of TnT and TnI contain differing amino acid sequences, monoclonal antibodies can be raised against cardiac-specific epitopes. This allowed for the development of sensitive immunoassays for cardiac troponins that have a far greater specificity than other markers. For example, detection of cTnI was specific for cardiac injury even in acute muscle disease, chronic muscle disease, chronic renal failure, and following intense exercise, such as running a marathon.[38] Additionally, measurement of plasma troponin levels allows for the detection of myocardial cell injury in syndromes, such as acute ischemic syndrome or myocarditis, that is undetectable using other markers.[39]

Finally, troponins offer additional advantages due to the timing of their release. CK-MB levels elevate rapidly post-MI (4 to 6 hours) but return to baseline after 2 to 4 days; CK-MB can thus only be used within a short window of time after a suspected MI. Conversely, LD levels remain elevated for up to 1 week but are not detectable until 24 to 48 hours post-MI (Fig. 26-4). Cardiac troponins, on the other hand, are detectable in the plasma at 3 to 12 hours after myocardial injury, peaking at 12 to 24 hours and remaining elevated for more than 1 week: 8 to 21 days for TnT and 7 to 14 days for TnI (Fig. 26-4).[39] Cardiac troponins thus offer the widest window for detection post-MI, and with the highest sensitivity and specificity.

Taken together, the characteristics of specific, sensitive, and rapid detection propelled cardiac troponins to the center of MI diagnosis, where they still remain. Cardiac troponin (I or T) is currently the preferred biomarker for myocardial necrosis, recognized to have nearly absolute myocardial tissue specificity as well as high clinical sensitivity, detecting even minor cardiac damage (as utilized in the universal definition of MI).[9] An elevated plasma cardiac troponin level is defined as a measurement greater than the 99th percentile of a normal reference value range, specified as the upper limit of the reference range (Fig. 26-4). Current guidelines recommend drawing blood for the measurement of troponin as soon as possible after onset of symptoms of a possible MI (universal definition of MI).[9] If troponin assays are not available, the next best alternative is CK-MB, and measurement of total CK is no longer recommended for the diagnosis of MI for the reasons outlined above (universal definition of MI).[9]

Other Markers of Cardiac Damage

In spite of the nearly universal use of troponin and CK-MB in diagnosing cardiac damage, it is worthwhile mentioning additional markers of cardiac damage that have been used in the past and/or proposed experimentally. These include **myoglobin, heart-type fatty acid–binding protein (H-FABP), ischemia-modified albumin (IMA), myeloperoxidase (MPO), C-reactive protein (CRP),**

CASE STUDY 26-2

A 59-year-old woman came to the emergency department of a local hospital complaining of pain and a feeling of heaviness in her abdomen for several days. She reported no weakness, chest pain, or left arm pain. She has no chronic health problems except for seasonal allergies and slightly elevated total cholesterol.

CARDIAC ENZYMES	8:30 PM, APRIL 11	6:30 AM, APRIL 12
Total CK (54–186 U/L)	170	106
CK-MB (0–5 ng/mL)	6.3	3.8
% CK-MB (<6%)	3.7	3.6
Myoglobin (<70 µg/L)	52	41
Troponin T (0–0.1 µg/L)	0.8	2.3

Questions

1. Do the symptoms and personal history of this patient suggest acute MI?

2. Based on the preceding laboratory data, would this diagnosis be acute MI?

3. Why or why not?

myeloid-related protein (MRP)-8/14, and pregnancy-associated plasma protein-A (PAPP-A). While their clinical utility has not been universally established, they are discussed frequently as potential alternatives, so they have been discussed here briefly.

Myoglobin

Myoglobin is an iron- and oxygen-binding protein found exclusively in the muscle and is normally absent from the circulation. The myoglobin found in the muscle forms pigments, giving the muscle its characteristic red color. The exact color of the muscle depends on the oxidation state of the iron atom in myoglobin and the amount of oxygen attached to it. Myoglobin is a small protein, which is released quickly when the muscle is damaged (see Fig. 26-4 for serum release pattern).[40] It has a very short half-life of 9 minutes.[41] Because myoglobin is released so quickly, it has been proposed as an adjunct marker for troponin or CK-MB in the early diagnosis of MI.[42] There are limitations to using myoglobin as a marker of cardiac damage. It is not specific for the heart, being elevated with any cause of skeletal muscle damage, and is cleared in an irregular pattern.[43] Recent studies have also shown that high sensitivity troponin assays can detect elevated troponin levels prior to elevations in myoglobin,[44-46] making myoglobin's use less attractive.

Heart-Type Fatty Acid–Binding Protein

H-FABP is a small protein, which behaves much like myoglobin in its kinetics and release. It is found in all muscles, but in contrast to myoglobin, H-FABP is found relatively more abundantly in the heart.[47] The utility of H-FABP has been described for the diagnosis of early acute MI. The sensitivity for the diagnosis of an acute MI has been reported to be higher than cardiac TnT (cTnT) or myoglobin.[48] However, cTnT has a higher specificity than H-FABP (94% vs. 52%) indicating that elevated H-FABP was found in patients without disease.[48] Recent studies have confirmed the utility of using both H-FABP and cTnI for the early diagnosis of MI/ACS.[49] Using both markers may also be a valuable rule-out test for patients presenting between 3 and 6 hours after chest pain,[49] though H-FABP is not used in the routine evaluation of chest pain.

Ischemia-Modified Albumin

In contrast to the markers described above that detect myocardial tissue damage, the IMA test does not. Instead it measures changes that occur in albumin in the presence of ischemia, giving it the advantage that it might detect ischemia before damage has occurred to the heart. The free radical formation that occurs during tissue ischemia is believed to modify albumin within minutes of ischemia and lasts for about 6 hours.[50-53] These modifications in albumin alter its ability to bind transition metals, such as cobalt, by its N-terminal domain.[52] The amount of IMA is measured by the spectrophotometric determination of albumin's binding to cobalt.[50] While IMA is not specific for cardiac damage, it does have a clinical sensitivity for ACS of 50% to 90%.[54,55] Additional studies will be necessary to determine the utility of IMA in the early diagnosis of ACS; its use will complement, not replace, troponin and CK-MB detection.

Novel Markers of Plaque Instability: MPO, CRP, MRP-8/14, and PAPP-A

MPO, CRP, MRP-8/14, and PAPP-A have been studied in international multicenter studies for their utility in the early diagnosis and risk stratification of acute MI in emergency departments in patients with acute chest pain.[56] The concentration of all four markers was significantly higher in patients with acute MI compared with patients with other diagnoses.[56] But these markers were all inferior to troponins in detecting acute MI.[56] MPO, MRP-8/14, and CRP were able to predict all-cause mortality and these provided independent prognostic information apart from clinical risk factors and high-sensitive cTnT; PAPP-A did not.[56] Interestingly, these plaque instability markers did not correlate with each other or myocardial cell death determined by troponin.[56] The exact mechanisms leading to plaque instability, plaque fissure, and subsequent rupture are not fully understood, but all are expressed in atherosclerotic plaques and contribute to vessel inflammation.[57-60]

CASE STUDY 26-3

An 83-year-old man with known severe coronary artery disease, diffuse small vessel disease, and significant stenosis distal to a vein graft from previous CABG surgery was admitted when his physician referred him to the hospital after a routine office visit. His symptoms included 3+ pedal edema, jugular vein distention, and heart sound abnormalities. Significant laboratory data obtained on admission were as follows:

Urea nitrogen (6–24 mg/dL)	53
Creatinine (0.5–1.4 mg/dL)	2.2
Total protein (6.0–8.3 g/dL)	5.8
Albumin (3.5–5.3 g/dL)	3.2
Glucose (60–110 mg/dL)	312
Calcium (4.3–5.3 mmol/L)	4.1
Phosphorus (2.5–4.5 mg/dL)	2.4
Total CK (54–186 U/L)	134
CK-MB (0–5 ng/L)	4
% CK-MB (<6%)	3
Myoglobin (<70 µg/L)	62
Troponin T (0–0.1 µg/L)	0.2

Questions

1. Do the symptoms of this patient suggest acute MI?

2. Based on the preceding laboratory data, would this diagnosis be acute MI? Why or why not?

3. Based on the preceding laboratory data, are there other organ system abnormalities present?

4. What are the indicators of these organ system abnormalities?

5. Is there a specific laboratory test that might indicate congestive heart failure in this patient?

CARDIAC INJURY OCCURS IN MANY DISEASE PROCESSES, BEYOND MI

The damage that occurs in the context of MI is due to cardiac muscle cell (myocyte) death. A spectrum of cell death occurs in myocytes, ranging from apoptosis to necrosis to a mixture between the two. Apoptotic cell death is characterized by decreasing cell size, membrane blebbing, nuclear aggregation of chromosomal DNA, and purposeful degradation of DNA. The resulting apoptotic bodies formed from the process of apoptosis are recognized by macrophage, which then remove the debris in an effort to minimize the immune response.[61] Apoptosis requires energy, so as ischemia progresses, the apoptotic process

stalls and necrosis occurs if energy supply fails to meet the energy demand, which occurs rapidly in the heart. Thus, a rapid clinical response to myocardial ischemia is essential to limiting the extent of necrosis that occurs and is a central tenet of treating MI. The faster cardiac interventions are performed to restore perfusion (along with oxygen) to the heart, the greater the reduction in infarct size. The strategies for reperfusion include percutaneous interventions using intravascular balloons and stents to clear coronary artery blockages and prevent their recurrence; coronary artery bypass grafting (CABG or "bypass surgery"); and the use of chemical thrombolytics, such as tissue plasminogen activator (aka tPA or tenecteplase).

Despite our focus here on the use of cardiac biomarkers in MI, a number of other causes of myocardial injury result in increased biomarker release. Like MI, these disease processes also have myocyte apoptosis and necrosis as part of their pathophysiology, which explains why these biomarkers may be elevated in these patients. Cell death, in the form of apoptosis and/or necrosis, is a key feature of cardiomyopathies due to genetic causes and/or stress-related causes and contributes to the worsening function that occurs with the disease[62-64] (Fig. 26-6). Cell death also occurs in decompensated heart failure and volume overload.[66] In the cardiac hypertrophy "pre-heart failure state," angiotensin II, catecholamine production, and cytokines release play a role in inducing cardiomyocyte apoptosis[67-69] (Fig. 26-6), which can lead to low level release of cardiac biomarkers. Cardiomyocyte cell death is also induced in myocarditis, whereby viruses and bacteria induce an autoimmune response, which recognizes cardiac-specific proteins as foreign and induces cardiac cells to die.[70] Similarly, bacterial toxins in sepsis can cause apoptosis and myocardial depression. Certain drugs are also capable of causing apoptosis and myocardial dysfunction, including doxorubicin and cyclophosphamide[71-73] (Fig. 26-6), as well as alcohol, cocaine, and methamphetamines.

THE LABORATORY WORKUP OF PATIENTS SUSPECTED OF HEART FAILURE AND THE USE OF CARDIAC BIOMARKERS IN HEART FAILURE

Heart failure is a pathological state in which the heart fails to adequately supply the metabolic needs of the body, typically due to a decrease in pumping function. The clinical manifestations of heart failure result largely from the retention of fluid, which is one of the body's maladaptive responses to decreased cardiac output. The most common symptoms of heart failure are shortness of breath, fatigue, and lower extremity edema.

The ACC/AHA/Heart Failure Society of America and the European Society of Cardiology have recommended specific laboratory and clinical tests for patients with suspected heart failure (see Table 26-4).[74-76]

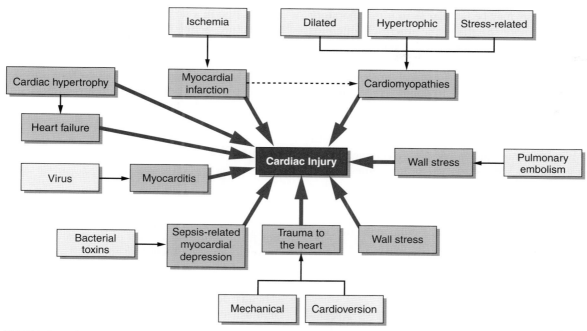

FIGURE 26-6 Common cardiac insults that result in cardiac injury and elevated cardiac biomarkers. Adapted from McLean and Huang.[65]

TABLE 26-4	AMERICAN COLLEGE OF CARDIOLOGY/AMERICAN HEART ASSOCIATION/ EUROPEAN SOCIETY OF CARDIOLOGY RECOMMENDED LABORATORY AND CLINICAL TESTS FOR PATIENTS WITH SUSPECTED HEART FAILURE

Complete blood count. A complete blood count can help determine if anemia or infection may be the cause of heart failure.

Serum electrolyte levels. An imbalance of electrolytes can cause fluid retention while it may play a role in the severity of heart failure.

BUN/creatinine. Determination of BUN/creatinine can determine if damage to the kidneys, due to hypo-perfusion, may be occurring secondary to heart failure.

Fasting glucose. Increased glucose levels in both diabetic patients and non-diabetic patients put them at an increased risk for heart failure.[77]

Liver function tests. Elevated liver enzymes (AST, ALT, and LD) may indicate if liver function is affected due to heart failure; congestion of the liver can occur secondary to the inefficiency with which the heart is able to move the venous circulation.

BNP/NT-proBNP levels. Both BNP and its precursor NT-proBNP are elevated after being released in the heart secondary to the stretch induced by heart failure. Their levels correlate closely with the severity of heart failure and can be used to differentiate cardiac causes of shortness of breath from primary lung disease.

ECG. A 12-lead ECG can detect ischemia, infarction, and arrhythmias as a cause for heart failure.

Urinalysis. Recent studies have described a relationship between the amount of protein excreted in urine and cardiovascular risk.[78] The specific relationship between urine protein and CV risk may be due to the common manifestation of vascular endothelial cell dysfunction.[79]

Lipid profile. The lipid profile, including total cholesterol, LDL, HDL, and triglyceride determination, should be performed to determine the risk of coronary heart disease.

TSH. Thyroid hormone function tests, in particular TSH levels, should be measured as both hyperthyroidism and hypothyroidism can be a primary cause of heart failure or can contribute to its severity.[74]

BUN, blood urea nitrogen; AST, aspartate aminotransferase; ALT, alanine aminotransferase; LD, lactate dehydrogenase; BNP, B-type natriuretic peptide; NT-proBNP, N-terminal pro-B–type natriuretic peptide; ECG, electrocardiogram; CV, cardiovascular; LDL, low-density lipoprotein; HDL, high-density lipoprotein; TSH, thyroid-stimulating hormone.

Many of these tests may be familiar as routine laboratory tests; others are more specific to the atherosclerotic process and compensatory cardiac function mechanisms.

The ACC/AHA recommendations also suggest determining a cTnI or cTnT if the clinical presentation is suggestive of an ACS; elevated troponin levels may also indicate the severity of the heart failure (discussed in the next section).[74-76] A chest x-ray, 2D echocardiographic analysis, and Doppler flow studies to identify ventricular and/or valvular abnormalities are also recommended in evaluating patients with suspected heart failure.[80,81] As CHD is the most common cause of heart failure, some evaluation for ischemic burden is indicated. To this end, coronary angiography or exercise stress testing may be used depending on the clinical scenario. Pulmonary function testing is generally not helpful in the diagnosis of heart failure as cardiogenic pulmonary edema and intrinsic lung disease can result in similar patterns of abnormalities.[76]

THE USE OF NATRIURETIC PEPTIDES AND TROPONINS IN THE DIAGNOSIS AND RISK STRATIFICATION OF HEART FAILURE

Though shortness of breath is the most common presentation of heart failure, it is a relatively non-specific symptom. Measurement of circulating B-type natriuretic peptide (BNP), or its precursor N-terminal pro-B–type natriuretic peptide (NT-proBNP), can be particularly helpful in distinguishing cardiac from non-cardiac causes of dyspnea and is widely used in emergency departments and other clinical settings.[74-76,82-85]

Natriuretic peptides are secreted from the heart in response to increased pressure and volume load. They play an important role in reducing intravascular volume by promoting natriuresis, diuresis, and vasodilation and inhibiting sympathetic nervous system signaling.[86,87] The pro-BNP is released by myocardial cells in response to increased volume, increased pressure, and cardiac hypertrophy; this precursor is cleaved by the protease enzyme furin into the active BNP and the inactive NT-proBNP. Both NT-proBNP and BNP are elevated in patients with ventricular dysfunction and strongly predict morbidity and mortality in patients with heart failure.[88-91] Multiple clinical studies have assessed the utility of both NT-proBNP and BNP for ruling out heart failure as a cause of dyspnea (shortness of breath) in the acute clinical setting.[91] Meta-analysis of these studies have found that the pooled estimates of sensitivity and specificity are equivalent for NT-proBNP and BNP. However, the optimum cutoff value for each peptide remains difficult to determine across all populations.[91]

Vasodilation and natriuresis are beneficial in the setting of heart failure, and thus BNP was pursued as a target for drug development. Scios (later Johnson & Johnson) developed recombinant BNP as Nesiritide.

It is the first in a new class of therapies designed to treat heart failure, acting as a neurohormonal suppressor just as endogenous BNP.[92] The importance of mentioning that recombinant BNP is used therapeutically is that it can be picked up by laboratory tests for BNP, but not NT-proBNP. Therefore, there are clinical situations wherein NT-proBNP may be the more appropriate test to use to follow heart failure patients.

Cardiac Troponins

While used primarily for the diagnosis of myocardial injury caused by ischemia, elevations of cTnT and cTnI levels were recognized in heart failure patients more than a decade ago.[93-95] The precise reason for elevated troponins in the non-ACS setting of heart failure is not clear. Ongoing cell death including apoptosis and necrosis may be one of the reasons, occurring as a result of increased myocardial wall stress[96] resulting in subendocardial ischemia due to increased myocardial oxygen demand. Diminished cardiac perfusion and oxygen delivery to the heart itself and impaired renal clearance of troponins may also contribute.[96]

While the detection of troponins in heart failure is not diagnostic, it has been reported to add prognostic value. In acute heart failure patients without ACS, elevations in cTnI occur more often than cTnT elevations, although increases in either were related to increased mortality.[96] Other studies have described a 2.6-fold increased risk of in-hospital mortality for heart failure patients with elevated troponin levels at the time of admission.[98] Elevated cardiac troponin has also been associated with lower systolic blood pressure and lower left ventricular ejection fraction at the time of admission,[98] both of which are markers for worse outcome. In outpatients with more severe chronic heart failure (New York Heart Failure Class III or IV), the presence of elevated cardiac troponin was also associated with lower ejection fraction and deteriorating clinical course.[95] Troponin levels were one of the strongest predictors of mortality, particularly if used in conjunction with BNP levels.[99] In general, concomitant elevations in multiple markers (cardiac troponin, high-sensitivity CRP [hsCRP], along with NT-proBNP) are associated with escalating risks of adverse events.[100] Few studies, however, have investigated how troponin levels may be helpful in the initial diagnosis of heart failure, so their current role in heart failure patients is limited to risk stratification.

MARKERS OF CHD RISK

C-Reactive Protein

Inflammation plays an important role in the development and progression of atherosclerosis and CHD. CRP is an acute marker of inflammation that is currently used

CASE STUDY 26-4

A 68-year-old man presented to the emergency department with sudden onset of chest pain, left arm pain, dyspnea, and weakness while away from home on a business trip. His prior medical history is not available, but he admits to being a 2-pack per day smoker for longer than 20 years.

Cardiac markers were performed at admission and 8 hours postadmission with the following results:

CARDIAC MARKERS	7:30 AM; SEPTEMBER 26	4:00 PM; SEPTEMBER 26
CK-MB (0–5 ng/L)	5.3	9.2
Myoglobin	76	124 (<70 µg/L)
Troponin T	<0.1	1.3 (0–0.1 µg/L)

Questions

1. Do these results indicate a specific diagnosis?

2. If so, what is the diagnosis?

3. What myoglobin, CK-MB, and TnT results would be expected if assayed at 4 PM on September 27?

4. Can any assumptions be made about the patient's lifestyle/habits/health that would increase his risk for this condition?

5. Are there any assays that might indicate his risk for further events of this type?

clinically in the evaluation of CVD risk. CRP is a pentameric protein consisting of five identical subunits that bind to specific ligands, such as LDL cholesterol, in a calcium-dependent manner. CRP is normally present in human plasma at levels less than 10 mg/L, but its rapid synthesis in the liver after stimulus from a variety of inflammatory cytokines may increase plasma levels by 1,000 fold, thus serving as a sensitive biomarker of systemic inflammation.[101] Because atherosclerosis and CHD derive largely from an inflammatory etiology, CRP has long been targeted as a biomarker for CHD, but it has recently gained widest acceptance as a marker of CHD risk.

CRP was first described in 1930 when physicians studying the serum from patients with pneumonia observed high seroreactivity with pneumococcal bacterial extracts.[102] After separating the extracts into discrete fractions, only one fraction—arbitrarily designated fraction C—was found to react heavily with serum from acutely ill patients. This fraction contained "non-protein material" that appeared "to be a carbohydrate common to the

Pneumococcus species," which was later called C polysaccharide.[102] Only serum from acutely ill patients reacted with the pneumococcal C polysaccharide, and this reactivity disappeared after resolution of their illness. In the early 1940s, a protein requiring calcium ions was identified to be present exclusively in the serum of acutely ill patients. This protein, called "reactive protein," was responsible for reactivity with C polysaccharide.[103,104]

Although first observed in patients afflicted with pneumococcal pneumonia, it became clear that serum CRP was present in many more pathological conditions, and elevated CRP became associated with systemic inflammation.[103] As a biomarker, CRP originally gained the widespread use as an index of acute rheumatic fever.[105] Its association with heart disease was first demonstrated in 1947 when the serum of patients with congestive heart failure was found to contain detectable CRP.[106] In the 1950s, the discovery of elevated CRP after MI supported the hypothesis that MI is associated with systemic inflammation,[107] as did the subsequent finding of elevated CRP in patients with CHD.[108] Despite these findings, interest in CRP as a marker of CVD did not develop until the 1980s, when it was shown that CRP levels correlated remarkably well not only with serum CK-MB post-MI but also with the symptoms of cardiac disease, such as chest pain,[109] unstable angina, and chronic atherothrombotic disease.[110] All of these findings helped support the long-held hypothesis that vascular injury and inflammation play important roles in CVD, but CRP failed to provide significant benefit over the other clinically used markers of CVD or MI.

In the 1990s, extensive analysis of epidemiological data revealed that CRP could be applied clinically in a prognostic manner, rather than as a serum biomarker post-MI. This prognostic value was evaluated through several prospective cohort studies that compared baseline CRP levels in healthy individuals with CRP levels after cardiac events.[111] The most influential data were extracted from the Physicians Health Study (PHS), which found that baseline CRP levels were significantly higher in individuals that eventually experienced MI than those who did not.[112] These results showed that baseline plasma levels of CRP in apparently healthy individuals could help predict the risk of first MI, thus demonstrating a novel and substantial application of CRP as a prognostic marker. CRP data from the PHS also demonstrated that the use of anti-inflammatory medication (aspirin) reduced the risk of vascular events, which supported the hypothesis that chronic inflammation contributes to atherosclerosis and CHD.[111] In the late 1990s, the Cholesterol and Recurrent Events (CARE) trial showed that lipid-lowering drugs, such as statins, reduce CRP levels in a largely LDL-dependent manner, suggesting that CRP evaluation may help determine the efficacy of pharmacologic interventions used to treat CVD.[113]

These studies demonstrated that CRP had immense clinical value as a potential novel biomarker for both cardiovascular risk and cardiovascular therapy management. Importantly, the CRP levels in these and later studies were baseline values that were orders of magnitude less than the CRP levels typically present during acute inflammation. Whereas CRP levels present during acute inflammation are readily detectible using common clinical laboratory methods, the levels of CRP reported in these studies were far below the threshold of detection in most standard clinical assays. Because these studies demonstrated substantial prognostic value of monitoring CRP values at baseline levels, it was thus necessary to develop more sensitive methods of CRP measurement. Specifically, it was necessary to measure CRP levels with extremely high sensitivity (hs), in the range of 0.15 and 10 mg/L.[101] In the early 2000s, such methods for hsCRP measurement were developed and validated,[101] and the first set of clinical guidelines for the use of hsCRP as a marker of cardiovascular risk prediction was published by the AHA and the Centers for Disease Control and Prevention in early 2003.[114] These guidelines recommended that hsCRP be the inflammatory marker of choice in the evaluation of cardiac heart disease risk, and they stated that hsCRP concentrations of <1, 1 to 3, and >3 correspond clinically to low, moderate, and high relative risk of CVD, respectively.[114]

Homocysteine

Homocysteine is a sulfur-containing amino acid formed in plasma from the metabolic demethylation of methionine, which is derived from dietary protein.[115] Plasma homocysteine circulates in four forms: (1) free thiol (homocysteine, Hcys; ~1%), (2) disulfide (homocystine; 5-10%), (3) mixed disulfide (Hcys-Cys; 5-10%), (4) protein-bound thiod groups (80-90%).[116] Total plasma homocysteine refers to the combined pool of all forms of homocysteine. Normal total plasma homocysteine ranges from 5 to 15 μmol/L, moderate is 16 to 30 μmol/L, intermediate is 31 to 100 μmol/L, and severe hyper-homocystinemia is >100 μmol/L.

Homocysteine was first isolated in 1932 but connections between homocysteine and vascular disease were not made until 1964, when a high incidence of vascular anomalies and arterial thromboses was observed in patients with homocystinuria.[117] Five years later, a physician studying vascular abnormalities in homocystinuria found an association between homocysteine and atherosclerosis, concluding that "elevated concentration of homocysteine, homocystine, or a derivative of homocysteine is the common factor leading to arterial damage."[118] Later studies demonstrated that premature vascular disease is extremely common in patients with homocystinuria, such that advanced atherosclerosis is frequently found in children with homocystinuria and

approximately 50% of patients experience thromboembolic events in their lifetime.[119]

These early studies demonstrated a clear link between extremely high levels of plasma homocysteine (>100 μmol/L [>13.5 mg/L]) and CVD, but mildly elevated homocysteine was later shown to pose a risk of CVD as well. A 1976 study found that "a reduced ability to metabolize homocysteine" may contribute to premature coronary artery disease,[120] and numerous cross-sectional, case–control, and prospective cohort studies further evaluated this relationship. Most, but not all, of these epidemiologic studies indicated that hyper-homocystinemia increases the risk of CVD, but the results varied significantly between studies and study type. Whereas cross-sectional and case–control studies consistently found that hyper-homocystinemia increases the risk of CVD, most prospective studies demonstrated little or no increased risk.[121] One meta-analysis, for example, found that case–control studies estimate approximately an 80% risk of developing CVD due to hyper-homocystinemia, whereas prospective cohort studies estimate only 20% risk.[122] Such variation in clinical and epidemiological data raised questions about what role, if any, homocysteine actually plays in the development of CVD.

Many of these questions have been addressed through a wide body of basic research investigating the mechanisms through which homocysteine may contribute to CVD. Potential mechanisms that have been proposed include homocysteine-induced damage to vascular endothelium,[123] accelerated thrombin formation,[124] promotion of lipid peroxidation,[125] vascular smooth muscle proliferation,[126] and attraction of monocytes to the vascular endothelium.[127] Animal models have shown that mild hyper-homocystinemia contributes to atherosclerotic lesion development and to early lipid accumulation in vascular endothelium.[128] And studies in rats have shown that hyper-homocystinemia stimulates the expression of vascular adhesion molecules, such as monocyte chemoattractant protein (MCP-1), vascular cell adhesion molecule 1, and E-selectin, which increases the binding of monocytes to the endothelium.[129] Treatment of cultured human endothelial and smooth muscle cells with homocysteine also induces the expression of MCP-1, as well as expression of IL-8, a T lymphocyte and neutrophil chemoattractant.[130] Homocysteine-induced expression of these chemokines promotes a pro-inflammatory state that may contribute to general vascular inflammation that drives atherosclerosis.[131] Together, evidence from in vitro and animal models supports the hypothesis that hyper-homocystinemia promotes atherosclerotic lesion development, thereby increasing the risk of CVD.

Collectively, there is a growing body of evidence implicating hyper-homocysteinemia as an independent risk factor of CVD. Clinically, it has been estimated that up to 40% of patients diagnosed with premature coronary artery disease, peripheral vascular disease, or recurrent venous thrombosis exhibit some extent of hyper-homocystinemia.[131] Several recent meta-analyses found that for every 5 µmol/L (0.7 mg/L) increase in serum homocysteine concentration, the risk of ischemic heart disease increased 20% to 30%[132,133] and that decreasing plasma homocysteine by 3 µmol/L (0.4 mg/L) (through folate supplementation) can reduce the risk of ischemic heart disease by 16%, deep vein thrombosis (DVT) by 25%, and stroke by 24%.[133] The clinical, epidemiological, and biochemical data support a role for homocysteine in the development of atherosclerosis and CVD, but further research will be necessary to delineate the exact mechanisms through which it exerts this effect.

MARKERS OF PULMONARY EMBOLISM

An embolus is a circulating mass of solid, liquid, or gas, and pulmonary embolism (PE) is an acute and serious condition in which an embolus becomes lodged within the pulmonary arteries, impairing blood flow through the pulmonary vasculature and increasing right ventricular pressure. The extent of pulmonary vascular occlusion and subsequent symptoms is a function of the size and location of the embolus. Although most pulmonary emboli involve a pulmonary vessel of second, third, or fourth order yielding mild or no clinical symptoms, extremely large emboli can lodge at the bifurcation of the main pulmonary artery to form *saddle emboli* that can rapidly block pulmonary circulation.[134] Saddle emboli and other emboli that occlude over 60% of the pulmonary circulation greatly increase the risk of right heart failure, cardiovascular collapse, and sudden death. The co-incidence of DVT and PE is quite high; approximately half of venous thromboemboli will develop into pulmonary emboli,[135] and approximately 95% of pulmonary emboli originate from deep veins of the legs[136] (Fig. 26-7).

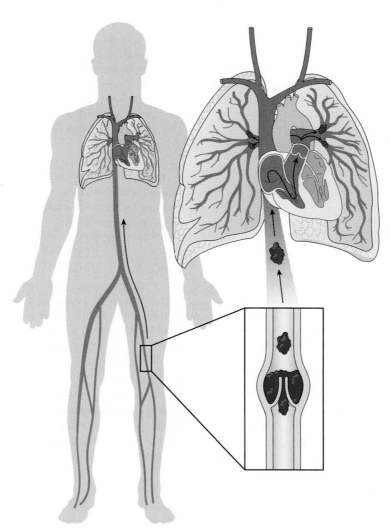

FIGURE 26-7 Thromboemboli originating from the deep veins of the legs travel through venous circulation through the heart and into the pulmonary vasculature, where they lodge in vessels of decreasing diameter and occlude blood flow. Adapted from Douma et al.[137]

The incidence of PE increases almost exponentially with age, ranging from approximately 5 per 100,000 in childhood to nearly 600 per 100,000 in persons over 75 years old[137] (Fig. 26-8). Women of reproductive age are at a greater risk for PE because of the associations between venous thromboembolism and pregnancy and the use of oral contraceptives. If left untreated, PE-related mortality can exceed 25%, but adequate treatment in the form of anticoagulation decreases this risk to approximately 5%.[139] Initial therapy after diagnoses of PE involves low molecular weight heparin, unfractionated heparin, or fondaparinux (trade name Arixtra), and long-term treatment includes oral vitamin K antagonists.[140]

Diagnosis of PE is inherently challenging because of the similarity of its symptoms to other more common conditions, such as ACS, and because signs and symptoms are frequently not present.[134] The classical presentation of a patient with PE includes chest pain, dyspnea, tachycardia, tachypnea, and coughing.[137] Unilateral leg swelling and redness may indicate DVT and increases the likelihood of PE. Syncope due to circulatory collapse is present in approximately 15% of patients with a large PE, and crackles or decreased breath sounds are common.[137] Vital signs may reveal tachycardia or mild hypoxia. Evidence of increased venous pressure, such as neck vein distension, or increased right ventricular pressure, such as a loud P2 (pulmonic valve closure sound), increases the diagnostic suspicion for PE.[137] Distinction between PE and ACS is particularly difficult because of their similar presentation, in particular chest pain, dyspnea, and ECG abnormalities.

Use of D-Dimer Detection in PE

The first step in the diagnostic workup of patients with suspected PE is determining the pretest clinical probability of PE using one of several decision rules.[137] The most widely used set of decision rules is the Wells score, which considers seven clinical variables obtained solely from medical history and physical examination, as well as the physician's judgment on the likelihood of PE versus other diagnoses.[141]

When the pretest probability of PE is low or intermediate, it is reasonable to order a D-dimer blood test.[137] D-Dimer is a product of plasmin-mediated fibrin degradation that consists of two D-domains from adjacent fibrin monomers that are cross-linked by activated factor XIII. Because D-dimer is derived from cross-linked fibrin, not fibrinogen, the presence of D-dimer in the bloodstream is indicative of current or recent coagulation and subsequent fibrinolysis. D-Dimer thus serves as an indirect marker of coagulation and fibrinolysis.[137] The choice of D-dimer assay is important as the sensitivity of various tests varies greatly. Enzyme-linked fluorescent assay, enzyme-linked immunosorbent assay (ELISA), and latex quantitative assay are highly sensitive quantitative assays for circulating D-dimer levels and are the tests of choice in the workup patients with suspected PE.[142]

D-Dimer levels are abnormal in approximately 90% of patients with PE,[143] and numerous studies have shown that a normal D-dimer results can rule out PE safely in patients with low or intermediate clinical probabilities.[137] However, D-dimer levels are normal in only 40% to 68% of patients without PE. Abnormal levels are often seen in patients with malignancy, recent surgery, renal dysfunction, or increased age.[143] The low specificity of D-dimer testing results in a poor positive predictive value and limited utility in patients with a high clinical probability of PE,[142] for whom CT and ventilation–perfusion scanning are reasonable initial diagnostic tests. However, the high sensitivity of the test translates to a valuable negative predictive value, meaning that D-dimer testing is most useful for excluding PE rather than diagnosing it. One study found that the sensitivity of the D-dimer (by high-sensitivity ELISA) for acute PE was 96.4% and the negative predictive value was 99.6%,[134] thus further evaluation of PE is not indicated for most patients with normal D-dimer levels.[134]

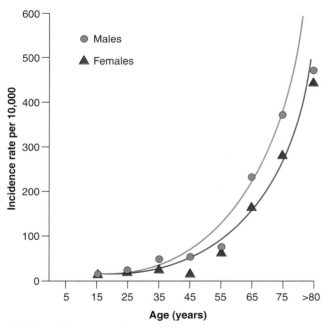

FIGURE 26-8 The incidence of pulmonary embolism (PE) as a function of age in the US population. Adapted from Anderson et al.[138]

Value of Assaying Troponin and BNP in Acute PE

A recent meta-analysis was performed to determine the prognostic value of elevated troponin levels in patients with acute PE.[144] Based on publications from January 1998 to November 2006, 122 of 618 patients were found to have elevated troponin levels (19.7%) compared with 51 of 1,367 patients with normal troponin levels.[144] An elevated troponin level was associated significantly with a short-term mortality (odds ratio 5.24), resulting from PE (odds ratio 9.44) and with adverse outcome events (odds ratio 7.03).[144] These results were consistent between TnI and TnT and in both prospective and retrospective studies. Therefore, an elevated troponin measurement in patients presenting with PE does appear to have utility in determining their short-term mortality outcome. This information can drive the clinician's clinical management as to whether a more aggressive management approach is necessary, such as the use of thrombolysis.

Similarly, BNP has been used as a predictor of adverse outcome in patients with PE. In a study of 110 consecutive patients with PE, the positive and negative predictive values of BNP levels were determined.[145] The risk of death related to PE if BNP > 21.7 pmol/L was 17%; the negative predictive value for uneventful outcome of a BNP < 21.7 pmol/L was 99%.[145] A larger meta-analysis of 12 studies, including 868 patients with acute PE, determined that elevated BNP levels were significantly associated with an increase in short-term mortality from all causes (odds ratio 6.57), and with death resulting from PE (odds ratio 6.10) or serious adverse events (odds ratio 7.47) with positive predictive values of 14% and negative predictive values of 95%.[146] Together these studies suggest a role for elevated BNP in helping to identify patients with acute PE at high risk for an adverse outcome, in order to drive a more aggressive management approach such as thrombolysis. The high negative predictive value of a normal BNP is also a particularly useful piece of data used to select patients with an uneventful clinical course.

SUMMARY

CHD is an extremely common condition that causes substantial morbidity and death worldwide. CHD is due in large part to atherosclerosis, which is best defined as a pro-inflammatory process in which cells, lipids, and connective tissue cause intimal thickening within large- and medium-sized arteries. This process impairs normal blood flow and may progress to occlude the entire vessel diameter. This narrowing of the coronary arteries leads to cardiac ischemia, which may manifest as activity-induced chest pain (stable angina), or ACS. Severe occlusion of coronary vessels causes

---

CASE STUDY 26-5

A 48-year-old woman was seen by her primary physician for a routine physical examination. Her father and his brother died before the age of 55 with acute MI and another uncle had CABG surgery at age 52. Because of this family history, she requested for any testing that might indicate a predisposition or increased risk factors for early cardiac disease. She does not smoke, does not have hypertension, is approximately 20 lb overweight, and exercises moderately. The following test results were obtained.

Total cholesterol (<200 mg/dL)	187 mg/dL
HDL cholesterol (30–75 mg/dL)	52 mg/dL
LDL cholesterol (60–130 mg/dL)	95 mg/dL
Lipoprotein(a) (<30 mg/dL)	34 mg/dL
Triglycerides (60–160 mg/dL)	203 mg/dL
Glucose (60–110 mg/dL)	83 mg/dL
Total CK (15–130 IU/L)	65 IU/L
CK-MB (<8 IU/L)	1.9 IU/L
% CK-MB (0–6%)	3
Homocysteine (<15 μmol/L)	18 μmol/L
Fibrinogen (2–4.5 mg/dL)	4.3 mg/dL
D-dimer (0–250 μg/mL)	160 μg/mL
hsCRP (0.016–0.76 mg/dL)	0.91 mg/dL

Questions

1. Do any of the results obtained indicate a high risk for development of cardiac disease? If so, which results?

2. Does this patient have risk factors for early cardiac disease that can be modified by diet or lifestyle modifications? If so, what changes can be made?

3. Is there any specific treatment that can be instituted to reduce this patient's risk?

4. How should this patient be monitored?

---

complete ischemia and subsequent necrosis of surrounding tissue, which is known as MI. The extent of MI and subsequent morbidity can vary tremendously, ranging from undetected infarction with little consequence to sudden death. Because of the physiological and pathological responses that take place within the myocardium immediately after infarction, rapid diagnosis is extremely important. Methods of rapidly diagnosing MI with a high sensitivity and specificity

TABLE 26-5	COMPARISON OF PAST AND PRESENT BIOMARKERS FOR CARDIAC DAMAGE AND FUNCTION WITH A SUMMARY OF THEIR CURRENT CLINICAL UTILITY				
MARKER	**CURRENTLY USED TO DIAGNOSE ACS/ ACUTE MI**	**CURRENTLY USED TO DIFFERENTIATE HEART FAILURE FROM LUNG DISEASE**	**CURRENTLY USED TO DIAGNOSE PULMONARY EMBOLISM/RISK STRATIFICATION**	**USED FOR CARDIOVASCULAR RISK STRATIFICATION**	**NO LONGER USED/USED LESS COMMONLY/ EXPERIMENTAL**
LD					X
CKMB	X				
Myoglobin					X
IMA					X
H-FABP					X
TnI, TnT	X		X	X	
hsTn	X				X
hsCRP				X	
Homocysteine				X	
BNP		X	X		
NT-proBNP		X	X		
D-Dimer			X		

LD, lactate dehydrogenase; CKMB, creatine kinase MB; IMA, ischemia-modified albumin; H-FABP, heart-type fatty acid–binding protein; TnI, troponin I; TnT, troponin T; hsTn, high-sensitive troponin; BNP, B-type natriuretic peptide; NT-proBNP, N-terminal pro-B–type natriuretic peptide.

are thus extremely important for the management and potentially the survival of a patient that presents with symptoms of MI.

Plasma biomarkers have become the centerpiece of evaluation and diagnosis of such patients (Table 26-5). AST, LD, and CK-MB were widely used biomarkers in the diagnosis of MI but have largely been replaced by high-sensitivity troponin assays. cTnI and cTnT assays have extremely high specificity to cardiac tissue, and detection methods are sensitive enough to pick up even very minor cardiac tissue damage. Current guidelines therefore recommend measurement of cardiac troponins

in the circulation as soon as possible after symptoms of MI. Other experimental markers, such as myoglobin, H-FABP, and IMA, lack the specificity of troponin testing but may be useful when assayed together with troponins.

Plasma biomarkers of cardiac disease risk are also an important factor in the management of patients at risk for CHD, in particular CRP and homocysteine, both of which indicate systemic inflammation and correlate with the elevated risk of CHD and MI. Similarly, the management and diagnosis of heart failure is facilitated by the analysis of circulating biomarkers, most importantly cardiac troponins and BNP.

For additional student resources please visit thePoint at http://thepoint.lww.com. **thePoint** ✳

QUESTIONS

1. A serum TnT concentration is of most value to the patient with an MI when
   a. The CK-MB has already peaked and returned to normal concentrations
   b. The onset of symptoms is within 3 to 6 hours of the sample being drawn
   c. The myoglobin concentration is extremely elevated
   d. The TnI concentration has returned to normal concentrations

2. A normal myoglobin concentration 8 hours after the onset of symptoms of a suspected MI will
   a. Essentially rule out an acute MI
   b. Provide a definitive diagnosis of acute MI
   c. Be interpreted with careful consideration of the TnT concentration
   d. Give the same information as a total CK-MB

3. Which of the following analytes has the highest specificity for cardiac injury?
   a. TnI
   b. CK-MB mass assays
   c. Total CK-MB
   d. AST

4. Which of the following newer markers of inflammation circulates in serum bound to LD and HDL?
   a. Lipoprotein-associated phospholipase A2
   b. CK-MB
   c. cTnI
   d. hsCRP

5. A person with a confirmed blood pressure of 125/87 would be classified as
   a. Prehypertension
   b. Normal
   c. Stage 1 hypertension
   d. Stage 2 hypertension

6. Rheumatic heart disease is a result of infection with which of the following organisms?
   a. Group A streptococci
   b. *Staphylococcus aureus*
   c. *Pseudomonas aeruginosa*
   d. *Chlamydia pneumoniae*

7. Which of the following defects is the most common type of congenital CVD encountered?
   a. Ventricular septal defects (VSD)
   b. Tetralogy of Fallot
   c. Coarctation of the aorta
   d. Transposition of the great arteries

8. Which of the following cardiac markers is the most useful indicator of congestive heart failure?
   a. BNP
   b. TnI
   c. CK-MB
   d. Glycogen phosphorylase isoenzyme BB

9. Which of the following is the preferred biomarker for the assessment of myocardial necrosis?
   a. CK
   b. AST
   c. CK-MB
   d. TnI

10. Which of the following is NOT a feature of an ideal cardiac marker?
    a. Ability to predict future occurrence of cardiac disease
    b. Absolute specificity
    c. High sensitivity
    d. Close estimation of the magnitude of cardiac damage

REFERENCES

1. Lindsell CJ, Anantharaman V, Diercks D, et al. The Internet Tracking Registry of Acute Coronary Syndromes (i*trACS): a multicenter registry of patients with suspicion of acute coronary syndromes reported using the standardized reporting guidelines for emergency department chest pain studies. *Ann Emerg Med.* December 2006;48(6):666-677, 677, e661-669.
2. Pope JH, Aufderheide TP, Ruthazer R, et al. Missed diagnoses of acute cardiac ischemia in the emergency department. *N Engl J Med.* April 2000;342(16):1163-1170.
3. Morrow DA. Clinical application of sensitive troponin assays. *N Engl J Med.* August 2009;361(9):913-915.
4. Runge MS, Ohman M, Stouffer GA. The history and physical exam. In: Runge MS, Stouffer GA, Patterson C, eds. *Netter's Cardiology.* 2nd ed. Philadelphia, PA: Saunders Elsevier; 2010.
5. Mosca L, Manson JE, Sutherland SE, Langer RD, Manolio T, Barrett-Connor E. Cardiovascular disease in women: a statement for healthcare professionals from the American Heart Association. Writing Group. *Circulation.* October 1997;96(7):2468-2482.
6. Douglas PS, Ginsburg GS. The evaluation of chest pain in women. *N Engl J Med.* May 1996;334(20):1311-1315.
7. Kudenchuk PJ, Maynard C, Martin JS, Wirkus M, Weaver WD. Comparison of presentation, treatment, and outcome of acute myocardial infarction in men versus women (the Myocardial Infarction Triage and Intervention Registry). *Am J Cardiol.* July 1996;78(1):9-14.
8. Braunwald E, Antman EM, Beasley JW, et al. ACC/AHA guidelines for the management of patients with unstable angina and non-ST-segment elevation myocardial infarction: executive summary and recommendations. A report of the American College of Cardiology/American Heart Association task force on practice guidelines (committee on the management of patients with unstable angina). *Circulation.* September 2000;102(10): 1193-1209.
9. Thygesen K, Alpert JS, White HD, et al. Universal definition of myocardial infarction. *Circulation.* November 2007;116(22): 2634-2653.
10. Glass CK, Witztum JL. Atherosclerosis. the road ahead. *Cell.* February 2001;104(4):503-516.
11. Lusis AJ. Atherosclerosis. *Nature.* September 2000;407(6801): 233-241.
12. Ross R. The pathogenesis of atherosclerosis—an update. *N Engl J Med.* February 1986;314(8):488-500.
13. Nakashima Y, Wight TN, Sueishi K. Early atherosclerosis in humans: role of diffuse intimal thickening and extracellular matrix proteoglycans. *Cardiovasc Res.* July 2008;79(1):14-23.
14. Skalen K, Gustafsson M, Rydberg EK, et al. Subendothelial retention of atherogenic lipoproteins in early atherosclerosis. *Nature.* June 2002;417(6890):750-754.
15. Moore KJ, Tabas I. Macrophages in the pathogenesis of atherosclerosis. *Cell.* April 2011;145(3):341-355.

16. Libby P. Changing concepts of atherogenesis. *J Intern Med.* March 2000;247(3):349-358.

17. Virmani R, Kolodgie FD, Burke AP, et al. Atherosclerotic plaque progression and vulnerability to rupture: angiogenesis as a source of intraplaque hemorrhage. *Arterioscler Thromb Vasc Biol.* October 2005;25(10):2054-2061.

18. Karmen A, Wroblewski F, Ladue JS. Transaminase activity in human blood. *J Clin Invest.* January 1955;34(1):126-131.

19. Ladue JS, Wroblewski F, Karmen A. Serum glutamic oxaloacetic transaminase activity in human acute transmural myocardial infarction. *Science.* September 1954;120(3117):497-499.

20. King J, Waind AP. Lactic dehydrogenase activity in acute myocardial infarction. *BMJ.* November 1960;2(5209):1361-1363.

21. Warburton FG, Bernstein A, Wright AC. Serum creatine phosphokinase estimations in myocardial infarction. *Br Heart J.* September 1965;27(5):740-747.

22. Wroblewski F, Gregory KF. Lactic dehydrogenase isozymes and their distribution in normal tissues and plasma and in disease states. *Ann N Y Acad Sci.* November 1961;94:912-932.

23. Vasudevan G, Mercer DW, Varat MA. Lactic dehydrogenase isoenzyme determination in the diagnosis of acute myocardial infarction. *Circulation.* June 1978;57(6):1055-1057.

24. Dreyfus JC, Schapira G, Resnais J, Scebat L. Serum creatine kinase in the diagnosis of myocardial infarct. *Rev Fr Etud Clin Biol.* April 1960;5:386-387.

25. Sobel BE, Shell WE. Serum enzyme determinations in the diagnosis and assessment of myocardial infarction. *Circulation.* February 1972;45(2):471-482.

26. French JK, White HD. Clinical implications of the new definition of myocardial infarction. *Heart.* January 2004;90(1):99-106.

27. Dillon MC, Calbreath DF, Dixon AM, et al. Diagnostic problem in acute myocardial infarction: CK-MB in the absence of abnormally elevated total creatine kinase levels. *Arch Intern Med.* January 1982;142(1):33-38.

28. Wagner GS, Roe CR, Limbird LE, Rosati RA, Wallace AG. The importance of identification of the myocardial-specific isoenzyme of creatine phosphokinase (MB form) in the diagnosis of acute myocardial infarction. *Circulation.* February 1973;47(2):263-269.

29. Malasky BR, Alpert JS. Diagnosis of myocardial injury by biochemical markers: problems and promises. *Cardiol Rev.* September-October 2002;10(5):306-317.

30. Robinson DJ, Christenson RH. Creatine kinase and its CK-MB isoenzyme: the conventional marker for the diagnosis of acute myocardial infarction. *J Emerg Med.* January-February 1999;17(1):95-104.

31. Scott BB, Simmons AV, Newton KE, Payne RB. Interpretation of serum creatine kinase in suspected myocardial infarction. *BMJ.* December 1974;4(5946):691-693.

32. Goldberg DM, Winfield DA. Diagnostic accuracy of serum enzyme assays for myocardial infarction in a general hospital population. *Br Heart J.* June 1972;34(6):597-604.

33. Goldberg DM. Clinical enzymology: an autobiographical history. *Clin Chim Acta Int J Clin Chem.* July 2005;357(2):93-112.

34. Cummins P, Perry SV. Troponin I from human skeletal and cardiac muscles. *Biochem J.* April 1 1978;171(1):251-259.

35. Adams JE 3rd, Abendschein DR, Jaffe AS. Biochemical markers of myocardial injury. Is MB creatine kinase the choice for the 1990s? *Circulation.* August 1993;88(2):750-763.

36. MacGeoch C, Barton PJ, Vallins WJ, Bhavsar P, Spurr NK. The human cardiac troponin I locus: assignment to chromosome 19p13.2-19q13.2. *Hum Genet.* November 1991;88(1):101-104.

37. Cummins B, Auckland ML, Cummins P. Cardiac-specific troponin-I radioimmunoassay in the diagnosis of acute myocardial infarction. *Am Heart J.* June 1987;113(6):1333-1344.

38. Adams JE 3rd, Bodor GS, Davila-Roman VG, et al. Cardiac troponin I. A marker with high specificity for cardiac injury. *Circulation.* July 1993;88(1):101-106.

39. Coudrey L. The troponins. *Arch Intern Med.* June 1998;158(11):1173-1180.

40. Kagen LJ. *Myoglobin: Biochemical, Physiological, and Clinical Aspects.* New York, NY: Columbia University Press; 1973.

41. Klocke FJ, Copley DP, Krawczyk JA, Reichlin M. Rapid renal clearance of immunoreactive canine plasma myoglobin. *Circulation.* June 1982;65(7):1522-1528.

42. McCord J, Nowak RM, McCullough PA, et al. Ninety-minute exclusion of acute myocardial infarction by use of quantitative point-of-care testing of myoglobin and troponin I. *Circulation.* September 2001;104(13):1483-1488.

43. Kagen L, Scheidt S, Butt A. Serum myoglobin in myocardial infarction: the "staccato phenomenon." Is acute myocardial infarction in man an intermittent event? *Am J Med.* January 1977;62(1):86-92.

44. Kavsak PA, MacRae AR, Newman AM, et al. Effects of contemporary troponin assay sensitivity on the utility of the early markers myoglobin and CKMB isoforms in evaluating patients with possible acute myocardial infarction. *Clin Chim Acta Int J Clin Chem.* May 2007;380(1-2):213-216.

45. Eggers KM, Oldgren J, Nordenskjold A, Lindahl B. Diagnostic value of serial measurement of cardiac markers in patients with chest pain: limited value of adding myoglobin to troponin I for exclusion of myocardial infarction. *Am Heart J.* October 2004;148(4):574-581.

46. Ilva T, Eriksson S, Lund J, et al. Improved early risk stratification and diagnosis of myocardial infarction, using a novel troponin I assay concept. *Eur J Clin Invest.* February 2005;35(2):112-116.

47. Van Nieuwenhoven FA, Kleine AH, Wodzig WH, et al. Discrimination between myocardial and skeletal muscle injury by assessment of the plasma ratio of myoglobin over fatty acid-binding protein. *Circulation.* November 1995;92(10):2848-2854.

48. Seino Y, Ogata K, Takano T, et al. Use of a whole blood rapid panel test for heart-type fatty acid-binding protein in patients with acute chest pain: comparison with rapid troponin T and myoglobin tests. *Am J Med.* August 2003;115(3):185-190.

49. McMahon CG, Lamont JV, Curtin E, et al. Diagnostic accuracy of heart-type fatty acid-binding protein for the early diagnosis of acute myocardial infarction. *Am J Emerg Med.* February 2012;30(2):267-274.

50. Bhagavan NV, Lai EM, Rios PA, et al. Evaluation of human serum albumin cobalt binding assay for the assessment of myocardial ischemia and myocardial infarction. *Clin Chem.* April 2003;49(4):581-585.

51. Christenson RH, Duh SH, Sanhai WR, et al. Characteristics of an albumin cobalt binding test for assessment of acute coronary syndrome patients: a multicenter study. *Clin Chem.* March 2001;47(3):464-470.

52. Bar-Or D, Curtis G, Rao N, Bampos N, Lau E. Characterization of the Co(2+) and Ni(2+) binding amino-acid residues of the N-terminus of human albumin. An insight into the mechanism of a new assay for myocardial ischemia. *Eur J Biochem.* January 2001;268(1):42-47.

53. Bar-Or D, Lau E, Winkler JV. A novel assay for cobalt-albumin binding and its potential as a marker for myocardial ischemia-a preliminary report. *J Emerg Med.* November 2000;19(4):311-315.

54. Roy D, Quiles J, Aldama G, et al. Ischemia Modified Albumin for the assessment of patients presenting to the emergency department with acute chest pain but normal or non-diagnostic 12-lead electrocardiograms and negative cardiac troponin T. *Int J Cardiol.* November 2004;97(2):297-301.

55. Sinha MK, Roy D, Gaze DC, Collinson PO, Kaski JC. Role of "Ischemia modified albumin", a new biochemical marker of myocardial ischaemia, in the early diagnosis of acute coronary syndromes. *Emerg Med J.* January 2004;21(1):29-34.

56. Schaub N, Reichlin T, Meune C, et al. Markers of plaque instability in the early diagnosis and risk stratification of acute myocardial infarction. *Clin Chem.* January 2012;58(1):246-256.

57. Nicholls SJ, Hazen SL. Myeloperoxidase and cardiovascular disease. *Arterioscler Thromb Vasc Biol.* June 2005;25(6):1102-1111.

58. Ionita MG, Vink A, Dijke IE, et al. High levels of myeloid-related protein 14 in human atherosclerotic plaques correlate with the characteristics of rupture-prone lesions. *Arterioscler Thromb Vasc Biol.* August 2009;29(8):1220-1227.

59. Bayes-Genis A, Conover CA, Overgaard MT, et al. Pregnancy-associated plasma protein A as a marker of acute coronary syndromes. *N Engl J Med.* October 2001;345(14):1022-1029.

60. Mueller C, Buettner HJ, Hodgson JM, et al. Inflammation and long-term mortality after non-ST elevation acute coronary syndrome treated with a very early invasive strategy in 1042 consecutive patients. *Circulation.* March 2002;105(12):1412-1415.

61. Krysko DV, Denecker G, Festjens N, et al. Macrophages use different internalization mechanisms to clear apoptotic and necrotic cells. *Cell Death Differ.* December 2006;13(12):2011-2022.

62. Yaoita H, Maruyama Y. Intervention for apoptosis in cardiomyopathy. *Heart Fail Rev.* June 2008;13(2):181-191.

63. Olivetti G, Abbi R, Quaini F, et al. Apoptosis in the failing human heart. *N Engl J Med.* April 1997;336(16):1131-1141.

64. Ibe W, Saraste A, Lindemann S, et al. Cardiomyocyte apoptosis is related to left ventricular dysfunction and remodelling in dilated cardiomyopathy, but is not affected by growth hormone treatment. *Eur J Heart Fail.* February 2007;9(2):160-167.

65. McLean AS, Huang SJ. Biomarkers of cardiac injury. In: Vaidya VS, Bonventre JV, eds. *Biomarkers: In Medicine, Drug Discovery, and Environmental Health.* eBook. New York, NY: John Wiley & Sons, Inc.; 2010:119-155.

66. Dent MR, Das S, Dhalla NS. Alterations in both death and survival signals for apoptosis in heart failure due to volume overload. *J Mol Cell Cardiol.* December 2007;43(6):726-732.

67. Anselmi A, Gaudino M, Baldi A, et al. Role of apoptosis in pressure-overload cardiomyopathy. *J Cardiovasc Med (Hagerstown).* March 2008;9(3):227-232.

68. Leri A, Claudio PP, Li Q, et al. Stretch-mediated release of angiotensin II induces myocyte apoptosis by activating p53 that enhances the local renin-angiotensin system and decreases the Bcl-2-to-Bax protein ratio in the cell. *J Clin Invest.* April 1998;101(7):1326-1342.

69. Colucci WS, Sawyer DB, Singh K, Communal C. Adrenergic overload and apoptosis in heart failure: implications for therapy. *J Card Fail.* June 2000;6(2 suppl 1):1-7.

70. Cooper LT, Jr. Myocarditis. *N Engl J Med.* April 2009;360(15):1526-1538.

71. Lai HC, Yeh YC, Ting CT, et al. Doxycycline suppresses doxorubicin-induced oxidative stress and cellular apoptosis in mouse hearts. *Eur J Pharmacol.* October 2010;644(1-3):176-187.

72. Shi J, Abdelwahid E, Wei L. Apoptosis in anthracycline cardiomyopathy. *Curr Pediatr Rev.* November 2011;7(4):329-336.

73. Asiri YA. Probucol attenuates cyclophosphamide-induced oxidative apoptosis, p53 and Bax signal expression in rat cardiac tissues. *Oxid Med Cell Longev.* September-October 2010;3(5):308-316.

74. Hunt SA, Abraham WT, Chin MH, et al. 2009 Focused update incorporated into the ACC/AHA 2005 guidelines for the diagnosis and management of heart failure in adults: a report of the American College of Cardiology Foundation/American Heart Association Task Force on practice guidelines developed in collaboration with the International Society for Heart and Lung Transplantation. *J Am Coll Cardiol.* April 2009;53(15):e1-e90.

75. Lindenfeld J, Albert NM, Boehmer JP, et al. HFSA 2010 comprehensive heart failure practice guideline. *J Card Fail.* June 2010;16(6):e1-194.

76. Dickstein K, Cohen-Solal A, Filippatos G, et al. ESC guidelines for the diagnosis and treatment of acute and chronic heart failure 2008: the Task Force for the Diagnosis and Treatment of Acute and Chronic Heart Failure 2008 of the European Society of Cardiology. Developed in collaboration with the Heart Failure Association of the ESC (HFA) and endorsed by the European Society of Intensive Care Medicine (ESICM). *Eur Heart J.* October 2008;29(19):2388-2442.

77. Haffner SJ, Cassells H. Hyperglycemia as a cardiovascular risk factor. *Am J Med.* December 2003;115(suppl 8A):6S-11S.

78. Buckalew VM Jr, Freedman BI. Effects of race on albuminuria and risk of cardiovascular and kidney disease. *Expert Rev Cardiovasc Ther.* February 2011;9(2):245-249.

79. Ochodnicky P, Henning RH, van Dokkum RP, de Zeeuw D. Microalbuminuria and endothelial dysfunction: emerging targets for primary prevention of end-organ damage. *J Cardiovasc Pharmacol.* 2006;47(suppl 2):S151-S162; discussion S172-S176.

80. Pinamonti B, Di Lenarda A, Sinagra G, Camerini F. Restrictive left ventricular filling pattern in dilated cardiomyopathy assessed by Doppler echocardiography: clinical, echocardiographic and hemodynamic correlations and prognostic implications. Heart Muscle Disease Study Group. *J Am Coll Cardiol.* September 1993;22(3):808-815.

81. Temporelli PL, Scapellato F, Eleuteri E, Imparato A, Giannuzzi P. Doppler echocardiography in advanced systolic heart failure: a noninvasive alternative to Swan-Ganz catheter. *Circulation. Heart Fail.* May 2010;3(3):387-394.

82. Maisel AS, Krishnaswamy P, Nowak RM, et al. Rapid measurement of B-type natriuretic peptide in the emergency diagnosis of heart failure. *N Engl J Med.* July 2002;347(3):161-167.

83. Januzzi JL Jr, Camargo CA, Anwaruddin S, et al. The N-terminal Pro-BNP investigation of dyspnea in the emergency department (PRIDE) study. *Am J Cardiol.* April 2005;95(8):948-954.

84. Maisel AS, McCord J, Nowak RM, et al. Bedside B-type natriuretic peptide in the emergency diagnosis of heart failure with reduced or preserved ejection fraction. Results from the Breathing Not Properly Multinational Study. *J Am Coll Cardiol.* June 2003;41(11):2010-2017.

85. Januzzi JL, van Kimmenade R, Lainchbury J, et al. NT-proBNP testing for diagnosis and short-term prognosis in acute destabilized heart failure: an international pooled analysis of 1256 patients: the International Collaborative of NT-proBNP Study. *Eur Heart J.* February 2006;27(3):330-337.

86. de Lemos JA, Morrow DA, Bentley JH, et al. The prognostic value of B-type natriuretic peptide in patients with acute coronary syndromes. *N Engl J Med.* October 2001;345(14):1014-1021.

87. McFarlane SI, Winer N, Sowers JR. Role of the natriuretic peptide system in cardiorenal protection. *Arch Intern Med.* December 2003;163(22):2696-2704.

88. Wang TJ, Larson MG, Levy D, et al. Plasma natriuretic peptide levels and the risk of cardiovascular events and death. *N Engl J Med.* February 2004;350(7):655-663.

89. Bibbins-Domingo K, Gupta R, Na B, Wu AH, Schiller NB, Whooley MA. N-terminal fragment of the prohormone brain-type natriuretic peptide (NT-proBNP), cardiovascular events, and mortality in patients with stable coronary heart disease. *JAMA.* January 2007;297(2):169-176.

90. Cowie MR, Jourdain P, Maisel A, et al. Clinical applications of B-type natriuretic peptide (BNP) testing. *Eur Heart J.* October 2003;24(19):1710-1718.

91. Worster A, Balion CM, Hill SA, et al. Diagnostic accuracy of BNP and NT-proBNP in patients presenting to acute care settings with dyspnea: a systematic review. *Clin Biochem.* March 2008;41(4-5):250-259.

92. Fonarow GC. B-type natriuretic peptide: spectrum of application. Nesiritide (recombinant BNP) for heart failure. *Heart Fail Rev.* October 2003;8(4):321-325.

93. Guler N, Bilge M, Eryonucu B, Uzun K, Avci ME, Dulger H. Cardiac troponin I levels in patients with left heart failure and cor pulmonale. *Angiology.* May 2001;52(5):317-322.

94. Logeart D, Beyne P, Cusson C, et al. Evidence of cardiac myolysis in severe nonischemic heart failure and the potential role of increased wall strain. *Am Heart J.* February 2001;141(2): 247-253.

95. La Vecchia L, Mezzena G, Zanolla L, et al. Cardiac troponin I as diagnostic and prognostic marker in severe heart failure. *J Heart Lung Transplant.* July 2000;19(7):644-652.

96. Nagarajan V, Tang WH. Biomarkers in advanced heart failure: diagnostic and therapeutic insights. *Congest Heart Fail.* July-August 2011;17(4):169-174.

97. Ilva T, Lassus J, Siirila-Waris K, et al. Clinical significance of cardiac troponins I and T in acute heart failure. *Eur J Heart Fail.* August 2008;10(8):772-779.

98. Peacock WFt, De Marco T, Fonarow GC, et al. Cardiac troponin and outcome in acute heart failure. *N Engl J Med.* May 2008;358(20):2117-2126.

99. Horwich TB, Patel J, MacLellan WR, Fonarow GC. Cardiac troponin I is associated with impaired hemodynamics, progressive left ventricular dysfunction, and increased mortality rates in advanced heart failure. *Circulation.* August 2003;108(7): 833-838.

100. Yin WH, Chen JW, Feng AN, Lin SJ, Young S. Multimarker approach to risk stratification among patients with advanced chronic heart failure. *Clin Cardiol.* August 2007;30(8):397-402.

101. Ledue TB, Rifai N. High sensitivity immunoassays for C-reactive protein: promises and pitfalls. *Clin Chem Lab Med.* November 2001;39(11):1171-1176.

102. Tillett WS, Francis T. Serological reactions in pneumonia with a non-protein somatic fraction of pneumococcus. *J Exp Med.* September 1930;52(4):561-571.

103. Abernethy TJ, Avery OT. The Occurrence during acute infections of a protein not normally present in the blood: I. Distribution of the reactive protein in patients' sera and the effect of calcium on the flocculation reaction with c polysaccharide of pneumococcus. *J Exp Med.* January 1941;73(2):173-182.

104. Macleod CM, Avery OT. The Occurrence during acute infections of a protein not normally present in the blood : II. Isolation and properties of the reactive protein. *J Exp Med.* January 1941;73(2):183-190.

105. Elster SK, Braunwald E, Wood HF. A study of C-reactive protein in the serum of patients with congestive heart failure. *Am Heart J.* April 1956;51(4):533-541.

106. Hedlund P. The appearance of acute phase protein in various diseases. *Acta Med Scand.* 1947;128(suppl 196):579-601.

107. Kroop IG, Shackman NH. Level of C-reactive protein as a measure of acute myocardial infarction. *Proc Soc Exp Biol Med.* May 1954;86(1):95-97.

108. Kroop IG, Shackman NH. The C-reactive protein determination as an index of myocardial necrosis in coronary artery disease. *Am J Med.* January 1957;22(1):90-98.

109. de Beer FC, Hind CR, Fox KM, Allan RM, Maseri A, Pepys MB. Measurement of serum C-reactive protein concentration in myocardial ischaemia and infarction. *Br Heart J.* March 1982;47(3):239-243.

110. Liuzzo G, Biasucci LM, Gallimore JR, et al. The prognostic value of C-reactive protein and serum amyloid a protein in severe unstable angina. *N Engl J Med.* August 1994;331(7):417-424.

111. Ridker PM. C-reactive protein: eighty years from discovery to emergence as a major risk marker for cardiovascular disease. *Clin Chem.* February 2009;55(2):209-215.

112. Ridker PM, Cushman M, Stampfer MJ, Tracy RP, Hennekens CH. Inflammation, aspirin, and the risk of cardiovascular disease in apparently healthy men. *N Engl J Med.* April 1997;336(14):973-979.

113. Ridker PM, Rifai N, Pfeffer MA, et al. Inflammation, pravastatin, and the risk of coronary events after myocardial infarction in patients with average cholesterol levels. Cholesterol and Recurrent Events (CARE) Investigators. *Circulation.* September 1998;98(9):839-844.

114. Pearson TA, Mensah GA, Alexander RW, et al. Markers of inflammation and cardiovascular disease: application to clinical and public health practice: a statement for healthcare professionals from the Centers for Disease Control and Prevention and the American Heart Association. *Circulation.* January 2003;107(3):499-511.

115. Abraham JM, Cho L. The homocysteine hypothesis: still relevant to the prevention and treatment of cardiovascular disease? *Cleve Clin J Med.* December 2010;77(12):911-918.

116. Hankey GJ, Eikelboom JW. Homocysteine and vascular disease. *Lancet.* July 1999;354(9176):407-413.

117. Gibson JB, Carson NA, Neill DW. Pathological Findings in Homocystinuria. *J Clin Pathol.* July 1964;17:427-437.

118. McCully KS. Vascular pathology of homocysteinemia: implications for the pathogenesis of arteriosclerosis. *Am J Pathol.* July 1969;56(1):111-128.

119. Nygard O, Nordrehaug JE, Refsum H, Ueland PM, Farstad M, Vollset SE. Plasma homocysteine levels and mortality in patients with coronary artery disease. *N Engl J Med.* July 1997;337(4):230-236.

120. Wilcken DE, Wilcken B. The pathogenesis of coronary artery disease. A possible role for methionine metabolism. *J Clin Invest.* April 1976;57(4):1079-1082.

121. Christen WG, Ajani UA, Glynn RJ, Hennekens CH. Blood levels of homocysteine and increased risks of cardiovascular disease: causal or casual? *Arch Intern Med.* February 2000;160(4):422-434.

122. Splaver A, Lamas GA, Hennekens CH. Homocysteine and cardiovascular disease: biological mechanisms, observational epidemiology, and the need for randomized trials. *Am Heart J.* July 2004;148(1):34-40.

123. Blundell G, Jones BG, Rose FA, Tudball N. Homocysteine mediated endothelial cell toxicity and its amelioration. *Atherosclerosis.* May 1996;122(2):163-172.

124. Loscalzo J. Homocysteine-mediated thrombosis and angiostasis in vascular pathobiology. *J Clin Invest.* November 2009;119(11):3203-3205.

125. Heinecke JW. Biochemical evidence for a link between elevated levels of homocysteine and lipid peroxidation in vivo. *Curr Atheroscler Rep.* September 1999;1(2):87-89.

126. Tsai JC, Perrella MA, Yoshizumi M, et al. Promotion of vascular smooth muscle cell growth by homocysteine: a link to atherosclerosis. *Proc Natl Acad Sci U S A.* July 1994;91(14): 6369-6373.

127. Sung FL, Slow YL, Wang G, Lynn EG, O K. Homocysteine stimulates the expression of monocyte chemoattractant protein-1 in endothelial cells leading to enhanced monocyte chemotaxis. *Mol Cell Biochem.* January 2001;216(1-2):121-128.

128. Chen Z, Karaplis AC, Ackerman SL, et al. Mice deficient in methylenetetrahydrofolate reductase exhibit hyperhomocysteinemia and decreased methylation capacity, with neuropathology and aortic lipid deposition. *Hum Mol Genet.* March 2001;10(5):433-443.

129. Wang G, Woo CW, Sung FL, Siow YL, O K. Increased monocyte adhesion to aortic endothelium in rats with hyperhomocysteinemia: role of chemokine and adhesion molecules. *Arterioscler Thromb Vasc Biol.* November 2002;22(11):1777-1783.

130. Poddar R, Sivasubramanian N, DiBello PM, Robinson K, Jacobsen DW. Homocysteine induces expression and secretion of monocyte chemoattractant protein-1 and interleukin-8 in human aortic endothelial cells: implications for vascular disease. *Circulation.* June 2001;103(22):2717-2723.

131. Austin RC, Lentz SR, Werstuck GH. Role of hyperhomocysteinemia in endothelial dysfunction and atherothrombotic disease. *Cell Death Differ.* July 2004;11(suppl 1):S56-S64.

132. Humphrey LL, Fu R, Rogers K, Freeman M, Helfand M. Homocysteine level and coronary heart disease incidence: a systematic review and meta-analysis. *Mayo Clin Proc.* November 2008;83(11):1203-1212.

133. Wald DS, Law M, Morris JK. Homocysteine and cardiovascular disease: evidence on causality from a meta-analysis. *BMJ.* November 2002;325(7374):1202.

134. Goldhaber SZ. Pulmonary embolism. *Lancet.* April 2004; 363(9417):1295-1305.

135. Silverstein MD, Heit JA, Mohr DN, Petterson TM, O'Fallon WM, Melton LJ 3rd. Trends in the incidence of deep vein thrombosis and pulmonary embolism: a 25-year population-based study. *Arch Intern Med.* March 1998;158(6):585-593.

136. Kumar V, Fausto N, Abbas A. *Robbins and Cotran Pathologic Basis of Disease.* 7th ed. Philadelphia, PA: W.B. Saunders Company; 2004.

137. Douma RA, Kamphuisen PW, Buller HR. Acute pulmonary embolism. Part 1: epidemiology and diagnosis. *Nat Rev Cardiol.* October 2010;7(10):585-596.

138. Anderson FA Jr, Wheeler HB, Goldberg RJ, et al. A population-based perspective of the hospital incidence and case-fatality rates of deep vein thrombosis and pulmonary embolism. The Worcester DVT Study. *Arch Intern Med.* May 1991;151(5): 933-938.

139. Douketis JD, Kearon C, Bates S, Duku EK, Ginsberg JS. Risk of fatal pulmonary embolism in patients with treated venous thromboembolism. *JAMA.* February 1998;279(6): 458-462.

140. van Es J, Douma RA, Gerdes VE, Kamphuisen PW, Buller HR. Acute pulmonary embolism. Part 2: treatment. *Nature Rev Cardiol.* November 2010;7(11):613-622.

141. Wells PS, Anderson DR, Rodger M, et al. Excluding pulmonary embolism at the bedside without diagnostic imaging: management of patients with suspected pulmonary embolism presenting to the emergency department by using a simple clinical model and d-dimer. *Ann Intern Med.* July 2001;135(2):98-107.

142. Agnelli G, Becattini C. Acute pulmonary embolism. *N Engl J Med.* July 2010;363(3):266-274.

143. Stein PD, Hull RD, Patel KC, et al. D-dimer for the exclusion of acute venous thrombosis and pulmonary embolism: a systematic review. *Ann Intern Med.* April 2004;140(8):589-602.

144. Becattini C, Vedovati MC, Agnelli G. Prognostic value of troponins in acute pulmonary embolism: a meta-analysis. *Circulation.* July 2007;116(4):427-433.

145. ten Wolde M, Tulevski, II, Mulder JW, et al. Brain natriuretic peptide as a predictor of adverse outcome in patients with pulmonary embolism. *Circulation.* April 2003;107(16): 2082-2084.

146. Coutance G, Le Page O, Lo T, Hamon M. Prognostic value of brain natriuretic peptide in acute pulmonary embolism. *Crit Care.* 2008;12(4):R109.

Renal Function

KARA L. LYNCH, ALAN H.B. WU

CHAPTER

27

CHAPTER OUTLINE

◆ **RENAL ANATOMY**
◆ **RENAL PHYSIOLOGY**
  Glomerular Filtration
  Tubular Function
  Elimination of Nonprotein Nitrogen Compounds
  Water, Electrolyte, and Acid–Base Homeostasis
  Endocrine Function
◆ **ANALYTIC PROCEDURES**
  Creatinine Clearance
  Estimated GFR
  Cystatin C
  β_2-Microglobulin

  Myoglobin
  Microalbumin
  Neutrophil Gelatinase–Associated Lipocalin
  Urinalysis
◆ **PATHOPHYSIOLOGY**
  Glomerular Diseases
  Tubular Diseases
  Urinary Tract Infection/Obstruction
  Renal Calculi
  Renal Failure
◆ **QUESTIONS**
◆ **REFERENCES**

Chapter Objectives

Upon completion of this chapter, the clinical laboratorian should be able to do the following:

- Diagram the anatomy of the nephron.
- Describe the physiologic role of each part of the nephron: glomerulus, proximal tubule, loop of Henle, distal tubule, and collecting duct.
- Describe the mechanisms by which the kidney maintains fluid and electrolyte balance in conjunction with hormones.
- Discuss the significance and calculation of glomerular filtration rate and estimated glomerular filtration rate.

- Relate the clinical significance of total urine proteins, microalbumin, myoglobin clearance, serum β_2-microglobulin, and cystatin C.
- List the tests in a urinalysis and microscopy profile and understand the clinical significance of each.
- Describe diseases of the glomerulus and tubules and how laboratory tests are used in these disorders.
- Distinguish between acute and chronic renal failure.
- Discuss the therapy of chronic renal failure with regard to renal dialysis and transplantation.

KEY TERMS

Acute renal failure
Aldosterone
Antidiuretic hormone (ADH)
Chronic kidney disease
Countercurrent multiplier system
Creatinine clearance
Cystatin C
Diabetes mellitus
Erythropoietin
Estimated glomerular filtration rate (eGFR)
Glomerular filtration rate (GFR)
Glomerulonephritis
Glomerulus
Hemodialysis

Hemofiltration
Loop of Henle
Microalbumin
β_2-Microglobulin (β2-M)
Myoglobin
Nephrotic syndrome
Prostaglandin
Renal threshold
Renin
Rhabdomyolysis
Tubular reabsorption
Tubular secretion
Tubule
Vitamin D

The kidneys are vital organs that perform a variety of important functions (Table 27-1). The most prominent functions are removal of unwanted substances from plasma (both waste and surplus); homeostasis (maintenance of equilibrium) of the body's water, electrolyte, and acid–base status; and participation in hormonal regulation. In the clinical laboratory, kidney function tests are used in the assessment of renal disease, water balance, and acid–base disorders and in situations of trauma, head injury, surgery, and infectious disease. This chapter focuses on renal anatomy and physiology and the analytic procedures available to diagnose, monitor, and treat kidney dysfunction.

RENAL ANATOMY

The kidneys are paired, bean-shaped organs located retroperitoneally on either side of the spinal column. Macroscopically, a fibrous capsule of connective tissue encloses each kidney. When dissected longitudinally, two regions can be clearly discerned—an outer region called the cortex and an inner region called the medulla (Fig. 27-1A). The pelvis can also be seen. It is a basin-like cavity at the upper end of the ureter into which newly formed urine passes. The bilateral ureters are thick-walled canals, connecting the kidneys to the urinary bladder. Urine is temporarily stored in the bladder until voided from the body by way of the urethra. Figure 27-1B shows the arrangement of nephrons in the kidney, functional units of the kidney that can only be seen microscopically. Each kidney contains approximately 1 million nephrons. Each nephron is a complex apparatus comprised of five basic parts, expressed diagrammatically in Figure 27-2.

- The glomerulus—a capillary tuft surrounded by the expanded end of a renal tubule known as Bowman's

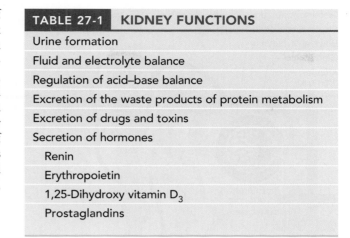

TABLE 27-1	KIDNEY FUNCTIONS
Urine formation	
Fluid and electrolyte balance	
Regulation of acid–base balance	
Excretion of the waste products of protein metabolism	
Excretion of drugs and toxins	
Secretion of hormones	
Renin	
Erythropoietin	
1,25-Dihydroxy vitamin D_3	
Prostaglandins	

capsule. Each glomerulus is supplied by an afferent arteriole carrying the blood in and an efferent arteriole carrying the blood out. The efferent arteriole branches into peritubular capillaries that supply the tubule.
- The proximal convoluted tubule—located in the cortex.
- The long loop of Henle—composed of the thin descending limb, which spans the medulla, and the ascending limb, which is located in both the medulla and the cortex, composed of a region that is thin and then thick.
- The distal convoluted tubule—located in the cortex.
- The collecting duct—formed by two or more distal convoluted tubules as they pass back down through the cortex and the medulla to collect the urine that drains from each nephron. Collecting ducts eventually merge and empty their contents into the renal pelvis.

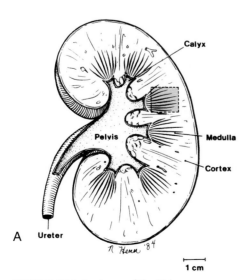

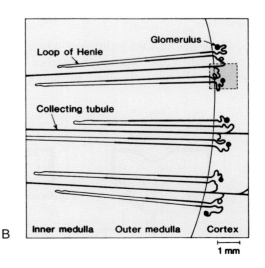

FIGURE 27-1 Anatomy of the kidney.

Distal convoluted tubule
Proximal convoluted tubule
Bowman's capsule
Glomerulus
Afferent arteriole

Efferent arteriole

Collecting tubule

Artery
Vein

Peritubular capillaries
Loop of Henle

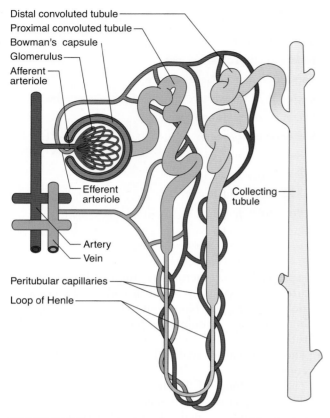

FIGURE 27-2 Representation of a nephron and its blood supply.

The following section describes how each part of the nephron normally functions.

RENAL PHYSIOLOGY

There are three basic renal processes:

1. Glomerular filtration
2. Tubular reabsorption
3. Tubular secretion

Figure 27-3 illustrates how three different substances are variably processed by the nephron. Substance A is filtered and secreted, but not reabsorbed; substance B is filtered and a portion reabsorbed; and substance C is filtered and completely reabsorbed.[1] The following is a description of how specific substances are regulated in this manner to maintain homeostasis.

Glomerular Filtration

The glomerulus is the first part of the nephron and functions to filter incoming blood. Several factors facilitate filtration. One factor is the unusually high pressure in the glomerular capillaries, which is a result of their position between two arterioles. This sets up a steep pressure difference across the walls. Another factor is the semi-permeable glomerular basement membrane, which has a molecular size cutoff value of approximately 66,000 Da, about the molecular size of albumin. This means that water, electrolytes, and small dissolved solutes, such as glucose, amino acids, low-molecular-weight proteins, urea, and creatinine, pass freely through the basement membrane and enter the proximal convoluted tubule. Other blood constituents, such as albumin; many plasma proteins; cellular elements; and protein-bound substances, such as lipids and bilirubin, are too large to be filtered. In addition, because the basement membrane is negatively charged, negatively charged molecules, such as proteins, are repelled. Of the 1,200 to 1,500 mL of blood that the kidneys receive each minute (approximately one-quarter of the total cardiac output), the glomerulus filters out 125 to 130 mL of an essentially protein-free, cell-free fluid, called *glomerular filtrate*. The volume of blood filtered per minute is the glomerular filtration rate (GFR), and its determination is essential in evaluating renal function, as discussed in the section on Analytic Procedures.

Tubular Function

Proximal Convoluted Tubule

The proximal tubule is the next part of the nephron to receive the now cell-free and essentially protein-free blood. This filtrate contains waste products, which are toxic to the body above a certain concentration, and substances that are valuable to the body. One function

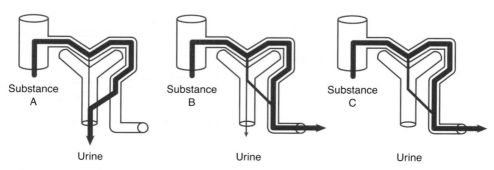

Substance A

Substance B

Substance C

Urine

Urine

Urine

FIGURE 27-3 Renal processes of filtration, reabsorption, and secretion.

of the proximal tubule is to return the bulk of each valuable substance back to the blood circulation. Thus, 75% of the water, sodium, and chloride; 100% of the glucose (up to the renal threshold); almost all of the amino acids, vitamins, and proteins; and varying amounts of urea, uric acid, and ions, such as magnesium, calcium, potassium, and bicarbonate, are reabsorbed. Almost all (98% to 100%) of uric acid, a waste product, is actively reabsorbed, only to be secreted at the distal end of the proximal tubule.

When the substances move from the tubular lumen to the peritubular capillary plasma, the process is called tubular reabsorption. With the exception of water and chloride ions, the process is active; that is, the tubular epithelial cells use energy to bind and transport the substances across the plasma membrane to the blood. The transport processes that are involved normally have sufficient reserve for efficient reabsorption, but they are saturable. When the concentration of the filtered substance exceeds the capacity of the transport system, the substance is then excreted in the urine. The plasma concentration above which the substance appears in urine is known as the renal threshold, and its determination is useful in assessing both tubular function and non-renal disease states. A renal threshold does not exist for water because it is always transported passively through diffusion down a concentration gradient. Chloride ions in this instance diffuse in the wake of sodium.

A second function of the proximal tubule is to secrete products of kidney tubular cell metabolism, such as hydrogen ions, and drugs, such as penicillin. The term tubular secretion is used in two ways: (1) tubular secretion describes the movement of substances from peritubular capillary plasma to the tubular lumen and (2) tubular secretion also describes when tubule cells secrete products of their own cellular metabolism into the filtrate in the tubular lumen. Transport across the membrane of the cell is again either active or passive.

Loop of Henle
The osmolality in the medulla in this portion of the nephron increases steadily from the corticomedullary junction inward and facilitates the reabsorption of water, sodium, and chloride. The hyperosmolality that develops in the medulla is continuously maintained by the loop of Henle, a hairpin-like loop between the proximal tubule and the distal convoluted tubule. The opposing flows in the loop, the downward flow in the descending limb, and the upward flow in the ascending limb are termed a countercurrent flow. To understand how the hyperosmolality is maintained in the medulla, it is best to look first at what happens in the ascending limb. Sodium and chloride are actively and passively reabsorbed into the medullary interstitial fluid along the entire length of the ascending limb. Because the ascending limb is relatively impermeable to water, little water follows and

the medullary interstitial fluid becomes hyperosmotic compared with the fluid in the ascending limb. The fluid in the ascending limb becomes hypotonic or dilute as sodium and chloride ions are reabsorbed without the loss of water, so the ascending limb is often called the diluting segment. The descending limb, in contrast to the ascending limb, is highly permeable to water and does not reabsorb sodium and chloride. The high osmolality of the surrounding interstitial medulla fluid is the physical force that accelerates the reabsorption of water from the filtrate in the descending limb. Interstitial hyperosmolality is maintained because the ascending limb continues to pump sodium and chloride ions into it. This interaction of water leaving the descending loop and sodium and chloride leaving the ascending loop to maintain a high osmolality within the kidney medulla produces hypoosmolal urine as it leaves the loop. This process is called the countercurrent multiplier system.[2]

Distal Convoluted Tubule
The distal convoluted tubule is much shorter than the proximal tubule, with two or three coils that connect to a collecting duct. The filtrate entering this section of the nephron is close to its final composition. About 95% of the sodium and chloride ions and 90% of water have already been reabsorbed from the original glomerular filtrate. The function of the distal tubule is to effect small adjustments to achieve electrolyte and acid–base homeostasis. These adjustments occur under the hormonal control of both antidiuretic hormone (ADH) and aldosterone. Figure 27-4 describes the action of these hormones.

Antidiuretic Hormone
ADH is a peptide hormone secreted by the posterior pituitary, mainly in response to increased blood osmolality; ADH is also released when blood volume decreases by more than 5% to 10%. Large decreases of blood volume will stimulate ADH secretion even when plasma osmolality is decreased. ADH stimulates water reabsorption. The walls of the distal collecting tubules are normally impermeable to water (like the ascending loop of Henle), but they become permeable to water in ADH. Water diffuses passively from the lumen of the tubules, resulting in more concentrated urine and decreased plasma osmolality.

Aldosterone
This hormone is produced by the adrenal cortex under the influence of the renin–angiotensin mechanism. Its secretion is triggered by decreased blood flow or blood pressure in the afferent renal arteriole and by decreased plasma sodium. Aldosterone stimulates sodium reabsorption in the distal tubules and potassium and hydrogen ion secretion. Hydrogen ion secretion is linked to bicarbonate regeneration and ammonia secretion, which also occur here. In addition to these ions, small amounts of chloride ions are reabsorbed.

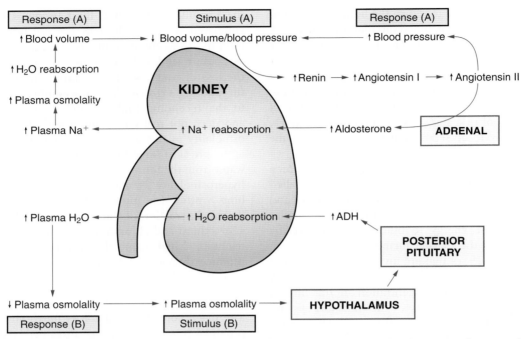

FIGURE 27-4 Antidiuretic hormone (ADH) and aldosterone control of the renal reabsorption of water and Na+. (Reprinted with permission from Kaplan A, et al. The kidney and tests of renal function. In: Kaplan A, Jack R, Orpheum KE, et al., eds. *Clinical Chemistry: Interpretation and Techniques.* 4th ed. Baltimore, MD: Williams & Wilkins; 1995:158, Figure 6.2.).

Collecting Duct

The collecting ducts are the final site for either concentrating or diluting urine. The hormones ADH and aldosterone act on this segment of the nephron to control reabsorption of water and sodium. Chloride and urea are also reabsorbed here. Urea plays an important role in maintaining the hyperosmolality of the renal medulla. Because the collecting ducts in the medulla are highly permeable to urea, urea diffuses down its concentration gradient out of the tubule and into the medulla interstitium, increasing its osmolality.[3]

Elimination of Nonprotein Nitrogen Compounds

Nonprotein nitrogen compounds (NPNs) are waste products formed in the body as a result of the degradative metabolism of nucleic acids, amino acids, and proteins. Excretion of these compounds is an important function of the kidneys. The three principal compounds are urea, creatinine, and uric acid.[4,5] For a more detailed treatment of their biochemistry and disease correlations, see Chapter 12.

Urea

Urea makes up the majority (more than 75%) of the NPN waste excreted daily as a result of the oxidative catabolism of protein. Urea synthesis occurs in the liver. Proteins are broken down into amino acids, which are then deaminated to form ammonia. Ammonia is readily

converted to urea, avoiding toxicity. The kidney is the only significant route of excretion for urea. It has a molecular weight of 60 Da and, therefore, is readily filtered by the glomerulus. In the collecting ducts, 40% to 60% of urea is reabsorbed. The reabsorbed urea contributes to the high osmolality in the medulla, which is one of the processes of urinary concentration mentioned earlier (see loop of Henle).

Creatinine

Muscle contains creatine phosphate, a high-energy compound for the rapid formation of adenosine triphosphate (ATP). This reaction is catalyzed by creatine kinase (CK) and is the first source of metabolic fuel used in muscle contraction. Every day, up to 20% of total muscle creatine (and its phosphate) spontaneously dehydrates and cycles to form the waste product creatinine. Therefore, creatinine levels are a function of muscle mass and remain approximately the same in an individual from day-to-day unless muscle mass or renal function changes. Creatinine has a molecular weight of 113 Da and is, therefore, readily filtered by the glomerulus. Unlike urea, creatinine is not reabsorbed by the tubules. However, a small amount of creatinine is secreted by the kidney tubules at high serum concentrations.

Uric Acid

Uric acid is the primary waste product of purine metabolism. The purines, adenine and guanine, are precursors of nucleic acids ATP and guanosine triphosphate, respectively. Uric acid has a molecular weight of 168 Da. Like creatinine, it is readily filtered by the glomerulus, but it then undergoes a complex cycle of reabsorption and secretion as it courses through the nephron. Only 6% to 12% of the original filtered uric acid is finally excreted. Uric acid exists in its ionized and more soluble form, usually sodium urate, at urinary pH > 5.75 (the first pK_a of uric acid). At pH < 5.75, it is undissociated. This fact has clinical significance in the development of urolithiasis (formation of calculi) and gout.

Water, Electrolyte, and Acid–Base Homeostasis

Water Balance

The kidney's contribution to water balance in the body is through water loss or water conservation, which is regulated by the hormone ADH. ADH responds primarily to changes in osmolality and intravascular volume. Increased plasma osmolality or decreased intravascular volume stimulates secretion of ADH from the posterior pituitary. ADH then increases the permeability of the distal convoluted tubules and collecting ducts to water, resulting in increased water reabsorption and excretion of more concentrated urine. In contrast, the major system regulating water intake is thirst, which appears to be triggered by the same stimuli that trigger ADH secretion.

In states of dehydration, the renal tubules reabsorb water at their maximal rate, resulting in production of a small amount of maximally concentrated urine (high urine osmolality, 1,200 mOsm/L).[6] In states of water excess, the tubules reabsorb water at only a minimal rate, resulting in excretion of a large volume of extremely dilute urine (low urine osmolality, down to 50 mOsm/L).[7,8] The continuous fine-tuning possible between these two extreme states results in the precise control of fluid balance in the body (Fig. 27-5).

Electrolyte Balance

The following is a brief overview of the notable ions involved in maintenance of electrolyte balance within the body. For a more comprehensive treatment of this subject, refer Chapter 16.

Sodium

Sodium is the primary extracellular cation in the human body and is excreted principally through the kidneys. Sodium balance in the body is controlled only through excretion. The renin–angiotensin–aldosterone hormonal system is the major mechanism for the control of sodium balance.

Potassium

Potassium is the main intracellular cation in the body. The precise regulation of its concentration is of extreme importance to cellular metabolism and is controlled chiefly by renal means. Like sodium, it is freely filtered by

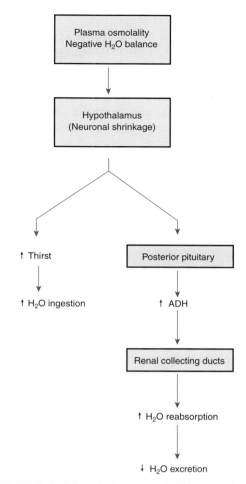

FIGURE 27-5 Antidiuretic hormone (ADH) control of thirst mechanism.

the glomerulus and then actively reabsorbed throughout the entire nephron (except for the descending limb of the loop of Henle). Both the distal convoluted tubule and the collecting ducts can reabsorb and excrete potassium, and this excretion is controlled by aldosterone. Potassium ions can compete with hydrogen ions in their exchange with sodium (in the proximal convoluted tubule); this process is used by the body to conserve hydrogen ions and, thereby, compensate in states of metabolic alkalosis.

Chloride

Chloride is the principal extracellular anion and is involved in the maintenance of extracellular fluid balance. It is readily filtered by the glomerulus and is passively reabsorbed as a counterion when sodium is reabsorbed in the proximal convoluted tubule. In the ascending limb of the loop of Henle, potassium is actively reabsorbed by a distinct chloride "pump," which also reabsorbs sodium. This pump can be inhibited by loop diuretics, such as furosemide. As expected, the regulation of chloride is controlled by the same forces that regulate sodium.[6,8]

Phosphate, Calcium, and Magnesium

The phosphate ion occurs in higher concentrations in the intracellular than in the extracellular fluid environments. It exists as either a protein-bound or a non–protein-bound form; homeostatic balance is chiefly determined by proximal tubular reabsorption under the control of parathyroid hormone (PTH). Calcium, the second-most predominant intracellular cation, is the most important inorganic messenger in the cell. It also exists in protein-bound and non–protein-bound states. Calcium in the non–protein-bound form is either ionized and physiologically active or nonionized and complexed to small, diffusible ions, such as phosphate and bicarbonate. The ionized form is freely filtered by the glomerulus and reabsorbed in the tubules under the control of PTH. However, renal control of calcium concentration is not the major means of regulation. PTH- and calcitonin-controlled regulation of calcium absorption from the gut and bone stores is more important than renal secretion or reabsorption. Magnesium, a major intracellular cation, is important as an enzymatic cofactor. Like phosphate and calcium, it exists in both protein-bound and ionized states. The ionized fraction is easily filtered by the glomerulus and reabsorbed in the tubules under the influence of PTH. See Chapter 24 for more detailed information.

Acid–Base Balance

Many nonvolatile acidic waste products are formed by normal body metabolism each day. Carbonic acid, lactic acid, ketoacids, and others must be continually transported in the plasma and excreted from the body, causing only minor alterations in physiologic pH. The renal system constitutes one of three means by which constant control of overall body pH is accomplished. The other two strategies involved in this regulation are the respiratory system and the acid–base buffering system.[9]

The kidneys manage their share of the responsibility for controlling body pH by dual means: conserving bicarbonate ions and removing metabolic acids. For a more in-depth examination of these processes, refer Chapter 17.

Regeneration of Bicarbonate Ions

In a complicated process, bicarbonate ions are first filtered out of the plasma by the glomerulus. In the lumen of the renal tubules, this bicarbonate combines with hydrogen ions to form carbonic acid, which subsequently degrades to carbon dioxide (CO_2) and water. This CO_2 then diffuses into the brush border of the proximal tubular cells, where it is reconverted by carbonic anhydrase to carbonic acid and then degrades back to hydrogen ions and regenerated bicarbonate ions. This regenerated bicarbonate is transported into the blood to replace what was depleted by metabolism; the accompanying hydrogen ions are secreted back into the tubular lumen, and from there, they enter the urine. Filtered bicarbonate is "reabsorbed" into the circulation, helping to return blood pH to its optimal level and effectively functioning as another buffering system.

Excretion of Metabolic Acids

Hydrogen ions are manufactured in the renal tubules as part of the regeneration mechanism for bicarbonate. These hydrogen ions, as well as others that are dissociated from nonvolatile organic acids, are disposed of by several different reactions with buffer bases.

Reaction with Ammonia (NH_3)

The glomerulus does not filter NH_3. However, this substance is formed in the renal tubules when the amino acid glutamine is deaminated by glutaminase. This NH_3 then reacts with secreted hydrogen ions to form ammonium ions NH_4^+), which are unable to readily diffuse out of the tubular lumen and, therefore, are excreted into the urine. This mode of acid excretion is the primary means by which the kidneys compensate for states of metabolic acidosis.

Reaction with Monohydrogen Phosphate (HPO_4^{-2})

Phosphate ions filtered by the glomerulus can exist in the tubular fluid as disodium hydrogen phosphate (Na_2HPO_4) (dibasic). This compound can react with hydrogen ions to yield dihydrogen phosphate (monobasic), which is then excreted. The released sodium then combines with bicarbonate to yield sodium bicarbonate and is reabsorbed. These mechanisms can excrete increasing amounts of metabolic acid until a maximum urine pH of approximately 4.4 is reached. After this, renal compensation is unable to adjust to any further decreases in blood pH and metabolic acidosis ensues. Few free hydrogen ions are excreted directly in the urine.

Endocrine Function

In addition to numerous excretory and regulatory functions, the kidney has endocrine functions as well. It is both a primary endocrine site, as the producer of its own hormones, and a secondary site, as the target locus for hormones manufactured by other endocrine organs. The kidneys synthesize renin, erythropoietin, 1,25-dihydroxy vitamin D_3, and the prostaglandins.

Renin

Renin is the initial component of the renin–angiotensin–aldosterone system. Renin is produced by the juxtaglomerular cells of the renal medulla when extracellular fluid volume or blood pressure decreases. It catalyzes the synthesis of angiotensin by cleavage of the circulating plasma precursor angiotensinogen. Angiotensin is converted to angiotensin II by angiotensin-converting enzyme. Angiotensin II is a powerful vasoconstrictor that increases blood pressure and stimulates release of aldosterone from the adrenal cortex. Aldosterone, in turn, promotes sodium reabsorption and water conservation.[7,8]

For a more detailed look at the complexities of this feedback loop, see Chapter 21.

Erythropoietin

Erythropoietin is a single-chain polypeptide produced by cells close to the proximal tubules, and its production is regulated by blood oxygen levels. Hypoxia produces increased serum concentrations within 2 hours. Erythropoietin acts on the erythroid progenitor cells in the bone marrow, increasing the number of red blood cells (RBCs). In chronic renal insufficiency, erythropoietin production is significantly reduced. Recently, recombinant human erythropoietin has been developed and is in routine use in chronic renal failure patients. Before this therapy, anemia was a clinical reality in these patients.[4,7] Erythropoietin concentrations in blood can be measured by immunoassays. Recombinant human erythropoietin has also been used in sports doping to stimulate erythrocyte production and increase the oxygen-carrying capacity in the blood of endurance athletes. Assays capable of detecting post-translational modifications on erythropoietin have been produced and are capable of distinguishing exogenous from endogenous erythropoietin.

1,25-Dihydroxy Vitamin D₃

The kidneys are the sites of formation of the active form of vitamin D, $1,25\text{-}(OH)_2$ vitamin D_3. This form of vitamin D is one of three major hormones that determine phosphate and calcium balance and bone calcification in the human body. Chronic renal insufficiency is, therefore, often associated with osteomalacia (inadequate bone calcification, the adult form of rickets), owing to the continual distortion of normal vitamin D metabolism.

Prostaglandins

The prostaglandins are a group of potent cyclic fatty acids formed from essential (dietary) fatty acids, primarily arachidonic acid. They are formed in almost all tissue and their actions are diverse. The prostaglandins produced by the kidneys increase renal blood flow, sodium and water excretion, and renin release. They act to oppose renal vasoconstriction due to angiotensin and norepinephrine.

ANALYTIC PROCEDURES

All laboratory methods used for the evaluation of renal function rely on the measurement of waste products in blood, usually urea and creatinine, which accumulate when the kidneys begin to fail. Renal failure must be advanced, with only about 20% to 30% of the nephrons still functioning, before the concentration of either substance begins to increase in the blood. The rate at which creatinine and urea are removed or cleared from the blood into the urine is termed clearance. Clearance is defined as that volume of plasma from which a measured amount of substance can be completely eliminated into the urine per unit of time expressed in milliliters per minute.[5] Calculation of creatinine clearance has become the standard laboratory method for determining the GFR. Urea clearance was one of the first clearance tests performed; however, it is no longer widely used since it does not accurately provide a full clearance assessment. Older tests used administration of insulin, sodium [¹²⁵I] iothalamate, or *p*-aminohippurate to assess glomerular filtration or tubular secretion. These tests are difficult to administer and are no longer common.

Creatinine Clearance

Creatinine is a nearly ideal substance for the measurement of clearance. It is an endogenous metabolic product synthesized at a constant rate for a given individual and cleared essentially only by glomerular filtration. It is not reabsorbed and is only slightly secreted by the proximal tubule. Serum creatinine levels are higher in males than in females due to the direct correlation with muscle mass. Analysis of creatinine is simple and inexpensive using colorimetric assays; however, different methods for assaying plasma creatinine, such as kinetic or enzymatic assays, have varying degrees of accuracy and imprecision (see Chapter 12).

Creatinine clearance is derived by mathematically relating the serum creatinine concentration to the urine creatinine concentration excreted during a period of time, usually 24 hours. Specimen collection, therefore, must include both a 24-hour urine specimen and a serum creatinine value, ideally collected at the midpoint of the 24-hour urine collection. The urine container must be kept refrigerated throughout the duration of both the collection procedure and the subsequent storage period until laboratory analysis can be performed. The concentration of creatinine in both serum and urine is measured by the applicable methods discussed in Chapter 12. The total volume of urine is carefully measured, and the creatinine clearance is calculated using the following formula:

$$\frac{U_{Cr}(mg/dL) \times V_{Ur}(mL/24\,hours)}{P_{Cr}\,(mg/dL) \times 1{,}440\ minutes/24\,hours} \times \frac{1.73}{A} \quad \text{(Eq. 27-1)}$$

where Cr is creatinine clearance, U_{Cr} is urine creatinine clearance, V_{Ur} is urine volume excreted in 24 hours, P_{Cr} is serum creatinine concentration, and $1.73/A$ is normalization factor for body surface area (1.73 is the generally accepted average body surface in square meters and A is the actual body surface area of the individual determined from height and weight). If the patient's body surface area varies greatly from the average (e.g., obese or pediatric patients), this correction for body mass must be included in the formula. Nomograms for the more exact determination of body surface area from weight and height values can be found in Appendix E. The reference range for creatinine clearance is lower in females compared with males and normally decreases with age.

Estimated GFR

The National Kidney Foundation recommends that estimated GFR (eGFR) be calculated each time a serum creatinine level is reported. (Additional information is available at the National Kidney Foundation web site at http://www.kidney.org/.) The equation is used to predict GFR and is based on serum creatinine, age, body size, gender, and race, without the need of a urine creatinine. Because the calculation does not require a timed urine collection, it should be used more often than the traditional creatinine clearance and result in earlier detection of chronic kidney disease (CKD). There are a number of formulas that can be used to estimate GFR on the basis of serum creatinine levels.

Cockcroft-Gault Formula

The Cockcroft-Gault formula is one of the first formulas used to estimate GFR. This formula predicts creatinine clearance and the results are not corrected for body surface area. This equation assumes that women will have a 15% lower creatinine clearance than men at the same level of serum creatinine.

$$GFR\ (mL/min) = \frac{(140-Age) \times Weight(kg)}{72 \times S_{Cr}(mg/dL)} \times$$
$$(0.85\ if\ female) \qquad \text{(Eq. 27-2)}$$

Modification of Diet in Renal Disease Formula

The modification of diet in renal disease (MDRD) formula was developed in the Modification of Diet in Renal Disease Study of chronic renal insufficiency. The study showed that the MDRD formula provided a more accurate assessment of GFR than the Cockcroft-Gault formula. The MDRD formula was validated in a large population that included European Americans and African Americans. It does not require patient weight and is corrected for body surface area. The MDRD formula is known to underestimate the GFR in healthy patients with GFRs over 60 mL/min and to overestimate GFR in underweight patients. The four-variable MDRD equation includes age, race, gender, and serum creatinine as variables.

$$GFR\ (mL/1.73\ m^2) = 186 \times S_{Cr}(mg/dL)^{-1.154} \times Age^{-0.203} \times (1.212\ if\ Black) \times (0.742\ if\ female) \qquad \text{(Eq. 27-3)}$$

CKD-EPI Formula

The CKD-EPI (Chronic Kidney Disease Epidemiology Collaboration) formula was published in 2009. It was developed in an effort to create a formula more accurate than the MDRD formula. Multiple studies have shown

the CKD-EPI formula to perform better and with less bias than the MDRD formula, especially in patients with higher GFR. Most laboratories still use the MDRD formula; however, some have converted to the CKD-EPI formula.

$$eGFR(mL/min/1.73\ m^2) = 141 \times min(S_{Cr}/k,1)^a \times max(S_{Cr}/k,1)^{-1.209} \times 0.993^{Age} \times (1.018\ if\ female) \times (1.159\ if\ Black) \qquad \text{(Eq. 27-4)}$$

k is 0.7 for females and 0.9 for males, a is −0.329 for females and −0.411 for males, min indicates the minimum of S_{Cr}/k or 1, and max indicates the maximum of S_{Cr}/k or 1.

Cystatin C

Cystatin C is a low-molecular-weight protein produced at a steady rate by most body tissues. It is freely filtered by the glomerulus, reabsorbed, and catabolized by the proximal tubule. Levels of cystatin C rise more quickly than creatinine levels in acute renal failure. Plasma concentrations appear to be unaffected by diet, gender, race, age, and muscle mass. Studies have shown measurement of cystatin C to be at least as useful as serum creatinine and creatinine clearance in detecting early changes in kidney function. A rise in cystatin C is often detectable before there is a measureable decrease in the GFR or increase in creatinine. Cystatin C can be measured by immunoassay methods.[11] Recent findings suggest that an equation that uses both serum creatinine and cystatin C with age, sex, and race would be better than equations that use only one of these serum markers.[12,13]

Biologic Variation

When the same test is performed on various individuals, we find that the mean of each person's results is not the same, showing that individual homeostatic setting points often vary. Biologic variation is defined as the random fluctuation around a homeostatic setting point.[14] This includes the fluctuation around the homeostatic setting point for a single individual, termed within-subject biologic variation, and differences between the homeostatic setting points of multiple individuals, termed between-subject biologic variation. In the case of creatinine, levels for an individual differ slightly over time, and the mean values of all individuals vary significantly from each other. Therefore, each individual's results span only a small portion of the population-based reference interval. This means that for creatinine, within-subject biologic variation is less than between-subject biologic variation. When this is true of a given analyte, the analyte is said to have marked individuality. Interestingly, the between-subject biologic variation is much smaller for cystatin C compared with creatinine, showing that population-based reference values are more useful for cystatin C compared with creatinine. However, the within-subject variation is greater for cystatin C compared with creatinine. As a result, creatinine is more helpful in monitoring renal function over time for a given individual, whereas cystatin C is potentially more useful for detecting minor renal impairment.

β₂-Microglobulin

β_2-Microglobulin (β2-M) is a small, nonglycosylated peptide (molecular weight, 11,800 Da) found on the surface of most nucleated cells. The plasma membrane sheds β2-M at a constant rate, as a relatively intact molecule. β2-M is easily filtered by the glomerulus and 99.9% is reabsorbed by the proximal tubules and catabolized. Elevated levels in serum indicate increased cellular turnover as seen in myeloproliferative and lymphoproliferative disorders, inflammation, and renal failure. Both blood and urine β2-M tests may be ordered to evaluate kidney damage and to distinguish between disorders that affect the glomeruli and the renal tubules. Measurement of serum β2-M is used clinically to assess renal tubular function in renal transplant patients, with elevated levels indicating organ rejection.

Myoglobin

Myoglobin is a low-molecular-weight protein (16,900 Da) associated with acute skeletal and cardiac muscle injury. Myoglobin functions to bind and transport oxygen from the plasma membrane to the mitochondria in muscle cells. Blood levels of myoglobin can rise very quickly with severe muscle injury. In rhabdomyolysis, myoglobin release from skeletal muscle is sufficient to overload the proximal tubules and cause acute renal failure. Early diagnosis and aggressive treatment of elevated myoglobin may prevent or lessen the severity of renal failure. Serum and urine myoglobin can be measured easily and rapidly by immunoassays.

Microalbumin

The term *microalbuminuria* describes small amounts of albumin in the urine. Urine microalbumin measurement is important in the management of patients with diabetes mellitus, who are at serious risk for developing nephropathy over their lifetime. In the early stages of nephropathy, there is renal hypertrophy, hyperfunction, and increased thickness of the glomerular and tubular basement membranes. In this early stage, there are no overt signs of renal dysfunction. In the next 7 to 10 years, there is progression to glomerulosclerosis, with increased glomerular capillary permeability. This permeability allows small (micro) amounts of albumin to pass into the urine. If detected in this early phase, rigid glucose control, along with treatment to prevent hypertension, can be instituted and progression to kidney failure prevented. Quantitative albumin-specific immunoassays, usually using nephelometry or immunoturbidimetry, are widely used. For a 24-hour urine collection, 30 to

300 mg of albumin is diagnostic of microalbuminuria. A 24-hour urine collection is preferred, but a random urine sample that uses a ratio of albumin to creatinine can also be used. An albumin to creatinine ratio of >30 mg/g is diagnostic of microalbuminuria.

Neutrophil Gelatinase–Associated Lipocalin

Neutrophil gelatinase–associated lipocalin (NGAL) is a 25-kDa protein expressed by neutrophils and epithelial cells including those of the proximal tubule. The gene encoding NGAL is upregulated in the presence of renal ischemia, tubule injury, and nephrotoxicity.[15] It can be measured in plasma and urine and is elevated within 2 to 6 hours of acute kidney injury (AKI). NGAL has been shown to be a useful early predictor of AKI and has prognostic value for clinical endpoints, such as initiation of dialysis and mortality. However, urinary NGAL excretion may also arise from systemic stress in the absence of AKI, limiting its specificity.

Urinalysis

Urinalysis (UA) permits a detailed, in-depth assessment of renal status with an easily obtained specimen. UA also serves as a quick indicator of an individual's glucose status and hepatic–biliary function. Routine UA includes assessment of physical characteristics, chemical analyses, and a microscopic examination of the sediment from a (random) urine specimen.

Specimen Collection

The importance of a properly collected and stored specimen for UA cannot be overemphasized. Initial morning specimens are preferred, particularly for protein analyses, because they are more concentrated from overnight retention in the bladder. The specimen should be obtained by a clean midstream catch or catheterization. The urine should be freshly collected into a clean, dry container with a tight-fitting cover. It must be analyzed within 1 hour of collection if held at room temperature or else refrigerated at 2°C to 8°C for not more than 8 hours before analysis. If not assayed within these time limits, several changes will occur. Bacterial multiplication will cause false-positive nitrite tests, and urease-producing organisms will degrade urea to ammonia and alkalinize the pH. Loss of CO_2 by diffusion into the air adds to this pH elevation, which, in turn, causes cast degeneration and red cell lysis.

Physical Characteristics
Visual Appearance
Color intensity of urine correlates with concentration: the darker the color, the more concentrated is the specimen. The various colors observed in urine are a result of different excreted pigments. Yellow and amber are generally due to urochromes (derivatives of urobilin, the end product of bilirubin degradation), whereas a yellowish-brown

to green color is a result of bile pigment oxidation. Red and brown after standing are due to porphyrins, whereas reddish-brown in fresh specimens comes from hemoglobin or red cells. Brownish-black after standing is seen in alkaptonuria (a result of excreted homogentisic acid) and in malignant melanoma (in which the precursor melanogen oxidizes in the air to melanin). Drugs and some foods, such as beets, may also alter urine color.

Odor
Odor ordinarily has little diagnostic significance. The characteristic pungent odor of fresh urine is due to volatile aromatic acids, in contrast to the typical ammonia odor of urine that has been allowed to stand. Urinary tract infections impart a noxious, fecal smell to urine, whereas the urine of diabetics often smells fruity as a result of ketones. Certain inborn errors of metabolism, such as maple sugar urine disease, are associated with characteristic urine odors.

Turbidity
The cloudiness of an urine specimen depends on pH and dissolved solids composition. Turbidity generally may be due to gross bacteriuria, whereas a smoky appearance is seen in hematuria. Thread-like cloudiness is observed when the specimen is full of mucus. In alkaline urine, suspended precipitates of amorphous phosphates and carbonates may be responsible for turbidity, whereas in acidic urine, amorphous urates may be the cause.[16]

Volume
The volume of urine excreted indicates the balance between fluid ingestion and water lost from the lungs, sweat, and intestine. Most adults produce from 750 to 2,000 mL every 24 hours, averaging about 1.5 L per person. Polyuria is observed in diabetes mellitus and insipidus (in insipidus, as a result of lack of ADH), as well as in chronic renal disease, acromegaly (overproduction of the growth hormone somatostatin), and myxedema (hypothyroid edema). Anuria or oliguria (<200 mL/d) is found in nephritis, urinary tract obstruction, AKI, and kidney failure.

Specific Gravity
The specific gravity (SG) of urine is the weight of 1 mL of urine in grams divided by the weight of 1 mL of water. SG gives an indication of the density of a fluid that depends on the concentration of dissolved total solids. SG varies with the solute load to be excreted (consisting primarily of NaCl and urea), as well as with the urine volume. It is used to assess the state of hydration/dehydration of an individual or as an indicator of the concentrating ability of the kidneys.

The most commonly encountered analytic method consists of a refractometer, or total solids meter. This operates on the principle that the refractive index of a urine specimen will vary directly with the total amount of dissolved solids in the sample. This instrument measures the refractive index of the urine as compared with water on a scale that is calibrated directly into the ocular

and viewed while held up to a light source. Correct calibration is vital for accuracy. Most recently, an indirect colorimetric reagent strip method for assaying SG has been added to most dipstick screens. Unlike the refractometer, dipsticks measure only ionic solutes and do not take into account glucose or protein.

The normal range for urinary SG is 1.003 to 1.035 g/mL. SG can vary in pathologic states. Low SG can occur in diabetes insipidus, pyelonephritis, and glomerulonephritis, in which the renal concentrating ability has become dysfunctional. High SG can be seen in diabetes mellitus, congestive heart failure, dehydration, adrenal insufficiency, liver disease, and nephrosis. SG will increase about 0.004 units for every 1% change in glucose concentration and about 0.003 units for every 1% change in protein. Fixed SG (isosthenuria) around 1.010 is observed in severe renal damage, in which the kidney excretes urine that is iso-osmotic with the plasma. This generally occurs after an initial period of anuria because the damaged tubules are unable to concentrate or dilute the glomerular filtrate.[16]

pH
Determinations of urinary pH must be performed on fresh specimens because of the significant tendency of urine to alkalinize on standing. Normal urine pH falls within the range of 4.7 to 7.8. Acidity in urine (pH < 7.0) is primarily caused by phosphates, which are excreted as salts conjugated to Na^+, K^+, Ca^{2+}, and NH_4^+. Acidity also reflects the excretion of the nonvolatile metabolic acids pyruvate, lactate, and citrate. Owing to the Na^+/H^+ exchange pump mechanism of the renal tubules, pH (H^+ concentration) increases as sodium is retained. Pathologic states, in which increased acidity is observed, include systemic acidosis, as seen in diabetes mellitus, and renal tubular acidosis (RTA). In RTA, the tubules are unable to excrete excess H^+ even though the body is in metabolic acidosis, and urinary pH remains around 6.

Alkaline urine (pH > 7.0) is observed postprandially as a normal reaction to the acidity of gastric HCl dumped into the duodenum and then into the circulation or following ingestion of alkaline food or medications. Urinary tract infections and bacterial contamination also will alkalinize pH. Medications such as potassium citrate and sodium bicarbonate will reduce urine pH. Alkaline urine is also found in Fanconi syndrome, a congenital generalized aminoaciduria resulting from defective proximal tubular function.

Chemical Analyses
Routine urine chemical analysis is rapid and easily performed with commercially available reagent strips or dipsticks. These strips are plastic coated with different reagent bands directed toward different analytes. When dipped into urine, a color change signals a deviation from normality. Colors on the dipstick bands are matched against a color chart provided with the reagents. Automated and semiautomated instruments that detect

by reflectance photometry provide an alternative to the color chart and offer better precision and standardization. Abnormal results are followed up by specific quantitative or confirmatory urine assays. The analytes routinely tested are glucose, protein, ketones, nitrite, leukocyte esterase, bilirubin/urobilinogen, and hemoglobin/blood.

Glucose and Ketones
These constituents are normally absent in urine. The clinical significance of these analytes and their testing methods are discussed in Chapter 14.

Protein
Reagent strips for UA are used as a general qualitative screen for proteinuria. They are primarily specific for albumin, but they may give false-positive results in specimens that are alkaline and highly buffered. Positive dipstick results should be confirmed by more specific chemical assays, as described in Chapter 11, or more commonly by microscopic evaluation to detect casts.

Nitrite
This assay semiquantitates the amount of urinary reduction of nitrate (on the reagent strip pad) to nitrite by the enzymes of gram-negative bacteria. A negative result does not mean that no bacteriuria is present. A gram-positive pathogen, such as *Staphylococcus*, *Enterococcus*, or *Streptococcus*, may not produce nitrate-reducing enzymes; alternatively, a spot urine sample may not have been retained in the bladder long enough to pick up a sufficient number of organisms to register on the reagent strip.[16]

Leukocyte Esterase
White blood cells (WBCs), especially phagocytes, contain esterases. A positive dipstick for esterases indicates possible WBCs in urine.

Bilirubin/Urobilinogen
Hemoglobin degradation ultimately results in the formation of the waste product bilirubin, which is then converted to urobilinogen in the gut through bacterial action. Although most of this urobilinogen is excreted as urobilin in the feces, some is excreted in urine as a colorless waste product. This amount is normally too small to be detected as a positive dipstick reaction. In conditions of prehepatic, hepatic, and posthepatic jaundice, however, urine dipstick tests for urobilinogen and bilirubin may be positive or negative, depending on the nature of the patient's jaundice. A more in-depth view of bilirubin metabolism and assay methods is given in Chapter 25. Reagent strip tests for bilirubin involve diazotization and formation of a color change. Dipstick methods for urobilinogen differ, but most rely on a modification of the Ehrlich reaction with *p*-dimethylaminobenzaldehyde.[16]

Hemoglobin/Blood
Intact or lysed RBCs produce a positive dipstick result. The dipstick will be positive in cases of renal trauma/injury, infection, and obstruction that result from calculi or neoplasms.

Sediment Examination
Centrifuged, decanted urine aliquot leaves behind a sediment of formed elements that is used for microscopic examination.

Cells
For cellular elements, evaluation is best accomplished by counting and then taking the average of at least 10 microscopic fields.

Red Blood Cells
Erythrocytes greater in number than 0 to 2/high-power field (HPF) are considered abnormal. Such hematuria may result simply from severe exercise or menstrual blood contamination. However, it may also be indicative of trauma, particularly vascular injury, renal/urinary calculi obstruction, pyelonephritis, or cystitis. Hematuria in conjunction with leukocytes is diagnostic of infection.

White Blood Cells
Leukocytes greater in number than 0 to 1/HPF are considered abnormal. These cells are usually polymorphonuclear phagocytes, commonly known as segmented neutrophils. They are observed when there is acute glomerulonephritis, urinary tract infection, or inflammation of any type. In hypotonic urine (low osmotic concentration), WBCs can become enlarged, exhibiting a sparkling effect in their cytoplasmic granules. These cells possess a noticeable Brownian motion and are called glitter cells, but they have no pathologic significance.

Epithelial Cells
Several types of epithelial cells are frequently encountered in normal urine because they are continuously sloughed off the lining of the nephrons and urinary tract. Large, flat, squamous vaginal epithelia are often seen in urine specimens from female patients, and samples heavily contaminated with vaginal discharge may show clumps or sheets of these cells. Renal epithelial cells are round, uninucleate cells and, if present in numbers greater than 2/HPF, indicate clinically significant active tubular injury or degeneration. Transitional bladder epithelial cells (urothelial cells) may be flat, cuboidal, or columnar and also can be observed in urine on occasion. Large numbers will be seen only in cases of urinary catheterization, bladder inflammation, or neoplasm.

Miscellaneous Elements
Spermatozoa are often seen in the urine of both males and females. They are usually not reported because they are of no pathologic significance. In males, however, their presence may indicate prostate abnormalities. Yeast cells are also frequently found in urine specimens. Because they are extremely refractile and of a similar size to RBCs, they can easily be mistaken under low magnification. Higher power examination for budding or mycelial forms differentiates these fungal elements from erythrocytes. Parasites found in urine are generally contaminants from fecal or vaginal material. In fecal contaminant category,

the most commonly encountered organism is *Enterobius vermicularis* (pinworm) infestation in children. In the vaginal contaminant category, the most common is the intensely motile flagellate, *Trichomonas vaginalis*. A true urinary parasite, sometimes seen in patients from endemic areas of the world, is the ova of the trematode *Schistosoma haematobium*. This condition will usually occur in conjunction with a significant hematuria.[16]

Bacteria

Normal urine is sterile and contains no bacteria. Small numbers of organisms seen in a fresh urine specimen usually represent skin or air contamination. In fresh specimens, however, large numbers of organisms, or small numbers accompanied by WBCs and the symptoms of urinary tract infection, are highly diagnostic for true infection. Clinically significant bacteriuria is considered to be more than 20 organisms/HPF or, alternatively, 10^5 or greater registered on a microbiologic colony count. Most pathogens seen in urine are gram-negative coliforms (microscopic "rods") such as *Escherichia coli* and *Proteus* spp. Asymptomatic bacteriuria, in which there are significant numbers of bacteria without appreciable clinical symptoms, occurs somewhat commonly in young girls, pregnant women, and patients with diabetes. This condition must be taken seriously because, if left untreated, it may result in pyelonephritis and, subsequently, permanent renal damage.

Casts

Casts are precipitated, cylindrical impressions of the nephrons. They comprise Tamm-Horsfall mucoprotein (uromucoid) from the tubular epithelia in the ascending limb of the loop of Henle. Casts form whenever there is sufficient renal stasis, increased urine salt or protein concentration, and decreased urine pH. In patients with severe renal disease, truly accurate classification of casts may require use of "cytospin" centrifugation and Papanicolaou staining for adequate differentiation. Unlike cells, casts should be examined under low power and are most often located around the edges of the coverslip.

Hyaline

The matrix of these casts is clear and gelatinous, without embedded cellular or particulate matter. They may be difficult to visualize unless a high-intensity lamp is used. Their presence indicates glomerular leakage of protein. This leakage may be temporary (as a result of fever, upright posture, dehydration, or emotional stress) or may be permanent. Their occasional presence is not considered pathologic.

Granular

These casts are descriptively classified as either coarse or finely granular. The type of embedded particulate matter is simply a matter of the amount of degeneration that the epithelial cell inclusions have undergone. Their occasional presence is not pathologic; however, large numbers may be found in chronic lead toxicity and pyelonephritis.

Cellular

Several different types of casts are included in this category. RBC or erythrocytic casts are always considered pathologic because they are diagnostic for glomerular inflammation that results in renal hematuria. They are seen in subacute bacterial endocarditis, kidney infarcts, collagen diseases, and acute glomerulonephritis. WBC or leukocytic casts are also always considered pathologic because they are diagnostic for inflammation of the nephrons. They are observed in pyelonephritis, nephrotic syndrome, and acute glomerulonephritis. In asymptomatic pyelonephritis, these casts may be the only clue to detection. Epithelial cell casts are sometimes formed by fusion of renal tubular epithelia after desquamation; occasional presence is normal. Many, however, are observed in severe desquamative processes and renal stases that occur in heavy metal poisoning, renal toxicity, eclampsia, nephrotic syndrome, and amyloidosis. Waxy casts are uniformly yellowish, refractile, and brittle appearing, with sharply defined, often broken edges. They are almost always pathologic because they indicate tubular inflammation or deterioration. They are formed by renal stasis in the collecting ducts and are, therefore, found in chronic renal diseases. Fatty casts are abnormal, coarse, granular casts with lipid inclusions that appear as refractile globules of different sizes. Broad (renal failure) casts may be up to two to six times wider than "regular" casts and may be cellular, waxy, or granular in composition. Like waxy casts, they are derived from the collecting ducts in severe renal stasis.

Crystals

Acid Environment

Crystals seen in urine with pH values of less than 7 include calcium oxalate, which are normal colorless octahedrons or "envelopes"; they may have an almost star-like appearance. Also seen are amorphous urates, normal yellow-red masses with a grain of sand appearance. Uric acid crystals found in this environment are normal yellow to red-brown crystals that appear in extremely irregular shapes, such as rosettes, prisms, or rhomboids. Cholesterol crystals in acid urine are clear, flat, rectangular plates with notched corners. They may be seen in nephrotic syndrome and in conditions producing chyluria and are always considered abnormal. Cystine crystals are also sometimes observed in acid urine; they are highly pathologic and appear as colorless, refractile, nearly flat hexagons, somewhat similar to uric acid. These are observed in homocystinuria (an aminoaciduria resulting in mental retardation) and cystinuria (an inherited defect of cystine reabsorption resulting in renal calculi).

Alkaline Environment

Crystals seen in urine with pH values greater than 7 include amorphous phosphates, which are normal crystals that appear as fine, colorless masses, resembling sand. Also seen are calcium carbonate crystals, which are normal forms that appear as small, colorless dumbbells or spheres. Triple phosphate crystals are also observed in alkaline urines; they are colorless prisms of three to six sides, resembling "coffin lids." Ammonium biurate crystals are normal forms occasionally found in this environment, appearing as spiny, yellow-brown spheres, or "thorn apples."

Other

Sulfonamide crystals are abnormal precipitates shaped like yellow-brown sheaves, clusters, or needles, formed in patients undergoing antimicrobial therapy with sulfa drugs. These drugs are seldom used today. Tyrosine/leucine crystals are abnormal types shaped like clusters of smooth, yellow needles or spheres. These are sometimes seen in patients with severe liver disease.[16]

PATHOPHYSIOLOGY

Glomerular Diseases

Disorders or diseases that directly damage the renal glomeruli may, at least initially, exhibit normal tubular function. With time, however, disease progression involves the renal tubules as well. The following syndromes have discrete symptoms that are recognizable by their patterns of clinical laboratory findings.

Acute Glomerulonephritis

Pathologic lesions in acute glomerulonephritis primarily involve the glomerulus. Histologic examination shows large, inflamed glomeruli with a decreased capillary lumen. Abnormal laboratory findings usually include rapid onset of hematuria and proteinuria (usually albumin and generally <3 g/d). The rapid development of a decreased GFR, anemia, elevated blood urea nitrogen (BUN) and serum creatinine, oliguria, sodium and water retention (with consequent hypertension and some localized edema), and, sometimes, congestive heart failure is typical. Numerous hyaline and granular casts are generally seen on UA. The actual RBC casts are regarded as highly suggestive of this syndrome. Acute glomerulonephritis is often related to recent infection by group A β-hemolytic streptococci. It is theorized that circulating immune complexes trigger a strong inflammatory response in the glomerular basement membrane, resulting in a direct injury to the glomerulus itself. Other possible causes include drug-related exposures, acute kidney infections due to other bacterial (and, possibly, viral) agents, and other systemic immune complex diseases, such as systemic lupus erythematosus and bacterial endocarditis.

Chronic Glomerulonephritis

Lengthy glomerular inflammation may lead to glomerular scarring and the eventual loss of functioning nephrons. This process often goes undetected for lengthy periods because only minor decreases in renal function occur at first and only slight proteinuria and hematuria are observed. Gradual development of uremia (or azotemia, excess nitrogen compounds in the blood) may be the first sign of this process.

Nephrotic Syndrome

Nephrotic syndrome (Fig. 27-6) can be caused by several different diseases that result in injury and increased permeability of the glomerular basement membrane. This defect almost always yields several abnormal findings, such as massive proteinuria (>3.5 g/d) and resultant hypoalbuminemia. The subsequent decreased plasma oncotic pressure causes a generalized edema as a result of the movement of body fluids out of vascular and into interstitial spaces. Other hallmarks of this syndrome are hyperlipidemia and lipiduria. Lipiduria takes the form of oval fat bodies in the urine. These bodies are degenerated renal tubular cells containing reabsorbed lipoproteins. Primary causes are associated directly with glomerular disease states.

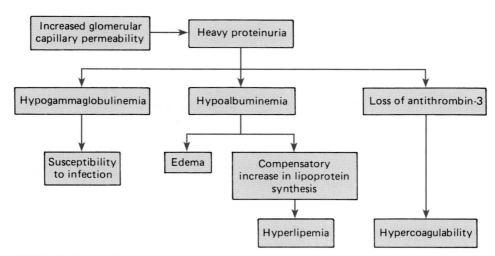

FIGURE 27-6 Pathophysiology of nephrotic syndrome.

Tubular Diseases

Tubular defects occur to a certain extent in the progression of all renal diseases as the GFR falls. In some instances, however, this aspect of the overall dysfunction becomes predominant. The result is decreased excretion/reabsorption of certain substances or reduced urinary concentrating capability. Clinically, the most important defect is RTA, the primary tubular disorder affecting acid–base balance. This disease can be classified into two types, depending on the nature of the tubular defect. In distal RTA, the renal tubules are unable to keep up the vital pH gradient between the blood and tubular fluid. In proximal RTA, there is decreased bicarbonate reabsorption, resulting in hyperchloremic acidosis. In general, reduced reabsorption in the proximal tubule is manifested by findings of abnormally low serum values for phosphorus and uric acid and by glucose and amino acids in the urine. In addition, there may be some proteinuria (usually <2 g/d).

Acute or chronic inflammation of the tubules and surrounding interstitium also may occur as a result of radiation toxicity, renal transplant rejection, viral–fungal–bacterial infections, and a reaction to medications. This is known as interstitial nephritis. Characteristic clinical findings in these cases are decreases in GFR, urinary concentrating ability, and metabolic acid excretion; leukocyte casts in the urine; and inappropriate control of sodium balance.[4,7]

Urinary Tract Infection/Obstruction

Infection

The site of infection may be either in the kidneys (pyelonephritis) or in the urinary bladder (cystitis). In general, a microbiologic colony count of more than 10^5 colonies/mL is considered diagnostic for infection in either locale. Bacteriuria (as evidenced by positive nitrite dipstick findings for some organisms), hematuria, and pyuria (leukocytes in the urine, as shown by positive leukocyte esterase dipstick) are all frequently encountered abnormal laboratory results in these cases. In particular, WBC (leukocyte) casts in the urine is considered diagnostic for pyelonephritis.[4,7,16]

Obstruction

Renal obstructions can cause disease in one of two ways. They may either gradually raise the intratubular pressure until nephrons necrose and chronic renal failure ensues or they may predispose the urinary tract to repeated infections.

Obstructions may be located in the upper or lower urinary tract. Blockages in the upper tract are characterized by a constricting lesion below a dilated collecting duct. Obstructions of the lower tract are evidenced by the residual urine in the bladder after cessation of micturition (urination); symptoms include slowness of voiding, both initially and throughout urination. Causes of obstructions can include neoplasms (e.g., prostate/bladder carcinoma or lymph node tumors constricting ureters), acquired diseases (e.g., urethral strictures or renal calculi), and congenital deformities of the lower urinary tract. The clinical symptoms of advancing obstructive disease include decreased urinary concentrating capability, diminished metabolic acid excretion, decreased GFR, and reduced renal blood flow. Laboratory tests useful in determining the nature of the blockage are UA, urine culture, BUN, serum creatinine, and CBC. Final diagnosis is usually made by radiologic imaging techniques.[5,8]

Renal Calculi

Renal calculi, or kidney stones, are formed by the combination of various crystallized substances, which are listed in Table 27-2. Of these, calcium oxalate stones are by far the most commonly encountered, particularly in the tropics and subtropics.

It is currently believed that recurrence of calculi in susceptible individuals is a result of several causes but mainly a reduced urine flow rate (related to a decreased fluid intake) and saturation of the urine with large amounts of essentially insoluble substances. Chemical analysis of stones is important in determining the cause of the condition. Specialized x-ray diffraction and infrared spectroscopy techniques are widely used for this purpose. Clinical symptoms are, of course, similar to those encountered in other obstructive processes: hematuria, urinary tract infections, and characteristic abdominal pain.[4,7,16]

TABLE 27-2	TYPES OF KIDNEY STONES
STONE COMPOSITION	**CAUSE OF STONE FORMATION**
Calcium oxalate	Hyperparathyroidism
	High urine calcium
	Vitamin D toxicity
	Sarcoidosis
	Osteoporosis
Magnesium ammonium phosphate	Infectious processes
Calcium phosphate	Excess alkali consumption
	Infection with urease-producing organisms
Uric acid	Gout
	High levels of uric acid in blood and urine
Cystine	Inherited cystinuria

Renal Failure

Acute Kidney Injury

Acute kidney injury is a sudden, sharp decline in renal function as a result of an acute toxic or hypoxic insult to the kidneys. AKI is a common and serious condition that occurs in approximately 5% of all hospitalized patients. The risk, injury, failure, loss of function, end-stage renal disease (RIFLE) and the Acute Kidney Injury Network definitions of AKI are based on changes in both serum creatinine and urinary output; however, both display poor specificity and sensitivity for the early detection of AKI.[17,18] Novel urine and plasma biomarkers, such as NGAL and Kidney injury molecule-1 (KIM-1), are emerging as excellent biomarkers for the early prediction and prognosis of AKI. AKI is subdivided into three types, depending on the location of the precipitating defect.

Prerenal AKI: The defect lies in the blood supply before it reaches the kidney. Causes can include cardiovascular system failure and consequent hypovolemia.

Intrinsic AKI: The defect involves the kidney. The most common cause is acute tubular necrosis; other causes include vascular obstructions/inflammations and glomerulonephritis.

Postrenal AKI: The defect lies in the urinary tract after it exits the kidney. Generally, acute renal failure occurs as a consequence of lower urinary tract obstruction or rupture of the urinary bladder.

Toxic insults to the kidney that are severe enough to initiate acute renal failure include hemolytic transfusion reactions, myoglobinuria due to rhabdomyolysis, heavy metal/solvent poisonings, antifreeze ingestion, and analgesic and aminoglycoside toxicities. These conditions directly damage the renal tubules. Hypoxic insults include conditions that severely compromise renal blood flow, such as septic/hemorrhagic shock, burns, and cardiac failure. The most commonly observed symptoms of acute renal failure are oliguria and anuria (<400 mL/d). The diminished ability to excrete electrolytes and water results in a significant increase in extracellular fluid volume, leading to peripheral edema, hypertension, and congestive heart failure. Most prominent, however, is the onset of the uremic syndrome or kidney failure, in which increased BUN and serum creatinine values are observed along with the preceding symptoms. The outcome of this disease is either recovery or, in the case of irreversible renal damage, progression to chronic renal failure.[4,7]

CASE STUDY 27-1

A 52-year-old man with a history of AIDS, hypertension, diabetes mellitus, and alcohol abuse was found unconscious in his home by his roommate. In the emergency department, he was hypotensive (103/60 mm Hg), febrile (temperature 101°F), and unresponsive. Computed tomography scan of the abdomen showed cholecystitis and gallstones. Laboratory data are listed.

The patient was diagnosed with acute renal failure. He was administered intravenous fluids; BUN fell to 68 mg/dL and creatinine fell to 2.2 mg/dL. The patient's blood culture report was positive for *E. coli*. He was treated with tobramycin and cefepime. The patient continued to deteriorate and died 5 days after admission. Cause of death was multiorgan failure secondary to AIDS, sepsis, and alcoholic cirrhosis.

Questions

1. What is the significance of the patient's elevated CK? Explain why the physician ordered a CK-MB and troponin level. What can you conclude about the patient's cardiac status?

2. What is the cause of his acute renal failure?

3. What is the significance of the patient's large urine hemoglobin?

4. How would you interpret this patient's liver function tests considering his clinical history?

Drugs of Abuse	Negative	Urinalysis	
Serum ethanol	84 mg/dL	Hemoglobin	Positive
		WBC	4 HPF (0–4)
		RBC	2 HPF (0–4)
CK	3,308 U/L (24–204)	BUN	71 mg/dL (8–21)
CK-MB	15 ng/mL (0–7.5)	Creatinine	4.1 mg/dL (0.9–1.5)
Troponin T	<0.01 ng/mL (0–0.4)	Alkaline phosphatase	443 U/L (45–122)
pH	7.50	Aspartate aminotransferase	305 U/L (9–45)
pCO_2	27 mm Hg	Alanine aminotransferase	78 U/L (8–63)
Total CO_2	15 mmol/L	Gamma glutamyl transpeptidase	724 U/L (11–50)
		Total bilirubin	2.7 mg/dL (0.2–1.0)
		Direct bilirubin	2.4 mg/dL (0–0.2)

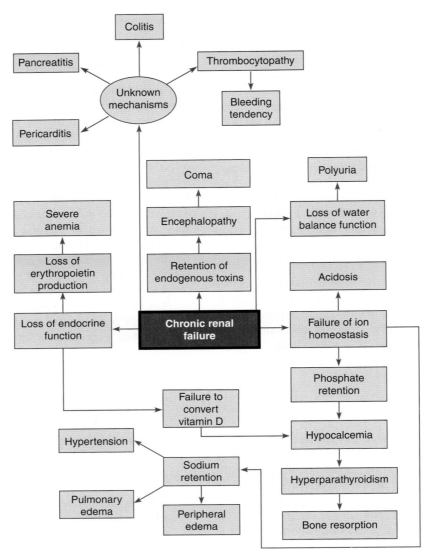

FIGURE 27-7 Pathophysiology of chronic kidney disease.

Chronic Kidney Disease

Chronic kidney disease is a clinical syndrome that occurs when there is a gradual decline in renal function over time (Fig. 27-7). According to the National Kidney Foundation, 1 in 11 U.S. adults has CKD and millions more are at risk (www.kidney.org). Early detection and treatment are needed to prevent progression to kidney failure and complications such as coronary vascular disease. The National Kidney Foundation has formulated guidelines for earlier diagnosis, treatment, and prevention of further disease progression. See Table 27-3 for the five stages of CKD. GFR and evidence of kidney damage based on measurement of proteinuria or other markers form the basis of the classifications.[19]

The conditions that can precipitate AKI also may lead to chronic renal failure. Several other causes for this syndrome are listed in Table 27-4.

Increasing Incidence of CKD

There is an increasing incidence of CKD in the United States due to the increase in diabetes, the aging population, obesity, and metabolic syndrome. Diabetes mellitus can have profound effects on the renal system. According to the National Kidney Foundation, diabetes is the leading cause of CKD and accounts for 45% of people diagnosed with kidney failure each year (www.kidney.org). The effects are primarily glomerular, but they may affect all kidney structures as well and are theorized to be caused by the abnormally hyperglycemic environment that constantly bathes the vascular system.[4,7]

Typically, diabetes affects the kidneys by causing them to become glucosuric, polyuric, and nocturic. These states are caused by the heavy demands made on the kidneys to diurese hyperosmotic urine. In addition, a mild proteinuria (microalbuminuria) often develops

TABLE 27-3	SYSTEMATIC CLASSIFICATION OF CHRONIC KIDNEY DISEASE STAGES	
STAGE	**DESCRIPTION**	**GFR (ML/MIN PER 1.73 m²)**
	At increased risk[a]	≥60 (with risk factors)
1	Kidney damage with normal or ↑GFR	>90
2	Kidney damage with normal or ↓GFR	60–89
3	Moderate ↓ GFR	30–59
4	Severe ↓ GFR	15–29
5	Kidney failure	<15

GFR, glomerular filtration rate; CKD, chronic kidney disease.

[a]At-risk patients should be screened. Stages 1–5 illustrate the progression of CKD.

Source: National Kidney Foundation. *K/DOQI Clinical Practice Guidelines for Chronic Kidney Disease: Executive Summary.* New York, NY: National Kidney Foundation, 2002:16.

between 10 and 15 years after the original diagnosis (see the section "Microalbumin"). Hypertension often manifests next, further exacerbating the renal damage. Eventually, chronic renal insufficiency or nephrotic syndrome may evolve, and each may be identified by their characteristic symptoms and laboratory findings. Early treatment of diabetes that focuses on tight control of blood glucose and prevention of high blood pressure may prolong the onset of chronic renal failure.

Aside from hypertension and diabetes, age is the key predictor of CDK. Due to the decline in fertility and increase in the average life span, the percentage of the population aged 65 years or older is projected to increase from 12.4% in 2000 to 19.6% in 2030, according to the U.S. Census Bureau. This continual rise, over the previous decade and those to come, contributes significantly to the increasing incidence of CKD.

TABLE 27-4	ETIOLOGY OF CHRONIC RENAL FAILURE
ETIOLOGY	**EXAMPLES**
Renal circulatory diseases	Renal vein thrombosis, malignant hypertension
Primary glomerular diseases	Systemic lupus erythematosus, chronic glomerulonephritis
Renal sequelae to metabolic disease	Gout, diabetes mellitus, amyloidosis
Inflammatory diseases	Tuberculosis, chronic pyelonephritis
Renal obstructions	Prostatic enlargement, calculi
Congenital renal deformity	Polycystic kidneys, renal hypoplasia
Miscellaneous conditions	Radiation nephritis

Epidemiologic evidence links obesity to CKD and kidney failure. However, diabetes mellitus and hypertension have potential confounding roles because obesity is a risk factor for diabetes and hypertension, the two most common causes of CKD and kidney failure. Recent studies show that obesity itself increases the risk of kidney injury.[20] As an individual gains weight, the nephron number remains the same; however, the GFR increases to meet the higher metabolic demands, which results in damage to the kidney.

The metabolic syndrome, characterized by the presence of at least three of the following risk factors—abdominal obesity, hypertension, low high-density lipoprotein cholesterol level, hypertriglyceridemia, or hyperglycemia—is a prevalent disorder in the United States. In a population study of a representative sample of the U.S. general population, the risk of CKD and microalbuminuria increased progressively with a greater number of components of metabolic syndrome.[21] Individuals with metabolic syndrome had a 2.6-fold increased risk of developing CKD compared with individuals without metabolic syndrome.[21] Interventions that target biochemical components of metabolic syndrome may reduce the risk of CDK.

Renal Hypertension

Renal disease–induced hypertension can be caused by decreased perfusion to all or part of the kidney (ischemia). Lack of perfusion may be caused by traumatic injury or narrowing of an artery or intrarenal arterioles. Chronic ischemia of any kind results in nephron dysfunction and eventual necrosis. The resulting changes in blood and body fluid volumes within the kidney trigger the activation of the renin–angiotensin–aldosterone system, setting off vasoconstriction that is manifested as persistent hypertension.

Renal hypertension can be evaluated by monitoring serum aldosterone, Na^+, and renin levels. As a result of the effect of aldosterone, there will be increased serum Na^+, decreased serum K^+, and increased urine K^+.

CASE STUDY 27-2

A 42-year-old man presented to the hospital admitting to have ingested 3 cups of antifreeze and a rodenticide product 10 hours prior. Upon arrival to the hospital, the patient was somnolent and afebrile and vitals were within normal limits. His chemistry results are shown below. Calcium oxalate crystals were found in his urine (pH 5). His urine toxicology screen was negative.

Na$^+$	139 mmol/L	Osmolality (serum)	416 mOsm/kg
K$^+$	4.3 mmol/L	Blood gases (arterial)	
Cl$^-$	94 mmol/L	pH	7.26
CO$_2$	10 mmol/L	pCO$_2$	13 mm Hg
BUN	9 mg/dL	pO$_2$	129 mm Hg
Creatinine	2.2 mg/dL	HCO$_3^-$	18 mmol/L
Glucose	167 mg/dL	Prothrombin time	12.8 s
Ca^{2+}	9.9 mg/dL	International normalized ratio	1.1
Albumin	4.5 g/dL		

Treatment with fomepizole (4-MP) was initiated to prevent further metabolism of ethylene glycol. The patient became agitated and was intubated for airway protection and placed on a propofol (sedative-hypnotic) drip. Nephrology was called and hemodialysis was started. Laboratory test results the morning after the first hemodialysis are listed below. The initial ethylene glycol level from time of presentation to the emergency room was received at this time and is included.

Na$^+$	143 mmol/L	Albumin	3.1 g/dL
K$^+$	4.1 mmol/L	Mg^{2+}	1.6 mg/dL
Cl$^-$	108 mmol/L	CK	405 U/L
CO$_2$	18 mmol/L	Osmolality	364 mOsm/kg
BUN	8 mg/dL	Blood gases (arterial)	
Creatinine	3.1 mg/dL	pH	7.4
Glucose	194 mg/dL	pCO$_2$	26 mm Hg
Ca^{2+}	7.7 mg/dL	pO$_2$	192 mm Hg
Ethylene glycol	499.4 mg/dL	HCO$_3^-$	15 mmol/L

The patient remained intubated and sedated. He continued to receive hemodialysis two times a day for 4 hours at a time. The patient also continued to receive fomepizole every 12 hours and following each round of hemodialysis. This treatment continued until the osmolar and anion gaps were normalized.

Questions

1. What caused the formation of the calcium oxalate crystals? What is the clinical significance of calcium oxalate crystal formation?

2. Calculate the anion and osmolar gaps for both sets of laboratory results. In this case, what is the cause of the anion and osmolar gaps? How are these values clinically significant?

3. What are other common drugs and toxins that can cause acute renal failure?

Therapy for AKI

Dialysis

In patients with AKI, uremic symptoms, uncontrolled hyperkalemia, and acidosis have traditionally been indications that the kidneys are unable to excrete the body's waste products and a substitute method in the form of dialysis was necessary. Dialysis is often instituted before this stage, however. Several forms of dialysis are available; however, they all use a semipermeable membrane surrounded by a dialysate bath.

In traditional hemodialysis (removal of waste from blood), the membrane is synthetic and outside the body. Arterial blood and dialysate are pumped at high rates (150 to 250 and 500 mL/min, respectively) in opposite directions. The blood is returned to the venous circulation and the dialysate discarded. The diffusion of low-molecular-weight solutes (<500 Da) into the dialysate is favored by this process, but mid-molecular-weight solutes (500 to 2,000 Da) are inadequately cleared. Creatinine clearance is about 150 to 160 mL/min.

In peritoneal dialysis, the peritoneal wall acts as the dialysate membrane and gravity is used to introduce and remove the dialysate. Two variations of this form are available, continuous ambulatory peritoneal dialysis (CAPD) and continuous cycling peritoneal dialysis; however, the process is continuous in both, being performed 24 hours a day, 7 days a week. This method is not as rigorous as the traditional method. Small solutes (e.g., potassium) have significantly lower clearance rates compared with the traditional method, but more large solutes are cleared and steady-state levels of blood analytes are maintained.

Continuous arteriovenous hemofiltration (ultrafiltration of blood), continuous venovenous hemofiltration, continuous arteriovenous hemodialysis, and continuous venovenous hemodialysis together make up the slow continuous renal replacement therapies developed to treat acute renal failure in critically ill patients in intensive care settings. In these methods, the semipermeable membrane is again outside the body. Solutes up to 5,000 Da (the pore size of the membranes) and water are slowly (10 mL/min) and continuously filtered from the blood in the first two methods, causing minimal changes in plasma osmolality. Volume loss can be replaced in the form of parenteral nutrition and intravenous medications. The final two methods are similar to the filtration methods, but a continuous trickle of dialysis fluid is pumped past the dialysis membrane, resulting in continuous diffusion and a doubling of the urea clearance.

Therapy for Kidney Failure

For patients with irreversible renal failure, dialysis and transplantation are the only two therapeutic options. Initiation of either treatment occurs when the GFR falls to 5 mL/min (10 to 15 mL/min in patients with diabetic nephropathy).

Dialysis

Traditional hemodialysis or its more recent, high-efficiency form and peritoneal dialysis are the available methods. The clinical laboratory used in conjunction with a hemodialysis facility must be able to adequately monitor procedural efficiency in a wide variety of areas. Renal dialysis has basic goals, and specific laboratory tests should be performed to evaluate the achievement of each goal.

Transplantation

The most efficient hemodialysis techniques provide only 10% to 12% of the small solute removal of two normal kidneys and considerably less removal of larger solutes. Even patients who are well dialyzed have physical disabilities and decreased quality of life. Kidney transplantation offers the greatest chance for full return to a healthy, productive life. However, this option is limited by the significant shortage of donor organs. For kidney failure patients, waiting for an organ donation can vary from several months to several years.

Renal transplantation is from a compatible donor to a recipient suffering from irreversible renal failure. The organ can be from a cadaver or a live individual (80% and 20%, respectively, of all kidney transplants in the United States). For this procedure to be successful, the body's immune response to the transplanted organ must be suppressed. Therefore, the donor and recipient are carefully

CASE STUDY 27-3

A 78-year-old woman with a history of hypertension, aortic thoracic graft, and esophageal reflux disease complained of fever (100°F) and weakness. She had been treated 3 weeks before at the hospital for a urinary tract infection. She was admitted to the hospital for a diagnostic workup and transfusion. Her laboratory results are as follows:

Na^+	129 mmol/L	Hct	25.6%
K^+	3.7 mmol/L	Hgb	8.5 g/dL
Cl^-	97 mmol/L	WBC	9,700
CO_2	19 mmol/L		
BUN	52 mg/dL		
Creatinine	3.2 mg/dL		

Urine culture was positive for *Citrobacter*. Urinalysis results are listed:

Color	Hazy/yellow
Specific gravity	1.015
pH	5
Blood	Large
Protein	2
Glucose	Negative
Ketones	Negative
Nitrates	Negative
RBC	>25
WBC	1–4
Casts	Granular, 1–4

The patient's renal function continued to decline, and she was put on hemodialysis. A renal biopsy was performed that showed end-stage crescentic glomerulonephritis. Two days later, the patient sustained a perforated duodenal ulcer, which required surgery and blood transfusion. Subsequently, she developed coagulopathy and liver failure. Her condition continued to deteriorate in the next few days, and she died following removal of life support.

Questions

1. Looking at the urinalysis, what is the significance of the results of 2+ protein and >25 RBCs?

2. What is the most likely cause of glomerulonephritis?

3. Why was the patient put on hemodialysis?

screened for ABO blood group, human leukocyte antigen (HLA) compatibility, and preformed HLA antibodies. The HLA system is the major inhibitor to transplantation.

Although kidney transplants have the capacity to function for decades, the mean half-life of a cadaveric transplant is approximately 7 years. The mortality rate is not significantly different from hemodialysis. Three-year graft survival figures vary from 65% to 85%, with live grafts doing better. It has been reported that there is no difference in patient survival among hemodialysis, CAPD, and cadaveric kidney transplantation. Live related-donor transplantation is associated with a better patient survival than other therapeutic options for kidney failure.

For additional student resources please visit thePoint at http://thepoint.lww.com. **thePoint**✳

QUESTIONS

1. Calculate creatinine clearance, given the following information: serum creatinine, 1.2 mg/dL; urine creatinine, 120 mg/dL; urine volume, 1750 mL/24 h; body surface area, 1.80 m².

2. Predict GFR in a 50-year-old woman who weighs 60 kg using the Cockcroft-Gault equation. Her serum creatinine level is 2.5 mg/dL.

3. The measurement of serum cystatin C, a small protein produced by nucleated cells, is useful for
   a. Detecting an early decrease in kidney function
   b. Calculating creatinine clearance
   c. Diagnosing end-stage renal disease
   d. Monitoring dialysis patients

4. Acute renal failure can be classified into three types. List each type and give an example of each.
   a. _____
   b. _____
   c. _____

5. The proximal tubule functions to
   a. reabsorb 75% of salt and water.
   b. concentrate salts.
   c. form the renal threshold.
   d. reabsorb urea.

6. Renal clearance is the
   a. volume of plasma from which a substance is removed per unit of time.
   b. volume of urine produced per day.
   c. amount of creatinine in urine.
   d. urine concentration of a substance divided by the urine volume per unit of time.

7. Renin release by the kidney is stimulated by
   a. a decrease in extracellular fluid volume or pressure.
   b. increased plasma sodium concentration.
   c. increased dietary sodium.
   d. renal tubular reabsorption.

8. The set of results that most accurately reflects severe renal disease is
   a. *serum creatinine, 3.7 mg/dL; creatinine clearance, 44 mL/min; BUN, 88 mg/dL*
   b. *serum creatinine, 1.0 mg/dL; creatinine clearance, 110 mL/min; BUN, 17 mg/dL*
   c. *serum creatinine, 2.0 mg/dL; creatinine clearance, 120 mL/min; BUN, 14 mg/dL*
   d. *serum creatinine, 1.0 mg/dL; creatinine clearance, 95 mL/min; BUN, 43 mg/dL*

9. Creatinine clearance results are corrected using a patient's body surface area to account for differences in
   a. muscle mass.
   b. age.
   c. dietary intake.
   d. sex.

10. A patient is suffering from an acute bleed. What is the most accurate way to describe the subsequent acute kidney injury?
   a. Prerenal acute kidney injury
   b. Renal acute kidney injury
   c. Postrenal acute kidney injury
   d. None of the above apply

REFERENCES

1. Vander A, Sherman JH, Luciano DS. *Human Physiology: The Mechanisms of Body Function*. 7th ed. New York, NY: McGraw-Hill; 1998:503, 508, 519.
2. Kaplan A, Szabo LL, Jack R, Opheim KE, Toivola B, Lyon AW. *Clinical Chemistry: Interpretation and Techniques*. 4th ed. Baltimore, MD: Williams & Wilkins; 1995:156-157.
3. Davies A, Blakely A, Kidd C. *Human Physiology*. London: Harcourt Publishers; 2001:747.
4. Rock RC, Walker WG, Jennings CD. Nitrogen metabolites and renal function. In: Tietz NW, ed. *Fundamentals of Clinical Chemistry*. 3rd ed. Philadelphia, PA: WB Saunders; 1987:669.
5. Russell PT, Sherwin JE, Obernolte R, et al. Nonprotein nitrogenous compounds. In: Kaplan LA, Pesce AJ, eds. *Clinical Chemistry: Theory, Analysis, and Correlation*. 2nd ed. St. Louis, MO: CV Mosby; 1989:1005.
6. Fraser D, Jones G, Kooh SW, et al. Calcium and phosphate metabolism. In: Tietz NW, ed. *Fundamentals of Clinical Chemistry*. 3rd ed. Philadelphia, PA: WB Saunders; 1987:705.
7. First MR. Renal function. In: Kaplan LA, Pesce AJ, eds. *Clinical Chemistry: Theory, Analysis, and Correlation*. 4th ed. St. Louis, MO: CV Mosby; 2003:477-491.
8. Kleinman LI, Lorenz JM. Physiology and pathophysiology of body water and electrolytes. In: Kaplan LA, Pesce AJ, eds. *Clinical Chemistry: Theory, Analysis, and Correlation*. 4th ed. St. Louis, MO: CV Mosby; 2003:441-461.
9. Sherwin JE, Bruegger BB. Acid-base control and acid-base disorders. In: Kaplan LA, Pesce AJ, eds. *Clinical Chemistry: Theory, Analysis, and Correlation*. 4th ed. St. Louis, MO: CV Mosby; 2003:462-476.
10. Levey AS, Stevens LA, Schmid CH, et al. A new equation to estimate glomerular filtration rate. *Ann Intern Med*. 2009;150:604-612.
11. Lab Tests Online. Cystatin C at a glance. http://www.labtestsonline.org/understanding/analytes/cystatin_c/glance.html
12. Stevens LA, Coresh J, Schmid CH, et al. Estimated GFR using serum cystatin C alone and in combination with serum creatinine: a pooled analysis of 3418 individuals with CKD. *Am J Kidney Dis*. 2008;51:395-406.
13. Schwartz GJ, Munoz A, Schneide MF, et al. New equations to estimate GFR in children with CKD. *J Am Soc Nephrol*. 2009;20:629-637.
14. Fraser CG. *Biological Variation: From Principles to Practice*. Washington, DC: AACC Press; 2001.
15. Haase M, Bellomo R, Haase-Fielitz A. Neutrophil gelatinase-associated lipocalin. *Curr Opin Crit Care*. 2010;16:526-532.
16. Kaplan LA, Pesce AJ. Examination of urine. In: Kaplan LA, Pesce AJ, eds. *Clinical Chemistry: Theory, Analysis, and Correlation*. 4th ed. St. Louis, MO: CV Mosby, 2003:1092-1109.
17. Bellomo R, Ronco C, Kellum JA, Mehta RL, Palevsky P. Acute renal failure—definition, outcome measures, animal models, fluid therapy and information technology needs: the Second International Consensus Conference of the Acute Dialysis Quality Initiative (ADQI) Group. *Crit Care*. 2004;8:R204-R212.
18. Mehta RL, Kellum JA, Shah SV, et al. Acute Kidney Injury Network: report of an initiative to improve outcomes in acute kidney injury. *Crit Care*. 2007;11:R31.
19. Mitchum C. Implementing the new kidney disease testing guidelines. *Clin Lab News*. 2002;September:14.
20. Kramer H, Luke A. Obesity and kidney disease: a big dilemma. *Curr Opin Nephrol Hypertens*. 2007;16:237-241.
21. Chen J, Muntner P, Hamm LL, et al. The metabolic syndrome and chronic kidney disease in U.S. adults. *Ann Intern Med*. 2004;140:167-174.

Pancreatic Function and Gastrointestinal Function

EDWARD P. FODY

CHAPTER OUTLINE

Chapter Objectives

Upon completion of this chapter, the clinical laboratorian should be able to do the following:

• Discuss the physiologic role of the pancreas in the digestive process.
• List the hormones excreted by the pancreas, together with their physiologic roles.
• Describe the following pancreatic disorders and list the associated laboratory tests that would aid in diagnosis:

acute pancreatitis, chronic pancreatitis, pancreatic carcinoma, cystic fibrosis, and pancreatic malabsorption.
• Describe the physiology and biochemistry of gastric secretion.
• List the tests used to assess gastric and intestinal function.
• Explain the clinical aspects of gastric analysis.
• Evaluate a patient's condition, given clinical data.

KEY TERMS

Cholecystokinin (CCK)
D-Xylose absorption test
Gastrin
Intrinsic factor
Islets of Langerhans

Lactose tolerance test
Pancreatitis
Pepsin
Secretagogues
Secretin
Steatorrhea
Zöllinger-Ellison syndrome

The gastrointestinal (GI) system is composed of the mouth, esophagus, stomach, small intestine, and large intestine. Digestion, which is primarily a function of the small intestine, is the process by which starches, proteins, lipids, nucleic acids, and other complex molecules are degraded to simple constituents (molecules) for absorption and use in the body. This chapter discusses the physiology and biochemistry of gastric secretion, intestinal physiology, pathologic aspects of intestinal function, and tests of gastric and intestinal function.

The pancreas is a large gland that is involved in the digestive process, but located outside of the GI system. It is composed of both endocrine and exocrine tissues. The liver is the other major external gland that is involved in the digestive process, and it is covered in Chapter 25. The endocrine functions of the pancreas include production of insulin and glucagon; both hormones are involved in carbohydrate metabolism. Exocrine function involves the production of many enzymes used in the digestive process. This chapter discusses the physiology of pancreatic function, diseases of the pancreas, and tests of pancreatic function.

PHYSIOLOGY OF PANCREATIC FUNCTION

As a digestive gland, the pancreas is only second in size to the liver, weighing about 70 to 105 g. It is located behind the peritoneal cavity across the upper abdomen at about the level of the first and second lumbar vertebrae, about 1 to 2 in. above the umbilicus. It is located in the curve made by the duodenum (Fig. 28-1). The pancreas is composed of two morphologically and functionally different tissues: endocrine tissue and exocrine tissue. The *endocrine* (hormone-releasing) component is by far the smaller of the two and consists of the **islets of Langerhans**, which are well-delineated, spherical or ovoid clusters composed of at least four different cell types. The islet cells secrete at least four hormones into the blood: insulin, glucagon, gastrin, and somatostatin. The larger, *exocrine* pancreatic (enzyme-secreting) component secretes about 1.5 to 2 L/d

of fluid, which is rich in digestive enzymes, into ducts that ultimately empty into the duodenum.

This digestive fluid is produced by pancreatic acinar cells (grape-like clusters), which line the pancreas and are connected by small ducts. These small ducts empty into progressively larger ducts, eventually forming one major pancreatic duct and a smaller accessory duct. The major pancreatic duct and the common bile duct open into the duodenum at the major duodenal papilla (Fig. 28-2). Normal, protein-rich, pancreatic fluid is clear, colorless, and watery, with an alkaline pH that can reach up to 8.3. This alkalinity is caused by the high concentration of sodium bicarbonate present in pancreatic fluid, which is used eventually to neutralize the hydrochloric acid in gastric fluid from the stomach as it enters the duodenum. The bicarbonate and chloride concentrations vary reciprocally so that they total about 150 mmol/L.

Pancreatic fluid has about the same concentrations of potassium and sodium as serum. The digestive enzymes, or their proenzymes secreted by the pancreas, are capable of digesting the three major classes of food substances (proteins, carbohydrates, and fats) and include (1) the proteolytic enzymes trypsin, chymotrypsin, elastase, collagenase,

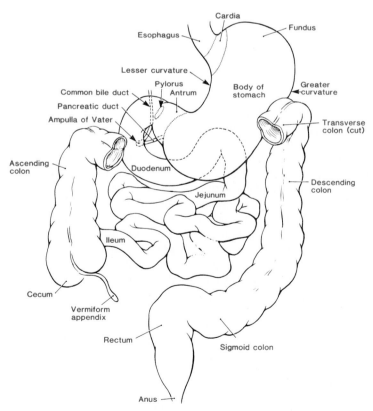

FIGURE 28-1 Peritoneum and mesenteries. The parietal peritoneum lines the abdominal cavity, and the visceral peritoneum covers abdominal organs. Retroperitoneal organs are covered by the parietal peritoneum. The mesenteries are membranes that connect abdominal organs to each other and to the body wall. (Reprinted with permission from Thompson JS, Akesson EJ, eds. *Thompson's Core Textbook of Anatomy.* 2nd ed. Philadelphia, PA: JB Lippincott; 1990:115.)

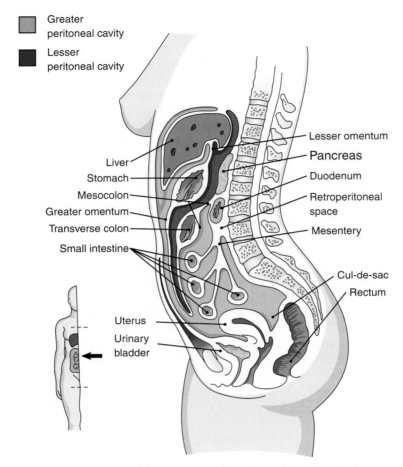

■ Greater
peritoneal cavity

■ Lesser
peritoneal cavity

Liver
Stomach
Mesocolon
Greater omentum
Transverse colon
Small intestine

Lesser omentum
Pancreas
Duodenum
Retroperitoneal
space
Mesentery

Cul-de-sac
Rectum

Uterus
Urinary
bladder

FIGURE 28-2 Diagram of the pancreas and its relationship to the duodenum.

leucine aminopeptidase, and some carboxypeptidases; (2) lipid-digesting enzymes, primarily lipase and lecithinase; (3) carbohydrate-splitting pancreatic amylase; and (4) several nucleases (ribonuclease), which separate the nitrogen-containing bases from their sugar-phosphate strands.

Pancreatic activity is under both nervous and endocrine control. Branches of the vagus nerve can cause a small amount of pancreatic fluid secretion when food is smelled or seen, and these secretions may increase as the bolus of food reaches the stomach. Most of the pancreatic action, however, is under the hormonal control of secretin and cholecystokinin (CCK; formerly called *pancreozymin*). Secretin is responsible for the production of bicarbonate-rich and, therefore, alkaline pancreatic fluid, which protects the lining of the intestine from damage. Secretin is synthesized in response to the acidic contents of the stomach reaching the duodenum. It can also affect gastrin activity in the stomach. This pancreatic fluid contains few digestive enzymes. CCK, in the presence of fats or amino acids in the duodenum, is produced by the cells of the intestinal mucosa and is responsible for release of enzymes from the acinar cells by the pancreas into the pancreatic fluid.

DISEASES OF THE PANCREAS

Other than trauma, only three diseases cause more than 95% of the medical attention devoted to the pancreas. If they affect the endocrine function of the pancreas, these diseases can result in altered digestion and nutrient metabolism. The role of the pancreas in diabetes mellitus is discussed in Chapter 14.

Cystic fibrosis (known by various other terms, such as *fibrocystic disease of the pancreas* and *mucoviscidosis*) is an inherited autosomal recessive disorder characterized by dysfunction of mucous and exocrine glands throughout the body. The disease is relatively common and occurs in about 1 of 1,600 live births. It has various manifestations and can initially present in such widely varying ways as intestinal obstruction of the newborn, excessive pulmonary infections in childhood, or, uncommonly, as pancreatogenous malabsorption in adults. The disease causes the small and large ducts and the acini to dilate and convert into small cysts filled with mucus, eventually resulting in the prevention of pancreatic secretions reaching the duodenum or, depending on the age of the patient, a plug that blocks the lumen of the bowel, leading to obstruction. As the disease progresses, there is increased destruction and fibrous scarring of the pancreas and a corresponding decrease in function. Cystic fibrosis is transmitted as an autosomal recessive disorder with a high degree of penetrance. It occurs primarily in persons of Northern European descent. The cystic fibrosis gene known as *CFTR* occurs on chromosome 7, and more than 900 mutations causing this disorder have been identified; however, some occur more commonly than others. In areas of high frequency, such as Brittany in Western France, more than 10% of the population may carry a cystic fibrosis mutation, and 1 in 3,000 infants may be affected, making it the most common genetic disorder in these populations. Genetic screening is now widely carried out.[1-3]

Pancreatic carcinoma is the fourth most frequent form of fatal cancer and causes about 38,000 deaths each year in the United States, which represents about 7% of all deaths from malignant neoplasms. The disease is slightly more common in males than females and in African Americans than whites. The 5-year survival rate is about 6% and most patients die within 1 year of diagnosis. Most pancreatic tumors arise as adenocarcinomas of the ductal epithelium. Because the pancreas has a rich supply of nerves, pain is a prominent feature of the disease. If the tumor arises in the body or tail of the pancreas, detection does not often occur until an advanced stage of the disease because of its central location and the associated vague symptoms. Cancer of the head of the pancreas is usually detected earlier because of its proximity to the common bile duct. Signs of these tumors are jaundice, weight loss, anorexia, and nausea. Jaundice is associated with signs of posthepatic hyperbilirubinemia (intrahepatic cholestasis) and low levels of fecal bilirubin, resulting in clay-colored stools. However, findings are not specific for pancreatic tumors, and other causes of obstruction must be ruled out.

Islet cell tumors of the pancreas affect the endocrine capability of the pancreas. If the tumor occurs in beta cells, hyperinsulinism is often seen, resulting in low blood glucose levels, sometimes followed by hypoglycemic shock. Pancreatic cell tumors, which overproduce gastrin, are called *gastrinomas*; they cause Zöllinger-Ellison syndrome and can be duodenal in origin. These tumors are associated with watery diarrhea, recurring peptic ulcer, and significant gastric hypersecretion and hyperacidity. Pancreatic cell glucagon-secreting tumors are rare; the hypersecretion of glucagon is associated with diabetes mellitus.

Pancreatitis, or inflammation of the pancreas, is ultimately caused by autodigestion of the pancreas as a result of reflux of bile or duodenal contents into the pancreatic duct. Pathologic changes can include acute edema, with large amounts of fluid accumulating in the retroperitoneal space and an associated decrease in effective circulating

blood volume; cellular infiltration, leading to necrosis of the acinar cells, with hemorrhage as a possible result of necrotic blood vessels; and intrahepatic and extrahepatic pancreatic fat necrosis. Pancreatitis is generally classified as acute (no permanent damage to the pancreas), chronic (irreversible injury), or relapsing/recurrent, which can also be acute or chronic. It commonly occurs in midlife. Painful episodes can occur intermittently, usually reaching a maximum within minutes or hours, lasting for several days or weeks, and frequently accompanied by nausea and vomiting. Pancreatitis is often associated with alcohol abuse or biliary tract diseases such as gallstones, but patients with hyperlipoproteinemia and those with hyperparathyroidism are also at a significantly increased risk for this disease.

Other etiologic factors associated with acute pancreatitis include mumps, obstruction caused by biliary tract disease, gallstones, pancreatic tumors, tissue injury, atherosclerotic disease, shock, pregnancy, hypercalcemia, hereditary pancreatitis, immunologic factors associated with postrenal transplantation, and hypersensitivity. Symptoms of acute pancreatitis include severe abdominal pain that is generalized or in the upper quadrants and often radiates toward the back or down the right or left flank. The etiology of chronic pancreatitis is similar to that of acute pancreatitis, but chronic excessive alcohol consumption appears to be the most common predisposing factor.

Laboratory findings include increased amylase, lipase, triglycerides, and hypercalcemia, which is often associated with underlying hyperparathyroidism. Hypocalcemia may be found and has been attributed to the sudden removal of large amounts of calcium from the extracellular fluid because of impaired mobilization or as a result of calcium fixation by fatty acids liberated by increased lipase action on triglycerides. Hypoproteinemia is attributable mainly to the notable loss of plasma into the retroperitoneal space. A shift of arterial blood flow from the inflamed pancreatic cells to less affected or normal cells causes oxygen deprivation and tissue hypoxia in the area of damage, including the surrounding organs and tissue.

All three conditions can result in severely diminished pancreatic exocrine function, which can significantly compromise digestion and absorption of ingested nutrients. This is the essence of the general malabsorption syndrome, which embodies abdominal bloating and discomfort; the frequent passage of bulky, malodorous feces; and weight loss. Failure to digest or absorb fats, known as steatorrhea, renders a greasy appearance to feces (more than 5 g of fecal fat per 24 hours). The malabsorption syndrome typically involves abnormal digestion or absorption of proteins, polysaccharides, carbohydrates, and other complex molecules, as well as lipids. Severely deranged absorption and metabolism of electrolytes, water, vitamins (particularly fat-soluble vitamins A, D, E, and K), and minerals can also occur. Malabsorption can involve a single substance, such as vitamin B_{12}, which results in a megaloblastic anemia (pernicious anemia), or lactose caused by a lactase deficiency. In addition to pancreatic exocrine deficiency, the malabsorption syndrome can be caused by biliary obstruction, which deprives the small intestine of the emulsifying effect of bile, and various diseases of the small intestine, which inhibit absorption of digested products.

TESTS OF PANCREATIC FUNCTION

Depending on etiology and clinical picture, pancreatic function may be suspect when there is evidence of increased amylase and lipase.[4-7] The reader is referred to Chapter 13 for an in-depth discussion of these enzymes. Other laboratory tests of pancreatic function include those used for detection of malabsorption (e.g., examination of stool for excess fat, D-xylose test, and fecal fat analysis), tests measuring other exocrine function (e.g., secretin, CCK, fecal fat, trypsin, and chymotrypsin), tests assessing changes associated with extrahepatic obstruction (e.g., bilirubin), and endocrine-related tests (e.g., gastrin, insulin, and glucose) that reflect changes in the endocrine cells of the pancreas.

Direct evaluation of pancreatic fluid may include measurement of the total volume of pancreatic fluid and the amount or concentration of bicarbonate and enzymes, which requires pancreatic stimulation. Stimulation may be accomplished using a predescribed meal or administration of secretin, which allows for volume and bicarbonate evaluation, or secretin stimulation followed by CCK stimulation, which adds enzymes to the pancreatic fluid evaluation. The advantage of these tests, both of which require intubation of the patient, is that the chemical and cytologic examinations are performed on actual pancreatic secretions. Cytologic examination of the fluid can often establish the presence, or at least the suspicion, of malignant neoplasms, although the precise localization of the primary organ of involvement (i.e., pancreas, biliary system, ampulla of Vater, or duodenum) is not possible by duodenal aspiration.

Because of advances in imaging techniques, these stimulation tests are used less often; none have proved especially useful in diagnosis of mild or acute pancreatic disease in which the acute phase has subsided. Most of the tests have found clinical utility in excluding the pancreas from diagnosis. The sweat test, used for screening cystic fibrosis, is not specific for assessing pancreatic involvement but, when used along with the clinical picture at the time of testing, can provide important diagnostic information. The following pancreatic function tests are reviewed briefly: secretin/CCK test, fecal fat

CASE STUDY 28-1

A 38-year-old man entered the emergency department with the complaint of severe, mid-abdominal pain of 6 hours' duration. A friend, who had driven him to the hospital, stated that the patient fainted three times as he was being helped into the automobile. The patient had a 15-year history of alcoholism and drank 1 to 2 pints of whiskey everyday. He had last been hospitalized for acute alcoholism 3 months ago, at which time he had relatively minor abnormalities of liver function. On this admission, his blood pressure was 80/40 mm Hg; pulse, 110 beats/min and thready; and respirations, 24 breaths per minute and shallow. Clinical laboratory test results are shown in Case Study Table 28-1.1.

Questions

1. What is the probable disease?

2. What is the cause for the low serum calcium?

3. What is the cause for the increased blood urea nitrogen?

CASE STUDY TABLE 28-1.1
LABORATORY RESULTS

Serum amylase	640 units (3.5–260 units)
Serum sodium	133 mmol/L (135–145 mmol/L)
Potassium	3.4 mmol/L (3.8–5.5 mmol/L)
Calcium	4.0 mmol/L (4.5–5.5 mmol/L)
Blood urea nitrogen	32 mg/dL (8–25 mg/dL)
White blood cell count	16,500/μL
Hemoglobin	12 g/dL

analysis, sweat chloride determinations, and amylase and lipase interpretation.

Secretin/CCK Test

The secretin/CCK test is a direct determination of the exocrine secretory capacity of the pancreas. The test involves intubation of the duodenum without contamination by gastric fluid, which would neutralize any bicarbonate. The test is performed after a 6-hour or overnight fast. Pancreatic secretion is stimulated by intravenously administered secretin in a dose varying from 2 to 3 U/kg of body weight, followed by CCK administration. If a simple secretin test is desired, the higher dose of secretin is given alone.

No single protocol has been uniformly established for the test. Pancreatic secretions are collected variously for 30, 60, or 80 minutes after administration of the stimulants, either as 10-minute specimens or as a single, pooled collection. The pH, secretory rate, enzyme activities (e.g., trypsin, amylase, or lipase), and amount of bicarbonate are determined. The average amount of bicarbonate excreted per hour is about 15 mmol/L for men and 12 mmol/L for women, with an average flow of 2 mL/kg. Assessment of enzymes must be taken in view of total volume output. Decreased pancreatic flow is associated with pancreatic obstruction and increase in enzyme concentrations. Low concentrations of bicarbonate and enzymes are associated with cystic fibrosis, chronic pancreatitis, pancreatic cysts, calcification, and edema of the pancreas.

CASE STUDY 28-2

A 56-year-old man who is an alcoholic presents with a 2-week history of mid-abdominal pain. He also describes clay-colored stools, mild icterus, nausea, vomiting, and a 10-lb weight loss. Laboratory findings are shown in Case Study Table 28-2.1.

Questions

1. What organ system is primarily involved?

2. What are the major diagnostic considerations?

3. What do the laboratory results mean? What additional laboratory tests would be useful in establishing a diagnosis?

4. What other studies or procedures might be required?

CASE STUDY TABLE 28-2.1
LABORATORY RESULTS

TEST	RESULT	REFERENCE RANGE
Serum bilirubin	4.2 mg/dL	0.3–1.0 mg/dL
Serum lactate dehydrogenase	625 IU/L	0–200 IU/L
Serum alanine aminotransferase	76 IU/L	0–46 IU/L
Serum alkaline phosphatase	462 IU/L	0–80 IU/L
Serum amylase	80 IU/L	0–85 IU/L
Urine bilirubin	3+	Negative

Fecal Fat Analysis

Fecal lipids are derived from four sources: unabsorbed ingested lipids, lipids excreted into the intestine (predominantly in the bile), cells shed into the intestine, and metabolism of intestinal bacteria. Patients on a lipid-free diet still excrete 1 to 4 g of lipid in the feces in a 24-hour period. Even with a lipid-rich diet, the fecal fat does not normally exceed about 7 g in a 24-hour period. Normal fecal lipid is composed of about 60% fatty acids; 30% sterols, higher alcohols, and carotenoids; 10% triglycerides; and small amounts of cholesterol and phospholipids. Although significantly increased fecal fat can be caused by biliary obstruction, severe steatorrhea is usually associated with exocrine pancreatic insufficiency or disease of the small intestine.

Qualitative Screening Test for Fecal Fat
Various screening tests have been devised for detecting steatorrhea. These tests commonly use fat-soluble stains (e.g., Sudan III, Sudan IV, Oil Red O, or Nile blue sulfate), which dissolve in and color lipid droplets. Of greater importance than the particular technical procedure is the level of experience and dependability of the clinical laboratorian performing the test.

Sudan Staining for Fecal Fat
Neutral fats (triglycerides) and many other lipids stain yellow-orange to red with Sudan III because the dye is much more soluble in lipid than in water or ethanol.[8,9] Free fatty acids do not stain appreciably unless the specimen is heated in the presence of the stain with 36% acetic acid. The slide may be examined warm or cool and the number of fat droplets assessed. As the slide cools, the fatty acids crystallize out in long, colorless, needle-like sheaves. Detection of meat fiber is accomplished by a third aliquot of fecal sample mixed on the slide with 10% alcohol and a solution of eosin stained for 3 minutes. The meat fiber should stain as rectangular cross-striated fibers. Splitting the sample and detecting neutral fats, fatty acids, and undigested meat fibers can provide diagnostic information. Increases in fats and undigested meat fibers are indicative of patients with steatorrhea of pancreatic origin. A representative fecal specimen is used for analysis.

Normal feces can have up to 40 or 50 small (1 to 5 mm), neutral lipid droplets per high-power microscope field. Steatorrhea is characterized by an increase in the number and size of stainable droplets, often with some fat globules in the 50- to 100-mm range. Fatty acid assessment greater than 100 stained small droplets, along with the presence of meat fiber, is expected in patients with steatorrhea.

Quantitative Fecal Fat Analysis
The definitive test for steatorrhea is the quantitative fecal fat determination, usually on a 72-hour stool collection, although the collection period may be increased to up to

5 days. Traditional methods for fecal fat determination are the gravimetric and titrimetric methods. Newer methods involve the use of infrared and nuclear magnetic resonance spectroscopy.[10,11] In the gravimetric method, fatty acid soaps (predominantly calcium and magnesium salts of fatty acids) are converted to free fatty acids, followed by extraction of most of the lipids into an organic solvent, which is then evaporated so that the lipid residue can be weighed. In titrimetric methods, lipids are saponified with hydroxide, and the fatty acid salts are converted to free fatty acids using acid. The free fatty acids, along with various unsaponified lipids, are then extracted with an organic solvent, and the fatty acids are titrated with hydroxide after evaporation of the solvent and redissolving of the residue in ethanol. The titration methods obviously measure only saponifiable fatty acids and, consequently, render results about 20% lower than those from gravimetric methods. A further objection is that titrimetric methods use an assumed average molecular weight for fatty acids to convert moles of fatty acids to grams of lipid.

At one time, it was common to measure the amount of free fatty acids as a percentage of total lipids on the presumption that a high percentage of free fatty acids indicates adequate pancreatic lipase activity. This method is no longer considered reliable because of spurious results, particularly caused by lipase produced by intestinal bacteria.

It is essential that patients be placed on a lipid-rich diet for at least 2 days before instituting the fecal collection. The diet must contain at least 50 g, and preferably 100 g, of lipids each day. Fecal collections should extend for 3 or more successive days.

There are various ways to express fecal lipid excretion. Expressing lipid excretion as a percentage of wet or dry fecal weight is open to serious challenge because of wide variations in both fecal water content and dry residue as a result of dietary intake. The most widely accepted approach is to report the grams of fecal fat excreted in a 24-hour period.

Gravimetric Method for Fecal Fat Determination
The entire fecal specimen is emulsified with water. An aliquot is acidified to convert all fatty acid soaps to free fatty acids, which are then extracted with other soluble lipids into petroleum ether and ethanol. After evaporation of the organic solvents, the lipid residue is weighed. All feces for a 3-day period are collected in tared containers. The containers *must not* have a wax coating. The specimen must be kept refrigerated.

Total lipid does not change significantly during 5 days' storage of the specimen at refrigerator temperatures. Patients must not ingest castor oil, mineral oil, or other oily laxatives and must not use rectal suppositories containing oil or lipid for 2 days before the test and during the test.

The reference range for fecal lipids in adults is 1 to 7 g per 24 hours.

Sweat Electrolyte Determinations

Measurement of the sodium and chloride concentration in sweat is the most useful test for the diagnosis of cystic fibrosis.[12-14] Significantly elevated concentrations of both ions occur in more than 99% of affected patients. The twofold to fivefold increases in sweat sodium and chloride are diagnostic of cystic fibrosis in children. Even in adults, no other condition causes increases in sweat chloride and sodium above 80 mmol/L. Sweat potassium is also increased, but less significantly so, and is not generally relied on for diagnosis. Contrary to some assertions, sweat electrolyte determinations do not distinguish heterozygote carriers of cystic fibrosis from normal homozygotes.

Older methods for acquiring sweat specimens required skilled technologists who frequently performed the test. Induction of sweat included applying plastic bags or wrapping the patient in blankets, which was fraught with serious risks of dehydration, electrolyte disturbances, and hyperpyrexia. In 1959, pilocarpine administration by iontophoresis was reported as an efficient method for sweat collection and stimulation. Iontophoresis uses an electric current that causes pilocarpine to migrate into a limited skin area, usually the inside of the forearm, toward the negative electrode from a moistened pad on the positive electrode. A collection vessel is then applied to the skin. The sweat is then analyzed for chloride. For confirmation, the test should be repeated. Commercially available surface electrodes that analyze the sweat chloride are readily available. For details, the reader is referred to Chapter 29.

It is widely accepted that sweat chloride concentrations greater than 60 mmol/L are diagnostic of cystic fibrosis in children. Sweat sodium and chloride concentrations in female patients undergo fluctuation with the menstrual cycle and reach a peak 5 to 10 days before the onset of menstruation but do not overlap with the ranges associated with cystic fibrosis.

Serum Enzymes

Amylase is the serum enzyme most commonly relied on for detecting pancreatic disease.[15,16] It is not, however, a function test. Amylase is particularly useful in the diagnosis of acute pancreatitis, in which significant increases in serum concentrations occur in about 75% of patients. Typically, amylase in serum increases within a few hours of the onset of the disease, reaches a peak in about 24 hours, and because of its clearance by the kidneys returns to normal within 3 to 5 days, often making urine amylase a more sensitive indicator of acute pancreatitis. The magnitude of the enzyme elevation cannot be correlated with the severity of the disease.

CASE STUDY 28-3

Parents brought their 7-year-old son to the pediatrician with the complaint of frequent fevers and failure to grow. The child had three bouts of pneumonia during the past 2 years and was bothered by chronic bronchitis, which caused him to cough up copious amounts of thick, yellow, mucoid sputum. Despite a big appetite, he had gained only 1 to 2 lbs in the past 2 years and was of short, frail stature. He especially liked salty foods. He usually had three or four bulky, foul-smelling bowel movements daily. A 9-year-old sister was in excellent health.

Questions

1. What is the most likely disease?
2. What clinical laboratory test would be most informative, and what results would be expected?
3. What other clinical laboratory tests would likely be abnormal?

Determination of the renal clearance of amylase is useful in detecting minor or intermittent increases in the serum concentration of this enzyme. To correct for diminished glomerular function, the most useful expression is the ratio of amylase clearance to creatinine clearance, as follows:

$$\frac{\text{\% Amylase clearance}}{\text{Creatinine}} = 100 \times \frac{\text{UA}}{\text{SA}} \times \frac{\text{SC}}{\text{UC}} \quad \text{(Eq. 28-1)}$$

where UA is urine amylase, SA is serum amylase, SC is serum creatinine, and UC is urine creatinine.

Normal values are less than 3.1%. Significantly increased values, averaging about 8% or 9%, occur in acute pancreatitis but may also occur in other conditions, such as burns, sepsis, and diabetic ketoacidosis.

The use of serum lipase in the clinical detection of pancreatic disease has been compromised in the past by technical problems inherent in the various analytic methods. Improved analytic methods appear to indicate that lipase increases in serum about as soon as amylase in acute pancreatitis and that increased levels persist somewhat longer than those of amylase. Consequently, some physicians consider lipase more sensitive than amylase as an indicator of acute pancreatitis or other causes of pancreatic necrosis.

Both amylase and lipase may be significantly increased in serum in many other conditions (e.g., opiate administration, pancreatic carcinoma, intestinal infarction, obstruction or perforation, and pancreatic trauma).

Amylase levels are also frequently increased in mumps, cholecystitis, hepatitis, cirrhosis, ruptured ectopic pregnancy, and macroamylasemia, which is a benign condition in which amylase binds to an immunoglobulin molecule, causing chronic elevation of serum amylase values but normal urine amylase levels. Lipase levels are often significantly increased in bone fractures and in association with fat embolism.

PHYSIOLOGY AND BIOCHEMISTRY OF GASTRIC SECRETION

Gastric secretion occurs in response to various stimuli[17]:

- Neurogenic impulses from the brain transmitted by means of the vagal nerves (e.g., responses to the sight, smell, or anticipation of food)
- Distention of the stomach with food or fluid
- Contact of protein breakdown products, termed secretagogues, with the gastric mucosa
- The hormone gastrin is the most potent stimulus to gastric secretion; it is secreted by specialized G cells in the gastric mucosa and the duodenum in response to vagal stimulation and contact with secretagogues.

Inhibitory influences include high gastric acidity, which decreases the release of gastrin by the gastric G cells. Gastric inhibitory polypeptide is secreted by K cells in the middle and distal duodenum and proximal jejunum in response to food products such as fats, glucose, and amino acids. Vasoactive intestinal polypeptide, produced by H cells in the intestinal mucosa, directly inhibits gastric secretion, gastrin release, and gastric motility.

Gastric fluid has a high content of hydrochloric acid, pepsin, and mucus. Hydrochloric acid is secreted against a hydrogen ion gradient as great as 1 million times the concentration in plasma (i.e., gastric fluid can reach a pH of 1.2 to 1.3 under conditions of augmented or maximal stimulation). Pepsin refers to a group of relatively weak proteolytic enzymes, with pH optima from about 1.6 to 3.6, that catalyze all native proteins except mucus. The most important component of gastric secretion in terms of body physiology is intrinsic factor, which greatly facilitates the absorption of vitamin B_{12} in the ileum.

CLINICAL ASPECTS OF GASTRIC ANALYSIS

Gastric analysis is used in clinical medicine mainly for the following purposes[18,19]:

- Gastric analysis was once widely used in clinical medicine but has now been largely replaced by fiberoptic endoscopy and improved radiologic procedures.
- Gastric analysis is used clinically mainly to detect hypersecretion characteristics of the *Zöllinger-Ellison syndrome*. This syndrome involves a gastrin-secreting neoplasm, usually located in the pancreatic islets, and exceptionally high plasma gastrin concentrations. Basal

1-hour secretion usually exceeds 10 mmol, and the ratio of basal 1-hour to maximal secretion usually exceeds 60% (i.e., the stomach is not really in the basal state but rather is pathologically stimulated by the high plasma gastrin level).

Gastric analysis is also used occasionally to evaluate pernicious anemia in adults. Gastric atrophy is present in this condition, and the stomach fails to secrete intrinsic factor, which binds to vitamin B_{12} to prevent its degradation by gastric acid. The pH of gastric fluid in this condition typically does not fall below 6, even with maximum stimulation. Rarely, gastric analysis may aid in determining the type of surgical procedure required for ulcer treatment.

Previously, various substances were used to stimulate gastric secretion (e.g., caffeine, alcohol, and test meals), but these are submaximal stimuli and obsolete. From 1953 until the late 1970s, histamine acid phosphate was used as a maximal stimulus to gastric secretion. Because of adverse effects, some of them severe, histamine has now been replaced by pentagastrin, which is a synthetic pentapeptide composed of the four C-terminal amino acids of gastrin linked to a substituted alanine derivative.

Normal gastric fluid is translucent, pale gray, and slightly viscous and often has a faintly acrid odor. Residual volume should not exceed 75 mL. Residual specimens occasionally contain flecks of blood or are green, brown, or yellow from reflux of bile during the intubation procedure. The presence of food particles is abnormal and indicates obstruction.

TESTS OF GASTRIC FUNCTION

Measuring Gastric Acid in Basal and Maximal Secretory Tests

After an overnight fast, gastric analysis is usually performed as a 1-hour basal test, followed by a 1-hour stimulated test subsequent to pentagastrin administration (6 μg/kg subcutaneously).[20,21] Test results reveal wide overlap among healthy subjects and diseased patients, except for anacidity (e.g., in pernicious anemia) and the extreme hypersecretion found in Zöllinger-Ellison syndrome. Gastric peptic ulcer is usually associated with normal secretory volume and acid output. Duodenal peptic ulcer is usually associated with increased secretory volume in both the basal and maximal secretory tests; considerable overlap occurs, nevertheless, with the normal range.

Measuring Gastric Acid

In stimulated secretion specimens, the ability of the stomach to secrete against a hydrogen ion gradient is determined by measuring the pH. The total acid output in a timed interval is determined from the titratable acidities and volumes of the component specimens. After intubation, the residual secretion is aspirated and retained. Secretion for the subsequent 10 to 30 minutes is discarded to allow for adjustment of the patient to the intubation procedure. Specimens are ordinarily obtained as 15-minute collections for a period of 1 hour.

The gastrin response to intravenous secretin stimulation may be used to investigate patients with mildly elevated serum gastrin levels. In this test, pure porcine secretin is injected intravenously, and gastrin levels are collected at 5-minute intervals for the next 30 minutes. In patients with Zöllinger-Ellison syndrome, the gastrin level increases at least 100 pg/mL over the basal level. Patients with ordinary peptic ulceration, achlorhydria, or other conditions show a slight decrease in gastrin concentration.

The volume, pH, and titratable acidity and the calculated acid output of each specimen are reported, as are the total volume and acid output for each test period (sum of the component specimens). There is considerable variation in gastric acid output among healthy subjects in both the basal and maximal secretory tests. Nevertheless, in the basal test, most healthy subjects secrete 0 to 6 mmol of acid in a total volume of 10 to 100 mL. In the maximal 1-hour test, using histamine or pentagastrin as the stimulus, most men secrete 1 to 40 mmol of acid in a total volume of 40 to 350 mL. Women and older persons usually secrete somewhat less acid than do young men.

Plasma Gastrin

Measurement of plasma gastrin levels is invaluable in diagnosing Zöllinger-Ellison syndrome, in which fasting levels typically exceed 1,000 pg/mL and can reach 400,000 pg/mL, compared with the normal range of 50 to 150 pg/mL.[22,23] Gastrin is usually not increased in simple peptic ulcer disease. Increased plasma gastrin levels do occur in most pernicious anemia patients but decrease toward normal when hydrochloric acid is artificially instilled into the stomach.

INTESTINAL PHYSIOLOGY

Digestion, predominantly a function of the small intestine, is the process in which starches, proteins, lipids, nucleic acids, and other complex molecules are degraded to monosaccharides, amino acids and oligopeptides, fatty acids, purines, pyrimidines, and other simple constituents. For most large molecules, digestion is necessary for absorption to occur. Each day, the duodenum receives about 7 to 10 L of ingested water and food and secretion from the salivary glands, stomach, pancreas, and biliary tract. The materials then enter the jejunum and ileum, where another 1 to 1.5 L of secretion is added. Ultimately, however, only about 1.5 L of fluid material

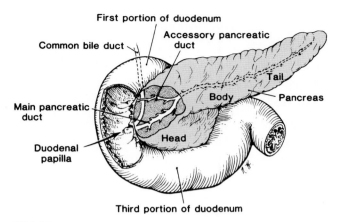

FIGURE 28-3 The abdominal structures of the alimentary tract.

reaches the *cecum*, which is the first portion of the colon or large intestines. This considerable absorptive capability is possible because the small intestine (about 20 feet long) has numerous mucosal folds, minute projections from the luminal surface called *villi*, and microscopic projections on the mucosal cells called *microvilli*, all of which greatly increase the secretory and absorptive surface to an estimated 200 m². Absorption takes place by passive diffusion for some substances and by active transport for others. In addition, the small intestine actively secretes electrolytes and other metabolic products. The large intestine (about 5 feet long) has two major functions: water resorption, in which the 1.5 L of fluid received by the cecum is reduced to about 100 to 300 mL of feces, and storage of feces before defecation. The abdominal structures that constitute the alimentary tract are shown diagrammatically in Figure 28-3.

CLINICOPATHOLOGIC ASPECTS OF INTESTINAL FUNCTION

Clinical chemistry testing of intestinal function focuses almost entirely on the evaluation of absorption and its derangements in various disease states. As discussed in the Pancreatic Function section of this chapter, diseases of the exocrine pancreas and biliary tract may also cause malabsorption. Intestinal diseases that may cause the malabsorption syndrome are highly varied in their etiology, pathogenesis, and severity. These intestinal diseases and disorders include tropical and nontropical or celiac sprue, Whipple's disease, Crohn's disease, primary intestinal lymphoma, small intestinal resection, intestinal lymphangiectasia, ischemia, amyloidosis, and giardiasis. In addition to the malabsorption syndrome, which ordinarily causes impaired absorption of fats, proteins, carbohydrates, and other substances, specific malabsorption states also occur (e.g., acquired deficiency of lactase, which prevents normal absorption of lactose, and Hartnup syndrome, a genetic disorder that involves deficient intestinal transport of phenylalanine and leucine).

CASE STUDY 28-4

A 34-year-old man was admitted for diagnostic evaluation with the complaint of epigastric pain of 2 years' duration, which was variously described as gnawing or burning. He had been diagnosed with a duodenal peptic ulcer 18 months ago; at that time, therapy of antacids and dietary revision provided considerable alleviation of symptoms. More recently, the pain had become more persistent and awakened the patient 4 to 6 times each night. Radiologic studies revealed a 2.5 cm ulcer crater in the first portion of the duodenum and a 0.5 cm ulcer in the antrum of the stomach. Serum electrolytes were normal. Hemoglobin was 8.3 g/dL with normal red blood cell indices. White blood count was 13,100. Gastric analysis revealed 640 mL of secretion in the basal hour, with an acid output of 38 mmol, and 780 mL of secretion in the 1-hour pentagastrin stimulation test, with an acid output of 48 mmol.

Questions

1. What is the probable disease?

2. In view of existing data, what other test would be virtually diagnostic for this disease?

3. What is the explanation for decreased hemoglobin and increased white blood cell count?

TESTS OF INTESTINAL FUNCTION

Lactose Tolerance Test

The disaccharidases, lactase (which cleaves lactose into glucose and galactose) and sucrase (which cleaves sucrose into glucose and fructose), are produced by the mucosal cells of the small intestine.[24,25] Congenital deficiencies of these enzymes are rare, but acquired deficiencies of lactase are commonly found in adults. Affected patients experience abdominal discomfort, cramps, and diarrhea after ingesting milk or milk products. About 10% to 20% of white Americans and 75% of African Americans are affected.

Lactose tolerance testing was used to establish this diagnosis, but the test is subject to many false-positive and false-negative results. This test has largely been replaced by hydrogen breath testing.

D-Xylose Absorption Test

D-Xylose is a pentose sugar that is ordinarily not present in the blood in any significant amount.[26,27] As with other monosaccharides, pentose sugars are absorbed unaltered in the proximal small intestine and do not require the intervention of pancreatic lytic enzymes. Therefore, the ability to absorb D-xylose is of value in differentiating malabsorption of intestinal etiology from that of exocrine pancreatic insufficiency. Because only about one-half of orally administered D-xylose is metabolized or lost by action of intestinal bacteria, significant amounts are excreted unchanged in the urine. Some protocols have used the measurement of only the D-xylose excreted in the urine during the 5 hours following ingestion of a 25-g dose by a fasting adult (0.5 g/kg in a child). Even with normal renal function, false-positive and false-negative results frequently occur. Blood levels measured one or more times after ingestion of D-xylose (e.g., at 30 minutes, 1 hour, or 2 hours) significantly improve the diagnostic reliability of the test. Some protocols use smaller doses of D-xylose to avoid abdominal cramps, intestinal hypermotility, and osmotic diarrhea that frequently accompany the 25-g dose.

D-Xylose Test

After ingestion of a specified solution of D-xylose, blood specimens are obtained and urine is collected for a 5-hour period to determine the extent of D-xylose absorption. The concentration of D-xylose is determined by heating protein-free supernates of urine and plasma to convert xylose to furfural, which is then reacted with *p*-bromoaniline to form a pink product, the absorbance of which is measured at 520 nm. Thiourea is added as an antioxidant to prevent the formation of interfering chromogens. After an overnight fast, the patient voids and drinks a D-xylose solution: 25 g of D-xylose in 250 mL of water for adults and 0.5 g/kg for children, or other dose as established. The patient drinks an equivalent amount of water during the next hour. No additional food or fluids are to be taken until the test is completed. Urine is collected for 5 hours after the D-xylose ingestion. A blood specimen is collected in potassium oxalate at 2 hours (commonly, 1 hour is chosen for children).

Normal blood concentrations of D-xylose in association with decreased urine excretion suggest impairment of renal function or incomplete urine collection. Aspirin therapy diminishes renal excretion of D-xylose, whereas indomethacin decreases intestinal absorption. After ingestion of a 25-g dose of D-xylose, healthy adults should excrete at least 4 g in the 5-hour period. For infants and children, the excretion following a dose of 0.5 g/kg for various ages expressed as percentages of ingested dose are shown in Table 28-1. Blood levels for healthy adults vary widely, but a blood concentration of less than 25 mg/dL at 2 hours should be considered abnormal after the 25-g dose. With the 0.5 g/kg dose, infants younger than 6 months should have a blood concentration of at least 15 mg/dL at 1 hour, infants older than 6 months and children should achieve levels of at least 30 mg/dL.

TABLE 28-1	D-XYLOSE RESULTS FOR PEDIATRIC PATIENTS[2,4]
AGE	**REFERENCE RANGE**
Younger than 6 mo	11–33%
6–12 mo	20–32%
1–3 y	20–42%
3–10 y	25–45%
Older than 10 y	25–50%

Serum Carotenoids

Carotenoids are various yellow to orange or purple pigments that are widely distributed vin animal tissue; they are synthesized by many plants and impart a yellow color to some vegetables and fruits. The major carotenoids in human serum are lycopene, xanthophyll, and beta carotene, the chief precursor of vitamin A in humans. Being fat soluble, carotenoids are absorbed in the small intestine in association with lipids. Malabsorption of lipids typically results in a serum concentration of carotenoids lower than the reference range of 50 to 250 mg/dL. Starvation, dietary idiosyncrasies, and fever also cause diminished serum concentrations. The test does not distinguish among the various etiologies of malabsorption.

Other Tests of Intestinal Malabsorption

Deficiencies of numerous analytes can occur in association with intestinal malabsorption. Measurement of these analytes is usually of value, not so much in confirming the diagnosis of malabsorption as in determining the extent of nutritional deficiency and, thus, the need for replacement therapy. Diminished appetite and dietary intake are usually more severe in patients who have malabsorption with an intestinal etiology. Body wasting or cachexia may be severe. Frequently, because loss of albumin into the intestinal lumen and diminished dietary intake of protein accompany the diminished absorption of oligopeptides and amino acids, a negative nitrogen balance occurs together with decreased serum total proteins and albumin. A serum albumin of less than 2.5 g/dL is much more characteristic of intestinal disease than of pancreatic disease. In association with severe disease of the small intestine, deficiencies of fat-soluble vitamins A, D, E, and K occur. Vitamin K deficiency, in turn, causes deficiencies of vitamin K–dependent coagulation factors II (prothrombin), VII (proconvertin), IX (plasma thromboplastin component), and X (Stuart-Prower factor), which are reflected in abnormal prothrombin time and partial thromboplastin time tests.

In severe small intestinal disease, such as tropical or celiac sprue, malabsorption of folate and vitamin B_{12} can occur, and megaloblastic anemia is rather common and is of some benefit in distinguishing intestinal from pancreatic disease. Absorption of iron is usually diminished, and the tendency toward low serum iron levels may be aggravated by intestinal blood loss. Intestinal absorption of calcium is often diminished as a result of calcium binding by unabsorbed fatty acids and accompanying vitamin D deficiency and decreased serum magnesium. Because sodium, potassium, water absorption, and metabolism may also be seriously deranged, serum sodium and potassium levels are decreased and dehydration occurs. Impaired absorption of carbohydrates in intestinal diseases, such as sprue, results in decreased to flat blood concentration curves in glucose, lactose, and sucrose tolerance tests.

CASE STUDY 28-5

A 26-year-old woman appeared in the outpatient clinic with the complaint of abdominal discomfort; diarrhea; and an 18-lb, unintentional weight loss during the past 2 to 3 years. She related a similar period of 5 or 6 years of abdominal distress and diarrhea in childhood, but this essentially disappeared when she was about 12 to 13 years old. She was now having three to five bowel movements daily, which were described as bulky, malodorous, and floating. She weighed 106 lbs and was 67 in. tall. She never had surgical procedures. Physical examination revealed poor skin turgor, general pallor, and a protuberant abdomen. Abnormal clinical laboratory values included those in Case Study Table 28-5.1.

Fecal examination revealed no ova or parasites, and bacteriologic culture revealed no pathogens.

Questions

1. What is the disease process?

2. What is the probable etiology in this case?

3. What is the cause of the abnormal coagulation tests?

4. What is the probable major cause for the anemia, and what are other possible contributing causes?

CASE STUDY TABLE 28-5.1
LABORATORY RESULTS

ANALYTE	RESULT
Hemoglobin	8.1 g/dL
Hematocrit	30%
RBC count	$4.1 \times 10^6/\mu L$
Serum sodium	134 mmol/L
Potassium	3.4 mmol/L
Serum carotenoids	14 µg/dL
Fecal fat	22 g/24 h
D-Xylose absorption test (25-g dose)	5-h excretion of 1.3 g and blood level at 2 h of 8 mg/dL
Prothrombin time	15.8 s (12–14 s)
Activated partial thromboplastin time	56 s (30–45 s)

For additional student resources please visit thePoint at http://thepoint.lww.com.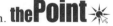

QUESTIONS

1. Laboratory findings in pancreatitis include all of the following EXCEPT
   a. Increased cortisol
   b. Increased amylase
   c. Increased lipase
   d. Increased triglycerides

2. Which of the following tests is a direct determination of the exocrine secretory capacity of the pancreas?
   a. Secretin/CCK test
   b. Amylase

   c. Quantitative fecal fat analysis
   d. D-Xylose test
   e. Lactose tolerance test

3. Which of the following statements concerning cystic fibrosis is NOT correct?
   a. Affects males and females about equally
   b. Occurs predominantly in populations of Northern European extraction
   c. Frequently diagnosed by measurement of sweat chloride

    d. Caused by a variety of mutations on chromosome 7

    e. Genetic screening is usually unsuccessful

4. The proper time period for the collection of a fecal fat specimen is
    a. 72 hours
    b. 24 hours
    c. 36 hours
    d. 48 hours
    e. 96 hours

5. Which of the following tests is only of the absorptive ability of the intestine?
    a. D-Xylose test
    b. Lactose tolerance test
    c. Fecal fat (72-hour collection)
    d. Serum carotenoids
    e. Serum albumin

6. A serum albumin of less than 2.5 g/dL would be most indicative of
    a. Intestinal disease
    b. Pancreatitis
    c. Peptic ulcer
    d. Pancreatic carcinoma

7. Which of the following is accurate when describing or diagnosing Zollinger-Ellison syndrome?

    a. Extreme hyposecretion of gastrin in the stomach
    b. Extreme hypersecretion of gastrin in the duodenum
    c. An increase in serum gastrin levels of 100 pg/mL following intravenous exposure to secretin
    d. A decrease in serum gastrin levels of 100 pg/mL following intravenous exposure to secretin
    e. Is confirmed when the hydrogen breath test is positive

8. The D-xylose absorption test is particularly helpful in differentiating malabsorption of intestinal etiology from exocrine pancreatic insufficiency because:
    a. D-Xylose is mostly absorbed in the stomach and then secreted via the kidney in its unaltered monosaccharide form.
    b. D-Xylose is mostly altered in the small intestine to facilitate its absorption across this membrane and metabolized by the liver so its metabolites may be excreted via the kidney.
    c. D-Xylose is mostly absorbed, not typically found in the blood, unaltered in the small intestine, and excreted unaltered via the kidney.
    d. None of the above describe why the D-xylose test is useful in identifying malabsorption diseases.

SUGGESTED READING

Berger HG, Buchler M, Kozarek R, et al. *An Integrated Textbook of Basic Science, Medicine and Surgery.* Indianapolis, IN: Wiley-Blackwell; 2008.

Feldman M, Friedman LS, Brandt LJ. *Sleisenger and Fordtran's Gastrointestinal and Liver Disease: Pathophysiology, Diagnosis, Management.* St. Louis, MO: WB Saunders; 2006.

REFERENCES

1. Scotet V, Gillet D, Dugueperoux I, et al. Spatial and temporal distribution of cystic fibrosis and of its mutations in Brittany, France: a retrospective study from 1960. *Hum Genet.* 2002;111:247-254.
2. Corbetta C, Seia M, Bassotti A, et al. Screening for cystic fibrosis in newborn infants: results of a pilot programme based on a two tier protocol (IRT/DNA/IRT) in the Italian population. *J Med Screen.* 2002;9:60-63.
3. Gregg AR, Simpson JL. Genetic screening for cystic fibrosis. *Obstet Gynecol Clin North Am.* 2002;29:329-340.
4. Walsh MK. Diagnosis, prognosis, and treatment of acute pancreatitis. *Am Fam Physician.* 2008;77:594.
5. Lankish PG. Chronic pancreatitis. *Curr Opin Gastroenterol.* 2007;23:502-507.
6. Schibli S, Corey M, Gaskin KJ, et al. Towards the ideal quantitative pancreatic function test: analysis of test variables that influence validity. *Clin Gastroenterol Hepatol.* 2006;4:90-97.
7. Leus J, Van Biervliet S, Robberecht E. Detection and follow up of exocrine pancreatic insufficiency in cystic fibrosis: a review. *Eur J Pediatr.* 2000;159:563-568.
8. Simko V. Sudan stain and quantitative fecal fat. *Gastroenterology.* 1990;98:1722-1723.
9. Huang G, Khouri MR, Shiau YF. Sudan stain of fecal fat: new insight into an old test. *Gastroenterology.* 1989;96(2 pt 1):421-427.
10. Kunz P, Künnecke B, Kunz I, et al. Natural abundance 13C-NMR spectroscopy for the quantitative determination of fecal fat. *Clin Biochem.* 2003;36:505-510.
11. Voortman G, Gerrits J, Altavilla M, et al. Quantitative determination of fecal fatty acids and triglycerides by Fourier transform infrared analysis with a sodium chloride transmission flow cell. *Clin Chem Lab Med.* 2002;40:795-798.
12. Baumer JH. Evidence based guidelines for the performance of the sweat test for the investigation of cystic fibrosis in the UK. *Arch Dis Child.* 2003;88:1126-1127.
13. Wang L, Freedman SD. Laboratory tests for the diagnosis of cystic fibrosis. *Am J Clin Pathol.* 2002;117(suppl):S109-S115.
14. De Boeck K, Wilschanski M, Castellani C, et al. Diagnostic Working Group. Cystic fibrosis: terminology and diagnostic algorithms. *Thorax.* 2006;61:627-635.
15. Matull WR, Pereira SP, O'Donohue JW. Biochemical markers of acute pancreatitis. *J Clin Pathol.* 2006;59:340-344.
16. Kylänpää-Bäck ML, Repo H, Kemppainen E. New laboratory tests in acute pancreatitis. *Addict Biol.* 2002;7:181-190.
17. Schubert ML. Gastric secretion. *Curr Opin Gastroenterol.* 2007;23:595-601.

18. Hung PD, Schubert ML, Mihas AA. Zollinger-Ellison syndrome. *Curr Treat Options Gastroenterol.* 2003;6:163-170.

19. Metz DC, Starr JA. A retrospective study of the usefulness of acid secretory testing. *Aliment Pharmacol Ther.* 2000;14:103-111.

20. Hirschowitz BI, Simmons J, Mohnen J. Long-term lansoprazole control of gastric acid and pepsin secretion in ZE and non-ZE hypersecretors: a prospective 10-year study. *Aliment Pharmacol Ther.* 2001;15:1795-1806.

21. Berger AC, Gibril F, Venzon DJ, et al. Prognostic value of initial fasting serum gastrin levels in patients with Zollinger-Ellison syndrome. *J Clin Oncol.* 2001;19:3051-3057.

22. Hung PD, Schubert ML, Mihas AA. Zollinger-Ellison syndrome. *Curr Treat Options Gastroenterol.* 2003;6:163-170.

23. Metz DC, Buchanan M, Purich E, Fein S. A randomized controlled crossover study comparing synthetic porcine and human secretins with biologically derived porcine secretin to diagnose Zollinger-Ellison syndrome. *Aliment Pharmacol Ther.* 2001;15:669-676.

24. Korpela R, Peuhkuri K, Poussa T. Comparison of a portable breath hydrogen analyser (Micro H2) with a Quintron MicroLyzer in measuring lactose maldigestion, and the evaluation of a Micro H2 for diagnosing hypolactasia. *Scand J Clin Lab Invest.* 1998;58:217-224.

25. Matthews SB, Waud JP, Roberts AG, Campbell AK. Systemic lactose intolerance: a new perspective on an old problem. *Postgrad Med J.* 2005;81:167-173.

26. Farrell RJ, Kelly CP. Diagnosis of celiac sprue. *Am J Gastroenterol.* 2001;96:3237-3246.

27. Uil JJ, van Elburg RM, van Overbeek FM, et al. Clinical implications of the sugar absorption test: intestinal permeability test to assess mucosal barrier function. *Scand J Gastroenterol Suppl.* 1997;223:70-78.

Body Fluid Analysis

KRISTY SHANAHAN, LILLIAN A. MUNDT

CHAPTER

29

CHAPTER OUTLINE

- ◆ AMNIOTIC FLUID
  Neural Tube Defects
  Hemolytic Disease of the Newborn
  Fetal Lung Maturity
  Phosphatidylglycerol
  Fluorescence Polarization
  Lamellar Body Counts
- ◆ CEREBROSPINAL FLUID

- ◆ SWEAT
- ◆ SYNOVIAL FLUID
- ◆ SEROUS FLUIDS
  Pleural Fluid
  Pericardial Fluid
  Peritoneal Fluid
- ◆ QUESTIONS
- ◆ REFERENCES

Chapter Objectives

Upon completion of this chapter, the clinical laboratorian should be able to do the following:

- Identify the source of amniotic fluid, cerebrospinal fluid, sweat, synovial fluid, pleural fluid, pericardial fluid, and peritoneal fluid.
- Describe the physiologic purpose of amniotic fluid, cerebrospinal fluid, sweat, synovial fluid, pleural fluid, pericardial fluid, and peritoneal fluid.

- Discuss the clinical utility of testing amniotic fluid, cerebrospinal fluid, sweat, synovial fluid, pleural fluid, pericardial fluid, and peritoneal fluid.
- Interpret the patient's status, given the results of a TDxFLM II test, L/S ratio, cerebrospinal fluid protein analysis, and sweat chloride test.
- Differentiate between a transudate and an exudate.

KEY TERMS

Amniocentesis
Amniotic fluid
Arachnoid villi/granulations
Ascites
Blood–brain barrier
Effusion
Exudate
Hypoglycorrhachia
L/S ratio
Oligoclonal banding

Otorrhea
Pericardial fluid
Peritoneal fluid
Pleural fluid
Respiratory distress syndrome
Rhinorrhea
Serous fluid
Surfactant
Synovial fluid
Thoracentesis
Transudate

This chapter is designed to acquaint the reader with several fluids that are often analyzed in the clinical chemistry laboratory. The source, method of collection, physiologic purpose, and clinical utility of laboratory measurements for each of these body fluids are emphasized.

AMNIOTIC FLUID

The amniotic sac provides an enclosed environment for fetal development. This sac is bilayered as the result of

a fusion of the amnionic (inner) and chorionic (outer) membranes at an early stage of fetal development. The fetus is suspended in amniotic fluid (AF) within the sac. The AF provides a cushioning medium for the fetus, regulates the temperature of the fetal environment, allows fetal movement, and serves as a matrix for influx and efflux of constituents such as glucose, sodium, and potassium.

Ultimately, the mother is the physiologic source for AF. Depending on the interval of the gestational period, the fluid may be derived from different sources. At the initiation of pregnancy, some maternal secretion across the amnion contributes to the volume. Shortly after formation of the placenta, embryo, and fusion of membranes, AF is largely derived by transudation across the fetal skin. In the last half of pregnancy, the skin becomes substantially less permeable, and fetal micturition, or urination, becomes the major volume source. The fate of the fluid also varies with the period of gestation. A bidirectional exchange is presumed to occur across the membranes and at the placenta. Similarly, during early pregnancy, the fetal skin is involved in exchange of AF. In the last half of pregnancy, the mechanism of fetal swallowing is the major fate of AF. There is a dynamic balance established between production and clearance; fetal urination and swallowing maintain this balance. The continual swallowing maintains intimate contact of the AF with the fetal gastrointestinal tract, buccal cavity, and bronchotracheal tree. This contact is evidenced by the sloughed material from the fetus that provides us with the "window" to fetal developmental and functional stages.

Cells found in the fluid originate within the fetus, and the chemical content reflects the continual swallowing and clearance of fluid. A sample of fluid is obtained by transabdominal amniocentesis (amniotic sac puncture), which is performed under aseptic conditions. Before an attempt is made to obtain fluid, the positions of the placenta, fetus, and fluid pockets are visualized using ultrasonography. Aspiration of anything except fluid could lead to erroneous conclusions, as well as possible harm to the fetus (Fig. 29-1).

Amniocentesis and subsequent AF analysis are performed to test for (1) congenital diseases, (2) neural tube defects (NTDs), (3) hemolytic disease, and (4) fetal pulmonary development. The first, diagnosis of genetic abnormality, can be accomplished by cell culture. Fluid obtained between 14 and 20 weeks of pregnancy is

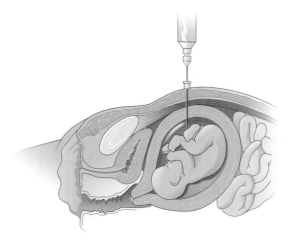

FIGURE 29-1 Amniocentesis. A sample is removed from the amniotic sac for fetal abnormality testing.

harvested for cells of fetal origin. The cells are cultured, collected for chromosomal analysis, and are lysed so that enzyme contents may be determined to evaluate for metabolic defects. This procedure has been largely supplanted by the use of chorionic villus sampling (CVS) and fluorescence in situ hybridization genetic analysis. CVS may pose a risk to the fetus, and first-trimester amniocentesis may provide a sample with less interfering substances.

Neural Tube Defects

Screening for NTDs is initially performed using maternal serum. The presence of elevated levels of α-fetoprotein (AFP) is primarily associated with NTDs such as spina bifida and anencephaly. Elevated maternal serum AFP can also be closely correlated with abdominal hernias into the umbilical cord, cystic hygroma, and poor pregnancy outcome. Low maternal serum AFP is associated with an increased incidence of Down's syndrome and other aneuploidies. The protocol for AFP testing is generally considered to include (1) maternal serum AFP, usually with the assay of hCG, unconjugated estriol, and inhibin A; (2) repeat, if positive; (3) diagnostic ultrasound; and (4) amniocentesis for confirmation. Interpretation of maternal serum AFP testing is complex, being a function of age, race, weight, gestational age, and level of nutrition. Testing of amniotic fluid α-fetoprotein (AFAFP) is the confirmatory procedure. AFP is a product of, first, the fetal yolk sac and, then, the fetal liver. It is released into the fetal circulation and presumably enters the AF by transudation. Entry into the maternal circulation could be by placenta crossover or from the AF. An open NTD (e.g., spina bifida) that causes an increase in AFAFP is accompanied by an increase in maternal serum AFP. Under normal conditions, AFAFP would be cleared by fetal swallowing and metabolism. An increased presence overloads this mechanism, causing AFAFP elevation. Both serum and AF are routinely analyzed using immunologic methods. Results are reported as multiples of the median. Because of the variety of demographics involved in determining normal values, each laboratory should establish its own median values for gestational weeks (usually weeks 15 to 21). Results can then be calculated using the formula:

$$MoM = \frac{\text{Specimen AFP concentration}}{\text{Median AFP concentration for gestational week}} \quad \text{(Eq. 29-1)}$$

Concern over the difficulty in interpreting AFP tests generated the need for a second test to confirm NTDs and abdominal wall defects. The method used is the assay for a central nervous system (CNS)–specific acetylcholinesterase (AChE). The NTD allows direct or, at least less difficult, passage of AChE into the AF. Analysis for CNS-specific AChE in the AF then offers a degree of confirmation for AFAFP. The methods used for CNS

AChE include enzymatic, immunologic, and electro-phoretic with inhibition. The latter includes the use of acetylthiocholine as substrate and BW284C51, a specific CNS inhibitor, to differentiate the serum pseudocholin-esterase from the CNS-specific AChE.

Hemolytic Disease of the Newborn

The analysis of AF to screen for hemolytic disease of the newborn (erythroblastosis fetalis) was the first recognized laboratory procedure performed on AF. Hemolytic disease of the newborn is a syndrome of the fetus resulting from incompatibility between maternal and fetal blood, because of differences in either the ABO or Rh blood group systems. Maternal antibodies to fetal erythrocytes cause a hemolytic reaction that can vary in severity. The resultant hemoglobin breakdown products, predominantly bilirubin, appear in the AF and provide a measure of the severity of the incompatibility reaction.

The most commonly used method is a direct spec-trophotometric scan of undiluted AF and subsequent calculation of the relative bilirubin amount. Classically, absorbance due to bilirubin is reported instead of a con-centration of bilirubin. The method consisted of scan-ning AF from 550 to 350 nm against a water blank. The resultant absorbances can be used differently to derive the necessary information. The common method, the method of Liley,[1] requires the plotting of the observations at 5 nm intervals against wavelength, using semilogarithmic paper. A baseline is constructed from 550 to 350 nm; the change at 450 nm is a result of bilirubin.

Care must be used in the interpretation of the spec-tra. A decision for treatment can be made based on the degree of hemolysis and gestational age. The rather lim-ited treatment options are immediate delivery, intrauter-ine transfusion, and observation. The transfusion can be accomplished by means of the umbilical artery and titrat-ed to the desired hematocrit. Several algorithms have been proposed to aid in decision making (Fig. 29-2). An example of an uncomplicated bilirubin scan is shown in Figure 29-3. To avoid interference in the spectro-photometric scan, specimens should be immediately centrifuged and the fluid separated from the sediment. This will prevent not only particulate interference but also the possibility of increased lysis of red blood cells in the specimen producing hemoglobin in the AF. As with all specimens for bilirubin analysis, AF specimens for bilirubin scans must be protected from light. Specimens are routinely collected in amber-colored tubes. Exposure to light results in the photo-oxidation of bilirubin to bili-verdin that will not be detected at 450 nm, resulting in underestimation of the hemolytic disease severity.

Examples of interferences, compared with a nor-mal specimen, are given in Figure 29-4. Each labora-tory should compile its own catalog of real examples for spectrophotometric analysis. The presence of hemoglobin

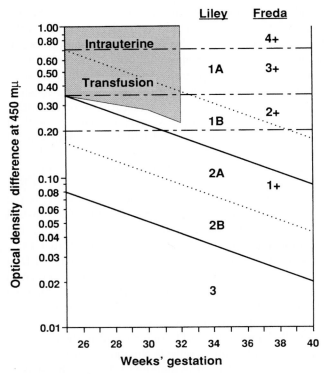

FIGURE 29-2 Assessment of fetal prognosis. Liley method: *1A, above broken line,* condition desperate, immediate delivery or transfusion; *1B, between broken and continuous lines,* hemoglobin > 8 g/100 mL, delivery or transfusion (*stippled area*) urgent; *2A, between continuous and broken lines,* hemoglobin 8 to 10 g/100 mL, delivery 36 to 37 weeks; *2B, between broken and continuous lines,* hemoglobin 11 to 13.9 g/100 mL, delivery 37 to 39 weeks; *3, below continuous line,* not anemic, delivery at term. Freda method: *4+, above upper horizontal line,* fetal death imminent, immediate delivery or transfusion; *3+, between upper and middle horizontal lines,* fetus in jeopardy, death within 3 weeks, delivery or transfu-sion as soon as possible; *2+, between middle and lower horizontal lines,* fetal survival for at least 7 to 10 days, repeat test, possible indication for transfusion; *1+, below lower horizontal line,* fetus in no immediate danger of death. (Adapted from Robertson JG. Evaluation of the reported methods of interpreting spectrophoto-metric tracings of amniotic fluid in rhesus isoimmunization. *Am J Obstet Gynecol.* 1966;95:120.)

is identified by its peak absorbance at 410 to 415 nm; the presence of urine is identified by the broad curve and confirmed by creatinine and urea analyses; and the pres-ence of meconium is identified by the distinctly greenish color of the AF and flat absorbance curve.

Fetal Lung Maturity

The primary reason for AF testing is the need to assess fetal pulmonary maturity. All the organ systems are at jeopardy from prematurity, but the state of the fetal lungs is a priority from the clinical perspective. The availability of laboratory tests that give an indication of maturity has also fostered this emphasis. Consequently, the labora-tory is asked whether sufficient specific phospholipids are reflected in the AF to prevent atelectasis (alveolar

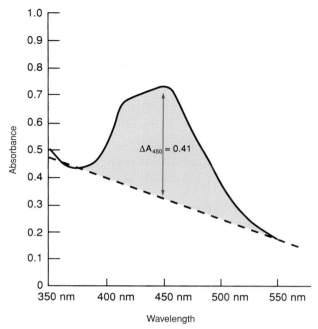

FIGURE 29-3 Change in $A_{450\ nm}$ from AF bilirubin scan.

collapse) if the fetus were to be delivered. This question is important when preterm delivery is contemplated because of other risk factors in pregnancy, such as preeclampsia and premature rupture of membranes. Risk factors to fetus or mother can be weighed against interventions, such as delay of delivery with steroid administration to

the mother to enhance fetal surfactant production, or against at-risk postdelivery therapies, such as exogenous surfactant therapy, high-frequency ventilation, and extracorporeal membrane oxygenation.

Alveolar collapse in the neonatal lung may occur during the changeover from placental oxygen to air as an oxygen source at birth if the proper quantity and type of phospholipid (surfactant) is not present. The ensuing condition, which may vary in the degree of severity, is called respiratory distress syndrome (RDS) . It has also been referred to as *hyaline membrane disease* because of the hyaline membrane found in affected lungs. Lung maturation is a function of differentiation, beginning near the 24th week of pregnancy, of alveolar epithelial cells (pneumocytes) into type I and type II cells. The type I cells form the alveolar–capillary membrane for exchange of gases. The type II cells produce and store the surfactants needed for alveolar stability in the form of lamellar bodies. As the lungs mature, increases occur in phospholipid concentration, particularly the compounds phosphatidylglycerol (PG) and lecithin[2] (Fig. 29-5). These two compounds, present in 10% and 70%, respectively, of total phospholipid concentration, are most important as surfactants. Their presence in high enough levels acts in concert to allow contraction

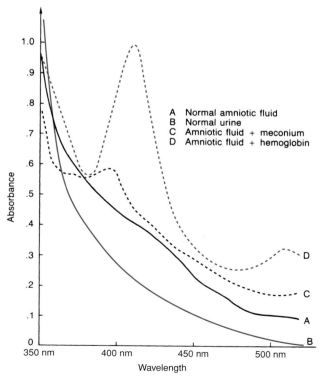

FIGURE 29-4 Amniotic fluid absorbance scans.

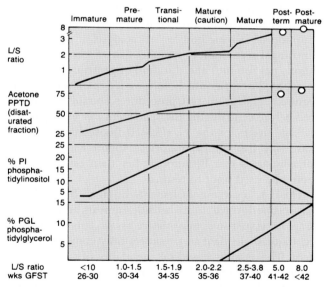

FIGURE 29-5 The form used to report the lung profile. The four determinations are plotted on the *ordinate*, and the weeks of gestation are plotted on the *abscissa* (as well as the *L/S ratio* as an "internal standard"). When plotted, these fall with a high frequency into a given grid that then identifies the stage of development of the lung as shown in the upper part of the form. The designation "mature (caution)" refers to patients other than those with diabetes who can be delivered *if necessary* at this time; if the patient has diabetes, she can be delivered with safety when the values fall in the "mature" grid. (Reprinted with permission from Kulovich MV, Hallman MB, Gluck L. The lung profile. I. Normal pregnancy. *Am J Obstet Gynecol.* 1979;135:57. Copyright 1977 by the Regents of the University of California.)

and re-expansion of the neonatal alveoli. To conceptualize their importance, remember the difficulty in blowing up a new toy balloon relative to a balloon that has been partially inflated. For the newborn, the normal amount of proper surfactant allows contraction of the alveoli without collapse. The next inspiration is the difference between a partially inflated versus a flattened new balloon. Insufficient surfactant allows alveoli to collapse, requiring a great deal of energy to re-expand the alveoli upon inspiration. This not only creates an extreme energy demand on a newborn but probably also causes physical damage to the alveoli with each collapse. The damage may lead to "hyaline" deposition, or the newborn may not have the strength to continue inspiration at the energy cost. The result of either can be fatal.

Tests for assessing FLM include functional assays and quantitative assays. Functional assays provide a direct physical measure of AF in an attempt to assess surfactant ability to decrease surface tension. These include the "bubble or shake" test and the foam stability index (FSI). Quantitative tests include the lecithin–sphingomyelin ratio (L/S ratio), PG, fluorescence polarization, and lamellar body counts.

Excessive force (anything greater than that needed to remove debris) can change the lipid profile by causing the lipids present to fractionate as a result of centrifugal force. The difference in ratios observed at 1,000 versus 3,000 g can radically alter clinical interpretation. Before adoption of any method for AF analysis, a protocol for centrifugal separation to include relative force (*not* revolutions per minute) and duration of centrifugation must be adopted and rigorously followed. Separation method requirements for all test procedures should be considered before centrifuging the specimen. For example, the package insert for the TDxFLM II fluorescent polarization assay (Abbott Laboratories, Abbott Park, IL) specifically states that filtration rather than centrifugation should be used prior to testing.

The FSI,[3] a variant of Clements' original "bubble test"[4] that was performed at the bedside, appears acceptable as a rapid, inexpensive, informative assay. This qualitative, technique-dependent test requires only common equipment. The assay is based on the ability of surfactant to generate a surface tension lower than that of a 0.47 mol fraction ethanol–water solution. If sufficient surfactant is present, a stable ring of foam bubbles remains at the air–liquid interface. As surfactant increases (fetal lung maturity probability increases), a larger mole fraction of ethanol is required to overcome the surfactant-controlled surface tension. The highest mole fraction used while still maintaining a stable ring of bubbles at the air–liquid interface is reported as the FSI (Table 29-1). The test is dependent on technique and can also be skewed by contamination of any kind in the AF (e.g., blood or meconium contamination). Interpretation of the FSI bubble patterns is difficult and technique dependent. Results

TABLE 29-1	FSI DETERMINATION		
	TUBE 1	TUBE 2	TUBE 3
Vol AF	0.50	0.50	0.50
Vol 95% EtOH	0.51	0.53	0.55
FSI	0.47	0.48	0.49

can vary among clinical laboratorians. Most laboratories have found that an FSI of 0.47 correlates well with an L/S ratio of 2.0.

The quantitative tests were given emphasis primarily by the work of Gluck et al.[5] The phospholipids of importance are PG, lecithin, and sphingomyelin (SP). Relative amounts of PG and lecithin increase dramatically with pulmonary maturity, whereas SP concentration is relatively constant and provides a baseline for the L/S ratio. Increases in PG and lecithin correspond to the larger amounts of surfactant being produced by the type II pneumocytes as fetal lungs mature.

The classic technique for separation and evaluation of the lipids involves thin-layer chromatography (TLC) of an extract of the AF. The extraction procedure removes most interfering substances and results in a concentrated lipid solution. Current practices use either one- or two-dimensional TLC for identification. Laboratory needs determine if a one-dimensional or a two-dimensional method is performed. An example of the phospholipids separation by one-dimensional TLC is shown in Figure 29-6.[6]

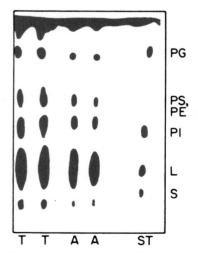

FIGURE 29-6 Thin-layer chromatogram of amniotic fluid phospholipids. Standard phospholipids (*ST*), total extract (*T*), and acetone-precipitable compounds (*A*) in amniotic fluid are shown. The phospholipid standards contained, per liter, 2 g each of lecithin and P1, 1 g each of PG and sphingomyelin, and 0.3 g each of PS and PE; 10 mL of the standard was spotted. (Reprinted with permission from Tsai MY, Marshall JG. Phosphatidylglycerol in 261 samples of amniotic fluid. *Clin Chem.* 25(5):683. Copyright 1979 American Association for Clinical Chemistry.)

The classic breakpoint for judgment of maturity has been an L/S ratio of 2. As a result of the time-consuming requirements of performing the L/S ratio, several additional tests have been developed to allow faster determination of FLM. The L/S ratio, however, remains the "gold standard" by which all methods are compared.

Phosphatidylglycerol

As mentioned previously, an additional phospholipid essential for FLM is PG that increases in proportion to lecithin. In the case of diabetic mothers, however, development of PG is delayed. Therefore, using an L/S ratio of 2.0 as an indicator of FLM cannot be relied upon to ensure that RDS will not occur unless PG is also included in interpretation of the L/S ratio. With the current trend toward less labor-intensive techniques, an immunologic assay using antibody specific for PG can be used to determine FLM.

The Aminostat-FLM (Irving Scientific, Santa Ana, CA) immunologic test is designed to measure the adequate presence of PG in AF. Because lecithin production is not affected in diabetic mothers and the levels of PG and lecithin rise at the same rate in unaffected pregnancies, the Aminostat-FLM can be used to determine whether adequate FLM is present. Good correlation has been shown compared with the L/S ratio. The antibody-specific immunologic assay offers the additional advantage, not present in other assays, of being unaffected by specimen debris such as meconium and blood.

CASE STUDY 29-1

A 28-year-old woman is pregnant for the second time, having miscarried a year ago. At the time she miscarried she was working as a volunteer in Haiti and did not seek medical care. Her doctor is concerned that the baby that she is carrying now may have hemolytic disease due to Rh incompatibility. She also has diabetes. She has an increase in optical density at 450 nm on her amniotic fluid screen with a Liley graph reading of 0.6 and is at approximately 34 weeks of gestation. Her L/S ratio was 2.1. The physician is considering inducing labor. Further testing of the amniotic fluid shows an FLM II reading of 55 mg surfactant/g of albumin.

Questions

1. What do the tests reveal? Why was the FLM II reading important in this case as she already had the L/S ratio results?

2. Why is the physician considering inducing labor?

3. Based on the FLM II results, is it safe for the physician to induce labor?

Fluorescence Polarization

The TDxFLM II Assay system (Abbott Laboratories) consists of a commercial reagent system that can be run on the versatile TDx automated polarizing instrument. The system compares the polarization of a fluorescent dye that combines with albumin and surfactant in the AF specimen. The concentration of albumin remains consistent throughout later gestation and serves as an internal standard similar to SP in the L/S ratio.

Dye molecules combined with albumin have restricted movement producing a high level of polarization and a reduced life span. In contrast, dye molecules combined with surfactant produce a lower level of polarization and have a longer life span. The polarizer separates the differences in polarization and determines the ratio of surfactant to albumin. The ratio of surfactant is expressed in milligrams of surfactant to grams of albumin and is achieved by instrumental comparison to a standard curve. A set of FLM II calibrators is run through the polarizer to develop the standard curve producing a range of 0 to 160 mg/g. The standard curve is stored in the polarizer.

Values of 55 mg surfactant per gram of albumin and higher are considered to indicate FLM. A value of 39 mg/g is considered immature, and values between 55 to 39 mg/g are considered borderline.

A protocol for interpretation based on gestational age has been reported.[7] The FLM II test correlates with an L/S ratio of 2.0.[8]

AF specimens must be filtered, not centrifuged, to avoid falsely decreased values for FLM. Filters and holders are provided with the assay system. Test interference can be caused by the presence of bilirubin, meconium, and blood.[9]

Lamellar Body Counts

The phospholipids are produced and secreted by the type II alveolar cells in the form of lamellar bodies. As FLM increases, these lamellated packets of surfactant also exhibit an increased presence in the AF. The fact that lamellar bodies are approximately the same size as platelets provides a convenient method to determine their concentration using the platelet channel on automated hematology analyzers.[10] Based on the model of analyzer used, the number of lamellar bodies needed to ensure FLM can vary. This variation occurs as a result of different instrumental methods used to detect the bodies. Acceptable counts must be correlated with the specific instrumentation.[11] A standardized protocol has been developed in an effort to make the assay transferable between laboratories.[12]

CEREBROSPINAL FLUID

Cerebrospinal fluid (CSF) is the liquid that surrounds the brain and spinal cord. The brain and spinal cord are covered by the meninges that consist of three layers: the dura mater, arachnoid, and pia mater (Fig. 29-7).

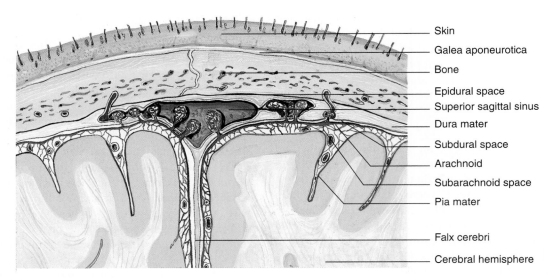

Skin
Galea aponeurotica
Bone
Epidural space
Superior sagittal sinus
Dura mater
Subdural space
Arachnoid
Subarachnoid space
Pia mater

Falx cerebri
Cerebral hemisphere

FIGURE 29-7 Meninges of the brain.

CSF flows between the arachnoid and the pia mater in an area referred to as the subarachnoid space. The three functions of the CSF are (1) physical support and protection, (2) provision of a controlled chemical environment to supply nutrients to the tissues and removal of wastes, and (3) intracerebral and extracerebral transport (Fig. 29-8).

The major and most obvious function of CSF is as a buoyant cushion for the brain. The denser brain floats in the less dense fluid, allowing movement within the skull. The significance of cushion function is demonstrated by the result of a blow to the head. The initial shock is transferred to the entire brain, instead of inflicting damage to one area. The brain may be bruised at the side opposite the blow, depending on the force imparted.

The second major function of CSF is the maintenance of a constant gross chemical matrix for the CNS. Serum components may vary greatly, but constituent levels of CSF are maintained within narrow limits.

The transport function is described as a neuroendocrine role. The CSF is involved in the distribution of hypophyseal hormones within the brain and the clearance of hormones from the brain to the blood.

The total CSF volume is about 150 mL or about 8% of the total CNS cavity volume. The fluid is formed predominantly at the choroid plexus deep within the brain and by the ependymal cells lining the ventricles. The endothelial cells of the choriod plexuses have very tight-fitting junctures to control the passage of substances across their membranes. This is termed the blood–brain barrier. Damage to the blood–brain barrier is frequently the reason for abnormal chemistry results in CSF analysis.

CSF is formed at an average rate of about 0.4 mL/min or 500 mL/d. Formation is a result of selective ultrafiltration of plasma and active secretion by the epithelial membranes. Absorption of CSF occurs at outpouchings

in the dura called arachnoid villi, also known as granulations, that protrude through the dura to the venous sinuses of the brain and into the bloodstream. The granulations act as one-way valves to maintain an excretion volume equal to the production volume.

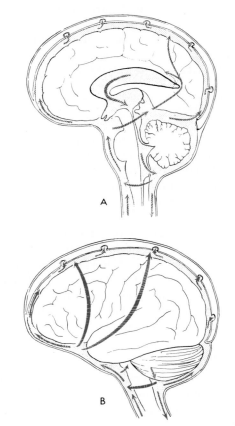

FIGURE 29-8 Major pathways of CSF. **(A)** Sagittal view. **(B)** Lateral view. (Reprinted with permission from Milhorat TH. *Hydrocephalus and the Cerebrospinal Fluid*. Baltimore, MD: Lippincott Williams & Wilkins; 1972:25.)

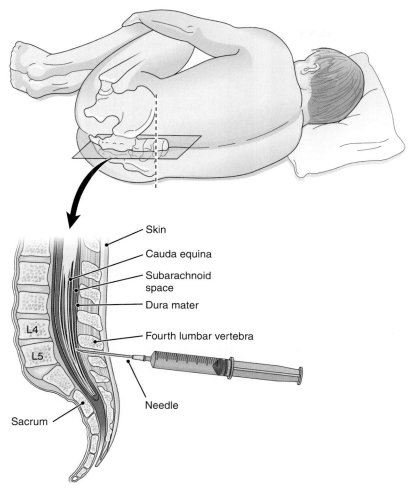

FIGURE 29-9 Placement of the needle for CSF collection.

Specimens of CSF are obtained by lumbar puncture, usually at the interspace of vertebrae L3-4 or lower, using aseptic technique (Fig. 29-9). The fluid obtained is usually separated into three numbered aliquots: (1) for chemistry and serology, (2) for microbiology, and (3) for hematology. It is paramount to remember that this specimen is of limited volume and should be analyzed immediately. Any remaining sample should be preserved because of its limited availability. The order of the tubes reflects the presumed order for minimalization of interference from less than optimal collection technique, with tube 3 presumably least contaminated by cells of intervening tissue.

Laboratory investigation of CSF is indicated for cases of suspected CNS infection, demyelinating disease, malignancy, and hemorrhage in the CNS. As with all patient samples entering the laboratory, visual examination of the specimen is the first and often the most important observation made. Normal CSF is clear, colorless, free of clots, and free of blood. Differences from these standards indicate a probable pathology and

merit further examination. Cloudy fluids usually require microscopic examination, with a yellow to brown or red color indicating the presence of blood.

The two most common reasons for blood and hemoglobin pigments to be found in CSF are traumatic tap and subarachnoid hemorrhage. Traumatic tap is the artifactual presence of blood or derivatives due to interdiction of blood vessels during the lumbar puncture. Hemorrhage results from a breakdown of the barrier of the CNS and circulatory system from trauma, for example. Because of the severity of hemorrhage, it must be differentiated from traumatic tap.

Blood cells may be introduced into a CSF specimen at the time of lumbar puncture. Therefore, careful differentiation must be made between traumatic tap and hemorrhage. If there is a significant difference in the amount of blood present between the first and last tubes collected (later tubes gradually clearing), then the puncture was traumatic. If all tubes collected show the same degree of blood, then a subarachnoid hemorrhage is most likely. Figure 29-10 demonstrates the difference in appearance

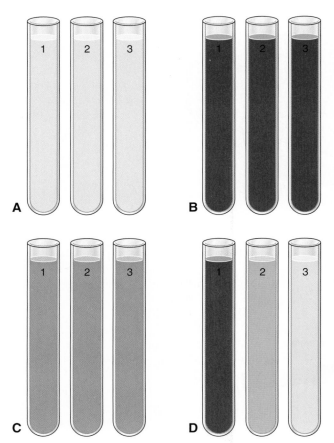

FIGURE 29-10 Comparison of CSF appearance between **(A)** normal CSF (all three tubes with the same clarity), **(B)** red CSF from fresh hemorrhage (all three tubes with the same red color and opaqueness), **(C)** xanthochromic CSF from old hemorrhage (all three tubes with the same yellow color and clear), and **(D)** CSF from a traumatic tap (decreasing amounts of redness in each successive tube). Note: Full color image on thePoint at http://thepoint.lww.com/.

of normal clear CSF, red CSF in hemorrhage, xanthochromic CSF from an old hemorrhage, and CSF from a traumatic tap.[13]

If lumbar puncture is performed within the first 4 hours after a subarachnoid hemorrhage, the CSF will appear pale pink to red, depending on the degree of hemorrhage. Red blood cells lyse in CSF due to the low level of proteins and lipids when compared with plasma. After hemolysis, the CSF will change from a cloudy or hazy pink–red to a clear pink–red and then through various shades of light orange, yellow, and amber (xanthochromia), as oxyhemoglobin changes to methemoglobin, and then after about 12 hours bilirubin is formed. Gradual decrease in CSF color occurs over the first 2 days, clearing in about 2 to 4 weeks.[14]

Biochemical (chemical) analysis of CSF has led to compilations of the scope of possible constituents. In clinical practice, however, the number of useful indicators becomes small. The tests of interest are glucose, protein (total and specific), lactate, and glutamine.

Most often used are glucose and proteins. Before any analysis, the fluid should be centrifuged to avoid contamination by cellular elements. The level of glutamine should reflect the level of CNS ammonia removed by glutamine formation from glutamate. This would be elevated in hepatic encephalopathy, as would occur in liver failure. The test has largely been supplanted by the relative ease and simplicity of reliable plasma ammonia determinations. The tests that have been most reliable diagnostically and accessible analytically are those for CSF glucose, total protein, and specific proteins. Glucose enters the spinal fluid predominantly via a facilitative transport compared with a passive (diffusional) or an active (energy-dependent) transport. It is carried across the epithelial membrane by a stereospecific carrier species. The carrier mechanism is responsible for transport of lipid-insoluble materials across the membrane into the CSF. Generally, this is a "downhill" process consistent with a concentration gradient. The CSF glucose concentration is about two-thirds that of plasma.

Because an isolated CSF glucose concentration may be misleading, it is recommended that a plasma sample be obtained 2 to 4 hours prior to the tap so that plasma and CSF glucose levels can equilibrate. Normal CSF glucose is considered to be 60% to 70% that of the blood glucose. Increased glucose levels are not clinically informative, usually providing only confirmation of hyperglycemia. With increasing blood glucose levels, the CSF glucose increases, but not proportionally. This is significant because it implies that the plasma/CSF glucose ratio decreases as gross hyperglycemia occurs.

The decreasing CSF/plasma glucose ratio as plasma glucose increases is consistent with a saturable carrier process. It would not be unusual for the ratio to be 0.4:0.6 with massive plasma glucose levels (more than 600 mg/dL), but a CSF glucose level of 80 mg/dL, with plasma level of 300 mg/dL, is clinically significant and would merit concern.

Decreased CSF glucose levels (hypoglycorrhachia) can be the result of (1) disorder in carrier-mediated transport of glucose into CSF, (2) active metabolism of glucose by cells or organisms, or (3) increased metabolism by the CNS. The mechanism of transport decrease remains under intense discussion, but it is speculated to be the cause in tuberculous meningitis and sarcoidosis. Acute purulent, amebic, fungal, and trichinosis meningitis are examples of glucose consumption by organisms, whereas diffuse meningeal neoplasia and brain tumor are examples of glucose consumption by CNS tissue. Consumption of glucose is usually accompanied by an increased lactate level due to anaerobic glycolysis by organisms or cerebral tissue.

An increased lactate level with a normal to decreased glucose level has been suggested as a readily accessible indicator for bacterial versus viral meningitis.[15] Analysis of glucose and lactate in CSF is easily accomplished by techniques used for plasma and serum. It is important that provision for the analysis of glucose or lactate in CSF be immediate or that the specimen be preserved with an antiglycolytic, such as fluoride ion.

Protein levels in CSF reflect the selective ultrafiltration of the CSF blood–brain barrier. All protein usually found in plasma is found in CSF, but at much lower levels. Total protein is about 0.5%, or 1%, that of plasma. The specific protein concentrations in CSF are not proportional to the plasma levels because of the specificity of the ultrafiltration process. Correlation is best accomplished using hydrodynamic ratios of the protein species rather than molecular weight. Because of the relationship of CSF proteins to serum, serum analysis should accompany specific CSF protein analysis. A decreased level of CSF total protein can arise from (1) decreased dialysis from plasma, (2) increased protein loss (e.g., removal of excessive volumes of CSF), or (3) leakage of CSF from a tear in the dura, otorrhea, or rhinorrhea. The last reason is most common. A dural tear can occur as a result of a previous lumbar puncture or from severe trauma. Otorrhea and rhinorrhea refer to the leakage of CSF from the ear or into the nose, respectively. Identification of CSF leakage is best done by an analysis for β-transferrin, a protein unique to the CSF.

An increased level of CSF total protein is a useful nonspecific indicator of pathologic states. Increases may be caused by (1) lysis of contaminant blood from traumatic tap, (2) increased permeability of the epithelial membrane, (3) increased production by CNS tissue, or (4) obstruction. Contamination from blood is significant because of the 200:1 concentration ratio. The presence of any amount of blood can elevate CSF protein levels. The blood–brain barrier becomes more permeable from bacterial or fungal infection or cerebral hemorrhage, whereas an increase in CNS production occurs in subacute sclerosing panencephalitis (SSPE) or multiple sclerosis (MS). There may also be combinations of permeability and production, with the collagen vascular diseases. An obstructive process, such as tumor or abscess, would also cause increased protein. Diagnostically more sensitive information can be obtained by analysis of the protein fractions present. A comparison to the serum pattern is necessary for accurate conclusions. Under normal conditions, prealbumin is present in CSF in higher concentration than in serum. Although the respective proteins can be determined in both serum and CSF, the proteins of greatest interest are albumin and immunoglobulin G (IgG). Because albumin is produced solely in the liver, its presence in CSF must occur by means of blood–brain barrier passage. IgG, however, can arise by local synthesis from plasma cells within the CSF. The measurement of albumin in both serum and CSF is then used to normalize the IgG values from each matrix to determine the source of the IgG.

To determine the integrity of the blood–brain barrier, a CSF/serum albumin index is calculated as follows:

$$\frac{\text{CSF albumin (mg/dL)}}{\text{Serum albumin (g/dL)}} = \frac{\text{CSF serum}}{\text{albumin index}} \quad \text{(Eq. 29-2)}$$

An index value less than 9 indicates an intact blood–brain barrier.

This index can then be used to calculate the IgG index to determine CNS synthesis of IgG to aid the diagnosis of demyelinating diseases, such as MS and SSPE. MS is the most common inflammatory demyelinating disease of the CNS:

$$\frac{\text{CSF IgG/serum IgG}}{\text{CSF albumin serum albumin}} = \frac{\text{CSF IgG}}{\text{index}} \quad \text{(Eq. 29-3)}$$

The normal value is <0.73

Increases in serum albumin cause increases in the CSF levels because of membrane permeability. However, increased CSF IgG, without concomitant CSF albumin increase, suggests local production (MS or SSPE). Increases in permeability and production are found with bacterial meningitis. Methods to analyze IgG and albumin CSF levels are the same as for serum but are optimized for the lower levels found.

Increased CSF protein levels or clinical suspicion usually indicates the need for electrophoretic separation of the respective proteins. At times, this separation demonstrates multiple banding of the IgG band. This observation is referred to as oligoclonal bands (a small number of clones of IgG from the same cell type with nearly identical electrophoretic properties). This occurrence is usually associated with inflammatory diseases and MS or SSPE. These types of disorders would stimulate the immunocompetent cells. The recognition of an oligoclonal pattern supersedes the report of normal protein levels and is a cause for concern if the corresponding serum separation does not demonstrate identical banding.

Another protein thought to be specific for MS is myelin basic protein (MBP). Initial reports suggested high specificity, but MBP has also been found in nondemyelinating disorders and does not always occur in demyelinating disorders. MBP levels are used to monitor therapy of MS. Current international guidelines for the diagnosis of MS recognize both an elevated IgG index and the presence of CSF oligoclonal bands that are not found in the serum as supporting evidence. Immunoassay procedures are available for analyzing MBP.[16]

SWEAT

The common eccrine sweat glands function in the regulation of body temperature. They are innervated by cholinergic nerve fibers and are a type of exocrine gland. Sweat has been analyzed for its multiple inorganic and organic contents but, with one notable exception,

CASE STUDY 29-2

A 31-year-old man was in good health until about 1 year ago, after he began working as an accountant. Within the last year, he began to notice episodic blurring of vision, diplopia, mild vertigo, and headache. He complained of sensory loss in his hands and a feeling of weakness after physical exertion but thought that was just "out of shape." He went to his physician after suffering leg and shoulder weakness accompanied by a feeling of paralysis, which was followed by a sensation of "pins and needles" in his left leg. Neurologic examination led to a spinal tap being performed for laboratory findings and a brain and spinal cord magnetic resonance imaging (MRI). His MRI showed demyelinating lesions, and other ancillary tests showed demyelinating damage to the auditory and visual pathway. The laboratory results were as follows:

CSF	Clear, colorless fluid, apparently free of debris; culture yields no growth
WBC	Normal
Glucose	60 mg/dL (plasma = 80 mg/dL)
Total protein	59 mg/dL
Albumin index	1.7
IgG index	0.97
Electrophoresis	Oligoclonal bands present

Questions

1. What is the significance of the albumin index? The IgG index?

2. What pathology is consistent with these results?

has not been proved as a clinically useful model. That exception is the analysis of sweat for chloride levels in the diagnosis of cystic fibrosis (CF). The sweat test is the single most accepted common diagnostic tool for the clinical identification of this disease. Normally, the coiled lower part of the sweat gland secretes a "presweat" upon cholinergic stimulation. As the presweat traverses the ductal part of the gland going through the dermis, various constituents are resorbed. In CF, the electrolytes, most notably chloride and sodium ions, are improperly resorbed owing to a mutation in the cystic fibrosis transmembrane conductance regulator (CFTR) gene, which controls a cyclic AMP–regulated chloride channel.

CF (mucoviscidosis) is an autosomal recessive inherited disease that affects the exocrine glands and causes electrolyte and mucous secretion abnormalities. This exocrinopathy is present only in the homozygous state.

The frequency of the carrier (heterozygous) state is estimated at 1 of 20 in the United States. The disease predominantly affects whites. The observed rate of expression ranks CF as the most common lethal hereditary disease in the United States, with death usually occurring by the third decade. The primary cause of death is pneumonia, secondary to the heavy, abnormally viscous secretion in the lungs. These heavy secretions cause obstruction of the micro-airways, predisposing the CF patient to repeated episodes of pneumonia. The third part of the diagnostic triad is pancreatic insufficiency. Again, abnormally viscous secretions obstruct pancreatic ducts. This obstruction ostensibly causes pooling and autoactivation of the pancreatic enzymes. The enzymes then cause destruction of the exocrine pancreatic tissue.

Diagnostic algorithms for CF continue to rely on abnormal sweat electrolytes, pancreatic or bronchial abnormalities, and family history. The use of blood immunoreactive trypsin, a pancreatic product, is now prevalent in newborn screening programs. The rapidly developing area of molecular genetics provides the definitive methodology. The gene defect causing CF has been localized on chromosome 7, and the most common mutations causing CF have been DNA "fingerprinted." As many as 1,550 mutations of the CFTR gene have been cataloged with the majority of patients found to be homozygous or heterozygous for the most common mutation. The sweat glands, although affected in their secretion, remain structurally unaffected by CF. Analysis of sweat for both sodium and chloride is valid but, historically, chloride was and is the major element, leading to use of the sweat chloride test. Because of its importance, a standard method has been suggested by the Cystic Fibrosis Foundation. This method is based on the pilocarpine nitrate iontophoresis method of Gibson and Cooke.[17] Pilocarpine is a cholinergic-like drug used to stimulate the sweat glands. The sweat is absorbed on a gauze pad during the procedure. After collecting sweat by iontophoresis, chloride analysis is performed. Many methods have been suggested, and all are dependent on laboratory requirements. Generally, the sweat is leached into a known volume of distilled water and analyzed for chloride (chloridometer). In general, values greater than 60 mmol/L are considered positive.

Other tests including osmolarity, conductivity, and chloride electrodes or patches placed on the skin are available but are considered screening tests with abnormal results followed by the Gibson-Cooke reference method. A variety of instrumentation is available for these screening tests.

Although a value of 60 mmol/L is generally recognized for the quantitative pilocarpine iontophoretic test, it is important to consider several factors in interpretation. Not only will there be analytic variation around the cutoff, an epidemiologic borderline area will also occur. Considering this, the range of 45–65 mmol/L for chloride would be more appropriate in determining the need for repetition. Some patients with *CFTR* mutations have been found to have values below 60 mmol/L. Other variables must be considered. Age generally increases the limit—so much so that it is increasingly difficult to classify adults. Obviously, the patient's state of hydration also affects sweat levels. Because the complete procedure is technically demanding, expertise should be developed before the test is clinically available. A complete description of sweat collection and analysis, including procedural justifications, is available for review.[18]

SYNOVIAL FLUID

Joints are classified as movable or immovable. The movable joint contains a cavity that is enclosed by a capsule; the inner lining of the capsule is synovial membrane (Fig. 29-11). This cavity contains synovial fluid, which is formed by ultrafiltration of plasma across the synovial membrane. The membrane also secretes a mucoprotein rich in hyaluronic acid into the dialysate, which causes the synovial fluid to be viscous. The membrane is composed of three different cell types: type A cells are rich in vacuoles and lysosomes and function as phagocytes; type B cells are rich in rough endoplasmic reticulum and presumed to be secretory in function; and type C cells appear to be hybrids of types A and B in appearance and function. Synovial fluid functions as a lubricant for the joints and as a transport medium for delivery of nutrients and removal of cell wastes. The volume of fluid found in a large joint, such as the knee, rarely exceeds 3 mL. Normal fluid is clear, colorless to pale yellow, viscous,

and nonclotting. Variations are indicative of pathologic conditions and are summarized in Table 29-2.

Collection of a synovial fluid sample is accomplished by arthrocentesis of the joint under aseptic conditions (Fig. 29-12). The sample should be collected in a heparin tube for culture, a heparin or liquid ethylenediamine-tetraacetic acid (EDTA) for microscopic analysis, and a fluoride tube for glucose analysis. Microscopic examination is the most useful in diagnostic significance.

Chemical analysis of synovial fluid includes the testing of several different analytes; most commonly used serum protein procedures can be used to measure synovial fluid protein. The normal range for synovial fluid protein is 1 to 3 g/dL. Increased synovial fluid protein levels are seen in ankylosing spondylitis, arthritis, arthropathies that accompany Crohn's disease, gout, psoriasis, Reiter syndrome, and ulcerative colitis. Synovial fluid glucose levels are interpreted using serum glucose levels after a 6- to 8-hour fast. Normally, synovial fluid glucose levels are less than 10 mg/dL lower than serum levels. Infectious disorders of the joint demonstrate large decreases in synovial fluid glucose and can be as much as 20 to 100 mg/dL less than serum levels. Other groups of joint disorders demonstrate a less of a decrease in synovial fluid glucose, 0 to 20 mg/dL.[19] The ratio of synovial fluid to plasma glucose (normally 0.9:1) remains the most useful. Decreased ratios are found in inflammatory (e.g., gout, rheumatoid arthritis [RA], and systemic lupus erythematosus) and septic (e.g., bacterial and viral arthritis) conditions. Standard methods for glucose analysis are applicable. Synovial fluid uric acid normally ranges from 6 to 8 mg/dL. The presence of uric acid in synovial fluid is helpful in diagnosing gout, especially at laboratories not able

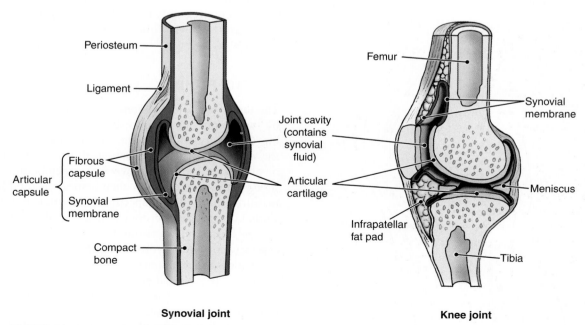

Synovial joint

Knee joint

FIGURE 29-11 Synovial joint and model.

TABLE 29-2	CLASSIFICATION OF SYNOVIAL FLUIDS						
GROUP	CATEGORY	VISUAL	VISCOSITY	MUCIN CLOT	CELL COUNT	GLUCOSE BLOOD: SF	OTHER
	Normal	Colorless—straw Clear	High	Good	<150 WBCs <25% neutrophils	0-10	
I	Noninflammatory	Yellow Slightly cloudy	Decreased	Fair	< −1,000 WBCs <30% neutrophils	0-10	
II	Inflammatory	White, gray, yellow Cloudy, turbid	Absent	Poor	<100,000 WBCs >50% neutrophils	0-4	
III	Septic	White, gray, yellow, or green Cloudy, purulent	Absent	Poor	50,000-200,000 WBCs >90% neutrophils	20-100	Positive cultures
IV	Crystal induced	White Cloudy, turbid, opaque, milky	Absent	Poor	500-200,000 WBCs <90% neutrophils	0-80	Crystals present
V	Hemorrhagic	Sanguinous, xanthochromic, red, or brown Cloudy	Absent	Poor	50-10,000 WBCs <50% neutrophils	0-20	RBCs present

Source: Mundt L, Shanahan K. *Graff's Textbook of Routine Urinalysis and Body Fluids.* 2nd ed. Philadelphia, PA: Lippincott Williams & Wilkins, 2011:268.

to perform crystal identification. Although rarely performed, lactic acid measurements can be helpful in diagnosing septic arthritis. Normally, synovial fluid lactate is less than 25 mg/dL but can be as high as 1,000 mg/dL in septic arthritis. Lactate dehydrogenase (LD) can be elevated in synovial fluid, while serum levels remain normal. Synovial fluid LD levels are usually increased in RA, infectious arthritis, and gout. Rheumatoid factor (RF) is an antibody to immunoglobulins. Most patients with RA have RF in their serum, whereas more than half of these patients will demonstrate RF in synovial fluid. Determining synovial fluid RF is important to diagnose cases where RF is only being produced by joint tissue. In these cases, synovial fluid RF may be positive while the serum RF is negative.[20]

SEROUS FLUIDS

The lungs, heart, and abdominal cavities are surrounded by two serous membranes: the parietal membrane lining the cavity wall and the visceral membrane lining the organs (Fig. 29-13). Serous fluids, an ultrafiltrate of plasma, are located between the membranes. When *serum* dialyzes across these membranes, the fluid formed is called serous fluid—specifically, pleural (lung), pericardial (heart), and peritoneal (abdominal) fluid.

The formation of serous fluid is a continuous process driven by the hydrostatic pressure of the systemic circulation and maintenance of oncotic pressure due to protein. The potential space is usually filled; that is, no gases are present. The fluid reduces or eliminates friction caused by expansion and contraction of the encased organs. A disturbance of the dynamic equilibrium that causes an increase in fluid is an abnormal state.

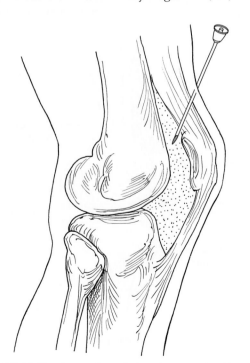

FIGURE 29-12 Placement of needle in arthrocentesis of knee joint.

CASE STUDY 29-3

A 57-year-old female has had joint pain for 4 years. Her joints are becoming progressively deformed with swelling. Her doctor orders a synovial fluid analysis cell count, differential, synovial fluid RF serology, protein, glucose, LD, serum glucose level, serum RF, and fluid crystal analysis. Her results are as follows:

Fluid appearance: Yellow/cloudy

WBC count, differential: >25,000 WBCs/µL, >50% segmented neutrophils (PMNs) with ragocytes seen

SYNOVIAL FLUID CHEMISTRIES	SERUM CHEMISTRIES
Protein: 3.7 g/dL	
Glucose: 81 mg/dL	Glucose: 100 mg/dL (ratio 0.81 fluid:1.0 serum)
LD: 100 mg/dL	
RF: positive	RF: positive
Crystals: None seen	

Questions

1. What do these results suggest that the patient has? Give evidence to support your answer.

2. If the patient had gout, what would her results typically show?

While body fluids vary in composition, they share some common characteristics. The critical roles of water and electrolytes are important determinants of any fluid composition and movement in the body. Water and electrolytes play crucial roles in many metabolic processes. Water enters the system through consumption of either water or food and also through cellular metabolic processes. For example, the water of oxidation can yield about 300 mL of water per day. Fluids of the body can be intracellular or extracellular, with about 55% of the water being intracellular and about 45% being extracellular.[21]

Extracellular fluid can be further divided into interstitial fluid, transcellular fluids in various body cavities, and plasma. Various forces control the movement of fluids within the body. Electrolyte and enzyme composition of intracellular fluid differs from extracellular fluids and knowledge of these differences can aid in understanding disease processes. For example, potassium levels are higher inside the cell than outside and sodium concentrations vary between the intracellular fluid and the extracellular fluid. Examining these biochemical differences, along with the examination of cellular elements, can assist in diagnosing and monitoring the patient's condition.[22]

Several forces, within and outside of the capillaries, work together to maintain fluid equilibrium. The tissue's colloidal osmotic pressure (interstitial fluid pressure), along with the capillary's hydrostatic pressure (filtration pressure), regulates the outward flow of fluid from the capillary. The colloidal osmotic pressure of the capillary and the tissue's hydrostatic pressure regulate the inward flow of fluid into the capillary from the tissue.[23]

Figure 29-14 illustrates the direction of these forces. The lymphatic system removes the fluids entering into the interstitial space. Figure 29-15 shows the normal flow of fluids among the bloodstream, tissues, and lymphatic vessels. An imbalance in pressures causes excessive egress of fluid into tissue spaces and can lead to accumulation of fluid in the body cavity. This accumulation of fluid is called an effusion. Effusions are further classified as transudate or exudate. Proper classification of effusions is critical to patient care.

A transudate may occur during various systemic disorders that disrupt fluid filtration, fluid reabsorption, or both. Conditions such as congestive heart failure, hepatic cirrhosis, and nephrotic syndrome are examples of systemic disorders that may result in the formation of

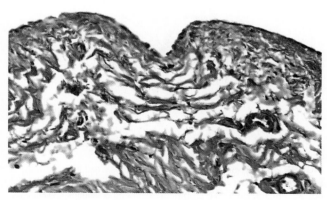

FIGURE 29-13 Mesothelial lining of serous body cavities.

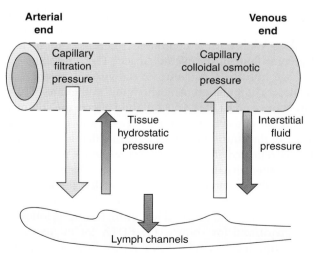

FIGURE 29-14 Forces governing the exchange of fluid at the capillary level.

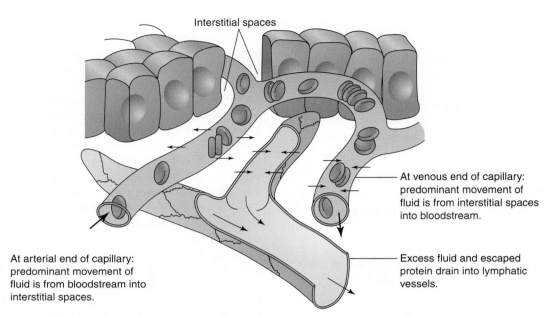

FIGURE 29-15 Exchanges through capillary membranes in the formation and removal of interstitial fluid.

transudates. Exudate effusions occur during inflammatory processes that result in damage to blood vessel walls, body cavity membrane damage, or decreased reabsorption by the lymphatic system. Infections, inflammations, hemorrhages, and malignancies are examples of pathologic processes that can cause the formation of exudates. The formation of transudates and exudates can damage tissues and body cavity membranes and alter lymphatic function.

Various laboratory tests are used to differentiate between transudates and exudates, including fluid appearance, specific gravity, amylase, glucose, LD, and proteins. Additional tests such as ammonia, lipids, and pH may be useful in confirming the cause of an effusion for specific body sites.

Pleural Fluid

The outer layer of the pleural sac, the parietal layer, is served by the systemic circulation and the inner layer, the visceral layer, by the bronchial circulation. Pleural fluid is essentially interstitial fluid of the systemic circulation. With normal conditions, there is 3 to 20 mL of pleural fluid in the pleural space. The fluid exits by drainage into the lymphatics of the visceral pleura and the visceral circulation. Any alteration in the rate of formation or removal of the pleural fluid affects the volume, causing an effusion. It is then necessary to classify the nature of the effusion by analysis of the pleural fluid. The fluid is removed from the pleural space by needle and syringe after visualization by radiology. This procedure is called thoracentesis; the fluid is called *thoracentesis fluid* or **pleural fluid** (Fig. 29-16). Specifically preserved aliquots of the fluid are used for future testing as follows: (1) heparinized for culture, (2) EDTA for microscopy, (3) sodium fluorescein (NaF) for glucose and lactate, and (4) nonanticoagulated for further biochemical testing.

Transudates are secondary to remote (nonpleural) pathology and indicate that treatment should begin elsewhere. An exudate indicates primary involvement of the pleura and lung, such as infection, and demands immediate attention. For example, any mechanical disturbance in the formation of fluid (e.g., hypoproteinemia causing decreased oncotic pressure) would increase the pleural fluid volume. This would be a transudative process. An exudative process involves damage to the membranes, allowing increased fluid entry such as would occur with infection or malignancy (Table 29-3). Further testing,

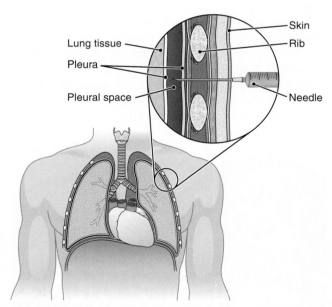

FIGURE 29-16 Thoracentesis. A needle is inserted into the pleural space to withdraw fluid. (From Cohen BJ. *Medical Terminology.* 4th ed. Philadelphia, PA: Lippincott Williams & Wilkins, 2004.)

TABLE 29-3	CAUSES OF PLEURAL EFFUSIONS
TRANSUDATIVE	**EXUDATIVE**
Congestive heart failure[a]	Bacterial pneumonia[a]
Nephrotic syndrome	Tuberculosis
Hypoproteinemia	Pulmonary abscess
Hepatic cirrhosis	Malignancy (lymphatic obstruction)
Chronic renal failure	Viral/fungal infection
	Pulmonary infarction
	Pleurisy
	Pulmonary malignancy
	Lymphoma
	Pleural mesothelioma

[a]Most common cause.

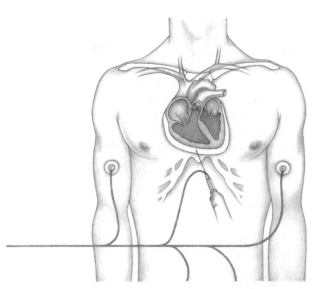

FIGURE 29-17 Aspirating pericardial fluid. In pericardiocentesis, a needle and a syringe are inserted through the chest wall into the pericardial sac (as shown below). Electrocardiographic monitoring, with a lead wire attached to the needle and electrodes placed on the limbs (right arm, left arm, and left leg), helps ensure proper needle placement and avoids damage to the heart. (From *Nursing Procedures.* 4th ed. Ambler, PA: Lippincott Williams & Wilkins; 2004.)

including chemical, microscopy, and culture, is then required to identify the etiology.

The assignment of fluid to either the transudate or exudate category had previously been based on the protein concentration of the fluid. This criterion has been replaced by the use of a series of fluid/plasma (F/P) ratios known as Light's criteria. Specifically, if the F/P ratio for total protein is greater than 0.5, if the ratio for LD is greater than 0.6, or if the pleural fluid LD/upper limit serum LD ratio reference interval is greater than 0.67, the fluid is an exudate. For pleural fluid, an additional characterization can be made by determining the pleural fluid cholesterol, the fluid-to-serum cholesterol ratio, and the fluid-to-serum bilirubin ratio. Exudates are indicated by fluid cholesterol greater than 60 mg/dL, fluid-to-serum cholesterol ratio greater than 0.3, and fluid-to-bilirubin ratio of 0.6 or higher.

Further characterization of the exudate by the chemistry laboratory may involve analysis for glucose, lactate, amylase, triglyceride, or pH. A decrease in glucose (increase in lactate) would suggest infection or inflammation. An increase in amylase compared with that of serum suggests pancreatitis. Grossly elevated triglyceride levels (2 to 10 × serum) could indicate thoracic duct leakage. The use of pH measurements, performed as one would perform a blood-gas level determination, has gained favor. Succinctly, pH less than 7.2 suggests infection, and pH close to 6.0 indicates esophageal rupture. The methodologies for these analyses are the same as those employed for the serum and blood constituents and, therefore, are feasible in the clinical laboratory.

Pericardial Fluid

The relationship of the pericardium, pericardial fluid, and the heart is similar to that with the lungs. Mechanisms of formation and drainage are the same. Pericardial effusions are an accumulation of fluid around the heart caused by damage to the mesothelium and are usually always exudates. Figure 29-17 illustrates the pericardium surrounding the heart. Normally, the pericardium contains less than 50 mL of fluid. The procedure for removing excess pericardial fluid, pericardiocentesis, is dangerous and therefore rarely performed (Fig. 29-17). However, this procedure is necessary to obtain a sample if cultures are needed to investigate an infection or if cytology is needed for suspected malignancy.[24]

Adenosine deaminase testing may be requested in suspected cases of tubercular effusions.

Peritoneal Fluid

Excess fluid (>50 mL) in the peritoneal cavity indicates disease. The presence of excess **peritoneal fluid** is called **ascites**, and the fluid is called *ascitic fluid*. The process of obtaining samples of this fluid by needle aspiration is *paracentesis* (Fig. 29-18). Usually, the fluid is visualized by ultrasound to confirm its presence and volume before paracentesis is attempted.

The same mechanisms that cause serous effusions in other body cavities are operative for the peritoneal cavity. Specifically, a disturbance in the rate of dialysis secondary to a primary, remote pathology is a transudate, compared with a primary pathology of the peritoneal membrane (an exudate). The multiple factors that apply to this large space, including renal function, tend

CASE STUDY 29-4

A 65-year-old female patient was admitted with a progressive increase in breathlessness, orthopnea, jugular venous distention, chest pain, ankle edema, sacral edema, swollen legs, arms, and hands over the previous 4 weeks. She suffered from dyspepsia, increasing over recent weeks, and the general practitioner had noted new heart murmurs. A pansystolic murmur was audible and inspiratory crackles were heard throughout both lung fields. Muffled heart sounds were heard, possibly due to the muffling effect of fluid surrounding the heart. She could not walk a block to the grocery store without being totally exhausted and short of breath. She was afebrile with rapid breathing, with a low volume pulse. Her sitting blood pressure was 100/60 mm Hg.

The ECG indicated sinus tachycardia with anterolateral Q waves indicating a previous infarction. Chest X-ray indicated cardiomegaly, interstitial edema, and fluid in the lower lungs. Routine chemistry showed serum Na^+ 129 mmol/L, K^+ 5.9 mmol/L, creatinine 157 mmol/L, and urea 9.1 mmol/L. Brain natriuretic peptide was elevated and troponin level was unremarkable.

The physician suspected progressive systolic dysfunction after myocardial infarction. An abnormality of the ECG in a breathless patient is a supportive evidence for a cardiac cause of dyspnea, while a normal ECG usually suggests another diagnosis.[25] Also radiological cardiomegaly most often represents significant ventricular dilatation or hypertrophy. A complication is the presence of increased pericardial fluid. Echocardiography provides definitive diagnosis. Echocardiography showed a dilated heart (left ventricular end diastolic distension [LVEDD]) with apical dilatation, compatible with previous anterior infarction, and with increased pericardial fluid.

Questions

1. Is this pericardial fluid most likely an exudate or a transudate? Under what conditions will the physician want to perform a pericardiocentesis to collect the fluid?

2. What condition does the patient most likely have?

to cloud the distinction. The most common cause of ascites with a normal peritoneum is portal hypertension. Obstructions to hepatic flow, such as cirrhosis, congestive heart failure, and hypoalbuminemia for any reason, demonstrate the highest incidence.

The exudative causes of ascites are predominantly metastatic ovarian, prostate, and colon cancer and infective peritonitis. The recommended method for determining transudates and exudates is the serum-ascites albumin gradient (SAAG). The SAAG is calculated by subtracting the fluid albumin level from the serum albumin level. A gradient of 1.1 g/dL or more used to indicate portal hypertension is the most accepted measurement. A neutrophil count greater than 250 cells/μm indicates peritonitis. Measurement of the tumor markers CEA and CA125 is indicated in suspected cases of malignancy.

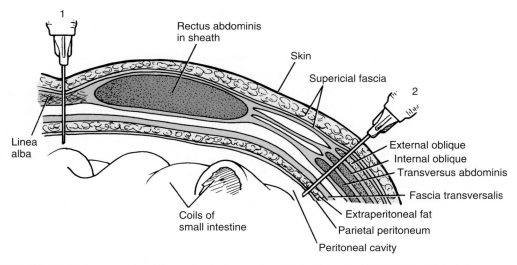

FIGURE 29-18 Paracentesis of the abdominal cavity in midline. (From Snell, MD, PhD, *Clinical Anatomy.* 7th ed. Philadelphia, PA: Lippincott Williams & Wilkins; 2003.)

CASE STUDY 29-5

A 47-year-old man was brought to the hospital by the police after falling to the pavement and being unable to rise. His admission laboratory values revealed the following:

LABORATORY VALUES

Sodium 133 mmol/L (135–146 mmol/L)	A nonreactive acute hepatitis panel
Potassium 3.1 mmol/L (3.6–5.2 mmol/L)	Ammonia level 71 μmol/L (9–35 μmol/L).
Chloride 93 mmol/L (96–110 mmol/L)	White blood cell count was $6.9 \times 10^3/\mu L$ ($4.5–11 \times 10^3/\mu L$)
Creatinine 0.7 mg/dL (0.8–1.5 mg/dL),	Platelet count $101 \times 10^3/\mu L$ ($130–400 \times 10^3/\mu L$)
Blood urea nitrogen < 5 mg/dL (7–25 mg/dL)	Hemoglobin and hematocrit 13.4 g/dL (13.5–17.5 g/dL) and 38.7% (40–51%),
Glucose 128 mg/dL (65–99 mg/dL)	Prothrombin time of 14.3 s (9.5–12.5 s), with an INR of 1.3 (0.9–1.1)
Total protein 6.9 g/dL (6–8 g/dL)	Normal partial thromboplastin time of 31.6 s
Albumin 2.4 g/dL (3.4–5.4 g/dL)	Alkaline phosphatase 241 U/L (20–120 U/L)
Total bilirubin of 8.0 mg/dL (<1.3 mg/dL)	AST 103 U/L (<45 U/L)
Acetaminophen level < 10 μg/mL (10–20 μg/mL)	ALT 40 U/L (<46 U/L)

An abdominal ultrasound was significant for the presence of ascites and a cirrhotic-appearing liver. The patient was admitted to the hospital for further evaluation and subsequent treatment of alcohol withdrawal and decompensated cirrhosis. He was put on a salt and protein-restricted diet and diuretics to manage ascites (accumulated fluid in the peritoneal cavity). He was treated with benzodiazepines and lactulose and placed on a diuretic regimen of furosemide 40 mg orally daily along with spironolactone 100 mg orally daily.

Ascitic fluid should be sampled in all inpatients and outpatients with new onset ascites. If uncomplicated cirrhotic ascites is suspected, the initial specimen of ascitic fluid should be sent for cell count and differential, albumin, and total protein concentration. With the results of the above tests, the SAAG can be calculated.

PERITONEAL FLUID

White blood cell count of 8/μL with 26% segmented neutrophils	Total protein less than 3.0 g/dL
Albumin of less than 1.0 g/dL	Fluid culture = no growth

Alcoholic hepatitis is a syndrome of progressive inflammatory liver injury associated with long-term heavy intake of ethanol. Patients who are severely affected present with subacute onset of fever, hepatomegaly, leukocytosis, marked impairment of liver function (e.g., jaundice and coagulopathy), and manifestations of portal hypertension (e.g., ascites, hepatic encephalopathy, and variceal hemorrhage). However, milder forms of alcoholic hepatitis often may not cause any symptoms.

Questions

1. What lab tests are abnormal?

2. What will the SAAG value be, and how is it calculated?

3. How will diuretics reduce this excess fluid?

4. Why is her diet salt restricted?

For additional student resources please visit thePoint at **http://thepoint.lww.com.**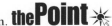

QUESTIONS

1. Laboratory testing for the assessment of fetal lung maturity includes all of the following tests **except**
   a. Acetylcholinesterase
   b. L/S ratio
   c. Fluorescence polarization
   d. Foam stability
   e. Lamellar body count

2. Amniotic fluid
   a. Provides a cushion for the fetus and is a mixture of maternal and fetal fluids
   b. Provides a cushion for the fetus
   c. Is a mixture of maternal and fetal fluids
   d. Is assessed by umbilical catheterization
   e. Provides a cushion for the fetus, is a mixture of maternal and fetal fluids, and is assessed by umbilical catheterization

3. Lamellar body counts reflect
   a. Surfactant phospholipid packets
   b. Platelet count of the fetus
   c. Platelet count of the mother
   d. Meconium count of the fetus
   e. All of these

4. A xanthochromic CSF indicates
   a. Cerebral hemorrhage
   b. Traumatic tap
   c. Bacterial meningitis
   d. Viral meningitis
   e. Multiple sclerosis

5. CSF glucose is measured to assess
   a. Infection
   b. Transport efficiency
   c. Diabetes
   d. Traumatic tap
   e. Hemochromatosis

6. An IgG index of 0.8 is indicative of
   a. Multiple sclerosis
   b. CSF leakage
   c. Fungal infection
   d. Malignancy
   e. Normal CSF

7. CF is characterized by
   a. Elevated sweat chloride levels
   b. Homozygous expression of an autosomal recessive trait
   c. Pancreatic insufficiency

   d. All of these
   e. None of these

8. Synovial fluid
   a. Is formed by plasma ultrafiltration and is rich in hyaluronic acid
   b. Is formed by plasma ultrafiltration
   c. Lubricates the pneumocytes
   d. Is rich in hyaluronic acid
   e. All of these

9. Serous fluids
   a. Are derived from serum
   b. Provide lubrication and protection
   c. Fill the potential space
   d. Are derived from serum and provide lubrication and protection only
   e. All of these

10. Pleural fluid exudates
    a. Are characterized by a total protein F/P ratio of 0.7
    b. Reflect primary involvement of the pleura
    c. Are characterized by an increased LD F/P ratio
    d. Are characterized by an increased cholesterol F/P ratio
    e. All of these

11. Analysis of paracentesis fluid is performed to
    a. Determine the cause of fluid presence and assess infection risk
    b. Determine the cause of fluid presence
    c. Assess infection risk
    d. Determine lung involvement
    e. All of these

12. The most common cause of ascites is
    a. Portal hypertension
    b. Venous return
    c. Parietal cell differentiation
    d. Eccrine infection
    e. Malignancy

13. When assessing the lipid profile to determine fetal lung maturity, it is critical to
    a. Centrifuge the amniotic fluid at low speeds to properly avoid fractionation of the lipids.
    b. Centrifuge the amniotic fluid at high speeds to properly fractionate the lipids.
    c. Avoid centrifugation of amniotic fluid for this test.

d. Centrifuge the amniotic fluid using a measure of revolutions per minute, not relative force.

14. Pulmonary maturity for the fetus is characterized by
    a. Increases in PG and lecithin, while sphingomyelin is constant.
    b. Decreases in PG and lecithin, while sphingomyelin is constant.
    c. Increases in PG and lecithin, while sphingomyelin decreases.
    d. Decreases in PG and lecithin, while sphingomyelin increases.

REFERENCES

1. Liley AW. Liquor amnil analysis in the management of the pregnancy complicated by rhesus sensitization. *Am J Obstet Gynecol.* 1961;82:1359.
2. Kulovich MV, Hallman MB, Gluck L. The lung profile. I. Normal pregnancy. *Am J Obstet Gynecol.* 1979;135:57.
3. Statland BE, Freer DE. Evaluation of two assays of functional surfactant in amniotic fluid: surface-tension lowering ability and the foam stability index test. *Clin Chem.* 1979;25:1770.
4. Clements JA, Plataker ACG, Tierney DF, et al. Assessment of the risk of the respiratory distress syndrome by a rapid test for surfactant in amniotic fluid. *N Engl J Med.* 1972;286:1077.
5. Gluck L, Kulovich MV, Borer RC Jr, et al. Diagnosis of the respiratory distress syndrome by amniocentesis. *Am J Obstet Gynecol.* 1971;109:440.
6. Tsai MY, Marshall JG. Phosphatidylglycerol in 261 samples of amniotic fluid from normal and diabetic pregnancies, as measured by one-dimensional thin layer chromatography. *Clin Chem.* 1979;25:682.
7. Kaplan LA, Chapman JT, Bock JL, et al. Prediction of respiratory distress syndrome using the Abbot FLM II amniotic fluid assay. *Clin Chim Acta.* 2002;326:61-68.
8. Winn-McMillan T, Karon B. Comparison of the TDx-FLM II and lecithin to sphingomyelin ratio assays in predicting fetal lung maturity. *Am J Obstet Gynecol.* 2005;193:778-762.
9. TDxFLx fetal Lung Maturity II (FLM II) package insert, reference 7A76. Abbott Park, IL: Abbott Laboratories, Diagnostic Division; 2003.
10. Khazardoost H, Yakazadeh S, Borna F, et al. Amniotic fluid lamellar body count and its sensitivity and specificity evaluating fetal lung maturity. *J Obstet Gynecol.* 2005;25:257-259.
11. Szallasi A, Gronowski AM, Eby CS. Lamellar body count in amniotic fluid: a comparison of four different hematology analyzers. *Clin Chem.* 2003;49:994-997.
12. Neerhof ME, Dohnal JC, Ashwood ER, et al. Lamellar body counts: a consensus on protocol. *Obstet Gynecol.* 2001;97:318-320.
13. Brunzel NA. *Fundamentals of Urine and Body Fluid Analysis.* 2nd ed. Philadelphia, PA: Saunders; 2004:327-328.
14. McBride LJ. *Textbook of Urinalysis and Body Fluids: A Clinical Approach.* New York, NY: Lippincott; 1998:200-201.
15. Bailey EM, Domenico P, Cunha BA. Bacterial or viral meningitis. *Postgrad Med.* 1990;88:217.
16. Okta M, Okta K, et al. Clinical and analytical evaluation of an enzyme immunoassay for myelin basic protein in cerebrospinal fluid. *Clin Chem.* 2000;46:1336-1330.
17. Gibson LE, Cooke RE. A test for concentration of electrolytes in cystic fibrosis of the pancreas utilizing pilocarpine by iontophoresis. *Pediatrics.* 1959;23:545.
18. Clinical Laboratory Standards Institute. *Sweat Testing: Sample Collection and Quantitative Analysis Approved Guidelines.* Villanova, PA: Clinical Laboratory Standards Institute, reaffirmed 2005. (CLSI document C34-A2.)
19. McBride LJ. *Textbook of Urinalysis and Body Fluids: A Clinical Approach.* Philadelphia, PA: Lippincott; 1998:234-235.
20. Ross DL, Neeley AE. *Textbook of Urinalysis and Body Fluids.* New York, NY: Appleton-Century-Crofts; 1983:255-256.
21. Calbreath DF. *Clinical Chemistry: A Fundamental Textbook.* Philadelphia, PA: Saunders; 1992:370.
22. Calbreath DF. *Clinical Chemistry: A Fundamental Textbook.* Philadelphia, PA: Saunders; 1992:371.
23. Ross DL, Neeley AE. *Textbook of Urinalysis and Body Fluids.* New York, NY: Appleton-Century-Crofts; 1983: 275.
24. Ross DL, Neeley AE. *Textbook of Urinalysis and Body Fluids.* New York, NY: Appleton-Century-Crofts; 1983: 280.
25. Davie AP, Francis CM, Love MP, et al. Value of the electrocardiogram in identifying heart failure due to left ventricular systolic dysfunction. *Br Med J.* 1996;312:222-224.

Specialty Areas of Clinical Chemistry

Therapeutic Drug Monitoring

DEBORAH E. KEIL, NADIA AYALA

CHAPTER 30

CHAPTER OUTLINE

- ◆ ROUTES OF ADMINISTRATION
- ◆ ABSORPTION
- ◆ DRUG DISTRIBUTION
- ◆ FREE VERSUS BOUND DRUGS
- ◆ METABOLISM
- ◆ DRUG ELIMINATION
- ◆ PHARMACOKINETICS
- ◆ SAMPLE COLLECTION
- ◆ PHARMACOGENOMICS
- ◆ CARDIOACTIVE DRUGS
  - Digoxin
  - Quinidine
  - Procainamide
  - Disopyramide
- ◆ ANTIBIOTICS
  - Aminoglycosides
  - Vancomycin
- ◆ ANTIEPILEPTIC DRUGS
  - First-Generation AEDs
- ◆ PSYCHOACTIVE DRUGS
  - Lithium
  - Tricyclic Antidepressants
  - Clozapine
  - Olanzapine
- ◆ IMMUNOSUPPRESSIVE DRUGS
  - Cyclosporine
  - Tacrolimus
  - Sirolimus
  - Mycophenolic Acid
- ◆ ANTINEOPLASTICS
  - Methotrexate
- ◆ QUESTIONS
- ◆ SUGGESTED READINGS
- ◆ REFERENCES

Chapter Objectives

Upon completion of this chapter, the clinical laboratorian should be able to do the following:

- Discuss the characteristics of a drug that make therapeutic drug monitoring essential.
- Identify the factors that influence the absorption of an orally administered drug.
- Relate the factors that influence the rate of drug elimination.
- Define drug distribution and the factors that influence it.
- Calculate volume of distribution, elimination constant, and drug half-life.
- Relate the concentration of a circulating drug to pharmacokinetic parameters.
- Name the therapeutic category of each drug presented in this chapter.
- Describe the major toxicities of the drugs presented in this chapter.
- Identify the features of each drug presented in this chapter that may influence its serum drug concentration.

KEY TERMS

Absorption
Bioavailability
Distribution
Elimination
Peak drug level

Pharmacogenomics
Pharmacokinetics
Standard dosage
Therapeutic drug monitoring
Therapeutic range
Trough drug levels

Therapeutic drug monitoring (TDM) involves the coordinated effort of several health professionals to measure and monitor circulating drug levels primarily in serum, plasma, or whole blood. After the physician has ordered TDM, laboratory personnel involved in the timing of blood collection, the measurement of drug levels, and reporting of these data play a critical role in achieving safe and effective patient drug therapy. The purpose of TDM is to (1) ensure that a given drug dosage is within a range that produces maximal therapeutic benefit and (2) identify when the drug is above or below a therapeutic range which may lead to either inefficacy or toxicity. For most drug therapies, dosage regimens that are safe and effective in most of the population have been established and therefore TDM is unneeded. With certain drugs, however, there is a narrow window between therapeutic effects or toxic outcomes. Therefore, careful patient monitoring with appropriate dosage adjustments is necessary.

The standard dosage is statistically derived from observations in a healthy population. Disease states may produce altered physiologic conditions in which the standard dose does not produce the predicted concentration in circulation. Patient age, gender, genetics, recent food consumption, prescription drugs, self-administered over-the-counter drugs, and even naturopathic agents may also influence drug levels and efficacy. In these cases, establishing a rational dosage regimen to fit individual situations is achieved with TDM.

The following are common indications for TDM:

* Identifying non-compliance in patients.
* Preventing the consequences of overdosing and underdosing.
* Maximizing therapeutic effect, particularly when there is a narrow dose range between a therapeutic and toxicity.
* Optimizing a dosing regimen based on drug–drug interactions or a change in the patient's physiologic state that may unpredictably affect circulating drug concentrations.

The basis of TDM includes consideration of the route of administration, rate of absorption, distribution of drug within the body, and rate of elimination (Fig. 30-1). There are many factors that influence each of these steps. Consequently, this path from drug administration to efficacy is by no means straightforward. This chapter introduces these concepts and how they influence circulating concentrations of a drug. The remainder of the chapter surveys selected drugs commonly subject to TDM.

ROUTES OF ADMINISTRATION

To achieve a therapeutic benefit, a drug must meet an appropriate concentration at its site of action. For instance, a cardioactive drug might need to reach myocytes at a

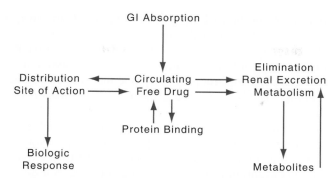

FIGURE 30-1 Overview of factors that influence the circulating concentration of an orally administered drug. GI, gastrointestinal.

dosage level that is effectively maintained in a therapeutic range for days to weeks. Intravenous (IV) administration into the circulatory system offers the most direct route with effective delivery to their sites of action. The unchanged fraction of the administered dose as it enters systemic circulation and eventually reaches its site of action defines its bioavailability. In addition to IV, drugs can be administered by several other routes. Each presents with different characteristics that influence circulating concentrations. Drugs can be injected directly into muscles (intramuscular [IM]) or just under the skin (subcutaneous [SC]). They can also be inhaled or absorbed through the skin (transcutaneous). Rectal delivery (suppository) is commonly used in infants and in situations in which oral delivery is unavailable. Oral administration is the most common route of delivery. The current discussion focuses on oral and IV administration.

ABSORPTION

For orally administered drugs, the efficiency of absorption from the gastrointestinal tract to its bioavailability in the bloodstream is dependent on many factors including (1) dissociation from its administered form, (2) solubility in gastrointestinal fluids, and (3) diffusion across gastrointestinal membranes. Tablets and capsules require dissolution before being absorbed. Liquid solutions have a tendency to be more rapidly absorbed. Some drugs are subject to uptake by active transport mechanisms intended for dietary constituents; however, most are absorbed by passive diffusion from the gastrointestinal tract to the bloodstream. This process requires that the drug be in a hydrophobic (nonionized) state. Because of gastric acidity, weak acids are efficiently absorbed in the stomach. Weak bases are preferentially absorbed in the intestine, where the pH is more basic. For most drugs, absorption from the gastrointestinal tract occurs in a predictable manner in healthy people. However, changes in intestinal motility, pH, inflammation, as well as the presence of food or other drugs may dramatically alter absorption rates. For instance, if the integrity of the gastrointestinal tract is compromised in a patient with inflammatory bowel syndrome, then the absorption of a drug may be altered. Gut absorption is also affected by coadministered drugs such as antacids, kaolin, sucralfate, cholestyramine, and anti-ulcer medications. Morphine may also slow gut motility, thereby influencing the rate of absorption of drugs.

Additionally, many of the absorptive characteristics of a drug may change with age, pregnancy, or pathologic conditions. In these instances, predicting the final circulating concentration in blood from a standard oral dose can be difficult. With the use of TDM, however, effective oral dosage regimens can be determined.

DRUG DISTRIBUTION

The free fraction of circulating drugs is subject to diffusion out of the vasculature into interstitial and intracellular spaces. The ability to leave circulation is largely dependent on the lipid solubility of the drug. Drugs that are highly hydrophobic can easily traverse cellular membranes and partition into lipid compartments, such as adipose and nerve cells. Drugs that are polar but not ionized also cross cell membranes but do not sequester into lipid compartments. Ionized species diffuse out of the vasculature but at a slow rate. The volume of distribution (V_d) index is used to describe the distribution characteristics of a drug. It is expressed mathematically as follows:

$$V_d = D/C \qquad \text{(Eq. 30-1)}$$

where V_d is volume of distribution (in liters), D is an IV injected dose (milligrams [mg] or grams [g]), and C is concentration in plasma (mg/L or g/L).

Drugs that are hydrophobic can have a large V_d due to partitioning into hydrophilic compartments. Substances that are ionized or are primarily bound in plasma have small V_d values due to sequestration in the vasculature.

FREE VERSUS BOUND DRUGS

Most drugs in circulation are subject to binding with serum constituents. Although many potential species may be formed, most are drug–protein complexes. An important aspect regarding drug dynamics is that typically the free fraction can interact with its site of action and result in a biologic response. This free drug fraction is also termed active. At a standard dose, total plasma content may be within the therapeutic range, but the patient experiences toxic adverse effects (high free fraction) or does not realize a therapeutic benefit (low free fraction). This may occur secondary to changes in serum protein content. Changes in serum-binding proteins may occur during inflammation, malignancies, pregnancy, hepatic disease, nephrotic syndrome, malnutrition, and acid–base disturbances. Albumin represents the majority of the protein constituents in serum and changes in its levels may affect the free versus bound status of many drugs. Additionally, increases in serum alpha-1-acid glycoprotein during acute phase reactions will lead to increased binding of drugs such as propranolol, quinidine, chlorpromazine, cocaine, and benzodiazepines. The serum fraction of free drug may also be influenced by the concentration of substances that compete for binding sites, which may be other drugs or endogenous substances, such as urea, bilirubin, or hormones. Free drug measurements should be considered for drugs that are highly protein bound and for which clinical signs are inconsistent with total drug concentrations.

METABOLISM

All substances absorbed from the intestine (except the rectum) enter the hepatic portal system. In this system, circulating blood from the gastrointestinal tract is routed through the liver before it enters into general circulation. Certain drugs are subject to significant hepatic uptake and metabolism during passage through the liver. This process is known as first-pass metabolism. Liver metabolism may not be the same process in every patient as this may be influenced by an individual's genetics. These variations are examined in the discipline of pharmacogenomics. In addition to genetic variation, a patient with a fatty or cirrhotic liver may have reduced capacity to metabolize drugs. This may be a particularly important consideration if the efficacy of a drug depends on a metabolic process generating a therapeutically active metabolite. This enzymatic process in the liver is referred to as biotransformation. Second, this patient may require reduced dosages of the drug as the rate of metabolism and the subsequent elimination process may be slowed.

Most drugs are xenobiotics. Xenobiotics are exogenous substances, yet they are capable of entering biochemical pathways intended for endogenous substances. There are many potential biochemical pathways in which drugs can be acted on or biotransformed. The biochemical pathway responsible for a large portion of drug metabolism is the hepatic mixed-function oxidase (MFO) system. The basic function of this system involves taking hydrophobic substances and, through a series of enzymatic reactions, converting them into water-soluble substances. These products are then either transported into the bile or released into the general circulation for elimination by renal filtration.

There are many enzymes involved in the MFO system. They are commonly divided into two functional groups or phases. Phase I reactions produce reactive intermediates. Phase II reactions conjugate functional groups to these reactive sites, the products of which are water soluble. The reactive intermediates can be conjugated with various functional groups; glutathione, glycine, phosphate, and sulfate are common. The MFO system is a nonspecific system that allows many different endogenous and exogenous substances to go through this series of reactions. Although there are many potential substrates for this pathway, the products formed from an individual substance are specific. For example, acetaminophen is a substrate for MFO ultimately leading to the formation of a glutathione conjugate following phase II reactions. In the presence of too much acetaminophen as in the case of an overdose, the MFO system may be overwhelmed and ineffective in metabolizing this drug to a safe, water-soluble end product for elimination by the kidneys. In this case, if the conjugating group for a given drug becomes depleted in phase II reactions, an accumulation of phase I products occurs. Excessive phase I products may result in toxic effects, and in the case of acetaminophen, irreversible damage to hepatocytes may occur.

It is also noteworthy that the MFO system is inducible. This is seen as an increase in the synthesis and activity of the rate-limiting enzymes within this pathway. The most common inducers are xenobiotics that are substrates for this pathway. Thus, certain drugs may stimulate their own rate of elimination. Due to biologic variability in the degree of induction, TDM could again assist in establishing an appropriate dosage regimen.

Because many potential substrates can enter the MFO system, many drug–drug interactions occur within this pathway. Competitive and noncompetitive interactions may occur. This results in altered rates of elimination of the involved drugs. Interactions are not limited to drug–drug, but may also include drug–food (i.e., grapefruit) or drug–beverage (i.e., alcohol and caffeine). For example, metabolism of acetaminophen by the hepatic MFO system is altered, rendering it more toxic in the presence of alcohol consumption. In most instances, the degree of alteration is unpredictable. Again, the value of TDM is apparent.

Implied in this discussion are that changes in hepatic status can result in changes in the concentration of circulating drugs eliminated by this pathway. Induction of the MFO system typically results in accelerated clearance and a corresponding shorter half-life. In the opposite manner, hepatic disease states characterized by a loss of functional tissue may result in slower rates of clearance and corresponding longer half-lives. For example, cirrhosis results in irreversible damage and fibrosis of the liver, rendering hepatocytes non-functional. Consequently, xenobiotics may not be effectively metabolized by the hepatic MFO system, thereby reducing the rate of metabolism and elimination while increasing the opportunity for toxicity. In these situations, TDM aids in dosage adjustment.

For some drugs, there is considerable variance in the rate of hepatic and nonhepatic drug metabolism within a normal population. This results in a highly variable rate of clearance, even in the absence of disease. Establishing dosage regimens for these drugs is, in many instances, aided by the use of TDM. With the use of molecular genetics, it is now possible to identify common genetic variants of some drug-metabolizing pathways. Identification of these individuals may assist in establishing an individualized dosage regimen.

DRUG ELIMINATION

Drugs can be cleared from the body by various mechanisms. The plasma free fraction of a parent drug or its metabolites is subject to glomerular filtration, renal secretion, or both. For those drugs not secreted or subject to reabsorption, the elimination rate of free drug directly relates to the glomerular filtration rate. Decreases in glomerular filtration rate directly result in increased serum half-life and concentration. The aminoglycoside antibiotics and cyclosporine are examples of drugs with this behavior.

Independent of the clearance mechanism, decreases in the serum concentration of drugs most often occur as a first-order process (exponential rate of loss). This implies that the rate of change of drug concentration over time varies continuously in relation to the concentration of the drug. First-order elimination follows the following general equation:

$$\Delta C/\Delta T = -kC \qquad \text{(Eq. 30-2)}$$

This equation defines how the change in concentration per unit time ($\Delta C/\Delta T$) is directly related to the concentration of drug (C) and the constant (k). The k value is a simple proportionality factor that describes the percentage change (negative because it is decreasing) per unit time; it is commonly referred to as the elimination constant or the rate of elimination. The graphic solution to this equation is an exponential function that declines in the predicted curvilinear manner, asymptotically approaching zero (Fig. 30-2). The graph shown in Figure 30-2 illustrates a large change at high drug concentrations and a smaller change at low drug concentrations. However, the rate (percent lost) remains the same. Plotting it in semilogarithmic dimensions (Fig. 30-3) can linearize this function.

Hepatic metabolism or renal filtration, or a combination of the two, eliminates most drugs. For certain drugs, elimination by these routes is highly variable. In addition, functional changes in these organs may result in changes in the rate of elimination. In these situations, information regarding elimination rate and estimating the circulating concentration of a drug after a given time period are important factors in establishing

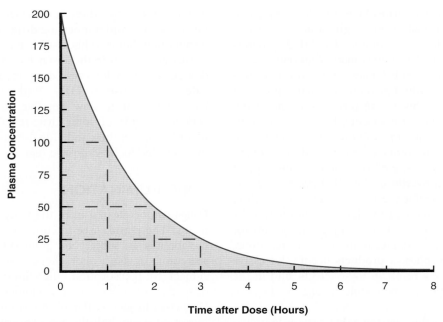

FIGURE 30-2 First-order drug elimination. This graph demonstrates exponential rate of loss on a linear scale. *Hash-marked lines* are representative of half-life.

an effective and safe dosage regimen. Equation 30-2 and Figures 30-2 and 30-3 are useful in determining the rate of elimination and the concentration of a drug after the time period. The following equation illustrates how the equation is used. Integration of Equation 30-2 yields the following:

$$C_T = C_0 e^{-kT} \qquad \text{(Eq. 30-3)}$$

where C_0 is the initial concentration of drug, C_T is the concentration of drug after the time period (T), k is the elimination constant, and T is the time period evaluated.

This is the most useful form of the elimination equation; from it, we can calculate the elimination constant or, if k is known, we can determine the amount of drug that will be present after a certain time period.

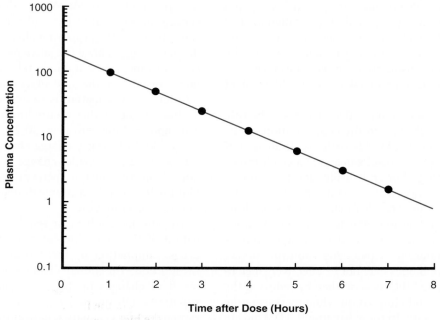

FIGURE 30-3 Semilogarithmic plot of exponential rate of drug elimination. The slope of this plot is equal to the rate of elimination (k).

Example:

The concentration of gentamicin is 10 μg/mL at 12:00. At 16:00, the gentamicin concentration is 6 μg/mL. What is the elimination constant (k) for gentamicin in this patient? Using Equation 30-3

$$C_T = C_0 e^{-kT}$$

$$C_0 = 10, \; C_T = 6, \; T = 4 \text{ hours}$$

Substituting these values into the equation produces

$$6 = 10_0 e^{-k \,(4 \text{ hours})}$$

Dividing both sides by 10 produces

$$0.6 = e^{-k \,(4 \text{ hours})}$$

To eliminate the exponential sign, we would take the natural logarithm of both sides:

$$\ln 0.6 = \ln(e^{-k \,(4 \text{ hours})})$$

Solving the natural log:

$$-0.51 = -k \,(4 \text{ hours})$$

Multiplying through by –1:

$$0.51 = k \,(4 \text{ hours})$$

Dividing both sides by 4 hours,

$$0.13/h = k$$

This calculated value for k indicates the patient is eliminating 13% of serum gentamicin per hour.

In this same patient on the same day, what would be the predicted serum concentration of gentamicin at midnight (24:00)?

For C_0, we can use either the 12:00 or 16:00 value as long as the correct corresponding time value is used. In this example, we will use the 16:00 value of 6 μg/mL.

$$C_0 = 6 \text{ μg/mL}, \; T = 8 \text{ hours}, \; k = 0.13/h$$

Substituting into Equation 30-3

$$C_T = 6e^{-0.13/h \,(8 \text{ hours})}$$

Solving for the exponent

$$C_T = 6e^{-1.04}$$

Note that the time unit (hours) has canceled. Solving for the exponent

$$C_T = 6 \,(0.35)$$
$$C_T = 2.1 \text{ μg/mL}$$

Note that the concentration units have carried through.

Although the elimination constant (k) is a useful value, it is not common nomenclature in the clinical setting. Instead, the term *half-life* is used. This represents the time needed for the serum concentration to decrease by one-half. It can be determined graphically (Fig. 30-2) or by conversion of the elimination constant (k) to half-

life (T) using the formula given in Equation 30-4. Of these two methods, the calculation provides an easy and accurate way to determine half-life. Thus, from the just-cited example, the half-life of gentamicin in this patient would be calculated as follows:

$$T_{1/2} = 0.693/k$$

$$T_{1/2} = (0.693)/(0.13/h) \qquad \text{(Eq. 30-4)}$$

$$T_{1/2} = 5.331 \text{ hours}$$

PHARMACOKINETICS

Pharmacokinetics is defined as the activity of a drug(s) in the body as influenced by absorption, distribution, metabolism, and excretion. This process assists in establishing or modifying a dosage regimen. It takes into consideration all factors that determine the concentration of a serum drug and its rate of change. Figure 30-3 is an idealized plot of elimination after an IV bolus. It assumes there is no distribution of this drug. A drug that does distribute outside of vascular space would produce an elimination graph such as in Figure 30-4. The rapid rate of change seen immediately after the initial IV bolus is a result of distribution and elimination. The rate of elimination (k) can be determined only after distribution is complete. Figure 30-5 is a plot of serum concentration as it would appear after oral administration of a drug. As absorbed drug enters the circulation, it is subject to simultaneous distribution and elimination. Serum concentrations rise when the rate of absorption exceeds distribution and elimination. The concentration declines as the rate of elimination and distribution exceeds absorption. The rate of elimination can only be determined after absorption and distribution are complete.

Most drugs are not administered as a single bolus but are delivered on a scheduled basis (e.g., once every 8 hours). With this type of administration, serum concentration of a drug oscillates between a maximum (peak drug level) and a minimum (trough drug level). The goal of a multiple-dosage regimen is to achieve a trough and peak in the therapeutic range and ensure that the peak is not in the toxic range. Evaluation of this oscillating function cannot be done immediately after initiation of a scheduled dosage regimen. Approximately 5 to 7 doses are required before a steady-state oscillation is acquired. The basis of this number (5 to 7 doses) is demonstrated in Figure 30-6.

After the first oral dose, absorption and distribution occur, followed only by elimination. Before the concentration of drug drops significantly, the second dose is given. The peak of the second dose is additive to what remained from the first dose. Because elimination is first order, the higher concentration results in a larger amount eliminated. The third through seventh scheduled doses

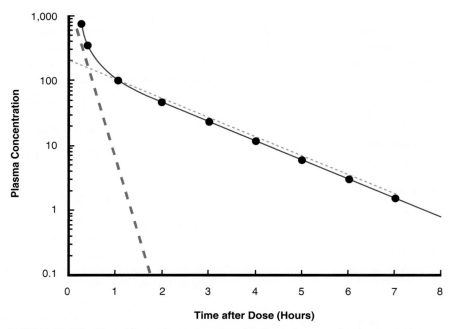

FIGURE 30-4 Semilogarithmic elimination plot of a drug subject to distribution. Initial rate of elimination is influenced by distribution *(dashed line)* and terminal elimination rate *(dotted line)*. After distribution is complete (1.5 h), elimination is first order.

all have the same effect, increasing serum concentration and the amount eliminated. By the end of the seventh dose, the amount of drug administered in a single dose is equal to the amount eliminated during the dosage period. At this point, steady state is established and peak and trough concentrations can be evaluated.

SAMPLE COLLECTION

Timing of specimen collection is the single most important factor in TDM. In general, trough concentrations for most drugs are drawn right before the next dose; peak concentrations are drawn 1 hour after an orally administered

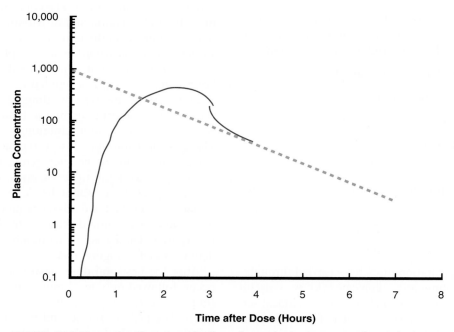

FIGURE 30-5 Plasma concentration of a drug after oral administration. After oral administration at time 0, serum concentration increases *(solid line)* after a brief lag period. Plasma concentrations peak when rate of elimination and distribution exceed rate of absorption. First-order elimination *(dotted line)* occurs when absorption and distribution are complete.

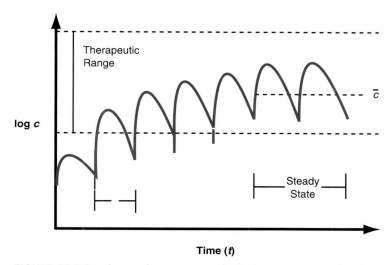

FIGURE 30-6 Steady-state kinetics in a multiple-dosage regimen. The character τ indicates the dosage interval. Equal doses at this interval reach steady state after six or seven dosage intervals. $\bar{c}$ mean drug concentration.

dose. This rule of thumb must always be used within the clinical context of the situation. A commonly used drug that is an exception to this rule is digoxin. In this situation, drugs that are absorbed slowly may require several hours before peak drug levels can be evaluated. In all situations, determination of serum concentrations should be done only after steady state has been achieved.

Serum or plasma is the specimen of choice for the determination of circulating concentrations of most drugs. Care must be taken that the appropriate container is used when collecting these specimens. Certain drugs have a tendency to be absorbed into the gel of certain serum separator collection tubes; it is necessary to follow vendor recommendations when this preanalytical effect is possible. Failure to do so may result in falsely low values. Heparinized plasma is suitable for most drug analysis. The calcium-binding anticoagulants add a variety of anions and cations that may interfere with analysis or cause a drug to distribute differently between cells and plasma. As a result, ethylenediaminetetracetic acid (EDTA), citrated and oxalated plasma are not usually acceptable specimens.

PHARMACOGENOMICS

The effectiveness of a drug over the population that uses it can be divided into categories of patients defined as responders and nonresponders. *Responders* are the patients benefiting from the therapeutic and desired effects of the drug, while *nonresponders* do not demonstrate a beneficial and desired therapeutic effect from the initiation of a given drug regimen. The therapeutic effectiveness of drugs in responders and nonresponders has recently been attributed to the interindividual variation in the genetic polymorphisms of the patients' drug metabolism pathways.

One of the most prominent gene families that affect drug metabolism is the cytochrome P450 (CYP450) family. It is a family of enzymes within the MFO system previously described. The variations in the enzymes (as a result of genetic polymorphism) are attributed to the differences in rates of drug metabolism over a population. The three most often linked to differences in degrees of drug metabolism are CYP2D6, CYP2C9, and CYP3A4. This information can then be used to personalize drug doses to the degree that is appropriate for the CYP450 profile of the patient. For example, if the patient's CYP450 profile indicates he or she has genes known to metabolize more slowly, they would be given lower doses of the drug to avoid toxic serum concentrations. In the opposite manner, if a patient's CYP450 profile indicates he or she has genes predisposing the patient to an increased rate of metabolism, he or she would need an increased dose to maintain therapeutic serum drug concentrations. Pharmacogenetic profiling can be used to predict drug–drug interactions or as an indicator if the drug will provide any therapeutic benefit at all.[1]

CARDIOACTIVE DRUGS

Many cardiac conditions are treated with drugs. Of these drugs, only a few require TDM. The cardiac glycosides and the antiarrhythmics are two classes of drugs for which assessment of serum concentration aids in decisions regarding their dosage regimen.

Digoxin

Digoxin is a cardiac glycoside used in the treatment of congestive heart failure. It functions by inhibiting membrane Na^+, K^+-ATPase. This causes a decrease in intracellular potassium, resulting in increased intracellular calcium in cardiac myocytes. The increased calcium improves cardiac contractility (inotropic effect). This effect is seen in the serum concentration range of 0.8 to 2 ng/mL (1.0 to 2.6 nmol/L).[2] Higher serum concentrations (3 ng/mL [3.8 nmol/L]) decrease the rate of ventricular depolarization. Although this level can be used to control ventricular tachycardia, it is infrequently used because of toxic adverse effects that become apparent at serum concentrations of greater than 2 ng/mL; these include nausea, vomiting, and visual disturbances. Cardiac effects, such as premature ventricular contractions (PVCs) and atrioventricular node blockage, are also common.

Absorption of orally administered digoxin is variable, and it is influenced by dietary factors, gastrointestinal motility, and formulation of the drug. In circulation, about 25% is protein bound. The nonbound (free) form of serum digoxin is sequestered into muscle cells. At equilibrium, the tissue concentration is 15 to 30 times greater than that of plasma. Elimination of digoxin occurs primarily by renal filtration of the plasma free form. The remainder is metabolized to several products by the liver. The half-life of plasma digoxin is 38 hours in an average adult. The major contributing factor to the extended half-life is the slow release of tissue digoxin back into circulation.

Because of variable gastrointestinal absorption of digoxin, establishing a dosage regimen usually requires assessment of serum concentrations after initial dosing to ensure that effective and nontoxic serum concentrations are achieved. In addition, changes in glomerular filtration rate can have a dramatic effect on serum concentration; frequent dosage adjustments, in conjunction with serum levels, need to be done in patients with renal disease. The therapeutic actions and toxicities of digoxin can be influenced by the concentration of serum electrolytes. Low serum potassium and magnesium potentiate digoxin actions.[2] In these conditions, adjustment of serum concentrations below the therapeutic range may be necessary to avoid toxicity. Thyroid status may also influence the actions of digoxin. Hyperthyroid patients display a resistance to digoxin actions; hypothyroid patients are more sensitive.[3]

The timing for evaluation of peak digoxin levels is crucial. In an average adult, serum levels peak between 2 and 3 hours after an oral dose. However, uptake into tissue is a relatively slow process. As a result, peak serum concentrations do not correlate with tissue concentrations. It has been established that the serum concentration 8 to 10 hours after an orally administered dose correlates with tissue concentration. Peak levels are usually evaluated at this time. Peak levels collected before this time are misleading and not valid.

Immunoassay is used to measure total digoxin concentration in serum.[2] With most commercial assays, cross-reactivity with hepatic metabolites is minimal;

however, newborns, pregnant women, and patients with uremia or late-stage liver disease produce an endogenous substance that cross-reacts with the antibodies used to measure serum digoxin. In patients with these digoxin-like immunoreactive substances, falsely elevated concentrations are common and should be considered along with the clinical context.

Quinidine

Quinidine is a naturally occurring drug that can be used to treat various cardiac arrhythmic situations. The two most common formulations are quinidine sulfate and quinidine gluconate. Oral administration is the most common route of delivery. Gastrointestinal absorption is complete and rapid for the sulfate. Peak serum concentrations are reached about 2 hours after an oral dose of the sulfate. The gluconate is a slow-release formulation.[2] Peak serum concentration is reached 4 to 5 hours after an oral dose. The most predominant toxic adverse effects of quinidine are nausea, vomiting, and abdominal discomfort. Cardiovascular toxicity, such as PVCs, may be seen at twice the upper limit of the therapeutic range. In most instances, monitoring of quinidine involves only determination of the trough level to ensure it is within the therapeutic range. Peak assessment is performed only when symptoms of toxicity are present. Because of its slow rate of absorption, trough levels of the gluconate are usually drawn 1 hour after the last dose.

Absorbed quinidine is about 70% to 80% bound to serum proteins.[2] Most is eliminated by hepatic metabolism. Induction of this system, such as by barbiturates, increases the clearance rate. Impairment of this system, as seen in late-stage liver disease, may extend the half-life of this drug. Plasma quinidine concentrations can be determined by chromatography or immunoassay. The production of quinidine may contain active contaminants such as dihydroquinidine. Early immunoassay detected quinidine only. Most current immunoassays cross-react with these bioactive contaminants. This provides for assessment of total quinidine potential.

Procainamide

Like quinidine, procainamide is used to treat cardiac arrhythmia. Oral administration is the most common. Gastrointestinal absorption is rapid and complete. Peak plasma concentrations occur at about 1 hour.[2] Absorbed procainamide is about 20% bound to plasma proteins. It is eliminated by a combination of renal filtration and hepatic metabolism. N-acetylprocainamide is a hepatic metabolite of the parent drug, with antiarrhythmic activity similar to procainamide. The total antiarrhythmic potential of this drug must take into consideration the parent drug and this metabolite. Alteration in either renal or hepatic function may lead to increased serum

CASE STUDY 30-1

A patient with congestive heart failure has been successfully treated with digoxin for several years. Laboratory records indicate semiannual peak digoxin levels have all been in the therapeutic range. This patient recently developed renal failure, and admission testing was performed. Selected serum or blood laboratory results from this specimen are shown in Case Study Table 30-1.1. Although serum digoxin is high, the physician indicates the patient is not exhibiting signs or symptoms of toxicity.

Questions

1. If these results were derived from a random specimen, how may the time since the last dose affect the interpretation of the digoxin results?

2. Other than time, what additional factors should be taken into consideration when interpreting the digoxin results?

3. What additional laboratory test would aid in the interpretation of this case?

CASE STUDY TABLE 30-1.1
LABORATORY RESULTS

TEST	RESULT	REFERENCE RANGE
Sodium	129	135–145 mmol/L
Potassium	5.5	3.5–5 mmol/L
Chloride	113	97–107 mmol/L
Blood pH	7.25	7.35–7.45
tCO$_2$	16	21–31 mmol/L
Urea nitrogen	180	5–20 mg/dL
Creatinine	4.5	0.6–1 mg/dL
Osmolality	275	282–300 mOsm/kg
Digoxin	2.5	0.9–2 ng/mL

concentration of the parent drug and its metabolites. Increased concentration results in myocardial depression and arrhythmia. Both procainamide and its active metabolite can be measured by immunoassay.

Disopyramide

Disopyramide (Norpace) is another drug used to treat cardiac arrhythmias. It is commonly used as a quinidine substitute when quinidine adverse effects are excessive. It is most commonly administered as an oral preparation. Gastrointestinal absorption is complete and rapid, with serum concentrations peaking at about 1 to 2 hours.[2] It

CASE STUDY 30-2

A patient is receiving procainamide for treatment of cardiac arrhythmia. An IV loading dose resulted in a serum concentration of 6.0 µg/mL. The therapeutic range for procainamide is 4 to 8 µg/mL, and its half-life is 4 hours. Four hours after the initial loading dose, another equivalent dose was given as an IV bolus. This resulted in a serum concentration of 7.5 µg/mL.

Questions

1. Does the serum concentration after the second dose seem appropriate? If not, what would be the predicted serum concentration at this time?

2. What factors would influence the rate of elimination of this drug?

binds to several plasma proteins. Binding is highly variable between individuals and is concentration dependent: as serum concentration increases, so does the percentage free. As a result, it is difficult to correlate total serum concentration with therapeutic benefit and toxicity. In most patients, total serum concentrations in the range of 3 to 7.5 µg/mL (8.8 to 22.1 µmol/L) have been determined to be effective and nontoxic; however, interpretation of disopyramide results should take the clinical perspective into consideration. The primary toxicities of disopyramide are dose dependent.[2] Anticholinergic effects, such as dry mouth and constipation, may be seen at serum concentrations greater than 4.5 µg/mL (13.3 µmol/L). Cardiac effects, such as bradycardia and atrioventricular node blockage, are usually seen at serum concentrations greater than 10 µg/mL (29.5 µmol/L). Disopyramide is primarily eliminated by renal filtration and, to a lesser extent, by hepatic metabolism. In conditions with low glomerular filtration rate, the half-life is prolonged and serum concentrations rise. Plasma disopyramide concentration can be determined by chromatography or immunoassay.

ANTIBIOTICS

Aminoglycosides

Aminoglycosides are a group of chemically related antibiotics used for the treatment of infections with gram-negative bacteria that are resistant to less toxic antibiotics. There are many individual agents within this classification. The most commonly encountered in a clinical setting are gentamicin, tobramycin, amikacin, and kanamycin. All share a common mechanism of action but vary in effectiveness against different strains of bacteria. All share a common nephrotoxicity and ototoxicity. The ototoxic effect involves disruption of inner ear cochlear and vestibular membranes, which results in hearing and balance impairment. These effects are irreversible. Cumulative effects may be seen with repeated high-level exposure. Nephrotoxicity is also of major concern. Aminoglycosides impair the function of proximal tubules of the kidney, which may result in electrolyte imbalance and possibly proteinuria. These effects are usually reversible; however, extended high-level exposure may result in necrosis of these cells and subsequent renal failure.[4] Toxic concentrations are usually considered as any concentration above the therapeutic range.

Because aminoglycosides are not well absorbed from the gastrointestinal tract, administration is limited to the IV or IM route; therefore, these drugs are not used in an outpatient setting. Aminoglycosides are eliminated by renal filtration. In patients with compromised renal function, appropriate adjustments must be made based on serum concentrations. Chromatography and immunoassay are the primary methods used for aminoglycoside determinations.

Vancomycin

Vancomycin is a glycopeptide antibiotic that is effective against gram-positive cocci and bacilli. Because of poor oral absorption, vancomycin is administered by IV infusion. Unlike other drugs, a clear relationship between serum concentration and toxic adverse effects has not been firmly established. Indeed, many of the toxic effects occur in the therapeutic range (5 to 10 µg/mL [3.45 to 6.9 µmol/L]).[4] The major toxicities of vancomycin are red man syndrome, nephrotoxicity, and ototoxicity. Red man syndrome is characterized by an erythemic flushing of the extremities. The renal and hearing effects are similar to those of the aminoglycosides. It appears that the nephrotoxic effects occur more frequently at trough concentrations that are greater than 10 µg/mL (6.9 µmol/L). The ototoxic effect occurs more frequently when peak serum concentrations exceed 40 µg/mL (27.6 µmol/L). Because vancomycin has a long distribution phase, in most instances, only trough levels are monitored to ensure the serum drug concentration is within the therapeutic range. Vancomycin is primarily eliminated by renal filtration and secretion. It is assayed by immunoassay and chromatographic methods.

ANTIEPILEPTIC DRUGS

Epilepsy, convulsions, and seizures are prevalent neurologic disorders. Because these drugs are used as prophylactics, therapeutic ranges are considered guidelines and should be interpreted in accordance with the presenting clinical context.[5] Effective concentrations are determined as the concentration that works, with no or acceptable adverse effects. In recent years, a second generation of antiepileptic drugs (AEDs) have been introduced in clinical practice as supplemental therapy to the more traditional drugs (i.e., phenobarbital and phenytoin). Unlike first-generation AEDs, optimal concentration ranges have not been firmly established. For these drugs, though, TDM may be indicated in initially establishing individual baseline concentrations at which the patient is responding well.[5] It is important to take these individual reference ranges into account, especially as physiologic conditions may be altered (age related, pregnancy, kidney or liver disease, etc.), and in reassessing these concentrations as other AEDs are added to an established regimen.[5] Most AEDs are analyzed by immunoassay or chromatography and measure the free or bound drug in a serum or plasma sample. In a normal physiologic state, the total drug concentration may be sufficient. A free drug measurement may only be necessary when there is cause for alteration in patient plasma protein, such as in the later stages of pregnancy, in late-stage renal or hepatic disease, malnutrition, or when a known drug–drug interaction may occur.[6] As with all TDM, sampling time must be consistent and the most preferred specimen is the trough serum concentration, collected at the end of the dosing interval.[6]

First-Generation AEDs

Phenobarbital

Phenobarbital is a slow-acting barbiturate that effectively controls several types of seizures. Absorption of oral phenobarbital is slow but complete. For most patients, peak serum concentration is reached about 10 hours after an oral dose. Circulating phenobarbital is 50% protein bound. It is eliminated primarily by hepatic metabolism. However, renal filtration is also significant. With compromised renal or hepatic function, the rate of elimination is decreased. The half-life of serum phenobarbital is 70 to 100 hours. Because of the slow absorption and long half-life, serum concentrations do not change dramatically within a dosing interval. Therefore, only trough levels are usually evaluated unless toxicity is suspected. Toxic adverse effects of phenobarbital include drowsiness, fatigue, depression, and reduced mental capacity.

Phenobarbital clearance occurs by the hepatic MFO system. It is noteworthy that it is also a potent inducer of this system. After initiation of therapy, dose adjustment is usually required after the induction period is complete. For most individuals, this is 10 to 15 days after the first dose.

Primidone is an inactive proform of phenobarbital. After absorption of an oral dose, this drug is rapidly converted to its active form, phenobarbital. Primidone

CASE STUDY 30-3

A child, who has been successfully treated for seizure disorders with oral phenytoin for several years, has had severe diarrhea for the past 2 weeks. Subsequent to this, the patient had a seizure. Evaluation of serum phenytoin at the time of the seizure revealed a low value. The dose was increased until serum concentrations were within the therapeutic range. The diarrhea was resolved. Several days after this, the patient had another seizure.

Questions

1. What is the most probable cause of the initial low serum phenytoin?

2. Would determination of free serum phenytoin aid in resolving the cause of the initial seizure?

3. What assays other than the determination of serum phenytoin would aid in this situation?

4. What is the most probable cause of the seizure after the diarrhea has been resolved?

is used in preference of phenobarbital when steady-state kinetics need to be established quickly. Primidone is rapidly absorbed and converted to the active drug. Both primidone and phenobarbital need to be measured to assess the total potential amount of phenobarbital in circulation.

Phenytoin

Phenytoin (Dilantin) is a commonly used treatment for seizure disorders. It is also used as a short-term prophylactic agent in brain injury to prevent loss of functional tissue. Phenytoin is primarily administered as an oral preparation. Gastrointestinal absorption is variable and sometimes incomplete. Circulating phenytoin has a high but variable degree of protein binding (87% to 97%) and can be easily displaced by other highly protein-bound drugs.[7] Like most drugs, the unbound (free) fraction is the biologically active portion of total serum concentration. Reduced protein binding may occur with anemia, with hypoalbuminemia, and in the coadministration of other drugs with similar binding properties. Thus, toxicity may be observed when the total serum drug concentration is within the therapeutic range. The major toxicity of phenytoin is initiation of seizures. Thus, seizures in a patient being treated with phenytoin may be a result of subtherapeutic or toxic concentrations. Additional adverse effects of phenytoin include hirsutism, gingival hyperplasia, vitamin D deficiency, and folate deficiency.

Phenytoin is eliminated by hepatic metabolism. At therapeutic concentrations, this elimination pathway may become saturated (zero-order kinetics). Therefore, relatively small changes in dosage or elimination may have dramatic effects on plasma concentration.

For most patients, total serum concentrations of 10 to 20 g/mL (39.6 to 79.2 × 10⁶ μmol/L) are effective. In many situations, however, the effective range of total serum concentration must be individualized to suit the clinical situation. It is also an inducer of the hepatic MFO pathway, which reduces the half-life of concurrently administered drugs that are eliminated by this pathway.[5] The therapeutic range for free serum phenytoin is 1 to 2 μg/mL (4.0 to 7.9 μmol/L). This has been well correlated with the pharmacologic actions of this drug. In patients with altered serum protein binding, determination of the free fraction aids in dosage adjustment.

Fosphenytoin is an injectable proform of phenytoin that is rapidly metabolized in serum, releasing the parent drug. It takes about 75 minutes for this conversion to take place. Most immunoassays for phenytoin do not detect this proform. Thus, peak levels should be evaluated only after the conversion to the active drug is complete.

Valproic Acid

Valproic acid is used as a monotherapy for the treatment of petit mal and absence seizures.[7] It is administered as an oral preparation. Gastrointestinal absorption is rapid and complete. Circulating valproic acid is highly protein bound (93%). The percentage bound decreases in renal failure, in late liver disease, and with coadministration of other drugs that may compete for its binding site. It is eliminated by hepatic metabolism, which may be induced by numerous coadministered AEDs but is inhibited by coadministration of felbamate (another AED).[7] The therapeutic range for valproic acid is relatively wide (50 to 120 μg/mL [347 to 832 μmol/L]). Determination of serum concentration is primarily done to ensure that toxic levels (>120 μg/mL) are not present. Nausea, lethargy, and weight gain are the most common adverse effects. Pancreatitis, hyperammonemia, and hallucinations have been associated with high serum levels (>200 μg/mL [>1387 μmol/L]). Hepatic dysfunction occasionally occurs in some patients even at therapeutic serum concentrations; therefore, hepatic indicators should be checked frequently for the first 6 months after initiation of therapy. Many factors may influence the nonbound (free) fraction of total serum valproic acid. Therefore, determination of the free fraction provides a more reliable index of therapeutic and toxic concentrations.

Carbamazepine

Carbamazepine (Tegretol) is an effective treatment in various seizure disorders. Because of its serious toxic adverse effects, it is less frequently used, except when patients do not respond to other drugs. Orally administered carbamazepine is absorbed with a high degree of variability. Circulating carbamazepine is 70% to 80% protein bound. It is eliminated primarily by hepatic metabolism. Many forms of liver dysfunction may result in serum accumulation. Carbamazepine is an inducer of its own metabolism. Thus, frequent plasma levels must be analyzed on initiation of therapy until the induction period has come to completion.

Carbamazepine toxicity is diverse and variable. Certain effects occur in a dose-dependent manner; others do not. There are several idiosyncratic effects of carbamazepine, which affect a portion of the population at therapeutic concentrations, including rashes, leukopenia, nausea, vertigo, and febrile reactions. Of these, leukopenia is the most serious. Leukocyte counts are commonly done during the first 2 weeks of therapy to detect this possible toxic effect. Liver function testing is also done during this period. Mild, transient liver dysfunction is commonly seen during this period. Large and persistent increases in liver indices or a significant leukopenia commonly result in discontinuation of the drug. The therapeutic range for carbamazepine is 4 to 12 μg/mL (16.9 to 50.8 μmol/L). Plasma concentrations greater than 15 μg/mL (63.5 μmol/L) are associated with hematologic dyscrasias and possible aplastic anemia.

Ethosuximide

Ethosuximide (zarontin) is used for controlling petit mal seizure. It is administered as an oral preparation. The therapeutic range is 40 to 100 μg/mL (283 to 708 μmol/L). The toxicities associated with high plasma concentrations are rare, tolerable, and self-limiting. TDM of ethosuximide is done to ensure that serum concentrations are in the therapeutic range.

Felbamate

Felbamate is an orally administered drug that is nearly completely absorbed by the gastrointestinal tract, and peak serum concentrations are reached within 1 to 4 hours.[8] In circulation, it is 30% bound to serum proteins and is eliminated by renal and hepatic metabolism. Felbamate is known for its toxicity and is primarily indicated in severe epilepsies such as in children with the mixed seizure disorder Lennox-Gastaut syndrome (refractory to all other AEDs) and in adults with refractory epilepsy.[5-7] When administered as a monotherapy, the half-life of the drug is 14 to 22 hours in adults. In comparison, clearance has been reported to be higher in children and reduced in the elderly. Renal impairment will increase the half-life to 27 to 34 hours. Felbamate therapy is contradicted in patients with hepatic dysfunction.[8] Metabolism of the drug is enhanced by enzyme inducers including phenobarbital, primidone, phenytoin, and carbamazepine, resulting in a decreased half-life.

TDM may be indicated due to the narrow therapeutic range and can be considered after steady state has been reached. In patients receiving therapeutic doses, the serum concentrations have been measured in the range of 30 to 60 μg/mL (126 to 252 μmol/L).[8] Adverse side effects have been documented and include fatal aplastic anemia and hepatic failure.[5,7]

Gabapentin

Gabapentin is administered orally with a maximum bioavailability of 60% and is reduced when antacids are administered concurrently. This drug may be indicated as monotherapy or in conjunction with other AEDs in patients suffering from complex partial seizures with or without generalized seizures.[5,7] It does not bind to serum proteins and is not metabolized hepatically. Gabapentin is eliminated unchanged by the kidneys and has a half-life of approximately 5 to 9 hours in patients with normal renal function.[8] Children require a 30% larger than normal dose to maintain a comparable half-life, as they eliminate the drug more quickly than does the normal adult. Due to the exclusive renal clearance of this drug, impaired kidney function increases half-life of the circulating drug in a linear manner.[8] Therapeutic concentration has been documented at 12 to 20 μg/mL (70.1 to 116.8 μmol/L), although a wide range of serum concentrations have been reported in association with seizure control. Multiple daily doses may be the preferred regimen as excessively high blood concentrations may lead to adverse drug effects, while low-level trough concentrations may lead to breakthrough seizures.[5] Gabapentin may be the most likely treatment consideration in patients with liver disease and in treating partial-onset seizures in patients with acute intermittent porphyria.[5]

Lamotrigine

Lamotrigine is orally administered and is rapidly and completely absorbed from the gastrointestinal tract. Its use is indicated in patients with partial and generalized seizures.[5] Once in circulation, it is approximately 55% protein bound.[8] Hepatic metabolism accounts for the majority of elimination.[7,8] In patients undergoing monotherapy, the half-life of lamotrigine is 15 to 30 hours. Its rate of elimination is highly dependent on patient age and physiologic condition. Younger infants tend to metabolize more slowly than do older infants. Children tend to metabolize on the order of twice as quickly as normal adults. There have been marked increases in clearance as pregnancy progresses, peaking at the 32nd week.[5]

Lamotrigine clearance is also influenced by the recognized enzyme-inducing AEDs such as phenobarbital, primidone, phenytoin, and carbamazepine. In a very opposite manner, valproic acid is an inhibitor of lamotrigine metabolism and may increase its half-life to 60 hours. The above drug–drug interactions justify a need for TDM during therapy. Individual therapeutic ranges do vary, but a concentration range of 2.5 to 15 µg/mL has been noted as efficacious and increasing concentration seems to correlate with increasing risk of toxicity.[8] Tailoring dose and serum concentration is advisable because therapeutic results have been observed in concentrations greater than previously noted therapeutic range (in lieu of toxic side effects).[8]

Levetiracetam

Levetiracetam is an orally administered AED that is nearly entirely bioavailable.[5,7,8] Its use is indicated in partial and generalized seizures. It does not bind to serum proteins. Its half-life is 6 to 8 hours, although the rate of elimination is increased in children and pregnant women and decreased in the elderly. Levetiracetam's rate of clearance correlates well with glomerular filtration rate, which may be of use in monitoring patients with renal impairment. The need for TDM of levetiracetam is not as pronounced as in other AEDs (due to its lack of pharmacokinetic variability) but may be useful in monitoring compliance and fluctuating levels during pregnancy.[5] Therapeutic concentrations have been reported at 8 to 26 µg/mL.

Oxcarbazepine

Oxcarbazepine is a prodrug that is almost immediately metabolized to licarbazepine.[7,8] It is indicated for the monotherapy of partial seizures and in secondarily generalized tonic–clonic seizures. Its protein binding is approximately 40%. Its peak concentration is at about 8 hours. It is metabolized by the liver into two pharmacologically active, equipotent enantiomers via keto reduction followed by glucuronide conjugation of the active licarbazepine derivative.[7,8] Its half-life is 8 to 10 hours in normal adults. In children, there is a higher clearance rate; therefore, a need exists for a higher dosing regimen to obtain the optimal serum concentration per kilogram of body weight compared with adults. The opposite scenario is seen in the elderly as their drug clearance is reduced by 30%.[8] The clearance of the drug and its metabolite is reduced in patients with marked renal dysfunction. The metabolism of licarbazepine is sensitive to enzyme inducers such as phenytoin and phenobarbital, which decreases the blood concentration by 20% to 40%.[8] TDM may be indicated until established steady state has been reached, at therapeutic failure, when there may be drug–drug interactions, and during pregnancy. Although not well defined, therapeutic effects of licarbazepine have been reported at serum concentrations of 12 to 35 µg/mL.

Tiagabine

Tiagabine absorption is rapid and nearly complete as circulating concentration peaks at 0.5 to 2 hours. It is approximately 96% protein bound, and its half-life is variable in the range of 4 to 13 hours. It is highly metabolized by the hepatic mixed-function oxidase pathway.[5,8] It is indicated in treating partial seizures.[7] Due to its significant protein binding, the ratio of free to bound drug is affected by other protein-binding drugs such as valproic acid, naproxen, and salicylates and by pregnancy.[8] Hepatic dysfunction also prolongs the half-life of the drug. TDM may be indicated due to intraindividual and interindividual variations. Therapeutic benefits of the drug have been observed at concentrations of 20 to 100 ng/mL.[8] Dose titration may be the most effective method in balancing therapeutic effects with adverse central nervous system (CNS) side effects of the drug. These side effects include symptoms of confusion, difficulty in speaking clearly (stuttering), mild sedation, and a tingling sensation in the body's extremities (paresthesia), especially in the hands and fingers.[5,9]

Topiramate

Topiramate is nearly completely bioavailable after oral administration, and peak concentration is reached within 1 to 4 hours.[7,8] It is 15% protein bound. The serum half-life is 20 to 30 hours. The majority of topiramate is eliminated by renal filtration; the remainder is eliminated by hepatic metabolism. Topiramate is indicated in partial and generalized seizures.[5] The dose–to–serum concentration ratio in children is less than that of adults per kilogram of body mass such that they require a higher dose to maintain serum topiramate concentrations comparable to adults.[8] Serum concentrations are increased secondary to renal insufficiency but may be decreased when used with other enzyme-inducing AEDs (listed in previous sections). Dose titration may also be the most effective method in balancing therapeutic effects with adverse CNS side effects; these include change of taste with particular foods (e.g., diet soda and beer) and a sensation of "pins and needles" in the extremities.[5,9] TDM may be indicated at steady state to provide the clinician with an effective individual baseline concentration, at therapeutic failure, and to monitor drug–drug interactions.[8]

Zonisamide

Zonisamide is orally administered and absorbed from the gastrointestinal tract on the order of 65% or higher. Peak serum concentrations are reached at 4 to 7 hours, and the drug is approximately 60% protein bound and accumulates extensively in erthyrocytes.[8] The majority is metabolized by the liver via glucuronide conjugation, acetylation, and oxidation and then renal excretion. Its use is implicated in the therapy of partial and generalized seizures. The half-life of zonisamide is 50 to 70 hours in patients receiving monotherapy and may reduce to 25 to 35 hours when other enzyme-inducing AEDs are being administered concurrently.[8] Children require higher doses to achieve effective serum concentrations comparable to that of an adult.[8] Clinicians treating patients with liver or kidney disease and using this drug should exercise caution as serum concentrations may increase proportionally with the level and type of organ impairment. There is documented overlap in zonisamide blood concentrations between those experiencing therapeutic effectiveness and those experiencing toxic side effects.[8] TDM may be indicated to establish a baseline level after steady state has been achieved, to detect drug–drug interactions, and at therapeutic failure. Therapeutic doses have been reported in patients with serum concentrations of 10 to 38 μg/mL.

PSYCHOACTIVE DRUGS

Lithium

Lithium is an orally administered drug used to treat manic depression (bipolar disorder). Absorption is complete and rapid. Lithium is a cationic metal that does not bind to proteins. Distribution is uniform throughout total body water. It is eliminated predominately by renal filtration and is subject to reabsorption. Compromises in renal function usually result in accumulation. Correlations between serum concentration and therapeutic response have not been well established. However, serum concentrations in the range of 0.5 to 1.2 mmol/L are effective in a large portion of the patient population.[10] The purpose of TDM for lithium is to avoid serum concentrations associated with toxic effects. Serum concentrations in the range of 1.5 to 2 mmol/L may cause apathy, lethargy, speech difficulties, and muscle weakness.[10] Serum concentrations greater than 2 mmol/L are associated with muscle rigidity, seizures, and possible coma. Determination of serum lithium is commonly done by ion-selective electrode. Flame emission photometry and atomic absorption are also viable methods. It is relatively inexpensive to monitor serum lithium in avoiding toxic side effects. Thus, it is prudent to do so for patients on such a regimen.[10]

Tricyclic Antidepressants

Tricyclic antidepressants (TCAs) are a class of drugs used to treat depression, insomnia, extreme apathy, and loss of libido. From a clinical laboratory perspective, imipramine, amitriptyline, and doxepin are the most relevant.[10] Desipramine and nortriptyline are active metabolic products of imipramine and amitriptyline, respectively, and must also be included. The TCAs are orally administered drugs with a varying degree of absorption. In many patients, they slow gastric emptying and intestinal motility, which significantly slows the rate of absorption. As a result, peak serum concentrations are reached in the range of 2 to 12 hours. The TCAs are highly protein bound (85% to 95%). For most TCAs, the therapeutic effects are not seen for the first 2 to 4 weeks after initiation of therapy. The correlations between serum concentration and therapeutic effects of

most TCAs are moderate to weak. They are eliminated by hepatic metabolism. Many of the metabolic products formed have therapeutic actions. The rate of metabolism of these agents is variable and influenced by a wide variety of factors. As a result, the half-life of TCAs varies considerably among patients. The rate of elimination can also be influenced by the coadministration of other drugs that are eliminated by hepatic metabolism. The toxicity of TCAs is dose dependent. At serum concentrations about twice the upper limit of the therapeutic range, drowsiness, constipation, blurred vision, and memory loss are common adverse effects. Higher levels may cause seizure, cardiac arrhythmia, and unconsciousness.

Because of the high variability in half-life and absorption, plasma concentrations of the TCAs should not be evaluated until a steady state has been achieved. At this point, therapeutic efficacy is determined from clinical evaluation of the patient, and potential toxicity is determined by serum concentration. Many of the immunoassays for TCAs use polyclonal antibodies, which cross-react among the different TCAs and their metabolites and are used for TCA screening rather than blood concentration monitoring and TDM.[10] In this analytic system, the results are reported out as "total tricyclics." Other immunoassays use an extraction step to separate parent drugs from the metabolites. Interpretation of these results after extraction requires an in-depth understanding of the assay. Chromatographic methods provide simultaneous evaluation of both the parent drugs and metabolites, which provides a basis for unambiguous interpretation of results.[10]

Clozapine

Clozapine is an atypical antipsychotic used to treat otherwise treatment-refractory schizophrenia, including its negative symptoms, suicidal tendencies, and various types of cognitive deficiencies associated with the disease. Research has found that although there is not a well-established clinical serum concentration, beneficial effects of the drug have been demonstrated at 350 to 420 ng/mL. TDM may be indicated to check for compliance and in patients with altered pharmacokinetics. TDM may also be used in avoiding symptoms of toxicity and overdosing, which may present with seizures.[11]

Olanzapine

Olanzapine is a thienobenzodiazepine derivative that effectively treats schizophrenia, acute manic episodes, and the recurrence of bipolar disorders.[11] It can be administered as a fast-acting IM injection at a dose of 2.5 to 10 mg per injection. Olanzapine is more likely administered orally and is 85% absorbed, although it is approximately 40% inactivated by first-pass metabolism. Women and nonsmokers tend to have lower clearance and thus a higher serum concentration of olanzapine compared with men and smokers.[11] There is indication that plasma concentration correlates well with clinical outcomes. TDM may help to optimize clinical response while balancing it with adverse affects with a therapeutic range of 20 to 50 ng/mL.[11]

IMMUNOSUPPRESSIVE DRUGS

Transplantation medicine is a rapidly emerging discipline within clinical medicine. The clinical laboratory plays many important roles that determine the success of any transplantation program. Among these responsibilities, monitoring of the immunosuppressive drugs used to prevent rejection is of key concern. Most of these drugs require establishment of individual dosage regimens to optimize therapeutic outcomes and minimize toxicity.

Cyclosporine

Cyclosporine is a cyclic polypeptide that has potent immunosuppressive activity. Its primary clinical use is suppression of host-versus-graft rejection of heterotopic transplanted organs. It is administered as an oral preparation. Absorption of cyclosporine is in the range of 5% to 50%. Because of this high variability, the relationship between oral dose and blood concentration is poor; therefore, TDM is an important part of establishing an initial dosage regimen. Circulating cyclosporine sequesters in cells, including erythrocytes.[12] Erythrocyte content is highly temperature dependent; therefore, evaluation of plasma concentration requires rigorous control of specimen temperature. To avoid this preanalytic variable, whole blood is the specimen of choice. Correlations have been established between whole blood concentration and therapeutic and toxic effects. Cyclosporine is eliminated by hepatic metabolism to inactive products.

Immunosuppression requirements differ depending on the organ transplanted. Cardiac, liver, and pancreas transplants have the highest requirement (300 ng/mL [250 nmol/L]). Whole blood concentrations in the range of 350 to 400 ng/mL (291 to 333 nmol/L) have been associated with toxic effects. The toxic effects of cyclosporine are primarily renal tubular and glomerular dysfunction, which may result in hypertension.[13] Several immunoassays are available for the determination of whole blood cyclosporine concentration. Many cross-react with inactive metabolites. Chromatographic methods are available; they provide separation and quantitation of the parent drug from metabolites.[14]

Tacrolimus

Tacrolimus (FK-506) is an orally administered immunosuppressive drug that is 100 times more potent than cyclosporine; therefore, the dosage is far less than that of cyclosporine.[15] Early use of tacrolimus suggested a

low degree of toxicity compared with cyclosporine at therapeutic concentrations. However, after extensive use in clinical practice, it has been demonstrated that both have comparable degrees of nephrotoxicity at therapeutic concentrations. At concentrations above therapeutic, tacrolimus has been associated with thrombus formation.

Many aspects of tacrolimus pharmacokinetics are similar to those of cyclosporine. Gastrointestinal uptake is highly variable. Whole blood concentrations correlate well with therapeutic and toxic effects. Tacrolimus is eliminated almost exclusively by hepatic metabolism. Metabolic products are primarily secreted into the bile. Increases in immunoreactive tacrolimus may be seen in cholestasis as a result of cross-reactivity with several of these products. Because of the high potency of tacrolimus, circulating therapeutic concentrations are low. This limits the methodologies capable of measuring whole blood concentrations. The most common method is high-performance liquid chromatography–mass spectrometry; however, several immunoassays are also available.

Sirolimus

Sirolimus (rapamycin) is an antifungal agent with immunosuppressive activity. It is U.S. Food and Drug Administration approved for patients receiving kidney transplants. Sirolimus is extremely potent and requires TDM due to its inherent toxicity. Adverse events include thrombocytopenia, anemia, leukopenia, infections, and hyperlipidemia.[16,17] It is commonly used in conjunction with cyclosporine or tacrolimus.[14,16] Sirolimus is rapidly absorbed after once-daily oral administration, with peak blood levels at about 1 hour. The oral bioavailability is 15% when taken in conjunction with cyclosporine.[17]

Serum concentration is affected extensively by intestinal and hepatic first-pass metabolism. It has a long half-life of 62 hours. Intraindividual and interindividual variability demonstrates the need for TDM as serum concentration is affected by individual differences in absorption, distribution, metabolism, and excretion. It binds more highly to lipoproteins than to serum protein; therefore, whole blood is the ideal specimen for analysis.[17] TDM commences using a trough level specimen obtained 5 to 7 days after initiation of therapy. Trough specimens are then drawn on a weekly basis for the first month following a biweekly sampling pattern in the second month and can be analyzed to establish a safe and effective therapeutic range. The therapeutic range is 4 to 12 µg/L when it is used in conjunction with cyclosporine and 12 to 20 µg/L if cyclosporine therapy is discontinued.[17] It is assayed using chromatography.[14,16]

Mycophenolic Acid

Mycophenolate mofetil is a prodrug that is rapidly converted in the liver to its active form of mycophenolic acid

(MPA).[13] It is a lymphocyte proliferation inhibitor.[18] It is used most commonly as supplemental therapy with cyclosporine and tacrolimus in renal transplant patients. As with the other antirejection drugs, low trough levels increase the risk of acute rejection, while high levels imply toxicity. It is an orally administered drug that is absorbed under neutral pH conditions in the intestine.[18] Interindividual variation of gastrointestinal tract physiology influences the degree of absorption of MPA. Once in circulation, it is 95% protein bound. The degree to which MPA is protein bound varies both intraindividually and interindividually and is dependent on circulating albumin concentration, renal function, and the concentration of other drugs that may be competitively binding to serum albumin.[18] Therapeutic serum concentrations have been documented at 1.0 to 3.5 µg/mL. MPA and its metabolites can be assayed using plasma specimen as the most likely sample of choice when using chromatography. Immunoassay is a less specific, yet common, method in assaying plasma MPA.[18] As with most immunoassay methods, cross-reactivity between MPA and its active metabolite (AcMPAG) should be taken into account and interpreted flexibly in the clinical picture as each demonstrates varying pharmacokinetics.

ANTINEOPLASTICS

Assessment of the therapeutic benefit and toxicity of most antineoplastic drugs is not aided by TDM, because correlations between plasma concentration and therapeutic benefit are hard to establish. Many of these agents are rapidly metabolized or incorporated into cellular macromolecular structures within seconds to minutes of their administration. In addition, the therapeutic range for many of these drugs includes concentrations associated with toxic effects. Considering that most antineoplastic agents are administered IV as a single bolus, the actual delivered dose is more important than circulating concentrations.

Methotrexate

Methotrexate is one of the few antineoplastic drugs in which TDM offers benefits to a therapeutic regimen. High-dose methotrexate followed by leucovorin rescue has been shown to be an effective therapy for various neoplastic conditions.[19] The basis of this therapy involves the relative rate of mitosis of normal versus neoplastic cells. In general, neoplastic cells divide more rapidly than do normal cells. Methotrexate inhibits DNA synthesis in all cells. Neoplastic cells, as a result of their rapid rate of division, have a higher requirement for DNA and are susceptible to depravation of this essential constituent before normal cells. The efficacy of methotrexate therapy is dependent on a controlled period of inhibition, one that is selectively detrimental to neoplastic cells. This is accomplished by administration of leucovorin, which reverses the actions of methotrexate at a specific time after methotrexate infusion. This is referred to as *leucovorin rescue*. Failure to stop methotrexate actions results in cytotoxic effects to most cells. Evaluation of serum methotrexate concentration, after the inhibitory time period has passed, is used to determine how much leucovorin is needed to counteract many of the toxic effects of methotrexate.[19]

The basic principles of TDM, which address absorption, distribution, and elimination, can also be applied to nontherapeutic substances that have entered the body. Indeed, the use of these concepts is central to the study of poisons.

For additional student resources please visit thePoint at http://thepoint.lww.com. **thePoint**

QUESTIONS

1. Drug X has a half-life ($T_{1/2}$) of 2 days. The concentration at noon today is 10 µg/mL. What would be the expected concentration of drug X at noon tomorrow?
   a. 7 µg/mL
   b. 7.5 µg/mL
   c. 5 µg/mL
   d. 3.5 µg/mL

2. Salicylic acid is a common component of many over-the-counter drugs. In a patient suffering from gastric achlorhydria, what would be the predicted serum concentration of this drug after a standard dose?
   a. Less than expected
   b. Greater than expected
   c. No change

3. Of the following, what would be the most appropriate time for evaluation of a peak digoxin level after oral administration?
   a. 8 hours after a dose
   b. Immediately before the next dose

c. Immediately after a dose

d. 3 days after a dose

4. Of the following statements concerning procainamide, which is TRUE?

    a. The primary toxicity of procainamide is bone marrow suppression.

    b. Procainamide is an antibiotic.

    c. *N*-Acetylprocainamide is an active product of procainamide metabolism.

    d. All of these are true.

    e. Procainamide is an antibiotic, and the primary toxicity of procainamide is bone marrow suppression.

5. Of the following statements concerning lithium, which is TRUE?

    a. Lithium is used as a drug to treat depression and mania.

    b. Lithium is an element.

    c. Lithium concentration in serum is most commonly evaluated by ion-specific electrode.

    d. All of these are true.

    e. Lithium is an element, and the lithium concentration in serum is most commonly evaluated by ion-specific electrode.

6. What is the purpose for determining serum concentrations of the antineoplastic drug methotrexate?

    a. All of these

    b. To ensure that serum concentrations are in the therapeutic range

    c. To ensure that serum concentrations are not in the toxic range

    d. To determine the amount of leucovorin needed to halt methotrexate action

    e. To ensure that serum concentrations are in the therapeutic range and to determine the amount of leucovorin needed to halt methotrexate action

7. A patient who has been successfully receiving gentamicin for the past 2 weeks has suddenly developed a renal condition in which glomerular filtration rate has significantly decreased. What would be the expected adjustment in dosage in response to this?

    a. The drug should be discontinued.

    b. The dosage should be increased.

    c. The time interval between dosages should be increased.

    d. Phenobarbital should be coadministered to stimulate hepatic metabolism.

    e. No dosage adjustment is required.

8. Salicylate and bilirubin compete for the same binding site on serum albumin. What effect would prehepatic jaundice have on salicylate?

    a. A decrease in the pharmacologic response to salicylate

    b. An increase in the rate of clearance of salicylate

    c. An increase in the free concentration of salicylate

    d. All of these

    e. An increase in the rate of clearance of salicylate and an increase in the free concentration of salicylate

9. Twenty milligrams of a drug is injected IV. One hour after injection, blood is drawn and assayed for the drug. The concentration in this specimen was 0.4 mg/L. What is the volume of distribution for this drug?

    a. 0.8 L

    b. 8 L

    c. 20 L

    d. 50 L

    e. Unable to determine with the data provided

10. A new orally administered drug has been introduced in your institution. It is unclear whether TDM is needed for this drug. What factors should be taken into consideration when addressing this question?

    a. Proximity of toxic range to therapeutic range

    b. Consequences of a subtherapeutic concentration in circulation

    c. Severity of toxic adverse effects

    d. Predictability of serum concentrations after a standard oral dose

    e. All of the above should be taken into consideration

SUGGESTED READINGS

Birkett DJ. *Pharmacokinetics Made Easy.* New York: McGraw-Hill; 2003.

Broussard L, Tuckler V. The value of TDM, toxicology. *Adv Admin Clin Lab.* 2004;13:32.

Graham K. Lab limelight: TDM: applications for pharmacogenetics. *Adv Admin Clin Lab.* 2007:16:81.

Hardman JG, Limbird LE, Gillman AG, eds. *Goodman & Gilman's The Pharmacological Basis of Therapeutics.* 10th ed. New York: Pergamon Press; 2002.

REFERENCES

1. Abbot A. With your genes? Take one of these, three times a day. *Nature*. 2003;425:760-762.
2. Campbell TJ, Williams MK. Therapeutic drug monitoring: antiarrhythmic drugs. *Br J Clin Pharmacol*. 2001;52:21S-34S.
3. Jurgens G, Graudal NA, Kampmann JP. Therapeutic drug monitoring of antiarrhythmic drugs. *Clin Pharmacokinet*. 2003;42:647-663.
4. Winston L, Benowitz N. Once-daily dosing of aminoglycosides: how much monitoring is truly required? *Am J Med*. 2003;114: 239-240.
5. Perucca E. An introduction to antiepileptic drugs. *Epilepsia*. 2005;46:31-37.
6. Eadie MJ. Therapeutic drug monitoring—antiepileptic drugs. *Br J Clin Pharmacol*. 2001;52:11S-19S.
7. Israni RK, Kasbekar N, Haynes K, Berns JS. Use of antiepileptic drugs in patients with kidney disease. *Semin Dial*. 2006;19: 408-416.
8. Johannessen SI, Tomson T. Pharmacokinetic variability of newer antiepileptic drugs. *Clin Pharmacokinet*. 2006;45:1061-1075.
9. Wikipedia Online. Searched Tiagabine. http://en.wikipedia.org/wiki/Tiagabine. Accessed February 17, 2008.
10. Mitchell PB. Therapeutic drug monitoring of psychotropic medications. *Br J Clin Pharmacol*. 2001;52:45S-54S.
11. Mauri MC, Volonteri LS, Colasanti A, Fiorentini A, De Gaspari IF, Bareggi SR. Clinical pharmacokinetics of atypical antipsychotics. *Clin Pharmacokinet*. 2007;46:359-388.
12. Masuda S, Inui K. An update review on individualized dosage of calcineurin inhibitors in organ transplant recipients. *Pharmacol Ther*. 2006;112:184-198.
13. Taylor AL, Watson CJE, Bradley JA. Immunosuppressive agents in solid organ transplantation: mechanisms of action and therapeutic efficacy. *Crit Rev Oncol Hematol*. 2005;56:23-46.
14. Johnston A, Holt DW. Immunosuppressant drugs—the role of therapeutic drug monitoring. *Br J Clin Pharmacol*. 2001;52:61S-73S.
15. Baraldo M, Furlanut M. Chronopharmacokietics of cyclosporine and tacrolimus. *Clin Pharmacokinet*. 2006;45:775-788.
16. Wong SHY. Therapeutic drug monitoring for immunosuppressants. *Clin Chim Acta*. 2001;313:241-253.
17. Stenton SB, Partovi N, Ensom MHH. Sirolimus: the evidence for clinical pharmacokinetic monitoring. *Clin Pharmacokinet*. 2005;44:769-786.
18. Elbarbry FA, Shoker AS. Therapeutic drug measurement of mycophenolic acid derivatives in transplant patients. *Clin Biochem*. 2007;40:752-764.
19. Lennard L. Therapeutic drug monitoring of cytotoxic drugs. *Br J Pharmacol*. 2001;52:75S-87S.

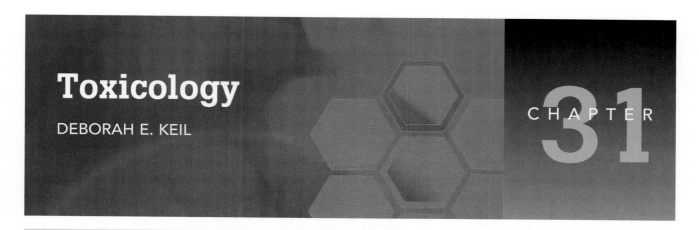

Toxicology

DEBORAH E. KEIL

CHAPTER 31

Chapter Objectives

Upon completion of this chapter, the clinical laboratorian should be able to do the following:

- Define the term *toxicology*.
- List the major toxicants.
- Define the pathologic mechanisms of the toxicants discussed in the chapter.

- Discuss the laboratory methods used to evaluate toxicity.
- Explain the difference between quantitative and qualitative tests in toxicology.
- Critically evaluate clinical laboratory data in poisoning cases and provide recommendations for further testing.
- Define the role of the clinical laboratory in the evaluation of exposure to poisons.

KEY TERMS

Bioaccumulation
Body burden
Dose–response relationship
Drugs of abuse
Individual dose–response relationship

LD_{50}
Poison
Quantal dose–response relationship
Toxicokinetics
Toxicology
Toxin
Xenobiotic

Toxicology is the study of the adverse effects of xenobiotics in humans. Xenobiotics include chemicals and drugs that are not normally found or produced in the body. The scope of toxicology is very broad. There are three major disciplines within toxicology: mechanistic, descriptive, and regulatory toxicology. *Mechanistic toxicology* elucidates the cellular, molecular, and biochemical effects of xenobiotics within the context of a dose–response relationship between the xenobiotic and the adverse effect. Mechanistic studies provide a basis for rational therapy design and the development of tests to assess the degree of exposure in individuals. *Descriptive toxicology* uses the results from animal experiments to predict what level of exposure will cause harm in humans. This process is known as *risk assessment*. In *regulatory toxicology*, interpretation of the combined data from mechanistic and descriptive studies is used to establish standards that define the level of exposure that will not pose a risk to public health or safety. Typically, regulatory toxicologists work for, or in conjunction with, government agencies. The Food and Drug Administration oversees human safety issues associated with therapeutic drugs, cosmetics, and food additives. The U.S. Environmental Agency has regulatory oversight with regard to pesticides, fungicides, rodenticides, and industry-related chemicals that may threaten safe drinking water and clean air. The Occupational Safety and Health Administration (OSHA) is responsible for ensuring safe and healthy work environments. The Consumer Product Safety Commission regulates household chemicals, while the Department of Transportation oversees transporting of chemical hazards. Additionally, there are a number of specialties in toxicology, including forensic, clinical, and environmental. *Forensic toxicology* is primarily concerned with the medicolegal consequences of exposure to chemicals or drugs. A major focus of this area is establishing and validating the analytic performance of the methods used to generate evidence in legal situations, including the cause of death. *Clinical toxicology* is the study of interrelationships between xenobiotics and disease states. This area emphasizes not only diagnostic testing but also therapeutic intervention. *Environmental toxicology* includes the evaluation of environmental chemical pollutants and their impact on human health. This is a growing area of concern as we learn more about the mechanisms of action of these chemicals, monitor occupational health, and increase public health biomonitoring efforts nationwide.

Within the organizational scheme of a typical medical laboratory, toxicology is usually considered a specialty of clinical chemistry, mainly because the qualitative and quantitative methodologies applied to measure xenobiotics overlap with this discipline. However, appropriate diagnosis and management of patients with acute poisoning or chronic exposures to xenobiotics require an integrated approach from all sections of the clinical laboratory.

XENOBIOTICS, POISONS, AND TOXINS

Definitions of the terms, xenobiotics, poisons, and toxins overlap, yet there are some important distinctions. To provide some clarity regarding their most appropriate use, the following definitions are provided. Xenobiotics, as previously discussed above, are defined as exogenous agents that may have an adverse effect on a living organism. This term is more often used to describe environmental chemicals or drug exposures. Examples include antibiotics, anti-depressants, and environmental exposures of concern such as perfluorinated and brominated compounds. Similarly, poisons are also agents that have an adverse effect on a biological system. This term is more often used when describing animal, plant, mineral, or gas poisons. Examples include venom from poisonous snakes, poison hemlock, arsenic, or carbon monoxide poisonings, respectively. Toxins, however, are substances that are biologically synthesized either in living cells or in microorganisms. Examples include botulinum toxin produced from the microorganism, *Clostridium botulinum*, hemotoxins produced from venomous snakes, and mycotoxins produced from fungus. Should the terms toxicant or toxic be used, this applies to a substance not produced within a living cell or microorganism. It is common for environmental chemicals to be referred to as toxicants or toxic substances.

From a clinical standpoint, about 50% of poisoning cases are intentional suicide attempts. Accidental exposure accounts for about 30% of cases. The remaining cases are a result of homicide or occupational exposure. Of these, suicide has the highest mortality rate. Accidental exposure occurs most frequently in children; however, an accidental drug overdose of either therapeutic or illicit drugs is relatively common in adolescents and adults. Occupational exposure to toxicants primarily occurs in industrial and agricultural settings. Adverse health effects due to environmental toxicant exposure, however, are an expanding area of concern as we learn more about the role of these agents in contributing to disease.

ROUTES OF EXPOSURE

Toxins can enter the body via several routes, with ingestion, inhalation, and transdermal absorption being the most common ones. Of these, ingestion of toxins is most often observed in the clinical setting. For most toxins to exert a systemic effect, they must be absorbed into circulation. Absorption of toxins from the gastrointestinal tract occurs via several mechanisms. Some are taken up by processes intended for dietary nutrients. However, most are absorbed by passive diffusion. This process requires that the substance cross the cellular barriers. Hydrophobic substances have the ability to diffuse across cell membranes and, therefore, can be absorbed anywhere along the gastrointestinal tract. Ionized substances cannot passively diffuse across membranes. Weak acids can become protonated in gastric acid. The result is a nonionized species, which can be absorbed in the stomach. In a similar manner, weak bases favor absorption in the intestine, where the pH is largely neutral or slightly alkaline. Other factors can influence absorbance of toxins from the gastrointestinal tract, including the rate of dissolution, gastrointestinal motility, resistance to degradation in the gastrointestinal tract, and interaction with other substances. Toxins that are not absorbed from the gastrointestinal tract do not produce systemic effects but may produce local effects, such as diarrhea, bleeding, and malabsorption of nutrients, which may cause systemic effects secondary to toxin exposure.

DOSE–RESPONSE RELATIONSHIP

The concept that any substance has the potential to cause harm if given at the correct dosage (even water) is a central theme in toxicology. Paracelsus (1493 to 1591) pioneered the use of chemicals in medicine and coined the term "the dose makes the poison." Understanding this dose–response relationship is fundamental and relevant to modern toxicology. There is a need to establish an index of the relative toxicity of substances to allow assessment of their potential to cause pathologic effects. Several systems are available. Most correlate the dose of a xenobiotic that will result in a harmful response. One such system correlates a single acute oral dose range with the probability of a lethal outcome in an average 70-kg man (Table 31-1). This is a useful system to compare the relative toxicities of substances. The predicted response in this system is death, which is valid. However, most xenobiotics can express pathologic effects other than death at lower degrees of exposure; therefore, other indices have been developed.

A more in-depth characterization can be acquired by evaluating data from a cumulative frequency histogram of toxic responses over a range of doses. This experimental approach is typically used to evaluate several responses over a wide range of concentrations. One response monitored is the toxic response. This is the response that has been associated with an early pathologic effect at lower than lethal doses. This response has been determined to be an indicator of the toxic effects specific for that toxin. For a substance that exerts early toxic effects by damaging liver cells, the response monitored may be increases in serum alanine aminotransferase (ALT) or γ-glutamyltransferase (GGT) activity. The dose–response

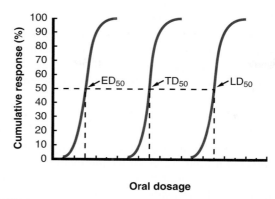

FIGURE 31-1 Dose–response relationship. Comparison of responses of a therapeutic drug over a range of doses. The ED_{50} is the dose of drug in which 50% of treated individuals will experience benefit. The TD_{50} is the dose of drug in which 50% of individuals will experience toxic adverse effects. The LD_{50} is the dose of drug in which 50% of individuals will result in mortality.

relationship implies that there will be an increase in the toxic response as the dose is increased. It should be noted that not all individuals display a toxic response at the same dose. The population variance can be seen in a cumulative frequency histogram of the percentage of people producing a toxic response over a range of concentrations (Fig. 31-1). The TD_{50} is the dose that would be predicted to produce a toxic response in 50% of the population. If the monitored response is death, the LD_{50} is the dose that would predict death in 50% of the population. Similar experiments can be used to evaluate the doses of therapeutic drugs. The ED_{50} is the dose that would be predicted to be effective or have a therapeutic benefit in 50% of the population. The therapeutic index is the ratio of the TD_{50} (or LD_{50}) to the ED_{50}. Drugs with a large therapeutic index have few toxic adverse effects when the dose of the drug is in the therapeutic range.

Dose–response relationships may apply to an individual or a population. The individual dose–response relationship pertains to changing health effects based on the change in xenobiotic exposure levels. Quantal dose–response relationships describe the change in health effects of a defined population based on changes in the exposure to xenobiotics.

Acute and Chronic Toxicity

Acute toxicity and *chronic toxicity* are terms used to relate the duration and frequency of exposure to observed toxic effects. Acute toxicity is usually associated with a single, short-term exposure to a substance, the dose of which is sufficient to cause immediate toxic effects. Chronic toxicity is usually associated with repeated frequent exposure for extended periods for greater than 3 months and possibly years, at doses that are insufficient to cause an immediate acute response. In many instances, chronic exposure

TABLE 31-1	TOXICITY RATING SYSTEM
TOXICITY RATING	**LETHAL ORAL DOSE IN AVERAGE ADULT**
Super toxic	<5 mg/kg
Extremely toxic	5–50 mg/kg
Very toxic	50–500 mg/kg
Moderately toxic	0.5–5 g/kg
Slightly toxic	5–15 g/kg
Practically nontoxic	>15 g/kg

Adapted from Klaassen CD. Principles of toxicology. In: Klaassen CD, Amdur MO, Doull J, eds. *Toxicology: The Basic Science of Poisons.* 3rd ed. New York, NY: Macmillan, 1986:13.

is related to an accumulation of the toxicant or the toxic effects within the individual. Chronic toxicity may affect different systems than those associated with acute toxicity. Therefore, dose–response relationships may differ for acute and chronic exposures for the same xenobiotic.

ANALYSIS OF TOXIC AGENTS

Toxicology testing may include both routine screening and targeted testing. Targeted testing includes examples such as when environmental risk of exposure is known, to support the investigation of a known exposure (e.g., spill, suicide attempt, and fire), to comply with occupational regulations or guidelines (e.g., OSHA), and to confirm clinical suspicions of poisoning. Due to nonspecific signs and symptoms of toxicity, as well as the fact that the duration and extent of exposure are often not known, diagnosis of most toxic element exposures depends on laboratory testing.

In general, toxicology testing is performed with urine or blood. In selecting the best specimen for a selected test, it is important to recognize that toxic agents exhibit unique absorption, distribution, metabolism, and elimination kinetics. As such, the predicted toxicokinetics of the individual element(s) involved must be coordinated with the selection of specimen, and timing of specimen collection, relative to the time of exposure. An exposure could be missed entirely if testing is performed with an inappropriate specimen. For example, an exposure to methylmercury could be missed if testing is performed with urine. An exposure to arsenic could be missed if testing is performed with blood collected a few days after the exposure.

Preanalytical variables such as elimination patterns, analyte stability, and specimen collection procedures must be considered. For urine testing, 24-hour collections are common, to compensate for elimination patterns that vary throughout a day. Normalizing results per gram of creatinine is also common. Random urine collections may not provide the most accurate profile of exposure when compared with the 24-hour collection, but they are useful for screening and qualitative detection of exposure to several potentially toxic agents. Any elevated result that is inconsistent with clinical expectations should be confirmed by testing a second specimen, or a second specimen type.

Several aspects of specimen collection, handling, and storage can introduce external contamination. Common sources of external contamination include patient clothing, skin, hair, the collection environment (e.g., dust, aerosols, and antiseptic wipes), and specimen handling variables (e.g., container, lid, and preservatives). Concentrated acids have commonly been used as urine preservatives. However, contaminants may be introduced in either the acid itself or in the process used to

add the acid to the urine (e.g., pipette tips). Specific sample collection containers (and lids) should be void of contaminating organic or inorganic agents that may interfere with analytical testing. For example, certified "trace element–free" collection tubes are available (royal blue top, for most elements; tan, for lead) for testing metals in blood. This is followed with consideration such as using acid-washed pipette tips, containers, and other supplies during handling of biological specimens for metals testing. Laboratories may also need to exercise precautions to prevent loss of toxic agents due to in vitro volatilization and metabolism. For instance, mercury and arsenic are particularly vulnerable to loss and metabolism, respectively, during sample processing and storage. These scenarios represent a fraction of the many toxicology specimen handling considerations necessary to reduce preanalytical error.

Analysis of toxic agents in a clinical setting is typically a two-step procedure. The first step is a screening test, which is a rapid, simple, qualitative procedure intended to detect specific substances or classes of toxicants. In general, these procedures have good analytic sensitivity but lack specificity. A negative result can rule out a drug or toxicant; however, a positive result should be considered a presumptive positive until confirmed by a second, more specific method. A variety of analytic methods can be used for screening and confirmatory testing. Immunoassays are commonly used to screen for drugs. In some instances, these assays are specific for a single drug (e.g., tetrahydrocannabinol [THC]). In most cases, however, drugs within general classes are detected (e.g., barbiturates and opiates). Thin-layer chromatography is a relatively simple, inexpensive method of detecting various drugs and other organic compounds. Gas chromatography (GC) is a widely used, well-established technique for the qualitative and quantitative determination of many volatile substances. The reference method for the quantitative identification of most organic compounds is GC, using a mass spectrometer as the detector. Inorganic compounds, including speciation, may be quantitated using inductively coupled plasma-mass spectrometry (ICP-MS) or atomic absorption (AA) methods.

TOXICOLOGY OF SPECIFIC AGENTS

Many chemical agents encountered on a regular basis have potential for toxicity. The focus of this section is to survey the commonly encountered nondrug toxins seen in a clinical setting, as well as those that present as medical emergencies with acute exposure.[1]

Alcohol

The toxic effects of alcohol are both general and specific. Exposure to alcohol, like exposure to most volatile organic solvents, initially causes disorientation, confusion, and euphoria, which can progress to unconsciousness, paralysis, and, with high-level exposure, even death. Most alcohols display these effects at about equivalent molar concentrations. This similarity suggests a common depressant effect on the central nervous system (CNS) that appears to be mediated by changes in membrane properties. In most cases, recovery from CNS effects is rapid and complete after cessation of exposure.

Distinct from the general CNS effects are the specific toxicities of each type of alcohol, which are usually mediated by biotransformation of alcohols to toxic products. There are several pathways by which short-chain aliphatic alcohols can be metabolized. Of these, hepatic conversion to an aldehyde, by alcohol dehydrogenase (ADH), and further conversion to an acid, by hepatic aldehyde dehydrogenase (ALDH), is the most significant.

$$\text{Alcohol} \xrightarrow{\text{ADH}} \text{Aldehyde} \xrightarrow{\text{ALDH}} \text{Acid} \qquad \text{(Eq. 31-1)}$$

Ethanol exposure is common.[2] Excessive ethanol consumption, with its associated consequences, is a leading cause of economic, social, and medical problems throughout the world. The economic impact is estimated to exceed $100 billion per year in terms of lost wages and productivity. Many social and family problems are associated with excessive ethanol consumption. The burden to the health-care system is significant. Ethanol-related disorders are consistently one of the top 10 causes of hospital admissions. About 20% of all hospital admissions have some degree of alcohol-related problems. It is estimated that 80,000 Americans die each year, either directly or indirectly, as a result of abusive alcohol consumption. This correlates to about a fivefold increase in premature mortality. In addition, consumption of ethanol during pregnancy may lead to fetal alcohol syndrome or fetal alcohol effects, both of which are associated with delayed motor and mental development in children.

Correlations have been made between blood alcohol concentration and the clinical signs and symptoms of acute intoxication. A blood alcohol level in the range of 80 mg/dL has been established as the statutory limit for operation of a motor vehicle in the United States. This is associated with a diminution of judgment and motor performance. The determination of blood ethanol concentration by the laboratory in cases of drunk driving requires an appropriate chain of custody, documentation of quality control, and proficiency testing records. About one-half of the 40,000 to 50,000 annual automobile-related fatalities in the United States involve alcohol as a factor.

Besides the short-term effects of ethanol, most pathophysiologic consequences of ethanol abuse are associated with chronic consumption over a long period. In an average adult, this correlates to the consumption of about 50 g of ethanol per day for about 10 years. Consumption to this degree has been associated with compromised function in various organ, tissue, and cell types. However, the liver is the most sensitive organ. The pathologic sequence starts with the accumulation of lipids in hepatocytes. With continued consumption, this may progress to alcoholic hepatitis. About 20% of individuals with long-term, high-level intake develop this form of toxic hepatitis. Of those who do, progression to cirrhosis is common. Cirrhosis can be characterized as fibrosis leading to a loss of functional hepatic mass. Progress through this sequence is associated with changes in many laboratory tests related to hepatic function. Several laboratory indicators of excessive ethanol consumption have sufficient diagnostic sensitivity and specificity to identify excessive ethanol consumption as the cause of a disease state. Most are related to the progression of ethanol-induced liver disease. Table 31-2 lists common laboratory indicators of prolonged hazardous consumption.

Several mechanisms have been proposed to mediate the pathologic effects of long-term ethanol consumption. Of these, adduct formation with acetaldehyde appears to play a key role. Hepatic metabolism of ethanol is a two-step enzymatic reaction. The final product is acetic acid. Acetaldehyde is a reactive intermediate in this pathway. Most ethanol is converted to acetic acid in this pathway;

TABLE 31-2	COMMON INDICATORS OF ETHANOL ABUSE
TEST	**COMMENTS**
GGT	Increases can be seen before the onset of pathologic consequences
	Increases in serum activity can occur in many non–ethanol-related conditions
AST	Increases in serum activity can occur in many non–ethanol-related conditions
AST/ALT ratio	A ratio of greater than 2.0 is highly specific for ethanol-related liver disease
HDL	High serum HDL is specific for ethanol consumption
MCV	Increased erythrocyte MCV is commonly seen with excessive ethanol consumption
	Increases are not related to folate or vitamin B_{12} deficiency

GGT, γ-glutamyltransferase; AST, aspartate aminotransferase; ALT, alanine aminotransferase; HDL, high-density lipoprotein; MCV, mean cell volume.

however, a significant portion of the intermediate is released in the free state.

$$\text{Ethnol} \rightarrow \text{Acetaldehyde} \rightarrow \text{Acetate}$$
$$\rightarrow \text{Acetaldehyde adducts} \quad \text{(Eq. 31-2)}$$

Extracellular acetaldehyde is a transient species as a result of rapid adduct formation with amine groups of proteins. Formation of acetaldehyde adducts has been shown to change the structure and function of various proteins. Many of the pathologic effects of ethanol have been correlated with the formation of these adducts.

Methanol is a common solvent. It may be ingested accidentally as a component of many commercial products or as a contaminant of homemade liquors. Methanol is initially metabolized by hepatic ADH to the intermediate formaldehyde. Formaldehyde is rapidly converted to formic acid by hepatic ALDH. The formation of formic acid causes severe acidosis, which may lead to death. Formic acid is also responsible for an optic neuropathy that may lead to blindness.

Isopropanol, also known as rubbing alcohol, is commonly available. It is metabolized by hepatic ADH to acetone, which is its primary metabolic end product. Both isopropanol and acetone have CNS depressant effects similar to ethanol. However, acetone has a long half-life. Intoxication with isopropanol, therefore, may result in severe acute-phase ethanol-like symptoms that may persist for an extended period.

Ethylene glycol (1,2-ethanediol) is a common component of hydraulic fluid and antifreeze. Ingestion by children is relatively common because of its sweet taste. The immediate effects of ethylene glycol ingestion are similar to those of ethanol. However, metabolism by hepatic ADH and ALDH results in the formation of several toxic species, including oxalic acid and glycolic acid, which results in severe metabolic acidosis. This is complicated by the rapid formation and deposition of calcium oxalate crystals in renal tubules. With high levels of consumption, calcium oxalate crystal formation may result in renal tubular damage.

Determination of Alcohols

From a medicolegal perspective, determination of blood ethanol concentration must be accurate and precise. Serum, plasma, and whole blood are acceptable specimens. Correlations have been established between ethanol concentration in these specimens and impairment of psychomotor function. Because ethanol uniformly distributes in total body water, serum, which has a greater water content than whole blood, has a higher concentration per unit volume. Most states have standardized the acceptable specimen types admissible as evidence. Some jurisdictions mandate a certain method (often GC) for legal ethanol determination.

When acquiring a specimen for ethanol determination, several preanalytical considerations are required

---

CASE STUDY 31-1

A patient with a provisional diagnosis of depression was sent to the laboratory for a routine workup. The complete blood cell count was unremarkable except for an elevated erythrocyte mean cell volume. Results of urinalysis were unremarkable. The serum chemistry testing revealed slightly increased aspartate aminotransferase, total bilirubin, and high-density lipoprotein levels. All other chemistry results, including glucose, urea, creatinine, cholesterol, pH, pCO_2, ALT, sodium, and potassium, were within the normal reference range. The physician suspects ethanol abuse; however, the patient claims to be a nonconsumer. Subsequent testing revealed a serum GGT three times the upper limit of normal. No ethanol was detected in serum. Screening tests for infectious forms of hepatitis were negative.

Questions

1. Are these results consistent with a patient who is consuming hazardous quantities of ethanol?

2. Is further testing needed to rule ethanol abuse in or out? If so, what tests would you recommend?

---

to ensure the integrity of this sample. The venipuncture site should be cleaned with an alcohol-free disinfectant. Because of the volatile nature of short-chain aliphatic alcohols, specimens must be capped at all times to avoid evaporation. Sealed specimens can be refrigerated or stored at room temperature for up to 14 days without loss of ethanol. Nonsterile specimens or those intended to be stored for long periods of time should be preserved with sodium fluoride to avoid increases in ethanol content that result from contamination due to the presence of bacterial fermentation.

Several analytic methods can be used for the determination of ethanol in serum. Among these, the enzymatic, GC, and osmometric methods are those most commonly used. When osmolarity is measured by freezing point depression, increases in serum osmolarity correlate well with increases in serum ethanol concentration. The degree of increase in osmolality due to ethanol is expressed as the difference between the measured and the calculated osmolality; the difference is called the *osmolar gap*. Serum osmolality increases by about 10 mOsm/kg for each 60 mg/dL increase in serum ethanol.

$$\text{Osmolar gap} = \text{measured osmolarity}$$
$$- \text{calculated osmolarity} \quad \text{(Eq. 31-3)}$$

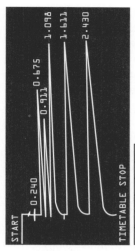

Retention Time (Minutes)	Analyte
0.675	Methanol
0.911	Acetone
1.098	Ethanol
1.611	Isopropanol
2.430	*n*-Propanol

FIGURE 31-2 Headspace gas chromatography of alcohol. The concentration of each alcohol can be determined by comparison to the response from the internal standard *n*-propanol.

This relationship is not specific for ethanol. Increases in the osmolar gap can also occur with certain metabolic imbalances; therefore, use of the osmolar gap for the determination of serum or blood ethanol concentration lacks analytic specificity. However, it is a useful screening test.

GC is the reference method for ethanol determination. This method can simultaneously quantitate other alcohols, such as methanol and isopropanol. This analysis starts with dilution of the serum or blood sample with a saturated solution of sodium chloride in a closed container. Volatiles within the liquid specimen partition into the air space (head space) of the closed container. Sampling of this head space provides clean specimens with little or no matrix effect. Quantitation of peaks can be done by constructing a standard curve or based on relative changes in proportion to an internal standard (*n*-propanol) as shown in Figure 31-2.

Enzymatic methods for the determination of ethanol are common. The enzyme used in this assay is a nonhuman form of ADH. This enzyme oxidizes ethanol to acetaldehyde with reduction of NAD^+ to NADH.

$$\text{Ethanol} + NAD^+ \xrightarrow{\text{ADH}} \text{Acetaldehyde} + \text{NADH}$$

(Eq. 31-4)

The NADH produced can be monitored directly by absorbance at 340 nm or can be coupled to an indicator reaction. This form of ADH is relatively specific for ethanol (Table 31-1). Intoxication with methanol or isopropanol produces a negative or low result; therefore, a negative result by this method does not rule out ingestion of other alcohols. There is good agreement between the enzymatic reactions of ethanol and GC. The enzymatic reactions can be fully automated and do not require specialized instrumentation.

Carbon Monoxide

Carbon monoxide is produced by incomplete combustion of carbon-containing substances. The primary environmental sources of carbon monoxide include gasoline engines, improperly ventilated furnaces, and wood or plastic fires. Carbon monoxide is a colorless, odorless, and tasteless gas that is rapidly absorbed into blood from inspired air.

When carbon monoxide binds to hemoglobin, it is called *carboxyhemoglobin (COHb)*. The affinity of carbon monoxide for hemoglobin is 200 to 225 times greater than for oxygen.[3,4] Air is about 20% oxygen by volume. If inspired air contained 0.1% carbon monoxide by volume, this would result in a 50% carboxyhemoglobinemia at equilibrium. For this reason, carbon monoxide is considered a very toxic substance. Because both carbon monoxide and oxygen compete for the same binding site, exposure to carbon monoxide results in a decrease in the concentration of oxyhemoglobin.

Carbon monoxide expresses its toxic effects by causing a leftward shift in the oxygen–hemoglobin dissociation curve, resulting in a decrease in the amount of oxygen delivered to the tissue.[3] The net effect of carbon monoxide exposure is a decrease in the amount of oxygen delivered to the tissue, producing hypoxia. The major toxic effects of carbon monoxide exposure are seen in organs with high oxygen demand, such as the brain and heart. The concentration of COHb (expressed as the percentage of COHb present to the capacity of the specimen to form COHb) and the corresponding symptoms are detailed in Table 31-3. The only treatment for carbon monoxide poisoning is 100% oxygen therapy.

TABLE 31-3	SYMPTOMS OF CARBOXYHEMOGLOBINEMIA
COHB (%)	**SYMPTOMS AND COMMENTS**
0.5	Typical in nonsmokers
5–15	Range of values seen in smokers
10	Shortness of breath with vigorous exercise
20	Shortness of breath with moderate exercise
30	Severe headaches, fatigue, impairment of judgment
40–50	Confusion, fainting on exertion
60–70	Unconsciousness, respiratory failure, death with continuous exposure
80	Immediately fatal

COHB, **carboxyhemoglobin.**

In severe cases, hyperbaric oxygen may be used. In a patient breathing 100% oxygen who has a normal respiratory function, the half-life of COHb is about 60 to 90 minutes.

Several methods are available for the evaluation of carbon monoxide poisoning. COHb has a cherry-red appearance. This is the basis of a spot test for excessive carbon monoxide exposure; 5 mL of 40% NaOH is added to 5 mL of aqueous dilution of whole blood. Persistence of a pink solution is consistent with a COHb level of 20% or greater. There are two primary quantitative assays for COHb: differential spectrophotometry and GC.

GC is an accurate and precise reference method for the determination of COHb. Carbon monoxide is released from hemoglobin after treatment with potassium ferricyanide. After analytic separation, carbon monoxide is detected by changes in thermal conductivity. Spectrophotometric methods work on the principle that different forms of hemoglobin present with different spectral absorbancy curves. By measuring absorbance at four to six different wavelengths, the concentration of the different species of hemoglobin (including COHb) can be determined by calculation. This is the most common method used and is the basis for several automated systems.

Caustic Agents

Caustic agents are found in many household products and occupational settings. Even though any exposure to a strong acid or alkaline substance is associated with injury, aspiration and ingestion present the greatest hazard. Aspiration is usually associated with pulmonary edema and shock, which can rapidly progress to death. Ingestion produces lesions in the esophagus and gastrointestinal tract, which may produce perforations. This results in hematemesis, abdominal pain, and possibly shock. The onset of metabolic acidosis or alkalosis occurs rapidly after ingestion. Corrective therapy for ingestion is usually by dilution.

Cyanide

Cyanide is classified as a supertoxic substance that can exist as a gas or solid or in solution. Exposure can occur by inhalation, ingestion, or transdermal absorption. Cyanide is used in many industrial processes. It is also a component of some insecticides and rodenticides. Cyanide is also produced as a pyrolysis product from the burning of some plastics, including urea foams used as insulation in homes. Thus, carbon monoxide and cyanide exposure may account for a significant portion of the toxicities associated with smoke inhalation. Ingestion of cyanide is a common suicide agent.

Cyanide expresses toxicity by binding to heme iron. Binding to mitochondrial cytochrome oxidase causes an uncoupling of oxidative phosphorylation. This results in rapid depletion of cellular adenosine triphosphate as a result of the inability of oxygen to accept electrons. Increases in cellular oxygen tension and venous po_2 occur as a result of lack of oxygen utilization. At low levels of exposure, patients experience headaches, dizziness, and respiratory depression, which can rapidly progress to seizure, coma, and death at slightly greater doses. Cyanide clearance is primarily mediated by rapid enzymatic conversion to thiocyanate, a nontoxic product rapidly cleared by renal filtration. Cyanide toxicity is associated with acute exposure at concentrations sufficient to exceed the rate of clearance by this enzymatic process.

Evaluation of cyanide exposure requires a rapid turnaround time. There are several methods available. Ion-specific electrode methods and photometric analysis following two-well microdiffusion separation are those most common. Chronic low-level exposure can be evaluated by the determination of urinary thiocyanate concentration.

Metals and Metalloids

Arsenic

Arsenic is a metalloid that may exist bound to or as a primary constituent of many different organic and inorganic compounds. It exists in both naturally occurring and manmade substances; therefore, exposure to arsenic may occur in various settings. Environmental exposure through air and water is prevalent in many industrialized areas. Occupational exposure occurs in agriculture and the smelting industries. It is also a common homicide and suicide agent. Ingestion of less harmful organic forms of arsenic such as arsenobetaine and arsenocholine can occur with seafood and include bivalves (clams, oysters, scallops, and mussels), crustaceans (crabs and lobsters), and some bottom feeding finfish.

Toxicity of arsenic is largely dependent on the valence state, solubility, and rate of absorption and elimination. The three major groups for arsenic include arsine gas (arsine trioxide), inorganic forms (trivalent and pentavalent), and organic forms (arsenobetaine and arsenocholine). Absorption of arsenic depends on the form of the compound. Inhalation of arsine gas demonstrates the most acute toxicity. Organic arsenic-containing compounds, such as those found in seafood, are rapidly absorbed by passive diffusion in the gastrointestinal tract. Other forms are absorbed at a slower rate. Clearance of arsenic is primarily by renal filtration of the free, ionized state. Arsenic is rapidly cleared from the blood, such that blood levels may be normal even when urine levels remain markedly elevated. The "fish arsenic" such as arsenobetaine and arsenocholine are cleared in urine within 48 hours. However, the initial half-life of inorganic arsenic is approximately 10 hours. Approximately 70% of inorganic arsenic is secreted in urine, of which 50% of excreted inorganic arsenic has been transformed to the organic form. However, these patterns may vary with the dose and clinical status of the patient. Chronic toxicity of arsenic can be due to low level, persistent exposure that may lead to bioaccumulation, or increased body burden of this metal. Arsenic expresses toxic effects by high-affinity binding to the thiol groups in proteins; therefore, this can reduce the portion available for renal filtration and elimination. Arsenic binding to proteins often results in a change in structure and function.[5] Because many proteins are capable of binding arsenic, the toxic symptoms of arsenic poisoning are nonspecific. Many cellular and organ systems are affected. Fever, anorexia, and gastrointestinal distress are seen with chronic or acute ingestion at low levels. Peripheral and central damage to the nervous system, renal effects, hemopoietic effects, and vascular disease leading to death are associated with high levels of exposure.

Analysis of arsenic is most commonly done by atomic absorption spectrophotometry (AAS). For arsenic, most forms are detectable in the blood for only a few hours. However greater than 90% of an arsenic exposure is recovered in the urine within 6 days, making urine the specimen of choice for an exposure that had occurred in the previous week.

Hair and fingernails are potential routes of elimination for toxins. For this reason, long-term exposure to toxins may be assessed in these tissues. Toxins may bind sulfhydryl groups in keratin found in hair and fingernails. Hair and fingernails are potential routes of elimination and concentrates in these tissues due to binding sulfhydryl groups in keratin. Typically, toxic element deposition in hair and fingernails is demonstrated 2 weeks after an exposure. In poisoning cases, distinct white lines of arsenic can be observed in the fingernails and this is referred to as Mees' lines.

Cadmium

Cadmium is a metal found in many industrial processes, with its main use being in electroplating and galvanizing. It is commonly encountered during the mining and processing of many metals. Cadmium is a pigment found in paints and plastics and is the cathodal material of nickel–cadmium batteries. Due to its widespread industrial applications, this element has become a significant environmental pollutant. In the environment, cadmium binds strongly to organic matter where it is immobilized in soil and taken up by the plant life and agricultural crops. Since tobacco leaves accumulate cadmium from the soil, regular use of tobacco-containing products is a common route of human cadmium exposure. Smoking is estimated to at least double the lifetime body burden of cadmium exposure. For nonsmokers, human exposure to cadmium is largely through the consumption of shellfish, organ meats, lettuce, spinach, potatoes, grains, peanuts, soybeans, and sunflower seeds.

Cadmium expresses its toxicity primarily by binding to proteins; however, it can also bind to other cellular constituents. Cadmium distributes throughout the body but has a tendency to accumulate in the kidney, where most of its toxic effects are expressed. An early finding of cadmium toxicity is manifested by renal tubular dysfunction. Tubular proteinuria, glucosuria, and aminoaciduria are typically seen. In addition to renal dysfunction, concomitant parathyroid dysfunction and vitamin D deficiency may also occur. *Itai itai* disease is characterized by severe osteomalacia and osteoporosis from the long-term consumption of cadmium-contaminated rice. Elimination of cadmium is very slow, as the biological half-life of cadmium is 10 to 30 years. Evaluation of excessive cadmium is most commonly accomplished by the determination of whole blood or urinary content using AAS.

Lead

Lead is a by-product or component of many industrial processes, which has contributed to its widespread presence in the environment. It was a common constituent of household paints before 1972 and is still found in commercial and art paints. Plumbing constructed of lead pipes or joined with leaded connectors has contributed to the lead concentration of water. Gasoline contained tetraethyl lead until 1978. This long-term utilization of leaded gasoline, lead-based paint, and lead-based construction materials has resulted in airborne lead, contaminated soil, and leaded dust.

The lead content of foods is highly variable. In the United States, the average daily intake for an adult is between 75 and 120 μg/d. This level of intake is not associated with overt toxicity. Because lead is present in all biological systems and because no physiologic or biochemical function has been found, the key issue is identifying the threshold dose that causes a toxic effect. Susceptibility to lead toxicity is dependent primarily on age. Adults are largely tolerant to the effects of lead compared with children.

Exposure to lead can occur by any route; however, ingestion of contaminated dietary constituents accounts for most exposures.[5] Gastrointestinal absorption of lead is influenced by various factors. Adults absorb 5% to 15% of ingested lead. Children have a greater degree of absorption. Infants absorb 30% to 40%. Factors controlling the rate of absorption are unclear. Absorbed lead binds with high affinity to many macromolecular structures. It distributes throughout the body. Lead distributes into two theoretical compartments. One is bone, which is the largest pool. Lead combines with the matrix of bone and can persist in this compartment for a long period. The half-life of lead in bone is longer than 20 years. The other theoretical compartment is soft tissue. The half-life of lead in this compartment is

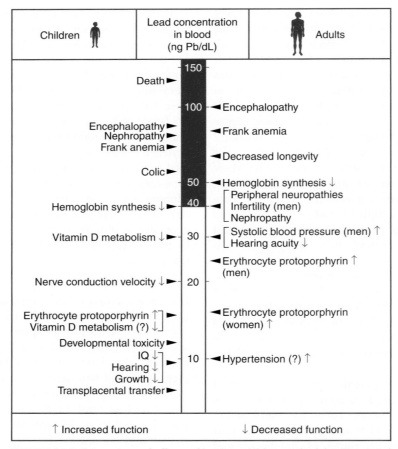

FIGURE 31-3 Comparison of effects of lead on children and adults. (Reprinted from Royce SE, Needleman HL, eds. *Case Studies in Environmental Medicine: Lead Toxicity.* Washington, DC: U.S. Public Health Service, ATSDR; 1990.)

somewhat variable; the average half-life in soft tissue is 120 days.

Elimination of lead occurs primarily by renal filtration. Because only a small fraction of total body lead presents in circulation, the elimination rate is slow. Considering the relatively constant rate of exposure and the slow elimination rate, total body lead accumulates over a lifetime. The largest accumulation occurs in bone. Significant accumulation also occurs in the kidney, bone marrow, circulating erythrocytes, and peripheral and central nerves.

Lead toxicity is multifaceted and occurs in a dose-dependent manner (Fig. 31-3). Abdominal or neurological symptoms manifest after acute exposure only. The neurologic effects of lead are of particular importance. Lead exposure causes encephalopathy characterized by a cerebral edema and ischemia. Severe lead poisoning can result in stupor, convulsions, and coma. Lower levels of exposure may not present with these symptoms. However, low-level exposure may result in subclinical effects typified by behavioral changes, hyperactivity, attention deficit disorder, and a decrease in intelligence

quotient (IQ) scores. Higher levels of exposure have been associated with demyelinization of peripheral nerves, which results in a decrease in nerve conduction velocity.

Children appear particularly sensitive to these effects and are now evaluated for lead poisoning before entry into school. The normal threshold for blood lead levels (BLL) set by the Centers for Disease Control and Prevention is 10 µg/dL. However, many states have lowered the upper limit of normal to 5 µg/dL. Growth deficits are seen in children with BLL greater than 10 µg/dL and anemia may occur at a BLL of 20 µg/dL. Children with a BLL less than 10 µg/dL have been reported to suffer from permanent IQ and hearing deficits. Currently, a threshold identifying permanent effects of lead poisoning is not known.

Lead is a potent inhibitor of many enzymes; this inhibition mediates many toxic effects. Noteworthy are the effects on vitamin D metabolism and the heme synthetic pathway. This results in changes in bone and calcium metabolism and in anemia. Decreased serum concentrations of both 25-hydroxy and 1,25-dihydroxy vitamin D are seen in excessive lead exposure. The anemia is primarily caused by an inhibition of the heme synthetic pathway, which results in increases in the concentration of several intermediates in this pathway, including aminolevulinic acid and protoporphyrin. Increases in protoporphyrin result in high concentrations of zinc protoporphyrin in circulating erythrocytes. Zinc protoporphyrin is a highly fluorescent compound. Measurement of this fluorescence has been used to screen for lead toxicity. Increased urinary aminolevulinic acid is a highly sensitive and specific indicator of lead toxicity that correlates well with blood levels. Another hematologic finding is the presence of basophilic stippling in erythrocytes as a result of inhibition of erythrocytic pyrimidine nucleotidase. This enzyme is responsible for the removal of residual DNA after extrusion of the nucleus. Basophilic stippling is a sensitive indicator of lead exposure.

Excessive lead exposure has also been associated with hypertension, carcinogenesis, birth defects, and compromised immunity. Lead causes several toxic renal effects. Early stages are associated with tubular dysfunction, resulting in glycosuria, aminoaciduria, and hyperphosphaturia. Late stages are associated with tubular atrophy and glomerular fibrosis. The fibrosis may result in a decreased glomerular filtration rate.

Treatment of lead poisoning involves removal from exposure and treatment with therapeutic chelators, such as ethylenediaminetetraacetic acid and dimercaptosuccinic acid. These substances are capable of removing lead from soft tissue and bone by forming low molecular weight, high-affinity complexes that can be cleared by renal filtration. The efficacy of this therapy is determined by monitoring the urinary concentration of lead.

The assessment of total body burden of lead poisoning is best evaluated by the quantitative determination of lead concentration in whole blood. The use of urine is also valid but correlates closer to the level of recent exposure. Care must be taken during specimen collection to ensure that the specimen does not become contaminated from exogenous sources. Lead-free containers are recommended for this purpose.

Several methods can be used to measure lead concentration. Chromogenic reactions and anodic stripping voltametry methods have been used, but they lack clinical utility because they lack analytic sensitivity. Point of care units have employed these methodologies to screen for lead exposure in children or adults in the workplace. X-ray fluorescence is a methodology used to measure screening for environmental levels of lead in nonbiological samples such as soil and foods. Whereas graphite furnace AAS has been used to confirm whole BLLs, a new standard of measurement has been set with quantitative ICP-MS.

Mercury

Mercury is a metal that exists in three forms: elemental (liquid at room temperature), inorganic salts, and as a component of organic compounds. Exposure occurs primarily by inhalation and ingestion. Consumption of contaminated foods is the major source of exposure in the general population. Inhalation and accidental ingestion of inorganic and organic forms in industrial settings is the most common reason for toxic levels. Each form of mercury has different toxicologic characteristics. Elemental mercury (Hg^0) can be ingested without significant effects. Inhalation of elemental mercury is insignificant because of its low vapor pressure. Cationic mercury (Hg^{2+}) is moderately toxic. Organic mercury, such as methyl mercury (CH_3Hg^+), is very toxic. Considering that the most common route of exposure to mercury is via ingestion, the primary factor that determines toxicity is gastrointestinal absorbance.

Elemental mercury is largely not absorbed because of its viscous liquid nature. Inorganic mercury is only partially absorbed. Although not significantly absorbed, inorganic mercury still has significant local toxicity in the gastrointestinal tract. The portion that is absorbed distributes uniformly throughout the body. The organic forms of mercury are rapidly and efficiently absorbed by passive diffusion. Systemic organic mercury partitions into hydrophobic compartments. This results in high concentrations in the brain and peripheral nerves.[5] In these lipophilic compartments, organic mercury is biotransformed to the divalent state, allowing it to bind to neuronal proteins. Elimination of systemic mercury occurs primarily via renal filtration of bound low molecular weight species or the free (ionized) state. Considering that most mercury is bound to protein, the elimination rate is slow. Therefore, chronic exposure exerts a cumulative effect.

Mercury toxicity is a result of protein binding, which results in a change of structure and function. The most significant result of this interaction is the inhibition of many enzymes. Binding to intestinal proteins after ingestion of inorganic mercury results in acute gastrointestinal disturbances. Ingestion of moderate amounts may result in severe bloody diarrhea because of ulceration and necrosis of the gastrointestinal tract. In severe cases, this may lead to shock and death. The absorbed portion of ingested inorganic mercury affects many organs. Clinical findings include tachycardia, tremors, thyroiditis, and, most significantly, a disruption of renal function. The renal effect is associated with glomerular proteinuria and loss of tubular function. Organic mercury may also have a renal effect at high levels of exposure. However, neurologic symptoms are the primary toxic effects of this hydrophobic form. Low levels of exposure cause tremors, behavioral changes, mumbling speech, and loss of balance. Higher levels of exposure result in hyporeflexia, hypotension, bradycardia, renal dysfunction, and death. Analysis of mercury is by AA, using whole blood or an aliquot of a 24-hour urine specimen or an anodal stripping voltametry. Analysis of mercury by AA requires special techniques as a result of the volatility of elemental mercury.

Pesticides

Pesticides are substances that have been intentionally added to the environment to kill or harm an undesirable life form. Pesticides can be classified into several categories, such as insecticides and herbicides. These agents have been applied for the control of vector-borne disease and urban pests and to improve agricultural productivity. Pesticides can be found in occupational settings and in the home; therefore, there are frequent opportunities for exposure. Contamination of food is the major route of exposure for the general population. Inhalation, transdermal absorption, and ingestion as a result of hand-to-mouth contact are common occupational and accidental routes of exposure.

Ideally, the actions of pesticides would be target specific. Unfortunately, most are nonselective and result in toxic effects to many nontarget species, including humans. Pesticides come in many different forms with a wide range of potential toxic effects. The health effects of short-term, low-level exposure to most of these agents have yet to be well elucidated. Extended low-level exposure to low levels may result in chronic disease states. Of primary concern is high-level exposure, which may result in acute disease states or death. The most common victims of acute poisoning are people who are applying pesticides and do not take appropriate precautions to avoid exposure. Ingestion by children at home is also common. Pesticide ingestion is also a common suicide vehicle.

There is a wide variation in the chemical configuration of pesticides, ranging from simple salts of heavy metals to complex high molecular weight organic compounds. Insecticides are the most prevalent of pesticides. Based on chemical configuration, the organophosphates, carbamates, and halogenated hydrocarbons are the most common insecticides. Organophosphates are the most abundant pesticides and are responsible for about one-third of all pesticide poisonings.

Organophosphates and carbamates function by inhibition of acetylcholinesterase, an enzyme present in both insects and mammals. In mammals, acetylcholine is a neurotransmitter found in both central and peripheral nerves. It is also responsible for the stimulation of muscle cells and several endocrine/exocrine glands. The actions of acetylcholine are terminated by the actions of membrane-bound, postsynaptic acetylcholinesterase. Inhibition of this enzyme by this agent results in the prolonged presence of acetylcholine on its receptor, which produces a wide range of systemic effects. Low levels of exposure are associated with salivation, lacrimation, and involuntary urination and defecation. Higher levels

of exposure result in bradycardia, muscular twitching, cramps, apathy, slurred speech, and behavioral changes. Death due to respiratory failure may also occur.

Absorbed organophosphates bind with high affinity to several proteins, including acetylcholinesterase. Protein binding prevents the direct analysis of organophosphates. Thus, exposure is evaluated indirectly by the measurement of acetylcholinesterase inhibition. Inhibition of this enzyme has been found to be a sensitive and specific indicator of organophosphate exposure. Because acetylcholinesterase is a membrane-bound enzyme, serum activity is low. To increase the analytic sensitivity of this assay, erythrocytes that have high surface activity are commonly used. Evaluation of erythrocytic acetylcholinesterase activity for detection of organophosphate exposure, however, is not commonly performed in reference laboratories because of low demand and the lack of an automated method.

An alternative test that has become commonly available is the measurement of serum pseudocholinesterase (SChE) activity. This enzyme is inhibited by organophosphates in a similar manner to the erythrocytic enzyme. Unlike the erythrocytic enzyme, however, changes in the serum activity of SChE lack sensitivity and specificity for organophosphate exposure. Pseudocholinesterase is found in the liver, pancreas, brain, and serum. The biological function of this enzyme is not well defined. Decreased levels of SChE can occur in acute infection, pulmonary embolism, hepatitis, and cirrhosis. There are also several variants of this enzyme that demonstrate diminished activity. Thus, decreases in SChE are not specific for organophosphate poisoning. The normal reference range for SChE is between 4,000 and 12,000 U/L. The intraindividual variation (the degree of variance within an average individual) is about 700 U/L. Symptoms associated with organophosphate toxicity occur at about a 40% reduction in activity. An individual whose normal SChE is on the high side of the normal reference range and who has been exposed to toxic levels of organophosphates may still have SChE activity in the normal reference range. Because of these factors, determination of SChE activity lacks sensitivity in the diagnosis of organophosphate poisoning. Therefore, SChE is considered a screening test, and clinical context must be taken into consideration when interpreting the results. Immediate antidotal therapy can be initiated in cases of suspected organophosphate poisoning with a decreased activity of SChE. However, continuation of therapy and documentation of such poisoning should be confirmed by testing of the erythrocytic enzyme.

TOXICOLOGY OF THERAPEUTIC DRUGS

Many overdose situations are the result of accidental or intentional excessive dosage of pharmaceutical drugs. All drugs are capable of toxic effects at the right dosage. This discussion focuses on the therapeutic drugs most commonly seen in clinical overdose situations.

Salicylates

Aspirin (acetylsalicylic acid) is a commonly used analgesic, antipyretic, and anti-inflammatory drug. It functions by decreasing thromboxane and prostaglandin formation through the inhibition of cyclooxygenase. At recommended doses, there are several noteworthy adverse effects, including interference with platelet aggregation and gastrointestinal function. There is also an epidemiologic relationship between aspirin, childhood viral infections (e.g., varicella and influenza), and the onset of Reye's syndrome.

Acute ingestion of high doses of aspirin is associated with various toxic effects through several different mechanisms.[1] Because it is an acid, excessive salicylate ingestion is associated with a metabolic acidosis. Salicylate is also a direct stimulator of the respiratory center. The hyperventilation produces a respiratory alkalosis. In many instances, the net result is an immediate mixed acid–base disturbance. Salicylates also inhibit the Krebs cycle, resulting in excess conversion of pyruvate to lactate. In addition, at high levels of exposure, salicylates stimulate mobilization and use of free fatty acid, resulting in excess ketone body formation. All these factors contribute to a metabolic acidosis that may lead to death. Treatment for overdose involves neutralizing and eliminating the excess acid and maintaining electrolyte balance.

Correlations have been established between serum concentrations of salicylates and toxic outcomes. Several methods are available for the quantitative determination of salicylate in serum. GC or liquid chromatography methods provide the highest analytic sensitivity and specificity but have not found clinical use because of equipment expense and technical difficulty. Several immunoassay methods are available; the most common method is a chromogenic assay known as the Trinder reaction, which reacts salicylate with ferric nitrate to form a colored complex that is then evaluated spectrophotometrically.

Acetaminophen

Acetaminophen, either solely or in combination with other compounds, is a commonly used analgesic drug. In healthy subjects, therapeutic dosages have few adverse effects. Overdose of acetaminophen, however, is associated with a severe hepatotoxicity (Fig. 31-4).

Absorbed acetaminophen is bound with high affinity to various proteins, resulting in a low free fraction. Thus, renal filtration of the parent drug is minimal. Most is eliminated by hepatic uptake, biotransformation, conjugation, and excretion. Acetaminophen can

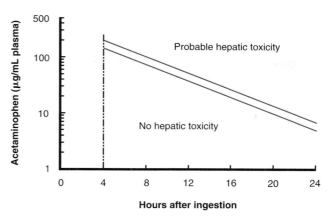

FIGURE 31-4 Rumack-Matthew nomogram. Prediction of acetaminophen-induced hepatic damage based on serum concentration. (Reprinted with permission from Rumack BH, Matthew H. Acetaminophen poisoning and toxicity. *Pediatrics*. 1975;55:871.)

follow several different pathways through this process, each forming a different product. The pathway of major concern is the hepatic mixed-function oxidase system. In this system, acetaminophen is first transformed to reactive intermediates, which are then conjugated with reduced glutathione. In overdose situations, glutathione can become depleted, yet reactive intermediates continue to be produced. This results in an accumulation of reactive intermediates inside the cell. Because some intermediates are free radicals, this results in a toxic effect to the cell that leads to necrosis of the liver, the organ in which these reactions are occurring.

The time frame for the onset of hepatocyte damage is relatively long. In an average adult, serum indicators of hepatic damage do not become abnormal until 3 to 5 days after ingestion of a toxic dose. The initial symptoms of acetaminophen toxicity are vague, nonspecific, and not predictive of hepatic necrosis.[6] The serum concentration of acetaminophen that results in depletion of glutathione has been determined for an average adult. Unfortunately, acetaminophen is rapidly cleared from serum and determination of serum acetaminophen is often made many hours after ingestion. In these situations, it is unknown whether toxic concentrations of acetaminophen were present at some previous time. To aid in this situation, nomograms (Fig. 31-4) are available that predict hepatotoxicity based on serum concentrations of acetaminophen at a known time after ingestion. It is also noteworthy that chronic, heavy consumers of ethanol metabolize acetaminophen at a more rapid rate than average, resulting in a more rapid formation of reactive intermediates and an increased possibility of depleting glutathione. Therefore, alcoholic patients are more susceptible to acetaminophen toxicity, and using the nomogram for interpretation in these patients is inappropriate.

The reference method for the quantitation of acetaminophen in serum is high-performance liquid chromatography. This method, however, is not widely used in clinical settings because of expense and technical difficulty. Immunoassay is currently the most common analytic method used for serum acetaminophen determination. Competitive enzyme or fluorescence polarization immunoassay systems are most frequently used.

TOXICOLOGY OF DRUGS OF ABUSE

Assessment of drug abuse is of medical interest for many reasons. In drug overdose, it is essential to identify the responsible agent to ensure appropriate treatment. In a similar manner, identification of drug abuse in nonoverdose situations provides a rationale for the treatment of addiction. For these reasons, testing for drugs of abuse is commonly done. This typically involves screening of a single urine specimen for many substances by qualitative screening procedures. In most instances, this procedure only detects recent drug use; therefore, with abstinence of relatively short duration, many abusing patients may not be identified. In addition, a positive drug screen cannot discriminate between single casual use and chronic abuse. Identification of chronic abuse usually involves several positive test results in conjunction with clinical evaluation. In a similar manner, a positive drug screen does not determine the time frame or dose of the drug taken. Drug abuse or overdose can occur with prescription, over-the-counter, or illicit drugs. The focus of this discussion is on substances with addictive potential.

The use of drugs for recreational or performance enhancement purposes is relatively common. The National Institute on Drug Abuse reports that about 30% of the population older than high school age have used an illicit drug. Testing for drug abuse has become commonplace in professional, industrial, and athletic settings. The potential punitive measures associated with this testing may involve or result in civil or criminal litigation. Therefore, the laboratory must ensure that data are legally admissible and defendable. This requires the use of analytic methods that have been validated as accurate and precise. It also requires documentation of specimen security. Protocols and procedures must be established that prevent and detect specimen adulteration and that may prevent drug detection. Measurement of urinary temperature, pH, specific gravity, and creatinine is commonly done to ensure that these specimens have not been diluted or treated with substances that may interfere with testing. Specimen collection should be monitored and a chain of custody established to guard against specimen exchange.

Testing for drugs of abuse can be done by several methods. A two-tiered approach of screening and confirmation is usually used. Screening procedures should be simple, rapid, inexpensive, and capable of being automated. They are often referred to as *spot tests*. In general, screening procedures have good analytic sensitivity with marginal specificity; a negative result can rule out an analyte with a reasonable degree of certainty. These methods usually detect classes of drugs based on similarities in chemical configuration. This allows the detection of parent compounds and congeners that have similar effects. Considering that many designer drugs are modified forms of established drugs of abuse, these methods increase the scope of the screening process. A drawback to this type of analysis is that it may also detect chemically related substances that have no or low abuse potential; therefore, interpretation of positive test results requires integration of clinical context and further testing. Confirmation testing uses methods that have high sensitivity and specificity; many of these tests provide quantitative as well as qualitative information. Confirmatory testing requires the use of a method different from that used in the screening procedure. GC–mass spectrophotometry (GC/MS) is the reference method for confirmation of most analytes.

There are several general analytic procedures commonly used for the analysis of drugs of abuse. Chromogenic reactions, the generation of a colored product usually by a chemical reaction, are occasionally used as screening procedures. Immunoassay-based procedures are widely used as both screening and confirmatory assays. In general, immunoassays offer a high degree of sensitivity and are easily automated. A wide variety of chromatography techniques are used for the qualitative identification and quantitation of drugs. Thin-layer chromatography is an inexpensive method for the screening of many drugs and has the advantage that no instrumentation is required. GC and liquid chromatography allow complex mixtures of drugs to be separated and quantitated. These methods are generally labor intensive and not well suited to screening.

Many drugs have the potential for abuse. Trends in drug abuse vary geographically and between different socioeconomic groups. For a clinical laboratory to provide an effective service requires knowledge of the drug or drug groups likely to be found within the patient population it serves. Fortunately, the process of selecting which drugs to test for has been aided by national studies that have identified the drugs of abuse most commonly seen in the population (Table 31-4). This provides the basis for test selection in most situations. The following discussion focuses on select drugs with a high potential for abuse.

Amphetamines

Amphetamine and methamphetamine are therapeutic drugs used for narcolepsy and attention deficit disorder. These drugs are stimulants with a high abuse potential. They produce an initial sense of increased mental and

TABLE 31-4	PREVALENCE OF COMMON DRUGS OF ABUSE
SUBSTANCE	**PREVALENCE (%)**
Alcohol	58
Marijuana	16
Cocaine	2–3
Benzodiazepines	?
Barbiturates	?
Opiates (heroin only)	0.2
Phencyclidine	0
MDMA	1
Amphetamines	0.1–1
Other stimulants	1.3
Other sedatives–hypnotics	0.2

MDMA, methylenedioxymethylamphetamine.

This table provides approximate frequencies of relevant drugs of abuse as surveyed from national data. The percentage values estimate the prevalence of use in individuals aged 18–25, the most common users, who by survey claim to have used drugs within the past 30 d. (Adapted from Department of Health and Human Services, Substance Abuse and Mental Health Administration, and Office of Applied Studies. Results from the 2006 National Survey on Drug Use and Health: national findings. Retrieved February 8, 2008, from http://www.drugabusestatistics.samhsa.gov/nsduh/2k6nsduh/2k6Results.pdf.)

CASE STUDY 31-2

An emergency department patient with a provisional diagnosis of overdose with an over-the-counter cold medicine undergoes a drug screen. Test results from immunoassay screening were negative for opiates, barbiturates, benzodiazepines, THC, and cocaine but positive for amphetamines. The salicylate level was 15 times the upper limit of the therapeutic range. Results for acetaminophen and ethanol were negative.

Questions

1. What would be the expected results of arterial blood gas analysis?

2. What would be the expected results of a routine urinalysis?

3. What are some of the possible reasons the amphetamine screen is positive?

physical capacity along with a perception of well-being. These initial effects are followed by restlessness, irritability, and possibly psychosis. Abatement of these late effects is often countered with repeated use. Tolerance and psychological dependence develop with chronic use. Overdose, although rare in experienced users, results in hypertension, cardiac arrhythmias, convulsions, and possibly death. Various compounds chemically related to amphetamines are components of over-the-counter medications, including ephedrine, pseudoephedrine, and phenylpropanolamine. These amphetamine-like compounds are common in allergy and cold medications.

Identification of amphetamine abuse involves analysis of urine for the parent drugs. Immunoassay systems are commonly used as the screening procedure. Because of variable cross-reactivity with over-the-counter medications that contain amphetamine-like compounds, a positive result by immunoassay is considered presumptive. Confirmation of immunoassay-positive tests is most commonly made with liquid chromatography or GC.

Methylenedioxymethylamphetamine

Methylenedioxymethylamphetamine (MDMA) is an illicit amphetamine derivative that is commonly referred to as "ecstasy."[7,8] Although it had been associated with club culture in the 1990s, its use has continued to grow.

It has a high potential for abuse. There are also as many as 200 "designer" analogues that have been developed to produce effects comparable to those of MDMA. MDMA and its analogues are primarily administered orally in tablets of 50 to 150 mg. Other, less-frequent routes of administration are inhalation, injection, or smoking. Its circulating half-life is 8 to 9 hours. The majority of the drug is eliminated by hepatic metabolism, although 20% is eliminated unchanged in the urine.

The onset of effect is 30 to 60 minutes and duration is about 3.5 hours. The desired effects include hallucinations, euphoria, empathic and emotional responses, and increased visual and tactile sensitivity. Its adverse effects include headaches, nausea, vomiting, anxiety agitation, impaired memory, violent behavior, tachycardia, hypertension, respiratory depression, seizures, hyperthermia, cardiac toxicity, liver toxicity, and renal failure. The presenting symptoms along with patient behavior and history must be taken into account as routine drug screening by immunoassay of a urine specimen will usually not test positive. Further analysis and confirmation of MDMA use are completed with GC/MS.

Anabolic Steroids

Anabolic steroids are a group of compounds related chemically to the male sex hormone testosterone. These artificial substances were developed in the 1930s as a therapy for male hypogonadism. It was soon discovered that the use of these compounds in healthy subjects increases muscle mass. In many instances, this results in an improvement in athletic performance. Recent studies have reported that 6.5% of adolescent boys and 1.9% of girls reported the use of steroids without a prescription.

Most illicit steroids are obtained through the black market from underground laboratories and foreign sources. The quality and purity of these drugs are highly variable. In most instances, the acute toxic effects of these drugs are related to inconsistent formulation, which may result in high dosages and impurities. A variety of both physical and psychological effects have been associated with steroid abuse. Chronic use of steroids has been associated with a toxic hepatitis. Chronic use has also been associated with accelerated atherosclerosis and abnormal aggregation of platelets, both of which predispose to stroke and myocardial infarction. In addition, steroid abuse causes an enlargement of the heart. In this condition, heart muscle cells develop faster than the associated vasculature. This may lead to ischemia of heart muscle cells, which predisposes to cardiac arrhythmias and possible sudden death. In males, chronic steroid use is associated with testicular atrophy, sterility, and impotence. In females, it causes the development of masculine traits, breast reduction, and sterility.

Evaluation of anabolic steroid use can be challenging. Until recently, the primary forms abused were animal derived or synthetic forms. There are several, well-established methods for the detection of the parent drug and its metabolite for the majority of these. The newer forms are very difficult or may be difficult to detect. To address this and related issues, the ratio of testosterone to epitestosterone is commonly used as a screening test. High ratios are associated with exogenous testosterone administration.[9]

Cannabinoids

Cannabinoids are a group of psychoactive compounds found in marijuana. Of these, THC is the most potent and abundant. Marijuana, or its processed product, hashish, can be smoked or ingested. A sense of well-being and euphoria is the subjective effect of exposure. It is also associated with an impairment of short-term memory and intellectual function. Effects of chronic use have not been well established. Overdose has not been associated with specific physiologic toxic outcomes. Tolerance and a mild dependence may develop with chronic use. THC is a lipophilic substance, which is rapidly removed from circulation by passive distribution into hydrophobic compartments, such as brain and fat. This results in slow elimination as a result of redistribution back into circulation and subsequent hepatic metabolism.

The half-life of THC in circulation is 1 day after a single use and 3 to 5 days in chronic, heavy consumers. Hepatic metabolism of THC produces several products that are primarily eliminated in urine. The major urinary metabolite is 11-nor-tetrahydrocannabinol-9-carboxylic acid (THC-COOH). This metabolite can be detected in urine for 3 to 5 days after a single use or for up to 4 weeks in a chronic, heavy consumer after abstinence. Immunoassay for THC-COOH is the basis of the screening test for marijuana consumption. GC/MS is used for confirmation. Both methods are sensitive and specific. Because of the low limit of detection of these methods, it is possible to find THC-COOH in urine as a result of passive inhalation. Urinary concentration standards have been established that can discriminate between passive and direct inhalation.

Cocaine

Cocaine is an effective local anesthetic with few adverse effects at therapeutic concentrations. At higher circulating concentrations, it is a potent CNS stimulator that elicits a sense of excitement and euphoria. Cocaine is an alkaloid salt that can be administered directly (e.g., by insufflation or intravenous injection) or inhaled as a vapor when smoked in the free-base form (crack). It has a high abuse potential. The half-life of the circulating cocaine is brief: 0.5 to 1 hour. Acute cocaine toxicity is associated with hypertension, arrhythmia, seizure, and myocardial infarction. Both subjective and toxic effects are expressed when circulating concentrations are rising. Because of its short half-life, maintaining the subjective effects over a single extended period requires repeated dosages of increasing quantity; therefore, correlations between serum concentration and the subjective or toxic effects cannot be established. Because the rate of change is more important than the serum concentration, a primary factor that determines the toxicity of cocaine is the dose and route of administration. Intravenous administration presents with the greatest hazard, closely followed by smoking.

Cocaine's short half-life is a result of rapid hepatic hydrolysis to inactive metabolites. This is the major route of elimination. Only a small portion of the parent drug can be found in urine after an administered dose. The primary product of hepatic metabolism is benzoylecgonine, which is primarily eliminated in urine. The half-life of benzoylecgonine is 4 to 7 hours. The presence of this metabolite in urine is a sensitive and specific indicator of cocaine use. It can be detected in urine for up to 3 days after a single use. In chronic heavy abusers, it can be detected in urine for up to 20 days after the last dose. The primary screening procedure for identification of cocaine use is the detection of benzoylecgonine in urine by immunoassay. Confirmation testing is done by GC/MS.

Opiates

Opiates are a class of substances capable of analgesia, sedation, and anesthesia. All are derived from or chemically related to substances derived from the opium poppy. The naturally occurring substances include opium, morphine, and codeine. Heroin, hydromorphone (Dilaudid), and oxycodone (Percodan) are chemically modified forms of the naturally occurring opiates. Meperidine (Demerol), methadone (Dolophine), propoxyphene (Darvon), pentazocine (Talwin), and fentanyl (Sublimaze) are the common synthetic opiates. Opiates have a high abuse potential. Chronic use leads to tolerance with physical and psychological dependence. Acute overdose presents with respiratory acidosis due to depression of respiratory centers, myoglobinuria, and possibly an increase in serum indicators of cardiac damage (e.g., CKMB and troponin). High-level opiate overdose may lead to death caused by cardiopulmonary failure. Treatment of overdose includes the use of the opiate antagonist naloxone.

Laboratory testing for opiates usually involves initial detection (screening) by immunoassay. Most immunoassays are primarily designed to detect morphine and codeine. However, cross-reactivity as a result of similarities in chemical structure allows detection of many of the opiates: naturally occurring, chemically modified, and synthetic. GC/MS is the confirmatory method of choice.

Phencyclidine

Phencyclidine (PCP) is an illicit drug with stimulant, depressant, anesthetic, and hallucinogenic properties. It has a high abuse potential. Adverse effects are commonly noted at doses that produce the desired subjective effects, such as agitation, hostility, and paranoia. Overdose is associated with stupor and coma. PCP can be ingested or inhaled by smoking PCP-laced tobacco or marijuana. It is a lipophilic drug that rapidly distributes into fat and brain. Elimination is slow as a result of redistribution into circulation and hepatic metabolism.

About 10% to 15% of an administered dose is eliminated unchanged in urine. Hepatic metabolism forms various products. Identification of PCP abuse is by detection of the parent drug in urine. In chronic heavy users, PCP can be detected 7 to 30 days after abstinence. Immunoassay is used as the screening procedure. GC/MS is the confirmatory method.

Sedatives–Hypnotics

Many therapeutic drugs can be classified as sedatives–hypnotics or tranquilizers. All members of this class are CNS depressants. They have a wide range of therapeutic roles and are commonly used. Most of these drugs have abuse potential, ranging from high to low. These drugs become available for illegal use through diversion from approved sources. Barbiturates and benzodiazepines are the most common types of sedative hypnotics abused. Although barbiturates have a higher abuse potential, benzodiazepines are more commonly found in abuse and overdose situations. This appears to be a result of availability. There are many individual drugs within the barbiturate and benzodiazepine classification. Secobarbital, pentobarbital, and phenobarbital are the more commonly abused barbiturates. Diazepam (Valium), chlordiazepoxide (Librium), and lorazepam (Ativan) are commonly abused benzodiazepines. Overdose with sedatives–hypnotics initially presents with lethargy and slurred speech, which can rapidly progress to coma. Respiratory depression is the most serious toxic effect of most of these agents. Hypotension can occur with barbiturates. The toxicity of many of these agents is potentiated by ethanol.

Immunoassay is the most common screening procedure for both barbiturates and benzodiazepines. Broad cross-reactivity within members of each group allows for the detection of many individual drugs. GC or liquid chromatography can be used for confirmatory testing.

For additional student resources please visit thePoint at **http://thepoint.lww.com. thePoint** ✴

QUESTIONS

1. Compound A is reported to have an oral LD$_{50}$ of 5 mg/kg body weight. Compound B is reported to have an LD$_{50}$ of 50 mg/kg body weight. Of the following statements regarding the relative toxicity of these two compounds, which is TRUE?

   a. Ingestion of low amounts of compound A would be predicted to cause more deaths than an equal dose of compound B.

   b. Ingestion of compound B would be expected to produce nontoxic effects at a dose greater than 100 mg/kg body weight.

   c. Neither compound A nor compound B is toxic at any level of oral exposure.

   d. Compound A is more rapidly adsorbed from the gastrointestinal tract than compound B.

   e. Compound B would be predicted to be more toxic than compound A if the exposure route were transdermal.

2. Which of the following statements best describes the TD_{50} of a compound?
   a. The dosage of a substance that would be predicted to cause a toxic effect in 50% of the population
   b. The dosage of a substance that is lethal to 50% of the population
   c. The dosage of a substance that would produce therapeutic benefit in 50% of the population
   d. The percentage of individuals who would experience a toxic response at 50% of the lethal dose
   e. The percentage of the population who would experience a toxic response after an oral dosage of 50 mg

3. Of the following analytic methods, which is most commonly used as the confirmatory method for identification of drugs of abuse?
   a. GC with mass spectrometry
   b. Scanning differential calorimetry
   c. Ion-specific electrode
   d. Immunoassay
   e. Nephelometry

4. A weakly acidic toxin ($pK_a = 4.0$) that is ingested will
   a. Be passively absorbed in the stomach ($pH = 3.0$)
   b. Not be absorbed because it is ionized
   c. Not be absorbed unless a specific transporter is present
   d. Be passively absorbed in the colon ($pH = 7.5$)
   e. Be absorbed only if a weak base is ingested at the same time

5. What is the primary product of methanol metabolism by the ADH and ALDH system?
   a. Formic acid
   b. Acetone
   c. Acetaldehyde
   d. Oxalic acid
   e. Formaldehyde

6. Which of the following statements concerning cyanide toxicity is TRUE?
   a. Inhalation of smoke from burning plastic is a common cause of cyanide exposure, and cyanide expresses its toxicity by inhibition of oxidative phosphorylation.
   b. Inhalation of smoke from burning plastic is a common cause of cyanide exposure.
   c. Cyanide is a relatively nontoxic compound that requires chronic exposure to produce a toxic effect.

   d. Cyanide expresses its toxicity by inhibition of oxidative phosphorylation.
   e. All of these are true.

7. Which of the following laboratory results would be consistent with acute high-level oral exposure to an inorganic form of mercury (Hg^{2+})?
   a. All of these
   b. High concentrations of mercury in whole blood and urine
   c. Proteinuria
   d. Positive occult blood in stool
   e. None of these

8. A child presents with microcytic, hypochromic anemia. The physician suspects iron-deficiency anemia. Further laboratory testing reveals a normal total serum iron and iron-binding capacity; however, the zinc protoporphyrin level was very high. A urinary screen for porphyrins was positive. Erythrocytic basophilic stippling was noted on the peripheral smear. Which of the following laboratory tests would be best applied to this case?
   a. Whole blood lead
   b. Urinary thiocyanate
   c. COHb
   d. Urinary anabolic steroids
   e. Urinary benzoylecgonine

9. A patient with suspected organophosphate poisoning presents with a low SChE level. However, the confirmatory test, erythrocyte acetylcholinesterase, presents with a normal result. Excluding analytic error, which of the following may explain these conflicting results?
   a. The patient has late-stage hepatic cirrhosis, or the patient has a variant of SChE that displays low activity.
   b. The patient has late-stage hepatic cirrhosis.
   c. The patient was exposed to low levels of organophosphates.
   d. The patient has a variant of SChE that displays low activity.
   e. All of these are correct.

10. A patient enters the emergency department in a coma. The physician suspects a drug overdose. Immunoassay screening tests for opiates, barbiturates, benzodiazepines, THC, amphetamines, and PCP were all negative. No ethanol was detected in serum. Can the physician rule out drug overdose as the cause of this coma with these results?
   a. No
   b. Yes
   c. Maybe

REFERENCES

1. Eldridge DL, Holstege CP. Utilizing the laboratory in the poisoned patient. *Clin Lab Med.* 2006;26:13-30.
2. Thorne D, Kaplan KJ. Laboratory indicators of ethanol consumption. *Clin Lab Sci.* 1999;120:343.
3. Kao LW, Nanagas KA. Toxicity associated with carbon monoxide. *Clin Lab Med.* 2006;26:99-125.
4. Widdop B. Analysis of carbon monoxide. *Ann Clin Biochem.* 2002;39:378-391.
5. Ibrahim D, Froberg B, Wolf A, Rusyniak DE. Heavy metal poisoning: clinical presentations and pathophysiology. *Clin Lab Med.* 2006;26:67-97.
6. Rowden AK, Norvell J, Eldridge DL, Kirk MA. Acetaminophen poisoning. *Clin Lab Med.* 2006;26:49-65.
7. Haroz R, Greenberg MI. New drugs of abuse in North America. *Clin Lab Med.* 2006;26:147-164.
8. Nyberg Karlsen S, Spigset O, Slordal L. The dark side of ecstasy: neuropsychiatric symptoms after exposure to 3,4-methylenedioxy-methamphetamine. *Basic Clin Pharmacol Toxicol.* 2007;102: 15-24.
9. Green G. Doping control for the team physician: a review of drug testing procedures in sport. *Am J Sports Med.* 2006;34: 1690-1698.

Circulating Tumor Markers: Basic Concepts and Clinical Applications

CHRISTOPHER R. MCCUDDEN, MONTE S. WILLIS

CHAPTER **32**

CHAPTER OUTLINE

- ◆ TYPES OF TUMOR MARKERS
- ◆ APPLICATIONS OF TUMOR MARKER DETECTION
  Screening and Susceptibility Testing
  Prognosis
  Monitoring Effectiveness of Therapy and Disease
  Recurrence
- ◆ LABORATORY CONSIDERATIONS FOR TUMOR
  MARKER MEASUREMENT
  Immunoassays
  High-Performance Liquid Chromatography
  Immunohistochemistry and Immunofluorescence
  Enzyme Assays

- ◆ FREQUENTLY ORDERED TUMOR MARKERS
  α-Fetoprotein
  Cancer Antigen 125
  Carcinoembryonic Antigen
  Human Chorionic Gonadotropin
  Prostate-Specific Antigen
- ◆ FUTURE DIRECTIONS
- ◆ QUESTIONS
- ◆ SUGGESTED READING
- ◆ REFERENCES

Chapter Objectives

Upon completion of this chapter, the clinical laboratorian should be able to do the following:

- Discuss the incidence of cancer in the United States.
- Explain the role of tumor markers in cancer management.
- Identify the characteristics or properties of an ideal tumor marker.

- State the major clinical value of tumor markers.
- Name the major tumor types and their associated markers.
- Describe the major properties, methods of analysis, and clinical use of α-fetoprotein, cancer antigen 125, carcinoembryonic antigen, β-human chorionic gonadotropin, and prostate-specific antigen.
- Explain the use of enzymes and hormones as tumor markers.

KEY TERMS

Cancer
Neoplasm
Oncofetal antigen

Oncogene
Staging
Tumor marker

Cancer is the second leading cause of mortality in developed countries, accounting for more than 2.7 million deaths annually. It is estimated that 45% of males and 38% of females will develop invasive cancer in their lifetime; males have a lifetime risk of dying from cancer of 23% whereas females have a 19% risk.[1] The age standardized rates for cancer incidence in North America are 326/100,000. Cancer is a broad term used to describe more than 200 different malignancies that affect more than 50 tissue types. Despite considerable efforts to reduce the incidence of malignancies, it is estimated that there will be more than 1.6 million new cases of cancer in the United States in 2012 (Table 32-1). Current global cancer statistics can be found at http://globocan.iarc.fr/factsheet.asp.

Biologically, *cancer* refers to the uncontrolled growth of cells that often forms a solid mass or tumor (neoplasm) and spreads to other areas of the body. The formation (*tumorigenesis*) and spreading (*metastasis*) of tumors are caused by a complex combination of inherited and acquired genetic mutations (for comprehensive reviews, see references 2 and 3). During tumorigenesis, these mutations include activation of growth factors (e.g., epidermal growth factor) and oncogenes (e.g., K-ras), in combination with inhibition of apoptosis, tumor suppressor, and cell cycle regulation genes (e.g., *BRCA1*, *p53*, and cyclins). As cancer progresses toward metastasis, additional genetic changes are required, such as loss of cell adhesion proteins (e.g., β-catenin and E-cadherin) and activation of angiogenesis genes (e.g., vascular

TABLE 32-1	ESTIMATED NEW CASES OF CANCER AND DEATHS FROM CANCER IN THE UNITED STATES					
	MALES			**FEMALES**		
TISSUE	**INCIDENCE (%)**	**DEATH (%)**	**TISSUE**	**INCIDENCE (%)**	**DEATHS (%)**	
Genital system	30	10	Breast	29	14	
Digestive system	18	27	Digestive system	16	22	
Respiratory system	15	30	Respiratory system	14	27	
Urinary system	12	7	Genital system	11	11	
Skin[a]	6	3	Endocrine system	6	1	
Lymphoma	5	4	Urinary system	6	4	
Oral cavity and pharynx	3	2	Lymphoma	5	3	
Leukemia	3	4	Skin[a]	4	1	
Other and unspecified primary sites	2	8	Leukemia	3	4	
Endocrine system	2	0	Other and unspecified primary sites	2	8	
Brain and other nervous system	1	3	Oral cavity and pharynx	1	1	
Myeloma	1	2	Brain and other nervous system	1	2	
Soft tissue (including heart)	1	1	Myeloma	1	2	
Breast	<1	<1	Soft tissue (including heart)	1	1	
Bones and joints	<1	<1	Eye and orbit	<1	<1	
Eye and orbit	<1	<1	Bones and joints	<1	<1	
Total cases	*848,170*	*301,820*		*790,740*	*275,370*	

[a]Excludes basal cell and squamous cell skin cancers.
Based on 2012 data from the American Cancer Society (http://www.cancer.org/).

endothelial growth factor) (Fig. 32-1). An understanding of these genetic mechanisms is the basis for many current and future cancer treatments.

Cancer severity is generally classified by a combination of several factors. Depending on the type of cancer, these factors include tumor size, histology, regional lymph node involvement, and presence of metastasis. For most solid tumors (e.g., breast, lung, and kidney), cancer is broadly classified (using roman numerals I to IV) into four stages (Fig. 32-2). These stages correlate with disease severity, where higher stages are indicative of significant spreading and severe systemic disease. As disease progresses, both proliferation and metastasis occur at the expense of normal organ processes, which is usually the ultimate cause of cancer-associated morbidity and mortality.

TYPES OF TUMOR MARKERS

Cancer can be detected and monitored using biologic tumor markers. Tumor markers are produced either directly by the tumor or as an effect of the tumor on healthy tissue (*host*). Tumor markers encompass an array of diverse molecules such as serum proteins, oncofetal antigens, hormones, metabolites, receptors, and enzymes.

A variety of enzymes are elevated nonspecifically in tumors (Table 32-2). These elevated enzymes are largely a result of the high metabolic demand of these proliferative cells. Accordingly, enzyme levels tend to correlate with tumor burden, making them clinically useful for monitoring the success of therapy. Serum proteins, such as β_2-microglobulin and immunoglobulins,

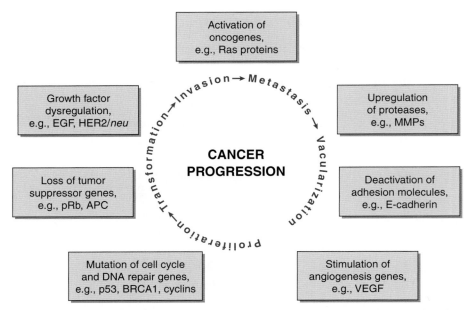

FIGURE 32-1 Genetic changes associated with cancer. A combination of acquired and/or hereditary defects causes tumor formation and metastasis. These processes begin with unregulated proliferation and transformation, followed by invasion and loss of cellular adhesion. A rich vascular supply of oxygen and nutrients is necessary to facilitate growth of a tumor larger than 100 to 200 μm. APC, familial adenomatous polyposis coli, mutated in colorectal cancers; BRCA1, breast cancer susceptibility gene; E-cadherin, adhesion molecule; EGF, epithelial growth factor; MMP, matrix metalloproteinase; p53, cell cycle regulator, mutated in 50% of cancers; pRB, retinoblastoma protein, mutated in many cancers; Ras, small G protein, mutated in many cancers; TIMP, tissue inhibitor of metalloproteinase; VEGF, vascular endothelial growth factor, drug target for inhibin of angiogenesis.

Cancer Staging and Progression

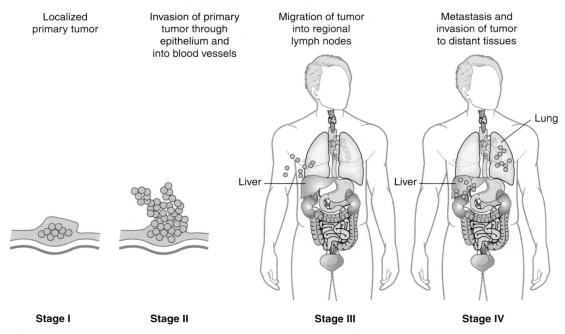

FIGURE 32-2 Generalized cancer staging and progression. Numerous factors are used in combination to define cancer stage; these include tumor size, extent of invasion, lymph node involvement, metastasis, and histologic assessments (basis for the TNM staging system). In this simplified diagram, stage is presented as a function of invasion and spreading regionally and to other tissues; the primary tumor is not shown.

TABLE 32-2	ENZYME TUMOR MARKERS			
TUMOR MARKER	**TUMOR TYPE**	**METHOD**	**SPECIMEN**	**CLINICAL UTILITY**
Prostate-specific antigen	Prostate cancer	IA	Serum	Prostate cancer screening, therapy monitoring, and recurrence
Lactate dehydrogenase	Hematologic malignancies	EA	Serum	Prognostic indicator; elevated non-specifically in numerous cancers
Alkaline phosphatase	Metastatic carcinoma of bone, hepatocellular carcinoma, osteo-sarcoma, lymphoma, leukemia	EA	Serum	Determination of liver and bone involvement; nonspecific elevation in many bone-related and liver cancers
Neuron-specific enolase	Neuroendocrine tumors	RIA, IHC	Serum	Prognostic indicator and monitoring disease progression for neuroendocrine tumors

EA, enzyme assay; IA, immunoassay; IHC, immunohistochemistry; RIA, radioimmunoassay.

are also used to monitor cancer therapy (Table 32-3). β_2-Microglobulin is found on the surface of all nucleated cells and can therefore be used as a nonspecific marker of the high cell turnover that is often observed in tumors. Immunoglobulins provide a more specific measure of plasma cell production of monoclonal proteins observed in hematologic malignancies such as multiple myeloma. Hormones and hormone metabolites are widely used as specific markers of secreting tumors (Table 32-4). Hormones are particularly valuable in diagnosing neuroblastomas, as well as pituitary and adrenal adenomas. One of the first classes of tumor markers discovered was the oncofetal antigens. Oncofetal antigens such as carcinoembryonic antigen (CEA) and α-fetoprotein (AFP) are expressed transiently during normal development and are then turned on again in the formation of tumors (see Table 32-5 for use of oncofetal antigens). Other tumor markers include monoclonal defined antigens, which were directly identified from human tumor extracts or cell lines. These are directed toward specific carbohydrate or cancer antigens and are best used for monitoring treatment of tumors that secrete these epitopes (Table 32-6). Finally, receptors are used to classify tumors for therapy (Table 32-7). These "nonserologic" markers are outside the scope of the chapter, but they are an important example of the diversity of tumor markers. Prototypic examples of such a marker are estrogen and progesterone receptors. When solid tumor biopsies are positive for these markers, tamoxifen chemotherapy is more likely to be effective.

Tumor markers are an invaluable set of tools that health care providers can use for a variety of clinical modalities. Depending on the marker and the type of malignancy, tumor markers may be used for screening, diagnosis, prognosis, therapy monitoring, and detecting recurrence (Fig. 32-3).

APPLICATIONS OF TUMOR MARKER DETECTION

The ideal tumor marker would be tumor specific, absent in healthy individuals, and readily detectable in body fluids. Unfortunately, all of the presently available tumor markers do not fit this ideal model. However, numerous

TABLE 32-3	SERUM PROTEIN TUMOR MARKERS			
TUMOR MARKER	**TUMOR TYPE**	**METHOD**	**SPECIMEN**	**CLINICAL UTILITY**
Serum M-protein	Plasma cell dyscrasias	SPE/IFE	Serum	Diagnosis, therapeutic monitoring of plasma cell malignancies
Serum-free light chains	Plasma cell dyscrasias	IA	Serum	Diagnosis, therapeutic monitoring of plasma cell malignancies
β_2-Microglobulin	Hematologic malignancies	IA	Serum	Prognostic marker for lymphoproliferative disorders

IA, immunoassay; IFE, immunofixation electrophoresis; SPE, serum protein electrophoresis.

TABLE 32-4	ENDOCRINE TUMOR MARKERS			
TUMOR MARKER	**TUMOR TYPE**	**METHOD**	**SPECIMEN**	**CLINICAL UTILITY**
ACTH	Pituitary adenoma, ectopic ACTH-producing tumor	IA	Serum	Diagnosis of ectopic ACTH-producing tumor
ADH	Posterior pituitary tumors	IA	Serum	Diagnosis of SIADH
C-peptide	Insulin-secreting tumors	ELISA, IA	Serum	Diagnosis of insulinoma
Calcitonin	MTC and neuroendocrine tumors	IA	Serum	Screening,[a] response to therapy, and monitoring recurrence of MTC
Chromogranin A	Pheochromocytoma, neuroblastoma, carcinoid tumors, small cell lung cancers	ELISA, RIA	Serum	Aid in diagnosis of carcinoid tumors, pheochromocytomas, and neuroblastomas
Cortisol	Adrenal tumors	IA	Serum or urine	Diagnosis of Cushing's syndrome, adrenal adenoma
Gastrin	Neuroendocrine tumor	IA	Serum	Zollinger-Ellison syndrome; gastrinoma
GH	Pituitary adenoma, ectopic GH-secreting tumors	IA	Serum	Diagnosis and post monitoring of acromegaly
HVA	Neuroblastoma, pheochromocytoma, paraganglioma	HPLC	24-h urine	Diagnosis of neuroblastoma[b]
5-HIAA	Carcinoid tumors	HPLC	24-h urine	Diagnosis of carcinoid tumors
Metanephrines (fractionated)[c]	Pheochromocytoma, paraganglioma, neuroblastoma	HPLC	24-h urine or plasma	Screening and diagnosis of pheochromocytoma
PTH	Parathyroid adenoma	IA	Serum	Diagnosis and postsurgical monitoring of parathyroid adenoma
PRL	Pituitary adenoma	IA	Serum	Diagnosis and postsurgical monitoring of prolactinoma
VMA	Pheochromocytoma, paraganglioma, neuroblastoma	HPLC	24-h urine	Diagnosis of neuroblastoma[b]

ACTH, adrenocorticotropic hormone; ADH, antidiuretic hormone; GH, growth hormone; HVA, homovanillic acid; 5-HIAA, hydroxyindoleacetic acid; PTH, parathyroid hormone; PRL, prolactin; VMA, vanillylmandelic acid; ELISA, enzyme-linked immunosorbent assay; HPLC, high-performance liquid chromatography; IA, immunoassay; LC-MS/MS, liquid chromatography–TANDEM mass spectrometry; MTC, medullary thyroid carcinoma; RIA, radioimmunoassay; SIADH, syndrome of inappropriate antidiuretic hormone secretion.

[a]Screening family members for MTC.
[b]HVA and VMA are used in combination for diagnosis of neuroblastomas.
[c]Metanephrine, normetanephrine.

tumor markers have been identified that have a high enough specificity and sensitivity to be used on a targeted basis for screening diagnosis, prognosis, detection of recurrence, and monitoring the response to treatment (Fig. 32-3). Clinically, tumor markers are used in combination with clinical signs, symptoms, and histology to facilitate clinical decision-making.

Screening and Susceptibility Testing

With the possible exception of prostate-specific antigen (PSA), no tumor marker identified to date can be used to effectively screen asymptomatic populations. This is because most of the clinically used tumor markers are found in normal cells and benign conditions in addition to

TABLE 32-5	USE OF SERUM α-FETOPROTEIN AND HUMAN CHORIONIC GONADOTROPIN FOR TESTICULAR CANCER CLASSIFICATION		
	GERM CELL TUMOR	**AFP**	**HCG**
Nonseminomatous tumors	Yolk sac tumor (endodermal sinus tumor)	Increased	No
	Choriocarcinoma	No	Increased
	Embryonal carcinoma	Increased	±
	Teratoma	No	No
Seminoma		Not elevated in pure tumors	±

AFP, α-fetoprotein; hCG, human chorionic gonadotropin.

cancer. Screening asymptomatic populations would therefore result in detection of false positives (patients without disease with detectable tumor marker), leading to undue alarm and risk to patients (e.g., unnecessary imaging, biopsy, and surgery). Presently, only a few tumor markers are used to screen populations with high incidence.

Susceptibility to cancer can be determined using molecular diagnostics in patients with breast, ovarian, or colon cancer by identifying germline mutations in patients with a family history of these diseases. Screening for susceptibility to breast and ovarian cancers is done by identifying germline *BRCA1* and *BRCA2* mutations. Similarly, familial colon cancers can be identified by the presence of the adenomatous polyposis coli gene (*APC*); >99% of people with familial APC develop colon cancer by the age of 40 years, such that prophylactic colectomy is performed. While gene testing can be done from blood samples, these are not really considered circulating tumor markers and therefore not discussed further.

Prognosis

Tumor marker concentration generally increases with tumor progression, reaching their highest levels when tumors metastasize. Therefore, serum tumor marker levels at diagnosis can reflect the aggressiveness of a tumor and help predict the outcome for patients. High concentrations of a serum tumor marker at diagnosis might indicate the presence of malignancy and possible metastasis, which is associated with a poorer prognosis. In other instances, the mere presence or absence of a particular marker may be valuable. Such is the case with some of the receptors used to base chemotherapeutic treatment in breast cancer, where certain therapy is indicated only in the presence of a given marker.

Monitoring Effectiveness of Therapy and Disease Recurrence

One of the most useful and common applications of tumor markers is monitoring therapy efficacy and detecting disease recurrence. After surgical resection, radiation, or drug therapy of cancer (chemotherapy), tumor markers are routinely followed serially. In patients with elevated tumor markers at diagnosis, effective therapy results in a dramatic decrease or disappearance of the tumor marker. If the initial treatment is effective, the appearance of circulating tumor markers can then be used as a highly sensitive marker of recurrence; many markers have a lead time of several months before disease would be detected by other modalities, allowing identification and treatment earlier during relapse.

LABORATORY CONSIDERATIONS FOR TUMOR MARKER MEASUREMENT

The unique characteristics and concentrations of tumor makers require special laboratory considerations. Two of the main considerations are the wide concentration range of tumor markers and the variability in tumor concentration between different manufacturers (lack of harmonization and standardization).

TABLE 32-6	CARBOHYDRATE AND CANCER ANTIGEN TUMOR MARKERS			
TUMOR MARKER	**TUMOR TYPE**	**METHOD**	**SPECIMEN**	**CLINICAL UTILITY**
CA 19-9	Gastrointestinal cancer and adenocarcinoma	Immunoassay	Serum	Monitoring pancreatic cancer
CA 15-3	Metastatic breast cancer	Immunoassay	Serum	Response to therapy and detecting recurrence
CA 27-29	Metastatic breast carcinoma	Immunoassay	Serum	Response to therapy and detecting recurrence
CA-125	Ovarian cancer	Immunoassay	Serum	Monitoring therapy

CA, cancer antigen.

TABLE 32-7	RECEPTOR TUMOR MARKERS			
TUMOR MARKER	**TUMOR TYPE**	**METHOD**	**SPECIMEN**	**CLINICAL UTILITY**
Estrogen receptor	Breast cancer	IHC	Biopsy	Hormonal therapy indicator
Progesterone receptor	Breast cancer	IHC	Biopsy	Hormonal therapy indicator
Her-2/*neu*	Breast, ovarian, gastrointestinal tumors	IHC, FISH, ELISA	Biopsy	Prognostic and hormonal therapy indicator
Epidermal growth factor receptor	Head, neck, ovarian, cervical cancers	IHC	Biopsy	Prognostic indicator

ELISA, enzyme-linked immunosorbent assay; FISH, fluorescence in situ hybridization; IHC, immunohistochemistry.

Lack of standardization makes comparison of serial patient results using different assays treacherous. There are multiple reasons why these assays are not comparable, including differences in antibody specificity, analyte heterogeneity, assay design, lack of standard reference material, calibration, kinetics, and variation in reference ranges. To most accurately monitor tumor marker concentrations in a patient, it is important to use the same methodology (or kit). It is also important to perform diligent quality control during lot changes. This includes careful comparison of QC material and patient samples because detection of tumor markers can vary widely between reagent lots; this is particularly a concern where polyclonal antibodies are used as reagents.

The other main consideration for tumor marker measurement is the wide concentration. Tumor markers often vary in concentrations by orders of magnitude, making accurate measurement challenging compared with routine chemistry analytes (e.g., concentration extremes for sodium are between 120 and 160 mmol/L, whereas human chorionic gonadotropin [hCG] may vary between 10 and 10,000,000 mIU/mL!). Handling these ranges requires careful attention to dilution protocols and the risk of antigen excess. These consideration are discussed in the context of specific methodology in the following sections.

Immunoassays

Immunoassays are the most commonly used method to measure tumor markers. There are many advantages to this method, such as the ability to automate testing and relative ease of use. Many tumor markers are amenable to automation and relatively rapid analysis using large

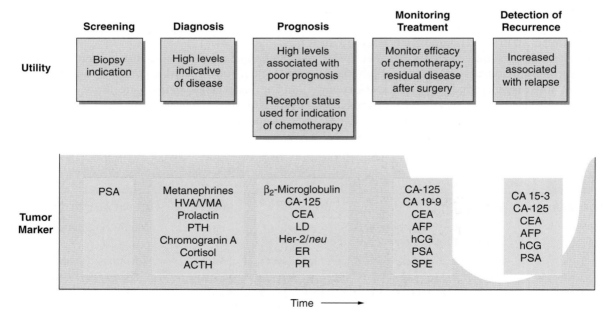

FIGURE 32-3 Tumor markers are used for screening, prognosis, treatment monitoring, and detecting recurrence of several types of cancer. Whereas few markers are used for screening, many are used to monitor therapy. Endocrine and hormone metabolite markers are often used to aid in diagnosis of secreting tumors. List is not comprehensive but provides examples of the most commonly used markers. Note: PSA screening remains controversial, see text.

COMMON CANCER TERMS

Angiogenesis: Development of new blood vessels to supply oxygen and nutrients to cells

Apoptosis: Programmed cell death

Cell cycle: Phases of cell activity divided into G, S, and M (growth, DNA synthesis, and mitosis, respectively)

Neoplasm: Synonymous with "tumor," it refers to uncontrolled tissue growth; it may be cancerous (malignant) or non-cancerous (benign). Derived from Greek meaning "new formation."

Oncogene: Encodes a protein that, when mutated, promotes uncontrolled cell growth

Tumor suppressor gene: Encodes a protein involved in protecting cells from unregulated growth

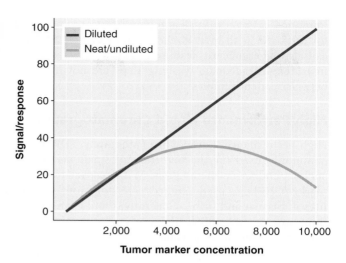

FIGURE 32-4 Hook effect (antigen excess) can occur with tumor markers because they may be found at very high concentrations. When reagents are depleted by excess antigen (the tumor marker), falsely low results may occur (represented by the "neat" curve). Dilution of samples can be used to detect and account for hook effect (represented by the "diluted" line).

immunoassay or integrated chemistry test platforms. However, there are some unique factors to be considered when using immunoassays to measure tumor markers? These factors include assay linearity, antigen excess (hook effect), and the potential for heterophile antibodies.

Linearity

The *linear range* is the span of analyte concentrations over which a linear relationship exists between the analyte and signal. Linearity is determined by analyzing (in replicates) specimens spanning the reportable range. Guidelines for this determination are outlined in the Clinical Laboratory Improvement Amendments (CLIA) guidelines for linearity.[4] Samples exceeding the linear range, which is much more likely to occur in the detection of tumor markers, need to be systemically diluted to determine values within the reportable linear range. Excessively high tumor marker concentrations can result in falsely low measurements, a phenomenon known as *antigen excess* or *hook effect*.

Hook Effect

When analyte concentrations exceed the analytical range excessively, there is potential for *antigen excess* or *hook effect*. When very high antigen concentrations are present, capture and/or label antibodies can be saturated, resulting in a lack of "sandwich" formation and thus in a significant decrease in signal. The name hook effect refers to the shape of the concentration–signal curve when the reagents are saturated with excess antigen (Fig. 32-4). Essentially, hook effect causes the actual tumor marker concentration to be grossly underestimated. If clinical suspicion is high for an elevated tumor marker, it can be identified by the laboratory with dilution and repeat testing. Samples displaying hook effect will yield higher (accurate) values on dilution (Fig. 32-4).

Heterophile Antibodies

Significant interference can be seen in immunoassays if an individual has circulating antibodies against human or animal immunoglobulin reagents. A subset of heterophilic antibodies are human anti-animal antibodies or human anti-mouse antibodies (HAMAs). HAMAs are most commonly encountered in patients who have been given mouse monoclonal antibodies for therapeutic reasons or who have been exposed to mice,[5] but they may be idiopathic. In patients, these antibodies can cause false-positive or, less commonly, false-negative results by cross linking the capture/label antibody (see Chapter 8). To confirm that heterophilic antibodies are present, samples are diluted and the linearity of the dilutions is analyzed (similar to eliminating hook effect). Samples with heterophilic antibodies do not give linear results upon dilution. The presence of anti-animal immunoglobulins can also be detected directly. Non-immune animal serum is often added to immunoassays to minimize the effects of heterophilic antibodies, and there are commercial blocking reagents that can be used to remove HAMAs. Many monoclonal therapeutic agents are now derived to include only fragments of an antibody to avoid the development of heterophilic antibodies. In the laboratory, heterophile antibodies can be detected by investigating results that are inconsistent with history and clinical scenario.

Common Analytical Concerns Applied to Tumor Marker Immunoassays

Immunoassays for tumor markers can be affected by interference from icterus, lipemia, hemolysis, and antibody cross-reactivity in the same manner as other immunoassays. As with all automated tests, the potential for carryover with high levels of tumor marker analytes can also be a concern, leading to falsely elevated levels in patients if adequate washing steps are not included between patient samples.

High-Performance Liquid Chromatography

High-performance liquid chromatography (HPLC) is commonly used for the detection of small molecules, such as endocrine metabolites. With respect to tumor markers, HPLC is used to detect catecholamine metabolites in plasma and urine. Generally, there is an extraction process, by which the analytes of interest are separated from either plasma or urine. Extractions are applied to a column where they are separated by their physical characteristics (charge, size, and polarity). Catecholamines and catecholamine metabolites are used to help diagnose carcinoid tumors, pheochromocytoma, and neuroblastoma. Neuroblastoma is a common malignant tumor occurring in approximately 7.5% of children under 15 years of age. Neuroblastoma is diagnosed by the detection of high levels of plasma epinephrine, norepinephrine, and dopamine (catecholamines). Pheochromocytoma, a rare tumor associated with hypertension, is diagnosed by detecting elevated plasma metanephrines (along with urine vanillylmandelic acid and free catecholamines). Carcinoid tumors are serotonin-secreting tumors that arise from the small intestine, appendix, or rectum leading to a host of symptoms (carcinoid syndrome), including pronounced flushing, bronchial constriction, cardiac valve lesions, and diarrhea. The diagnosis of carcinoid tumors involves the detection of 5-hydroxyindole-acetic acid, which is a serotonin metabolite. In all of these cases, HPLC is used to detect the hormones and metabolites secreted by these tumors for diagnosis, therapeutic monitoring, and recurrence. HPLC is not subject to hook effect, lot-to-lot antibody variation, and heterophile antibodies, but is more labor intensive and requires more experience and skill than automated immunoassays.

Immunohistochemistry and Immunofluorescence

While not found in circulation, it is important for laboratorians to be familiar with solid tissue tumor markers. These are identified in tissue sections typically from fine-needle aspirate or biopsy samples. Specific antibodies (and the proper control antibodies) are incubated with tissue sections to detect the presence (or absence) of antigens using colorimetric or fluorescent secondary antibodies. In many ways, this is similar to detection by immunoassay, but the added value is the ability to determine whether the antigen in question is in a particular cell type (such as a tumor), in the specific subcellular location. A good example of the use of a tumor marker that is detected by immunohistochemistry is the identification of estrogen and progesterone receptors in breast cancer. When breast tumors are positive for estrogen and progesterone receptors at the cell surface, they tend to respond to hormonal therapy, while tumors lacking these receptors are treated with other chemotherapeutic modalities. There has also been a recent guideline update on the use of hormone receptors as prognostic indicators.[6]

Enzyme Assays

The detection of elevated circulating enzymes generally cannot be used to identify a specific tumor or site of tumor. One key exception to this is the PSA, which is in fact an enzyme; PSA is a serine protease of the kallikrein family, found in both diseased and benign prostate glands. Before the widespread use of immunoassays and the discovery of oncofetal antigens, enzyme detection use was widespread. Because enzymes are found in much higher concentrations intracellularly, release into the system resulted when cells necrosed or underwent changes in permeability. Examples of enzymes that have been used as tumor markers include alkaline phosphatase (bone, liver, leukemia, and sarcoma), creatine kinase–BB (prostate, small cell lung, breast, colon, and ovarian), lactate dehydrogenase (liver, lymphomas, leukemia, and others), and of course PSA (prostate). Enzyme activity assays (see also Chapter 13) are used to quantify all of these enzymes, with the exception of PSA, which is measured by immunoassay.

FREQUENTLY ORDERED TUMOR MARKERS

α-Fetoprotein

AFP is an abundant serum protein normally synthesized by the fetal liver that is re-expressed in certain types of tumors. This re-expression during malignancy classifies AFP as a carcinoembryonic protein. AFP is often elevated in patients with hepatocellular carcinoma (HCC) and germ cell tumors.

Regulation and Physiology

AFP is a 70-kD glycoprotein related to albumin that normally functions as a transport protein. Like albumin, it is involved in regulating oncotic pressure in the fetus. During development, AFP peaks at approximately one tenth the concentration of albumin at 30 weeks of gestation. The upper normal limit for serum AFP is approximately 15 ng/mL (reference intervals are method dependent) in healthy adults. Infants initially have high serum AFP values that decline to adult levels at an age of 7 to 10 months.[7]

Clinical Application and Interpretation

AFP is used for the diagnosis, staging, prognosis, and treatment monitoring of HCC. Also known as hepatoma, HCC is a tumor that originates in the liver, often due to chronic disease such as hepatitis and cirrhosis. Patients with HCC frequently have elevated serum AFP; however, as with most tumor markers, AFP is not completely specific. For example, AFP can also be increased in benign conditions such as pregnancy and liver disease, as well as other types of malignancies such as testicular cancer.

Although it is not widely used for screening in Europe and North America, AFP has been used to detect HCC in populations with high disease prevalence such as in China. When used for screening high-risk populations, AFP has a sensitivity ranging from 40% to 65% and specificity of 80% to 95% (at cutoffs ranging from 20 to 30 ng/mL).[8] Very high levels of AFP (>500 ng/mL) in high-risk individuals are considered diagnostic of HCC.[9] Several expert groups, including the National Comprehensive Cancer Network, National Academy of Clinical Biochemistry, and the British Society of Gastroenterology, now recommend that AFP be used in conjunction with ultrasound imaging every 6 months in patients at high risk for developing HCC. This includes patients with hepatitis B virus– and/or hepatitis C virus–induced liver cirrhosis.[10]

High levels of AFP in HCC are associated with poor prognosis and are exemplified in individuals who do not respond to therapy or have residual disease following surgery. Correspondingly, a decrease in circulating AFP levels after treatment is associated with prolonged survival rates. It is therefore recommended that serial measurements of AFP be used to monitor treatment and postsurgery in patients with HCC.

The other major use for AFP as a tumor marker is for classification and monitoring therapy for testicular cancer. Testicular cancer includes several subtypes broadly classified into seminomatous and nonseminomatous tumors. Seminomatous tumors form directly from malignant germ cells, whereas nonseminomatous tumors differentiate into embryonal carcinoma, teratoma, choriocarcinoma, and yolk sac tumors (endodermal sinus tumor).[11] AFP is used in combination with β-human chorionic gonadotropin (β-hCG) to classify nonseminomatous tumors (Table 32-5). Serum AFP is also useful for tumor staging; AFP is increased in 10% to 20% of stage I tumors, 50% to 80% of stage II tumors, and 90% to 100% of stage III nonseminomatous testicular cancer. As with HCC, AFP can be used serially to monitor therapy efficacy and disease progression.

Methodology

AFP is measured using any of a variety of commercially available automated immunoassays. These assays are typically sandwich immunoassays relying on monoclonal or polyclonal antibodies directed toward different regions of AFP. Serial monitoring of AFP should be done using the same laboratory and assay to ensure changes (or lack of change) are due to the tumor and not assay variation. As with other glycoproteins, AFP displays some heterogeneity where certain isoforms are preferentially produced by malignant cells. Antibodies against these isoforms produced by malignant cells may in the future be used to improve the specificity of AFP immunoassays.

Application and Pathophysiology

The primary applications of AFP as a tumor marker are for HCC and nonseminomatous testicular cancer. AFP is typically used as a marker to monitor therapy, detect residual tumor, or detect relapse.

Cancer Antigen 125

Cancer antigen 125 (CA-125) was first defined by a murine monoclonal antibody raised against a serous ovarian carcinoma cell line.[10] CA-125 may be useful for detecting ovarian tumors at an early stage and for monitoring treatments without surgical restaging.

Regulation and Physiology

CA-125 is expressed in the ovary, in other tissues of müllerian duct origin, and in human ovarian carcinoma cells. The CA-125 gene encodes a high molecular weight (200,000 to 1,000,000 kDa) mucin protein containing a putative transmembrane region and a tyrosine phosphorylation site.[12] Although it is not usually found in serum, CA-125 may be elevated in patients with endometriosis, during the first trimester of pregnancy, or during menstruation.

Clinical Application and Interpretation

CA-125 is a serologic marker of ovarian cancer. Ovarian cancer accounts for approximately 3% of the newly diagnosed malignancies in women and is among the top five causes of cancer-related death (Table 32-1). Ovarian cancer includes a broad range of categories, including sex cord tumors, stromal tumors, germ cell tumors, and, most commonly, epithelial cell tumors. As with most other tumor markers, CA-125 should not be used to screen for ovarian cancer in asymptomatic individuals. However, CA-125 is elevated in a high percentage of ovarian tumors and is recommended as an annual test for women with a family or prior history of ovarian cancer. CA-125 levels also correlate with ovarian cancer stage. CA-125 is elevated in 50% of patients with stage I disease, 90% of patients with stage II, and more than 90% of patients with stage III or IV.

Other tumor markers for ovarian cancer have been developed. Human epididymis protein 4 (HE4) is another Food and Drug Administration FDA)–cleared test for ovarian cancer. HE4 offers improved specificity over CA-125, where it is less frequently elevated in non-malignant conditions, such as endometriosis. Tumor

CASE STUDY 32-1

A 33-year-old man with a history of chronic liver disease presents with edema, abdominal pain, and recent weight loss. Laboratory examination reveals a low platelet count, hypoalbuminemia, and prolonged prothrombin time and partial thromboplastin time.

Questions

1. Which tumor marker may aid in diagnosing this patient?

2. What additional laboratory tests would be useful in diagnosing this patient?

3. The patient is treated with surgery; how should tumor markers be used to determine the success of surgery?

markers are an active area of research, such that more new markers can be expected in the future.

Methodology

CA-125 can be detected by immunoassays that use OC125 and M11 antibodies. These monoclonal antibodies recognize distinct nonoverlapping regions of the CA-125 epitope. CA-125 is available on many automated platforms. However, results from different platforms are not interchangeable due to differences between reagent detection methods. The upper normal limit for serum CA-125 is 35 U/mL.

Application and Pathophysiology

CA-125 is predominantly used to monitor therapy and to distinguish benign masses from ovarian cancer.[13] For example, in postmenopausal women with a palpable abdominal mass, a high level (>95 U/mL) of CA-125 has a 90% positive predictive value for ovarian cancer. For therapy monitoring, CA-125 is useful both for predicting the success of surgery (debulking procedures) and for determining efficacy of chemotherapy. Therefore, patients with elevated CA-125 following either treatment modality have a poor prognosis. Prognosis is also associated with CA-125 half-life; a CA-125 half-life of less than 20 days is associated with longer survival; the average half-life of CA-125 is 4.5 days.[14,15]

Carcinoembryonic Antigen

CEA was discovered in the 1960s and is a prototypical example of an oncofetal antigen; it is expressed during development and then re-expressed in tumors. CEA is the most widely used tumor marker for colorectal cancer and is also frequently elevated in lung, breast, and gastrointestinal tumors. CEA can be used to aid in the diagnosis, prognosis, and therapy monitoring of colorectal

cancer. Although high levels of CEA (>10 ng/mL) are frequently associated with malignancy, high levels of CEA are not specific for colorectal cancer and therefore CEA is not used for screening.

Regulation and Physiology

CEA is a large heterogeneous glycoprotein with a molecular weight of approximately 200 kDa. It is part of the immunoglobulin superfamily and is involved in apoptosis, immunity, and cell adhesion. Because of its role in cell adhesion, CEA has been postulated to be involved in metastasis. Akin to other serologic tumor markers, CEA may be elevated nonspecifically because of impaired clearance or through increased production. Increased CEA concentrations have been observed in heavy smokers and in some patients following radiation treatment and chemotherapy. CEA may also be elevated in patients with liver damage due to prolonged clearance. The upper normal range for serum CEA is 2.5 to 5 ng/mL depending on the assay.

Clinical Application and Interpretation

The main clinical use of CEA is as a marker for colorectal cancer. In colon cancer, CEA is used for prognosis, in postsurgery surveillance, and to monitor response to chemotherapy. For prognosis, CEA can be used in combination with histology and the TNM (see definition box) staging system to establish the need for adjuvant therapy (addition of chemotherapy or treatment after surgery). Adjuvant therapy is indicated in patients with stage II disease (i.e., tumor has spread beyond immediate colon but not to lymph nodes) who have high levels of CEA.[16]

Methodology

Although CEA assays historically used polyclonal antibodies, these have largely been replaced by the use of monoclonal anti-CEA antibodies. CEA is available on numerous commercial automated platforms. Due to the high heterogeneity of CEA, it is essential that the same assay method be used for serial monitoring.

Application and Pathophysiology

Before surgical resection, baseline CEA values are typically obtained to confirm successful removal of the tumor burden. After surgery and during chemotherapy, it is recommended that CEA levels be serially monitored

TNM STAGING SYSTEM

T—tumor size and involvement/invasion of nearby tissue
N—regional lymph nodes involvement
M—metastasis; extent of tumor spreading from one tissue to another

every 2 to 3 months to detect recurrence and determine therapy efficacy; the half-life of CEA is approximately 2 to 8 days depending on the assay and the individual. If treatment is successful, CEA levels should drop into the reference interval in 1 to 4 months. CEA is not recommended for screening asymptomatic individuals for colorectal cancer. While there are no specific guidelines recommending the use of CEA in other types of cancer, it may be of value for detecting recurrence of antigen-positive breast and gastrointestinal cancers and medullary thyroid carcinoma, and to aid in the diagnosis of non–small cell lung cancer.

Human Chorionic Gonadotropin

hCG is a dimeric hormone normally secreted by trophoblasts to promote implantation of the blastocyst and the placenta to maintain the corpus luteum through the first trimester of pregnancy. Some types of tumor invasion is actually similar to uterine implantation, except that implantation in pregnancy is regulated and limited. hCG is elevated in trophoblastic tumors, mainly choriocarcinoma, and germ cell tumors of the ovary and testis.

Regulation and Physiology

hCG is a 45-kD glycoprotein consisting of α- and β-subunits. A unique aspect of hCG is that it is degraded into multiple fragments. In serum, this results in the presence of the intact molecule, nicked hCG, the free β-subunit (β-hCG), and a hyperglycosylated intact form. Either intact hCG or the free β-subunit may be elevated in malignancies, and most assays detect multiple fragments of hCG.

CASE STUDY 32-2

A 65-year-old man presents to the emergency department after he had abnormally tarry-colored stool on multiple occasions. He has had gastrointestinal discomfort and has felt increasingly tired during the past 2 months. Physical examination reveals a guaiac-positive stool. A subsequently colonoscopy identified a circumferential mass in the sigmoid colon. A biopsy was performed, which identified the mass as an adenocarcinoma. CEA level was obtained as part of the presurgery workup.

Questions

1. Is the CEA test useful as a screening test for colon carcinoma?

2. What other conditions can result in elevated CEA levels?

3. How is CEA used to monitor patients after surgery for colon cancer?

Clinical Application and Interpretation

hCG has several clinical applications as a tumor marker. It is a prognostic indicator for ovarian cancer, a diagnostic marker for classification of testicular cancer, and the most useful marker for detection of gestational trophoblastic diseases (GTDs).[2] GTDs include four distinct types of tumors (hydatidiform mole, persistent/invasive gestational trophoblastic neoplasia, choriocarcinoma, and placental site trophoblastic tumors) that are classified by clinical history, ultrasound, histology, and hCG levels. hCG is invariably elevated in women with GTDs[17] and is often found at higher levels than are observed in normal pregnancy (i.e., >100,000 mIU/mL). It is particularly a helpful marker for monitoring GTD therapy, as levels of hCG correlate with tumor mass and prognosis; hCG is not actually cleared by the FDA for use as a tumor marker despite its widespread utility.

Methodology

hCG can be measured by using any of a variety of widely available automated immunoassays. Typical assays use monoclonal capture and tracer antibodies targeted toward epitopes in the β-subunit and intact hCG. Total β-hCG assays are the most useful assays because they detect both intact hormone and free β-hCG. Due to the variability in hCG assays,[18] it is imperative that patients be monitored with the same technique. It is also important for laboratories to be aware of the relative cross-reactivity of their assay with different hCG isoforms; because hCG assays are designed to detect pregnancy, they are not all equivalent for application as tumor markers.

Application and Pathophysiology

In testicular cancer, the free β-hCG subunit is elevated in 60% to 70% of patients with nonseminomas. hCG can be used in combination with AFP and biopsies to diagnose subtypes of testicular cancer (Table 32-5). Ectopic β-hCG is also occasionally elevated in ovarian cancer and some lung cancers. It is generally accepted that free β-hCG is sensitive and specific for aggressive neoplasms; the free β-hCG is not detectable in the serum of healthy subjects.

Prostate-Specific Antigen

PSA is a 28-kD glycoprotein produced only in the epithelial cells of the acini and ducts of the prostatic ducts in the prostate. It is a serine protease of the kallikrein gene family. It functionally regulates seminal fluid viscosity and is instrumental in dissolving the cervical mucus cap, allowing sperm to enter.

Regulation and Physiology

In healthy men, low circulating levels of PSA can be detected in the serum. There are two major forms of PSA that are found circulating in the blood: (1) free and (2)

CASE STUDY 32-3

A 25-year-old man with a history of testicular cancer is followed postsurgery over the course of 10 months, with β-hCG and AFP monitored. The patient is treated with radiation at 2 months, followed by chemotherapy (taxol, ifosfamide, and cisplatin) from months 6 through 9 (see Case Study Fig. 32-3.1).

Questions

1. What type of germ cell tumor might this patient have based on the serum AFP and β-hCG levels?

2. Explain the pattern of AFP and hCG observed in the graph.

3. Can a final diagnosis be made based only on the tumor marker findings? If not, why not?

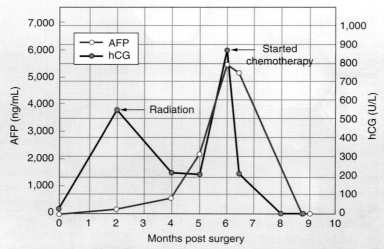

CASE STUDY FIGURE 32-3.1 Time course of hCG and AFP in patient with testicular cancer. The patient was treated with radiation at 2 mo, and then again with chemotherapy (taxol, ifosfamide, and cisplatin) from months 6 through 9. Reference range for AFP is less than 10 μg/L and that for hCG is less than 5 U/L.

complexed. Most of the circulating PSA is complexed to α_1-antichymotrypsin or α_2-macroglobulin. Assays to detect total and free PSA have been developed. While the detection of total PSA has been used in screening for and in monitoring of prostate cancer, evidence for the usefulness in detecting free PSA as a fraction of total has been identified. Patients with malignancy have a lower percentage of free PSA. As with other tumor markers, PSA is not entirely specific. Men with benign prostatic hyperplasia (BPH) and prostatitis can also have high PSA levels. Additional markers, such as prostate cancer gene-3 (PCA-3), are starting to be used to address this lack of specificity.

Clinical Application and Interpretation

Although controversial, annual PSA testing is recommended by the American Cancer Society and American Urological Association for men over 50 to detect prostate cancer.[19] Men at higher risk (first-degree relative with prostate cancer or African American) should begin screening at ages 40 to 45 years. A 2-year screening interval may be appropriate for men with PSA levels less than 2.0 ng/mL. Screening should always include a digital rectal examination (DRE). Screening utility decreases with age and is not appropriate for men with less than a 10-year life expectancy. In addition to the use of standard cutoff values of total PSA (<4 ng/mL is generally considered normal), other measurements of PSA have been used to test for prostate malignancy; age-adjusted cutoff values of PSA, PSA velocity (rate of rise over time), and free PSA/total PSA ratios have been used to increase the accuracy of PSA testing.[20] Patients with a total PSA greater than 4 ng/mL and/or a clinical suspicion of cancer by DRE undergo biopsy to confirm the presence of prostate cancer and they are followed closely over time.

Prostate infection, irritation, and BPH (enlargement) can result in increased PSA. Moreover, recent ejaculation or DRE can also lead to increases in circulating PSA.[21-25] It has also been recognized that cancer can be present at all concentrations of PSA (Table 32-8).[26,27] Taken together, these studies urge the interpretation of PSA in the context of the clinical picture (including DRE, imaging, and family history).

TABLE 32-8	PREVALENCE OF PROSTATE CANCER AT DIFFERENT PROSTATE-SPECIFIC ANTIGEN CONCENTRATIONS

PSA CONCENTRATION (ng/mL)	PREVALENCE OF PROSTATE CANCER (%)
<1	6–10
1–4	17–25
4–10	20–30
>20	>80

There remains controversy over the use of PSA as a screening test for the general population. While some randomized controlled studies have shown that PSA screening reduces prostate cancer mortality,[28,29] another large trial showed no benefit.[30] In addition, PSA screening causes many men to receive unnecessary treatment, which carries its own risks. With conflicting data come conflicting guidelines for PSA screening. Recommendations range from not screening at all to obtaining baseline PSA values in all men beginning at 40 years. Collectively, guidelines encourage patients to be informed as to the pros and cons of testing. In addition, many guidelines support targeted testing, where patients are at higher risk for disease based on their family history and age in combination with other clinical information. The use of PSA for prostate cancer screening is likely to remain controversial for some time.

Methodology
PSA is measured by immunoassay, which detects both free PSA and PSA complexed with α_1-antichymotrypsin but not α_2-macroglobulin. Most immunoassays commercially available use enzyme, fluorescence, or chemiluminescence on an automated immunoassay platform. Because antibodies recognizing different epitopes may recognize the multiple forms of PSA variably, there can be some discrepant PSA results between manufacturers. Known interferences that have been reported for PSA include both the Hook effect[31] and HAMAs.[32,33]

Application and Pathophysiology
The best clinical use and first clinical application of PSA testing was to monitor for the progression of prostate cancer after therapy. After radical prostatectomy, serum PSA should become undetectable if the cancer is localized. In a series of men treated by radical prostatectomy from 1982 through 1997, biochemical recurrence was found to proceed any evidence of metastatic disease by nearly 8 years.[34] This use of PSA to monitor cancer progression has also been found useful after radiation or endocrine therapy.[35]

CASE STUDY 32-4

A 52-year-old man presented for an annual physical, where a screening PSA and DRE were performed. A serum PSA of 7.0 was detected, and on DRE, asymmetric nodules were detected (see Case Study Fig. 32-4.1). A transrectal biopsy, the gold standard for prostate cancer diagnosis, revealed the presence of carcinoma. A radical prostatectomy was performed a month later, where the preoperative PSA level was 7.1.

Questions

1. Was a prostatectomy performed on this patient because of an elevated PSA?

2. Is there any evidence for residual disease or recurrence in this patient?

3. Why was PSA testing delayed for 1 month after the prostatectomy?

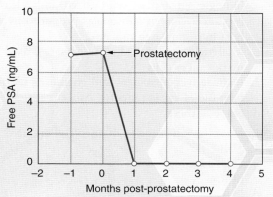

CASE STUDY FIGURE 32-4.1 Time course of serum PSA after radical prostatectomy. Because PSA is produced exclusively in the prostate gland, radical prostatectomy in this patient resulted in PSA levels below the level of detection of the assay. The half-life of PSA is 2 to 3 d, which generally requires approximately 1 mo for this drop to occur. At 3 mo after prostatectomy, this patient's PSA levels were undetectable (generally <0.1–0.3 ng/mL), indicating that residual disease was not present. After the first year of surgery, PSA levels should be taken every 3 mo (as shown). During the second year, it will be taken every 4 mo, and after that, every 6 mo. Any increase in PSA strongly indicates the recurrence of disease, with a delay in clinical symptoms 1 to 5 y.

FUTURE DIRECTIONS

Serological tumor markers provide an adjunct to clinical findings and imaging studies for diagnosis, monitoring, and treatment of cancer. Individual markers are not sufficiently sensitive or specific enough to be used in isolation. Tumor markers are an area of active research, such that laboratorians should remain aware of new guidelines and the development of new tests.

For additional student resources please visit thePoint at http://thepoint.lww.com. **thePoint**✳

QUESTIONS

1. What percentage of women will have invasive cancer at some time in their life?
   a. 33%
   b. 25%
   c. 50%
   d. 75%

2. Tumor marker tests are used to
   a. All of these
   b. Aid in staging of cancer
   c. Monitor response to therapy
   d. Detect recurrent disease

3. Tumor markers may be defined as
   a. Biologic substances synthesized and released by cancer cells or substances produced by the host in response to cancer cells
   b. Analytic tests (e.g., immunoassays) used to mark cancer cells
   c. Radioactive substances and chemicals used to help the physician identify cancer cells
   d. None of these

4. Which of the following is an oncofetal antigen?
   a. AFP
   b. CA-125
   c. β-hCG
   d. PSA

5. What are the major limitations of tumor markers?
   a. Sensitivity and specificity
   b. Cost
   c. Turnaround time
   d. Imprecision

6. The major clinical use for CA-125 is monitoring treatment response of
   a. Ovarian carcinoma
   b. Colorectal cancer
   c. Prostatic cancer
   d. Breast cancer

7. The most common immunoassays used to measure PSA detect which form of the enzyme?
   a. Total PSA
   b. Free PSA
   c. PSA complexed with α1-antichymotrypsin
   d. PSA complexed with α2-macroglobulin

8. Which of the following enzymes is commonly used as a tumor marker?
   a. LD
   b. Lipase
   c. Aldolase
   d. Catalase

9. A tumor marker used in the assessment of choriocarcinoma or hydatidiform mole is
   a. β-hCG
   b. CEA
   c. AFP
   d. IgG

10. A serum PSA is used for all of the following except
    a. Diagnosis
    b. Screening
    c. Monitoring response
    d. Detecting recurrence

11. The following serum PSA measurements were obtained from two male patients that were being monitored over an 18-week period.

	Week 1	Week 6	Week 10	Week 15	Week 18
Patient A	21 ng/mL	26 ng/mL	46 ng/mL	79 ng/mL	78 ng/mL
Patient B	14 ng/mL	46 ng/mL	89 ng/mL	120 ng/mL	110 ng/mL

Which of the following statements most accurately describes these data?
   a. Patient A may have a more aggressive prostate cancer based on the velocity of these measurements.
   b. Patient A is most likely to have benign prostate cancer.
   c. Patient B is most likely to be experiencing an inflammatory reaction and this is largely contributing to the elevated PSA above 100 ng/mL.
   d. Patient B may have a more aggressive prostate cancer based on the velocity of these measurements.
   e. Answers *a* and *c* most accurately describe these data.

12. When measuring tumor markers in the clinical laboratory, which of the following has been reported to contribute to 30% to 70% of the total amount of measurement error?
    a. Preanalytical errors
    b. Analytical errors
    c. Hook effect
    d. Using different immunoassay methods
    e. Not comparing lot numbers between ELISA kits

SUGGESTED READING

Diamandis EP, Fritsche HA, Lilja H, et al. *Tumor Markers: Physiology, Pathobiology, Technology, and Clinical Applications.* Washington, DC: AACC Press; 2002.

Wu JT. *Circulating Tumor Markers of the New Millennium: Target Therapy, Early Detection, and Prognosis.* Washington, DC: AACC Press; 2002.

REFERENCES

1. National Cancer Institute, Statistical Research and Applications Branch. DevCan: probability of developing or dying of cancer software version 6.1.0. http://srab.cancer.gov/devcan/. Accessed October 20, 2008.
2. Abeloff MD, Armitage JO, Niederhuber JE, Kastan MB, McKenna WG, eds. *Abeloff's Clinical Oncology.* 4th ed. Philadelphia, PA: Churchill Livingstone; 2008.
3. Hanahan D, Weinberg RA. The hallmarks of cancer. *Cell.* 2000;100:57-70.
4. Clinical and Laboratory Standards Institute. Standards and guidelines for clinical laboratories. www.clsi.org. Accessed October 20, 2008.
5. Klee GG. Human anti-mouse antibodies. *Arch Pathol Lab Med.* 2000;124:921-923.
6. Harris L, Fritsche H, Mennel R, et al. American Society of Clinical Oncology 2007 update of recommendations for the use of tumor markers in breast cancer. *J Clin Oncol.* 2007;25:5287-5312.
7. Bader D, Riskin A, Vafsi O, et al. Alpha-fetoprotein in the early neonatal period—a large study and review of the literature. *Clin Chim Acta.* 2004;349:15-23.
8. Gupta S, Bent S, Kohlwes J. Test characteristics of alpha-fetoprotein for detecting hepatocellular carcinoma in patients with hepatitis C. A systematic review and critical analysis. *Ann Intern Med.* 2003;139:46-50.
9. Wu JT. Serum alpha-fetoprotein and its lectin reactivity in liver diseases: a review. *Ann Clin Lab Sci.* 1990;20:98-105.
10. Diamandis EP, Hoffman BR, Sturgeon CM. National Academy of Clinical Biochemistry laboratory medicine practical guidelines for the use of tumor markers. *Clin Chem.* 2008;54:1935-1939.
11. Raghavan D. *Germ Cell Tumors.* London and Ontario: BC Decker; 2003.
12. Yin BW, Lloyd KO. Molecular cloning of the CA125 ovarian cancer antigen: identification as a new mucin, MUC16. *J Biol Chem.* 2001;276:27371-27375.
13. Duffy MJ, Bonfrer JM, Kulpa J, et al. CA125 in ovarian cancer: European Group on Tumor Markers guidelines for clinical use. *Int J Gynecol Cancer.* 2005;15:679-691.
14. Bast RC Jr, Xu FJ, Yu YH, et al. CA 125: the past and the future. *Int J Biol Markers.* 1998;13:179-187.
15. Verheijen RH, von Mensdorff-Pouilly S, van Kamp GJ, Kenemans P. CA 125: fundamental and clinical aspects. *Semin Cancer Biol.* 1999;9:117-124.
16. Duffy MJ, van Dalen A, Haglund C, et al. Clinical utility of biochemical markers in colorectal cancer: European Group on Tumour Markers (EGTM) guidelines. *Eur J Cancer.* 2003;39:718-727.
17. Bower M, Rustin G. Serum tumor markers and their role in monitoring germ cell cancers of the testis. In: Vogelzang N, Scardino P, Shipley W, Coffey D, eds. *Comprehensive Textbook of Genitourinary Oncology.* 2nd ed. Philadelphia, PA: Lippincott Williams & Wilkins; 2000:931.
18. Cole LA, Sutton JM, Higgins TN, Cembrowski GS. Between-method variation in human chorionic gonadotropin test results. *Clin Chem.* 2004;50:874-882.
19. Smith RA, Cokkinides V, Eyre HJ. American Cancer Society guidelines for the early detection of cancer, 2006. *CA Cancer J Clin.* 2006;56:11-25; quiz 49-50.
20. Loeb S, Catalona WJ. Prostate-specific antigen in clinical practice. *Cancer Lett.* 2007;249:30-39.
21. Herschman JD, Smith DS, Catalona WJ. Effect of ejaculation on serum total and free prostate-specific antigen concentrations. *Urology.* 1997;50:239-243.
22. Crawford ED, Schutz MJ, Clejan S, et al. The effect of digital rectal examination on prostate-specific antigen levels. *JAMA.* 1992;267:2227-2228.
23. Chybowski FM, Bergstralh EJ, Oesterling JE. The effect of digital rectal examination on the serum prostate specific antigen concentration: results of a randomized study. *J Urol.* 1992;148:83-86.
24. Collins GN, Martin PJ, Wynn-Davies A, et al. The effect of digital rectal examination, flexible cystoscopy and prostatic biopsy on free and total prostate specific antigen, and the free-to-total prostate specific antigen ratio in clinical practice. *J Urol.* 1997;157:1744-1747.
25. Tarhan F, Orcun A, Kucukercan I, et al. Effect of prostatic massage on serum complexed prostate-specific antigen levels. *Urology.* 2005;66:1234-1238.
26. Thompson IM, Goodman PJ, Tangen CM, et al. The influence of finasteride on the development of prostate cancer. *N Engl J Med.* 2003;349:215-224.
27. Thompson IM, Pauler DK, Goodman PJ, et al. Prevalence of prostate cancer among men with a prostate-specific antigen level < or =4.0 ng per milliliter. *N Engl J Med.* 2004;350:2239-2246.
28. Schröder FH, Hugosson J, Roobol MJ, et al. Screening and prostate-cancer mortality in a randomized European study. *N Engl J Med.* March 2009;360(13):1320-1328.
29. Schröder FH, Hugosson J, Roobol MJ, et al. Prostate-cancer mortality at 11 years of follow-up. *N Engl J Med.* 2012;366(11):981-990.
30. Andriole GL, Crawford ED, Grubb RL, et al. Mortality results from a randomized prostate-cancer screening trial. *N Engl J Med.* March 2009;360(13):1310-1319.
31. Akamatsu S, Tsukazaki H, Inoue K, Nishio Y. Advanced prostate cancer with extremely low prostate-specific antigen value at diagnosis: an example of high dose hook effect. *Int J Urol.* 2006;13:1025-1027.
32. Park S, Wians FH Jr, Cadeddu JA. Spurious prostate-specific antigen (PSA) recurrence after radical prostatectomy: interference by human antimouse heterophile antibodies. *Int J Urol.* 2007;14:251-253.
33. Descotes JL, Legeais D, Gauchez AS, et al. PSA measurement following prostatectomy: an unexpected error. *Anticancer Res.* 2007;27:1149-1150.
34. Pound CR, Partin AW, Eisenberger MA, et al. Natural history of progression after PSA elevation following radical prostatectomy. *JAMA.* 1999;281:1591-1597.
35. Roach M 3rd, Hanks G, Thames H Jr, et al. Defining biochemical failure following radiotherapy with or without hormonal therapy in men with clinically localized prostate cancer: recommendations of the RTOG-ASTRO Phoenix Consensus Conference. *Int J Radiat Oncol Biol Phys.* 2006;65:965-974.

Nutrition Assessment

LINDA S. GORMAN, MARIA G. BOOSALIS

CHAPTER
33

CHAPTER OUTLINE

- ◆ **NUTRITION CARE PROCESS: OVERVIEW**
- ◆ **NUTRITION ASSESSMENT**
- ◆ **BIOCHEMICAL MARKERS: MACRONUTRIENTS**
  Protein
  Fat
  Carbohydrate
- ◆ **BIOCHEMICAL MARKERS: MISCELLANEOUS**
  Parenteral Nutrition
  Electrolytes

  Urine Testing
  Organ Function
- ◆ **BIOCHEMICAL MARKERS: MICRONUTRIENTS**
  Vitamins
  Conditionally Essential Nutrients
  Minerals
  Trace Elements
- ◆ **QUESTIONS**
- ◆ **REFERENCES**

Chapter Objectives

Upon completion of this chapter, the clinical laboratorian should be able to do the following:

- Discuss the contribution of individual nutrient classes to human metabolism.
- Discuss therapeutic nutrition support by enteral and parenteral routes.
- List biochemical parameters used to monitor nutritional status.
- Describe the biochemical roles of vitamins.
- Correlate alterations in vitamin status with circumstances of increased metabolic requirements, age-related physiologic changes, or pathologic conditions.

- Describe drug–nutrient interactions that influence vitamin status.
- Delineate laboratory procedures used in the assessment of vitamin status.
- Discuss the role of the laboratory in nutritional assessment and monitoring.
- List the populations at risk for malnutrition.
- Identify the plasma protein changes as a result of stress.
- Describe some of the electrolyte and mineral abnormalities associated with total parenteral nutrition.

KEY TERMS

Body mass index (BMI)
Dietary Reference Intake (DRI)
Essential nutrients
Hypervitaminosis
Hypovitaminosis

Kwashiorkor
Malnutrition
Marasmus
Nitrogen balance
Nutrient
Parenteral nutrition
Vitamin

NUTRITION CARE PROCESS: OVERVIEW

The *nutrition care process (NCP)* is defined as "a systemic problem-solving method that dietetic professionals use to critically think and make decisions to address nutrition-related problems and provide safe and effective quality nutrition care."[1] In other words, this process is the systematic approach used by the registered dietitian (RD)

to identify, diagnose, and treat any nutrition-related problems or disorders.

There are four components to the NCP: nutrition assessment; nutrition diagnosis; nutrition intervention, and nutrition monitoring and evaluation.[1]

The focus of this chapter is the first component of the NCP, specifically nutrition assessment. *Nutrition assessment* is defined as a "systematic process of obtaining, verifying, and interpreting data in order to make decisions about the nature and cause of nutrition-related problems."[1] Nutrition assessment includes the "A–Es of assessment."[2]

> A—anthropometric or body composition measurements
>
> B—biochemical analyses, the prime focus of this chapter
>
> C—clinical examination usually performed by the physician or other health-care provider
>
> D—dietary analysis and assessment to determine usual food intake generally performed by the RD
>
> E—environmental assessment, which includes a consideration of all the other aspects of the individual's environment that may affect his/her ability to purchase, prepare, and consume food.

NUTRITION ASSESSMENT

A. Anthropometric measurements include, at a minimum, the measurement of height and weight and from those two measurements the calculation of the body mass index (BMI). The BMI "describes relative weight for height, is significantly correlated with total body fat content" and should be "used to assess overweight and obesity and to monitor changes in body weight."[3]

Other measurements in this category that are helpful, especially when assessing an individual, include a weight history (amount or percentage of gain vs. loss; intentional vs. unintentional) and possibly a waist circumference measurement (to help identify additional comorbidity risk and the presence of metabolic syndrome).

Other anthropometric or body composition measurements that belong in this category include skinfold thickness, hydrostatic weighing, air-displacement plethysmography, dual-energy x-ray absorptiometry, and bioelectrical impedance analysis, all of which are beyond the scope of this chapter. All of these different types of measurements are used to determine the percentage of fat, lean body muscle, water, and/or bone mineral density in the human body.

Until this epidemic of overweight/obesity lessens, approximately two of every three adults measured may be either overweight (BMI 25 to 29.9 kg/m^2) or obese (BMI $\geq$ 30 kg/m^2) by the National Heart, Lung, and Blood Institute (NHLBI) standards. On the other side of the spectrum is the adult who may be malnourished/undernourished and possibly also underweight (BMI < 18.5 kg/m^2).

B. Biochemical assessment/markers are divided into macronutrients and micronutrients. The macronutrients include markers of carbohydrate, protein, and fat metabolism and utilization. How these markers change during inflammation and disease can be important to

know if treatment is to be effective. Health-care providers appreciate the clinical laboratory assessment of these markers and expect to receive the results in a timely manner. Micronutrient measurements are often more difficult to obtain and yet may hold the key to why a patient straddles the fence between health and illness. Insufficient or excessive vitamins and/or minerals can have a serious impact on the enzymes and biochemistry of the human body. In particular, trace elements or minerals are especially important to many biologically significant metabolic reactions.

There is a close interrelationship between the function of certain organs in the body and nutrient balance/imbalance, both positive and negative. Liver function will be affected if there is insufficient protein and excess fats. Liver function within normal limits is critical to the adequate processing of ingested protein and fats and the packaging/storage of certain vitamins and minerals. An excessive intake of protein may also be harmful to kidney function due to the excess of nonprotein nitrogen compounds formed that must then be removed. On the other hand, normal renal function is critical to the amount of protein, sodium, and fluids that can be consumed. Other nutrient imbalances can affect the heart (fats, water imbalances, vitamin deficiencies or excesses, selenium, etc.), pancreas, and/or other glands. The thyroid in particular not only requires adequate iodine and tyrosine levels for hormone synthesis but also requires adequate iron levels as enzyme cofactors for the formation and degradation of T_4 and T_3.[4]

In addition, during hospitalization, biomarkers enable the health-care team to monitor and detect acute stress and other systemic inflammatory conditions. The acute-phase reactant proteins and other circulating vitamins and/or minerals that are monitored can help pinpoint patients at risk and in need of nutritional intervention and aid in the identification of the systemic inflammatory response syndrome.[5,6,7-11] In addition, signs of a chronic inflammatory state can be ascertained with the aid of clinical laboratory tests.[12]

Assessing the biomarkers in a nutrition assessment is the responsibility of the clinical laboratory professional. These are discussed individually in a later section of this chapter.

C. The clinical component of the nutrition assessment consists of the history of present illness, the past medical history, and an inquiry into the family history. It also includes the physical examination and a careful review of systems looking for signs of disease/illness. It includes a measurement of blood pressure as well as presence of any physical limitations/restrictions regarding physical movement/activity.

For example, the *review of systems* is a head-to-toe examination looking for signs of malnutrition and/or disease. For instance, ease of pluckability of hair (>8 to

10 hairs at one time) may indicate a protein deficiency that requires biochemical verification via measurement of circulating proteins such as albumin and transthyretin. Changes in vision such as night blindness or Bitot's spots may indicate a deficiency of vitamin A.

Metabolic syndrome is defined by utilizing information derived from the first three components (A–C) of a nutrition assessment. Specifically, the presence of three or more of any of the following parameters defines the presence of the metabolic syndrome in an individual according to the American Heart Association and the NHLBI.[13] These parameters include the following:

1. An elevated waist circumference. In women, ≥35 in. (88 cm); in men, ≥40 in. (102 cm)
2. Elevated triglyceride levels, i.e., ≥150 mg/dL
3. Elevated fasting glucose, i.e., ≥100 mg/dL
4. Reduced high-density lipoprotein (HDL) cholesterol. In women, <50 mg/dL; in men, <40 mg/dL
5. Elevated blood pressure, i.e., ≥130/85 mm Hg

D. The dietary component of the nutritional assessment strives to determine the adequacy of the usual day's intake with respect to nutritional recommendations that are specific for an individual's age, gender, level of physical activity, and particular health conditions. In addition, if there are any specific dietary needs that must be met, an assessment to determine whether these needs are met must also be included. There are several ways to assess adequacy of intake—by general food groupings and respective servings using the USDA Food Guidance System ChooseMyPlate eating plans[14] or via specific nutrients compared with the Dietary Reference Intake (DRI) recommendations (Recommended Dietary Allowance [RDA], Adequate Intake [AI], and/or Tolerable Upper Limits [UL]).[15] Examples of tools used by the RD to determine dietary adequacy include the 24-hour recall, the 3-day food record or diary, and/or the food frequency questionnaire. Again, specific details of each methodology are beyond the scope of this chapter.

E. The environmental assessment takes into consideration all aspects of an individual's environment or living conditions that may affect his or her ability to purchase, prepare, and/or consume food.

For example, it includes financial status to determine if money is a limiting factor to obtaining one's nutritional needs/adequate nutrition.

An individual's physical living conditions (e.g., adequate cooking skills, preparation supplies, and running water), social support system, and religious beliefs (especially if it prevents the individual from consuming certain food groups) are other types of information included.

This assessment also evaluates the highest level of education attained to tailor educational materials and message. In essence, any aspect of the environment that may affect the ability to purchase, prepare, and/or consume food is included in this evaluation.

The information obtained from all A–E aspects of a complete nutrition assessment is then summarized and reviewed by the RD or other health-care professional to determine a nutrition diagnosis, the next step in the NCP. Once the nutrition diagnosis is made, a plan for the nutrition intervention is designed and implemented followed by monitoring and evaluation as the last component of the NCP.

BIOCHEMICAL MARKERS: MACRONUTRIENTS

Protein

The primary objective is to identify the patient who is malnourished and then, through nutritional therapy, to preserve or replenish the protein component of the body. Laboratory nutrition assessment is best accomplished by monitoring selected serum proteins that ideally have a short biologic half-life and reflect changes in protein status by measuring their concentration changes in the serum. These concentrations of protein markers are affected by protein malnutrition associated with end-stage liver and renal disease and severe infection and, most significantly, by stress injury. Because the effect of the inflammatory response is closely associated with the decline of essential transport proteins, a separation of the inflammatory state from protein malnutrition can be problematic, except by using an acute-phase reactant, such as C-reactive protein (CRP). The prognostic inflammatory nutritional index, using the ratio of the CRP–orosomucoid (α_1-acid glycoprotein) product to the albumin–transthyretin product, is intended to resolve this issue.[16] Table 33-1 offers detailed information about these protein markers.

Albumin
Albumin has long been used in the assessment of hospitalized patients. The albumin concentration in the body is influenced by albumin synthesis, degradation, and distribution. Low levels of serum albumin may reflect low hepatic production or loss from transfer of albumin between the extravascular and the vascular compartment. The long biologic half-life of albumin (approximately 20 days) allows changes in the serum concentration only after long periods of malnutrition. Low albumin levels have been identified as a predictor of mortality in patients in long-term-care facilities. Hospitalized patients with low serum albumin levels experience a fourfold increase in morbidity and a sixfold increase in mortality.[17,18]

Serum albumin is not a good indicator of short-term protein and energy deprivation; however, albumin levels are good indicators of chronic deficiency. Traditionally,

TABLE 33-1	CHARACTERISTICS OF PLASMA PROTEINS OF NUTRITIONAL INTEREST		
PROTEIN	**MOLECULAR WEIGHT (κD)**	**HALF-LIFE**	**REFERENCE RANGE**
Albumin	65,000	20 d	33–48 g/L
Fibronectin	250,000	15 h	220–400 mg/L
Prealbumin (transthyretin)	54,980	48 h	160–350 mg/L
Retinol-binding protein	21,000	12 h	30–60 mg/L
Insulin-like growth factor 1	7,650	2 h	0.10–0.40 mg/L
Transferrin	76,000	9 d	1.6–3.6 g/L

albumin has been used to help determine two important nutritional states. First, it helps identify chronic protein deficiency under conditions of adequate non–protein-calorie intake, which leads to marked hypoalbuminemia. This may result from the net loss of albumin from both the intravascular and extravascular pools, causing kwashiorkor. Second, albumin concentrations may help define marasmus, a deficiency of calories with adequate protein status. In this condition, the serum albumin level remains normal despite considerable loss of body weight. Studies have classified various levels of malnutrition by using albumin levels. Serum albumin levels of ≥35 g/L are considered normal. Albumin levels of 28–30 to 35 g/L indicate mild malnutrition, levels of 23–25 to 28–30 g/L indicate moderate malnutrition, and levels less than 23 to 25 g/L indicate severely depleted albumin. Serum albumin is an accurate marker of the catabolic stress of infection. A level of ≤32 g/L indicates that if a patient is in the hospital for up to 10 days, there is a 75% risk of developing decubitus ulcers. Serum albumin levels of less than 25 g/L can be used as an accurate measure of predicting survival prognosis in 90% of critically ill patients.

Transferrin

Transferrin is a glycoprotein with a biologic half-life of approximately 9 days (shorter than albumin). It is synthesized in the liver and binds and transports ferric iron. Transferrin synthesis is regulated by iron stores. When hepatocyte iron is absent or low, transferrin levels rise in proportion to the deficiency. It is an early indicator of iron deficiency, and the elevated transferrin is the last analyte to return to normal when iron deficiency is corrected.

The half-life of transferrin is approximately one-half that of albumin, and the body pool is smaller than that of albumin; therefore, transferrin is more likely to indicate protein depletion before serum albumin concentration changes. The usefulness of transferrin in diagnosis of subclinical, marginal, or moderate malnutrition is questionable, however, because a wide range of values have been reported in various studies. Transferrin levels can be lowered by factors other than protein or energy deficiency, such as nephrotic syndrome, liver disorders, anemia, and neoplastic disease.

In hospital and nursing home settings, transferrin levels have been used as indices of morbidity and mortality.[19] Information shows, however, that serum transferrin concentrations are not sufficiently sensitive to detect a change in nutritional status that occurs after 2 weeks of total parenteral nutrition.[20] In addition to being responsive to serum iron concentrations, transferrin is uniquely sensitive to some antibiotics and fungicides.

Transthyretin

Transthyretin is sometimes called thyroxine-binding prealbumin or prealbumin because it migrates ahead of albumin in the customary electrophoresis of serum or plasma proteins. In normal situations, each transthyretin subunit contains one binding site for retinol-binding protein (RBP). Transthyretin and RBP are considered the major transport proteins for thyroxine and vitamin A, respectively.

Because of its short half-life and small body pool, transthyretin is a better indicator of visceral protein status and positive nitrogen balance than albumin and transferrin.[20] Transthyretin is a superior indicator for monitoring short-term effects of nutritional therapy. The concentration of transthyretin and RBP complex, greatly decreased in protein-energy malnutrition,[21] returns toward normal values after nutritional replenishment. Transthyretin has a low pool concentration in the serum, a half-life of 2 days, and a rapid response to low energy intake, even when protein intake is inadequate for as few as 4 days.[22] Serum transthyretin concentrations are decreased postoperatively by 50 to 90 mg/L in the first week, with the ability to double in 1 week or at least increase 40 to 50 mg/L in response to adequate nutritional support. If the transthyretin response increases less than 20 mg/L in 1 week as an outcome measure, this indicates either inadequate nutritional support or inadequate response.[20,23]

When transthyretin decreases to levels of less than 80 mg/L, severe protein-calorie malnutrition develops; however, nutritional support can cause a daily increase in transthyretin of up to 10 mg/L.[20] These concentrations do not appear to be significantly influenced by fluctuations in the hydration state. Although end-stage liver disease appears to affect all protein levels in the body, liver disease does not affect transthyretin as early or to the same extent as it affects other serum protein markers, particularly RBP. Although transthyretin levels may be elevated in patients with renal disease, if a trend in the direction of change is noted, the changes are likely to reflect alteration in nutritional status and nitrogen balance. Steroids can cause a slight elevation in transthyretin, but the nutritional trend can still be followed because transthyretin responds to both overfeeding and underfeeding.

Transthyretin is also used as an indicator of the adequacy of a nutritional feeding plan[20] because changes in plasma protein are correlated with nitrogen balance. Transthyretin concentrations increase in patients with positive nitrogen balance and decrease in patients with negative nitrogen balance. When the transthyretin level is ≥180 mg/L, this correlates with a positive nitrogen balance and indicates a return to adequate nutritional status. It has been shown in both the pediatric and neonate population to be a highly accurate and relatively inexpensive marker for nutritional status[24,25] and has been found to be the most sensitive and helpful indicator when looking at the nutritional status of very ill patients.[26]

In summary, transthyretin effectively demonstrates an anabolic response to feeding and is a good marker for visceral protein synthesis in patients receiving metabolic or nutritional support.[26-28]

Retinol-Binding Protein

RBP has been used in monitoring short-term changes in nutritional status.[29-31] Its usefulness as a metabolic marker is based on its biologic half-life of 12 hours and its small body pool size. As a single polypeptide chain, RBP interacts strongly with plasma transthyretin and circulates in the plasma as a 1:1 mol/L transthyretin–RBP complex.[32] A potential problem exists in using RBP as a nutritional marker, however. Although RBP has a shorter half-life than transthyretin (12 hours, compared with 2 days), it is excreted in the urine, and its concentration increases more significantly than transthyretin in patients with renal failure. In contrast to RBP, transthyretin concentration is only moderately elevated in advanced chronic renal insufficiency.

Insulin-Like Growth Factor 1

Insulin-like growth factor 1 (IGF-1) (formerly termed somatomedin C) is important for stimulation of growth. The molecular size and structure of IGF-1 is similar to proinsulin.[33] IGF-1 serum concentrations are regulated by growth hormone and nutritional intake. Growth hormone stimulates the liver to produce IGF-1, which circulates bound to IGF-BP3. IGF-BP3 modulates the biologic effect of IGF-1 in the stress response, causing both decreases and increases in biologic activity. IGF-1 has been used as a nutritional marker in adults and children,[34-36] although not routinely.

Fibronectin

Fibronectin is an opsonic glycoprotein with a half-life of about 15 hours in humans. This protein has repeating blocks of a homogeneous sequence of amino acids and is an α_2-glycoprotein that serves important roles in cell-to-cell adherence and tissue differentiation, wound healing, microvascular integrity, and opsonization of particulate matter. It is considered the major protein regulating phagocytosis. Synthesis sites include endothelial cells, peritoneal macrophages, fibroblasts, and the liver. Fibronectin concentrations may decrease after physiologic damage caused by severe shock, burns, or infection. Levels return to normal on recovery. Fibronectin is of interest because it is not exclusively synthesized in the liver,[37] and it is an indicator of sepsis in burn patients. Fibronectin levels have been shown to decrease during infection or severe stress, partly due to its opsonic property. The infection or trauma, however, does not significantly decrease fibronectin concentration.[38] Fibronectin only increases in severe infection, in which it remains flat and does not increase as soon as IGF-1. It is not routinely used as a nutritional marker.

Nitrogen Balance

Another nutritional evaluation tool, nitrogen balance, is the difference between nitrogen intake and nitrogen excretion. It is one of the most widely used indicators of protein change and/or adequacy of feeding in a controlled setting. In the healthy adult population, anabolic and catabolic rates are in equilibrium, and the nitrogen balance approaches zero. During stress, trauma, or burns, the nutritional intake decreases, and due to an increase in catabolism, nitrogen losses increase and may exceed intake, leading to a negative nitrogen balance. During recovery from illness, the nitrogen balance should become positive with either enteral or parenteral nutrition (PN) support. In humans, 90% to 95% of the daily nitrogen loss is accounted for by elimination through the kidneys. About 90% of this loss is in the form of urea. Therefore, the determination of 24-hour urinary urea nitrogen (UUN) is a method for estimating the amount of nitrogen excretion. The nitrogen balance is calculated as follows[39]:

$$\text{Nitrogen balance} = \frac{24 \text{ hour protein intake(g)}}{6.25}$$

$$- (24 \text{ hour UUN (g)} + 4\text{g}) \quad \textbf{(Eq. 33-1)}$$

Protein intake includes grams of protein that are provided by intravenous amino acids or by enteral feeding. Protein intake (in grams) is converted into grams of nitrogen by dividing by 6.25. The factor of 4 in the equation represents an estimation of nonurinary losses of nitrogen (e.g., from skin, feces, hair, and nails).[39] Nitrogen balance, as calculated by this equation, is not valid in patients with severe stress or sepsis, as can be seen in critical care areas or in patients with renal disease. Determining the validity of this equation in other clinical conditions involving normally high nitrogen losses may be difficult or even incorrect.

C-Reactive Protein

CRP is an acute-phase protein that increases dramatically under conditions of sepsis, inflammation, and infection. CRP can increase dramatically up to 1,000 times after tissue injury, which are more than two or three orders of magnitude greater than any other acute-phase reactant. CRP rises in concentration 4 to 6 hours before other acute-phase reactants begin to rise.[5,10,12,40,41]

The flow phase of marked catabolism presents clinically with tachycardia, fever, increased respiratory rate, and increased cardiac output. During this time, synthesis rates of CRP and other acute-phase proteins increase and albumin and prealbumin decrease.[5] Even with this increase in acute-phase proteins, a significant negative nitrogen balance usually occurs secondary to the greater protein catabolism.[43] Whether this catabolic state produces a clinically defined malnutrition or a separate entity is unknown, but it certainly produces weight loss with decreased albumin and prealbumin levels.

High-sensitivity CRP is an additional marker for inflammation and has been applied as a predictor of cardiac disease and other cholesterol-related atherosclerotic disorders.

Cytokines

Nutrition research has recently focused on cytokines, in particular the interleukins, a complex group of proteins and glycoproteins that can exert pleiotropic effects on several different target cells. Most interleukins are produced by macrophages and T-lymphocytes, in response to antigenic or mitogenic stimulation, and affect primary T-lymphocyte function. Most nutritional investigations regarding cytokines have been performed on interleukin-1 (IL-1), IL-6, and tumor necrosis factor-α (TNF-α). In addition to these cytokines released by the immune system, adipose cells (adipocytes) release similar compounds, including IL-6 and TNF-α as well as other adipokines such as leptin, resistin, visfatin, and adiponectin, to mention a few. These cytokines and adipokines are subsequently involved in many reactions and body systems that are beyond the scope and purpose of this chapter.

Fat

Fat is a macronutrient that, in appropriate amounts, is needed for a balanced diet. Alterations in fat intake may also affect circulating lipid levels and lipid metabolism.

Laboratory markers for total cholesterol as well as triglycerides enable us to assess some of these lipid changes. Excess fat and/or kilocalorie intake and the repercussions from such a diet can be assessed by looking at HDL and low-density lipoprotein cholesterol levels as well as various lipoproteins. These markers are further discussed in Chapter 15.

Carbohydrate

Nutrition assessment for type 1 and type 2 diabetes mellitus comes into play after diagnosis and requires periodic laboratory assessment for patient compliance/monitoring of treatment. Patients with diabetes have a chronic illness that can be regulated by medication and diet, if they are willing to change many of their habits and eating preferences. Dietitians and physicians rely on laboratory assessment of patient compliance by looking at glucose markers of blood glucose, glycosylated hemoglobin/proteins, and fructosamine. As the diabetic patient has long-term health issues with their disease, additional laboratory tests for renal function such as microalbumin and estimated glomerular filtration rate will also be requested. The partnership between the laboratory and those treating the diabetic patient is needed to assist the diabetic patient in attaining the highest quality of good health. These laboratory markers are further discussed in Chapter 14.

BIOCHEMICAL MARKERS: MISCELLANEOUS

Parenteral Nutrition

Parenteral nutrition is a widely used means of intense nutritional support for patients who are malnourished or in danger of becoming malnourished because they are unable to consume required amounts of nutrients or to take nutrients enterally (i.e., by mouth). PN therapy involves administering appropriate amounts of carbohydrate, amino acid, and lipid solutions, as well as electrolytes, vitamins, minerals, and trace elements, to meet the caloric, protein, and nutrient requirements while maintaining water and electrolyte balance.[44] PN can be provided peripherally or centrally, the latter being more frequently used. These central PN preparations are usually administered through a subclavian catheter. Preferably, an individual will eat by mouth or a feeding tube that is placed either in the stomach or ideally the upper duodenum. These aforementioned tube feedings deliver nutrients. Patients may also have gastrointestinal surgery to have a feeding gastrostomy or jejunostomy catheter put in place during the surgical procedure. Because PN administration bypasses normal absorption and circulation routes, careful laboratory monitoring of these patients is critical. The goal is to provide optimal nutritional status by whatever routes nutrients are administered. An unintended weight loss of more than

10% to 12% leads to suspicion of either disease or malnutrition. The patient's height, age, and activity level are also considered.[45]

It is important to monitor the PN patient to avoid possible complications. Such laboratory monitoring provides necessary information needed to properly administer PN therapy.

Electrolytes

Sodium regulation is a problem in children during PN. Daily sodium requirements may vary depending on renal maturity and the ability of the child's body to regulate sodium. Factors that increase the amount of sodium necessary to maintain normal serum sodium concentrations in both children and adults are glycosuria, diuretic use, diarrhea or other excessive gastrointestinal losses, and increased postoperative fluid losses.

Hyperkalemia is a common problem in children when blood is obtained by heel stick. The squeezing of the heel may cause red cell hemolysis, resulting in falsely high serum potassium levels. Although adequate nutrition may be supplied to promote anabolism, hypokalemia may develop as the extracellular supply is used for cell synthesis.

The primary function of chloride is osmotic regulation. Hyperchloremia metabolic acidosis is a problem when crystal amino acid solutions are used, but such acidosis can be prevented or treated by altering the amount of chloride salt in the PN solution. Supplying some of the sodium and potassium requirements as acetate or phosphate salts can reduce the required amount of chloride. The reformulation of synthetic amino acid solutions by commercial manufacturers has helped to avoid this serious complication. If hyperchloremia metabolic acidosis does occur, treatment with sodium and potassium acetate solutions is used because acetate is metabolized rapidly to bicarbonate. Acetate salts are compatible with all other common PN components and are ideal to use when acidosis is present. Sodium bicarbonate cannot be used in PN solutions containing calcium because calcium carbonate readily precipitates. The use of acetate not only increases serum bicarbonate but also decreases the amount of chloride delivered to the patient.

Urine Testing

In small premature infants, glycosuria during the early phase of PN is a signal that glucose infusion is too rapid. If glucose appears in the urine of small infants after glucose tolerance has been established, however, the clinician should question the presence of respiratory disease, sepsis, or cardiovascular changes.

Organ Function

In order to successfully feed an individual, whether by mouth or parenterally, the major organ systems need to function properly, including the liver that metabolizes nutrients and/or the kidneys that excrete nutrient waste products. For this reason, health/nutrition professionals measure various markers such as circulating enzymes and proteins to determine adequate organ function.

BIOCHEMICAL MARKERS: MICRONUTRIENTS

Vitamins

Vitamins have a wide range of functions in biologic tissue, serving as cofactors in many enzymatic reactions, so that these enzymes have low catalytic activity in cellular reactions if vitamins are not present. These compounds and their biologically inactive precursors must be partially obtained from food sources and, in some instances, from bacterial synthesis. When cellular vitamin and activity levels from diet or intestinal absorption are inadequate, it is termed vitamin deficiency. The term *vitamin* has an historical basis in deficiency states that were relieved by specific food intake. The most notable examples are scurvy (vitamin C, sailors and lime consumption, limeys); rickets (vitamin D in the early industrial age); beriberi (alcoholics and thiamine); pellagra (niacin) and night blindness (vitamin A); megaloblastic anemia (folic acid or vitamin B_{12}); spina bifida (folic acid); and pernicious anemia with neuropathy (vitamin B_{12}). Abnormal increases of metabolism requiring high supplies of one of these cofactors may be termed *vitamin insufficiency* or *vitamin dependency*, depending on the level of supply demanded for physiologic function.[46,47]

Variabilities in clinical expression of vitamin abnormalities result from differences in any of the following: in specific cause, degree, and duration of vitamin inadequacy, the simultaneous presence of nutritional insufficiencies, and/or the increased metabolic demands imposed by conditions such as pregnancy, infection, and cancer. The clinical symptoms of vitamin deficiencies are usually nonspecific in early stages and in mild, chronic deficiency states. A combination of dietary history, physical examination, and laboratory measurements is often required to diagnose vitamin deficiency. Vitamin metabolism is complex and vitamin supplementation of foods is common. It is not unusual to find vitamin toxicities from inappropriate use of vitamin supplementation.

For simplicity, vitamins of diverse chemical structure are classified as either water soluble or fat soluble. Fat-soluble vitamins include A, D, E, and K. Those vitamins soluble in water include the B complex of vitamins—thiamine, riboflavin, niacin, vitamins B_6 and B_{12}, biotin, folate, and vitamin C. Water-soluble vitamins are readily excreted in the urine and are less likely than fat-soluble vitamins to accumulate to toxic levels in the body. Vitamins, classified as fat or water soluble, and the symptoms usually seen in deficiency states are shown in Table 33-2.[48,49]

TABLE 33-2 VITAMIN AND DEFICIENCY STATES

VITAMIN NAME	CLINICAL DEFICIENCY
FAT-SOLUBLE VITAMINS	
Vitamin A_1	Night blindness, growth retardation, abnormal taste response, dermatitis, recurrent infections
Vitamin E	Mild hemolytic anemia (newborn), red blood cell fragility, ataxia
Vitamin D	Rickets (young), osteomalacia (adult)
Vitamin K	Hemorrhage (ranging from easy bruising to massive bruising), especially post-traumatic bleeding
WATER-SOLUBLE VITAMINS	
Vitamin B_1	Infants: dyspnea, cyanosis, diarrhea, vomiting Adults: beriberi (fatigue, peripheral neuritis), Wernicke-Korsakoff syndrome (apathy, ataxia, visual problems)
Vitamin B_2	Angular stomatitis (mouth lesions), dermatitis, photophobia, neurologic changes
Vitamin B_6	Infants: irritability, seizures, anemia, vomiting, weakness Adults: facial seborrhea
Niacin/niacinamide	Pellagra (dermatitis, mucous membrane inflammation, weight loss, disorientation)
Folic acid	Megaloblastic anemia
Vitamin B_{12}	Megaloblastic anemia, neurologic abnormalities
Vitamin C	First, vague aches and pains; if long term, scurvy (hemorrhages into skin, alimentary and urinary tract, anemia, wound healing delayed)

Investigating the dietary deficiency of vitamins (hypovitaminosis) is sustained primarily from knowledge of dietary sources and dietary practices that produce inadequate intake or absorption. In the early 1990s, the Food and Nutrition Board of the Institute of Medicine began the process of reviewing the previous nutritional recommendations known as RDAs to also include the prevention of chronic diseases. In addition, besides the RDA, there are additional categories such as estimated average requirement, AI, and tolerable upper intake level (UL).[49-51]

Chemical determination of human vitamin states has been approached in the following ways:

- Measurement of active cofactors or precursors in biologic fluids or blood cells
- Measurement of urinary metabolites of the vitamin
- Measurement of a biochemical function requiring the vitamin (e.g., enzymatic activity), with and without in vitro addition of the cofactor form
- Measurement of urinary excretion of vitamin or metabolites after a test load of the vitamin
- Measurement of urinary metabolites of a substance, the metabolism of which requires the vitamin after administration of a test load of the substance

Reduced serum concentrations of a vitamin do not always indicate a deficiency that interrupts cellular function. Conversely, values within the reference interval do not always reflect adequate function. Interpretation of laboratory values must be done with knowledge of the biochemistry and physiology of vitamins.[52-54]

Fat-Soluble Vitamins

Vitamin A

Retinol and retinoic acid are derived directly from dietary sources, primarily as retinyl esters, or from metabolism of dietary carotenoids (provitamin A), primarily beta carotene. Major dietary sources of these compounds include animal products and pigmented fruits and vegetables (carotenoids). Vitamin A is stored in the liver and transported in the circulation complexed to RBP and transthyretin. Vitamin A and related retinoic acids are a group of compounds essential for vision, cellular differentiation, growth, reproduction, and immune system function. A clearly defined physiologic role for retinol is in vision. Retinol is oxidized in the rods of the eye to retinal, which, when complexed with opsin, forms rhodopsin, allowing dim-light vision. This vitamin and vitamin D act through specific nuclear receptors in the regulation of cell proliferation. Vitamin A deficiency leads to night blindness (nyctalopia) and, when prolonged, may cause total blindness. In vitamin A deficiency states, epithelial cells (cells in the outer skin layers and cells in the lining of the gastrointestinal, respiratory, and urogenital tracts) become dry and keratinized. Fruits and vegetables contain carotene, which is a precursor of retinol. Carotenes provide more than one-half of the retinol requirements in the American diet. Vitamin A deficiency is most common among children living in nonindustrialized countries and is usually a result of insufficient dietary intake. Deficiency may also occur because of chronic fat malabsorption or impaired liver function or may be associated with severe stress and protein malnutrition. Premature infants are born with lower serum retinol and RBP levels, as well as lower hepatic stores of retinol; therefore, these newborns are treated with vitamin A as a preventive measure.[54,56]

When ingested in high doses, either chronically or acutely, vitamin A causes many toxic manifestations and may ultimately lead to liver damage due to hypervitaminosis. High doses of vitamin A may be obtained from excessive ingestion of vitamin supplements or large amounts of liver or fish oils, which are rich in vitamin A. Carotenoids, however, are not known to be toxic because of a reduced efficiency of carotene absorption at high doses and limited conversion to vitamin A. The RDA of vitamin A is 900 μg retinol activity equivalent (RAE) per day for adult males and 700 μg RAE per day for adult females.[49] Measurement of retinol is the most common means of assessing vitamin A status in the clinical setting. Retinol is most commonly measured by high-performance liquid chromatography (HPLC). Toxicity is usually assessed by measuring retinyl ester levels in serum rather than retinol, which is accomplished by HPLC.[56]

Vitamin E
Vitamin E is a powerful antioxidant and the primary defense against potentially harmful oxidations that cause disease and aging, protecting unsaturated lipids from peroxidation (cleavage of fatty acids at unsaturated sites by oxygen addition across the double bond and formation of free radicals). The role of vitamin E in protecting the erythrocyte membrane from oxidant stress is presently its major documented role in human physiology. It has been shown to strengthen cell membranes and augment such functions as drug metabolism, heme biosynthesis, and neuromuscular function. The generic name for vitamin E is tocopherol, which includes several biologically active isomers.[57] Alpha-tocopherol is the predominant isomer in plasma and the most potent isomer by current biologic assays. About 40% of ingested tocopherol is absorbed, affected mainly by the amount and degree of unsaturated dietary fat, largely determining the physiologic requirement. Absorbed vitamin E is associated with circulating chylomicrons, very-low-density lipoprotein, and chylomicron remnants. Dietary sources of tocopherols include vegetable oil, fresh leafy vegetables, egg yolk, legumes, peanuts, and margarine. Diets suspect

for vitamin E deficiency are those low in vegetable oils, fresh green vegetables, or unsaturated fats.

The major symptom of vitamin E deficiency is hemolytic anemia. Although the use is still controversial, premature newborns are commonly supplemented with vitamin E to stabilize red blood cells and prevent hemolytic anemia. There is evidence for preventive roles of vitamin E in retrolental fibroplasia, intraventricular hemorrhage, and mortality of small, premature infants. Premature infants receiving vitamin E in amounts that sustain serum levels above 30 mg/L have an increased incidence of sepsis and necrotizing enterocolitis.[57]

Patients with conditions that result in fat malabsorption, especially cystic fibrosis and abetalipoproteinemia, are also susceptible to vitamin E deficiency.[55] A relationship exists between vitamin E deficiency and progressive loss of neurologic function in infants and children with chronic cholestasis.[55] Absorption of dietary vitamin E is most efficient in the jejunum, where it combines with lipoproteins and is transported through the lymphatics. Vitamin E is stored in the liver and other tissues with high lipid content and excreted principally in the feces. Assessment of vitamin E status is, therefore, primarily indicated in newborns, patients with fat malabsorption states, and patients receiving synthetic diets. Synergistic with two other essential nutrients, selenium and ascorbic acid, vitamin E is also necessary for the maintenance of normal vitamin A levels.[55] This vitamin deficiency commonly occurs in two groups: premature, very-low-birth-weight infants and patients who do not absorb fat normally. Although megadoses of vitamin E do not produce toxic effects, high doses have no proven health benefit; the RDA is 15 mg/d for adult males and/or females.[49] The most widely distributed and most biologically active form of vitamin E is alpha-tocopherol, which is the form commonly measured in the laboratory using HPLC methods.[57]

Vitamin D
Vitamin D refers to a group of related metabolites used for proper skeleton formation and mineral homeostasis. Exposure of the skin to sunlight (ultraviolet light) catalyzes the formation of cholecalciferol from 7-dehydrocholesterol. The other major form of vitamin D is ergocalciferol (vitamin D_2). Vitamin D occurs in foods as cholecalciferol or ergocalciferol. The most active metabolite of vitamin D is $1,25(OH)_2D_3$. It stimulates intestinal absorption of calcium and phosphate for bone growth and metabolism and, together with parathyroid hormone, stimulates bone to increase the mobilization of calcium and phosphate. $1,25(OH)_2D_3$ has an important proapoptotic effect, acting through a vitamin D hormonal system, that depends on binding of the active ligand to a vitamin D receptor. This led to important drug discovery developments in which calcium and phosphate release is minimized and proliferative and

anti-inflammatory effects of D-analogues are modulated.[55]

In northern climates, it is difficult to receive enough ultraviolet exposure to fully meet minimum requirements (2 h/d). Major dietary sources of vitamin D include irradiated foods and commercially prepared milk. Small amounts are found in butter, egg yolks, liver, sardines, herring, tuna, and salmon. The RDA of vitamin D for adults is 15 to 20 µg/d, depending on age.[56] Absorbed in the small intestine, vitamin D requires bile salts for absorption. It is stored in the liver and excreted in the bile. Severe deficiency in children causes a failure to calcify cartilage at the growth plate in metaphysical bone formation, leading to the development of rickets. In adults, the deficiency leads to undermineralization of bone matrix in remodeling, resulting in osteomalacia. Low levels of vitamin D are reported with the use of anticonvulsant drugs and in small bowel disease, chronic renal failure, hepatobiliary disease, pancreatic insufficiency, and hypoparathyroidism. Vitamin D can be toxic, especially in children. Elevated levels of vitamin D are present in hyperparathyroidism and hypophosphatemia and during pregnancy. Excess vitamin D produces hypercalcemia and hypercalciuria, which can lead to calcium deposits in soft tissue and irreversible renal and cardiac damage.[55]

It is important to measure the metabolic form of vitamin D [$1,25(OH)_2D_3$], parathyroid hormone, and calcium levels when diagnosing primary hyperparathyroidism and different types of rickets, when monitoring patients with chronic renal failure, and when assessing patients on $1,25(OH)_2D_3$ therapy. Two forms are most commonly measured in the clinical laboratory: $25(OH)D_3$ and $1,25(OH)_2D_3$. $25(OH)D_3$ is the major circulating form of vitamin D; its measurement is a good indicator of vitamin D nutritional status, as well as vitamin D intoxication. The reference range is 22 to 42 ng/mL for $25(OH)$ D_3 and 30 to 53 pg/mL for $1,25(OH)_2D_3$. Quantitation of the metabolites of vitamin D should be performed using radioimmunoassay (RIA) or HPLC in conjunction with competitive protein binding.[12,58]

Vitamin K

Vitamin K (from the German word "Koagulation") is the group of substances essential for the formation of prothrombin and at least five other coagulation proteins, including factors VII, IX, and X and proteins C and S. The quinone-containing compounds are a generic description for menadione and derivatives exhibiting this activity. Vitamin K helps convert precursor forms of these coagulation proteins to functional forms; this transformation occurs in the liver. Dietary vitamin K is absorbed primarily in the terminal ileum and, possibly, the colon. Vitamin K is synthesized by intestinal bacteria; this synthesis provides 50% of the vitamin K requirement. Major dietary sources are cabbage, cauliflower,

CASE STUDY 33-1

A 4-year-old boy is brought to an Alaskan children's clinic by the Social Services System of Alaska. The child was living in a foster home. Infrequently outdoors, his diet consisted of few green vegetables, dairy products, or meats. He began walking at 14 months; his legs showed some bowing. There is tetany or convulsions. He is small for his age: 27 lb; 90.6 cm tall; third percentile. His laboratory test results are shown in Case Study Table 33-1.1.

CASE STUDY TABLE 33-1.1
LABORATORY RESULTS

TEST	RESULT	REFERENCE RANGE
Hgb	14.1 g/dL	12.0–18.0 g/dL
Hct	46%	34.0–52.0%
WBC	8.4 × 10³/µL Normal differential	4.0–11.0 µL
URINALYSIS		
Specific gravity	1.010	1.003–1.030
pH	6.8	5.0–9.0
Glucose	Negative	Negative
Protein	Negative	Negative
Microscopic	Negative	Negative
Amino acid screen	Negative	Negative
SERUM		
Na	140 mmol/L	132–143 mmol/L
K	4.0 mmol/L	3.2–5.7 mmol/L
Cl	101 mmol/L	98–116 mmol/L
CO_2	24 mmol/L	23–29 mmol/L
Ca	7.0 mg/dL	8.9–10.3 mg/dL
Phosphate	1.1 mg/dL	3.4–5.9 mg/dL
Alkaline phosphatase	23 units	15–20 units
Total protein	6.6 g/dL	5.6–7.7 g/dL
Albumin	3.4 g/dL	3.1–4.8 g/dL

Questions

1. What is the most likely diagnosis and reason for this disorder?

2. What can be done to prevent this disorder/condition?

spinach and other leafy vegetables, pork, liver, soybeans, and vegetable oils. Uncomplicated dietary vitamin K deficiency is considered rare in healthy children and adults.

Vitamin K deficiency may be caused by antibiotic therapy, which results from decreased synthesis of the vitamin by intestinal bacteria. When vitamin K antagonists, such as warfarin sodium (Coumadin), are used for anticoagulant therapy, anticoagulant factors II, VII, IX, and X are synthesized but nonfunctional. An apparent vitamin K deficiency may lead to a hemorrhagic episode or may result when anticoagulants, such as warfarin sodium, are used.[59,60,61]

Prothrombin time (velocity of clotting after addition of thromboplastin and calcium to citrated plasma) determination is an excellent index of prothrombin adequacy. Prothrombin time is prolonged in vitamin K deficiency and in liver diseases characterized by decreased synthesis of prothrombin. Vitamin K deficiency also results in prolongation of the partial thromboplastin time, but the thrombin time is within the reference interval.

Toxicity from vitamin K is not commonly seen in adults. Large doses in infants may result in hyperbilirubinemia. The adult AI for vitamin K is 120 µg/d for males and 90 µg/d for females.[49] In most laboratories, vitamin K is not assayed; however, prothrombin time is used as a functional indicator of vitamin K status.[61] The normal prothrombin time is 11 to 15 seconds, which varies with the method. With a vitamin K deficiency, the prothrombin time is prolonged. Several herbal supplements (e.g., garlic, gingko, and ginseng) may enhance the effects of Coumadin or interact with platelets, increasing the risk of bleeding.

Water-Soluble Vitamins

Thiamine

Thiamine (vitamin B_1) or thiamin acts as a coenzyme in decarboxylation reactions in major carbohydrate pathways and in branched-chain amino acid metabolism. It is rapidly absorbed from food in the small intestine and excreted in the urine. The clinical condition associated with chronic thiamine deficiency is beriberi. Although usually occurring in underdeveloped countries of the world, beriberi may be found in the United States among persons with chronic alcoholism. Decreased intake, impaired absorption, and increased requirements all appear to play a role in the development of thiamine deficiency in persons with alcoholism. The RDA of thiamine is 1.2 mg/d for adult males and 1.1 mg/d for adult females.[49] Thiamine functional activity is best measured by erythrocyte transketolase activity, before and after the addition of thiamine pyrophosphate (TPP). Thiamine deficiency is present if the increase in activity after the addition of TPP is greater than 25%.[62]

Riboflavin

Riboflavin (vitamin B_2) functions primarily as a component of two coenzymes, flavin mononucleotide and flavin adenine dinucleotide. These two coenzymes catalyze various oxidation–reduction reactions. Dietary riboflavin is absorbed in the small intestine. The body stores of a well-nourished person are adequate to prevent riboflavin deficiency for 5 months. Excess riboflavin is excreted in the urine and has no known toxicity. Foods high in riboflavin include milk, liver, eggs, meat, and leafy vegetables. Riboflavin deficiency occurs with other nutritional deficiencies, alcoholism, and chronic diarrhea and malabsorption. Certain drugs antagonize the action or metabolism of riboflavin, including phenothiazine, oral contraceptives, and tricyclic antidepressants.[63] The RDA of riboflavin is 1.3 mg/d for adult males and 1.1 mg/d for adult females.[49] Reduced glutathione reductase activity greater than 40% is an indication of deficiency.

Pyridoxine

Pyridoxine (vitamin B_6) is ubiquitous. Vitamin B_6 is three related compounds: pyridoxine, occurring mainly in plants, and pyridoxal and pyridoxamine, which are present in animal products. The major dietary sources of vitamin B_6 are meat, poultry, fish, potatoes, and vegetables; dairy products and grains contribute lesser amounts. Readily absorbed from the intestinal tract, vitamin B_6 is excreted in the urine in the form of metabolites.[64] Vitamin B_6 deficiency rarely occurs alone; it is more commonly seen in patients deficient in several B vitamins. Those particularly at risk for deficiency are patients with uremia, liver disease, absorption syndromes, malignancies, or chronic alcoholism. High intake of proteins increases the requirements for vitamin B_6. Deficiency is associated with hyperhomocysteinemia. Vitamin B_6 has low toxicity because of its water-soluble nature; however, extremely high doses may cause peripheral neuropathy. The RDA of vitamin B_6 is 1.3 to 1.7 mg/d for adult males and 1.3 to 1.5 mg/d for adult females, depending on age.[49]

Niacin

The requirement for niacin in humans is met, to some extent, by the conversion of dietary tryptophan to niacin. Niacin is the generic term for both nicotinic acid and nicotinamide. Niacin functions as a component of the two coenzymes nicotinamide adenine dinucleotide and nicotinamide adenine dinucleotide phosphate, which are necessary for many metabolic processes, including tissue respiration, lipid metabolism, fatty acid metabolism, and glycolysis. Reduction of the coenzyme yields dihydronicotinamide (NADH or NADPH), which has a strong absorption at 340 nm, a feature widely used in assays of pyridine nucleotide–dependent enzymes.

Niacin is absorbed in the small intestine, and excess is excreted in the form of metabolites in the urine.[65] Pellagra, the clinical syndrome resulting from niacin deficiency, is associated with diarrhea, dementia, dermatitis, and death. Niacin deficiency may result from alcoholism. To decrease lipid levels, pharmacologic doses of nicotinic acid are given therapeutically. The toxicity of niacin is low. When large doses are ingested, however, as often occurs during lipid-lowering therapies, flushing of the skin and vasodilation may occur. The RDA of niacin is 16 mg/d for adult males and 14 mg/d for adult females.[49] Blood or urinary niacin levels are of value in assessing niacin nutritional status.

Folate

Folate is the generic term for components nutritionally and chemically similar to folic acid. Folate functions metabolically as coenzymes involved in various one-carbon transfer reactions. Folate and vitamin B_{12} are closely related metabolically. The hematologic changes that result from deficiency of either vitamin are indistinguishable. Folate in the diet is absorbed in the jejunum, and the excess is excreted in the urine and feces. Large quantities of folate are also synthesized by bacteria in the colon. Structural relatives of pteroylglutamic acid (folic acid) are metabolically active compounds usually referred to as folates. Food folates are primarily found in green and leafy vegetables, fruits, organ meats, and yeast. Boiling food and using large quantities of water result in folate destruction. The average American diet may be inadequate in folate for adolescents and for pregnant or lactating women.[66]

The major clinical symptom of folate deficiency is megaloblastic anemia. Laboratory indices of deficiency are, in order of occurrence, low serum folate, hypersegmentation of neutrophils, high urinary formiminoglutamic acid (a histidine metabolite accumulating in the absence of folate), low erythrocyte folate, macro-ovalocytosis, megaloblastic marrow, and anemia. Serum folate levels, although an early index of deficiency, can frequently be low despite normal tissue stores. Because most folate storage occurs after the vitamin B_{12}–dependent step, erythrocyte folate can also be reduced in deficiency of either vitamin B_{12} or folate. Despite this overlap, erythrocyte folate concentration is accepted as the best laboratory index of folate deficiency.[67] Most physicians order both serum and erythrocyte folate levels because serum levels indicate circulating folate and erythrocyte levels better approximate stores. Homocysteine elevation in serum and urine occurs in folate deficiency.[68] Total homocysteine is generally measured, which is the sum of all homocysteine species, both free and protein-bound forms.[69]

Folate requirement is increased during pregnancy and especially during lactation. The increase during lactation results, in part, from the presence of high-affinity folate binders in milk. Dietary supplementation of folate in pregnant women reduces the incidence of fetal neural tube defects. Other instances of increased folate requirement include hemolytic anemia, iron deficiency, prematurity,

and multiple myeloma. Patients receiving dialysis treatment rapidly lose folate. Clinical conditions[69,70] associated with folate deficiency include megaloblastic anemia, alcoholism, malabsorption syndrome, carcinoma, liver disease, chronic hemodialysis, and hemolytic and sideroblastic anemia. Certain anticonvulsants and other drugs that interfere with folate metabolism include sulfasalazine, isoniazid, and cycloserine. Folate deficiency of dietary origin commonly occurs in older persons. Phenytoin (Dilantin) therapy accelerates folate excretion and interferes with folate absorption and metabolism. Alcohol interferes with folate's enterohepatic circulation, and methotrexate, a chemotherapeutic agent, inhibits the enzyme dihydrofolate reductase (Table 33-3). Low levels of serum folate can occur with use of oral contraceptives.

There are no known cases of folate toxicity; the RDA is 400 µg/d for adult males and females.[49] In women of childbearing age, 400 µg/d of folate is recommended to prevent or reduce the incidence of neural tube defects.[56]

Reference ranges are as follows:

Serum: 3 to 16 ng/mL (6.8 to 36.3 nmol/L)

Erythrocyte: 130 to 630 ng/mL (294.5 to 1,427.5 nmol/L)

Deficient stores: <140 ng/mL (<317.3 nmol/L)

TABLE 33-3	ACTIONS OF DRUGS AND ORAL CONTRACEPTIVES ON VITAMINS
DRUG OR NUTRIENT	
Pyridoxine—antagonized by isoniazid, steroids, penicillamine	
Riboflavin—antagonized by phenothiazines, some antibiotics	
Folate—antagonized by phenytoin, alcohol, methotrexate, trimethoprim	
Ascorbate—antagonized by (increased excretion) aspirin, barbiturates, hydantoins	
Ascorbate excess—interferes with actions of aminosalicylic acid, tricyclic antidepressants, anticoagulants; may cause "rebound scurvy" on withdrawal	
ORAL CONTRACEPTIVE AGENTS CAUSE	
Increased serum vitamin A, retinol-binding protein	
Decreased requirement for vitamins K and C	
Decreased vitamin B_6 status indices	
Decreased riboflavin use	
Increased niacin pathway of tryptophan	
Decreased induction of thiamin deficiency	
Decreased serum folate (cycle-day dependent)	
Decreased induction of cervical folate deficiency	

Folate levels may be measured in serum using a microbiologic assay with *Lactobacillus casei* or a competitive protein-binding assay for levels in serum and erythrocytes. When folate deficiency develops, serum levels fall first, followed by a decrease in erythrocyte folate levels and ultimately hematologic manifestation.[69,70] Measuring both serum and erythrocyte levels is helpful because serum levels indicate circulating folate and erythrocyte levels better approximate stores.[67]

Serum contains endogenous binding proteins that can bind folate and result in falsely low serum folate concentration measurements. Although measurement of red blood cell folate concentration has advantages over the serum assay for the diagnosis of megaloblastic anemia, analytic problems may result from the various forms of folate in erythrocytes. Folate in the serum is almost exclusively present in the monoglutamate form; however, in red blood cells, it is in the polyglutamate form and as high-molecular-weight complexes.[69,70]

Vitamin B12

Vitamin B_{12} (cobalamin) refers to a large group of cobalt-containing compounds. Intestinal absorption of vitamin B_{12} takes place in the ileum and is mediated by a unique binding protein called intrinsic factor, which is secreted by the stomach. Vitamin B_{12} participates as a coenzyme in enzymatic reactions necessary for hematopoiesis and fatty acid metabolism. Excess vitamin B_{12} is excreted in the urine. Vitamin B_{12} bears a corrin ring (containing pyrroles similar to porphyrin) linked to a central cobalt atom. Different corrinoid compounds, or cobalamins, are distinguished by the substituent linked to the cobalt. The active cofactor forms of vitamin B_{12} are methylcobalamin and deoxyadenosylcobalamin. The primary dietary sources for vitamin B_{12} are from animal products (e.g., meat, eggs, and milk). Therefore, total vegetarian diets are likely to be deficient or low in vitamin B_{12}. Animals derive vitamin B_{12} from intestinal microbial synthesis. The average daily diet contains 3 to 30 μg of vitamin B_{12}, of which 1 to 5 μg is absorbed. The frequency of dietary deficiency increases with age, occurring in more than 0.5% of people older than 60,[70] although the symptoms resulting from dietary deficiency are rare.

Most vitamin B_{12} absorption occurs through a complex with intrinsic factor, a protein secreted by gastric parietal cells. This intrinsic factor–B_{12} complex binds with specific ileal receptors. "Blocking" intrinsic factor antibodies prevents binding of vitamin B_{12} to intrinsic factor, and "binding" antibodies can combine with either free intrinsic factor or the intrinsic factor–B_{12} complex, preventing attachment of the complex to ileal receptors and intestinal uptake of the vitamin. Parietal cell antibodies have also been identified as a cause of pernicious anemia. After release from the intrinsic factor complex within the mucosal cell, vitamin B_{12} circulates in plasma bound to specific transport proteins and is deposited in liver, bone marrow, and other tissues. There is a significant enterohepatic circulation of vitamin B_{12}. Plasma contains both types of transport proteins, transcobalamins, and the three forms of vitamin B_{12} (hydroxocobalamin, methylcobalamin, and deoxyadenosylcobalamin).

In the Schilling test, the patient receives a small, oral dose of radiolabeled vitamin B_{12}. Parenteral B_{12} is given simultaneously to saturate binding sites. Serum and urine are collected at intervals, and labeled B_{12} is measured in the specimens. Patients who cannot absorb vitamin B_{12} (usually a deficiency of intrinsic factor, as in pernicious anemia)[70] cannot absorb the labeled B_{12} and, therefore, have low levels in the blood and urine.

The term *pernicious anemia* is now most commonly applied to vitamin B_{12} deficiency resulting from lack of intrinsic factor. Antibodies to intrinsic factor and parietal cells are common in patients with pernicious anemia, their healthy relatives, and patients with other autoimmune disorders. Deficiency of B_{12} can occasionally occur in strict vegetarians because of dietary deficiency. A loss of vitamin B_{12} also occurs in individuals infected with fish tapeworm or because of malabsorption diseases, such as sprue or celiac disease. Low vitamin B_{12} levels occur with folate deficiency, and a vitamin B_{12} deficiency can be masked by large doses of folate. Toxicity of vitamin B_{12} has not been reported. The RDA of vitamin B_{12} for adults is 2.4 μg/d.[49] Assay methods for B_{12} are either microbiologic assay using *Lactobacillus leichmannii* competitive protein-binding RIA or an enzyme immunoassay.

Deficiency of vitamin B_{12} causes two major disorders—megaloblastic anemia (pernicious anemia) and a neurologic disorder called combined systems disorder.[69] The neurologic manifestations are variable and may be subtle. For this reason, vitamin B_{12} deficiency should be considered a cause of any unexplained macrocytic anemia or neurologic disorder, especially in an elderly person. Serum vitamin B_{12} may be used in the initial assessment.[69] Methylmalonic acid levels may be more definitive because the lower reference limit of B_{12} is unclear. Patients with pernicious anemia usually have atrophic gastritis and have an increased incidence of gastric carcinoma. The reference range for vitamin B_{12} is 110 to 800 pg/mL (81.2 to 590.4 pmol/L).[69,70] The most common methods for determination of vitamin B_{12} are the competitive protein-binding RIAs, which are based on the principle that vitamin B_{12} released from endogenous binding proteins can be measured by its competition with colabeled B_{12} for a limited amount of specific binding protein. The binding proteins typically used are animal intrinsic factors. Special measures must be taken to eliminate interference caused by other, nonspecific protein binders of vitamin B_{12}. Several nonradioisotopic assays for vitamin B_{12} have been developed for routine laboratory use.

CASE STUDY 33-2

A 65-year-old woman was admitted to the hospital with mild congestive heart failure. She had been seen in the family practice clinic with complaints of numbness, tingling in the calves and feet, and weight loss. The physical examination revealed a slightly confused, depressed, pale woman. Her blood pressure was 110/70 mm Hg. Faint scleral icterus was present. There was 1+ pitting and ankle edema. The neurologic examination revealed loss of vibratory sensation in both legs, with exaggerated ankle and knee reflexes. Initial laboratory results are shown in Case Study Table 33-2.1.

CASE STUDY TABLE 33-2.1 LABORATORY RESULTS

TEST	RESULT	REFERENCE RANGE
Hgb	9.3 g/dL	12–16 g/dL
Hct	28%	38–47%
MCH	35 pg	27–31 pg
MCV	108 fL	80–96 fL
MCHC	32.4 g/dL	32–36 g/dL
Na	141 mmol/L	136–145 mmol/L
K	4.2 mmol/L	3.5–5.3 mmol/L
Cl	102 mmol/L	96–106 mmol/L
CO_2	26 mmol/L	22–29 mmol/L
Ca	9.7 mg/dL	8.4–10.3 mg/dL
Glucose	100 mg/dL	70–110 mg/dL
BUN	14 mg/dL	10–20 mg/dL
Creatinine	1.0 mg/dL	0.4–1.4 mg/dL
Serum B_{12}	130 pg/mL	180–900 pg/mL
Serum folate	6 ng/mL	5–12 ng/mL
RBC folate	105 ng/mL	200–700 ng/mL

Questions

1. What is a biologically active form of cobalamin in plasma?
2. Where is intrinsic factor made in the body?
3. What is the binding protein for vitamin B_{12}?
4. List food substances that contain vitamin B_{12}.
5. List food substances that contain folate.

Biotin

Biotin is a coenzyme for several enzymes that transport carboxyl units in tissue and plays an integral role in gluconeogenesis, lipogenesis, and fatty acid synthesis.[71] Dietary biotin is absorbed in the small intestine, but it is also synthesized in the gut by bacteria. Numerous foods contain biotin, although no food is especially rich (up to 20 µg/100 g). The dietary intake of biotin, while low in the neonatal period, increases as newborns switch from colostrum to mature breast milk. Biotin deficiency can be produced by ingestion of large amounts of avidin, found in raw egg whites that bind to biotin. Biotin deficiency has been noted in patients receiving long-term PN and in infants with genetic defects of carboxylase and biotinidase enzymes. The AI for biotin is 30 µg/d.[49]

Reference ranges of 200 to 500 pg/mL (0.82 to 2.05 nmol/L) have been established in whole blood and serum.[71,72] Assays had been performed using microbiology functional assay and the *Lactobacillus* organism. Newer methods of isotopic dilution, chemiluminescent, and photometric assays are now available but rarely used in hospital laboratories. Specimens are usually sent to a reference laboratory for analysis.[72]

Pantothenic Acid

A growth factor occurring in all types of animal and plant tissue was first designated as vitamin B_3 and later named *pantothenic acid* (from Greek for "everywhere"). Dietary sources include liver and other organ meats, milk, eggs, peanuts, legumes, mushrooms, salmon, and whole grains. Approximately 50% of pantothenate in food is available for absorption. Pantothenate is metabolically converted to 4′-phosphopantetheine, which becomes covalently bound to either serum acyl carrier protein or coenzyme A. Coenzyme A is a highly important acyl-group transfer coenzyme involved in many reaction types. The AI for pantothenic acid in adults is 5 mg/d.[49] Whole blood pantothenate of less than 100 µg/dL and urinary excretion of less than 1 mg/d are regarded as indicative of deficiency.[73] Reference range for urine is 1 to 15 mg/d or 5 to 68 µmol/d. Assays using a load test look for excretion of the acetylated *p*-aminobenzoic acid that is formed.[73]

Ascorbic Acid

The most commonly discussed vitamin, ascorbic acid (vitamin C), is a strong reducing compound that has to be acquired via dietary ingestion. Major dietary sources include fruits (especially citrus) and vegetables (e.g., tomatoes, green peppers, cabbage, leafy greens, and potatoes). Ascorbic acid is important in formation and stabilization of collagen by hydroxylation of proline and lysine for cross-linking and conversion of tyrosine to catecholamines (by dopamine β-hydrolase). It increases the absorption of certain minerals, such as iron, and is absorbed in the upper small intestine and distributed throughout the water-soluble compartments of the body.[74] The deficiency state, known as scurvy, is characterized by hemorrhagic disorders, including swollen, bleeding gums and impaired wound healing and anemia.[74,75]

Although urine is the primary route of excretion, measurement of urinary ascorbate is not recommended for status assessment. Drugs known to increase urinary excretion of ascorbate include aspirin, aminopyrine, barbiturates, hydantoin, and paraldehyde. Ascorbic acid requirements are more increased with acute stress injury and chronic inflammatory states, but are also increased with pregnancy and oral contraceptive use. Excessive intake may interfere with vitamin B_{12} metabolism and drug actions (e.g., aminosalicylic acid, tricyclic antidepressants, and anticoagulants).[74,75]

The most widely used assay for ascorbic acid is the 2,4-dinitrophenylhydrazine method. In this procedure, ascorbic acid is first oxidized to dehydroascorbic acid and 2,3-diketogulonic acid with the formation of a colored product that absorbs at 520 nm. This method measures the total vitamin C content of the sample because ascorbic acid, dehydroascorbic acid, and diketogulonic acid are also measured, and it is subject to interference from amino acids and thiosulfates. HPLC has been developed to give increased sensitivity and specificity. The reference range for ascorbic acid is 0.4 to 0.6 mg/dL (23 to 34 µmol/L).[75] The RDA for vitamin C is 90 mg/d for adult males and 75 mg/d for adult females.[49]

Conditionally Essential Nutrients

Carnitine

Carnitine, which includes l-carnitine and its fatty acid esters (acylcarnitine), is described as a conditionally essential nutrient.[76] Meat, poultry, fish, and dairy products are the major dietary sources. Foods of plant origin generally contain little carnitine, except for peanut butter and asparagus.[76] Normal diets provide more than half the human requirement, but strict vegetarian diets provide only 10% of the total carnitine needed by humans.[76] Synthesis occurs in liver, brain, and kidney. l-carnitine facilitates entry of long-chain fatty acids into mitochondria for oxidation and energy production.[76] The major signs of carnitine deficiency are muscle weakness and fatigue. Total carnitine is measured after hydrolysis of ester forms to free carnitine. Human deficiency can be either hereditary or acquired—by inadequate intake, increased requirement (pregnancy and breastfeeding), or increased urinary loss (valproic acid therapy). Infants and patients following a course of long-term PN and those on hemodialysis are most vulnerable to deficiency.[76]

CASE STUDY 33-3

A 27-year-old man was diagnosed with a carcinoid tumor in the lower portion of the small intestine. The tumor was debulked, with removal of a portion of the lower section of the small intestine. His recovery course was somewhat complicated by weight loss. Seven months after surgery, he underwent a laparotomy, which showed that the carcinoid tumor had not been entirely removed; more of the small bowel was removed because of the obstructing adhesions. He recovered from the second surgery, and tube feeding was discontinued. He came back to the clinic 18 months after the initial surgery slightly pale and stating that he was having trouble maintaining weight. His laboratory evaluation showed slight hypochromic, macrocytic anemia, normal renal function, and normal liver function. A stool specimen was negative for ova, parasites, and enteric pathogens. He was readmitted for intravenous fluid and electrolyte replacement.

CASE STUDY TABLE 33-3.1
LABORATORY RESULTS

TEST	RESULT	REFERENCE RANGE
Albumin	3.4 g/dL	3.5–5 g/dL
Prealbumin	15 mg/dL	18–40 mg/dL
Na	139 mmol/L	136–145 mmol/L
K	3.7 mmol/L	3.5–5 mmol/L
Cl	101 mmol/L	99–109 mmol/L
Bicarbonate	23 mmol/L	22–28 mmol/L
Ca	8.6 mg/dL	8.5–10.5 mg/dL
Mg	1.7 mg/dL	1.5–2.5 mg/dL
Phosphate	3 mg/dL	2.8–4 mg/dL
Prothrombin time	17 s	10–14 s
Ferritin	22 ng/mL	20–250 ng/mL
Vitamin A	207 µg/L	300–800 mg/L
Vitamin D	6 ng/mL	30–53 ng/mL
Vitamin E	2 mg/L	5–18 mg/L
Vitamin C	0.4 mg/dL	0.4–0.6 mg/dL
Vitamin B_{12}	100 pg/mL	110–800 pg/mL
Fecal fat	30 g/d	<6 g/d (72 h)

Questions

1. What biochemical evidence exists for fat malabsorption?

2. What nutritional parameters would be affected by fat malabsorption?

3. Identify the fat-soluble vitamins.

4. What condition results from vitamin B_{12} deficiency?

Minerals

Calcium/Phosphorus

One of the most important aspects of PN monitoring is determining deficiencies and excesses of calcium, phosphorus, and magnesium. When regulated inadequately, these minerals not only affect bone mass but can also precipitate life-threatening situations. Calcium and phosphorus are related closely in the important role of bone mineralization. Calcium is present in serum in two forms—protein bound, or nondiffusible, and ionized diffusible calcium. Ionized calcium is the physiologically active form and constitutes only 25% of total serum calcium. Regardless of total serum calcium, a decrease in ionized calcium may result in tetany. Decreased ionized calcium is often caused by an increase in blood pH (alkalosis). It is important to monitor ionized serum calcium and blood pH, especially in a patient on PN who is receiving calcium supplementation along with ingredients in the PN solution that may alter blood pH. Although calcium imbalance is frequent in newborns undergoing PN, it is much less common in adolescents and adults. Hypercalciuria with nephrolithiasis has been reported, however, as a complication in patients on long-term PN.

A reciprocal relationship exists between calcium and phosphorus. Intracellular phosphate is necessary to promote protein synthesis and other cellular functions. Calcium and phosphorus must be monitored carefully to maintain the correct balance between these two minerals. Severe hypophosphatemia has been reported in patients undergoing prolonged PN.[77,78] Magnesium, as a PN solution additive, is closely related to calcium and phosphorus. A reciprocal relationship exists between magnesium and calcium and, in certain situations, between magnesium and phosphorus. Low levels of magnesium can cause tetany, whereas high levels can increase cardiac atrioventricular conduction time. Certain electrolyte and mineral abnormalities associated with PN are shown in Table 33-4.

Given the emergence of osteoporosis and osteopenia as women's health issues, new emphasis has been given to assessment of calcium and vitamin D. Postmenopausal women lack the estrogen levels that previously helped to maintain bone structure. In addition, they may also lack adequate vitamin D and calcium intakes that could maintain bone without estrogen assistance.

Iron

Iron plays a crucial role in respiration and transfer of oxygen to body tissues. The importance of iron in the nutritional sense has to do with its importance to several enzymes, as well as the fact that excess iron has been associated with increasing the amount of free radicals and infection in patients. Enzymes requiring iron cofactor include aconitase, succinate dehydrogenase, and isocitrate dehydrogenase from the tricarboxylic acid cycle. Catalase for the breakdown of both hydrogen peroxide and myeloperoxidase found in neutrophils requires iron as cofactor. The ribonucleotide reductase and xanthine oxidase involved in RNA and DNA metabolism both require iron as cofactor. Besides the enzymes part of the cytochrome P-450 mechanism, iron is also needed by tryptophan hydroxylase (production of serotonin), phenylalanine hydroxylase, homogentisic acid oxidase, and tyrosine hydroxylase (formation of L-DOPA catecholamine precursor).[79,80] There are many other enzymes that require iron, and without sufficient quantities, these enzymes are prevented from performing as they

TABLE 33-4	ELECTROLYTE AND MINERAL ABNORMALITIES ASSOCIATED WITH PARENTERAL NUTRITION	
ABNORMALITY	**MANIFESTATIONS**	**USUAL CAUSES**
Hypernatremia	Edema, hypertension, thirst, intracranial hemorrhage	Inappropriate sodium intake
	Weakness, hypotension, oliguria, tachycardia	Inadequate sodium intake relative to water
Hyperkalemia	Weakness, paresthesia, cardiac arrhythmias	Acidosis, renal failure, excessive potassium intake
	Weakness, alkalosis, cardiac abnormalities	Insufficient potassium intake associated with protein anabolism
Hyperchloremia	Metabolic acidosis	Excessive chloride intake, amino acid solutions with high chloride content
Hypocalcemia	Tetany, seizures, rickets, bone demineralization	Inadequate calcium, phosphorus, and/or vitamin D intake
Hypophosphatemia	Weakness, bone pain, bone demineralization	Insufficient phosphorus intake
Hypomagnesemia	Seizure, neuritis	Inadequate intake of magnesium

should in energy metabolism, growth and proliferation, biotransformations of drugs, myelinogenesis, cell differentiation, and nutrient absorption. Deficiencies of iron are associated with not only anemia but also akathisia, or "restless leg syndrome." Increasing the iron supplies to these patients has led to improvement and a reduction in symptoms.[80,81]

Iron absorption by the gastrointestinal system will be affected by the level of iron present in the body and in ferritin storage form. Low levels of serum or body iron enhance absorption from the intestinal cells as the ferritin levels are low and the apotransferrin levels are high. Other absorption enhancers of iron include vitamin C, copper, cobalt, and manganese when present in the intestine. Inhibitors of absorption besides excess ferritin in mucosal cells include phytic acid, polyphenols of tea and wine, and calcium.[79,81]

Measurements of iron, transferrin, and ferritin have already been discussed elsewhere in this book. The nutritional assessment of iron uses these same methods and reference ranges.

The RDA for iron is 8 mg/d for adult males and adult females over 51 years of age and 18 mg/d for adult females 19 to 50 years of age.[49]

CASE STUDY 33-4

A 66-year-old postmenopausal woman complained of severe weakness and dyspnea during the past 6 months on exertion. She noted that her appetite had decreased, with resultant weight loss. Her past medical history revealed ulcers. On admission to the hospital, she had normal blood pressure and pulse. Skin, conjunctiva, and mucous membranes were pale. Lungs were clear at auscultation. A grade 3/6 systolic murmur was present, heard best at the lower left sternal border and radiating to the carotids and axilla. Stool guaiac examination was 2+. Nail beds were pale, with no pedal edema. Laboratory data on admission are shown in Case Study Table 33-4.1.

Questions

1. This patient's anemia is probably best explained by
   a. dietary habits.
   b. chronic blood loss.
   c. chronic intravascular hemolysis.
   d. chronic inflammatory disease.

2. What are the clinical manifestations of her anemia?

3. The bone marrow iron stores are
   a. reduced.
   b. normal.
   c. absent.
   d. increased but present only in reticuloendothelial cells.

4. If the correct treatment for this anemia is with oral ferrous sulfate, the treatment should
   a. be stopped as soon as the hematocrit returns to normal.
   b. be continued indefinitely, even if the cause of the deficiency has been corrected.
   c. be continued for 3 to 6 months after the hematocrit returns to normal to replace body iron stores.
   d. be continued only until there is a brisk response in the reticulocyte index and hematocrit.

CASE STUDY TABLE 33-4.1
LABORATORY RESULTS

TEST	RESULT	REFERENCE RANGE
CBC		
Hct	15%	36–48%
Hb	3.8 g/dL	12–16 g/dL
RBC	2.79×10^6/mL	$3.6–5.0 \times 10^6$/mL
MCV	53.8 fL	82–98 fL
MCHC	25.3 g/dL	31–37 g/dL
WBC	8.2×10^3/mL	$4.0–11.0 \times 10^3$/mL
Neutrophil	80%	40–80%
Lymph	20%	15–40%
Reticulocyte count	5.5%	0.5–1.5%
Reticulocyte index	0.8%	>3%
CHEMISTRY		
BUN	15 mg/dL	7–18 mg/dL
Glucose	150 mg/dL	Fasting 70–100 mg/dL
		Nonfasting 70–150 mg/dL
ELECTROLYTES	**NORMAL**	
Bilirubin	1.0 mg/dL	0.2–1 mg/dL
Direct	0.4 mg/dL	0–0.2 mg/dL
T_3 and T_4	Normal	
Serum Fe	15 µg/dL	30–150 µg/dL
TIBC	439 µg/dL	241–421 µg/dL

Trace Elements

Copper

This metal is essential for a number of biochemical reactions as it is an essential element to enzymes critical to these reactions. The enzyme cytochrome oxidase has a copper component and is involved in reactions in the electron transport system where ATP energy is generated. Copper is part of the enzyme dopamine monooxygenase, which is necessary for neuron activity and transmission of impulse. A lack of copper at this crucial juncture can lead to neurologic problems. The enzyme superoxide dismutase is involved in reaction to reduce the free radical superoxide. Copper is an essential part of this enzyme, so its function as a free radical scavenger is related to the superoxide dismutase activity. A deficiency of copper sizable enough to affect the superoxide dismutase activity leaves the patient's cells open to free radical damage and cellular destruction. Ceruloplasmin is the fourth enzyme listed here that requires copper for activity. Eight copper atoms, four covalently bound and four loosely bound, are needed for ceruloplasmin to convert iron from the 3 plus state to the absorbed 2 plus state. Ceruloplasmin is viewed as an acute-phase reactant protein,[82] but it has a biochemical action as an enzyme that converts iron atoms to an ingestible state.

Because copper has such a large impact on many biochemical reactions, it is understandable that the liver contains high levels of copper. The turnover of copper from the liver is closely regulated, with excesses excreted through the bile leaving the liver. Deficiencies of copper are rare due to the liver's close regulation of copper levels. However, preterm babies, Menkes disease, and deficiency due to high dietary intake of zinc, iron, or vitamin C can be potential causes of copper deficiencies. PN can also lead to deficiency of copper. The diets of most patients on PN must be supplemented to maintain optimal levels of several trace elements; these elements must also be monitored to prevent deficiency or toxicity. Copper and zinc are the most common trace elements added to PN solutions. Pallor, decreased pigmentation, vein enlargement, and rashes resembling seborrheic dermatitis are the major clinical signs of copper deficiency, which at times go unnoticed. Some other abnormalities include recurrent leukopenia (white blood cell count, less than 5×10^9/L) and neutropenia (neutrophils, less than 1.5×10^9/L).

The diagnosis of copper deficiency is confirmed when both serum copper and ceruloplasmin (the copper-binding glycoprotein) are low. It is difficult to make this diagnosis in premature infants, however, because their serum copper levels remain depressed until about 9 weeks of age. Low copper levels have also been reported in malabsorption syndrome, protein-wasting intestinal diseases, nephrotic syndrome, severe trauma, and burns. The anemia seen in copper deficiencies is related to the low ceruloplasmin activity and thus lack of iron absorption into the patient.

Menkes disease is an X-linked recessive disease in which copper transport is adversely affected. Lack of copper absorption leads to low liver and serum levels of copper. The symptoms for Menkes disease include kinky hair, mental retardation, seizures, arterial aneurysms, and bone demineralization.[82]

The opposite of copper deficiency is copper toxicity. RDs may be asked to help a patient with Wilson's disease reduce their intake of copper. Although Wilson's disease is a deficiency of ceruloplasmin protein, the copper that should be attached is in the serum and liver leading to a toxic copper state. Patients with Wilson's disease have blockages of copper excretion from the liver to bile or serum. This accumulation of copper in the liver can go into hepatitis, then a fibrosis, and then a cirrhosis if not treated with chelation and diet restricted in copper content. Copper toxicity to brain leads to tremors, dysphasia, chorea, and drooling. Patients with Wilson's disease need lifelong monitoring and chelation treatment.

Indirect copper measurements are attained by measuring the ceruloplasmin levels. Ceruloplasmin serum levels are 123 to 230 mg/L.[83] The RDA for copper in adults is 900 µg/d.[49]

Zinc

Zinc is an essential metal for over 200 enzymes in humans. Metalloenzymes using zinc include carbonic anhydrase, alkaline phosphatase, thymidine kinase, alcohol dehydrogenase, and RNA and DNA polymerases. The range of biochemical functions of zinc-containing metalloenzymes includes protein synthesis, gene expression, transport processes, immunologic reactions, and wound healing, to name a few. Carbonic anhydrase needs zinc to foster the reactions it catalyzes between carbon dioxide and water. When zinc is deficient, carbonic anhydrase activity is lower in the blood, stomach, and intestines of affected patients. Patients with sickle cell anemia are especially at risk for adverse affects due to the lack of zinc for the carbonic anhydrase reaction as well as insufficient zinc for their red cells.

The role of zinc in wound healing and immune function is the primary reason that this trace metal needs to be monitored when assessing nutritional adequacy in hospitalized patients. The biosynthesis of connective tissues and ability to fight off infections after surgery can be positively affected if the patient's nutritional status is monitored and zinc levels are kept within the therapeutic range.

Patients on PN may develop acute zinc deficiency.[84,85] They initially suffer from a massive urinary loss of zinc during phases of catabolism. When weight gain begins, the zinc-deficient patient may experience diarrhea, perioral dermatitis, and alopecia. Premature newborns are particularly predisposed to zinc deficiency because zinc normally is acquired at the rate of about 500 mg/d during the final month of gestation. To compensate for this deficiency, zinc supplements for the premature newborn should be 50% higher than those for the full-term newborn. This concentration is then gradually decreased until it is the same as for a full-term infant.

Zinc should be monitored even more frequently in patients with ongoing gastrointestinal losses, even if they are receiving zinc supplements in their parenteral solutions.[86] Normal zinc absorption is only 30% to 40% of dietary intake. This means that while the duodenum and proximal jejunum are sites of active transport of zinc absorption, this absorption area limits zinc intake. Given the competition between zinc and copper absorption, interference of other metals for the metalloprotein needed to transport zinc can further limit the level of zinc intake and absorption. Deficiency of zinc can thus be a problem in normal people, let alone one who has a compromised immune system and surgical trauma.

Zinc transport in serum uses albumin primarily and α_2-macroglobulin. Some zinc may be transported by transferrin and amino acids, but this is not significant in most patients. Excretion of zinc is via the feces, with 25% of the excreted zinc leaving with pancreatic secretions. Urinary loss of zinc is about 5% of dietary intake of zinc. Sweat and semen can also be routes of zinc loss from humans.

Zinc is required for vision, taste, and smell functions. It promotes tissue repair, connective tissue synthesis, bone growth, and insulin synthesis. Zinc is involved in carbohydrate, protein, and phosphorus metabolism. Its role in antibody production and white blood cell well-being fosters the finding that zinc is needed for immune functions.

Malnutrition, infertility, inflammation, and hair loss are often treated with zinc supplementation because it has such a wide array of body functions.

Deficiencies of zinc are usually due to lack of absorption. Whether dietary fiber prevents zinc absorption or a conflicting metal prevents zinc uptake, a deficiency of zinc can be seen in the array of its known functions. Wound healing is reduced or lacking, appetite is lost, skin lesions develop secondary infections, fertility declines, and RNA and DNA synthesis is hampered.

In addition to the direct methods for zinc assessment discussed in Chapter 18, the indirect methods look at the effects of zinc on proteins and metalloenzymes. Specimen collection without contamination has been hard to achieve, making zinc measurements higher than actual values. Red cells contain zinc, so hemolysis elevates zinc plasma values.[87] The RDA for zinc is 11 mg/d for adult males and 8 mg/d for adult females.[49]

Selenium

Selenium (Se) as a trace mineral is reported to have an influence on cancer, cardiovascular diseases (CVDs), diabetes, and arthritis. Trace amounts of selenium in humans necessitate a daily RDA for selenium in adults of

CASE STUDY 33-5

A young woman 33 years old complains to her family physician that she is always tired and cannot get her weight to a normal level. Her father has type 2 diabetes and her grandmother is being treated for cardiovascular disease (CVD) post myocardial infarction. Her mother and brother are on medication for high blood pressure. Her physician performs a physical examination and determines that her waist circumference is increased at 90 cm. Her blood pressure is 135/90 mm Hg. Blood is drawn and the results are listed in Case Study Table 33-5.1.

CASE STUDY TABLE 33-5.1
LABORATORY RESULTS

TEST	RESULT	REFERENCE RANGE
Albumin	3.4 g/dL	3.5–5 g/dL
Total protein	7.1 g/dL	6.0–8.0 g/dL
Na	141 mmol/L	136–145 mmol/L
K	3.7 mmol/L	3.5–5 mmol/L
Cl	103 mmol/L	99–109 mmol/L
Bicarbonate	23 mmol/L	22–28 mmol/L
Glucose	120 mg/dL	80–100 mg/dL
BUN	19 mg/dL	7–18 mg/dL
Creatinine	1.1 mg/dL	0.5–1.1 mg/dL
Total cholesterol	196 mg/dL	<200 mg/dL
LDL cholesterol (calc)	127 mg/dL	<100 mg/dL
HDL cholesterol	35 mg/dL	>50 mg/dL (women)
Triglycerides	167 mg/dL	<150 mg/dL
AST	40 U/L	5–30 U/L
ALT	45 U/L	6–37 U/L
ALP	41 U/L	30–90 U/L

Questions

1. Given the information in this case study, the suspected disease is
   a. Diabetes type 2
   b. Metabolic syndrome
   c. Cirrhosis
   d. Atherosclerosis leading to CVD

2. Of the indicators seen in this case, which ones indicate to you that your choice in question 1 is correct. Why?

3. What treatment modality is required for this patient? How will the laboratory contribute to that treatment plan?

55 µg/d,[49] but most texts indicate a daily intake of over 100 mg. Selenium functions as an essential cofactor to the antioxidant enzyme glutathione peroxidase, which is involved in neutralizing hydrogen peroxide formed during lipid oxidation in cells. Free radicals like hydrogen peroxide need to be removed if cell membranes and DNA are to remain intact.[88,89] Selenium incorporation into proteins and enzymes occurs through the selenocysteine dietary form, but a secondary selenomethionine also comes from dietary sources. Selenomethionine is not advantageous as it may interfere with normal methionine incorporation into proteins. The selenocysteine form is desirable and its positive effects are seen in the enzyme glutathione peroxidase as well as other selenium-containing enzymes.

Functions of selenium in humans include antiatherogenic effect, anticancer effect, antioxidant, improved fertility, and increasing the immune response.[90] Deficiency of selenium, obviously, will lead to decreased capabilities in these areas. Incidence of CVD and cancer seems to rise in populations lacking adequate selenium. Furthermore, cell damage and susceptibility to infections also increase when selenium is deficient. Cancer increases as well as cell damage and the susceptibility to infections when selenium is deficient. Fertility issues affected include low sperm motility and an increase in female miscarriages. Adequate levels of selenium promote white blood cell production, improved thyroid metabolism, and healthy eye lens, skin, and hair. Besides the heart, thyroid, and skin, selenium helps maintain normal liver function and aids in slowing down the aging process.[91]

Selenium deficiency decreases function of selenium-dependent enzymes like glutathione peroxidase. This compromises vitamin E actions in cell membranes and can lead to increased levels of free radicals like hydrogen peroxide. The damage that the free radicals cause to heart, liver, and other organ tissue can leave them susceptible to cancer, viral and bacterial infections, and even cell death and organ failure. The cardiovascular damage due to selenium deficiency has resulted in juvenile cardiomyopathy (Keshan's disease) and chondrodystrophy (Kashin-Beck disease).[91] Other effects of selenium deficiency associated with heart disease and stroke include cataracts, anemia, increased cancer risk, diabetes, arthritis, early aging, infertility, and decreased immune function.

The cardiomyopathy effects of selenium deficiency are seen in home PN (HPN). A case report describes a 46-year-old man who developed an enlarged heart and a myopathy.[92] The findings reported include that selenium-derived deficiency adversely affected the red blood cell selenium levels and the glutathione peroxidase levels. Red cells were then susceptible to the oxidative stress without a way to neutralize those compounds. Recognition of the problem resulted in the patient being started on selenium. In a month, he improved, once selenium was added to his HPN solutions. A second earlier study on selenium

CASE STUDY 33-6

An 18-year-old female of small bone frame comes to her physician complaining about feeling tired and fatigued. She has had a recent severe cold and took various over-the-counter medications including zinc-containing cold lozenges to get some relief. She thinks her cold has made her weak, but after a month and half she decides she needs a doctor to check her out for other infections. Her blood work is shown in Case Study Table 33-6.1.

CASE STUDY TABLE 33-6.1
LABORATORY RESULTS

TEST	RESULT	REFERENCE RANGE
CBC		
Hct	25%	36–48%
Hb	7.8 g/dL	12–16 g/dL
RBC	3.1×10^6/mL	$3.6–5.0 \times 10^6$/mL
MCV	67 fL	82–98 fL
MCHC	25.3 g/dL	31–37 g/dL
WBC	7.2×10^3/mL	$4.0–11.0 \times 10^3$/mL
Neutrophil	56%	40–80%
Lymph	20%	15–40%
Reticulocyte count	2.5%	0.5–1.5%
Reticulocyte index	1.7%	>3%
CHEMISTRY		
BUN	15 mg/dL	7–18 mg/dL
Glucose	110 mg/dL	Fasting 70–100 mg/dL
		Nonfasting 70–150 mg/dL
ELECTROLYTES	**NORMAL**	
Bilirubin	1.6 mg/dL	0.2–1 mg/dL
Direct	0.5 mg/dL	0–0.2 mg/dL
T_3 and T_4	Normal	
Serum zinc	125 µg/dL	60–120 µg/dL
Ceruloplasmin	15 mg/dL	17–54 mg/dL

Questions

1. What type of anemia does this patient exhibit?

2. Why do you think her ceruloplasmin value is decreased?

3. What do you think her physician will recommend for this patient?

deficiency looked at patients with significant dilated cardiomyopathy.[88] The results indicated no significant difference in the patient group with the disease versus the age- and gender-matched control group without disease. While both groups had lower than normal selenium levels, the question as to why some developed disease while others did not remained an unresolved scientific question.

Excessive selenium levels can occur with excessive supplementation. Effects of excess includes fatigue, irritability, loss of hair and nails, vomiting, nerve damage, skin rashes, and brittle bones.[91,92] Specifically, a recent review found that indiscriminant use of selenium supplementation above RDA had adverse effects in individuals with diabetes.[93]

For additional student resources please visit thePoint at http://thepoint.lww.com. **thePoint** ✳

QUESTIONS

1. Which of the following describes the correct source, function, and deficient state of the vitamin listed?
   a. Thiamine (B$_1$)—whole grains, carbohydrate metabolism, beriberi
   b. Vitamin E—plant tissues, antioxidant, osteomalacia
   c. Niacin—meat, oxidation–reduction reactions, scurvy
   d. Folic acid—dairy products, myelin formation

2. Which vitamin would be affected if a patient was diagnosed with a disorder involving fat absorption?
   a. Vitamin K
   b. Vitamin B$_{12}$
   c. Ascorbic acid
   d. Thiamine

3. Which vitamin is a powerful antioxidant, protects the erythrocyte membrane from oxidative stress, and is found primarily in vegetable oils?
   a. Vitamin E
   b. Vitamin K
   c. Vitamin C
   d. Folic acid

4. A 70-year-old man presented to his physician with a broken arm. Laboratory work indicated an elevated prothrombin time, with all other laboratory results being normal. The man was also taking an antibiotic for an earlier respiratory infection. Which, if any, of the following vitamins might be involved?
   a. Vitamin K
   b. Vitamin D
   c. Biotin
   d. None of these

5. The most commonly used method for determination of vitamin B$_{12}$ is

   a. Competitive protein-binding RIA
   b. Chemiluminescence assay
   c. Magnetic separation immunoassay
   d. HPLC

6. The term describing patients who are chronically calorie malnourished and lose both adipose and muscle tissue, but who do not demonstrate a protein deficiency, is
   a. Marasmus
   b. Kwashiorkor
   c. Debilitated
   d. None of these

7. Metabolic syndrome is a complex disorder with many parameters to measure. Which of the following is NOT needed to assess metabolic syndrome?
   a. Elevated HDL cholesterol
   b. Elevated triglyceride levels
   c. Elevated fasting glucose
   d. Elevated blood pressure

8. Which of the following nutritional markers has been found to be the most sensitive and helpful indicator of nutritional status in very ill patients?
   a. Transthyretin
   b. Transferrin
   c. Albumin
   d. Somatomedin C

9. Laboratory monitoring of the patient on TPN therapy is important to avoid possible complications. Which of the following trace elements should be monitored on a weekly basis?
   a. Copper
   b. Selenium
   c. Molybdenum
   d. Chromium

REFERENCES

1. Lacey K, Pritchett E. Nutrition Care Process and Model: ADA adopts road map to quality care and outcomes management. *J Am Dietetic Assoc.* 2003;103:1061-1072.
2. Sebastian JG, Boosalis MG. Nutritional aspects of home health care. In: Martinson IM, Widmer AG, Portillo CJ, eds. *Home Health Care Nursing.* 2nd ed. Philadelphia, PA: WB Saunders, 2002:140-179.
3. NHLBI. Obesity Education Initiative electronic textbook: treatment guidelines. http://www.nhlbi.nih.gov/guidelines/obesity/e_txtbk/txgd/40.htm. Accessed August 1, 2012.
4. Dillman E, Gala C, Green W, et al. Hypothermia in iron deficiency due to altered triiodo-thyroxine metabolism. *Am J Physiol.* 1980;239:377-381.
5. Boosalis MG, Ott L, Levine AS, et al. The relationship of visceral proteins to nutritional status in chronic and acute stress. *Crit Care Med.* 1989;17:741-747.
6. Boosalis MG, McCall JT, Solem LD, et al. Serum copper and ceruloplasmin and urinary copper levels in thermal injury. *Am J Clin Nutr.* 1986;44:899-906.
7. Boosalis MG, Solem LD, Ahrenholz DH. Serum and urinary selenium levels in thermal injury. *Burns Incl Therm Inj.* 1986;12:236-240.
8. Boosalis MG, McCall JT, Solem LD, et al. Serum and urinary silver levels in thermal injury. *Surgery.* 1987;101:40-43.
9. Boosalis MG, McCall JT, Solem LD, et al. Serum zinc response in thermal injury. *J Am Coll Nutr.* 1988;7:69-76.
10. Boosalis MG, Gray D, Walker S, et al. The acute phase response in autologous bone marrow transplantation. *J Med.* 1992;23:175-193.
11. Boosalis MG, Stiles NJ. Nutritional assessment in elders: biochemical analyses. *Clin Lab Sci.* 1995;8:31-33.
12. Boosalis MG, Snowdon DA, Tully CL, et al. The acute phase response and plasma carotenoid concentrations in older women: findings from the Nun Study. *Nutrition.* 1996;12:475-478.
13. National Heart, Lung, Blood Institute, NHLBI. http://www.nhlbi.nih.gov/health/health-topics/topics/ms/diagnosis.html. Accessed August 1, 2012.
14. USDA. ChooseMyPlate. http://www.choosemyplate.gov. Accessed August 1, 2012.
15. USDA Agricultural Research Service. http://www.ars.usda.gov/News/docs.htm?docid=9265. Accessed August 1, 2012.
16. Royle GT, Kettlewell MGW. Liver function tests in surgical infection and malnutrition. *Ann Surg.* 1980;192:459.
17. Apelgren KN, Rombeau JL, Twomey PL, et al. Comparison of nutritional indices and outcome in critically ill patients. *Crit Care Med.* 1982;10:305.
18. Ingenbleek Y, Van Den Schrieck H-G, De Nayer P, et al. Albumin, transferrin and thyroxine-binding prealbumin/retinol-binding protein (TBPA-RBP) complex in assessment of malnutrition. *Clin Chim Acta.* 1975;63:61.
19. Georgieff MK, Amarnath UM, Murphy EL, et al. Serum transferrin levels in the longitudinal assessment of protein-energy status in preterm infants. *J Pediatr Gastroenterol Nutr.* 1989;8:234.
20. Ingenbleek Y, De Visscher M, De Nayer P. Measurement of prealbumin as an index of protein-calorie malnutrition. *Lancet.* 1972;2:106.
21. Smith FR, Goodman DS, Zaklama MS, et al. Serum vitamin A, retinol-binding protein, and prealbumin concentrations in protein calorie malnutrition. I. Functional defect in hepatic retinol release. *Am J Clin Nutr.* 1973;26:973.
22. Bernstein LH, Leukhardt-Fairfield CJ, Pleban W, et al. Usefulness of data on albumin and prealbumin concentrations in determining effectiveness of nutritional support. *Clin Chem.* 1989;35:271.
23. Large S, Neal G, Glover J, et al. The early changes in retinol-binding protein and prealbumin concentrations in plasma of protein-energy malnourished children after treatment with retinol and an improved diet. *Br J Nutr.* 1980;43:393.
24. Georgieff MK, Sasanow SR, Pereira GR. Serum transthyretin levels and protein intake as predictors of weight gain velocity in premature infants. *J Pediatr Gastroenterol Nutr.* 1987;6:775.
25. Giacoia GP, Watson S, West K. Rapid turnover transport proteins, plasma albumin, and growth in low birth weight infants. *J Parenter Enteral Nutr.* 1984;8:367.
26. Moskowitz SR, Pereira G, Spitzer A, et al. Prealbumin as a biochemical marker of nutritional adequacy in premature infants. *J Pediatr.* 1983;102:749.
27. Church JM, Hill GL. Assessing the efficacy of intravenous nutrition in general surgical patients: dynamic nutritional assessment with plasma proteins. *J Parenter Enteral Nutr.* 1987;11:135.
28. Tuten MB, Wogt S, Dasse F, et al. Utilization of prealbumin as a nutritional parameter. *J Parenter Enteral Nutr.* 1985;9:709.
29. Cavarocchi NC, Au FC, Dalal FR, et al. Rapid turnover proteins as nutritional indicators. *World J Surg.* 1986;10:468.
30. Carlson DE, Cioffi WG Jr, Mason AD Jr, et al. Evaluation of serum visceral protein levels as indicators of nitrogen balance in thermally injured patients. *J Parenter Enteral Nutr.* 1991;15:440.
31. Ingenbleek Y, Van Den Schrieck HG, De Nayer P, et al. The role of retinol-binding protein in protein-calorie malnutrition. *Metabolism.* 1975;24:633.
32. Smith FR, Suskind R, Thanangkul O, et al. Plasma vitamin A, retinol-binding protein and prealbumin concentrations in protein-calorie malnutrition. III. Response to varying dietary treatments. *Am J Clin Nutr.* 1975;28:732.
33. Baxter RC. The somatomedins: insulin-like growth factors. *Adv Clin Chem.* 1986;25:49.
34. Isley WL, Lyman B, Pemberton B. Somatomedin-C as a nutritional marker in traumatized patients. *Crit Care Med.* 1990;18:795.
35. Clemmons DR, Underwood LE, Dickerson RN, et al. Use of plasma somatomedin-C/insulin-like growth factor I measurements to monitor the response to nutritional repletion in malnourished patients. *Am J Clin Nutr.* 1985;41:191.
36. Unterman TG, Vazquez RM, Slas AJ, et al. Nutrition and somatomedin. XIII. Usefulness of somatomedin-C in nutritional assessment. *Am J Med.* 1985;78:228.
37. Mosher DF. Physiology of fibronectin. *Annu Rev Med.* 1984;35:561.
38. Saba TM, Blumenstock FA, Shah DM, et al. Reversal of opsonic deficiency in surgical, trauma, and burn patients by infusion of purified human plasma fibronectin. *Am J Med.* 1986;80:229.
39. Russell MK, McAdams MP. Laboratory monitoring of nutritional status. In: Matarese LE, Gottschlich MM, eds. *Contemporary Nutrition Support Practice: A Clinical Guideline.* Philadelphia, PA: WB Saunders; 1998:54.
40. Deodhar SD. C-reactive protein: the best laboratory indicator available for monitoring disease activity. *Cleve Clin J Med.* 1989;56:126.
41. Hokama Y, Nakamura RM. C-reactive protein: current status and future perspectives. *J Clin Lab Anal.* 1987;1:15.
42. Wilmore DW, Black PR, Muhlbacher F. Injured man: trauma and sepsis. In: Winters RW, Greene M, eds. *Nutritional Support of the Seriously Ill Patient.* New York, NY: Academic Press; 1983:33-52.
43. Cerra FB. Hypermetabolism, organ failure, and metabolic support. *Surgery.* 1987;101:1.
44. Dudrick SJ. A clinical review of nutritional support of the patient. *J Parenter Enteral Nutr.* 1979;3:444.
45. Howard L, Meguid MM. Nutritional assessment in total parenteral nutrition. *Clin Lab Med.* 1981;1:611.
46. Briggs MH, ed. *Vitamins in Human Biology and Medicine.* Boca Raton, FL: CRC Press; 1981.
47. Food and Nutrition Board. *Recommended Dietary Allowances.* 10th ed. Washington, DC: National Academy of Science; 1989.
48. Otten JJ, Hellwig JP, Meyers LD, eds. *Dietary Reference Intakes: The Essential Guide to Nutrient Requirements.* Washington, DC:

Institute of Medicine, National Academies Press; 2006. http://www.nap.edu/catalog.php?record_id=11537. Accessed August 1, 2012.

49. Boosalis MG. Vitamins. In: Matarese LE, Gottschlich MM, eds. *Contemporary Nutrition Support Practice: A Clinical Guideline.* Philadelphia, PA: WB Saunders; 1998:145-162.

50. Boosalis MG. Micronutrients. In: Boosalis MG, ed. *The Science and Practice of Nutrition Support: A Case-Based Core Curriculum.* Dubuque, IA: Kendall/Hunt Publishing; 2001:85-106.

51. Otten JJ, Hellwig JP, Meyer LD, eds. *Dietary Reference Intakes: The Essential Guide to Nutrient Requirements.* Washington DC: National Academies Press; 2006:5-19.

52. Ensminger AH, Ensminger ME, Konlande JE, et al. *Foods and Nutrition Encyclopedia.* 2nd ed. Boca Raton, FL: CRC Press; 1994:2257-2260.

53. Sauberlich HE. *Laboratory Tests for the Assessment of Nutritional Status,* 2nd edition. Boca Raton, FL: CRC Press; 1999:11-280.

54. Book LS. Fat soluble vitamins and essential fatty acids in total parenteral nutrition. In: Lebenthal E, ed. *Total Parenteral Nutrition: Indications, Utilization, Complications.* New York, NY: Raven Press; 1986:59-81.

55. Institute of Medicine, Food and Nutrition Board. *Dietary Reference Intakes for Calcium and Vitamin D.* Washington, DC: National Academies Press; 2010. http://books.nap.edu/openbook.php?record_id=13050&page=1106. Accessed February 28, 2012.

56. Underwood BA. Methods for assessment of vitamin A status. *J Nutr.* 1990;120(suppl 11):1459-1463.

57. Bieri JG, Evarts RP, Thorp S. Factors affecting the exchange of tocopherol between red cells and plasma. *Am J Clin Nutr.* 1977;30:686.

58. Holick MF. The use and interpretation of assays for vitamin D and its metabolites. *J Nutr.* 1990;120(suppl 11):1464-1469.

59. Suttie, J.W. Vitamin K. In: Diplock AD, ed. *Fat-Soluble Vitamins: Their Biochemistry and Applications.* London: Heinemann; 1985:225-311.

60. Hazell K, Baloch KH. Vitamin K deficiency in the elderly. *Gerontol Clin.* 1970;12:10-17.

61. Sitren H. Vitamin K. In: Baumgartner TG, ed. *Clinical Guide to Parenteral Micronutrition.* New York, NY: Fujizawa USA; 1991:411-430.

62. Sitren HS, Bailey LB, Cerda JJ, Anderson CR. Thiamin (vitamin B₁). In: Baumgartner TG, ed. *Clinical Guide to Parenteral Micronutrition.* New York, NY: Fujizawa USA; 1991:431-449.

63. Sitren HS, Bailey LB, Cerda JJ, Anderson CR. Riboflavin (vitamin B₂). In: Baumgartner TG, ed. *Clinical Guide to Parenteral Micronutrition.* New York, NY: Fujizawa USA; 1991:451-468.

64. Bailey LB. Pyridoxine (vitamin B₆). In: Baumgartner TG, ed. *Clinical Guide to Parenteral Micronutrition.* New York, NY: Fujizawa USA; 1991:521-539.

65. Sitren HS, Bailey LB, Cerda JJ, Anderson CR. Niacin (vitamin B₃). In: Baumgartner TG, ed. *Clinical Guide to Parenteral Micronutrition.* New York, NY: Fujizawa USA; 1991:469-486.

66. Bailey LB. Folic acid. In: Baumgartner TG, ed. *Clinical Guide to Parenteral Micronutrition.* New York, NY: Fujizawa USA; 1991:573-590.

67. Bailey LB. Folate status assessment. *J Nutr.* 1990;120(suppl 11):1508-1511.

68. Ueland PM, Refsum H, Stabler SP, et al. Total homocysteine in plasma or serum: methods and clinical applications. *Clin Chem.* 1993;39:1764-1779.

69. Steinkamp RC. Vitamin B₁₂ and folic acid: clinical and pathophysiological considerations. In: Brewster MA, Naito IIK, eds. *Nutritional Elements and Clinical Biochemistry.* New York, NY: Plenum; 1980:169-240.

70. Bailey LB. Cobalamine (vitamin B₁₂). In: Baumgartner TG, ed. *Clinical Guide to Parenteral Micronutrition.* New York, NY: Fujizawa USA; 1991:541-572.

71. Roth KS. Biotin in clinical medicine: a review. *Am J Clin Nutr.* 1981;34:1967.

72. Zempleni J, Mock DM. Advanced analysis of biotin metabolites in body fluids allows a more accurate measurement of biotin bioavailability and metabolism in humans. *J Nutr.* 1999;129:494S-497S.

73. McCormick DB, Greene HL. Vitamins. In: Burtis CA, Ashwood ER, eds. *Tietz Textbook of Clinical Chemistry.* 3rd ed. Philadelphia, PA: WB Saunders; 1999:999-1029.

74. Englard S, Seifter S. The biochemical functions of ascorbic acid. *Annu Rev Nutr.* 1986;6:265-304.

75. Jacob RA. Assessment of human vitamin C status. *J Nutr.* 1990;120(suppl 11):1480-1485.

76. Tanphaichitr V, Leelahagul P. Carnitine metabolism and human carnitine deficiency. *Nutrition.* 1993;9:246-254.

77. Takala J, Neuvonen P, Klossner J. Hypophosphatemia in hypercatabolic patients. *Acta Anaesthesiol Scand.* 1985;29:65.

78. Tovey SJ, Benton KGF, Lee HA. Hypophosphatemia and phosphorus requirements during intravenous nutrition. *Postgrad Med.* 1977;53:289.

79. Ghosh K. Non-haematological effects of iron deficiency: a perspective. *Indian J Med Sci.* 2006;60:30-37.

80. Willis WT, Gohil K, Brooks GA, Dallman PR. Iron deficiency: improved exercise performance within 15 hours of iron treatment in rats. *J Nutr.* 1990;120:909-916.

81. Nuttall KL, Klee GG. Iron. In: Burtis CA, Ashwood ER, eds. *Tietz Fundamentals of Clinical Chemistry.* 5th ed. Philadelphia, PA: WB Saunders; 2001:596-601.

82. O'Dell BL. Copper. In: Ziegler EF, Filer EF Jr, eds. *Present Knowledge in Nutrition.* 7th ed. Washington, DC: ILSI Press; 1996:261-267.

83. Lockitch G, Godophin W, Pendray MR, et al. Serum zinc, copper, retinol-binding protein, prealbumin and ceruloplasmin concentrations in infants receiving intravenous zinc and copper supplement. *J Pediatr.* 1983;102:304.

84. Bogden JD, Klevay LM. *Clinical Nutrition of Essential Trace Elements and Minerals.* Totowa, NJ: Humana Press; 2000.

85. Gordon EF, Gordon RC, Passal DB. Zinc metabolism: basic clinical and behavioral aspects. *J Pediatr.* 1981;99:341.

86. Jeejeebhoy KN. Zinc and chromium in parenteral nutrition. *Bull N Y Acad Med.* 1984;60:118.

87. ARUP Lab. Zinc, serum. http://www.aruplab.com/guides/ug/tests/0020097.jsp. Accessed August 1, 2012.

88. Fawzy ME, Yazigi AE, Stefadouros MA, et al. The role of selenium deficiency in dilated cardiomyopathy in Saudi Arabia. *Ann Saudi Med.* 1999;19:20-22.

89. Hussein O, Rosenblat M, Refael G, et al. Dietary selenium increases cellular glutathione peroxidase activity and reduces the enhanced susceptibility to lipid peroxidation of plasma and low density lipoprotein in kidney transplant recipients. *Transplantation.* 1997;63:679-685.

90. Girodon F, Galan P, Monget AL, et al. Impact of trace elements and vitamin supplementation on immunity and infections in institutionalised elderly patients. *Arch Intern Med.* 1999;159:748-754.

91. Fleet JC, Mayer J. Dietary selenium repletion may reduce cancer incidence in people at high risk who live in areas with low soil selenium. *Nutr Rev.* 1997;55:277-279.

92. Wamique YS. Cardiomypathy in association with selenium deficiency: a case report. *J Parenter Enteral Nutr.* 2002;26:63-66.

93. Boosalis MG. The role of selenium in chronic disease. *Nutr Clin Pract.* 2008;23(2):152-160.

Clinical Chemistry and the Geriatric Patient

LAURA M. BENDER, JACK M. McBRIDE

CHAPTER OUTLINE

Chapter Objectives

Upon completion of this chapter, the clinical laboratorian should be able to do the following:

- Define aging, apoptosis, atherosclerosis, free radical, geriatrics, gerontology, homeostasis, menopause, and osteoporosis.
- Discuss the impact of geriatric patients on the clinical laboratory.
- Describe the current theories of aging.
- Appraise the physiologic changes that occur with the aging process.

- Identify the age-related changes in clinical chemistry analytes.
- Explain the problems associated with establishing reference intervals for the elderly.
- Describe the effects of medication on clinical chemistry results in the elderly.
- Discuss the effects of exercise and nutrition on chemistry results in the elderly.
- Correlate age-related physiologic changes and laboratory results with pathologic conditions.

KEY TERMS

Free radical
Geriatrics

Gerontology
Menopause
Osteoporosis

The number and proportion of older individuals in the total population is increasing rapidly in the United States and other developed nations. There are a number of physiological and metabolic changes unique to aging that may affect clinical laboratory values. In addition, aging is often accompanied by multiple medical conditions requiring diverse medications, which can also affect clinical laboratory values. This chapter will summarize the issues that should be given special consideration with regard to clinical chemistry in the geriatric patient.

THE AGING OF AMERICA

In 2010, there were over 40 million individuals in the United States aged 65 years and older, making up 13% of the population. Not only was this the largest number of

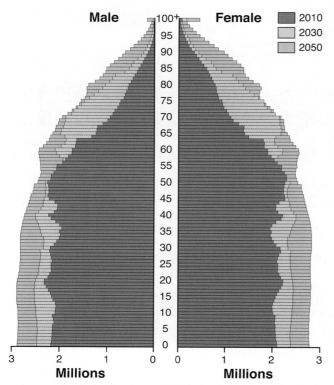

FIGURE 34-1 Data taken from the US Census Bureau 2008 display the age/gender structure of the population in this country and the projected changes that are expected to occur over the next 40 years. There is an anticipated shift in the age structure for the 13% of the population falling into the subclass of 65 or older. The distribution is expected to increase to nearly 20% by the year 2030.[4] (Source: U.S. Census Bureau, 2008.)

aged individuals and the largest percentage of the population ever reported in a US Census, this segment of the population grew much more rapidly than the US population as a whole. The number of Americans over 65 years of age grew 15.1% over the preceding 10 years, compared with 9.7% for all Americans. Within this group of "seniors" there were almost 5.5 million individuals aged 85 years and older and while they only made up 1.78% of the US population, this subset was growing at the remarkable rate of almost 30% over the previous 10 years.[1]

The first "baby boomers," individuals born during the post–World War II surge from 1946 to 1964, started turning 65 in 2011. Additionally, life expectancy has increased significantly in the United States, and in 2010 the average female was expected to live to 80.8 years while the average male was expected to live to 75.7.[2] Approximately 10,000 boomers will turn 65 each day for the next two decades, more than doubling the number of Americans 65 years of age or older to 88.5 million by 2050.[3] Figure 34-1, taken from the U.S. Census Bureau 2008: "The Next Four Decades: The Older Population in the United States," categorizes the age structure of the American population and the projected changes over the next 40 years. These changes are largely due to the aging of the baby boomers along with immigration trends.[4] Complementary data from the 2010 census document illustrates and characterizes the increase in the population numbers over the past 110 years.[1] Depending on immigration, fertility and longevity rates, these seniors are expected to constitute over 20% of the total US population by 2050 (Fig. 34-2).[4,5] The total population

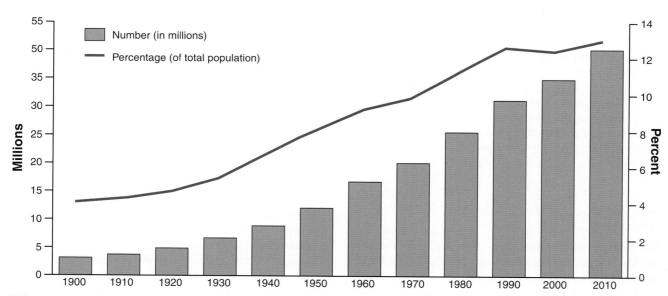

FIGURE 34-2 Population 65 years and older by size and percent of total population: 1900 to 2010. This figure shows the age growth over the past 110 years in the United States. Currently over 40.3 million people are over age 65. This was an additional increase of 5.3 million over the numbers in the 2000 census. Additionally, the percentage of the population over age 65 has increased from 12.4% in 2000 to 13% in 2010. Further, the percentage of the US population >85 years is expected to continue to increase, and in 2050, this age range is expected to make up over 20% of the US population. (Source: U.S. Census Bureau, decennial census of population, 1900 to 2000; *2010 Census Summary File 1*.)

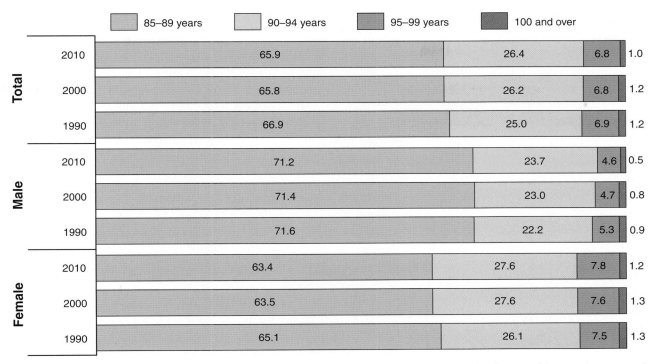

FIGURE 34-3 Projected population of Americans over the age of 65 by age and sex. The percent distribution of the population over the age of 85 is further broken down according to gender.[4] The largest percentage increase during the previous 20 years was in the 90 to 94 year age group, which saw an increase of 1.4% between the years 1990 and 2010. Females contribute a larger percentage to the oldest-old calculation compared with the male data. (Source: U.S. Census Bureau, *1990 Census Summary File 2C, Census 2000 Summary File 1,* and *2010 Summary File 1.*)

over the age of 65 (Fig. 34-3) is expected to reach 19 million in the United States by 2050, almost 4.5% of the total population.[4] With the burden of medical illness and medication use falling disproportionately on the elderly, a dramatic increase in the utilization of health care services, including clinical chemistry, is inevitable.

AGING AND MEDICAL SCIENCE

Gerontology, the study of aging, and geriatrics, the subspecialty of clinical medicine that focuses on care of the aged, have much to tell us about normal aging, as well as the unique features of common illnesses in the elderly. The differentiation of "normal" or "healthy" aging versus the accumulation of multiple medical problems with age is an area of active research and debate. There are several analytical measurements that change when comparing a diseased individual to a healthy one, but because there are also a number of biochemical changes that occur as a consequence of normal aging, it can be difficult to differentiate between abnormal physiological changes and normal signs of aging in geriatric patients.

One important principle is that aging is extremely heterogeneous. The extent of differences between individuals of the same age is often quite significant. Indeed, an individual's overall health status and expected longevity are more closely related to their functional status than

their chronologic age. By that we mean that an 86-year old jet-setting international attorney looks very unlike a 60-year old nursing home patient bedbound with dementia. Another issue that arises with respect to caring for the elderly is that older adults may mistake a health symptom for a normal part of aging, and therefore not seek medical attention as early as they should.[6]

An important consideration is the concept of diminished physiological reserve. While an aged person usually has the same adaptive mechanisms to stress as a younger person, those adaptations may not be as rapid or as robust. Therefore, with diminished reserve, an aged individual may encounter adverse health effects much more quickly than a younger person. For example, an elderly person undergoing diuretic therapy for hypertension would not be able to withstand a long period of vomiting and diarrhea compared with a younger person. Age-associated decrease in total body water would favor dehydration and development of hypernatremia and delirium.[7]

While age-dependent changes in concentrations of analytes have been shown to be important in a number of areas of chemistry, there are also several examples of chemistry values that are unchanged as a consequence of age.[8] Table 34-1 outlines some of the age-specific changes that occur in regard to certain chemistry analytes, and some of these changes will be specifically addressed in the coming section outlining physiologic changes with

TABLE 34-1	CHANGES IN SELECTED CLINICAL CHEMISTRY ANALYTES WITH AGE[9-29]	
INCREASE	**DECREASE**	**UNCHANGED**
ANP		ACTH
Alk phosphatase (females)	ADH	Calcium
Calcitonin	Albumin	Chloride
C-reactive protein		Cortisol
EPO	Aldosterone	Creatinine
Ferritin	Vitamin B$_{12}$	HDL-C
Fibrinogen	LDL-C	Insulin
Folic acid	Cholesterol	Sodium
FSH	DHEA-S	Total T4
Free T4	Estrogen	pH or slight decrease
Gamma globulins	Ferritin	
Homocysteine	Growth hormone	
Insulin	IGF-1	
Lactate	po$_2$	
Parathyroid hormone	Progesterone	
Potassium	Testosterone	
TBG	T3	
TSH (slight)	Total protein	
Transferrin	Uric acid	
Triglycerides	Vitamin D	
GGT		

ANP, atrial natriuretic peptide; ACTH, adrenocorticotropic hormone; ADH, antidiuretic hormone; EPO, erythropoietin; HDL-C, high-density lipoprotein cholesterol; LDL-C, low-density lipoprotein cholesterol; FSH, follicle-stimulating hormone; DHEA-S, sulfated dehydroepiandrosterone; IGF-1, insulin-like growth factor-1; TBG, thyroid binding globulin; TSH, thyroid-stimulating hormone; GGT, γ-glutamyl transferase; T3, triiodothyronine.

age. Ideally, the changes that impact laboratory results would be classified in age-specific reference ranges, but since these are not readily available changes in analyte level over time can help to manage patient treatment.[8]

GENERAL PHYSIOLOGIC CHANGES WITH AGING

The aging process involves both biochemical and physiological changes and can be subdivided into various organ systems. The systems continue to function appropriately unless they are subjected to excess stress. With increasing age, an individuals' ability to respond to stress decreases. This leads to an age-associated increase in the prevalence of pathological conditions. Table 34-2 outlines some of the more common factors impacting the interpretation of clinical laboratory results.

Muscle

Total body muscle mass typically decreases with age, but the rate and extent of loss have a strong genetic component. This age-related decline (sarcopenia) results in a decrease in lean body mass and a decrease in total creatinine production, such that serum creatinine is no longer reliable for assessment of renal function in the aged.[9]

Bone

Total bone density and mass decreases with age in both men and women, though the changes are much more dramatic in women after menopause.[10] Serum calcitonin levels typically rise with age, but ionized calcium levels remain stable.[11] Parathyroid hormone (PTH) levels increase in post-menopausal women and this increase is associated with changes in bone metabolism.[12]

Gastrointestinal System

The incidence of atrophic gastritis increases with age, with a consequent increase in vitamin B12 deficiency from poor absorption.[13] The incidence of achlorhydria (low or absent gastric acid production) also increases

TABLE 34-2	FACTORS IMPACTING INTERPRETATION OF CLINICAL LABORATORY RESULTS FOR THE ELDERLY[6,20,21,30-35]

Exercise
   Duration
   Type
Medications
   Polypharmacy
Mobility
   Immobility
   Posture
Nutritional status
Personal habits
   Alcohol use
   Smoking
Presence of chronic or subclinical disorders
Validity of reference intervals
Specimen collection variables
   Site
   Trauma
   Volume

CASE STUDY 34-1

A healthy 65-year-old man entered the hospital to have his appendix removed. Preoperative laboratory results are shown in Case Study Table 34-1.1.

CASE STUDY TABLE 34-1.1 LABORATORY RESULTS

TEST	RESULT	REFERENCE RANGE
Albumin	25 g/L	35–50 g/L
BUN	35 mg/dL	8–26 mg/dL
Creatinine	1.7 mg/dL	0.9–1.5 mg/dL
Serum osmolality	280 mOsm/kg	275–295 mOsm/kg
Sodium	140 mmol/L	135–145 mmol/L

Question

1. What is the BUN/Creatinine ratio for this patient?

2. What do these data suggest?

3. Which test results support this conclusion?

with age, which can result in decreased calcium and iron absorption, as well as an increased incidence of bacterial overgrowth in the small intestine.[14] Albumin levels decrease, and the incidence of malnutrition, leading to higher mortality rates, also increases.[36]

Kidney/Urinary System

The number of functional glomeruli decreases with age, resulting in a decrease in kidney size and weight. Glomerular filtration rate (GFR) declines, and renal blood flow is even more reduced, such that filtration fraction (GFR/renal plasma flow) actually increases.[16] Additionally, the kidney's concentrating ability declines. The result of all these changes is that acid/base, water, and electrolyte levels remain normal under optimal conditions, but physiologic reserve is diminished. The secretion of erythropoietin (epo), the glycoprotein hormone that controls red blood cell production increases with age, and the level of serum renin, an enzyme that regulates blood pressure, decrease. Renal responsiveness to atrial natriuretic peptide (ANP) decreases, and serum levels of ANP and brain natriuretic peptide increase with age.[17,37] Structural, neurological, and immune changes result in an increased incidence of urinary tract infection in the elderly, especially in women.[18]

Immune System

The thymus shrinks with age, causing a decrease in thymosin levels and T-cell function. B-cell function slowly declines, as well, such that cellular and humoral immune responses are less vigorous and slower in the aged than in younger individuals.[19] Autoimmune antibody (antinuclear antibody [ANA]) levels increase,[38] and hematopoietic stem cell numbers decrease.[39] Examples of the consequences of declining cellular immunity in the elderly include reactivation of latent tuberculosis and herpes varicella zoster virus (HVZ). HVZ is the virus responsible for the chicken pox, but in an adult reactivation is termed shingles and presents as a painful, blistering skin rash. The prevalence of shingles in the United States is about a million cases per year, and susceptibility to shingles increases at the age of 50 years. This increase has led to the development of a live vaccine for elderly adults.[40]

Endocrine System

Serum adrenocorticotropic hormone and cortisol levels typically do not change with age, though response to stress may be delayed. Pulsatile secretion of growth hormone typically diminishes with age, resulting in a decrease in lean body mass/fat ratio, as well as loss of overall body mass. The peak but not the basal levels of melatonin secretion decrease with age, which may contribute to sleep cycle disorders as well as diminished protection from free radicals.[41] Norepinephrine secretion generally increases, which contributes to systemic vasoconstriction and decrease in myocardial relaxation; epinephrine levels remain stable. Aldosterone levels may decline, which can contribute to orthostatic hypotension, or a drop in blood pressure upon standing.[42] Thyroid hormone levels are typically well preserved or slightly increased into very old age.[43,44]

Sex Hormones

Although menopause in women typically occurs prior to the earliest ages considered "geriatric," the reduction in gonadal production of estrogen and progesterone and secondary increase in hypothalamic gonadotropin-releasing hormone persist through the remainder of a woman's life.[45] Testosterone levels in men typically exhibit a gradual decrease with increasing age—the term "andropause" has been used to describe this observation in analogy to menopause, but the decline in serum levels of sex hormone is not abrupt and not as significant in degree for men as it is for women, and in these authors' opinion the term is best avoided. The distinction between a normal serum testosterone level for age and hypogonadism in an aged man is a point of some contention and includes consideration of sexual function, general perception of well-being by the individual, and other clinical factors in addition to the value of the serum testosterone level.[46] Dehydroepiandrosterone (DHEA), sulfated DHEA, and pregnenolone all decrease with age.

Glucose Metabolism

Insulin secretion is unchanged, though there are age-related changes at the cellular level in insulin sig-naling, receptors, and glucose transporters. An individual with the genetic predisposition to type II diabetes mellitus is more likely to manifest clinical illness with increasing age, body mass index, and lack of exercise. The combination of an aging population, increasing obesity, and an increasing number of individuals from racial/ethnic groups at increased risk of diabetes (African American, Hispanic American, American Indian) has resulted in a dramatic increase in the number of older adults with diabetes.[47] Many of these individuals will also suffer some of the consequences of diabetes, including damage to the eyes, kidneys, nerves, and blood vessels.

EFFECTS OF AGE ON LABORATORY TESTING

Basic biochemical and physiological changes accompany the aging process, and these changes can impact an individual's clinical laboratory test results. It is important that laboratorians understand how these changes can impact specific tests. It has been suggested that the presence of age-specific changes may warrant separate reference intervals for the elderly,[44,48] but these are not readily available. In addition, consideration of preanalytical variables must be factored into the interpretation of laboratory results. How does the aging process affect interpretations of drug levels in the elderly? What are the effects of exercise and nutrition on chemistry results? Table 34-3 describes some of the factors that laboratorians should consider when interpreting test results for the elderly and defines some of the laboratory values that are impacted by these changes.

TABLE 34-3	EFFECTS OF AGE ON LABORATORY TESTING[10,17,19,37,38,43-46,49-56]	
	NORMAL PHYSIOLOGICAL CHANGES WITH AGE	**LABORATORY VALUES THAT CORRELATE**
Muscle	↓ Muscle mass	↓ Creatinine
Bone	↓ Mineral content of bone, ↓ cartilage	↑ PTH (females), ↓ calcium, and calcitonin
GI	↓ Gastric motility, vitamin absorption, and drug absorption	↓ Vitamin B12, calcium, and Fe absorption
Kidney	↓ Renal function	↑ Serum ANP, BNP, epo, and GFR, creatinine ↓ Renin
Immune	↑ Hematopoietic stem cells, bone marrow activity, thymosin, and T-cell function ↓ Autoimmune antibodies	↑ ANAs
Endocrine	↑ Cancer incidence	↓ Aldosterone ↑ Norepinephrine
Reproductive	↓ Sex hormones	↓ Testosterone, estrogen, progesterone, DHEA-S, and pregnenolone ↑ GnRH

PTH, parathyroid hormone; GI, gastrointestinal; ANP, atrial natriuretic peptide; BNP, brain natriuretic peptide; EPO, erythropoietin; GFR, glomerular filtration rate; ANA, antinuclear antibody; DHEA-S, sulfated dehydroepiandrosterone; GnRH, gonadotropin-releasing hormone.

Muscle

As muscles age, they begin to decrease in number and size. Creatinine levels correlate with both muscle mass and renal function. In the geriatric population, a decrease in muscle mass coupled with the decrease in renal function keeps the creatinine level nearly the same or slightly increased.

Bone

Adequate calcium intake and sufficient vitamin D are important in maintaining bone mass and density. Osteoporosis incidence is high in the elderly population, and this leads to increased risk of fracture. In addition, osteoporosis incidence coincides with increased risk of vitamin D deficiency. Vitamin D helps with absorption of dietary calcium from the intestine, thus decreased vitamin D levels can impact the amount of dietary calcium that is absorbed. Additionally, vitamin D deficiency leads to inadequate absorption of calcium, which leads to low serum levels and increased PTH levels. This increased PTH then causes increased calcium loss from the bone which increases alkaline phosphatase levels.[20]

Gastrointestinal System

The gastrointestinal system includes the digestive tract and accessory organs including the pancreas and the liver. There are a number of age-related changes with respect to the liver analytes. C-reactive protein, an acute phase reactant, has been shown to be elevated in the elderly.[57] This elevation is thought to be a non-specific indicator of inflammation, and typically is a poor prognostic indicator.[30] Gamma-glutamyl transferase (GGT) levels tend to increase with age in a gender-specific manner. Men do not show this age-related increase, but men tend to have higher levels of GGT than women. Fibrinogen, an acute phase reactant, is frequently elevated in geriatric patients, and this increase coincides with inflammatory disease, stroke, coronary dysfunction, and cancer.[21,31]

Ferritin levels can be low in the elderly population, and when this is seen, it is usually due to iron deficiency anemia, similar to younger people. Transferrin levels can be reduced due to iron-deficient anemia or as a result of acute or chronic stress. Albumin levels are frequently decreased in the elderly population as a result of inflammation, malnutrition, and liver disease. Levels can be high in dehydration, but elevations above the upper limits of normal rarely occur in the elderly due to the prevalence of other health conditions that mask alterations.[22] Total protein levels are also frequently decreased in the elderly for the same reasons that albumin levels are low.

Urinary System

Serum creatinine levels tend to be lower in the elderly. Again, this decreased serum level is associated with decreased muscle mass.

Immune System

As age increases, infection-induced morbidity and mortality rise. This is in part due to a weakened immune system. The innate immune system, commonly referred to as the "first line of defense," is the non-specific antigen activation that confers short-term protection from a pathogen. Adaptive immune system, on the other hand, is activated by the innate system and refers to the protection from antigen that an individual develops throughout the life. Both the innate and adaptive immune systems become damaged and dysfunctional as individuals age, leading to increased prevalence of infection, and potentially also autoimmune disease and cancer.[58] Gastroenteritis is more frequently observed as individuals' age, but the increased frequency is thought to be a result of a weakened immune system.[23] Pathogenic bacteria can enter and infect the digestive tract and contribute to presentation. Additionally, there is an increase in antinuclear antibody production, which correlates with incidence of arthritis.[32]

Endocrine System

There are a variety of age-related changes to endocrine hormone regulation. These can be subclassified according to whether the hormone level increases or decreases.

CASE STUDY 34-2

A healthy 70-year-old woman is seen by her primary care physician for an annual check-up. She complains of muscle weakness, drowsiness and confusion. Her laboratory results are shown in Case Study Table 34-2.1.

CASE STUDY TABLE 34-2.1 LABORATORY RESULTS

TEST	RESULT (MG/DL	REFERENCE RANGE
Calcium	12.0	8.5–10.2 mg/dL
Parathyroid hormone	111	12–72 pg/mL

Questions

1. Based on the laboratory data, how might the PTH test be interpreted?
2. Should any additional testing be done?

Increased Hormone Level

Elevated levels of cortisol, though rarely present, have been reported to be associated with decreased cognitive function and memory loss.[49] A slight increase in thyroid-stimulating hormone (TSH) has been observed, but again, this is not profound.[43,44] Follicle-stimulating hormone (FSH) levels increase with aging, but with this increase, there is a downregulation of FSH receptors, such that in menopause, there are no longer circulating cells with FSH receptors and thus no responsiveness to the high level of hormone. ANP levels increase with age and the levels have been shown to be nearly fourfold higher in healthy elderly individuals than in younger people.[50] Anemia is common in the elderly population, and EPO, a marker for anemia, rises in elderly patients.[24] PTH levels are slightly higher in older individuals than gender-matched pairs.[51]

Decreased Hormone Level

In contrast to the finding with cortisol, DHEA levels have been shown to decrease by 40% to 60%.[25] Estrogen and progesterone levels decrease with age, and the reduction in estrogen further upregulates FSH levels. IGF-1 and GH levels decrease with age. Secretion rates and serum concentrations of aldosterone decrease with age, and this decrease is a consequence of a decreased level of renin.[52,59] Pituitary function declines with age and hypothalamic antidiuretic hormone (ADH) levels are increased.

Sex Hormones

Levels of expression of all sex hormone diminish with age. Testosterone levels decrease with age, as do estrogen and progesterone levels.[46]

Glucose Metabolism

Insulin sensitivity decreases with age. As a result of this decreased sensitivity, there is an increase in the prevalence of type 2 diabetes, with the incidence reaching a peak between the ages of 60 and 74.[60]

ESTABLISHING REFERENCE INTERVALS FOR THE ELDERLY

Most laboratory tests have "gender-specific" reference ranges and/or "age-specific" reference ranges. The broad categories for the age ranges are very wide, and the adult reference range includes individuals between 18 and about 50 years. As people live longer, age-related criteria for the analysis and interpretation of test results become increasingly important. Because of the need to establish reference ranges in a healthy population, and the increased prevalence of at least one health condition in the aged, there are little data on more appropriate age-specific reference ranges for older adults. Based on this lack of data, there has been an increased interest

in determining age-related reference ranges in order to more effectively identify individuals with early stage disease.[53,61,62] While the idea has a lot of merit, there are currently no publications establishing age-appropriate reference ranges for the elderly.

Certain analyte fluctuations that are seen as individual's age are clearly the result of aging organs, but other analytes do not lend themselves to such apparent delineation.[63] In addition, coincident medical conditions can further complicate the issue. The requirement that reference values be obtained from healthy, normal individuals unfortunately limits a large number of geriatric patients from contributing to establishing these references. As a result of exclusion criteria, the geriatric population is also vastly underrepresented in most randomized clinical trials, which further precludes contribution to reference range generation.[64] In addition, there is a wide intraindividual variability among the various analytes, which has been seen as a major obstacle for determining age-appropriate reference ranges among the elderly. Instead, the current clinical approach that has been increasingly implemented is careful documentation of laboratory values and paying closer attention to changes over time instead of where the values fit in with the remainder of the population. This is not feasible among all elderly, as there is a small subset that resists treatment and thus does not see a medical professional on a regular basis.[65] A lack of baseline measurements coupled with the lack of age-specific reference ranges continues to make diagnosis challenging. Currently, most physicians that care for the geriatric patient population rely on established patient care, frequent routine examinations, and following changes in laboratory values over time as an early indicator of a problem.

PREANALYTICAL VARIABLES UNIQUE TO GERIATRIC PATIENTS

There are a number of factors that contribute to the accuracy and validity of test results in any population, but several of these factors have a greater impact in the geriatric patient. These include sample collection, sample handing, and physiological variables. Geriatric patients can present a challenge to phlebotomists due to disease, malnutrition, or dehydration.[66] With increased age there is a reduction in healing rate and an increased risk of acquiring infection due in part to a gradual loss in the capacity of the immune system to fight off infections.[67] Further, the skin and veins are less elastic and can be injured more easily during venipuncture. The decrease in muscle mass and collagen leads to a decrease in vascular stability of veins and a subsequent decrease in blood flow. Physiological changes in the patient may impact laboratory results due to unavoidable issues that arise at the time of collection. Increased hemolysis or insufficient volume can ultimately impact the validity of the result. Other factors that may influence normal laboratory values in geriatric patients include diet, medications, exercise, smoking, alcohol consumption, physical activity, and body composition. While these factors influence results independent of age, geriatric patients are more likely to have one or several of these causing variations in test results. Caution should always be exercised when reporting results in a geriatric patient, but clearly an absurd result (one not compatible with life) should be investigated to identify potential causes of the discrepancy.

DISEASES PREVALENT IN THE ELDERLY

There are many diseases that are especially common in the elderly. Table 34-4 outlines the prevalence of some of these conditions in Americans 65 years and older as reported in the 2007 to 2008 National Health Interview Survey, a self-reported statistically valid sample of the US population.[68] The overall prevalence of these diseases is inadequately understood due to poor documentation and the presence of multiple conditions warranting many medications. There have been attempts to classify disease prevalence in the elderly population based upon pharmacy databases.[69] Classification in this population has been difficult due to inaccuracies related to misidentification of conditions or diseases, or incomplete medical records. Approaches to classify individuals at an earlier stage of disease have led clinicians and laboratorians to begin to analyze the use of combination drug therapies as markers of disease. A list of drugs that patients are prescribed is available in a pharmacy database, and with this list, statistics can be generated calculating nationwide averages for disease prevalence.

The majority of the diseases noted in Table 34-5 are degenerative conditions, and there is a concern that increased life expectancy will increase the number of years with declining health. Health is defined as the state of being free from illness or injury, and deteriorating health is the number one reason that elderly leave their

TABLE 34-5	LEADING CAUSES OF DEATH IN THE ELDERLY[86]
Heart disease	
Cancer	
Cerebrovascular disease	
Chronic obstructive pulmonary disease	
Pneumonia	
Diabetes	
Influenza	
Septicemia	
Nephritis	
Alzheimer's	

homes and enter retirement facilities.[70] Unfortunately, without baseline measurement, it can be difficult to identify noteworthy changes in analyte levels.

Menopause is defined as the time when the primary function of the human ovaries is permanently terminated. This time is variable for each individual, but typically it begins between the ages of 35 and 58 years. This wide age range is based in part on the fact that functional disorders affecting the reproductive system can speed the transition to menopause. For instance, women with cancer of the reproductive tract, polycystic ovary syndrome, or endometriosis typically transition to menopause earlier than women without these conditions.[71-73] The precise definition of menopause is lack of menses for >1 year. This transitional phase from reproductive to non-reproductive typically lasts about a year to a year and a half, and during this period of time, there is a gradual decline in ovarian function, thus a decrease in ovarian hormone production.[73] The changes that occur are caused by reduced estrogens that result from loss of the granulosa and interstitial cells lining the follicles.[74] The placenta normally produces hCG during pregnancy, but in addition to placental production, hCG can also arise from the pituitary. In perimenopausal women, hCG levels are often detected in the absence of pregnancy as a result of ovarian failure.[54] Pituitary hCG is more commonly detected in women ≥55 years, and marked elevations in this age group are most commonly associated with cancer.[75]

Osteoporosis, a bone disease that is prevalent in the elderly, leads to increased risk of bone fracture. Two types of tissue form bone, compact and spongy (trabecular). Compact bone accounts for 80% of the total bone mass of an adult, while trabecular bone accounts for the remaining 20%. Trabecular bone is highly porous (30% to 90%), while compact bone has a porosity of 5% to 30%. The risk of fracture is highest in bones with more compact tissue,

TABLE 34-4	DISEASES PREVALENT IN THE ELDERLY: 2007–2008 NATIONAL HEALTH INTERVIEW SURVEY[68]
Hypertension	55.7%
Arthritis	49.5%
Heart disease	31.9%
Cancer	22.5%
Diabetes	18.6%
Asthma	10.4%
Chronic bronchitis/emphysema	9.0%
Stroke	8.8%

which functions in whole body support. Bone mineral density (BMD) is reduced with age, and the World Health Organization has defined osteoporosis as BMD 2.5 standard deviations below peak bone mass.[76] This decreased density and an observed reduction in a number of bone-associated proteins both contribute to the weakened condition. Classifications of osteoporosis include primary type 1, primary type 2, and secondary (also known as type 3).[77] While primary type 1 is more frequently seen in elderly females, there is a growing precedence of osteoporosis in men. Secondary osteoporosis occurs in women or men that are older than 70 years of age and is typically associated with decreased bone formation and decreased renal production of dihydroxy vitamin D. Vitamin D deficiency causes decreased calcium absorption, which increases the PTH levels and promotes calcium mobilization from the bones, resulting in a further diminished level of calcium. Type 3 osteoporosis is the only form of osteoporosis that affects individuals of any age. Most cases of type 3 osteoporosis are due to drug treatment or medication use, such as steroids,[78] and type 3 is not common in the elderly. Laboratory testing surrounding osteoporosis includes monitoring serum calcium, phosphate, creatinine, alkaline phosphatase, and 25-hydroxy vitamin D, and in men, testing also includes testosterone.[79]

Dementia is a syndrome defined as impairment of memory and at least one other cognitive domain (language, perceptual skills, attention, constructive abilities, orientation, and problem solving) that is severe enough to significantly impair day-to-day function.[80] Dementia is common in the elderly—approximately 10% of individuals over 65 years suffer from the syndrome; this rises to as high as 50% of those over 85 years.[81] Mild cognitive impairment (MCI) is a term used to describe similar cognitive problems that are not severe enough to significantly impair day-to-day function, but between 6% and 25% of individuals with MCI will go on to develop dementia in 1 year.

Dementia can be described in a number of ways, including the area of the brain that is most affected (cortical vs. subcortical), whether the etiology is known or unknown (secondary vs. primary), age of onset (pre-senile vs. senile), or by clinical syndrome. Many types of dementia can only be definitively diagnosed by pathological examination of brain tissue, which is obviously not helpful to the individual suffering from the illness, and correlation between the clinical syndromes and pathologic findings has historically been fairly poor. Recent advances in imaging and neurochemistry have improved this somewhat.[82]

Alzheimer's disease (AD) is the most common form of dementia, responsible for approximately 70% of cases.[81] The pathologic findings of AD include amyloid plaques (made of beta amyloid) and neurofibrillary tangles (made of tau protein). Individuals with AD typically have a fairly slow but steady progression of impairment.

Vascular dementia is the second most common form of dementia and may be caused either by multiple clinically evident strokes (multi-infarct dementia) or by ischemic changes in the deep white matter of the brain. Individuals with vascular dementia typically have a "stuttering" or "stair-step" progression of impairment, but the speed of progression and specific manifestations may vary widely, depending on which areas of the brain are damaged.[82-84]

Dementia with Lewy bodies (DLB) is the third most common form of dementia and is characterized by prominent visual hallucinations, significant fluctuations in mental status, and parkinsonism (motor symptoms similar to those of Parkinson's disease). Lewy bodies are collections of alpha-synuclein protein inside neurons, but whether they are a cause or an effect of the illness is unclear, and Lewy bodies are also seen in Parkinson's disease, as well as in some cases of Alzheimer's. DLB typically progresses more quickly than AD.

There are also less common types of dementia including Pick's disease, frontotemporal dementia, Creutzfeldt-Jakob disease, normal pressure hydrocephalus, Huntington's disease, and Wernicke-Korsakoff syndrome. Typically diagnosis of dementia is based on the patient's history and physical examination. Brain imaging and clinical laboratory testing may be performed to confirm or eliminate suspicion of specific clinical abnormalities.[85]

AGE-ASSOCIATED CHANGES IN DRUG METABOLISM

As adults age, changes occur that impact how the body metabolizes and utilizes drug compounds. Absorption, distribution, metabolism, and excretion of the drugs are impacted by the normal aging process. The prevalence of multiple health conditions in this subset of the population has highlighted the issue of polypharmacy[33] and the importance of therapeutic drug monitoring. Such testing in the laboratory helps prevent overdose and adverse drug reactions. Calculation of the actual in situ drug level is a key factor when looking at the results and metabolic rate, and elimination of these compounds needs to be considered for optimal dosing.[87]

Absorption

The rate of drug absorption from the small intestine slows with aging, leading to a lower peak serum concentration and a decrease in the time to reach peak. Typically, the total amount of drug absorbed (bioavailability) is the same in younger and older patients.[88] An exception arises due to an age-related decrease in hepatic function. Drugs that undergo extensive first-pass metabolism (such as nitrates) tend to have greater serum concentrations or greater bioavailability than drugs involved in conjugation or acetylation reactions.

Varying disease states or other drugs administered concurrently to the elderly may also cause changes in absorption. For example, calcium carbonate is frequently recommended for bone health in the elderly. This calcium salt requires gastric acid for absorption and should therefore be taken with food to stimulate gastric acid secretion. Patients with achlorhydria from natural causes or from acid-suppressing medications such as proton pump inhibitors or H2 blockers should instead take calcium citrate, the absorption of which does not require gastric acid.[89]

Distribution

Volume of distribution (V_d) is the volume of plasma into which a fixed concentration of drug is dissolved. The larger the V_d, the greater the distribution of the compound. Older adults typically have less body water and lean body mass as a percent of total body mass—or in other words have more fat as a percent of total body mass. Drugs such as ethanol and lithium which are water soluble (*hydrophilic*) have a lower volume of distribution in the elderly. Highly water-soluble drugs tend to be more concentrated in elderly individuals due to decreased body water. Additionally, drugs such as benzodiazepines and barbiturates which are fat-soluble (*lipophilic*) have higher volumes of distribution in the elderly due to increased body fat and decreased lean body mass.[90] The extent to which a drug binds to plasma proteins also impacts its volume of distribution. Many drugs bind to albumin, which is often decreased in the elderly. The unbound (free) portion of the drug is the pharmacologically active portion, and many drug assays measure total (bound and unbound) drug concentrations. Elderly patients with "normal" total drug levels may have excessive levels of free drug and exhibit signs of toxicity due in part to decreased albumin levels. Digoxin and phenytoin are examples of drugs that are significantly protein bound[91]—geriatricians will typically aim for the low end of the therapeutic range because of this issue.[92]

Metabolism

The liver is responsible for the majority of drug metabolism, and both hepatic blood flow and hepatic mass decrease with age. Phase I pathways of drug metabolism (hydroxylation, oxidation, dealkylation, and reduction) result in metabolites that may be of lesser, equal, or greater pharmacologic effect than the parent drug. In contrast, phase II pathways (glucuronidation, conjugation, or acetylation) result in inactive metabolites. Therefore, drugs metabolized by phase II pathways are generally preferred for the elderly because of decreased incidence of toxicity—for example, lorazepam is preferred over diazepam when benzodiazepine therapy is required in the elderly. The half-life of diazepam is extremely long, and as a result of this prolonged half-life, its metabolites accumulate to unexpectedly high levels in the elderly with repeated dosing. Because of this, lorazepam is preferred in this patient population.[93]

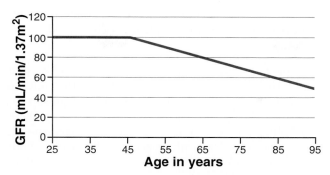

FIGURE 34-4 Rate of GFR decline in normal individuals with age. The course of GFR decline with normal aging was based on a cross-sectional study of iothalamate clearance in patients aged 17 to 70 years.[94] (Modified from Hebert L, Cody R, Slivka A, Sedmak D. Hypertension-induced kidney, heart, and central nervous system disease, diagnosis and management of renal disease and hypertension. 1994.)

Elimination

Kidney mass and blood flow decrease with age which results in gradual decline in GFR. Figure 34-4 graphically represents this gradual, age-related decline over time. Further, the current estimates of the prevalence of chronic kidney disease in individuals over age 60 years are nearly 40%.[94,95] This decrease in GFR impairs elimination of therapeutic drugs and increases toxicity and adverse outcomes.[96,97] Therapeutic drug monitoring is an important consideration to ensure that compounds ingested are being metabolized and excreted appropriately. The gold standard for determining GFR is a measurement of creatinine in a 24-hour urine sample, though measurement of creatinine in a random serum sample is more commonly tested due to ease of collection. A number of formulas exist to calculate GFR, and no formula is ideal for all patient populations. The three equations used to estimate renal function are the Modification of Diet in Renal Disease (MDRD) equation, the Cockcroft-Gault equation (CG), and the Chronic Kidney Disease Epidemiology Collaboration equation (CKD EPI).[98-100] All three formulas use serum creatinine levels in combination with other factors to estimate GFR. The Food and Drug Administration traditionally uses the CG equation in its recommendations on appropriate dosing of therapies.[101] Most clinical laboratories estimate renal function using the MDRD equation because this equation requires serum creatinine, age, race, and gender, but not weight. There have been studies to assess the best equation for different demographics and patient populations. The findings of these studies have been contradictory and based on the mixed results there is no consensus equation used in the elderly patient population.[102,103] Different GFR results can change the dose of drug administered, thus there has been effort to find alternate methods to achieve the best estimation of GFR. There have been various methods proposed and tested, but none has been widely incorporated into clinical laboratory testing, and creatinine measurement remains as the most frequently used method.

Example 1: Diazepam

Diazepam is highly lipophilic—it is quickly and efficiently absorbed and accumulates with multiple doses. It is metabolized by phase I mechanisms to N-desmethyldiazepam and temazepam. Both of these metabolites are further metabolized to oxazepam—all three metabolites are pharmacologically active. Both temazepam and oxazepam are inactivated by glucuronidation (a phase II process) and eliminated via the kidney. Elimination half-life increases by approximately 1 hour for each year of age beginning with a half-life of 20 hours at 20 years of age.[104] This appears to be due to an increase in volume of distribution with age and a decrease in clearance. Consequently, the elderly may have lower peak concentrations, and on multiple dosing higher trough concentrations. It will also take longer to reach steady state.[13]

Example 2: Morphine Sulfate

Parenteral morphine has a smaller volume of distribution, higher plasma concentration, and slower clearance in elders compared with young adults. Older adults experience at least equivalent levels of pain relief with half the dose of intramuscular morphine sulfate as younger adults and the relief lasts longer. It is not clear if this is entirely due to age-related changes in pharmacokinetics, or if there are age-related changes in pharmacodynamics at work here, as well. In any event, morphine should be administered at lower doses and longer intervals in the elderly, at least initially, to avoid toxicity.[88]

ATYPICAL PRESENTATIONS OF COMMON DISEASES

There are a number of medical problems that can occur in any age, but these conditions may present differently in the elderly. Differences in presentation or biological responsiveness to common conditions will typically be most evident to physicians or nursing staff who interact one-on-one with patients[6]; however, there are some unusual presentations that can be represented by the laboratory values. These are outlined below:

- Apathetic hyperthyroidism—hyperthyroidism with a paradoxical symptom of fatigue/apathy, instead of typical anxiety and hyperactivity. Thyroid disease in the elderly appears traditionally in the typical manner. Apathetic hyperthyroidism, a rare form of Graves' disease, presents in an unusual way in elderly patients. Unlike younger patients with Graves', older patients generally present with low to normal TSH. Before the advent of ultrasensitive TSH testing, the moderate variation in TSH made diagnosis difficult, but today

laboratories routinely use ultrasensitive TSH tests, which make diagnosis of these patients more straightforward.[105,106]

- Acute myocardial infarction (AMI) is the leading cause of morbidity in the United States.[107] The incidence of myocardial infarction (MI) increases with age, and manifestations of MI can be unique. While the majority of younger patients (less than age 65) present with chest pain, the most common alternate AMI symptom in the elderly patient is shortness of breath.[108] The age-related respiratory changes, including shallow breathing and decreased respiratory rate, can complicate the diagnosis in some cases.

Geriatric Syndromes

There are a number of common constellations of symptoms in the elderly that are considered "geriatric syndromes." This concept emphasizes that certain issues commonly observed in the elderly population typically result from multiple coexisting and interacting problems. Since clinical training outside geriatrics tends to emphasize "Occam's razor"—looking for the simplest explanation for a patient's problems—the approach to geriatric syndromes requires a change in the diagnostic logical process.[109] Multiple parallel lines of investigation, rather than a single linear approach, are often required for adequate evaluation of these syndromes. The American Geriatric Society considers the conditions in Table 34-6 to be geriatric syndromes. The identification of a geriatric syndrome cannot be made with a specific laboratory test, but some tests can help explore the underlying cause of the symptoms that lead to patient presentation.

TABLE 34-6   GERIATRIC SYNDROMES[110]

- Difficulty swallowing
- Malnutrition
- Sleep problems
- Bladder control problems
- Delirium
- Dementia
- Vision problems
- Hearing problems
- Dizziness
- Fainting
- Difficulty walking
- Falls
- Osteoporosis
- Pressure ulcers

THE IMPACT OF EXERCISE AND NUTRITION ON CHEMISTRY RESULTS IN THE ELDERLY

Research indicates that regular exercise can increase the lifespan and improve the quality of life among geriatric patients. Maintaining physical activity improves physical strength and fitness, as well as balance. Exercise helps prevent depression, and manage and defend against diseases such as diabetes, heart disease, breast and colon cancer, and osteoporosis.[34,111,112] Physical activity also improves endurance, flexibility sleep, mood, and self-esteem.[113] Increased physical activity may prevent more rapid deterioration. Fitness-related activities can reduce the risk of falling, and incorporation of exercise into lifestyle has been shown to be one of the best ways to improve bone mass throughout the life.[114] There have also been data linking the positive effects of exercise and long-term maintenance of cognitive function.[115] More importantly, lack of physical activity was shown to be a better predictor of all-cause mortality than being overweight or obese.[116]

The successful management of aging requires proper nutrition in addition to regular exercise. It is reported that 10% to 40% of hospitalized older adults suffer from malnutrition, which can be defined as any disorder of nutrition status resulting from a deficiency of nutrient intake, impaired metabolism, or overnutrition.[117] The difficulty recognizing the problem makes treatment a challenge.[36] Some of the laboratory values that can indicate undernutrition are low albumin and low pre-albumin. There are a number of issues with the identification of malnutrition in the elderly. Based on this, there is increasing interest in establishing nutritional assessment tools for identification of undernourished individuals.[118]

Clearly, geriatric dietary intake is a concern in the area of undernourishment, but excessive calorie intake, resulting in obesity and increased prevalence of type 2 diabetes, is also a worry.[47] Based on increasing incidence of diabetes with aging, and the previously discussed benefits of physical activity, increasing numbers of elderly people are being encouraged to become active. Clinicians and laboratorians will need a better understanding of how exercise is likely to impact test results of older individuals. This will require closer attention to baseline measurements and observations of changes over time.

For additional student resources please visit thePoint at **http://thepoint.lww.com.**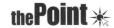

QUESTIONS

1. Which of the following occurs in an infant immediately after birth?
   a. Closure of the ductus arteriosus and adult respiration
   b. Normal hepatic function and bilirubin metabolism
   c. Adult rates of glomerular filtration by the kidneys
   d. Normal water homeostasis

2. How much blood should be drawn at any one time from a 7-lb baby?
   a. No more than 2.5 mL
   b. No more than 10 mL
   c. No more than 20 mL
   d. No more than 1.0 mL

3. When choosing a chemistry analyzer for a pediatric laboratory, it is necessary to
   a. Be able to analyze from small volumes
   b. Have rapid turnaround
   c. Have an extensive menu
   d. Have front-end automation

4. High blood ammonia levels result in
   a. Respiratory acidosis
   b. Metabolic acidosis
   c. Metabolic alkalosis
   d. Respiratory alkalosis

5. Point-of-care testing is helpful when
   a. Results are needed quickly
   b. Only small sample sizes are available
   c. The device can be linked to the hospital LIS
   d. Quality control samples are not needed

6. Which of the following immunoglobulins is provided to a new baby by the mother?
   a. IgG
   b. IgD
   c. IgM
   d. IgA

7. The pituitary secretes which of the following hormones (more than one answer is possible)?
   a. Growth hormone
   b. Testosterone

   c. Insulin-like growth factor
   d. Thyroid-stimulating hormone

8. Tandem mass spectrometry can be used to detect
   a. 25 to 30 metabolic diseases
   b. Cystic fibrosis
   c. Combined immune deficiency
   d. Panhypopituitarism

9. Aminoglycoside drug levels, such as gentamicin, should be measured
   a. 30 minutes after a dose
   b. 3 hours after a dose
   c. At steady state
   d. At any time

10. Which condition is least likely to be associated with increased alkaline phosphatase levels?
   a. Osteoporosis
   b. Paget's disease
   c. Hyperparathyroidism
   d. Osteomalacia

11. Which could account for drug toxicity following a normally prescribed dose?
   a. All of these
   b. Decreased renal clearance by the kidney
   c. Altered serum protein binding
   d. Liver impairment

12. Hearing loss is common among the elderly and may cause embarrassment. What should be done to facilitate the specimen collection process?
   a. Adjust your position to speak into the ear with the best hearing.
   b. Speak very loud and forcefully.
   c. Don't speak at all. Just give the patient printed instructions.
   d. Use a microphone.

13. Given the following information, calculate the creatinine clearance using the Cockcroft-Gault formula:
   Age = 85; weight = 70 kg; sex = male
   Serum creatinine = 1.0 mg/dL
   a. 53
   b. 72
   c. 47
   d. 35

14. Glucose intolerance, abnormal cholesterol level, high blood pressure, and upper body obesity are characteristics of
   a. Insulin resistance
   b. Chronic inflammatory disease
   c. Coronary heart disease
   d. Cerebrovascular disease

REFERENCES

1. Werner CA. The Older Population: 2010. http://www.census.gov/prod/cen2010/briefs/c2010br-09.pdf. Accessed August 26, 2012.
2. 2010 Average Life Expectancyby Gender, Race and Country. suite101.com. http://suite101.com/article/2010-life-expectancy-longevity-factors-and-the-latest-news-a284558. Accessed August 26, 2012.
3. Passell JA, Cohn D. *U.S. Population Projections: 2005-2050.* Washington, DC: Pew Research Center; 2008. http://pewhispanic.org/files/reports/85.pdf. Accessed August 26, 2012.
4. Vincent GK, Velkoff VA. *The Next Four Decades: The Older Population in the United States: 2010 to 2050.* Washington, DC: US Census Bureau; 2008. http://www.census.gov/prod/2010pubs/p25-1138.pdf. Accessed August 26, 2012.
5. Martin P, Midgley E. Immigration: shaping and reshaping America. *Popul Bull.* 2006;61:3-27.
6. Gray-Vickrey P. Gathering "pearls" of knowledge for assessing older adults. *Nursing.* 2010;40:34-42.
7. Gerber A. Navigating in evidence-poor waters—how much hydration is needed at the end of life? The recommendations of a Swiss expert group (Bigorio Group). *Ther Umsch.* 2012;69:91-92.
8. Faulkner WR. *Geriatric Clinical Chemistry Reference Values.* Washington, DC: American Association for Clinical Chemistry; 1993.
9. Burks TN, Cohn RD. One size may not fit all: anti-aging therapies and sarcopenia. *Aging (Albany, NY).* 2011;3:1142-1153.
10. Uusi-Rasi K, Sievänen H, Pasanen M, Kannus P. Age-related decline in trabecular and cortical density: a 5-year peripheral quantitative computed tomography follow-up study of pre- and postmenopausal women. *Calcif Tissue Int.* 2007;81: 249-253.
11. Phillips K, Aliprantis A, Coblyn J. Strategies for the prevention and treatment of osteoporosis in patients with rheumatoid arthritis. *Drugs Aging.* 2006;23:773-779.
12. Lombardi G, Di Somma C, Vuolo L, et al. Role of IGF-I on PTH effects on bone. *J Endocrinol Invest.* 2010;33:22-26.
13. Hausman DB, Johnson MA, Davey A, et al. The oldest old: red blood cell and plasma folate in African American and white octogenarians and centenarians in Georgia. *J Nutr Health Aging.* 2011;15:744-750.
14. Bhutto A, Morley JE. The clinical significance of gastrointestinal changes with aging. *Curr Opin Clin Nutr Metab Care.* 2008;11: 651-660.
15. Tan JC, Workeneh B, Busque S, et al. Glomerular function, structure, and number in renal allografts from older deceased donors. *J Am Soc Nephrol.* 2009;20:181-188.
16. Tanner GA. Kidney function. In: Rhoades RA, Bell DR, eds. *Medical Physiology: Principles for Clinical Medicine.* 4th ed. Philadelphia, PA: Lippincott Williams and Wilkins; 2012:399-426. http://www.lww.com/webapp/wcs/stores/servlet/product_Medical-Physiology_11851_-1_12551_Prod-9781451110395
17. Baylis C, Schmidt R. The aging glomerulus. *Semin Nephrol.* 1996;16:265-276.
18. Matthews SJ, Lancaster JW. Urinary tract infections in the elderly population. *Am J Geriatr Pharmacother.* 2011;9:286-309.
19. Foster AD, Sivarapatna A, Gress RE. The aging immune system and its relationship with cancer. *Aging Health.* 2011;7:707-718.

20. Winzenberg T, van der Mei I, Mason RS, Nowson C, Jones G. Vitamin D and the musculoskeletal health of older adults. *Aust Fam Physician.* 2012;41:92-99.

21. Makarewicz-Wujec M, Kozlowska-Wojciechowska M. Nutrient intake and serum level of gamma-glutamyltransferase, MCP-1 and homocysteine in early stages of heart failure. *Clin Nutr.* 2011;30:73-78.

22. Llewellyn DJ, Langa KM, Friedland RP, Lang IA. Serum albumin concentration and cognitive impairment. *Curr Alzheimer Res.* 2010;7:91-96.

23. del Val JH. Old-age inflammatory bowel disease onset: a different problem? *World J Gastroenterol.* 2011;17:2734-2739.

24. Vanasse GJ, Berliner N. Anemia in elderly patients: an emerging problem for the 21st century. *Hematology Am Soc Hematol Educ Program.* 2010;2010:271-275.

25. Laughlin GA, Barrett-Connor E. Sexual dimorphism in the influence of advanced aging on adrenal hormone levels: The Rancho Bernardo Study. *JCEM.* 2000;85:3561-3568.

26. Carlsson L, Lind L, Larsson A. Reference values for 27 clinical chemistry tests in 70-year-old males and females. *Gerontology.* 2010;56:259-265.

27. Lapin A, Böhmer F. Laboratory findings in elderly patients: a forgotten aspect of laboratory medicine? *Z Gerontol Geriatr.* 1999;32:41-46.

28. Millán-Calenti JC, Sánchez A, Lorenzo-López L, Maseda A. Laboratory values in a Spanish population of older adults: a comparison with reference values from younger adults. *Maturitas.* 2012. doi:10.1016/j.maturitas.2012.01.005.

29. Tietz NW, Shuey DF, Wekstein DR. Laboratory values in fit aging individuals—sexagenarians through centenarians. *Clin Chem.* 1992;38:1167-1185.

30. Kushner I. C-reactive protein elevation can be caused by conditions other than inflammation and may reflect biologic aging. *Cleve Clin J Med.* 2001;68:535-537.

31. Breitling LP, Claessen H, Drath C, Arndt V, Brenner H. Gamma-glutamyltransferase, general and cause-specific mortality in 19,000 construction workers followed over 20 years. *J Hepatol.* 2011;55:594-601.

32. Rutger Persson G. Rheumatoid arthritis and periodontitis—inflammatory and infectious connections. Review of the literature. *J Oral Microbiol.* 2012;4:2066-2074.

33. Terrie YC. Understanding and managing polypharmacy in the elderly. 2004 . http://www.pharmacytimes.com/publications/issue/2004/2004-12/2004-12-9094. Accessed August 26, 2012.

34. Marks BL, Katz LM, Smith JK. Exercise and the aging mind: buffing the baby boomer's body and brain. *Phys Sportsmed.* 2009;37:119-125.

35. High-Normal Uric Acid Linked with Mild Cognitive Impairment in the Elderly. 2077. http://www.apa.org/news/press/releases/2007/01/uric-cognition.aspx. Accessed August 26, 2012.

36. Tsutsumi R, Tsutsumi YM, Horikawa YT, et al. Decline in anthropometric evaluation predicts a poor prognosis in geriatric patients. *Asia Pac J Clin Nutr.* 2012;21:44-51.

37. Sim V, Hampton D, Phillips C, et al. The use of brain natriuretic peptide as a screening test for left ventricular systolic dysfunction— cost-effectiveness in relation to open access echocardiography. *Fam Pract.* 2003;20:570-574.

38. Weksler ME, Goodhardt M. Do age-associated changes in "physiologic" autoantibodies contribute to infection, atherosclerosis, and Alzheimer's disease? *Exp Gerontol.* 2002;37:971-979.

39. Tuljapurkar SR, McGuire TR, Brusnahan SK, et al. Changes in human bone marrow fat content associated with changes in hematopoietic stem cell numbers and cytokine levels with aging. *J Anat.* 2011;219:574-581.

40. Zussman J, Young L. Zoster vaccine live for the prevention of shingles in the elderly patient. *Clin Interv Aging.* 2008;3:241-250.

41. Gooneratne NS, Edwards AY, Zhou C, et al. Melatonin pharmacokinetics following two different oral surge-sustained release doses in older adults. *J Pineal Res.* 2011. doi:10.1111/j.1600-079X.2011.00958.x.

42. Rockwood MRH, Howlett SE, Rockwood K. Orthostatic hypotension (OH) and mortality in relation to age, blood pressure and frailty. *Arch Gerontol Geriatr.* 2012. doi:10.1016/j.archger.2011.12.009.

43. Huber KR, Mostafaie N, Stangl G, et al. Clinical chemistry reference values for 75-year-old apparently healthy persons. *Clin Chem Lab Med.* 2006;44:1355-1360.

44. Bremner AP, Feddema P, Leedman PJ, et al. Age-related changes in thyroid function: a longitudinal study of a community-based cohort. *J Clin Endocrinol Metab.* 2012. doi:10.1210/jc.2011-3020.

45. Shaw ND, Srouji SS, Histed SN, Hall JE. Differential effects of aging on estrogen negative and positive feedback. *Am J Physiol Endocrinol Metab.* 2011;301:E351-355.

46. Barron AM, Pike CJ. Sex hormones, aging, and Alzheimer's disease. *Front Biosci (Elite Ed).* 2012;4:976-997.

47. Morley JE. Diabetes and aging: epidemiologic overview. *Clin Geriatr Med.* 2008;24:395-405.

48. Kokotas H, Grigoriadou M, Petersen MB. Age-related macular degeneration: genetic and clinical findings. *Clin Chem Lab Med.* 2011;49:601-616.

49. Lupien SJ, de Leon M, de Santi S, et al. Cortisol levels during human aging predict hippocampal atrophy and memory deficits. *Nat Neurosci.* 1998;1:69-73.

50. Davis KM, Fish LC, Minaker KL, Elahi D. Atrial natriuretic peptide levels in the elderly: differentiating normal aging changes from disease. *J Gerontol A Biol Sci Med Sci* 1996;51:M95-101.

51. Sherman SS, Hollis BW, Tobin JD. Vitamin D status and related parameters in a healthy population: the effects of age, sex, and season. *J Clin Endocrinol Metab.* 1990;71:405-413.

52. Bauer JH. Age-related changes in the renin-aldosterone system. Physiological effects and clinical implications. *Drugs Aging.* 1993;3:238-245.

53. Ueda M, Araki T, Shiota T, Taketa K. Age and sex-dependent alterations of serum amylase and isoamylase levels in normal human adults. *J Gastroenterol.* 1994;29:189-191.

54. Cole LA, Khanlian SA, Muller CY. Normal production of human chorionic gonadotropin in perimenopausal and menopausal women and after oophorectomy. *Int J Gynecol Cancer.* 2009;19:1556-1559.

55. Mulkerrin E, Epstein FH, Clark BA. Aldosterone responses to hyperkalemia in healthy elderly humans. *J Am Soc Nephrol.* 1995;6:1459-1462.

56. Glassock RJ, Winearls C. Ageing and the glomerular filtration rate: truths and consequences. *Trans Am Clin Climatol Assoc.* 2009;120:419-428.

57. Evrin PE, Nilsson SE, Oberg T, Malmberg B. Serum C-reactive protein in elderly men and women: association with mortality, morbidity and various biochemical values. *Scand J Clin Lab Invest.* 2005;65:23-31.

58. Castle SC. Clinical relevance of age-related immune dysfunction. *Clin Infect Dis.* 2000;31:578-585.

59. Flood C, Gherondache C, Pincus G, et al. The metabolism and secretion of aldosterone in elderly subjects. *J Clin Invest.* 1967;46:960-966.

60. Cowie CC, Rust KF, Ford ES, et al. Full accounting of diabetes and pre-diabetes in the U.S. population in 1988-1994 and 2005-2006. *Diabetes Care.* 2008;32:287-294.

61. Drion I, Joosten H, van Hateren KJ, et al. Employing age-related cut-off values results in fewer patients with renal impairment in secondary care. *Ned Tijdschr Geneeskd.* 2011;155:A3091.

62. Coin A, Giannini S, Minicuci N, et al. Limb fat-free mass and fat mass reference values by dual-energy X-ray absorptiometry

(DEXA) in a 20-80 year-old Italian population. *Clin Nutr. (Edinburgh, Scotland)*. 2012. doi:10.1016/j.clnu.2012.01.012.

63. Garry PJ. *Laboratory Medicine and the Aging Process. Joseph A. Knight*. Chicago, IL: ASCP Press; 1996:420 pp., $45.00, ISBN 0–89189-397–0. *Clin Chem*. 1997;43:2444-2444.

64. Clinical Trials Neglect the Elderly. The New Old Age Blog. 2011. http://newoldage.blogs.nytimes.com/2011/08/19/clinical-trials-neglect-the-elderly/. August 26, 2012.

65. Mayo Clinic Staff. Caring for the elderly: dealing with resistance. *Mayo Foundation for Medical Education and Research (MFMER)* MY01436. 2010.

66. Isaac RM. Nutrition support makes more than sense/cents. *J Can Diet Assoc*. 1988;49:89-91.

67. Vukmanovic-Stejic M, Rustin MHA, Nikolich-Zugich J, Akbar AN. Immune responses in the skin in old age. *Curr Opin Immunol*. 2011;23:525-531.

68. Patricia M, Barnes MA, Barbara Bloom MPA, Nahin RL. National Health Statistics Reports. 2008.

69. Naughton C, Bennett K, Feely J. Prevalence of chronic disease in the elderly based on a national pharmacy claims database. *Age Ageing*. 2006;35:633-636.

70. Deteriorating Health Top Reason to Leave Home, Seniors Say. McKnight's. 2008. http://www.mcknights.com/deteriorating-health-top-reason-to-leave-home-seniors-say/article/110638/. Accessed August 26, 2012.

71. Pamuk ON, Dönmez S, Cakir N. Increased frequencies of hysterectomy and early menopause in fibromyalgia patients: a comparative study. *Clin Rheumatol*. 2009;28:561-564.

72. Hermes GL, McClintock MK. Isolation and the timing of mammary gland development, gonadarche, and ovarian senescence: implications for mammary tumor burden. *Dev Psychobiol*. 2008;50:353-360.

73. Racho D, Teede H. Ovarian function and obesity—interrelationship, impact on women's reproductive lifespan and treatment options. *Mol Cell Endocrinol*. 2010;316:172-179.

74. McConnell DS, Stanczyk FZ, Sowers MR, Randolph JF, Jr, Lasley BL. Menopausal transition stage-specific changes in circulating adrenal androgens. *Menopause (New York, NY)*. 2012. doi:10.1097/gme.0b013e31823fe274.

75. Cole LA. HCG variants, the growth factors which drive human malignancies. *Am J Cancer Res*. 2012;2:22-35.

76. World Health Organization. Assessment of fracture risk and its application to screening for postmenopausal osteoporosis. Report of a WHO Study Group. *World Health Organ Tech Rep Ser*. 1994;843:1-129.

77. Koda-Kimble MA, Young LY, Alldredge BK. *Applied Therapeutics: The Clinical Use of Drugs*. Philadelphia, PA: Lippincott Williams & Wilkins; 2004.

78. Gourlay M, Franceschini N, Sheyn Y. Prevention and treatment strategies for glucocorticoid-induced osteoporotic fractures. *Clin Rheumatol*. 2007;26:144-153.

79. Lee J, Vasikaran S. Current recommendations for laboratory testing and use of bone turnover markers in management of osteoporosis. *Ann Lab Med*. 2012;32:105-112.

80. Buell JS, Dawson-Hughes B, Scott TM, et al. 25-Hydroxyvitamin D, dementia, and cerebrovascular pathology in elders receiving home services. *Neurology*. 2010;74:18-26.

81. Alzheimer's Association—Latest Facts & Figures Report. 2012. http://www.alz.org/alzheimers_disease_facts_and_figures.asp. Accessed August 26, 2012.

82. de la Torre JC. A turning point for Alzheimer's disease? *BioFactors (Oxford, England)*. 2012. doi:10.1002/biof.200.

83. Engelborghs S, De Vreese K, Van de Casteele T, et al. Diagnostic performance of a CSF-biomarker panel in autopsy-confirmed dementia. *Neurobiol Aging*. 2008;29:1143-1159.

84. Garcia A, Zanibbi K. Homocysteine and cognitive function in elderly people. *CMAJ*. 2004;171:897-904.

85. Homocysteine: One of the Best Objective Markers of Your Health Status. 2012. http://www.drbenkim.com/articles-homocysteine.html. Accessed August 26, 2012.

86. Top 10 Causes of Death Among Adults Over Age 65. About.com Senior Health. 2010. http://seniorhealth.about.com/od/deathand-dying/tp/cause_death.htm. Accessed August 26, 2012.

87. Ruiz JG, Array S, Lowenthal DT. Therapeutic drug monitoring in the elderly. *Am J Ther*. 1996;3:839-860.

88. Villesen HH, Banning AM, Petersen RH, et al. Pharmacokinetics of morphine and oxycodone following intravenous administration in elderly patients. *Ther Clin Risk Manage*. 2007;3:961-967.

89. Bo-Linn GW, Davis GR, Buddrus DJ, et al. An evaluation of the importance of gastric acid secretion in the absorption of dietary calcium. *J Clin Invest*. 1984;73:640-647.

90. Hughes SG. Prescribing for the elderly patient: why do we need to exercise caution? *Br J Clin Pharmacol*. 1998;46:531-533.

91. Dasgupta A. Clinical utility of free drug monitoring. *Clin Chem Lab Med*. 2002;40:986-993.

92. Tjia J, Field TS, Fischer SH, et al. Quality measurement of medication monitoring in the "meaningful use" era. *Am J Manage Care*. 2011;17:633-637.

93. Kraemer G. *Epilepsy in the Elderly: Clinical Aspects and Pharmacotherapy*. Stuttgart, Germany: Thieme; 1999.

94. Hebert L, Cody R, Slivka A, Sedmak D. Hypertension-induced kidney, heart, and central nervous system disease, diagnosis and management of renal disease and hypertension. 1994.

95. Busko M. Prevalence of CKD in the US Continues to Rise. Medscape.com. 2007. http://www.medscape.com/viewarticle/553492. Accessed August 26, 2012.

96. Glassock RJ. The GFR decline with aging: a sign of normal senescence, not disease. *Nephrol Times*. 2009;2:6-8.

97. Euans DW. Renal function in the elderly. *Am Fam Physician*. 1988;38:147-150.

98. Levey AS, Bosch JP, Lewis JB, et al. A more accurate method to estimate glomerular filtration rate from serum creatinine: a new prediction equation. Modification of Diet in Renal Disease Study Group. *Ann Intern Med*. 1999;130:461-470.

99. Cockcroft DW, Gault MH. Prediction of creatinine clearance from serum creatinine. *Nephron*. 1976;16:31-41.

100. Levey AS, Stevens LA, Schmid CH, et al. A new equation to estimate glomerular filtration rate. *Ann Intern Med*. 2009;150:604-612.

101. Nacif MS, Arai AA, Lima JA, Bluemke DA. Gadolinium-enhanced cardiovascular magnetic resonance: administered dose in relationship to United States Food and Drug Administration (FDA) guidelines. *J Cardiovasc Magn Reson*. 2012;14:18.

102. Carter JL, Stevens PE, Irving JE, Lamb EJ. Estimating glomerular filtration rate: comparison of the CKD-EPI and MDRD equations in a large UK cohort with particular emphasis on the effect of age. *QJM*. 2011. doi:10.1093/qjmed/hcr077.

103. Gill J, Malyuk R, Djurdjev O, Levin A. Use of GFR equations to adjust drug doses in an elderly multi-ethnic group—a cautionary tale. *Nephrol Dial Transplant*. 2007;22:2894-2899.

104. Drug Safety Labeling Changes—Valium (diazepam) Tablets 2009. http://www.fda.gov/Safety/MedWatch/SafetyInformation/Safety-RelatedDrugLabelingChanges/ucm119276.htm. Accessed August 26, 2012.

105. Hyperthyroidism: Thyroid Disorders: Merck Manual Professional. 2012. http://www.merckmanuals.com/professional/endocrine_and_metabolic_disorders/thyroid_disorders/hyperthyroidism.html. Accessed August 26, 2012.

106. Reuben DB, Yoshikawa TT, Besdine RW, eds. *Geriatric Review Syllabus*. 3rd ed. Washington DC: American Geriatrics Society; 1996:296-297.

107. Smolina K, Wright FL, Rayner M, Goldacre MJ. Determinants of the decline in mortality from acute myocardial infarction in England between 2002 and 2010: linked national database study. *BMJ*. 2012;344:d8059.

108. Woon VC, Lim KH. Acute myocardial infarction in the elderly—the differences compared with the young. *Singapore Med J*. 2003;44:414-418.

109. Drachman DA. Occam's razor, geriatric syndromes, and the dizzy patient. *Ann Intern Med*. 2000;132:403-404.

110. Inouye SK, Studenski S, Tinetti ME, Kuchel GA. Geriatric syndromes: clinical, research, and policy implications of a core geriatric concept. *J Am Geriatr Soc*. 2007;55:780-791.

111. American College of Sports Medicine Position Stand. Exercise and physical activity for older adults. *Med Sci Sports Exerc*. 1998;30:992-1008.

112. Rose DJ, Hernandez D. The role of exercise in fall prevention for older adults. *Clin Geriatr Med*. 2010;26:607-631.

113. Sarah Kovatch MFA, Melinda Smith MA, Segal J. Senior exercise and fitness tips. Helpguide.org, 2012.

114. Gómez-Cabello A, Ara I, González-Agüero A, Casajús JA, Vicente-Rodríguez G. Effects of training on bone mass in older adults: a systematic review. *Sports Med (Auckland, NZ)*. 2012. doi:10.2165/11597670-000000000-00000.

115. Kraft E. Cognitive function, physical activity, and aging: possible biological links and implications for multimodal interventions. *Neuropsychol Dev Cogn B Aging Neuropsychol Cogn*. 2012;19:248-263.

116. van Dam RM, Li T, Spiegelman D, Franco OH, Hu FB. Combined impact of lifestyle factors on mortality: prospective cohort study in US women. *BMJ*. 2008;337:a1440.

117. Milne AC, Potter J, Vivanti A, et al. Protein and energy supplementation in elderly people at risk from malnutrition. The Cochrane Library. 2009. http://onlinelibrary.wiley.com/doi/10.1002/14651858.CD003288.pub3/abstract. Accessed August 26, 2012.

118. López-Contreras M-J, Torralba C, Zamora S, Pérez-Llamas F. Nutrition and prevalence of undernutrition assessed by different diagnostic criteria in nursing homes for elderly people. *J Hum Nutr Diet*. 2012. doi:10.1111/j.1365-277X.2012.01237.x.

Clinical Chemistry and the Pediatric Patient

DEAN C. CARLOW, MICHAEL J. BENNETT

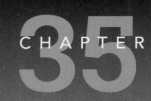

CHAPTER 35

CHAPTER OUTLINE

Chapter Objectives

Upon completion of this chapter, the clinical laboratorian should be able to do the following:

• Define the adaptive changes that occur in the newborn.
• Describe the developmental changes that occur throughout childhood.
• Discuss the problems associated with collecting blood from small children.
• Understand the role of point-of-care testing in pediatric settings.

• Summarize the changes that occur in children with regard to electrolyte and water balance, endocrine function, liver function, and bone metabolism.
• Explain how drug treatment and pharmacokinetics differ between children and adults.
• Discuss the procedures used to diagnose inherited metabolic diseases.
• Describe the development and disorders of the immune system.

KEY TERMS

Drug metabolism
Endocrine system
Genetic disease

Growth
Immunity
Physiologic development

Point-of-care testing
Sexual maturation
Tandem mass spectrometry

720

DEVELOPMENTAL CHANGES FROM NEONATE TO ADULT

Pediatric laboratory medicine provides many unique opportunities to study how the homeostatic and physiologic mechanisms that control normal human development evolve. With these opportunities to study development comes a completely new set of challenges, many based on failure of some component of the normal development process and resulting disease. With this scenario in mind, it becomes clear that the environment for the specialist pediatric laboratorian is different from the environment encountered in adult practice, in which physiologic development is not a major issue. The diseases encountered in pediatric practice, therefore, differ considerably from those in adult situations. Moreover, the nature of body size and, hence, available blood volume create additional problems for the analyst with regard to choice of instrumentation and testing menu.

The greatest pediatric challenge relates to the birth of an infant. There is a requirement at this time for rapid adaptation from intrauterine life, in which homeostasis is maintained by maternal and placental means, to the self-maintenance needed to adapt to extrauterine life. Issues related to this adaptation are further complicated by prematurity or intrauterine growth retardation (IGR), when many organ systems have not reached sufficient maturity to enable the newborn to adapt to the necessary changes at the time of delivery.[1]

Respiration and Circulation

At birth, the normal infant rapidly adapts by initiating active respiration. The stimuli for this process include clamping of the umbilicus, cutting off maternal delivery of oxygen, and the baby's first breath. Initiation of breathing requires the normal expression of surfactant in the lungs. Surfactant is necessary for the normal expansion and contraction of alveoli and allows gaseous exchange to take place.

Initiation of respiration and expansion of lung volume cause increased pulmonary blood flow and reduced blood pressure. This, in turn, results in closure of the ductus arteriosus and a shift in blood flow through the heart that allows newly oxygenated blood from the lungs to be directed through the left side of the heart to the body. Blood flow now goes from the right side of the heart to the lungs for oxygenation. Closure of the ductus arteriosus is essential for this process to take place.

Growth

A normal baby delivered at term weighs about 3.2 kg. A baby weighing less than 2.5 kg at term is regarded as small for gestational age, which is usually a result of IGR. Babies of low birth weight born before term are regarded as premature. In the first days of life, weight loss is a result of insensible water loss through the skin. This is generally offset by weight gain of 6 g/kg/d as feeding is initiated. An infant's body weight will double in 4 to 6 months. Premature babies tend to grow at a slower rate and often still weigh less than a term baby at the equivalent of term.

Organ Development

Most organs are not fully developed at birth. Glomerular filtration rate (GFR) of the kidney and renal tubular function mature during the first year of life at which point laboratory markers of renal function approximate adult values. Liver function can take 2 to 3 months to fully mature. Motor function and visual acuity develop during the first year of life. This development is accompanied by changes in the electroencephalogram until the normal "adult" picture is seen. There are dramatic changes in hematopoiesis as the switch from fetal hemoglobin to adult hemoglobin takes place. This coincides with significant hyperbilirubinemia as fetal hemoglobin is broken down, coincident with immature hepatic pathways of bilirubin metabolism. Bone growth in the rapid growth phases in the first few years of life and at puberty results in cyclical changes in bone growth markers. Sexual maturation results in significant endocrine changes, particularly of the hypothalamic–pituitary–gonadal hormone pathway, which eventually lead to the constitutive development of adult secondary sexual characteristics and eventually to the adult.

Problems of Prematurity and Immaturity

Intrauterine development is programmed for a normal 38- to 40-week gestation.[1] Many organs are not fully ready to deal with extrauterine life before this time. This organ immaturity results in many of the clinical problems that we see associated with prematurity, which include respiratory distress (lung immaturity), electrolyte and water imbalance (kidney immaturity), and excessive jaundice (liver immaturity). Infants born before their due date constitute a major burden on the laboratory. They not only have abnormal biochemical parameters that require frequent blood drawing but also have small blood volumes from which to draw on.

PHLEBOTOMY AND CHOICE OF INSTRUMENTATION FOR PEDIATRIC SAMPLES

Phlebotomy

Blood collection from infants and young children is complicated by the patient's size and frequently by the ability of the patient to communicate with the phlebotomist. The small blood volume of small patients dictates both the number of tests that can safely be performed on the

TABLE 35-1	IMPLICATIONS OF A 10 ML BLOOD DRAW IN AN INFANT POPULATION	
AGE	**WEIGHT (KG)**	**TOTAL BLOOD VOLUME (%)**
26 wk gestation	0.9	9.0
32 wk gestation	1.6	5.5
34 wk gestation	2.1	4.0
Term	3.4	2.5
3 mo	5.7	2.0
6 mo	7.6	1.6
12 mo	10.1	1.4
24 mo	12.6	1.0

TABLE 35-2	RECOMMENDED BLOOD DRAW VOLUMES FOR PEDIATRIC PATIENTS		
WEIGHT (KG)	**MAXIMUM VOLUME FOR A SINGLE BLOOD DRAW (ML)**	**WEIGHT (KG)**	**MAXIMUM VOLUME FOR A SINGLE BLOOD DRAW (ML)**
2	4	30	60
4	8	32.5	65
6	12	35	70
8	16	37.5	75
10	20	40	80
12.5	25	42.5	85
15	30	45	90
17.5	35	47.5	95
20	40	50	100
22.5	45	52.5	105
25	50	55	110
27.5	55		

Courtesy of Dr. David Friedman, Children's Hospital of Philadelphia, Philadelphia, Pennsylvania.

patient and the number of times that blood can safely be drawn for repeat analysis.[2] Table 35-1 shows the percentage of total body blood that is drawn from an individual with a 10 mL blood draw. This volume is standard in adult laboratory medicine but the table clearly shows that this amount of blood represents about 5% of total blood volume in a premature neonate. Clearly, frequent blood draws of this nature will quickly lead to anemia and the need for blood transfusion. Table 35-2 shows the guidelines for blood volume collection developed at the Children's Hospital of Philadelphia. It is necessary on occasion to advise the physician that a particular set of orders may result in excessive blood depletion and transfusion requirement.

Infants and children have smaller veins than adults; to ensure that small veins do not collapse, narrow-gauge needles are generally used for venipuncture. Smaller needles increase the risk of hemolysis and hyperkalemia.

Frequently, good access to veins is impossible in a pediatric patient with intravenous and central lines in place. Capillary samples are often collected when suitable veins are not available. However, capillary blood obtained by skin puncture is usually contaminated, at least to some extent, by interstitial fluid and tissue

debris. The concentration of protein (and protein-bound constituents) is approximately three times lower in interstitial fluid than in plasma. Table 35-3 highlights the major differences in analyte composition between venous serum and capillary serum. The lower concentrations of protein, bilirubin, and calcium in capillary specimens likely reflect mixing (and dilution) with interstitial fluid. Capillary samples, by either heel or thumb stick, should be collected by phlebotomists with pediatric expertise. The heel should be warmed and well perfused to "arterialize" the capillaries. This can be achieved by gently rubbing the area or by immersion in warm water. The lancet puncture should be in an area of the heel away from bone. Stabbing into bone may result in osteomyelitis, which is a very difficult to treat infection of the

TABLE 35-3	DIFFERENCES IN COMPOSITION OF CAPILLARY AND VENOUS SERUM			
CAPILLARY VALUE GREATER THAN VENOUS VALUE (%)		**NO DIFFERENCE BETWEEN CAPILLARY AND VENOUS VALUES**	**CAPILLARY VALUE LESS THAN VENOUS VALUE (%)**	
Glucose	1.4	Phosphorous	Bilirubin	5.0
Potassium	0.9	Urea	Calcium	4.6
			Chloride	1.8
			Sodium	2.3
			Total protein	3.3

Source: Burtis CA, Ashwood ER, eds. *Tietz Fundamentals of Clinical Chemistry.* 5th ed. Philadelphia, PA: WB Saunders; 2001.

bone. Excessive squeezing or milking of the lancet site can result in both hemolysis and factitious hyperkalemia from tissue fluid leakage.

Preanalytic Concerns

There is a growing trend toward complete front-end automation in clinical chemistry laboratories. The clear advantage with automation of sample handling is that traditional bottlenecks at sites of data entry and centrifugation are removed and turnaround times are reduced. Several issues have retarded the introduction of full-scale automation in pediatrics. A typical pediatric chemistry laboratory receives samples in tubes of many different sizes, varying from standard adult tubes to small "peditubes." While several of the large chemistry analyzers can directly sample from small pediatric tubes, as of this time, no manufacturer of laboratory equipment has developed a fully automated system that can handle this range of tubes.

However, there have been reports in the literature from individual laboratories that have modified existing robotic instrumentation to allow complete automation of the testing process using pediatric tubes.[3,4]

A second important issue relates to evaporation of sample from open tubes. Most automated sample handling systems require open-topped tubes for processing. With large sample volumes, the effect of evaporation is minimal. With small volumes that have relatively large surface areas to total volume, evaporation can be significant and may effect results by as much as 10%.

Choice of Analyzer

Careful inspection and choice of analytic systems remain crucial for handling pediatric samples. Until recently, only a few analyzers were capable of performing multiple analytic procedures on small sample volumes (5 to 50 µL). Today, most analyzers can perform this function. Choice of analyzer becomes dependent on issues such as the following:

1. How much dead volume is there in the system? The smaller the dead volume, the greater is the number of tests that can be run.
2. Does clot or bubble detection allow for salvage of sample? All analyzers can detect a clot, but not all will allow retrieval of sample.
3. Is the system truly random access? This allows selectivity of menu for a given sample.

Typically, sample throughput time is less of an issue, as pediatric facilities tend to run fewer samples than busy adult services.

POINT-OF-CARE ANALYSIS IN PEDIATRICS[5]

Point-of-care testing (POCT), or near-patient testing, plays an important and expanding role in pediatric practice.[5] Testing devices that are portable and easy to use,

require small specimen volume, do not require sample preparation, and provide rapid results at the bedside are providing the momentum for increased POCT. To provide cost-effective and appropriate quality assurance for POCT, several factors need to be addressed.

1. Does the analyte really require immediate turnaround for optimal patient management? Analyzers are becoming available that measure increasing numbers of different analytes at the patient's bedside. Typically, the cost of POCT measurement is higher than the traditional laboratory measurement. The idea of instant results is so seductive that nonlaboratorian users often discount economic factors. In the author's institution, the clinical laboratory has played a leading role in determining which POCT assays will be available and in which clinical settings they have real value (Table 35-4).
2. Who chooses the POCT device? As the field of POCT expands, the number of devices on the market is also increasing. The clinical laboratory should be the setting in which POCT devices for institutional use should be first evaluated. The laboratory should make choices for instrumentation. Important features of a good POCT device should include the following:

- The ability to lock out untrained users. Only individuals accredited to use the device should be allowed access via a personal code.

TABLE 35-4	IMPORTANT PEDIATRIC POINT-OF-CARE TESTS AND TESTING SITES
TEST	
Blood gas	
Electrolyte	
Glucose	
Activated clotting time	
Hemoglobin	
Glycated hemoglobin	
Pregnancy	
Urinalysis	
Prothrombin time	
Rapid *Streptococcus*	
TESTING SITES	
Coronary care unit/intensive care unit	
Trauma unit/emergency department	
Diabetes clinic	
Transport	
Surgery	
Extracorporeal membrane oxygenation sites	

- The device should not be allowed to proceed to patient sample analysis without running and validating appropriate quality assurance procedures.
- The data should be downloadable to the hospital laboratory information system (LIS) for evaluation by the hospital quality assurance officer. Downloading the data also allows for billing and data entry into patient charts, features readily lost when analyzers are used that cannot be linked to the LIS.

The data generated by POCT devices have limitations. Typical analytic performance is not as good as that with the main laboratory analyzer. POCT data are less precise and not suited to monitoring therapy in instances where small changes are important. The linear range for most POCT devices is not as broad as that of the main chemistry analyzer, and users need to be aware of these limitations. A prime example in the authors' institution is the use of POCT glucose analyzers. The instrument used for acute diabetic management loses linearity above 400 mg/dL, particularly in patients who are hemoconcentrated. We recommend that any POCT glucose level above 400 mg/dL be immediately checked in the main laboratory. Hypoglycemia is also particularly common in pediatrics and characteristically difficult to accurately quantitate using POCT devices. Low glucose levels should also be checked using a more sensitive main laboratory analyzer.

REGULATION OF BLOOD GASES AND pH IN NEONATES AND INFANTS

Primary maintenance of blood gas and pH homeostasis following birth requires that the lungs and kidneys are sufficiently mature to regulate acid and base metabolism. At about 24 weeks of gestation, the lung expresses two distinct types of cells: type 1 and type 2 pneumocytes. Type 2 pneumocytes are responsible for the secretion of surfactant, which contains the phospholipids lecithin and sphingomyelin. Surfactant is required for the lungs to expand and the transfer of blood gases following delivery. Oxygen crosses into the circulation, and carbon dioxide is removed and expired. Immaturity of the surfactant system as a result of prematurity or IGR results in respiratory distress syndrome (RDS). In RDS, there is failure to excrete carbon dioxide and, as a result, carbon dioxide levels rise, causing respiratory acidosis; oxygen levels are low and result in additional oxygen requirements for the baby.

The relative amounts of lecithin and sphingomyelin are critical for normal surfactant function. The measurement of amniotic fluid lecithin/sphingomyelin (L/S) ratio has been used for many years to predict fetal lung maturity. A ratio of less than 1.5 is considered indicative of surfactant deficiency.

TABLE 35-5	CAUSES OF ACIDOSIS AND ALKALOSIS IN NEONATES AND INFANTS
RESPIRATORY ACIDOSIS	**HYPOVENTILATION/CO$_2$ RETENTION**
Metabolic acidosis	Renal tubular bicarbonate wasting
	Anoxia
	Poor tissue perfusion
	Metabolic disease
Respiratory alkalosis	Hyperventilation
	High blood ammonia/ metabolic disease
Metabolic alkalosis	Pyloric stenosis/loss of gastric acid
	Excessive bicarbonate administration
	Low blood potassium

The fetal fibronectin (fFN) test is a promising new test designed to determine the likelihood of premature delivery and risk of fetal maturity.[6,7] fFN is a protein secreted uniquely by the fetus; toward term, it is found in maternal cervical fluid. A POCT device is available that has been designed for use in the obstetrician's office. It has a high predictive value for impending early delivery of the baby and can be used to alert the pediatrician to the potential for RDS.

The trauma and relative anoxia during delivery can also induce acidosis in the newborn. This is typically a metabolic acidosis associated with increased lactic acid production. Serum bicarbonate levels are reduced in this situation compared with the respiratory acidosis in RDS. Persistent metabolic acidosis in the newborn that is difficult to correct with bicarbonate replacement is an indication for further intensive evaluation for possible inborn error of metabolism or other etiologies that require differentiation (Table 35-5).

Alkalosis is an unusual finding in pediatric medicine. One important cause of alkalosis is hyperammonemia, which may be secondary to a number of etiologies, including liver disease and inborn errors of metabolism (Table 35-5).

Blood Gas and Acid–Base Measurement

Oxygen status can readily be measured using noninvasive transcutaneous monitoring. Good correlation has been demonstrated between the arterial pressure of oxygen and transcutaneous measurement. Transcutaneous carbon dioxide monitors are also in widespread use. The measurement of acid–base status requires blood sampling. Most blood gas/acid–base analyzers can be adapted to take the small capillary samples routinely collected in pediatric settings. It is important for the person drawing the capillary blood to do so anaerobically, which requires thorough warming of the capillary site and collection of a freely flowing blood sample from a lancet stick. The sample needs to be sealed to ensure minimal gas exchange. Analysis should be performed immediately to not compromise the sample integrity. The author's laboratory maintains a goal of a 10-minute turnaround time from the sample receipt.

Most blood gas analyzers measure pO_2, pCO_2, and pH by ion-specific electrodes and calculate bicarbonate concentration by the Henderson-Hasselbalch equation. The Henderson-Hasselbalch equation is less valid when pH is far outside the normal physiologic range (extreme acidosis or alkalosis). On these occasions, it may become important to measure the bicarbonate concentration using a direct measurement.

Many blood gas analyzers have been upgraded in recent years to measure additional analytes, including blood sodium, potassium, and chloride, using ion-specific electrodes and lactate and urea and several instruments measure bilirubin and creatinine. The major advantage of this type of analyzer in pediatrics is that whole blood can be used. The volumes are typically smaller than those required for the main chemistry analyzer, and the lack of need for centrifugation shortens the turnaround time. One disadvantage of using whole blood is that the analyst cannot detect whether a sample is hemolyzed.

REGULATION OF ELECTROLYTES AND WATER: RENAL FUNCTION

From the 35th week of gestation, the fetal kidneys develop rapidly in preparation for extrauterine life.[1] The kidneys, critical organs for the maintenance of electrolyte and water homeostasis, control the rate of salt and water loss and retention. At term, neither the glomeruli nor the renal tubules function at the normal rate. The GFR is about 25% of the rate seen in older children and does not reach full potential until age 2 years (Table 35-6).

TABLE 35-6	DEVELOPMENT OF GLOMERULAR FILTRATION IN THE NEWBORN	
GLOMERULAR FILTRATION RATE		
AGE	(mL/MIN PER 1.73 m² MEAN)	RANGE
1 d	24	3–38
2–8 d	38	17–60
10–22 d	50	32–68
37–95 d	58	30–86
1–2 y	115	95–135[a]

[a]Adult values.

Tubular function also develops at a similar rate. The maximal concentrating power of the kidney is only about 78% of that of the adult kidney at this time, although the tubular response to antidiuretic hormone appears to be normal. This gradual process of renal development in the newborn results in diminished filtration and impaired reabsorption of salt and water; therefore, in the newborn period and early infancy, large shifts in serum electrolyte levels can be observed. These problems are exacerbated in the preterm infant with renal function that is even less mature.

The kidneys also primarily maintain water loss and retention. However, in the newborn period, insensible water loss through the skin is also an important cause of water and electrolyte imbalance. Water loss and consequent hemoconcentration frequently result from the use of radiant heaters that are used to maintain body temperature. Increased water loss also occurs via respiration in children with RDS. Up to one-third of insensible water loss may occur through this route. The total body water content of a newborn is about 80%; 55% is intracellular fluid and 45% is extracellular fluid. The extracellular water is 20% plasma water and 80% interstitial. During the first month of extrauterine life, the total body water content decreases to about 60%, mostly a result of loss of the interstitial component.[1]

Disorders Affecting Electrolytes and Water Balance

The causes of hypernatremia (sodium, >145 mmol/L) and hyponatremia (sodium, <130 mmol/L) are listed in Table 35-7. Both disturbances can have dire outcomes,

TABLE 35-7	CAUSES OF HYPERNATREMIA AND HYPONATREMIA
HYPERNATREMIA	
Excessive loss of water through overhead heater	
Gastrointestinal fluid loss	
Fluid deprivation	
Renal loss of water/nephrogenic diabetes insipidus	
Administration of hypertonic fluids containing sodium	
HYPONATREMIA	
Inappropriate antidiuretic hormone secretion due to trauma or infection	
Administration of hypotonic fluids	
Renal tubular acidosis	
Salt-losing congenital adrenal hyperplasia (21-hydroxylase deficiency)	
Cystic fibrosis	
Diuretics	
Renal failure	

with a high risk of seizures. This is a result of the shift of water out of or into brain cells, with concurrent shrinkage or expansion of these cells. Hypernatremia results from hypotonic fluid loss, and hyponatremia results from hypertonic fluid loss. Hyponatremia may also be a result of excessive body water content and needs to be distinguished from hypertonic loss. Clinical evaluation and measurement of other components, including hematocrit, serum albumin, creatinine, and blood urea nitrogen, can be used to differentiate these etiologies. All of these compounds will be elevated with hemoconcentration. Clinically, it is usually possible to distinguish dehydration from excessive hydration.

Treatment of electrolyte and water loss is directed at replacing the loss to regain normal physiologic levels. Care must be taken to avoid too rapid a replacement, particularly with hypertonic dehydration. If water replacement is done too quickly, a rapid expansion of neuronal cell volume can occur, which results in seizures.

The causes of hyperkalemia and hypokalemia are listed in Table 35-8. The symptoms of hyperkalemia (serum potassium, >6.5 mmol/L) include muscle weakness and cardiac conduction defects that may lead to heart failure. In pediatrics, it is particularly important to recognize factitious hyperkalemia as a result of (a) hemolysis and bad capillary blood collection and (b) without hemolysis but with high potassium tissue leakage.

Because the situation regarding electrolyte and water homeostasis can change rapidly in small infants, it is important to monitor therapeutic intervention on a frequent basis.[1,2] The availability of POCT devices that use small volumes of whole blood helps with management of these imbalances, with the only caution being that it is impossible to detect hemolysis and factitious hyperkalemia on a whole blood sample.

TABLE 35-8	CAUSES OF HYPERKALEMIA AND HYPOKALEMIA
HYPERKALEMIA	
Fluid deprivation/dehydration causing tissue leakage	
Intravascular hemorrhage causing release from red cells	
Trauma/tissue damage	
Acute renal failure	
Salt-losing adrenal hyperplasia (see *hyponatremia*)	
Exchange transfusion using stored blood	
HYPOKALEMIA	
Inappropriate antidiuretic hormone secretion	
Diuretics, particularly furosemide	
Alkalosis	
Pyloric stenosis	
Renal tubular acidosis secondary to bicarbonate loss	

DEVELOPMENT OF LIVER FUNCTION

Physiologic Jaundice

The liver is an essential organ for many metabolic processes. The processing of many normal metabolic pathways and the metabolism of exogenous compounds, in particular, pharmacologic agents, proceed slower in neonates. The most striking effect of an immature liver, even in a normal-term baby, is the failure to adequately metabolize bilirubin. Bilirubin is an intermediate of the breakdown of the heme molecules, which accumulate as fetal hemoglobin is rapidly destroyed and replaced by adult hemoglobin. Normally, the liver conjugates bilirubin to glucuronic acid using the enzyme bilirubin UDP-glucuronoyltransferase. Conjugated bilirubin can be readily excreted in the bile or through the kidneys. At birth, this enzyme is too immature to complete the process and increased levels of unconjugated bilirubin and "physiologic" jaundice result. At this time, a normal baby may have a serum bilirubin level of up to 15 mg/dL, most of which is unconjugated. This level, which would be alarming in adult practice, should fall back to baseline by about 10 days of age. Because excessive jaundice can lead to kernicterus and result in severe brain damage, the measurement of blood conjugated and unconjugated bilirubin has an important role in pediatrics. An alternative means of reducing high unconjugated circulating bilirubin levels is phototherapy with ultraviolet light, which causes bilirubin to be converted to a potentially less toxic and more readily excreted metabolite. Severe cases may require an exchange transfusion. Complete absence of the bilirubin-conjugating enzyme results in severe persistent jaundice and Crigler-Najjar disease, a rare genetic disease. It is important to differentiate Crigler-Najjar from physiologic immaturity because treatment options vary considerably.

CASE STUDY 35-1

A newborn infant was born with a bilirubin level of 7 mg/dL (mostly unconjugated) that rose to 10 mg/dL by the third day of life. The infant was breastfed normally and the bilirubin levels returned to normal values within 2 weeks without treatment.

Questions

1. What is the most likely diagnosis? Are there likely to be any long-term adverse health effects?

2. What is the most likely biochemical cause of the elevated bilirubin level?

3. What other disorders can cause unconjugated hyperbilirubinemia in neonates?

Energy Metabolism

The liver plays an essential role in energy metabolism for the whole body (Table 35-9). Carbohydrates derived from the diet as disaccharides or polysaccharides form the bulk of our energy sources. They are broken down into simpler monosaccharides, which reach the liver via the portal blood system. The primary sugars in newborns and infants come from the breakdown of disaccharide lactose in milk. Lactose is broken down to glucose and galactose. When it reaches the hepatocytes, galactose is converted to glucose by a series of enzymic reactions that have unique pediatric significance. Genetic deficiency of any of the reactions results in failure to convert galactose to glucose and essentially reduce the energy content of milk by 50%. The most common cause of failure to convert galactose to glucose results in galactosemia or deficiency of galactose-1-phosphate uridyltransferase, a serious genetic disease of the newborn. In this disease, galactose-1-phosphate accumulates inside liver cells and causes hepatocellular damage and rapid liver failure. Other organs are also involved with this disease, including the renal tubules and the eyes. Galactose-1-phosphate accumulation causes acute renal tubular failure and tubular loss of glucose, phosphate, and amino acids. The loss of glucose in cooperation with the liver damage results in severe hypoglycemia. Accumulation of galactose in the eye results in cataract formation. A simple test that directs us to the diagnosis of galactosemia is the urine reducing substance test. This detects the presence of non–glucose-reducing sugars (galactose) in urine when a child is symptomatic. The clinical significance of establishing a diagnosis is clear; galactosemia is often fatal if undiscovered but completely treatable by dietary lactose restriction when diagnosis is made.

TABLE 35-9	IMPORTANT BIOCHEMICAL PATHWAYS IN THE LIVER
CATABOLIC	
Transamination	
Amino acid oxidation to make ketones and acetyl-CoA	
Fatty acid oxidation to make ketones	
Urea cycle to remove ammonia	
Bilirubin metabolism (hemoglobin breakdown)	
Drug and exogenous xenobiotic compounds metabolized	
ANABOLIC	
Albumin synthesis	
Clotting factor synthesis	
Lipoprotein synthesis, very-low-density lipoprotein	
Gluconeogenesis (synthesis of glucose)	
Bile acid synthesis	

Another critical pathway of carbohydrate energy metabolism in the newborn involves the pathway of gluconeogenesis. At birth, a term baby has sufficient liver glycogen stores to provide glucose as an energy source and maintain euglycemia. If the delivery is particularly stressful, these reserves of energy may become depleted prematurely. At this time, the normal physiologic role of gluconeogenesis, which essentially converts the amino acid alanine into glucose, becomes critical in maintaining glucose homeostasis. This pathway is not always mature at birth and suboptimal operation results in what is termed *physiologic hypoglycemia*. Newborns can survive blood glucose levels below 30 mg/dL, although adults would fall into rapid hypoglycemic coma and risk sudden death at these levels. Physiologic hypoglycemia usually corrects quickly as the enzyme systems mature or by simple intravenous glucose infusion. Persistent and severe hypoglycemia should alert the physician to a possible inborn error of metabolism, such as galactosemia, disorders of gluconeogenesis, or fatty acid oxidative metabolism.

Diabetes

Blood glucose homeostasis and hepatic metabolism of glucose are maintained by the concerted actions of several hormones.[8] Following a meal, the level of glucose in the circulation rises, which triggers increased synthesis and release of insulin by the pancreatic β-cells of the islets of Langerhans. Increased levels of insulin in the circulation cause glucose to be taken up by certain cells, such as hepatocytes and muscle cells, and to be converted into glycogen as a future source of energy. As a result of the insulin action, blood glucose levels begin to fall to the preprandial level. Glucagon, a hormone secreted by the α cells of the islets of Langerhans, has an opposing effect to that of insulin. It is generally believed that the insulin/glucagon ratio, rather than absolute amounts of either, is the primary endocrine modulator of circulating glucose levels. Other hormones, including cortisol, epinephrine, and insulin-like growth factor (IGF), can also affect glucose levels. These hormones are secreted in response to stress and can affect glucose measurement when samples are collected under stressful situations.

Diabetes mellitus, a condition in which the endocrine control of glucose metabolism is abnormal, is usually related to failure of the insulin regulatory pathway. Type 1 diabetes (insulin dependent) is the most common in pediatrics. This may be caused by failure of the pancreas to secrete insulin or by the presence of circulating insulin antibodies that reduce the ability for endocrine action. This type of diabetes can be further classified as immune mediated or idiopathic. In the immune-mediated form (the most common form), the insulin-secreting β-cells are destroyed by a T-cell–mediated autoimmune response. This form of diabetes was previously termed "juvenile diabetes" because it is the predominant form in children. A patient typically presents with diabetic keto-acidosis, with profound hyperglycemia and metabolic acidosis that result from the liver increasing fatty acid metabolism and producing excess ketone bodies.

The diagnostic criteria for diabetes mellitus have recently been updated and are currently diagnosed by demonstrating any of the following: fasting plasma glucose level ≥ 126 mg/dL (7.0 mmol/L), plasma glucose ≥ 200 mg/dL (11.1 mmol/L) 2 hours after a 75 g oral glucose load, symptoms of hyperglycemia and casual plasma glucose ≥ 200 mg/dL (11.1 mmol/L), glycated hemoglobin (Hb A1c) ≥ 6.5%.[9] A positive result on any of the above should be repeated on a different day prior to the diagnosis of diabetes.

Type 2 diabetes (non-insulin dependent) is normally associated with increased resistance to normally secreted insulin in obese individuals. Obesity, particularly of the central (abdominal) region, is the most important risk factor for developing type 2 diabetes as it is strongly associated with insulin resistance, which, when coupled with relative insulin deficiency, leads to the overt development of type 2 diabetes. During the past 30 years, the number of children diagnosed as being overweight has increased by >100% and this epidemic of childhood obesity is causing children to suffer from chronic complications that were previously only seen in adults.[10] Type 2 diabetes now accounts for a considerable proportion of newly diagnosed cases of diabetes in the pediatric population.

Urbanization, unhealthy diets, and increasingly sedentary lifestyles have contributed to increase the prevalence of childhood obesity, particularly in developed countries.[11] The metabolic syndrome is a combination of medical disorders that when occurring together greatly increase the risk of cardiovascular disease and diabetes. Several definitions of the metabolic syndrome exist, but generally include diabetes or impaired glucose resistance, hypertension, dyslipidemia (increased triglycerides and decreased high-density lipoprotein) and central obesity. The link between obesity, metabolic syndrome, and type 2 diabetes has been well characterized in adult populations, but has been increasingly observed in pediatric populations. In children and adolescents, a number of studies have demonstrated a link between childhood metabolic syndrome and elevated cardiovascular risk in later life.[11]

It is important to recognize diabetes as a cause of hyperglycemia in children and to distinguish it from other medical causes of high blood sugar, including acute pancreatic disease or hypersecretion of counterregulatory hormones such as growth hormone (GH), cortisol, or catecholamines. Chronic hyperglycemia can be readily distinguished from acute causes by simply measuring the blood concentration of glycated hemoglobin or hemoglobin A1c, a well-established marker for long-term hyperglycemia. This assay also has great value in monitoring diabetic compliance in patients on treatment and has recently been included as one of the diagnostic criteria of diabetes.[9]

Nitrogen Metabolism

The liver plays a central role in nitrogen metabolism. It is involved with the metabolic interconversions of amino acids and the synthesis of nonessential amino acids. The liver synthesizes many body proteins, including most proteins found in the circulation, such as albumin, transferrin, and the complement clotting factors. The liver does not synthesize immunoglobulins. The liver is also responsible for complete metabolism of the breakdown products of nitrogen turnover, such as ammonia and urea through the urea cycle and creatinine and uric acid from energy stores and nucleic acids, respectively. Blood ammonia levels are higher in the newborn period than in later life, presumably due to immaturity of urea cycle enzymes and the portal circulation. A blood ammonia level of 100 μmol/L in a newborn would be regarded as less significant than the same level in a 1-year-old. Persistently elevated ammonia levels should alert the investigator to possible liver damage and secondary failure of the urea cycle. High ammonia levels suggest a possible primary defect in the urea cycle, and patients should be evaluated for such a defect.

Nitrogenous End Products as Markers of Renal Function

In contrast to the high neonatal ammonia levels, creatinine and uric acid levels are lower in newborns. Both metabolites rise eventually to normal adult ranges. Creatinine concentrations in blood increase with muscle mass and are independent of diet. It is filtered at the glomerulus and not extensively reabsorbed by the renal tubules. Its measurement as a clearance ratio in blood and in a 24-hour urine sample has been used as a marker for the GFR for many years. Creatinine clearance is calculated from the creatinine concentration in the collected urine sample, the urine flow rate, and the plasma creatinine concentration. Creatinine clearance calculations are not commonly performed anymore due to the difficulties in collecting a complete 24-hour urine specimen and the fact that newer, more convenient methods to estimate the GFR using a single plasma creatinine value are commonly used.

While several different equations exist to estimate GFR from plasma creatinine values in adults, the most widely used is the Modification of Diet in Renal Disease formula.[12] The equation estimates GFR from the patient's serum creatinine (mg/dL), age, sex, and ethnicity as follows:

$$GFR \ (mL/min/1.73 \ m^2) = 175 \times S_{cr}^{-1.154}$$
$$\times \ (Age)^{-0.203} \times (0.742 \ \text{if female})$$
$$\times \ (1.212 \ \text{if African American}) \qquad \text{(Eq. 35-1)}$$

This equation has only been validated in patients greater than 18 years and since this equation does not adjust for body mass, it may underestimate estimated GFR for heavy people and overestimate it for underweight people. In children, the most widely used and extensively validated equation is the Schwartz equation,[13] which estimates GFR from serum creatinine (mg/dL), the child's height (cm), and a constant as follows:

$$\text{GFR (mL/min/1.73 m}^2) = (0.41 \times \text{Height in cm)/} \\ \text{Serum creatinine in mg/dL} \qquad \text{(Eq. 35-2)}$$

The use of both of the above equations requires the use of a creatinine assay that has been standardized and its calibration traceable to the gold standard measurement technique, isotope dilution mass spectrometry (IDMS).

The worldwide standardization of creatinine to a single gold standard methodology was a major undertaking by several of the world's leading clinical chemistry organizations, medical societies, and instrument manufacturers, with a goal of reducing the interlaboratory variation in creatinine assay calibration. This has allowed for more accurate estimations of GFR, which has allowed healthcare providers to better identify and treat chronic kidney disease and improve patient outcomes. As of 2012, virtually all manufacturers of creatinine assays have standardized their assays to the IDMS gold standard.

Serum cystatin C, a new and possibly more sensitive marker, has recently appeared on the market as a potential replacement for creatinine[14] since it is independent of muscle mass and recent meat ingestion. Cystatin C (an inhibitor of cysteine protease) is a ubiquitous protein secreted by most cells in the body. Cystatin C is freely filtered at the glomerulus and reabsorbed by the tubular epithelial cells, with only a very small amount being excreted in the urine. Several recent studies have proposed equations to relate cystatin C concentrations to GFR, and some of the proposed equations actually incorporate both creatinine and cystatin C values. A recent study proposed a modification of the Schwartz equation for use in children with chronic kidney disease; one that utilizes both serum creatinine and cystatin C.[15] However, this marker awaits further evaluation in pediatric populations, but it could potentially replace the creatinine clearance assay and remove the need for difficult 24-hour urine collections from children. Incomplete collections form the basis of most errors in this assay.

Liver Function Tests

As discussed, the liver is responsible for performing a large number of synthetic and catabolic processes, and normal liver function is central to maintaining body homeostasis. Several laboratory tests have emerged that are generally classified as liver function tests.

The measurements of serum albumin and total and conjugated bilirubin are true tests of liver function because they measure the synthetic and metabolic pathways for these compounds. In protein–calorie malnutrition, the reduced availability of amino acids for synthesis of new proteins results in diminished functional synthetic rate and low levels of newly synthesized proteins, such as albumin. Very low levels of albumin indicate a long exposure to protein restriction, and its measurement in blood is often used as a guide to nutritional status and chronic liver disease of other causes. Impaired hepatocellular function also results in reduced ability to conjugate bilirubin, with subsequent increase in the unconjugated form, which is normally barely detectable.

Other tests, such as measurement of liver enzymes, more truly reflect tests of liver cell integrity and are not strictly functional assays. Large elevations in serum aspartate aminotransferase and alanine aminotransferase indicate hepatocellular damage and subsequent leakage of cellular contents into the serum, and elevated ALP suggests hepatic biliary damage but gives little functional information.

CALCIUM AND BONE METABOLISM IN PEDIATRICS

Normal bone growth, which parallels body growth, requires integration of calcium, phosphate, and magnesium metabolism with endocrine regulation from vitamin D, parathyroid hormone (PTH), and calcitonin.[8] The active metabolite of vitamin D is 1,25-dihydroxy vitamin D. Hydroxylation of vitamin D from the diet takes place in the liver and in the kidneys and requires normal functioning of these organs. Absorption of vitamin D from the gastrointestinal tract, conversion to its active form in the kidney, and incorporation of calcium and phosphate into growing bone require normally active PTH. Secretion of PTH is, in turn, modulated by serum calcium and magnesium levels. Low levels of both divalent cations inhibit PTH secretion. Calcitonin has an antagonistic effect on PTH action.

Much recent attention has been given to the study of vitamin D deficiency and the role of vitamin D in maintaining optimal health. Vitamin D deficiency can result from inadequate nutritional intake of vitamin D coupled with inadequate sunlight exposure or use of sunscreens, disorders that limit vitamin D absorption and conditions that impair the conversion of vitamin D into active metabolites including certain liver and kidney diseases. Deficiency results in impaired bone mineralization and leads to bone softening diseases including rickets in children and osteoporosis and osteomalacia in adults. According to numerous recent studies, vitamin D may be helpful in preventing other diseases, including several types of cancer, diabetes, multiple sclerosis, obesity, and hypertension.[16]

Vitamin D deficiency is common in children, and the American Academy of Pediatrics has recently doubled the amount of vitamin D recommended for all infants (beginning in the first few days of life) from 200 to 400 IU/d.[16] This dose is required to prevent rickets and possibly help prevent other chronic diseases. The serum concentration of 25-hydroxyvitamin D is typically used to determine vitamin D status. It reflects vitamin D produced in the skin as well as that acquired from the diet and has a fairly long circulating half-life.

Several assay manufacturers produce immunoassays that are convenient for hospital-based clinical laboratories; however, the gold standard reference method is liquid chromatography coupled with tandem mass spectrometry. There have been ongoing issues with variability in results of 25-hydroxyvitamin D levels measured by different methods and immunoassays produced by different manufacturers. Recently, a standard reference material was produced and made commercially available. This should allow assay manufacturers and laboratories to better standardize their assays. In addition, several new proficiency schemes have been developed to help ensure consistency between laboratories.

The rapid bone growth that occurs during infancy, and later during puberty, requires optimal coordination of mineral absorption, transport, and endocrine-controlled incorporation of the minerals into growing bone. Approximately 98% of total body calcium content is present in bone and less than 1% is measurable in the blood. Serum calcium is present as the unbound ionized fraction (about 50% of total in blood), with the rest bound to protein (40%) or chelated to anions in the circulation, such as phosphate and citrate. Serum ionized and bound calcium levels are highly regulated and maintained within strict homeostatic limits. Abnormalities in any of the regulatory components have profound clinical effects on children.

Hypocalcemia and Hypercalcemia

Hypocalcemia is defined as total serum calcium below 7.0 mg/dL (1.75 mmol/L) or ionized calcium below 3.0 mg/dL (0.75 mmol/L). In the newborn and particularly the immature newborn, these levels may be commonly encountered with few symptoms. However, hypocalcemia can result in irritability, twitching, and seizures. Serum calcium is usually measured in infants with seizures of unknown etiology. Prolonged hypocalcemia can result in reduced bone growth and rickets. The causes of hypocalcemia are listed in Table 35-10. Hypomagnesemia frequently occurs with hypocalcemia. Because low levels of serum magnesium also inhibit PTH secretion, it is important to consider the possibility of concurrent hypomagnesemia in a child with hypocalcemic seizures and to correct any abnormalities that may be identified in the magnesium status as calcium is also corrected.

TABLE 35-10	CAUSES OF HYPOCALCEMIA
Prematurity	
Metabolic acidosis	
Vitamin D deficiency	
Liver disease (failure to activate vitamin D)	
Renal disease (failure to activate vitamin D)	
Hypoparathyroidism	
Low calcium intake	
High phosphorus intake	
Diuretic use	
Hypomagnesemia	
Exchange transfusion (anticoagulants in transfused blood)	

Hypercalcemia is defined as total serum calcium of greater than 11.0 mg/dL (2.75 mmol/L). This is an unusual finding in pediatrics (Table 35-11) but has potentially severe clinical implications. Patients with hypercalcemia have poor muscle tone, constipation, and failure to thrive and may develop kidney stones leading to renal failure.

ENDOCRINE FUNCTION IN PEDIATRICS

The field of endocrinology provides numerous examples of the "differences" that occur in clinical chemistry between children and adults.[2] The process of maturation from a prepubertal child into a sexually fertile adult, for example, requires a complex, endocrine-mediated, developmental process switching on during childhood. As addressed in the previous section, the bone growth that accompanies systemic growth also requires a complex process, which is also under endocrine control.

Hormone Secretion

The endocrine system relates to a group of hormones that are typically produced and secreted by one specialized cell type into the circulation, where the hormonal effect is exerted in other target cells through the binding of the hormones to specialized receptors. Some of these hormones are polypeptides; others are amino acid derivatives or steroids.

TABLE 35-11	CAUSES OF HYPERCALCEMIA
Hyperparathyroidism	
Acute renal failure	
Excessive intake of vitamin D	
Idiopathic hypercalcemia of infancy	
Hypercalcemia is less common than hypocalcemia in infants.	

Four major endocrine systems have been described, all of which play critical roles in normal human development. These systems all involve the hypothalamus as a major higher brain control center, the pituitary gland as a major secretor of hormones, and then various end organs, which have responsive elements for the pituitary hormone and affect many metabolic and developmental functions. These end organs include the thyroid gland, adrenal cortex, liver, and gonads. Each system involves regulated secretion of a tropic hormone by the hypothalamus, which in turn is transported to and controls endocrine secretion by the pituitary, and, occasionally, secondary hormonal secretion by the end organ, which then produces the appropriate cellular endocrine effect. There is feedback on the hypothalamus by the final product of the pathway (long-loop feedback) and also by the endocrine product of the pituitary (short-loop feedback). The feedback regulates hypothalamic control of the pathway. Clearly, there are many areas that can go wrong in each of these pathways, all of which result in disease. Certain disease conditions are uniquely pediatric and they are discussed further.

Hypothalamic–Pituitary–Thyroid System

The hypothalamus secretes thyrotropin-releasing hormone (TRH), a 3–amino acid peptide, into the portal blood system between the hypothalamus and the anterior pituitary.[8] TRH binds to a receptor on specialized cells in the anterior pituitary that stimulates the secretion of thyroid-stimulating hormone (TSH), a polypeptide made up of two chains (α and β). The α-chain is common to human chorionic gonadotrophin, follicle-stimulating hormone (FSH) and luteinizing hormone (LH) and the β-chain confers specificity to all of these hormones. TSH is released into the circulation and targets its end organ, the thyroid gland. Unique TSH receptors on the thyroid gland, when occupied by a TSH molecule, cause the follicular cells of the thyroid gland to synthesize and release thyroid hormones into the circulation. The synthesis of thyroid hormone involves several complex steps in which iodine is trapped within the thyroid tissue and is used to iodinate tyrosine residues on a prohormone thyroglobulin, which is then cleaved to release the iodinated amino acid triiodothyronine (T_3) and tetraiodothyronine (T_4). Thyroid hormones in the circulation are greater than 99% bound to specific transporter proteins called *thyroid-binding globulins*. Free thyroid hormone, in particular free T_3, is the active form of the hormone and reacts with receptors on many peripheral tissues to cause increased metabolism and simulate normal growth and development. T_4, T_3 (long loop), and TSH (short loop) levels feed back on the hypothalamus to regulate TRH production.

Two major areas of dysfunction in this endocrine pathway need consideration in pediatrics: primary hypothyroidism and secondary hypothyroidism. Primary hypothyroidism results from any defect that causes failure of the thyroid gland to synthesize and secrete thyroid hormone. This results in a common disease known as *congenital hypothyroidism* (CH), which is present in 1 of 4,000 births and is screened for in all newborns in the Developed world. Untreated patients with this disease have severe mental retardation with unusual facial appearances. Treatment by thyroid replacement therapy is usually successful when diagnosis is established. The best diagnostic test is to measure TSH levels in blood spots from newborns or serum if CH is suspected in later childhood. TSH levels are high as a result of failure of the long feedback loop. Thyroid hormone levels, typically total T_4 but also free T_4, in untreated patients are very low.

Secondary hypothyroidism is a result of the failure of the pituitary gland to secrete TSH, which results in lack of thyroid gland stimulation and subsequent low production of thyroid hormone. The differential diagnosis is established by measuring low circulating TSH levels. Because the pituitary is involved with all major endocrine systems, it is important to study the other pituitary pathways to determine if hypothyroidism is the result of an isolated TSH defect or due to panhypopituitarism involving all other pathways. Panhypopituitarism is clinically complex and may include features of hypoglycemia, salt loss, poor somatic and bone growth, failure to thrive, and, in later childhood, failure to develop secondary sexual characteristics.

Hypothalamic–Pituitary–Adrenal Cortex System

This system is essential for regulating mineral and carbohydrate metabolism.[4] The hypothalamus secretes corticotrophin-releasing hormone, a 41–amino acid polypeptide, into the portal blood system, which binds to receptors on specialized anterior pituitary cells, resulting in the release of corticotrophin or adrenocorticotropic hormone (ACTH) into the circulation. ACTH binds to receptors on cells in the adrenal cortex, which are stimulated to secrete the steroid hormones, cortisol and aldosterone. This pathway is also stimulated by stress at the higher cerebral center. ACTH acts as a short-loop feedback control on the hypothalamus, while cortisol and aldosterone are long-loop regulators. Aldosterone functions in the kidneys to regulate salt and water homeostasis. Cortisol interacts in many peripheral tissues and has many metabolic functions involving the regulation of carbohydrate, protein, lipid, and overall energy metabolism. Cortisol also plays a poorly understood role in the provision of resistance to infection and inflammation that accounts for the therapeutic use of steroids in many clinical situations. As with all endocrine systems, diseases occur that result from hyperfunction

TABLE 35-12	CONGENITAL DISEASES OF THE ADRENAL CORTEX
	METABOLIC PROFILE
21-Hydroxylase*a*	↑ 17-Hydroxyprogesterone, ↓ cortisol
3β-Hydroxy dehydrogenase	↑ Dehydroepiandrosterone
11β-Hydroxylase	↑ 11-Deoxycortisol, ↓ cortisol
17α-Hydroxylase	↑ 17-Ketosteroids, ↓ testosterone
18-Hydroxylase	↓ Aldosterone, ↑ renin

*a*Common disorder screened for in all newborns.

or hypofunction of the hypothalamic–pituitary–adrenal pathway. Diseases may be primary, resulting from end-organ dysfunction, or secondary, resulting from pituitary or hypothalamic disease. Pediatric diseases associated with primary disorders of the adrenal cortex are shown in Table 35-12. Many of the disorders listed are rare genetic diseases. However, steroid 21-hydroxylase deficiency is sufficiently common (about 1 of 5,000 births) to merit whole population screening in most developed countries in the world by measurement of blood spot 17-hydroxyprogesterone levels. This disorder results in failure to adequately synthesize both aldosterone and cortisol. Aldosterone deficiency results in renal salt-losing crises, and patients in the newborn period can be profoundly hyponatremic and hyperkalemic. Failure to synthesize cortisol results in stress-induced hypoglycemia. Furthermore, intermediates of steroid metabolism, which build up as a result of the metabolic block, cause androgenization. Girls born with this disorder frequently have ambiguous genitalia and may be first classed as boys. Boys may not have such pronounced abnormalities at birth, but may still develop electrolyte crises.[17] Defects of the other enzymes in the steroid pathway result in a variety of clinical signs and symptoms including salt loss, androgenization, hypertension, and hypoglycemia and diagnosis frequently requires steroid profiling.

Growth Factors

The hypothalamus secretes two regulatory hormones that effect growth. GH-releasing hormone is a 40–amino acid polypeptide that stimulates release of GH from the anterior pituitary. GH-inhibiting factor, also known as *somatostatin*, inhibits GH secretion. Additional factors from higher cerebral centers (cerebral cortex), including catecholamines, serotonin, ghrelin and endorphins, have a positive effect on GH secretion. Inhibition of GH secretion also occurs when infants are socially deprived. The mechanism for this reversible inhibition is not known, but neglect and potential child abuse are major differentials in infants with retarded growth.

CASE STUDY 35-2

A 5-year-old boy is taken to his pediatrician because of growth delay. He was below the third percentile in height and weight. There was no history of trauma and any other pertinent family history or clinical findings. A randomly obtained growth hormone level was well below the normal value for this patient's age.

Questions

1. What conditions may be associated with growth delay?

2. Does the single growth hormone result confirm a diagnosis of growth hormone deficiency? If not, what additional testing should be performed to confirm a diagnosis?

3. If further testing reveals a deficiency in growth hormone, is the patient likely to respond to therapy?

GH is a 191–amino acid polypeptide, with the liver as its primary site of action. GH receptors on the liver that are occupied by a GH molecule cause the liver to secrete a group of related polypeptide hormones, called *IGFs*, and their binding proteins, called *IGF-binding proteins*. IGF-1 and IGF-BP3 are the most significant products of GH activity on the liver. IGF-1 has a molecular structure similar to insulin; however, it is a much more potent stimulator of linear growth and increased metabolism in infants.

This pathway probably represents the most important endocrine pathway responsible for normal childhood growth. Deficiencies of any component of the pathway are known to result in poor growth, resulting in short statured adults.

There are difficulties in measuring GH in serum, which result from diurnal variation of secretion and stress-related effectors including catecholamines. A single, low level of GH is not sufficient to confirm GH deficiency. It is important to determine true organic deficiency, caused by hypothalamic or pituitary disease, from emotional deficiency because only organic deficiency responds to expensive GH replacement therapy, while nonorganic GH deficiency will respond to emotional lifestyle changes. Trauma to the head may also cause failure of GH secretion by the pituitary through direct anoxic damage to the very sensitive specialized GH-secreting cells. This type of growth failure will respond to GH therapy. Several stimulation tests have been devised to test the absolute capacity of the pituitary to secrete GH. These stimulation tests include inducement of hypoglycemia with insulin, arginine, or clonidine or direct stimulation with glucagon. These tests require that up to five blood samples be collected in the 2 hours poststimulation and the peak level of GH secretion determined. If this is less than 7 ng/mL (7 μg/L), the patient has organic GH deficiency and is likely to respond to GH therapy.[18]

Downstream testing for serum IGF-1 and IGF-BP3 levels is available and shows great promise in the identification of GH deficiency because these compounds are not secreted by the liver in GH deficiency and their basal levels do not seem to have the large variation that occurs for GH. In addition, defects of both IGF and IGF-BP synthesis and secretion have been recognized as a cause of growth failure in certain infants. Individuals with these defects are unlikely to respond to GH replacement.

Endocrine Control of Sexual Maturation

The hypothalamus secretes a 10–amino acid peptide called *gonadotrophin-releasing hormone (GnRH)* into the portal blood system. GnRH binds to a specific receptor and causes the release of two larger polypeptide hormones, called *FSH* and *LH*, from the anterior pituitary in both males and females.

Baseline levels of the gonadotrophins FSH and LH are very low in infants and young children as a result of GnRH suppression.

FSH and LH have different effects in males and females, both before and during puberty. In males, the target hormonal activity is directed to the testis and causes the release of androgens, primarily the steroid hormones testosterone and androstenedione which are released into the circulation. In females, the primary site of action is the ovary and results in the secretion of a different family of steroid hormones—estrogens, primarily estradiol—into the circulation. Prior to puberty, the circulating levels of androgens and estrogens are very low. The measurement of pediatric gonadotrophin levels and sex steroid hormones provides excellent examples of the need for unique pediatric reference ranges for these biomarkers as the pediatric clinical laboratory is often requested to measure these hormones when a child appears to be going into premature puberty. Testosterone is particularly difficult to measure in prepubertal children as many commercial immunoassays detect an interfering compound, which results in false elevation of the hormone level. Measurement by mass spectrometry appears to overcome these interferences.

During puberty, the GnRH suppression is removed and there is a gradual increase in FSH and LH secretion, with concomitant increase in androgen levels in males and estrogen and progesterone levels in females. These changes result in the development of secondary sexual characteristics and onset of menarche in females. This period of childhood is also associated with a major surge in linear and bone mass growth until adult proportions are achieved.

Disorders of this endocrine pathway are associated with either premature or precocious puberty or delayed onset of puberty. The measurement of serum FSH, LH, testosterone, and estradiol levels is useful in evaluating disordered puberty. Often, disorders of other endocrine systems effect puberty. Congenital adrenal hyperplasia results in excess secretion of androgen-like steroids that can effect puberty. Disorders of the hypothalamus and pituitary can effect secretion of FSH and LH, which if reduced will result in delayed puberty.

DEVELOPMENT OF THE IMMUNE SYSTEM

In pediatric clinical facilities, the vast majority of hospital visits and admissions are related to complications arising from infectious diseases. At the same time, although the parents or caregivers may be exposed to the same infectious etiologies, they do not become so ill as to require medical attention. This is because the child does not have the same degree of immunity to disease at birth or during infancy.[1]

Basic Concepts of Immunity

The immune system is divided into two functional divisions: the innate immune system and the adaptive immune system. The innate immune system is the first line of defense, particularly in the newborn and infant not exposed to infection. The adaptive immune system generates a specific reaction following exposure to an infectious agent and provides greater immunity with subsequent exposure to that agent. Initially, however, the first response to exposure may be suboptimal and result in illness related to that exposure.

Components of the Immune System

Skin
The skin is normally an effective barrier to most microorganisms, although in premature babies this barrier is less well developed and can easily become a source of infection. Many newborns with congenital infections manifest profound skin lesions. Most infectious agents enter the body by the nasopharynx, gastrointestinal tract, lungs, or genitourinary tract. Normally, various physical and biochemical defenses protect the nonsurgical sites of entry. Lysozyme, an enzyme widely distributed in different secretions, for example, is capable of partially digesting a chemical bond in the membrane of many bacterial cell walls, thus reducing the infectivity. In premature babies, this pathway of defense is less effective. Surgical incisions and intravenous or central lines are also potential sites of entry for infectious agents.

Phagocytes
Phagocytes are present in many cell types. When a foreign organism such as a bacterium penetrates an epithelial surface, it encounters phagocytic cells, which are derived

from bone marrow and recruited into tissue in response to the organism. These cells engulf and digest particles. Phagocytic cells include polymorphonuclear cells, which are short lived in the circulation, and monocytes that, when exposed to a foreign particle, develop into macrophages that subsequently recognize the organism when the individual is re-exposed and mount a concerted defense that is typically more potent than that of the first exposure.

B Cells
B cells are lymphocytes that are characterized by the presence of surface immunoglobulins. These cells can differentiate into plasma cells that are able to respond to foreign antigens in the circulation by producing neutralizing antibodies. Activation, proliferation, and differentiation of B cells are assisted by cytokine secretion from T-cell lymphocytes, which do not produce antibodies. On binding antigen, antibodies can activate a cascade involving the complement pathway, which ultimately produces lysis and cellular death of foreign organisms.

Natural Killer Cells
Natural killer (NK) cells are leukocytes capable of recognizing cell-surface changes on host cells infected by viral particles. The NK cells bind to these target cells and can kill them and the virus. The NK cells respond to interferons, which are cytokine molecules produced by the host cells when infected by virus. Interferons are also part of the innate immune system capable of providing resistance to infection in host cells not virally infected.

Acute-Phase Proteins
Acute-phase proteins are defense proteins produced by the liver in response to infection, particularly bacterial infection. Certain proteins can increase in the serum by 2-fold to 100-fold. The most significant acute-phase protein is called *C-reactive protein (CRP)* because of its ability to bind to the C-protein of *pneumococci*. CRP bound to bacteria promotes the binding of complement that, in turn, aids phagocytosis. Serum CRP levels are routinely measured to determine the degree of infection

in pediatric patients. The required sensitivity of the CRP assay for this clinical purpose is less than that used for the high-sensitivity CRP assay used clinically as an independent risk factor for cardiac disease. In the pediatric application of this assay, rapid turnaround of results is most important. The complement system consists of at least 20 proteins, most of which are acute-phase proteins. They interact sequentially with each other, with antigen–antibody complexes, and with cell membranes in a coordinate manner to ultimately destroy bacteria and viruses. Clinically, the complement proteins that are measured most often are C3 and C4. Low levels of either of these proteins indicate poor ability to destroy foreign particles. For more detailed descriptions of acute-phase proteins, the reader is referred to Chapter 11.

Antibody Production
Immunoglobulins are classified into five major groups, based on structure and function: IgG, IgM, IgA, IgD, and IgE. Secreted by plasma cells derived from B lymphocytes, their properties are listed in Table 35-13. IgG is the major immunoglobulin subclass providing antibody response in adults and represents 70% to 75% of total immunoglobulin content. IgG is further broken down into four additional subclasses: IgG1–4. Each immunoglobulin is built from similar structural units, based on two heavy polypeptide chains (A, G, M, D, and E) and two light chains (κ and λ). The ability to recognize large numbers of foreign antigens is a result of the infinite ability of the genes for the so-called variable region of the immunoglobulin molecule to rearrange. This area recognizes foreign antigens, and a gene rearrangement with production of a unique antibody covers each new foreign antigen exposed to the body. Because of the large number of different immunoglobulin species within each subgroup, electrophoretic separation of these serum proteins on an isoelectric-focusing gel during serum protein electrophoresis analysis generates a region that is diffuse, unlike the albumin or transferrin bands, which are distinct bands.

TABLE 35-13	PROPERTIES OF IMMUNOGLOBULIN (Ig) CLASSES				
	IgG[a]	**IgA**	**IgM**	**IgD**	**IgE**
Mass (kD)	160	160	970	184	188
Percent of total Ig	70–75	10–15	5–10	<1	Trace
Crosses placenta	Yes	No	No	No	No
In breast milk	Yes	Yes	No	Unknown	Unknown
Activates complement	Yes	Yes	Yes	No	No
In secretions	No	Yes	No	No	No
Binds to mast cells	No	No	No	No	Yes

[a]Present as four subclasses (IgG1–4).

Neonatal and Infant Antibody Production

The human fetus is able to synthesize a small amount of IgM and, to a lesser degree, IgA. IgG has a lower molecular weight than IgM and is readily able to cross the placenta. IgG is also transferred from mother to baby in breast milk. Transplacental and breast milk–derived IgG offer the baby a passive immunologic protection until endogenous IgG production becomes a significant protective factor. The half-life of IgG is about 30 days, and with prolonged breastfeeding, the infant can derive additional protection. The process of antibody production in infants takes several years to complete when based on total serum levels of the immunoglobulin subclasses, which take up to 4 years to be attained and provide another example of how age-related reference ranges are particularly important in pediatric laboratory medicine. Premature babies have an even greater immunoglobulin deficit than term babies because of diminished transplacental delivery of antibodies.

Immunity Disorders

Given the complexity of the immune system, there are many stages at which acquired or genetically inherited defects can result in inappropriate infectious disease in the pediatric population.[19] Transient hypogammaglobulinemia of infancy may occur because of prematurity or, in certain infants, may be a result of delayed onset of immunoglobulin production of unknown etiology. These infants eventually develop a normal immune system but will be prone to repeated bouts of severe infection until this time. At the opposite end of the spectrum, complete absence of γ-globulins occurs in boys in an X-linked disorder known as *agammaglobulinemia*, or Bruton's disease. This disorder presents early in life, with recurrent febrile infections. Patients do not have B cells and have low levels of all endogenous immunoglobulin subclasses. The disease process probably begins the moment that any maternally derived immunoglobulins have been lost. The most common infections are of the upper and lower respiratory tracts, causing otitis, pneumonia, sinusitis, meningitis, sepsis, and osteomyelitis. Without early γ-globulin therapy, these children die from respiratory complications. Other immune pathways are normal in these children.

Severe Combined Immune Deficiency

One of the most graphic examples of unique pediatric disease comes from infants who lack both humoral and cellular pathways for killing bacteria and viruses. These children are at risk for severe infection each time they are exposed to an infectious agent. The vivid image is of the "boy in the bubble," existing in a completely sterile environment to avoid contact with any bacteria or virus particles. Severe combined immune deficiency (SCID) may be inherited as an X-linked disorder only seen in boys or it may be autosomal recessive and girls may also inherit the disease. There are several causes of SCID, including genetic diseases of purine metabolism and disorders of lymphocyte development and maturation, in which both T cells and B cells, if present, are nonfunctional. The most common purine disorder, adenosine deaminase deficiency, is responsible for 15% of SCID cases. It is diagnosed by measuring elevated levels of adenosine in body fluids. Establishing this diagnosis is important because enzyme replacement therapy using recombinant enzyme has been successfully used to treat the disorder.

GENETIC DISEASES

Analytic methods for the identification of genetic disease play an important part in the pediatric clinical chemistry laboratory.[1,20-22] The presentations of many genetic diseases are unique to the pediatric population and require physicians and clinical laboratorians who provide services to have specialized knowledge and training. Most diseases that present with clinical signs in infants and children are inherited in an autosomal recessive mode, which means that the patient has two disease-causing mutations in the gene for that disorder, one inherited maternally and one inherited paternally. Parents are almost always without any symptoms. Several examples of diseases with this inheritance pattern have already been introduced in this chapter, including galactosemia and congenital adrenal hyperplasia as a result of steroid 21-hydroxylase deficiency. Certain other diseases are recessive but are inherited on the X chromosome. Typically, boys inherit a mutated X chromosome from their mothers; because they do not inherit a paternal X chromosome, they show signs of disease with only one mutation. Girls carrying an X chromosome mutation may also demonstrate disease signs due to the fact that one of their X chromosomes becomes inactivated and if the active X chromosome carries the mutation they will have the disease. Dominantly inherited diseases, which can be inherited as a single mutation through either parental line, frequently tend not to present as unique childhood diseases. Examples include familial hypercholesterolemia, Huntington disease, and factor V Leiden thrombophilia, all of which are generally regarded as diseases of the adult population, although the mutation is inherited at birth. All of the examples described above are diseases of DNA that replicates in the cell nucleus. Mitochondria, the organelles responsible for generating cellular energy and other important metabolic pathways, also contain DNA (mtDNA), which encodes proteins involved in energy generation. mtDNA has a high rate of spontaneous mutation and results in a large number of energy-wasting diseases, many of which present with high blood lactate levels. Mitochondria are only inherited from the mother, so that mtDNA mutations that are not spontaneous can only come from the maternal lineage.

Cystic Fibrosis

Cystic fibrosis (CF) is one of the most commonly inherited genetic diseases encountered by pediatric clinical chemistry laboratories. The rate of this debilitating disease is 1 of 2,400 live births, which results from recessively inherited mutations in the cystic fibrosis transmembrane regulator (*CFTR*) gene. Patients may present in the newborn period with severe pancreatic insufficiency caused by accumulated thick mucous secretions in the pancreatic ducts, which inhibit the secretion of pancreatic digestive enzymes. These babies have steatorrhea and fail to thrive. Patients with CF do not always develop pancreatic symptoms; however, in most patients, the thick mucus that accumulates in the lungs causes respiratory disease and makes them particularly susceptible to rare infectious diseases, such as *Pseudomonas*. Although palliative therapies have improved over the past few generations because of the availability of better antibiotics, CF is still regarded as untreatable.

The gold standard diagnostic test for CF has been available for many years. It involves measurement of chloride content in sweat collected after pilocarpine iontophoresis. This type of testing is time consuming and requires specialist experience from the operator. The genetic basis for CF has been established. Although there are some mutations that are frequently encountered in the population, such as the ΔF508, there are hundreds of other mutations. The American College of Medical Genetics and the American College of Obstetrics and Gynecology recommended heterozygote screening in selected couples.[23] This recommendation poses an analytic challenge because of the large number of mutations and is dependent upon the availability of clinically and cost acceptable mutation detection technology (see Chapter 28).

Newborn Screening for Whole Populations

Certain inherited diseases are sufficiently common in the population to be considered candidates for whole population screening.[20,21] Phenylketonuria was the first genetic metabolic disorder to be screened in every baby born in the developed world. Other diseases that are readily treatable were added to the list in following years, including steroid 21-hydroxylase deficiency, sickle cell disease, CH and, in some states, galactosemia. These genetic diseases respond well to simple therapy, often dietary. In most states, this process takes place in the state screening laboratory, a facility that has the ability to easily follow up abnormal test results. The nature of the testing procedure requires a sensitive screening test that has few false-negative results. There should then be confirmation using a test that is more specific to rule out false-positive results.

Tandem mass spectrometric analysis allows many different biochemical genetic diseases to be screened on a single sample at the same time and the technology was introduced about a decade ago into many programs. This technique allows whole groups of similar compounds, in particular amino acids for the diagnosis of amino acid disorders and acylcarnitines for the diagnosis of fatty acid oxidation and some organic acid disorders, to be analyzed on small sample volumes without complex sample preparation (Table 35-14). The analytic time

TABLE 35-14	METABOLIC DISEASES DETECTABLE BY NEWBORN SCREENING USING TANDEM MASS SPECTROMETRY
AMINO ACIDS	
Phenylketonuria (PKU)	
Maple syrup urine disease (MSUD)	
Tyrosinemia, types 1 and 2	
Homocystinuria	
Hypermethioninemia	
UREA CYCLE	
Argininemia	
Citrullinemia	
Argininosuccinic aciduria (ASA)	
ORGANIC ACIDS	
Propionic acidemia (PA)	
Methylmalonic acidemia (MMA)	
Isovaleric acidemia (IVA)	
Glutaric acidemia, types 1 and 2 (GA1, GA2)	
β-Ketothiolase deficiency	
3-Hydroxy-3-methylglutaryl-CoA lyase (HMG-CoA lyase) deficiency	
3-Methylcrotonyl-CoA carboxylase(MCC) deficiency	
Malonyl-CoA decarboxylase deficiency	
2-Methyl-3-hydroxybutyryl-CoA dehydrogenase deficiency[a]—	
FATTY ACIDS	
Medium-chain acyl-CoA dehydrogenase (MCAD) deficiency	
Short-chain acyl-CoA dehydrogenase (SCAD)[b] deficiency	
Very-long-chain acyl-CoA dehydrogenase (VLCAD) deficiency	
Carnitine palmitoyltransferase, types 1A and 2 (CPT1A, CPT2)	
Carnitine acylcarnitine translocase (CAT) deficiency	
Long-chain 3-hydroxyacyl-CoA dehydrogenase (LCHAD) deficiency	
Mitochondrial trifunctional protein (MTP) deficiency	

[a]Clinical significance not established.
[b]Possibly a benign biochemical condition.

is about 2 minutes per sample, which means that it is possible to readily perform analysis for an entire state. The birth rate in the United States is approximately 4.2 million births per year. Tandem mass spectrometry has been shown to be capable of handling this workload and all states currently offer this program.

The present status of newborn screening for metabolic diseases comprises a panel of 29 recommended conditions, referred to as the uniform panel, of which 20 can presently be diagnosed using tandem mass spectrometry. The most common of these additional disorders is medium-chain acyl-CoA dehydrogenase (MCAD) deficiency, which is a defect of the pathway in which we derive energy from fatty acids during periods of fasting or high energy demand such as fever. Prior to including this defect in newborn screening programs, infants would develop fasting-induced hypoglycemia and liver failure often leading to death or neurological damage. Subsequent to screening by measurement of blood spot octanoylcarnitine (C8) and presymptomatic diagnosis with early management, the outcomes for children with MCAD deficiency have improved greatly. In addition to the core screening diseases, a number of secondary diseases can also be identified using tandem mass spectrometry, some of which are very rare and have less data to confirm sensitivity and specificity. Many additional metabolic diseases can be diagnosed by tandem mass spectrometry; however, the current evidence to support a substantial benefit at the population level by uniform screening is less strong. Methods to diagnose additional diseases by tandem mass spectrometry are constantly being developed and it is likely that routine population-based screening will be expanded in the near future. The next most likely group of conditions to be included in programs will be lysosomal storage diseases that were long considered to be untreatable and therefore unsuitable. However, treatment modalities are currently being investigated for many lysosomal storage diseases and it is likely that the most success will come from early instigation of treatment.

CASE STUDY 35-3

An infant presented to the pediatrician with failure to thrive, steatorrhea (foul-smelling, fatty stool), and persistent respiratory infections. An older sibling with the same clinical presentation has a confirmed genetic disease.

Questions

1. What is the likely diagnosis?

2. How is the disease inherited?

3. What is the molecular mechanism of this disease?

4. What is the gold standard diagnostic test?

Diagnosis of Metabolic Disease in the Clinical Setting

At the present time, the clinical laboratory is needed to confirm the diagnosis of newborns screened positive for the disorders listed in Table 35-14[24] and also for the rest of the 500 single-gene defects that result in biochemical genetic disease not presently detectable by tandem mass spectrometry. These inborn errors of metabolism can be broken down generally into two main types:

Large-Molecule Diseases

Large-molecule diseases have an accumulating intermediate of metabolism composed of large complex molecules; examples are listed in Table 35-15. Many of these diseases involve intracellular accumulation of the abnormal chemical with relatively small excretion in body fluids. In glycogen storage diseases, the glycogen accumulates in liver and muscle but cannot be seen in blood or urine samples. The histopathologist, using microscopic examination of tissue, often makes these diagnoses. A few, mostly urine, tests are available for gathering clues to large-molecule diseases, including glycosaminoglycan (mucopolysaccharide) analysis using high-voltage electrophoresis, to identify unusual metabolites associated with the mucopolysaccharide storage diseases. These tests are relatively insensitive, and confirmation of the diagnosis requires measurement of deficient enzyme activity in a body tissue. Fortunately, many enzymes that result in large-molecule storage diseases can be found in

TABLE 35-15	EXAMPLES OF LARGE-MOLECULE STORAGE DISORDERS
MUCOPOLYSACCHARIDE (MPS) OR GLYCOSAMINOGLYCAN STORAGE DISEASES	
Hurler disease (MPS, type I)	
Hunter disease (type II)	
Morquio disease (type IV)	
COMPLEX LIPID STORAGE	
Gaucher disease	
Tay-Sachs disease	
Niemann-Pick disease (types A, B, C)	
GLYCOGEN STORAGE DISEASES	
Von Gierke (type 1)	
Pompe (type 2)	
McArdle (type 5)	
PEPTIDE STORAGE	
Neuronal ceroid lipofuscinoses, types 1–10 (Batten disease)	
POST-TRANSLATIONAL PROTEIN MODIFICATION	
Carbohydrate-deficient glycoprotein syndromes	

white blood cells, enabling confirmation to be made on a blood sample. Enzymic confirmation can be difficult to establish in small babies because large blood samples are frequently required for diagnostic testing.

Small-Molecule Diseases

Small-molecule diseases result from defects in metabolic pathways of intermediary metabolism. Usually, the abnormal compounds that are present in these diseases are low-molecular-weight compounds that are readily excreted in body fluids; the types of pathways involved are listed in Table 35-16. Initially, the clinical chemistry laboratory had few diagnostic tools capable of identifying the large number of metabolic intermediates that may accumulate in these diseases, and a number of simple, colorimetric urine tests, such as the dinitrophenylhydrazine test for ketoacids, were developed to establish diagnosis. These methods lack both sensitivity and specificity and have no role to play in the modern clinical chemistry laboratory. They have been superseded by assays with greater sensitivity and specificity, often based on separation technology and mass spectrometry.

Small-molecule diseases have a variable clinical presentation and could present to almost any medical subspecialty with any organ system involved (Table 35-16 lists certain pathways that may be involved). Biochemical testing for these diseases is usually described in two phases. First, it is important to recognize the degree of tissue compromisation at presentation. This requires routine chemistry evaluation for blood gas status, if

TABLE 35-16	PATHWAYS INVOLVED WITH SMALL-MOLECULE METABOLIC DISEASE AND EXAMPLES
Amino acids—phenylketonuria	
Fatty acids—medium-chain acyl-CoA dehydrogenase deficiency	
Organic acids—propionic acidemia	
Urea cycle—citrullinemia	
Oxidative phosphorylation—mitochondrial DNA diseases	
Vitamin metabolism—pyridoxine responsive seizures	
Steroid biosynthesis and breakdown—21-hydroxylase deficient congenital adrenal hyperplasia	
Cholesterol synthesis—Smith-Lemli-Opitz syndrome	
Purine and pyrimidine metabolism—adenosine deaminase form of severe combined immunodeficiency	
Neurotransmitter metabolism—4-hydroxybutyric aciduria	
Plasmalogen synthesis—Zellweger syndrome	
Glutathione metabolism—pyroglutamic aciduria	
Oxalate metabolism—hyperoxaluria types 1 and 2	
Creatine metabolism—guanidinoacetic acidemia	

CASE STUDY 35-4

A normal appearing infant was identified with a positive newborn screen. Prior to the introduction of tandem mass spectrometry into the newborn screening program, a sibling had been born who, in association with a viral illness, developed profound hypoglycemia, liver failure leading to coma, and subsequent irreparable brain damage. The sibling was subsequently shown by clinical testing to have the same disorder that the newborn screened positively for.

Questions

1. What is the most likely diagnosis?

2. What biomarker would confirm this on the newborn screening process?

3. What is the likelihood that the newborn will follow the same clinical course as the older sibling?

4. What group of genetic diseases are likely to be incorporated into whole population screens next?

acidotic; anion gap measurement; liver function testing; analysis of skeletal and cardiac muscle markers, such as creatine kinase or troponin levels; lactic acid; and ammonia measurement. All of these analyses should be available stat and used to monitor management once a diagnosis is established. The second phase of analysis should be to look for metabolic markers that pinpoint the site of a defect. These tests involve a form of separation technology, such as ion-exchange chromatography or ultra-performance liquid chromatography for amino acids. The preferred material for amino acid analysis is serum because the renal tubules have efficient transport systems for reabsorbing filtered amino acids. It is possible to miss an amino acid abnormality if only urine is analyzed. Urine amino acid analysis is of value if a tubular defect such as cystinuria is suspected. The most useful test for detecting abnormal metabolic intermediates is organic acid analysis. This test is performed on urine and should only be performed using the technique of gas chromatography–mass spectrometry. It is a method that is capable of identifying metabolic markers for up to 200 genetic diseases. As mentioned earlier, tandem mass spectrometry is another technique seeing rapid growth in the metabolic disease diagnosis field. This technique is being applied to newborn screening and is playing an increasing role in analysis of multiple different metabolites, many of which were not easily measurable prior to the introduction of this technology.

TABLE 35-17	DRUGS WITH WELL-DEFINED THERAPEUTIC INDICES	
DRUG	**THERAPEUTIC RANGE**	**TOXICITY**
Phenytoin	10–20 mg/L (39.6–79.3 µmol/L)	>40 (159) causes seizures, ataxia
Phenobarbital	10–40 mg/L (43–172 µmol/L)	>40 (172) causes drowsiness; >60 (258) coma
Carbamazepine	4–10 mg/L (16.9–42.3 µmol/L)	>10 (42.3) causes drowsiness
Theophylline[a]	5–15 mg/L (27.8–83.3 µmol/L)	>20 (111) can cause cardiac arrhythmia
Caffeine[a]	5–15 mg/L (26–77 µmol/L)	Less toxic than theophylline
Methotrexate 61	Depends on therapy	High levels cause myelosuppression
Gentamicin	5–10 mg/L (peak)[b] (10.5–20.9 µmol/L)	>12 (25.1) ototoxic; renal toxicity

[a]Theophylline is metabolized to caffeine in neonates but not in adults. Used to treat apnea.
[b]Peak level should be drawn 30 min after last dose for aminoglycoside drugs. Children are particularly prone to hearing loss at toxic levels.

DRUG METABOLISM AND PHARMACOKINETICS

There are several important differences in the way that infants and children handle pharmacologic agents compared with adults.[1] This area of pediatric laboratory medicine provides many good examples of why children should not be regarded as "small adults." It is not clinically appropriate to prorate the amount of drug prescribed to a child based on relative body weight compared with an adult dose.

Drug metabolism depends on the following factors: absorption, circulation and volume of distribution, and metabolism and clearance. Often, the medium in which a drug is provided to a child differs from that in which an adult may take the same drug. Syrups, for instance, provide a more rapid release of a drug and greater availability for gastrointestinal absorption than tablets, which have the drug trapped in a solid matrix that requires digestion. Children are more likely to be given medication in a palatable form, such as syrup, and to require lower doses. The pH of gastric secretions differs in infants. At birth, the gastric pH is nearly neutral, not reaching the adult level of acidity for several years. This pH difference can affect the absorption of certain drugs, including some frequently prescribed penicillins. The distribution of drugs often differs between adults and children. Lipid-soluble drugs are taken up into lipid reserves and only slowly released into the circulation. Because infants have relatively little adipose tissue, these drugs are not stored as efficiently. The overall effect is that lipid-soluble drugs reach a higher level more quickly than in individuals with sizable fat stores; however, the drug is also cleared more rapidly. It becomes appropriate for drugs to be provided in smaller, more frequent doses to optimize the effect. Hepatic metabolism of many drugs is immature in young infants. This may delay the metabolic conversion to an active drug or increase the time in which an active drug is circulating. Good hepatic function is important for clearing those drugs metabolized by the liver, as good renal function is important for clearing drugs that have water-soluble end products.

Therapeutic Drug Monitoring

The principles of therapeutic drug monitoring remain the same in adult and pediatric clinical chemistry. It is important to measure the blood levels of various drugs if that information can provide important guidance to the physician with regard to optimal dosing. This is most important if a drug has a well-defined therapeutic index. This means that the drug is known to be ineffective if the blood level is below a certain value, that there is a well-defined therapeutic range over which the drug is effective, and that there is a higher level at which the drug becomes toxic. It is important to monitor levels of drugs with these characteristics. Table 35-17 lists drugs for which the importance of therapeutic monitoring is established.

Toxicologic Issues in Pediatric Clinical Chemistry

Issues related to the provision of a toxicologic service can be divided into two distinct groups in pediatrics. The first group involves infants and young children who unknowingly consume pharmacologic and other chemical agents. This usually involves the child finding access to medication belonging to another individual in the household and consuming the medication as if it were candy. It is relatively easy for the investigator to ascertain the nature of the medication by identifying what is available in the household. Toxicologic investigation can usually be restricted to a few specific tests.

A rare, but potentially dangerous condition is that of Munchausen syndrome by proxy. In this condition, mental illness in a caregiver causes them to give unnecessary and illness-causing drugs to an otherwise well child. This can go unrecognized and result in multiple hospitalizations and even death of the child. Clinical suspicion of this form of child abuse should involve performing a comprehensive drug screen to identify causative agents. Because of the intermittent nature of clinical presentation of

Munchausen syndrome by proxy, it can often be confused with metabolic disease. Metabolic studies, in addition to comprehensive toxicologic studies, may be necessary.

Because the likelihood of self-ingestion of street drugs of abuse is present in older children, pediatric clinical chemistry laboratories should make assays available for street drugs similar to those in adult practice.

For additional student resources please visit thePoint at http://thepoint.lww.com. **thePoint**✷

QUESTIONS

1. All of the following represent normal physiology of the newborn except
   a. Weight of 2.4 kg
   b. Immature liver function and inability to eliminate excess bilirubin
   c. Closure of the ductus arteriosus and a shift of blood flow through the heart
   d. 4 to 6 months for the infant's body weight to double

2. Which of the following choices is false concerning blood obtained by heel stick (capillary) and venipuncture (venous)?
   a. The chemical composition of the sera derived from each is identical.
   b. The capillary specimen is likely contaminated with interstitial fluid and tissue debris.
   c. Venous blood contains higher bilirubin and calcium concentrations.
   d. Capillary blood contains less concentrated proteins due to mixing with interstitial fluid.

3. Under normal conditions, what is the maximum amount of blood that should be drawn from a 30-kg child during a single blood draw?
   a. 60 mL
   b. 80 mL
   c. 40 mL
   d. 20 mL

4. When choosing a chemistry analyzer for a pediatric laboratory, it is necessary to
   a. Incorporate total laboratory automation
   b. Be able to analyze from small volumes
   c. Have a rapid turnaround time
   d. Ensure a minimum specimen dead volume

5. Which of the following is true regarding POCT?
   a. Results are generally available more rapidly than with traditional laboratory tests.
   b. POCT is usually less expensive than traditional laboratory measurements.

   c. The device cannot be linked to the hospital information system.
   d. Quality control samples are not needed.

6. Which of the following conditions are related to acidosis in the newborn?
   a. Anoxia and trauma during delivery
   b. Respiratory distress syndrome
   c. Hyperammonemia caused by liver disease
   d. Hyperventilation

7. Which of the following are characteristics of renal development and function during the neonatal period?
   a. Control the rate of salt and water loss and retention
   b. GFR about 50% of the rate seen in older children
   c. Completely developed by 24 weeks of gestation
   d. Have a maximum solute concentrating power of approximately 30% of an adult kidney

8. Which of the following statements about the neonatal thyroid system is true?
   a. Secondary hypothyroidism is usually diagnosed by measuring a low TSH level.
   b. Thyroid hormones (T_4 and T_3) are less than 50% bound to thyroid-binding globulins.
   c. CH is a very rare and untreatable disorder.
   d. A low measured TSH level may be due to a global pituitary gland dysfunction (panhypopituitarism).

9. Cystic fibrosis
   a. Is diagnosed by the measurement of elevated chloride concentration in sweat following iontophoresis
   b. Is a very uncommon genetic disease
   c. Is caused by only a single type of mutation in the CF transmembrane regulator (CFTR) gene
   d. Is characterized by thin, watery mucous secretions in the lungs and pancreatic ducts

REFERENCES

1. Green A, Morgan I, Gray J. *Neonatology and Laboratory Medicine.* London: ACB Venture Publications; 2003.
2. Soldin SJ, Rifai N, Hicks JMB, eds. *Biochemical Basis of Pediatric Disease.* Washington, DC: American Association for Clinical Chemistry; 1992.
3. Rautenberg MW, van Solinge WW, Heunks JJ, et al. Pediatric tube direct sampling by the Abbott Architect Integrated ci8200 Chemistry/Immunochemistry Analyzer. *Clin Chem.* 2006;52: 768-770.
4. Demir AY, van Solinge WW, Kemperman H. Handling of and direct sampling from primary barcode-labeled pediatric tubes on Vitros clinical chemistry analyzers integrated into an enGen work cell. *Clin Chem.* 2005;51:920-921.
5. Gill FN, Bennett MJ. Point of care testing in pediatrics. In: Price CP, St. John A, Hicks JM, eds. *Point of Care Testing.* 2nd ed. Washington, DC: American Association for Clinical Chemistry; 2004:341-352.
6. Honest H, Bachmann LM, Gupta JK, Kleijnen J, Khan KS. Accuracy of cervicovaginal fetal fibronectin test in predicting risk of spontaneous preterm birth: systematic review. *BMJ.* 2002;325: 301-311.
7. Goldenberg RL, Mercer BM, Iams JD. The preterm prediction study: patterns of cervicovaginal fetal fibronectin as predictors of spontaneous preterm delivery. *Am J Obstet Gynecol.* 1997;177:8-12.
8. Polak M, Van Vliet G. Disorders of the thyroid gland. In: Sargoglou K, Hoffman G, Roth K, eds. *Pediatric Endocrinology and Inborn Errors of Metabolism.* New York: McGraw-Hill; 2009: 353-382.
9. Summary of the Revisions for the 2010 Clinical Practice Recommendations. *Diabetes Care.* 2010;33(suppl 1):S3.
10. Hannon TS, Rao G, Arslanian SA. Childhood obesity and type 2 diabetes mellitus. *Pediatrics.* 2005;116(2):299-306.
11. Zimmet P, Alberti K, George MM, et al.; IDF Consensus Group. The metabolic syndrome in children and adolescents—an IDF consensus report. *Pediatr Diabetes.* 2007;8:299-306.
12. Levey AS, Coresh J, Greene T, et al. Chronic Kidney Disease Epidemiology Collaboration. Using standardized serum creatinine values in the modification of diet in renal disease study equation for estimating glomerular filtration rate. *Ann Intern Med.* August 2006;145(4):247-254.
13. Schwartz GJ, Work DF. Measurement and estimation of GFR in children and adolescents. *J Am Soc Nephrol.* November 2009;4(11):1832-1843.
14. Newman DJ. Cystatin C. *Ann Clin Biochem.* 2002;39:89-104.
15. Schwartz GJ, Munoz A, Schneider MF, et al. New equations to estimate GFR in children with CKD. *J Am Soc Nephrol.* 2009;20:629-637.
16. Wagner C, Greer FR. Prevention of rickets and vitamin D deficiency in infants, children, and adolescents. *Pediatrics.* 2008;122:1142.
17. Austin A, Finkielstein GP. Adrenal disorders. In: Dietzen DJ, Bennett MJ, Wong ECC, eds. *Biochemical and Molecular Basis of Pediatric Disease.* 4th ed. Washington, DC: AACC Press; 2010: 135-153.
18. Winter WE, Rosenbloom AL. Disorders of growth. In: Dietzen DJ, Bennett MJ, Wong ECC, eds. *Biochemical and Molecular Basis of Pediatric Disease.* 4th ed. Washington, DC: AACC Press; 2010; 171-194.
19. Loechelt BJ. Primary immunodeficiency diseases. In: Dietzen DJ, Bennett MJ, Wong ECC, eds. *Biochemical and Molecular Basis of Pediatric Disease.* 4th ed. Washington, DC: AACC Press; 2010: 409-427.
20. Valle D, Beaudet AL, Vogelstein B, Kinzler KW, Antonarakis SE, Ballabio A, eds. Online Metabolic and Molecular Bases of Inherited Disease (OMMBID). http://www.ommbid.com/. Accessed July 30, 2012.
21. Sargoglou K, Hoffman G, Roth K, eds. *Pediatric Endocrinology and Inborn Errors of Metabolism.* New York: McGraw-Hill; 2009.
22. Hommes FA, ed. *Techniques in Diagnostic Human Biochemical Genetics.* New York: Wiley-Liss; 1991.
23. American College of Obstetricians & Gynecologists, American College of Medical Genetics. *Preconception and Prenatal Carrier Screening for Cystic Fibrosis: Clinical and Laboratory Guidelines.* Washington, DC: American College of Obstetricians & Gynecologists; 2001.
24. Dietzen, DJ, Rinaldo P, Whitley RJ, et al. National Academy of Clinical Biochemistry Laboratory Medicine Practice Guidelines: follow-up testing for metabolic diseases identified by expanded newborn screening using tandem mass spectrometry; executive summary. *Clin Chem.* 2009;55:1615-1626. http://www.aacc.org/. Accessed July 30, 2012. members/nacb/lmpg/onlineguide/published-guidelines/newborn/pages/default.aspx#. Accessed July 30, 2012.

Index

RRS1211